PRINCIPLES AND PRACTICE
OF
CLINICAL BACTERIOLOGY

PRINCIPLES AND PRACTICE OF CLINICAL BACTERIOLOGY

Edited by

A.M. Emmerson
Queen's Medical Centre, Nottingham, UK

P.M. Hawkey
University of Leeds, UK

S.H. Gillespie
Royal Free Hospital School of Medicine, London, UK

JOHN WILEY & SONS
Chichester · New York · Weinheim · Brisbane · Singapore · Toronto

Other Wiley Editorial Offices

John Wiley & Sons, Inc., 605 Third Avenue,
New York, NY 10158-0012, USA

VCH Verlagsgesellschaft mbH, Pappelallee 3,
D-69469 Weinheim, Germany

Jacaranda Wiley Ltd, 33 Park Road, Milton,
Queensland 4064, Australia

John Wiley & Sons (Asia) Pte Ltd, 2 Clementi Loop #02-01,
Jin Xing Distripark, Singapore 129809

John Wiley & Sons (Canada) Ltd, 22 Worcester Road,
Rexdale, Ontario M9W 1L1, Canada

Library of Congress Cataloging-in-Publication Data

Principles and practice of clinical bacteriology / edited by A.M.
    Emmerson, P.M. Hawkey, and S.H. Gillespie.
        p. cm.
    Includes bibliographical references and index.
    ISBN 0-471-93617-0 (alk. paper)
    1. Medical bacteriology. I. Emmerson, A.M. II. Hawkey, P.M.
(Peter M.) III. Gillespie, S.H.
    [DNLM: 1. Bacteriological Techniques, QY 100 P957 1996]
QR46.P84 1996
616'.014–dc20
DNLM/DLC
for Library of Congress   95-39525
                                            CIP

British Library Cataloguing in Publication Data

A catalogue record for this book is available from the British Library

ISBN 0-471-93617-0

Typeset in 10/12pt Times by Mathematical Composition Setters, Salisbury
Printed and bound in Great Britain by Bookcraft (Bath) Ltd, Midsomer Norton
This book is printed on acid-free paper responsibly manufactured from sustainable forestation,
for which at least two trees are planted for each one used for paper production.

CONTENTS

CONTRIBUTORS

DLAWER A.A. ALA'ALDEEN   Department of Microbiology, University of Nottingham, University Hospital, Nottingham NG7 2UH, UK

STEPHEN D. ALLEN   Department of Clinical Microbiology, Indiana University, Indianapolis, IN 46223, USA

BURT E. ANDERSON   Viral Rickettsial Zoonoses Branch, Centre for Disease Control and Prevention, National Center for Infectious Diseases, 1600 Clifton Road NE MS-G13, Atlanta, GA 30333, USA

MICHAEL BARNHAM   Harrogate General Hospital, Knaresborough Road, Harrogate, HG2 7ND, UK

AFONSO L. BARTH   Division of Hospital Infection, Central Public Health Laboratory, 61 Colindale Avenue, London NW9 5HT, UK

CHRISTIANE C. BÉBÉAR   Laboratoire de Bacteriologie, Centre Hospitalier Universitaire de Bordeaux, Hôpital Pellegrin, Place Amémlie Raba Léon, 33076 Bordeaux Cédex, France

E. BERGOGNE-BÉRÉZIN   Department of Microbiology, Bichat-Claude University Hospital, 46 Rue Hucard, 75877 Paris Cedex 18, France

ROGER C.W. BERKELEY   Department of Pathology and Microbiology, School of Medical Sciences, University of Bristol, University Walk, Bristol BS8 1TD, UK

T. J. BLANCHARD   Department of Clinical Sciences, London School of Hygiene and Tropical Medicine, Keppel Street, London WC1E 7HT, UK

J.S. BRAZIER   PHLS Anaerobic Reference Unit, University Hospital of Wales, Heath Park, Cardiff CF4 4XW, UK

ALAN COCKAYNE   Department of Microbiology, University of Nottingham, University Hospital, Nottingham NG7 2UH, UK

BARRY D. COOKSON   Division of Hospital Infection, Central Public Health Laboratory, 61 Colindale Avenue, London NW9 5HT, UK

RAYMOND J. DATTWYLER   Department of Allergy Rheumatology and Clinical Immunology, SUNY at Stony Brook, Stony Brook, NY 11794-8161, USA

B.I. DAVIES   Department of Medical Microbiology, De Wever Ziekenhuis, Heerlen 5401 CX, The Netherlands

B. DRASAR   Department of Clinical Sciences, London School of Hygiene and Tropical Medicine, Keppel St, London WC1E 7HT, UK

B.I. DUERDEN   Department of Medical Microbiology and Public Health Laboratory, University of Wales College of Medicine, Heath Park, Cardiff CF4 4XN, UK

A.M. EMMERSON   Department of Microbiology, University Hospital, Queen's Medical Centre, Nottingham NG7 2UH, UK

ROGER G. FINCH   Department of Microbiology and Infectious Diseases, The City Hospital, Hucknall Road, Nottingham NG5 1PB, UK

W. FREDERIKSEN   Statens Seruminstitut, Artillerivej 5, 2300 Copenhagen, Denmark

STEPHEN H. GILLESPIE   Department of Microbiology, Royal Free Hospital School of Medicine, Pond Street, London NW3 2QG, UK

J.R.W. GOVAN   Department of Medical Microbiology, University of Edinburgh Medical School, Teviot Place, Edinburgh EH8 9AG, UK

RICHARD L. GUERRANT   University of Virginia School of Medicine, Charlottesville, VA 22908, USA

V. HALL   PHLS Anaerobic Reference Unit, University Hospital of Wales, Heath Park, Cardiff CF4 4XW, UK

J.M. HARDIE   Department of Oral Microbiology, London Hospital Medical College, Turner Street, London E1 2AD, UK

T.G. HARRISON   Division of Hospital Infection, Central Public Health Laboratory, 61 Colindale Avenue, London NW9 5HT, UK

C.A. HART   Department of Medical Microbiology, University of Liverpool, Duncan Building, Royal Liverpool Hospital, Liverpool L69 3BX, UK

PETER M. HAWKEY   Department of Microbiology, University of Leeds, Leeds LS2 9JT, UK

TONY J. HOWARD   Public Health Laboratory Service, University Hospital of Wales, Heath Park, Cardiff CF4 4XW, UK

CATHERINE A. ISON   Department of Medical Microbiology, St Mary's Hospital Medical School, London W2 1PG, UK

KEVIN G. KERR   Department of Microbiology, University of Leeds, Leeds LS2 9JT, UK

VOLKAN KORTEN   Section of Infectious Disease, Marmara University Hospital, Tophanelioglu C. No. 13-15, Altunizade, Istanbul 81190, Turkey

P.N. LEVETT   MRC Leptospirosis Laboratory, Enmore No 2, Lower Collymore Rock, St Michael, Barbados

NIALL A. LOGAN   Department of Biological Sciences, Glasgow Caledonian University, Cowcaddens Road, Glasgow G4 0BA, UK

BENJAMIN J. LUFT   Department of Medicine, Division of Infectious Diseases, SUNY at Stony Brook, Stony Brook, NY 11794-8161, USA

DAVID M. LYERLY   Department of Microbiology, Indiana University, Indianapolis IN 46223 USA

D.C.W. MABEY   Department of Clinical Sciences, London School of Hygiene and Tropical Medicine, Keppel Street, London WC1E 7HT, UK

W. MANNHEIM   Statens Seruminstitut, Artillerivej 5, 2300 Copenhagen, Denmark

R.C. MATTHEWS   Pertussis Reference Laboratory, University Department of Medical Microbiology, Clinical Sciences Building, Manchester Royal Infirmary, Manchester M13 9WL, UK

TIMOTHY D. MCHUGH   Department of Microbiology, Royal Free Hospital School of Medicine, Pond Street, London NW3 2QG, UK

S.E. MILLERSHIP   Consultant for Communicable Disease Control, North Essex Health Authority, Witham, Essex CM5 2TT, UK

S.D. MILLS   Department of Microbiology, University of Toronto, 100 College Street, Toronto, Ontario M5G 1L5, Canada

PHILIP G. MURPHY   Bacteriology Department, Belfast City Hospital, Belfast BT19 7AD, UK

BARBARA E. MURRAY   Division of Infectious Diseases, University of Texas Health Science centre, Houston Medical School, Houston TX 77225, USA

JAMES G. OLSON   Viral Rickettsial Zoonoses Branch, Center for Disease Control and Prevention, National Center for Infectious Diseases, 1600 Clifton Road NE MS-G13, Atlanta, GA 30333, USA

JAMES C. PATON   Department of Microbiology, Women's and Children's Hospital, North
                        Adelaide, SA 5006, Australia

CHARLES W. PENN   School of Biological Sciences, University of Birmingham, Birmingham
                        B15 2TT, UK

J.L. PENNER   Department of Microbiology, University of Toronto, 100 College Street,
                        Toronto, Ontario M5G 1L5, Canada

TYRONE L. PITT   Division of Hospital Infection, Central Public Health Laboratory, 61
                        Colindale Avenue, London NW9 5HT, UK

M. PRENTICE   Department of Medical Microbiology, St Bartholomew's Hospital, West
                        Smithfield, London EC1A 7BE, UK

NOEL W. PRESTON   Pertussis Reference Laboratory, University Department of Medical
                        Microbiology, Clinical Sciences Building, Manchester Royal Infirmary,
                        Manchester M13 9WL, UK

NATHAN M. THIELMAN   University of Virginia School of Medicine, Charlottesville, VA 22908,
                        USA

R.A. WHILEY   Department of Oral Microbiology, London Hospital Medical College,
                        Turner Street, London E1 2AD, UK

HELEN H.Y. WONG   School of Biological Sciences, University of Birmingham, Birmingham
                        B15 2TT, UK

E.J. YOUNG   Section of Infectious Diseases, Veterans Administration Medical Center,
                        Houston, TX 77030, USA

FOREWORD

The interface between the laboratory and the clinic is the domain of clinical bacteriology. Several decades ago it was widely believed that the availability of antimicrobial therapies would render the practice of clinical bacteriology and infectious diseases obsolete. Quite the contrary, we are dealing with the appearance of new pathogens that were previously unrecognized or unclassified, as well as the re-emergence of major bacterial pathogens that have become quite resistant to conventional treatment. A medical microbiology textbook of two decades ago would make no mention of organisms such as *Bartonella henselae (Rochalimea), Borrelia burgdorferi, Legionella pneumophila, Chlamydia pneumoniae*, or *Helicobacter pylori*. The identification and study of these new nosologic entities have truly been one of the most exciting and rewarding areas of modern science. Information about these pathogens "fills the gaps" in our knowledge about disease processes that were long suspected of being due to infectious agents. With the new knowledge that has been obtained, often through the application of molecular techniques, important gaps in our understanding of new and old infectious diseases have been filled.

While the study of new pathogens is clearly appropriate, the re-emergence of some of mankind's oldest infectious disease foes — including cholera, tuberculosis and diphtheria — poses persisting challenges.

It is not just the identity of new infectious agents that have underscored the importance of clinical bacteriology, With tremendous advances in molecular biology and instrumentation techniques, we now have remarkable methodologies for the detection and identification of microorganisms or their products. These identification strategies have attained levels of exquisite sensitivity. Nonetheless, for the active clinician and scientists working in busy clinical laboratories, considerable experience and high degrees of technical skills are still required for the conventional practice of identification and microbial speciation, serologic testing, and antimicrobial susceptibility testing. Emphasis must be placed on the accuracy of these new techniques, because sensitivity and rapidity are not necessarily desirable goals in themselves.

A better understanding of the host–parasite relationship has evolved from detailed studies of microbial pathogenesis. The molecular tools that have achieved unparalleled sensitivity have been invaluable in sophisticated epidemiologic studies and the measurement and detection of mechanisms by which some microbes cause disease. Molecular biology has provided a precise basis for studying the mechanisms of tissue damage by toxins, the acquisition of drug-resistance by common bacterial pathogens, and the trigger mechanisms for the unleashing of autoimmune diseases.

The authors of this text have done a remarkable job in compiling an encyclopaedic approach to the major bacterial pathogens with which clinicians and clinical bacteriologists must deal. Can a single text "tie together" divergent disciplines and meld new biological data into useful teaching concepts? Two approaches that have been adopted in many formal texts are the syndromic approach and the categoric one. The first is a patient-orientated approach and involves differential diagnosis factored by clinical findings. The other approach is more classic and has been retained by *Principles and Practice of Clinical Bacteriology*. This approach assumes identification of the pathogen and thereupon provides the reader with a comprehensive knowledge base. Thus, this is an invaluable reference source not only for the student, learning about the many causes of bacterial disease, but also for the clinician and laboratory worker, who seeks to learn more about an identified disease process.

For the student and specialist, both the syndromic approach and the categoric approach are valuable and, in the course of study and professional experience, must be integrated. Thus, this book serves as a bridge to further understanding of a complex and evolving medical science. The state-of-the-art information provided by the many authors in this volume will prove to be invaluable in both the formal study of bateriology and in the clinical application of state-of-the-art science to bedside medicine.

Lowell S. Young, M.D.
Director, Kuzell Institute for Arthritis & Infectious Diseases
California Pacific Medical Center
University of California, San Francisco

PREFACE

The production of *Principles and Practice in Clinical Bacteriology* was inspired by the success of the sister volumes in virology and mycology. There has been a perception among both the lay public and the medical profession that, particularly in the developed world, the battle between disease causing bacteria and man has been won. The massive advances in fundamental biology and diagnostic techniques in the last half of the 19th century and the first half of the 20th century laid the bedrock of diagnostic bacteriology. The discovery and introduction of a plethora of antimicrobial agents in the last fifty years seems to complete the victory over infectious diseases. Those involved in the diagnosis and management of infectious diseases acknowledge that the description of a whole range of either novel or under-recognized pathogens has expanded the subject considerably. Furthermore, the rapidly evolving problem of antimicrobial resistance in bacteria is challenging the assumption that all is well with the treatment of infection.

With this surge of interest in infectious diseases, we felt there was a need for a text which is of a sufficient size to provide comprehensive information for specialist and non-specialist alike, without being so large and comprehensive as to be confined to the shelves of the library. We placed particular emphasis on providing succinct, but comprehensive digests of molecular pathogenesis, appropriate diagnostic methods and the treatment of bacterial infections. The practising clinical microbiologist and infectious disease physician should be able to turn to the relevant chapter and find that extra bit of information to provide an authoritative description of an infection to clinical colleagues and trainees alike. The book should also be helpful to new entrants to bacteriology enabling them to get a firm grasp of the basic properties of pathogenic bacteria, from taxonomy to treatment.

A.M. Emmerson
P.M. Hawkey
S.H. Gillespie
February 1997

1

STREPTOCOCCI: INTRODUCTION

R.A. Whiley and J.M. Hardie

In the period of over 100 years since the streptococci were recognized as a genus, the classification of these bacteria has been the subject of considerable debate. From the early days following the pioneering work of Rebecca Lancefield in the 1920 to 1940s, when heavy reliance was placed on possession of group-specific antigens, through to the extensive biochemical and physiological characterization of strains in numerical taxonomic studies, application of modern chemotaxonomic techniques and nucleic acid studies, the genus *Streptococcus* has undergone major taxonomic revisions and is now, broadly speaking, divided into three species groups. These are usually referred to as the pyogenic, oral (viridans) and 'other' streptococci (Bentley *et al.*, 1991; Schleifer and Kilpper-Balz, 1987). The oral or viridans streptococci, with which Chapter 1a is mainly concerned, are usually found in the oral cavity and upper respiratory tract of man. Although these bacteria form part of the normal flora of the mouth they include several important opportunistic pathogens and are commonly associated with dental caries (the *S. mutans* group), infective endocarditis (most oral streptococcal species) and abscesses at both oral and non-oral sites (particularly the '*S. milleri* group').

Included within the α-haemolytic streptococci, but not usually associated with the human oral cavity, is the species *S. bovis*, which has been linked with colonic cancer. However, it should be emphasized that the haemolytic reaction is not a reliable taxonomic feature, with some isolates of the oral species producing β-haemolysis. In addition, the observed haemolytic reaction is often dependent on the source of blood (e.g. sheep or horse), incubation conditions and atmosphere, and composition of the growth medium. Within the pyogenic group of streptococci, which includes several important pathogenic species characteristically producing β-haemolysis, exceptions are also found. Thus while the type of haemolysis produced on blood agar may form a convenient descriptive criterion for discussion purposes, such divisions should be viewed as artificial and not necessarily reflecting the natural relationships between species.

Principles and Practice of Clinical Bacteriology. Edited by A.M. Emmerson, P.M. Hawkey and S.H. Gillespie
© 1997 John Wiley & Sons Ltd

1a

α-HAEMOLYTIC AND NON-HAEMOLYTIC STREPTOCOCCI

R.A. Whiley and J.M. Hardie

INTRODUCTION

The genus *Streptococcus* consists of Gram-positive cocci that are facultatively anaerobic, non-sporing and catalase negative, with cells arranged in chains or pairs. Nutritional requirements are complex and carbohydrates are fermented to produce L(+)-lactic acid as the major end product. A few species may grow as short rods on solid media. The streptococci include species that are important pathogens of man and domestic animals as well as several well-known opportunist pathogens (Skinner and Quesnel, 1978). The significance of the streptococci in sepsis was recognized by the end of the nineteenth century and some time later it was realized that these bacteria also had an important role as respiratory pathogens, notably in the case of Lancefield group A streptococci (*S. pyogenes*) as the major cause of sore throats and scarlet fever occurring within families and closed communities (Ross, 1990). Until the late 1980s the genus *Streptococcus* also included several species of benefit to man, such as *S. lactis*, *S. cremoris* and *S. diacetylactis* (the 'lactic group'), which are of importance to the dairy industry. The latter group, as well as enterococci,

have since been excluded from the streptococci (Schleifer and Kilpper-Bälz, 1987).

The continuing importance of the streptococci as a cause of infection ensures that these bacteria are the focus of considerable interest and effort from the clinical microbiologist and researcher alike. Advances continue to be made in several different areas including epidemiology, mechanisms of pathogenicity, interactions between host and bacterium, taxonomy and genetics, much of this progress being due to the application of molecular techniques to the study of streptococci. In this chapter emphasis is placed on those α-haemolytic streptococci that are of particular significance for humans (Table 1a.1). Further information about streptococci associated mainly with animals can be obtained from a review by Devriese (1991).

HISTORY

The latter part of the nineteenth century marked both the recognition of streptococci as the causative agents of sepsis and the use of the term *Streptococcus* in the generic sense. The first species to be named was *S. pyogenes* for chain-forming cocci isolated from acute suppurative lesions in

Principles and Practice of Clinical Bacteriology. Edited by A.M. Emmerson, P.M. Hawkey and S.H. Gillespie
© 1997 John Wiley & Sons Ltd

TABLE 1a.1   SPECIES OF α-HAEMOLYTIC STREPTOCOCCI CURRENTLY RECOGNIZED

Species	Source	Comments
S. acidominimus	Cattle (man)[a]	No Lancefield group antigen
S. adjacens	Man	Nutritionally variant streptococci (NVS)
S. anginosus	Man	'S. milleri group'
S. bovis	Ruminants, pigs, man	Usually Lancefield group D antigen; occasional cause of human endocarditis
S. constellatus	Man	'S. milleri group'
S. cricetus	Hamsters, (man)[a]	Formerly S. mutans serotype a
S. crista	Man	'Tufted fibril group'
S. defectivus	Man	NVS
S. equinus	Ruminants, (man)	Lancefield group D antigen; occasional cause of human endocarditis
S. gordonii	Man	Formerly S. sanguis
S. intermedius	Man	'S. milleri group'
S. mitis	Man	Redefined and new type strain recommended
S. mutans	Man	Includes serotypes c, e and f
S. oralis	Man	Has been known as 'S. mitior', 'S. mitis' and 'S. sanguis II'
S. parasanguis	Man	Atypical viridans streptococci formerly designated 'MGH' group, DNA homology groups III and IV
S. pneumoniae	Man	Closely related to S. oralis
S. rattus	Rats (man)	Formerly S. mutans serotype b
S. salivarius	Man	Closely related to S. thermophilus and S. vestibularis
S. sanguis	Man	Redefined
S. sobrinus	Man	Formerly S. mutans serotypes d and g
S. vestibularis	Man	Closely related to S. salivarius and S. thermophilus

[a] (Man): indicates that man rarely harbours these species.

man, and it is interesting to note that problems concerning the identity or non-identity of streptococcal 'types' found in different diseases were the subject of considerable debate from that early point onwards.

Streptococcal characteristics most frequently examined in early studies included macroscopic (colonial) and microscopic morphologies, cultural tests, virulence in rats and mice, agglutination tests and haemolysis. Later, these approaches were supplanted by a series of biochemical tests that had previously been used successfully to characterize streptococcal isolates from saliva and faeces. It was not until much later that the first systematic classification of streptococci from a wide range of clinical and environmental sources was produced (Sherman, 1937).

The haemolytic reaction on blood agar became a feature upon which great emphasis was placed for classifying streptococcal strains, particularly in view of the fact that many of the pathogenic species were observed to be strongly haemolytic on blood agar. β-Haemolysis, or complete haemolysis, refers to a clear zone around a colony in which no intact erythrocytes remain. α-Haemolysis is characterized by the partial clearing of red blood cells often accompanied by greening of the agar around the colony. Microscopic examination of the region around the colony will reveal the presence of clumps of intact erythrocytes. (The term 'haemolytic' alone usually refers to β-haemolysis whereas 'non-haemolytic' may be taken to include both α- and non-(γ)-haemolytic strains).

Serological grouping was, for many years, used as the main criterion in the classification of streptococcal strains, following the demonstration of the group-specific nature of carbohydrate antigens present in the cell walls of streptococci and its apparent correlation with species defined by other methods. A consequence of this reliance on serology was the acceptance of the Lancefield serological groups (particularly groups A−E and N) as distinct species, and research into biological and chemical aspects of the streptococci and their natural relationships did not progress for some years (Skinner and Quesnel, 1978).

CLASSIFICATION

Over the past 20−30 years the taxonomy of the streptococci has been developed using a wide variety of approaches, thereby reducing the emphasis previously placed on serology and haemolysis. Significant investigations contributing towards these advances have included cell wall composition, metabolic studies, numerical taxonomy and nucleic acid analyses such as transformation studies, G + C determination (DNA base composition, mol% guanine + cytosine), reassociation and base sequence comparisons (Skinner and Quesnel, 1978; Schleifer and Kilpper-Bälz, 1987; Hardie and Whiley, 1994). Data from these investigations, in particular the more recent involving DNA−DNA hybridization, rRNA cataloguing and comparative sequence analysis of small subunit (16S) rRNA have resulted in the extensive revision of the composition of the genus *Streptococcus*, allowing intrageneric (species−species) geneological relationships to be measured and the determination of the relationships between *Streptococcus* and other, closely and distantly related, genera. The major change to the composition of the genus has been the recognition that both the lactic and enterococcal groups constitute separate genera which have been named *Lactococcus* and *Enterococcus*, respectively (Schleifer and Kilpper-Bälz, 1987). Currently the genus *Streptococcus sensu stricto* includes 40 species which comprise mainly the pyogenic and oral groups together with a collection of species that do not readily form a discrete species group and which are often referred to as the 'other streptococci' (Hardie and Whiley, 1995). Recent developments in the taxonomy of the α-haemolytic streptococci are reviewed below.

Oral Streptococci

From the first systematic study of the genus (Sherman, 1937) the classification and identification of the oral or viridans streptococci was recognized as unsatisfactory. Consequently, many studies have been undertaken over the years to try and clarify the taxonomy of these bacteria, with the result that most of the new and amended species descriptions and nomenclatural changes within the genus *Streptococcus* have occurred in this group. A significant contribution to this area came from the studies undertaken by Colman and Williams (1972) that involved cell wall analyses, biochemical and physiological testing and genetic transformation. These authors described six species within the viridans streptococci – *S. mutans*, *S. sanguis*, *S. salivarius*, *S. milleri* and *S. mitior* together with *S. pneumoniae*, which could be differentiated on the basis of a short series of biochemical tests. Since then the increased use of genotypic approaches has resulted in the number of species recognized within the oral group being increased to a total of 22, including *S. pneumoniae* and *S. thermophilus* (the latter is a close relative of *S. salivarius*).

Initial emphasis was on DNA G + C determinations and DNA−DNA reassociation experiments, but the more recent application of approaches such as peptidoglycan analysis, multi-locus enzyme electrophoresis, DNA−rRNA hybridization, RNA cataloguing and 16S rRNA comparative sequence analysis has revealed that the oral streptococci comprise four main species groups centred on *S. mutans*, *S. salivarius*, *S. anginosus* ('*S. milleri*') and *S. oralis* or *S. mitis* ('*S. mitior*') (Schleifer and Kilpper-Bälz, 1987; Bentley *et al.*, 1991; Hardie and Whiley, 1994; Kawamura *et al.*, 1995a). These are considered in more detail below. A diagram showing the phylogenetic relationships between different groups of streptococci is reproduced in Figure 1a.1.

Mutans streptococci

This group of oral streptococci is associated with dental caries in man and animals and because of this has been the subject of extensive investigations. Their characteristics include the ability to produce both soluble and insoluble polysaccharides from

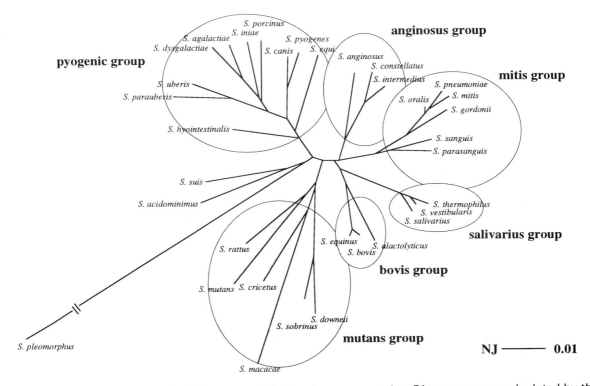

Figure 1a.1 Phylogenetic relationships among 34 *Streptococcus* species. Distances were calculated by the neighbour-joining (NJ) method. Reproduced from Kawamura *et al.* (1995) with permission.

sucrose which are important in the formation of dental plaque and in the pathogenicity (cariogenicity) of the organism. Following the original species description of *S. mutans* from carious teeth by Clarke (1924) and its isolation from a case of bacterial endocarditis shortly afterwards, little attention was paid to this species until the 1960s when it was demonstrated that caries could be experimentally induced and transmitted in animals. Similar caries-inducing streptococci were found to be present in the dental plaque of man. From that point onwards *S. mutans* became the focus of considerable attention for the application of extensive biochemical testing, serology (eight serotypes or serovars, designated a–h, have so far been demonstrated in species making up the mutans group), cell wall studies, comparative enzyme studies, electrophoretic separation of whole-cell derived polypeptides, membrane proteins, and intracellular proteins together with genotypic studies

(Hamada and Slade, 1980; Loesche, 1986). These studies revealed that isolates identified as *S. mutans* comprised a phenotypically and genetically heterogeneous taxon. As a result seven distinct species are currently recognized within the mutans group: *S. mutans* (serotypes c, e and f), *S. sobrinus* (serotypes d and g), *S. rattus* (serotype b), *S. downei* (serotype h), *S. cricetus* (serotype a), *S. ferus* (serotype c) and *S. macacae* (serotype c), although the taxonomic position of *S. ferus* is uncertain. Of these streptococci, *S. mutans* and *S. sobrinus* are commonly isolated from man whilst *S. cricetus* and *S. rattus* are occasionally recovered.

S. salivaris, S. vestibularis and S. thermophilus

Streptococcus salivarius, although not usually considered to be a significant pathogen, is commonly isolated from most areas within the oral cavity, particularly from the tongue and other mucosal surfaces and from whole saliva. This species is considered to be an important component of the oral ecosystem, because of the production of an extracellular polysaccharide (levan) from fructose and the production of urease by some strains. *S. salivarius* is a relatively easily identified species that was originally described in 1906 although the distinction between this and the much less clearly defined oral species, *S. mitis*, was later obscured by the use of inadequate phenotypic identification tests. This trend had important consequences for the classification and identification of the oral streptococci, because the name *S. mitis* was applied to a heterogeneous collection of non-haemolytic streptococci. The confusion and problems surrounding this latter species are detailed below. Notwithstanding these early difficulties, the definition of *S. salivarius* was later improved by further characterization particularly on the basis of biochemical, physiological and nutritional requirements. DNA–DNA reassociation experiments have since revealed that *S. salivarius* is closely related to *S. thermophilus* (a non-oral bacterium from dairy sources) and also to a more recently described oral species *S. vestibularis* which consists of α-haemolytic, urease-producing streptococci that are found mainly on the vestibular mucosa of the human mouth (Hardie and Whiley, 1994). The formation of a distinct species group by these three streptococci has been confirmed by 16S rRNA sequence comparisons (Bentley *et al.*, 1991; Kawamura *et al.*, 1995a).

S. anginosus, S. constellatus and S. intermedius (the 'Streptococcus milleri group')

These streptococci are common members of the oral flora and are clinically significant due to their association with purulent infections at oral and non-oral sites in man. The name '*S. milleri*' has been used for a biochemically and serologically heterogeneous collection of streptococci that recently have been shown to comprise three separate, albeit closely related species: *S. anginosus*, *S. constellatus*

and *S. intermedius* (Whiley and Beighton, 1991). The classification of these bacteria was confused for many years and this has been reflected in the number of different names that have been applied to them in the past: '*Streptococcus* MG', the minute colony-forming streptococci of Lancefield groups F and G, the haemolytic and non-haemolytic streptococci possessing the type antigens of Lancefield group F and '*S. milleri*'. The latter species epithet was used to include all these taxa on the basis of their overall biochemical and physiological similarity (Colman and Williams, 1972). However, on the other side of the Atlantic, the close resemblance between '*Streptococcus* MG' and streptococci previously named *S. anginosus*, *S. constellatus* and *S. intermedius* was recognized (Facklam, 1977). Rather than include all these non-haemolytic streptococci within a single species Facklam preferred to divide them on the basis of lactose fermentation into '*S. anginosus–constellatus*' (lactose non-fermenters) and '*S. MG–intermedius*' (lactose fermenters). The problems resulting from the use of conflicting identification schemes and nomenclatures gave rise to the suggestion for an alternative scheme in which non-haemolytic isolates should continue to be divided on the basis of lactose fermentation into *S. constellatus* (lactose −) and *S. intermedius* (lactose +) with β-haemolytic strains of Lancefield groups A, C, F, G or non-groupable designated *S. anginosus*. The answer to whether these streptococci represented a single species or not was further obscured by the conflicting data obtained in numerous studies using biochemical, serological or chemotaxonomic criteria. Evidence from DNA–DNA reassociation studies has also been in disagreement although this has been largely attributed to the inherent differences in the various methods employed. The weight of evidence from nucleic acid studies currently supports the recognition of three separate species – *S. anginosus*, *S. constellatus* and *S. intermedius* – and these have been published with amended species descriptions (Whiley and Beighton, 1991). As described later, these species definitions have allowed specific disease associations to be explored more accurately.

S. oralis, S. sanguis and closely related species

Clarification of the number of distinct species present within this group of streptococci and their accurate identification based on a robust classification has been achieved through the application of nucleic acid studies (Hardie and Whiley, 1992, 1994). The bacteria considered here form a group of species that currently includes *S. sanguis*, *S. gordonii*, *S. parasanguis*, *S. crista*, *S. oralis*, *S. mitis* and *S. pneumoniae*. In the case of several of these species, notably *S. sanguis*, *S. mitis* and *S. oralis*, combined taxonomic and nomenclatural changes have been the cause of considerable confusion. Part of this confusion arose from the emphasis placed on the possession of the Lancefield group H antigen, which was not well defined. The early literature includes descriptions of what were considered at the time to be biochemically similar isolates from the blood and heart vegetations of patients with bacterial endocarditis that were variously called '*Streptococcus* sbe', *S. sanguis* and the streptococci of Lancefield group H. Unfortunately the original strain used to raise the group H antiserum was not recorded and subsequent workers used other strains for the same purpose. Therefore the situation arose where the taxonomic position of strains carrying a 'group H antigen' could not be determined with any degree of certainty. The name *S. sanguis* was originally used for polysaccharide (dextran)-producing strains that were divided into serotypes I, II and I/II. However, Colman and Williams (1972) considered that both dextran-producing and non-producing strains should be included within this species whilst those strains unable to hydrolyse arginine and aesculin and which lacked rhamnose in their cell walls should be excluded. These latter strains were given the name '*S. mitior*' by these authors. An alternative nomenclature was proposed from the USA in which those streptococci corresponding to *S. sanguis* and '*S. mitior*' were designated *S. sanguis* biotype I, *S. sanguis* biotype II (raffinose fermenters) and *S. mitis* (raffinose non-fermenters) (Facklam, 1977). The confusion arising from the use of these alternative nomenclatural schemes

(which persist in the literature today) was not helped by the inclusion of the name *S. mitis* which, as mentioned previously, had traditionally been assigned to an ill-defined 'species' from the early days of streptococcal identification (*S. mitis* was the name given to a heterogeneous collection of α-haemolytic streptococci that could be differentiated from other recognized species on the basis of mainly negative criteria, notably by an inability to hydrolyse aesculin, ferment inulin or produce extracellular polysaccharide). Further confusion arose because the name '*S. mitior*' was not validly published and the name *S. oralis* was subsequently proposed for streptococci physiologically resembling '*S. mitior*'. Later investigations using DNA–DNA hybridization together with cell wall analyses and physiological testing demonstrated that the group of strains originally brought together within *S. oralis* were genetically as well as phenotypically heterogeneous, resulting in the redefinition of *S. oralis* (Kilpper-Bälz et al., 1985; Kilian et al., 1989). Another group of strains that possessed the same peptidoglycan type as *S. oralis* (Lys-direct) but differed in not containing ribitol teichoic acid within their cell walls was found to form a genetically distinct species and was assigned the name *S. mitis* (Kilian et al., 1989). At the time of writing both *S. oralis* and *S. mitis* are recognized according to the amended descriptions of Kilian et al. (1989).

Similar approaches have revealed that strains of *S. sanguis* comprise two distinct centres of variation and this has given rise to an amended description of *S. sanguis* and the recognition of another species, *S. gordonii* (Kilian et al., 1989).

Concurrent with the recent taxonomic developments within this group of species was the realization that the type strain NCTC 3165, that had been arbitrarily assigned to *S. mitis*, belonged to the newly described species *S. gordonii*. The result of this has been the replacement of NCTC 3165 by another strain, NCTC 12261, as the appropriate type strain of the species *S. mitis* as currently defined.

The long legacy of confusion that has stemmed from a poor definition of the Lancefield group H antigen and the emphasis placed on its possession seems hardly surprising in retrospect: antiserum raised against strain Blackburn (British group H) has been shown to react with some but not all strains of both *S. sanguis* and *S. gordonii*, while antiserum against strain F90A (American group H) reacts with some but not all strains of *S. gordonii* (Kilian *et al.*, 1989). Thus, no single antiserum appears to be species specific according to current taxonomic definitions.

Two further species have been described amongst streptococci resembling *S. sanguis*. The first, *S. parasanguis*, was originally isolated from clinical specimens (blood, throat and urine) and has been reported occasionally in bacterial endocarditis and from patients with Kawasaki disease (Hardie and Whiley, 1994). Strains are unable to ferment inulin, frequently unable to hydrolyse aesculin, do not produce extracellular polysaccharides but produce alkaline phosphatase and bind salivary amylase. The second, named *S. crista*, originally isolated from the human oral cavity and throat, is characterized by the presence of tufted fibrils on the cell surface and is able to hydrolyse arginine and weakly hydrolyse aesculin but is not able to ferment raffinose or produce alkaline phosphatase (Hardie and Whiley, 1995). The clinical importance, if any, of these two species has yet to be determined.

Nutritionally variant streptococci

This clinically important group of streptococci consists of two currently recognized species: *S. adjacens* and *S. defectivus*. They have been variously referred to in the literature as satelliting, thiol requiring, vitamin B_6 dependent, pyridoxal dependent or nutritionally deficient and require the addition of cysteine or one of the active forms of vitamin B_6 (pyridoxal hydrochloride or pyridoxamine hydrochloride) to complex media. The nutritionally variant streptococci (NVS) form part of the normal flora of the human throat, urogenital and intestinal tracts and are of clinical interest because of their association with bacterial endocarditis and other conditions including otitis media, abscesses of the brain and pancreas, wounds, pneumonia, osteomyelitis and cancer

(Bouvet *et al.*, 1989). These streptococci were originally thought to be closely related to '*S. mitior*' on the basis of physiological properties, the demonstration of a pH-dependent red chromophore together with the absence of rhamnose and the presence of ribitol teichoic acid in their cell walls. However, DNA–DNA hybridization studies demonstrated that the NVS comprised two separate species that were distinct from other recognized streptococcal species.

In a recent study based on 16S rRNA sequences, *S. adjacens* and *S. defectivus* were transferred to a new genus *Abiotrophia*, as *A. adiacens* and *A. defectiva* respectively (Kawamura *et al.*, 1995b).

Other α- and non-haemolytic streptococci

Several other species of α- and non-haemolytic streptococci are of clinical importance and deserve consideration here.

Streptococcus bovis was originally described as a bovine bacterium causing mastitis. Strains identified as *S. bovis* have also been isolated from patients with endocarditis and this species is also reported to be associated with colon cancer and other inflammatory bowel diseases in humans. Despite the recognition of the clinical significance of this organism its classification remains unsatisfactory. This may be because studies of these streptococci have concentrated either on collections of strains of bovine origin or of human strains, but not usually on both together. In addition the confusing array of biotypes that have been reported in the literature has made identification difficult. Originally described as a bovine bacterium able to ferment arabinose, raffinose, starch and inulin but not mannitol, *S. bovis* was considered to be distinct from another *Streptococcus* of bovine origin called *S. inulinaceus*. The latter species was characterized by its inability to ferment arabinose or starch and ability to ferment mannitol. However, the isolation of intermediate strains that were unable to ferment arabinose but which could hydrolyse starch eventually led to the inclusion of all of these strains within *S. bovis*. Strains of *S. bovis* from human sources are characterized as typically being able to ferment mannitol and inulin but not sorbitol or arabinose and producing copious amounts of extracellular polysaccharide (glucan) from sucrose or raffinose. In addition, a variant biotype from man has been recognized that is unable to ferment mannitol and does not produce glucan. The study of strains included within *S. bovis* by DNA–DNA hybridization has revealed a high degree of genetic heterogeneity at the species level although, as with the phenotypic studies, these have tended to concentrate either on strains from human sources or from animals but not on both (Coykendall, 1989). One study on mainly animal isolates revealed six DNA homology groups (Farrow *et al.*, 1984). Homology group 1 contained the type strains of both *S. bovis* and *S. equinus*, leading the authors to propose that the name *S. equinus* be given priority and that *S. bovis* be reduced to synonymity. Homology group 2 contained mannitol-fermenting strains from bovine mastitis together with one human strain, group 3 contained strains from dairy sources previously identified as *S. bovis* that were unusual in being unable to produce acetoin (VP negative), group 4 comprised strains from human sources as well as a strain from frozen peas, group 5 strains had been previously identified as *S. bovis* and were unusual in not producing acetoin and in producing acid from a wide range of carbohydrates (the name *S. saccharolyticus* was proposed for these streptococci), and group 6 comprised strains previously identified as *S. equinus* from pigs and chickens that characteristically were unable to ferment lactose (*S. alactolyticus* was the name proposed for these strains). Two other DNA homology-based studies concentrated mainly on strains from human sources and both indicated that phenotypically typical strains, together with some of the variant strains, belong to the same DNA homology group.

In summary, these streptococci include examples of both close (species level) and more distant genetic relationships between phenotypically diverse strains as well as low levels of DNA homology between strains separated by only a few biochemical differences. The classification of *S. bovis*, *S. equinus* and the other taxa mentioned above clearly needs further clarification through the study of a more fully representative collection of strains.

Streptococcus acidominimus was first described from bovine udders and consists of mainly α-haemolytic strains. Although not generally recognized as a human pathogen this species has, nevertheless, been isolated from cases of vaginosis and upper genital tract infection and should be noted here. The taxonomic position of *S. acidominimus* is uncertain and a recent study using 16S rRNA gene sequence comparisons placed this species outside the main species groups.

Identification and Strain Typing

The rapid and extensive taxonomic revision of the genus *Streptococcus*, including the demonstration of several new species and amended descriptions of others, has to some extent outpaced the availability of comprehensive schemes for routine identification. However, significant improvements to this situation have come about through the incorporation into identification schemes of fluorogenic and chromogenic substrates for the rapid detection of preformed enzyme activities. These test schemes combine tests for the detection of glycosidases and arylamidase reactions with more traditional tests such as carbohydrate fermentation, arginine dihydrolase and acetoin production. A further development has been the inclusion of these tests in a more standardized format in some commercially available test kits, which helps to reduce the degree of discrepancy between biochemical test results from different laboratories. Currently, a 32-test kit for identifying streptococci is available which takes into account most of the currently recognized species (ID 32 Strep system, bioMerieux). In an independent evaluation the kit gave correct identification of 95.4% (413/433) strains examined, including 109 strains that required some additional tests for complete identification. Sixteen strains remained unidentified and four were misidentified (Freney *et al.*, 1992). In another study the test kit gave correct identification of 87% of strains examined. However, *S. mitis* and *S. oralis* were not easily differentiated using this method (Kikuchi *et al.*, 1995). Other phenotypic tests that have been reported to be potentially useful, particularly for the oral streptococci, include acid and alkaline phosphatases, neuraminidase (sialidase), IgAl protease production, salivary amylase binding, extracellular polysaccharide production and the detection of hyaluronidase and chondroitin sulphate depolymerase activities. Several other approaches to species identification have been investigated such as pyrolysis–mass spectrometry, whole-cell derived polypeptide patterns by sodium dodecyl sulphate – polyacrylamide gel electrophoresis (SDS–PAGE) or other electrophoretic separation techniques and the analyses of long-chain fatty acids and cell wall components. However, these strategies have not been widely adopted and remain a part of the repertoire of the specialist research laboratory. Detailed procedures for identification of streptococcal isolates are given later in the section on Laboratory Diagnosis, with biochemical reactions shown in Table 1a.7.

Some progress has already been made towards the development of genetic-based approaches to species identification. DNA probes for this purpose have been described that utilize whole chromosomal preparations or cloned DNA fragments. However, as with most other groups of bacteria, by far the greatest promise for a genetically based identification approach lies in the exploitation of nucleotide sequence data derived from the small (16S) subunit gene of the ribosomal RNA (rRNA) cistron. Published studies have provided 16S rRNA gene sequence data for most, but not all, α- and non-haemolytic streptococci although the extension of this to the development of rDNA probes is still awaited (Bentley *et al.*, 1991; Kawamura *et al.*, 1995a). Species identification through the comparison of restriction fragment length polymorphism (RFLP) of whole chromosomal DNA has been attempted but has found limited use due largely to the complexity of the resulting patterns. The use of restriction fragment polymorphism analysis of rRNA genes (ribotyping) has proved to be a better approach and allows the recognition of *S. sanguis*, *S. oralis* and *S. gordonii* strains, although it appears not to differ-

entiate between *S. parasanguis* and *S. mitis* (Rudney and Larson, 1993).

The comparison of strains on the basis of whole chromosomal restriction digests or rRNA gene restriction patterns are the current methods of choice for differentiating between strains within a species (strain typing). The main disadvantage of the former lies in the complexity of the patterns, making comparisons between several strains potentially difficult. Since rRNA gene restriction patterns are simpler, this approach has found more favour for typing and has been used to investigate genetic diversity within several species of oral streptococci including the mutans group, the NVS and *S. sanguis*, *S. oralis* and close relatives. The number of studies where these techniques have been applied to particular clinical investigations is as yet small. However, in one recent study ribotyping was used to demonstrate the identity of blood culture and oral isolates of streptococci from two patients with endocarditis (Fiehn *et al.*, 1995).

Alternative typing methods that have been utilized for discriminating between oral streptococcal strains include conventional biotyping, plasmid profiling, serotyping and bacteriocin production. Bacteriocin typing, plasmid profiling and ribotyping of *S. mutans* strains have been used in investigations into the distribution of particular types within individuals and family groups as well as in the study of transmission of this species between mothers and offspring (Hardie and Whiley, 1992).

GENERAL PROPERTIES OF α-HAEMOLYTIC STREPTOCOCCI

Isolation and Cultural Features

The α- and non-haemolytic streptococci are fastidious organisms, having a complex nutritional requirement including the need for a carbohydrate source, amino acids, peptides and proteins, fatty acids, vitamins, purines and pyrimidines. These bacteria therefore need complex growth media commonly containing meat extract, peptone and blood or serum. Greater growth yields can be obtained in broth cultures by the use of buffered media which offer some protection from the otherwise rapid fall in pH that occurs due to the fermentation of carbohydrate. On solid media streptococci produce heavier growth when they are enriched with blood, serum or glucose. Colonies on blood agar are typically 1 mm or less in diameter after incubation for 24 hours at 37 °C, are non-pigmented and often appear translucent. Nutritionally variant streptococci require the addition of 0.001% pyridoxal HCl or pyridoxamine diHCl. As streptococci are facultative anaerobes incubation is best carried out routinely in an atmosphere of air + 10% carbon dioxide or in an anaerobic gas mix containing nitrogen (70–80%), hydrogen (10–20%) and carbon dioxide (10–20%). Some have an absolute requirement for carbon dioxide, particularly on initial isolation. The growth obtained in broth cultures varies between a diffuse turbidity to a granular appearance with clear supernatant depending on the strain and species. On blood agar the streptococci discussed here usually produce α-haemolysis or are non-haemolytic. However, as previously mentioned, the haemolytic reactions of different strains within a species may vary and can sometimes be influenced by the source (horse, sheep, etc.) of blood in the agar. The appearance of haemolysis can also be varied by preparing either pour plates or surface spread plates.

Several selective media are available for the isolation of oral streptococci and have been reviewed elsewhere (Skinner and Quesnel, 1978; Hardie and Whiley, 1992; Whiley et al., 1993). The two most commonly used (trypticase–yeast–cystine TYC and Mitis Salivarius agar MS) contain 5% sucrose to promote the production of extracellular polysaccharides resulting in the production of characteristic colonial morphologies as an aid to identification. TYC is available commercially from Lab M (Amersham, UK); MS agar is available commercially from Oxoid (Basingstoke, Hampshire, UK) and from Difco (Michigan, USA).

Some examples of colonial morphology on different culture media are illustrated in Figure 1a.2.

Colonial morphology on TYC agar

Streptococcus mutans   Colonies are 0.5–2.0 mm diameter, white, grey or occasionally yellow, rough, heaped and resemble frosted glass. Texture is crumbly although the whole colony can be easily detached from the surface of the agar. Water-soluble glucan may be produced in sufficient quantities to appear as a drop of clear liquid on the top of the colony or as a puddle around it.

Streptococcus sobrinus   Colonies are approximately 0.5 mm diameter, white, rough and irregular. A white halo or milky zone may be produced that surrounds the colonies.

Streptococcus sanguis and S. gordonii   Colonies are 1–2 mm in diameter, grey, white or colourless, smooth and rubbery. The colonies are usually strongly adherent to the surface of the agar and cannot be detached. Some strains of these species do not produce extracellular polysaccharide, in which case they produce soft, non-adherent colonies.

Streptococcus oralis   This species includes strains of two colonial types: (1) similar to S.

Figure 1a.2 Colonial appearance of α–haemolytic streptococci on blood agar (BA) and 5% sucrose containing agars (TYC, Mitis–Salivarius [M–S]): (a) S. anginosus (BA); (b) S. anginosus (TYC); (c) S. anginosus (M–S); (d) S. intermedius (BA) showing rough and smooth colony variants; (e) S. salivarius (BA); (f)–(g) S. salivarius (TYC) showing extracellular polysaccharide (ecp) production (fructan); (h) S. salivarius (M–S); (i) S. sanguis (BA); (j) S. sanguis (TYC) showing ecp production (glucan); (k) S. sanguis (M–S); (l) S. mutans (BA); (m) S. mutans (TYC) showing ecp production (glucan); (n) S. mutans (M–S); (o) S. bovis (BA); (p) S. bovis (M–S) showing ecp production (glucan). The authors gratefully acknowledge the help and advice given by Mr. R. Westran of the Department of Medical Microbiology, LHMC, in the preparation of this figure.

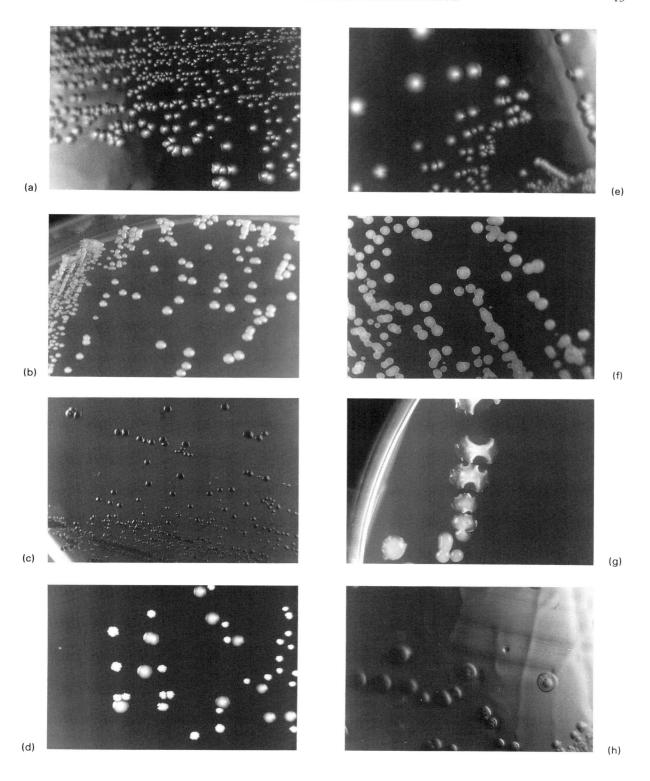

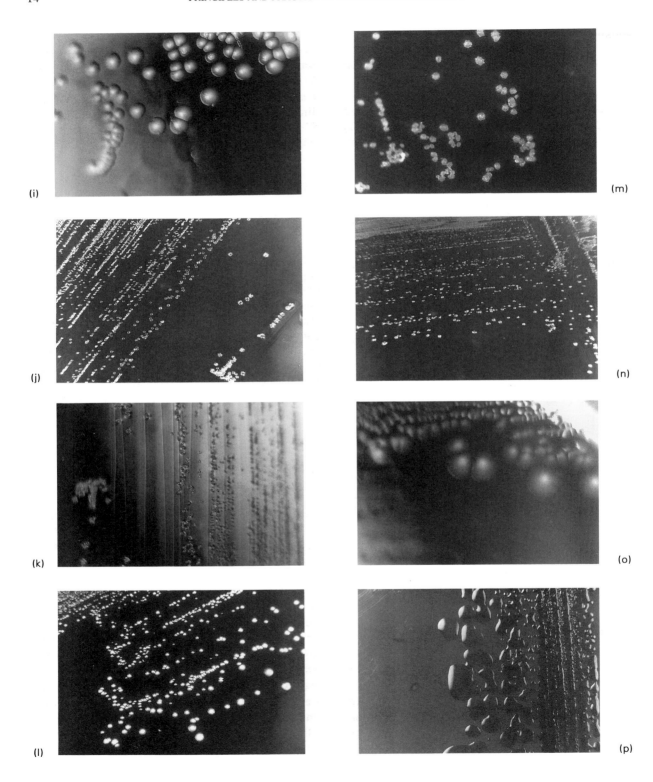

(i)

(m)

(j)

(n)

(k)

(o)

(l)

(p)

sanguis; (2) a 0.5–2.0 mm diameter, smooth, soft, non-adherent, grey, white or colourless. Some strains of this species do not produce extracellular polysaccharide.

Streptococcus anginosus, S. constellatus and S. intermedius Colonies are of two types: (1) 1–2 mm diameter grey or white, smooth and soft; (2) 0.5–1.0 mm diameter, grey or white, dry, crumbly and 'pinpointed'.

Streptococcus vestibularis Colonies are 1–2 mm diameter, smooth, soft and white. No extracellular polysaccharide is produced.

Streptococcus mitis and S. parasanguis Colonies are similar to the soft, non-polysaccharide-producing strains of *S. oralis*.

Streptococcus salivarius Colonies are 2–6 mm diameter, domed, smooth and mucoid although older colonies may become hard, pitting the agar.

Streptococcus bovis Colonies of glucan-producing strains are characterized by the presence of copious amounts of extracellular polysaccharide giving rise to watery/slimy growth that is maximized on incubation in air + 5% carbon dioxide.

When grown on MS agar *S. mutans* strains appear rough and resemble frosted glass, *S. salivarius* strains give either large (2–5 mm diameter), smooth, mucoid colonies or rough, irregular colonies, *S. sanguis* strains give <1.0 mm diameter, hard, rubbery, adherent colonies (zooglea) and *S. vestibularis* strains form 2–3 mm diameter, matt, colonies with undulate edges when grown anaerobically.

Other selective media

Streptococcus mutans Several selective media have been developed for the isolation of mutans streptococci. Two that are frequently used are based on TYC or MS agars and have the addition of bacitracin (0.1 or 0.2 units/ml) and an increased amount of sucrose (20%).

Streptococcus anginosus, S. constellatus and S. intermedius (the 'S. milleri group') Nalidixic acid–sulphamethazine agar (NAS) uses 40 g/l sensitivity agar 30 μg/ml nalidixic acid, 1 mg/ml sulphamethazine (4-amino-N-[4,6-dimethyl-2-pyrimidinyl]benzene sulphonamide) + 5% defibrinated horse blood. This medium is also selective for *S. mutans*.

Cellular morphology

Streptococci are usually spherical in shape with cells of approximately 1 μm diameter arranged in chains or pairs. The length of the chains may vary between a few cells only to over 50 cells depending on the strain. Streptococci stain positive in the Gram stain although older cultures may appear Gram variable. Some strains may appear as short rods under certain cultural conditions. It has also been reported that with the nutritionally variant streptococci the persistence of aberrant morphological forms can occur despite continued subculture on media supplemented with pyridoxal HCl and may therefore pose a problem during identification of clinical isolates.

Biochemical and metabolic characteristics

Under conditions of glucose excess streptococci ferment glucose to L-lactate by the glycolytic pathway. This is homolactic fermentation with approximately 95% of the sugar being converted to lactate. However, if growth is limited by the amount of glucose present then heterolactic fermentation takes place and the main end products of glucose metabolism are formate, acetate and ethanol, with only approximately 1% of the glucose being converted to lactate. Under glucose limitation streptococci possessing the arginine deaminase system will give an increased cell yield if arginine is added to the culture medium. A wide range of carbohydrates can be transported into the cell by phosphoenolpyruvate-mediated phosphotransferases (PEP–PTS) and thereby utilized. This ability forms the basis of many of the commonly used phenotypic tests that are included in identification schemes for these bacteria. Interestingly, PTS systems are usually repressed under acidic conditions although in the case of the acidogenic species *S. mutans* a low pH enhances the growth and production of acid due to the presence in these streptococci of an alternative sugar uptake system driven by the energy associated with the cell membrane (protonmotive force).

Several of these streptococci are characterized by the production of extracellular polysaccharides when grown in excess sucrose. These polysaccharides are composed of glucose subunits (glucans or dextrans) or of fructose subunits (fructans) and are formed directly from sucrose by glucosyltransferases and fructosyltransferases, respectively.

Antigenic complexity

As mentioned above the success obtained in producing a serological classification for the pyogenic streptococci was not extended to the α- and non-haemolytic species. Several early attempts to this end were unsatisfactory and failed to produce an all-encompassing scheme for these streptococci. The difficulties surrounding the serology of *S. sanguis*, *S. oralis* and related species have been referred to earlier. In retrospect these studies were probably frustrated by the unsatisfactory classification of the viridans streptococci at the time as well as by the numerous serological cross-reactions that characterize these species. Serological studies have also been undertaken on the '*S. milleri*-group' with the aim of developing a useful scheme for serotyping clinical isolates. In one study (Kitada *et al.*, 1992), 91 clinical isolates were tested for possession of a Lancefield group antigen and/or one of eight cell surface carbohydrate serotyping antigens (a–k). Unfortunately 19/91 isolates (21%) failed to react against any of the antisera, added to which the identity of the streptococci examined cannot be related to currently accepted species with any certainty.

Serological analysis of some of these streptococci has provided useful data with important consequences. Serological subdivisions within the mutans streptococci together with biochemical and genetic data led to the recognition of several distinct species of acidogenic oral bacteria and this is of considerable significance to studies of dental caries. There are currently eight serotypes (serovars) recognized within these streptococci (a–h) based on the possession of serotype specific cell wall polysaccharide antigens (Hamada and Slade, 1980): *S. mutans* (c, e and f), *S. sobrinus* (d and g), *S. cricetus* (a), *S. rattus* (b), *S. downei* (h), *S. ferus* (c) and *S. macacae* (c). Characterization of the antigenic composition of mutans streptococci, particularly *S. mutans* and *S. sobrinus*, has been central to the search for an effective and safe vaccine against dental caries. Earlier attempts to use crude whole cell or cell wall preparations for immunization were criticized over the potential for immunological cross-reactions with human tissue, particularly to heart tissue, and this led to a search for candidate antigens that would not result in such cross-reactivity. Further consideration is given below to the possibility of immunizing against dental caries.

INFECTIONS CAUSED BY α-HAEMOLYTIC AND NON-HAEMOLYTIC STREPTOCOCCI

As mentioned previously, these streptococci comprise a significant part of the normal commensal flora of the body. They are involved in a number of different types of infection described below, in which the source of the causative organisms is almost invariably endogenous, being derived from the host's microflora (Hardie and Whiley, 1992). The streptococcal species themselves are generally thought to be of relatively low virulence, not usually associated with acute, rapidly spreading infections such as those caused by *S. pyogenes*, although they clearly have phenotypic features which result in the production of disease under appropriate circumstances (Hardie and Whiley, 1994).

Since many of these streptococci are present in the mouth, upper respiratory tract, genitourinary tract and, to a lesser extent, gastrointestinal tract, they are sometimes involved in pathological processes at these sites, possibly following some local or systemic change in host susceptibility, or an alteration in local environmental conditions. Alternatively, the streptococci at a mucosal site may gain access to the bloodstream as a result of some local traumatic event and set up an infection at a distant location, such as the heart valve in endocarditis or in the brain, giving rise to a cerebral abscess.

Several major pathogenic species of bacteria have been shown to produce the enzyme IgAl protease, which may significantly enhance their ability to withstand this important immunoglobulin at mucosal surfaces. Amongst the known IgA protease producers are *Haemophilus influenzae*, *Neisseria gonorrhoeae* and *Streptococcus pneumoniae*, but this ability is also found in some of the α-haemolytic streptococci and has even been suggested as a useful discriminatory test for identification purposes (Kilian *et al.*, 1989). Streptococci known to produce IgA protease include several of the species which are associated with endocarditis and with abscesses, including *S. sanguis* and *S. oralis*. Although this property is not directly responsible for the pathogenic activities of these organisms, any factor which enables a potential pathogen to withstand the host's defence mechanisms is potentially a significant virulence determinant.

In the following sections, the main types of infection commonly associated with the viridans streptococci are described under the headings of infective endocarditis, dental caries, abscesses, and infections in immunocompromised patients. It is a feature of this group of microorganisms that there is no specific, named disease that is invariably and exclusively caused by any individual species. In contrast, most of these opportunistic infections are associated with several different streptococcal species and, in some cases, representatives of other genera.

Infective Endocarditis

Pathogenesis

Infective endocarditis involving α-haemolytic streptococci usually occurs in patients with pre-existing valvular lesions and is typically subacute, whereas the acute form of endocarditis which can occur in those with previously undamaged heart valves is associated with more virulent bacteria such as *Staphylococcus aureus*, *Streptococcus pyogenes* or *Streptococcus pneumoniae*. Patients at particular risk of developing subacute endocarditis include those with congenital heart defects affecting the valves, those with acquired cardiac lesions following rheumatic fever, and those who have undergone valve replacement surgery (Littler and Shanson, 1989). These predisposing conditions give rise to the development of non-infected platelet−fibrin vegetations (non-bacterial thrombotic vegetations) on the endocardium which may subsequently become infected by circulating microorganisms in the bloodstream during a transient bacteraemia (Freedman, 1987).

It is often difficult to pinpoint exactly the precipitating event which gives rise to the development of endocarditis because of the prolonged time period that may elapse between a particular episode of bacteraemia and the subsequent development of the disease. This time interval may be further extended as a result of the insidious onset of signs and symptoms which can make early diagnosis difficult. An important potential source of the organisms which cause bacteraemias is the oral cavity, although streptococci and other endocarditis-inducing bacteria can also enter the bloodstream from other body sites. Any surgical procedure in the mouth, especially tooth extraction, periodontal surgery, apicectomy and deep scaling, will almost invariably give rise to a transient bacteraemia, and patients with known predisposing cardiac lesions should always be protected with prophylactic antibiotics when undergoing such treatment. Even less invasive procedures, including restorative dentistry (fillings and crowns), impression taking and toothbrushing, may occasionally cause a bacteraemia, particularly in patients with poor oral hygiene and extensive periodontal disease.

When investigating the likely site of entry of bacteria in cases of endocarditis, it should not be forgotten that surgery or endoscopy in other parts of the body, such as the gastrointestinal, genitourinary and respiratory tracts, may also produce a transient bacteraemia. Entry through the skin is another potential route, but this is less likely to be the source of a bacteraemia due to α-haemolytic streptococci.

Although α-haemolytic streptococci are not the only organisms which get into the bloodstream from time to time, they do account for a large proportion of cases of endocarditis (see below). However, ability to cause infective endocarditis is certainly not confined to any particular genus or species, and cases reported in the literature indicate that almost any microorganism can, on occasions, be isolated from patients with this condition.

A number of features of streptococci isolated from endocarditis have been investigated as potential virulence determinants and some of these are listed in Table 1a.2. The ability of certain species, including *S. sanguis*, to aggregate human platelets, and attachment to extracellular matrix components (ECM) such as collagen, laminin and fibronectin, are among the factors which may be significant. The production of extracellular polysaccharides from sucrose by some streptococcal species has also been suggested as a relevant property, and a fimbriae-associated protein that may be involved in the attachment of *S. parasanguis* to platelet–fibrin

vegetations has been described. Several of these putative virulence factors have been tested experimentally, either *in vitro* or in animal experiments, and the ability to aggregate platelets certainly appears to be one of the factors of particular significance (Hardie and Whiley, 1994).

Epidemiology

It has been estimated that about 20 cases of infective endocarditis per million of the population per year can be expected in England and Wales, of whom, on past experience, about 20% are likely to die (Young, 1987). Between 1975 and 1987, around 200 (±30) deaths per year were recorded in these countries.

There have been many surveys of the causative agents in infective endocarditis over the years, but, despite some reported changes in the frequency of occurrence of different microorganisms, streptococci continue to be the most common group found, accounting for about 50% of cases in most published series (Littler and Shanson, 1989; Hardie and Whiley, 1992; Young, 1987).

In studies where the streptococci from cases of endocarditis have been identified to species level, virtually all of the known α-haemolytic species have been identified on at least some occasions. Most commonly, these have included *S. sanguis*, '*S. mitior*' (possibly corresponding to *S. oralis*) and *S. mutans*, with less frequent isolations of other species. It is sometimes difficult to equate the identity of the streptococci reported in earlier studies with the currently accepted classification and nomenclature, particularly with respect to

TABLE 1a.2 POTENTIAL VIRULENCE DETERMINANTS OF STREPTOCOCCI ASSOCIATED WITH INFECTIVE ENDOCARDITIS

Aggregation of platelets
Adherence to:
  platelets
  fibronectin
  fibrinogen
  laminin
  other extracellular matrix proteins
Production of extracellular polysaccharides (glucans and fructans)
Surface lipoteichoic acid (LTA)
Avoidance of host defences

---

strains identified as *S. sanguis*, '*S. mitior*', *S. mitis*, or simply '*S. viridans*'. In one recent study, 47 streptococcal isolates from 42 confirmed cases of infective endocarditis were identified by current taxonomic criteria showing that *S. sanguis* (representing three biotypes), *S. oralis* and *S. gordonii* were the most common species in this series (Douglas *et al.*, 1993). Smaller numbers of *S. bovis*, *S. parasanguis*, *S. mitis*, *S. mutans* and *S. salivarius* were also found. These data are shown in Table 1a.3, together with a composite summary of comparable results from previously published reports.

Clinical features

Infective endocarditis due to α-haemolytic streptococci is usually subacute and may be difficult to diagnose in the earlier stages because of the vagueness and non-specificity of the signs and symptoms. The patient often presents initially with fever, general malaise and a heart murmur, whilst other features such as emboli, cardiac failure, splenomegaly, finger clubbing, petechial haemor-

rhages and anaemia may also be seen at some stage. In addition to fever, rigours and malaise, patients may also suffer from anorexia, weight loss, arthralgia and confusion (Littler and Shanson, 1989). Because of the decline in the number of cases of rheumatic heart disease in some countries and the increase in other predisposing causes, the clinical presentation of infective endocarditis can vary considerably and may not conform to classical descriptions of the disease.

Laboratory diagnosis

Whenever there is clinical suspicion of infective endocarditis, it is important to take blood cultures as soon as possible, before antibiotic treatment is started. At least 20 ml of blood should be taken from adults on each sampling occasion, and it is usually recommended that three separate samples are collected during the 12–24-hour period following the initial provisional diagnosis. Most positive cultures are obtained from the first two sets of blood cultures. If antibiotic therapy has already been commenced it may be necessary to collect

TABLE 1a.3   STREPTOCOCCI ISOLATED FROM INFECTIVE ENDOCARDITIS

Species[a]	Isolation frequency (% of streptococcal isolates)	
	Earlier literature[b]	Douglas et al. (1993)[c]
S. sanguis	7–29	31.9[d]
S. oralis	7–30	29.8
S. gordonii	NR	12.7
S. bovis	5–17	ND
S. parasanguis	NR	4.2
S. mitis	NR	4.2
S. mutans	3–18	4.2
S. salivarius	1–4	4.2
'S. milleri group'	3–15	ND
NVS	8–17	ND
Enterococci	5–10	ND
Unidentified	1–33	2.1

NR, not recorded (may have been reported under different names); ND, not detected; NVS, nutritionally variant streptococci.
[a] Species names as currently recognized.
[b] From summary of earlier published studies in Hardie and Whiley (1992).
[c] data from Douglas *et al.* (1993).
[d] Three biotypes of *S. sanguis* reported.

several more blood cultures over a few days in order to increase the chances of obtaining positive cultures (Littler and Shanson, 1989).

Aseptically collected blood samples should, ideally, be inoculated into at least two culture bottles, to allow reliable isolation of both aerobic and anaerobic bacteria. The 'nutritionally variant streptococci' (*S. adjacens* and *S. defectivus*) require the addition of pyridoxal to the medium for successful isolation. Many laboratories now use semi-automated systems for processing blood culture specimens, but both these and conventional methods sometimes yield 'culture-negative' results from patients with suspected endocarditis. Such negative results may be due to previous antibiotic therapy, the presence of particularly fastidious bacteria, use of poor culture media or isolation techniques, or infection due to microorganisms other than bacteria. In these cases, serological evidence of infection may be helpful (Littler and Shanson, 1989).

Management

Effective management of infective endocarditis includes both treatment to control and eliminate the causative infectious agent and other measures to maintain the patient's life and well-being. Increasingly, cardiac surgery is carried out at a relatively early stage in order to replace damaged and ineffective heart valves.

The antimicrobial treatment depends upon maintaining sustained, high-dose levels of appropriate bactericidal agents, usually administered intravenously or intramuscularly, at least in the early stages. It is vital that the aetiological agent, once isolated from repeated blood cultures, be fully identified and tested for antibiotic sensitivity. In some cases, such as with the enterococci, sensitivity to synergistic mixtures of drugs as well as to single chemotherapeutic agents may be required. In addition to determining which antibiotics are most likely to be effective against the particular organisms isolated, the microbiology laboratory will also be required periodically to monitor that bactericidal levels of the selected drug(s) are being maintained in the patient's blood.

Clearly the choice of antimicrobial agents depends upon the identity of the causative agent. In the case of streptococcal endocarditis, the bacteria are usually sensitive to penicillin so that benzyl penicillin, together with probenecid (to reduce renal excretion of the penicillin), is often the drug of choice. For less sensitive streptococci, and invariably for enterococci, penicillin is given together with an aminoglycoside which has a synergistic effect. For patients who are allergic to penicillin, intravenous vancomycin is a possible alternative drug (BSAC, 1992).

Prevention

When patients are known to have predisposing cardiac lesions, great care should be taken to protect them from the risk of endocarditis whilst undergoing any dental, surgical or investigational procedures which might induce a transient bacteraemia. However, even if carried out perfectly, this approach is not likely to prevent all episodes of endocarditis because up to 50% of cases of the disease occur in individuals without previously diagnosed cardiac abnormalities (Littler and Shanson, 1989). For the identified 'at risk' groups, appropriate antibiotic prophylaxis should be given as summarized in Table 1a.4.

The main principle governing these prophylactic regimens is that a high circulating blood level of a suitable bactericidal agent should be achieved at the time when the bacteraemia occurs. It is definitely not desirable to start prophylaxis many hours (or even days) prior to dental surgery or other operative procedures since this will only encourage the selection of resistant strains amongst the resident microflora. In the case of bacteraemias arising during dental surgery, additional protection can be achieved by supplementing the use of systemic antibiotics with locally applied chlorhexidine gluconate gel (1%) or chlorhexidine gluconate mouthwash (0.2%), 5 minutes before the procedure. The actual dental procedures which require antibiotic prophylaxis include extractions, scaling, and surgery involving gingival tissues. A most important consideration for patients who are at risk of endocarditis is that their dental treatment be planned

TABLE 1a.4   RECOMMENDED ANTIBIOTIC PROPHYLAXIS FOR ENDOCARDITIS

(1)   Dental procedures under local or no anaesthetic (including those with prosthetic valve).
   (a)   Patients not allergic to penicillin and who have not received penicillin more than once in previous month
      Oral amoxycillin 3 g, 1 hour before procedure (under supervision)
      (child under 5 years, quarter of adult dose; 5–10 years, half adult dose)
   (b)   Patients who are allergic to penicillin or have received penicillin more than once in previous month
      Oral clindamycin 600 mg, 1 hour before procedure
      (child under 5 years, quarter of adult dose; 5–10 years, half adult dose)
   (c)   Patients who have had endocarditis
      Amoxycillin + gentamicin (as under general anaesthesia)
(2)   Dental procedures under general anaesthesia
   (a)   No special risk, not allergic to penicillin (or recent penicillin treatment)
      Either
      Amoxycillin 1 g i.m. or i.v. at induction, then oral amoxycillin 500 mg 6 hours later
      (child under 5 years, quarter of adult dose; 5–10 years, half adult dose)
      Or
      Oral amoxycillin 3 g + oral probenecid 1 g, 4 hours before procedure
   (b)   Special risk (prosthetic valve or previous episode of endocarditis)
      Amoxycillin 1 g i.m. or i.v. + gentamicin 120 mg i.m. or i.v. at induction, then oral amoxycillin 500 mg
      6 hours later
      (child under 5 years, quarter of adult dose of amoxycillin + gentamicin 2 mg/kg; 5–10 years, half adult
      dose of amoxycillin + gentamicin 2 mg/kg)
   (c)   Patients who are allergic to penicillin or have received penicillin more than once in previous month
      Either
      Vancomycin 1 g i.v. over at least 100 minutes, then gentamicin 120 mg i.v. at induction or 15 minutes
      before procedure
      (child under 10 years, vancomycin 20 mg/kg; gentamicin 2 mg/kg)
      Or
      Teicoplanin 400 mg i.v. + gentamicin 120 mg at induction or 15 minutes before procedure
      (child under 14 years, teicoplanin 6 mg/kg + gentamicin 2 mg/kg)
      Or
      Clindamycin 300 mg i.v. over at least 10 minutes at induction or 15 minutes before procedure then oral or
      i.v. clindamycin 150 mg 6 hours later
      (child under 5 years, quarter of adult dose; 5–10 years, half adult dose)
(3)   Upper respiratory tract procedures.
      As for dental procedures; postoperative dose may be given parenterally if swallowing is painful
(4)   Genitourinary tract procedures
      As for special-risk patients undergoing dental procedures under general anaesthesia, except that clinamycin is
      not given; if urine is infected, prophylaxis should also cover infecting organism
(5)   Obstetric, gynaecological and gastrointestinal procedures
      As for genitourinary procedures
      (prophylactic cover only recommended for patients with prosthetic valves or who have had endocarditis
      previously)

Information from British National Formulary (1994), based on Recommendations of Endocarditis Working Party of the British Society
for Antimicrobial Chemotherapy.

carefully to avoid the need for frequent antibiotic prophylaxis. Even more essential for these individuals is the application of good oral hygiene and other preventive techniques in order to avoid the need for bacteraemia-inducing operative procedures as far as possible.

As indicated in Table 1a.4, prophylaxis is also required for patients undergoing surgery or invasive investigative procedures involving other parts of the body (BSAC, 1992).

Dental Caries

Pathogenesis

Dental caries or dental decay is a disease that destroys the hard tissues of the teeth. If unchecked, the disease process may progress to involve the pulp of the tooth and, eventually, the periapical tissues surrounding the roots. Once the process has reached the periapical region, infection may either remain localized as an acute dental abscess or a chronic granuloma, or may spread more widely in various directions depending on its anatomical position. In some cases, such spreading infections arising from a carious tooth may give rise to a life-threatening situation, particularly if the airway is obstructed by submandibular swelling (as in Ludwig's angina) or if the infection spreads to the brain.

Although there have been many theories about the aetiology of dental caries over the centuries, it is generally accepted today that the disease is initiated by acid demineralization of the teeth. This occurs as a result of the metabolic activities of saccharolytic bacteria (such as streptococci) which are situated on the tooth surface as part of the complex microbial community known as dental plaque. Dental plaque accumulates rapidly on exposed tooth surfaces in the mouth (like biofilms in many other ecological situations where there are solid–liquid interfaces), and consists of a complicated mixture of bacteria and their products, including several streptococcal species. When an external source of carbohydrate becomes available, in the form of dietary carbohydrate (usually sucrose), streptococci and other bacteria rapidly utilize the fermentable sugars and release acidic metabolic end products, such as lactic acid. These can be detected almost immediately in dental plaque following sugar intake and result in a rapid drop in pH. If the pH drops below the level of about 5.5 the environment is sufficiently acidic to cause demineralization of the dental enamel (Hardie, 1992).

In practice, the development of dental caries at any particular site depends on several interrelated factors, including:

(1) the complexity of the dental plaque microflora:
   (a) several different acid-producing species present;
   (b) possible acid-neutralizing effects of metabolic activities of other plaque bacteria;
   (c) physical situation of potentially cariogenic species in relation to the tooth surface and other plaque bacteria;

(2) the influence of environmental factors:
   (a) type, amount and frequency of dietary sugar intake;
   (b) effects of fluorides and other chemicals;
   (c) oral hygiene procedures;
(3) host factors:
   (a) systemic and local immune responses;
   (b) susceptibility of teeth (affected by genetic, developmental and environmental factors);
   (c) composition and flow rate of saliva.

Another important aspect of the disease is the progression of caries from a small initial lesion at the tooth surface caused by acidogenic bacteria to a large cavity which may involve enamel, dentine, pulp and, ultimately, periapical tissues. Microbiologically, it is known that the particular bacteria involved at different stages of the process vary, providing an example of the phenomenon of microbial succession.

In the initial stages of caries, which are critical for possible preventive strategies, the bacteria involved (often referred to as cariogenic bacteria) are acidogenic species which are able to colonize the tooth surface. These include species within the genera *Streptococcus* and *Lactobacillus*, although most of the evidence favours streptococci in the earliest stages. Once a cavity has been produced and the lesion extends beyond the amelo-dentinal junction, a complex mixture of bacteria is found which comprises both Gram-positive and Gram-negative species, some of which are obligate anaerobes. In the less highly mineralized dentine, proteolytic activities of these bacteria may contribute significantly to the destructive process, whereas enamel dissolution is due almost entirely to the effects of acid.

The absolute necessity for bacteria in the production of dental caries was shown experimentally in germ-free animals in the late 1950s. Such animals (rats and hamsters) only developed caries when the mouth was inoculated with bacteria, even though they received a high-sugar, cariogenic diet. Similar experimental procedures have been employed subsequently by several investigators to demonstrate the cariogenic potential of different bacterial species and strains. Such studies have indicated that cariogenic potential is not confined to a single genus or species, but that several species of *Streptococcus*, *Lactobacillus* and *Actinomyces* may play a role in the disease (Hardie, 1992). However, species of the '*Streptococcus mutans* group', notably *S. mutans* and *S. sobrinus*, have usually been shown to be the most cariogenic organisms in such animal studies, both with regard to disease severity and the proportion of strains tested that are capable of inducing the disease (Hamada and Slade, 1980; Loesche, 1986).

Most detailed studies on the pathogenesis of dental caries have concentrated on the mutans streptococci, since these are widely regarded as the most significant initiators of the disease. Properties of these streptococci that are considered to be important in caries are listed in Table 1a.5. Mutant strains lacking one or more of these attributes have been shown to have reduced cariogenetic potential in gnotobiotic animals. As in other areas of microbial pathogenicity, increasing attention is now being given to the use of molecular genetics in studying the virulence determinants of cariogenic bacteria (Russell, 1994). Several genes coding for putative virulence factors in *S. mutans* have now been cloned and sequenced.

Epidemiology

Many cross-sectional studies have been reported in which the prevalence of caries, as determined by the number of decayed, missing and filled tooth surfaces (DMFS), is correlated with the levels of mutans streptococci (MS), either in saliva or in samples of dental plaque from the tooth surfaces. Such studies frequently reveal that there is indeed an association between these variables, but this does not necessarily prove a cause-and-effect relationship. Considerably

fewer longitudinal studies have been undertaken, since these are extremely costly and time consuming, but most of these have also tended to support the evidence which incriminates *S. mutans* and *S. sobrinus* as the most common aetiological agents in dental caries. However, the possible involvement of other bacteria, such as the lactobacilli, cannot be excluded on the basis of available epidemiological evidence (Bowden, 1991).

The observed associations between numbers of mutans streptococci (and lactobacilli) in saliva and caries are sometimes utilized as a method of assessing caries risk in individual patients. Thus, those with mutans streptococci levels of 2.5×10^5 cfu/ml or higher are regarded as being at 'high risk' with respect to dental caries and may require intensive dietary advice and other preventive measures. These counts can be performed by conventional viable counting methods, using media selective for mutans streptococci, or by a commercially available kit test ('Dentocult', Orion Diagnostica, Finland).

Considerable interest has been shown in the acquisition and transmission of *S. mutans*, since colonization of infants' mouths by this species may be related to their subsequent caries experience. Earlier studies using bacteriocin typing as a method for monitoring strains indicated that mothers were the most common source of the mutans streptococci acquired by infants, and these findings have been confirmed and extended more recently using other strain-typing methods, such as DNA restriction fragment polymorphism. It has been shown that mothers with high salivary mutans streptococci levels transmit these bacteria to their children at an earlier age than those with low mutans streptococci counts, and that these children are subsequently likely to experience more caries. It also appears that initial acquisition of mutans streptococci by infants

TABLE 1a.5   PROPERTIES OF MUTANS STREPTOCOCCI ASSOCIATED WITH CARIOGENICITY

Acidogenicity	Production of acid from carbohydrates
Aciduricity	Ability to survive at relatively low pH
Production of extracellular polysaccharides from sucrose	Glucans, dextrans
Production of intracellular polysaccharides	Glycogen-like storage products
Ability to colonize tooth surfaces	Survival and growth in dental plaque

may occur at specific times during growth and development (Caufield *et al.*, 1993). Such observations raise the interesting prospect of monitoring the oral microflora of pregnant and nursing mothers, with a view to recommending measures that may inhibit or delay the acquisition of mutans streptococci by their offspring.

Clinical features

The clinical presentation of caries depends upon a number of variables, including the stage and severity of the disease, the age of the patient and the type of tooth and tooth surface affected. In the earliest stages, carious lesions may appear as chalky, white spots on the enamel. Pits and fissures of posterior teeth may show colour changes and feel 'sticky' to the touch when probed with a dental explorer. Caries can also be initiated on the root surface in older patients with recession of the gingival tissues, producing lesions adjacent to the gingival margins of the teeth. At a slightly later stage, actual cavitation may be observed visually or detected by probing. For detection of early lesions between the posterior teeth, on the approximal surfaces, radiographs are required to aid diagnosis (Kidd and Joyston-Bechal, 1987).

As the disease advances, it becomes easier to detect because of the progressive destruction of tooth tissue. In rampant caries, all or most of the teeth may be destroyed, sometimes leaving nothing but a row of stumps in the mouth. A particular form of this is seen in infants ('nursing bottle caries') and is associated with the use of sweetened feeding bottles, comforters and dummies, resulting in the almost complete decay of the anterior teeth. Another form of rampant caries is sometimes seen in adult patients following loss of salivary gland secretions, particularly following radiotherapy of the head and neck region.

When dental caries are allowed to progress to the stage where the deeper dentine and pulp tissue are involved, patients may complain of pain, sometimes excruciating. At an earlier stage, before severe pulpal involvement, the tooth with a carious cavity may become sensitive to sweetness and temperature changes.

The final stage is reached when the pulp becomes necrotic and infected, and infection may then spread to the periapical region and beyond. At this point, clinical presentation depends on the actual tooth involved and the extent of spread of the infection.

Laboratory diagnosis

In practice, dental caries is invariably diagnosed by a combination of clinical observation and radiographs. Laboratory techniques can be used as a measure of 'caries risk', usually by estimating the salivary numbers of mutans streptococci and lactobacilli, as mentioned previously. Such 'caries activity tests' do have a useful place for monitoring the efficacy of preventive measures, such as restriction of dietary sugar intake, although they are not widely used in general dental practice in the UK.

Management

The treatment of dental caries depends upon the severity of the condition and the particular teeth and sites involved. In the very earliest stages of the disease, before actual cavitation of the tooth surface has occurred, it may be possible to arrest the carious process and achieve some degree of repair and remineralization of the enamel by topical application of fluorides.

Treatment of established carious lesions (cavities) in the enamel, dentine or cementum (in root surface caries) of the tooth is normally accomplished by removing the diseased dental tissue with rotary instruments (burs or drills) and various hand instruments, then restoring the tooth with appropriate filling or crowns materials (Kidd and Joyston-Bechal, 1987).

When the carious process is so advanced that the dental pulp and periapical tissues are involved, the tooth may either be extracted or, in some cases, saved by endodontic (root canal) treatment. The principle of the latter is to clean out and debride the root canal mechanically, treat with locally applied disinfectants or antibiotics to eliminate any residual microorganisms, and finally occlude the canal with an inert root filling.

Prevention

The main approaches to caries prevention include the control of dietary carbohydrates, particularly by reducing the frequency of sugar intakes, the use of fluorides (both systematically and topically), maintenance of good oral hygiene and plaque control, application of fissure sealants, and regular dental check-ups (Kidd and Joyston-Bechal, 1989). Attempts to control the microorganisms involved in caries by mechanical or chemical plaque control (such as with chlorhexidine gluconate gels or mouthwashes) have not generally been successful as a long term measure although they do have a place alongside the other preventive approaches, as a short-term expedient.

Considerable interest has been shown in the possibility of developing a caries vaccine directed against *S. mutans*, although this has not yet resulted in any tangible results in humans. Several types of vaccine have been developed and tested in laboratory animals, starting with whole bacterial cells and progressing to glucosyltransferase enzymes and various other specific purified protein antigens (Russell, 1992). A significant protective effect has been demonstrated in many of these studies, but it has not so far proved possible to transfer these encouraging experimental results to human clinical trials. This is partly due to concerns about potential safety risks, possibly arising from cross-reactions between streptococcal antigens and human heart tissues (claimed not to be found with the more highly purified protein preparations), and also because caries can effectively be prevented by other means.

One benefit of the attempts to prevent dental caries by active immunization has been a great increase in understanding about the mechanisms of mucosal immunity. Some workers have also been exploring the interesting possibility of passive immunization by oral administration of preformed monoclonal antibodies against a cell surface antigen of *S. mutans* (Russell, 1992).

Abscesses Caused by Alpha-Haemolytic Streptococci

Pathogenesis

Streptococci are frequently isolated from purulent infections in various parts of the body, including dental, brain and liver abscesses. Commonly there is a mixture of several organisms in the pus, which may contain obligate anaerobes as well as streptococci, and other facultative anaerobes. Thus, it is difficult to determine the contribution that any individual bacterial strain or species is making to the infectious process. The source of these bacteria is usually the patient's own commensal microflora and may be derived from the mouth, upper respiratory tract, gastrointestinal or genitourinary tract.

The species which comprise the '*S. milleri* Group' (*S. anginosus*, *S. intermedius* and *S. constellatus*) are often associated with abscesses and other purulent conditions. Researchers have started to look for possible virulence determinants in these species, including the production of hyaluronidase and a range of other hydrolytic enzymes which may contribute to the breakdown of host tissues.

Epidemiology

Until the recent clarification of the taxonomy of *S. anginosus*, *S. constellatus* and *S. intermedius*, it was not possible to study disease associations of these streptococci with any degree of precision. Now that the three species can be identified with confidence, such epidemiological investigations have become feasible. Examination of a large series of isolates from several different laboratories has been reported and appears to indicate that there are some associations between particular species and the site infected. Of special interest is the preponderance of isolates of *S. intermedius* from brain and liver abscesses, and the frequency of isolation of *S. anginosus* from infections of the genitourinary and gastrointestinal tracts (Whiley *et al.*, 1992).

Application of molecular typing methods, such

as ribotyping, should facilitate further studies to determine the sites of origin of these streptococcal species. Thus, for example, they could help to establish whether a particular strain isolated from a brain abscess was derived from the patient's mouth, alimentary tract, or some other body site. The selective medium described earlier could also be useful for more detailed ecological studies on the distribution of the 'S. milleri group' in different parts of the body (Whiley et al., 1993).

Clinical features

There are no particular features which clearly distinguish abscesses associated with α-haemolytic streptococci from those caused by other microorganisms. The actual presentation depends upon the site and extent of the abscess as well as the nature of the causative organisms. Since the infections are often mixed, sometimes with obligate anaerobes, streptococci may be isolated from foul-smelling, apparently anaerobic pus.

Laboratory diagnosis

Successful diagnosis depends to a large extent on obtaining adequate clinical samples that have not been contaminated with normal commensal bacteria from the skin or mucosal surfaces. Whenever possible, aspirated pus samples should be collected and inoculated onto appropriate culture media for aerobic, micro-aerophilic and anaerobic incubation. Isolates of presumptive streptococci can be identified as described elsewhere in this chapter.

Management

Clinical management of all abscesses, whether or not streptococci are involved, requires both surgical drainage and antimicrobial chemotherapy. Since the infection is frequently mixed, a combination of antimicrobial agents may be indicated to combat the different species present. For example, a combination of penicillin and metronidazole may be appropriate for abscesses caused by streptococci and one or more obligate anaerobes, as is often the case with infections around the head and neck.

Prevention

There are no specific methods for preventing abscesses, since these can occur at almost any body site and may be caused by many different types of microorganism. In the case of odontogenic abscesses, which can arise around the apex of teeth with necrotic pulps (periapical abscess) or from the periodontal pocket (periodontal abscess), the best method of prevention is early professional attention to predisposing conditions, such as dental caries, traumatic damage to teeth, and periodontal disease.

Streptococcal Infections in Immunocompromised Patients

It is apparent from numerous reports in the literature that α-haemolytic streptococci can cause serious opportunistic infections in patients who are immunocompromised, sometimes resulting in septicaemia or the adult respiratory distress syndrome (ARDS) (Hardie and Whiley, 1994). Several species have been identified from such patients, although the correct nomenclature for these isolates is sometimes uncertain from published reports. However, strains corresponding to S. oralis, S. mitis, S. sanguis and S. parasanguis have been found in some more recent studies on neutropenic patients (McWhinney et al., 1993; Beighton et al., 1994), and these findings are consistent with earlier reports. It has also been suggested that these species may be associated with Kawasaki disease, although a definite aetiological connection remains to be established (Ohkuni et al., 1993).

The site of entry of the streptococci which cause systemic infections in neutropenic and immunocompromised patients, including those with haematological or other malignancies, may not be easy to determine, but is likely to be the oral cavity or gastrointestinal tract in many cases. There is insufficient information available at present to suggest possible virulence determinants or pathogenic mechanisms involved in these infections. As mentioned later in the section on antimicrobial susceptibility, some streptococcal isolates from neutropenic patients are found to be relatively resistant to penicillin and other antibiotics.

LABORATORY DIAGNOSIS

Specimens

Alpha- and non-haemolytic streptococci can be isolated from a wide range of clinical specimens such as blood, pus, wounds, skin swabs, body fluids and biopsies as well as from dental plaque, saliva and other oral sites. When sampling oral sites for ecological studies it is often necessary to ensure that the area sampled is small enough to be representative of a discrete site rather than running the risk of obscuring the differences between sites through sampling too big an area. Within the mouth soft tissues can be swabbed and whole saliva collected in a sterile bottle, either unstimulated or after stimulation by chewing paraffin wax. A standardized disposable plastic loop can be used to obtain quantitatively similar results from the dorsal surface of the tongues of infants where conventional saliva collection is not possible. Dental plaque can be collected in several ways depending on the area of the tooth to be studied: the more accessible, smooth enamel surfaces can be sampled using a variety of rigid instruments, while the areas between teeth (approximal plaque) will necessitate the use of alternatives such as dental probes, scalers, dental floss or abrasive strips. For areas such as the pits and fissures of the teeth, and also for subgingival plaque, curettes, scalers, paper points and hyperdermic needles have been tried as sampling devices. Obtaining pus from an oral abscess is best done by direct aspiration using a hypodermic syringe rather than by swabbing, to reduce the risk of contaminating the sample with the oral flora, although in some cases (e.g. with infants) swab samples may be the only option available, unless the patient is undergoing a general anaesthetic.

Transport medium

Where the laboratory processing of a specimen will be delayed then the clinical sample is best held in a suitable reduced transport medium such as the one detailed below:

Reduced transport fluid (RTF)

	(ml/100 ml RTF)
Na_2CO_3 (8% solution)	0.5
0.1 M Ethylenediamine tetraacetate (EDTA)	1.0
1% DL-Dithiothreitol	2.0
0.6% K_2HPO_4 (sol. a)	7.5
0.6% KH_2PO_4, 1.2% NaCl, 1.2% $(NH_4)_2SO_4$, 0.24% $MgSO_4$ (sol. b)	7.5

Alpha-haemolytic streptococci are best isolated from clinical samples on a combination of non-selective and selective agar media. Non-selective examples include a variety of blood-containing complex media such as Blood agar no. 2 (Oxoid Ltd, Hants, UK), Columbia agar (Gibco BRL, Life Technologies, Paisley, UK), Fastidious Anaerobic agar (LabM, Amersham, UK), Brain Heart Infusion agar (Oxoid Ltd, Hants, UK) supplemented with 5% by volume defibrinated horse or sheep blood. Selective media have been described above.

Liquid culture of these streptococci can be carried out in a commercial broth such as Todd Hewitt broth or Brain Heart Infusion broth (Oxoid Ltd, Hants, UK). Alternatively an 'in-house' laboratory formulation can be used such as the example below (Strep. Base + 0.5% glucose), which has been used in the authors' laboratory for several years:

Strep. Base + 0.5% glucose broth

	(g/l)
Proteose peptone (Oxoid)	20.0
Yeast extract (Difco)	5.0
NaCl	5.0
Na_2HPO_4	1.0
Glucose	5.0

Adjust to pH 7.6, autoclave at 121 °C for 15 minutes.

Initial Screening Tests

Putative streptococci should be examined by Gram staining for Gram-positive cocci typically arranged in chains of varying length. Longer chains are produced when the organisms are grown in broth culture. Isolates should be tested for catalase reaction and only catalase-negative strains put through further streptococcal identification tests.

The clinical microbiologist should also be aware that, as a result of recent taxonomic studies, several other genera of facultatively anaerobic Gram-positive cocci have been proposed which may superficially resemble streptococci (see Hardie and Whiley, 1994). The scheme of tests shown in Table 1a.6 will allow the differentiation

of these genera on the basis of a few morphological, cultural and biochemical tests. In addition, it should be noted that the proposed genus, *Atopobium*, consists of Gram-positive cocci and rods and includes strains previously identified as *Lactobacillus minutus*, *Lactobacillus rimae* and *Streptococcus parvulus* (Collins and Wallbanks, 1992). The recognition of an increasing number of distinct genera amongst the Gram-positive cocci and coccobacilli means that great caution must be exercised in the interpretation of morphological observations.

TABLE 1a.6 DIFFERENTIAL CHARACTERISTICS OF *STREPTOCOCCUS* AND OTHER GRAM-POSITIVE, CATALASE NEGATIVE, FACULTATIVELY ANAEROBIC COCCUS GENERA

Genus	Cells arranged as	Pyr	Lap	6.5% NaCl	BE	Growth at: 10 °C	Growth at: 45 °C	Susceptibility to vancomycin	Haemolysis
Streptococcus	chains	−[a]	+	−[b]	−[c]	−	V	S	α,β,γ
Enterococcus[d]	chains	+	+	+	+	+	+	S[e]	α,β,γ
Lactococcus	chains	+	+	V	+	+	−[f]	S	α,γ
Vagococcus[d]	chains	+	+	+	+	+	−	S	α,γ
Globicatella	chains	+	−	+	−	−	−	S	α
Leuconostoc[g]	chains	−	−	V	V	+	V	R	α,γ
Pediococcus	tetrads	−	+	V	+	−	+	R	α
Aerococcus	tetrads	+	−	+	V	−	+	S	α
Tetragenococcus	tetrads	−	+	+	+	−	+	S	α
Gemella	tetrads	+	V	−	−	−	−	S	α,γ
Helcococcus	tetrads	+	−	+	+	−	−	S	γ

Abbreviations: Pyr, pyrrolidonyl amylamidase production; Lap, leucine aminopeptidase production; BE, reaction on bile-aesculin medium; α, α-haemolysis; β, β-haemolysis; γ, γ-haemolysis; +, ≥95% positive; −, ≥5% negative; V, variable reaction; R, resistant; S, susceptible.
[a] NVS and some group A streptococci are Pyr positive.
[b] Some β-haemolytic streptococci grow in 6.5 % NaCl broth.
[c] 5–10% of viridans streptococci are bile–aesculin positive.
[d] Some enterococci are motile; *Vagococcus* is motile (formerly called group N streptococci).
[e] Some strains are vancomycin resistant.
[f] Some strains grow very slowly at 45 °C.
[g] Gas is produced by *Leuconostoc* from glucose in Mann, Rogosa, Sharpe *Lactobacillus* broth (MRS).
Table adapted from Facklam and Sahm (1995).

TABLE 1a.7 DIFFERENTIAL CHARACTERISTICS OF α-HAEMOLYTIC STREPTOCOCCI OF MAN

	S. mutans	S. sobrinus	S. cricetus	S. rattus	S. intermedius	S. constellatus	S. anginosus	S. sanguis[a]
Acid from:								
Aesculin	+	−	+	+	NT	NT	NT	+(−)
Amygdalin	+(−)[b]	−	+	+	+(−)	−(+)	+	−
Arbutin	+	−	+	+	+	+	+	+
N-Acetylglucosamine	+	−	+	+	+	−(+)	−(+)	+
Inulin	+	+(−)	+	+	−	−	−	+
Lactose	+	+(−)	+(−)	+(−)	+	+(−)	+	+
Mannitol	+	+(−)	+	+	−	−	−(+)	+

continued

TABLE 1a.7 (CONTINUED)

	S. mutans	S. sobrinus	S. cricetus	S. rattus	S. intermedius	S. constellatus	S. anginosus	S. sanguis[a]
Melibiose	+(−)c	−	+	+	−	−	−	+(−)
Pullulan	−	−	NT	NT	+	−	+(−)	+(−)
Raffinose	+	−	+	+	−	−	−(+)	+(−)
Starch	−	−	−	−	NT	NT	NT	−(+)
Sorbitol	+	−(+)b	+	+	−	−	−	−(+)
Tagatose	+(−)	+	NT	NT	−	−	−	NT
Trehalose	+	+	+(−)	+	+	+(−)	+	+
Hydrolysis of:								
Aesculin	+	+(−)	+(−)	+	+	+d	+	+(−)
Arginine	−	−	−	+	+	+	+	+
Starch	+	NT	−	−	NT	NT	NT	+(−)
Production of:								
α-Galactosidase	+	−	NT	NT	−	−	−(+)	+(−)
β-Galactosidase	−	−	NT	NT	+	−	−(+)	−(+)
α-Glucosidase	+	+	NT	NT	+	+	−(+)	−
β-Glucosidase	+	−	NT	NT	−(+)	−	+	−(+)bd
N-Acetylgalactosaminidase	−	−	NT	NT	+	−	−	−
N-Acetylglucosaminidase	−	−	NT	NT	+	−	−	+(−)bd
α-L-Fucosidase	−	−	NT	NT	+	−	−	−
β-D-Fucosidase	−	−	NT	NT	+	−	−	−(+)b
Sialidase	−	−	NT	NT	+	−	−	−
Alkaline phosphatase	−	−	NT	NT	+	+	+	−
Extracellular polysaccharide	+	+	+	+	−	−	−	+
H_2O_2	−	+	−	−	−	−	−(+)	+
Hyaluronidase	−	−	NT	NT	+	+(−)	−	−
Acetoin (VP)	+	+	+	+	+	+	+	−
Urea	−	−	−	−	−	−	−	−

	S. gordonii[a]	S. parasanguis	S. crista	S. oralis	S. mitis[a]	S. pneumoniae	S. adjacens[a]	S. defectivus
Acid from:								
Aesculin	+	NT	NT	−	−(+)	NT	NT	NT
Amygdalin	+	−(+)	−	−	−	−	−	−
Arbutin	+	−(+)	+	−	−	−	NT	NT
N-Acetylglucosamine	+	+	+	+	+	+(−)	NT	NT
Inulin	+(−)	−	−	−	−(+)b	+	V	−
Lactose	+	+	+(−)	+	+	+	−	V
Mannitol	−	−	−	−	−b	−	−	−
Melibiose	−(+)	+(−)	−	+b	+(−)b	−b	−	−
Pullulan	−	NT	V	+	+(−)	NT	−	+
Raffinose	−(+)	+(−)	−	+(−)	+(−)b	+	−	V
Starch	−	−	NT	−b	−	−	−	+
Sorbitol	−	−	−	−	−	−	−	−
Tagatose	NT	NT	−	−(+)	−	−	+(−)	−
Trehalose	+	V	+	−(+)	−	+	−	+
Hydrolysis of:								
Aesculin	+	−(+)	−	−	−	−(+)b	NT	NT
Arginine	+	+	+(−)	−	+(−)	−	−	−
Starch	+(−)	+	NT	+	+(−)	+(−)	NT	NT
Production of:								
α-Galactosidase	−(+)	+	−	NT	+(−)	+	−	+
β-Galactosidase	+(−)bd	NT	−(+)	+b	+(−)bd	+	−	+b
α-Glucosidase	+(−)bd	+	−	+	+b	+	−	−
β-Glucosidase	+	−(+)	−	−	−	−(+)	+b	+b

continued

TABLE 1a.7 *(CONTINUED)*

	S. gordonii[a]	S. parasanguis	S. crista	S. oralis	S. mitis[a]	S. pneumoniae	S. adjacens[a]	S. defectivus
N-Acetylgalactosaminidase	+(−)	+	+	+	−	+	−	−
N-Acetylglucosaminidase	+	+	+	+	+	+(−)	+	−(+)
α-L-Fucosidase	+	−(+)	+	−	−	−(+)	+	+
β-D-Fucosidase	−	−(+)	−	+[d]	+	−(+)	−	−
Sialidase	−	−	−	+	−(+)	+	−(+)	+
Alkaline phosphatase	+	+(−)	−	+	V	−	−	−
Extracellular polysaccharide	+	−	NT	+(−)	−	−	−	NT
H₂O₂	+	+	+	+	+	+	NT	NT
Hyaluronidase	−	−	−	−	−	+	NT	NT
Acetoin (VP)	−	−	−	−	−	−	V	V
Urea	−	−	−	−	−	−	−	−

	S. salivarius	S. vestibularis	S. bovis I	S. bovis II/1	S. bovis II/2	S. equinus	S. acidominimus[e]
Acid from:							
Aesculin	+	NT	NT	NT	NT	NT	NT
Amygdalin	+	+(−)	NT	NT	NT	NT	NT
Arbutin	+	−(+)	NT	NT	NT	NT	NT
N-Acetylglucosamine	+	+(−)	NT	NT	NT	+	NT
Inulin	+(−)	−	+(−)	−	−	NT	NT
Lactose	+(−)	+(−)	+	−(+)	−	−	+(−)
Mannitol	−	−	+	−	−	−	−(+)
Melibiose	−	−	−	+(−)	−(+)	−	−
Pullulan	+	−	+	+(−)	−	−	−
Raffinose	−	−	+(−)	+(−)	+(−)	−	−
Starch	−	−	+	+(−)	−(+)	NT	NT
Sorbitol	−	−	−	−	−	−	−
Tagatose	−	−	−	−	−	−	−
Trehalose	−(+)	V	+	−(+)	+	−(+)	+(−)
Hydrolysis of:							
Aesculin	+	+(−)	+	+	+	+	−
Arginine	−	−	−	−	−	−	−
Starch	+	NT	+	−	−	NT	NT
Production of:							
α-Galactosidase	−	−	+(−)	+	+	−	−
β-Galactosidase	+(−)	+	−	−	+	−	−
α-Glucosidase	+	+(−)	NT	NT	NT	NT	NT
β-Glucosidase	+	−	+	+(−)	+	+	−
N-Acetylgalactosaminidase	−	−	NT	NT	NT	NT	NT
N-Acetylglucosaminidase	−	−	−	−	−(+)	−	−
α-L-Fucosidase	−	−	NT	NT	NT	NT	NT
β-D-Fucosidase	+(−)	−	NT	NT	NT	NT	NT
Sialidase	−	−	NT	NT	NT	NT	NT
Alkaline phosphatase	+	−	−	−	−	−	−
Extracellular polysaccharide	+	−	+	−	−	NT	NT
H₂O₂	−	+	NT	NT	NT	NT	NT
Hyaluronidase	−	−	NT	NT	NT	NT	NT
Acetoin (VP)	+(−)	−	+	+(−)	+	+	−
Urea	−(+)	+	−	−	−	−	−

Abbreviations: ecp, extracellular polysaccharide; alk P, alkaline phosphatase; VP, acetoin production in the Voges–Proskaeur; V, reported as 'variable'; NT, not tested.
[a] Some authors have described biotypes within these species (Kilian *et al.*, 1989; Beighton *et al.*, 1991).
[b] Reports vary between studies.
[c] Some strains do not ferment melibiose and less frequently ferment arbutin or produce α-glucosidase.
[d] Weak or slow reactions given by some strains.
[e] High final pH results in difficulty when reading tests.
Data from Kilian *et al.* (1989); Beighton *et al.* (1995); Hardie and Whiley (1995).

Identification to Species Level

Where the identification of isolates to species level is required this can be carried out using either laboratory-based biochemical test schemes or commercial identification kits with accompanying databases. Although species-level identification of α-haemolytic streptococci is not routinely carried out in many clinical laboratories, this may be deemed necessary in the case of suspected pneumococcal infection, isolates obtained from deep-seated abscesses, blood cultures and other normally sterile sites, specimens from endocarditis, or where pure cultures have been grown. Differential tests for the identification of α- and non-haemolytic streptococci are summarized in Table 1a.7. With some species, identification can be further complicated: one frequently quoted scheme divides *S. sanguis*, *S. gordonii* and *S. mitis* into four, three and two main biotypes respectively (Kilian *et al.*, 1989) whilst, in another, *S. sanguis* is divided into three biotypes (Beighton *et al.*, 1991). There is, however, only partial correspondence between the *S. sanguis* biotypes of these two studies.

A flow chart summarizing the procedures for characterization and identification of α-haemolytic streptococci is shown in Figure 1a.3.

ANTIMICROBIAL SUSCEPTIBILITY

Studies on α-haemolytic and non-haemolytic streptococci have generally shown them to be highly susceptible to penicillin and many other antimicrobial agents, although some resistant strains have been reported over the years (Phillips *et al.*, 1976; Hardie and Whiley, 1992). This has led to the widespread, but sometimes erroneous, view that these streptococci are unlikely to pose any problems for selection of appropriate antibiotics when treatment is indicated.

Some recent reports continue to show that most streptococcal isolates are sensitive to β-lactam antibiotics, although this probably depends on the sources of the strains. For example, one study on the isolates from cases of endocarditis in the Netherlands showed that most of the streptococci were highly susceptible to penicillin (van der Meer *et al.*, 1991). However, in contrast, an investigation on the antibiotic susceptibility of 211 viridans streptococci from blood cultures found that 38% of the isolates were at least partially resistant to penicillin (minimal inhibitory concentration (MIC) ≥ 0.25 mg/l). Tetracycline resistance, which has often been reported, was found in 41% of the strains and in 7% of these was combined with erythromycin resistance (Potgieter *et al.*, 1992). In the same study, several strains of *S. mitis* were found to have high levels of resistance to aminoglycosides and no evidence of synergy for combinations of penicillin and gentamicin against some of these could be demonstrated.

In a survey of antibiotic resistance amongst oral streptococci from dental patients at risk of endocarditis, resistance to amoxycillin and erythromycin was found in many isolates, although no strains had an MIC to amoxycillin greater than 24 mg/l (the expected mean serum concentration after a 3 g oral dose) (Longman *et al.*, 1991). The antibiotic-resistant strains were identified mainly as *S. sanguis* biotype II, according to the API-20 system (probably corresponding to *S. oralis*), but others were found to belong to *S. sanguis* biotype I, *S. mitis* and *S. salivarius*.

Antimicrobial resistance amongst streptococci from the blood of neutropenic patients is of particular significance, since infection with these relatively non-virulent organisms may be life threatening in such individuals. McWhinney *et al.* (1993) reported the occurrence of some resistance to benzylpenicillin and ceftazidime amongst 47 blood culture isolates from neutropenic patients who were receiving quinolone prophylaxis (ciprofloxacin). All strains were susceptible to vancomycin, teicoplanin and imipenem, and most to amoxycillin, co-amoxiclav, azlocillin, clarithromycin, erythromycin and azithromycin. Other studies on streptococci from neutropenic patients have shown up to 26% of strains to be resistant or partially resistant to penicillin, but susceptible to vancomycin, imipenem, meropenem and several cephalosporins.

From the increasing amount of published information, only some of which has been quoted here, it is clearly unsafe to assume that all isolates

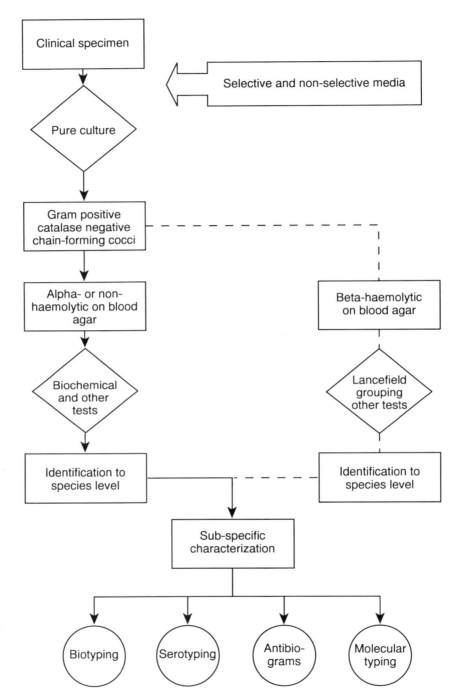

Figure 1a.3 Steps in the isolation, identification and further characterization of α-haemolytic and other streptococci.

of streptococci will be fully sensitive to penicillin and other commonly used antibiotics. In some series of cases, β-lactam resistance has quite frequently been observed, and resistance to erythromycin and tetracycline is also relatively common. It is therefore necessary to monitor the antibiotic resistance trends in streptococci, particularly amongst isolates associated with infections in neutropenic and immunocompromised patients (Potgieter *et al.*, 1992). Streptococci of the '*S. milleri* group', which are most often associated with purulent infections, do usually appear to be sensitive to penicillin and other β-lactams. However, resistance to erythromycin and clindamycin has been reported in over 10% of isolates, and tetracycline resistance is even more frequently encountered.

As discussed in Chapter 1c, there is considerable interest in the emergence of penicillin resistance in *S. pneumoniae*, which is related to the possession of low-affinity penicillin-binding proteins (PBPs) by resistant strains. It has recently been demonstrated that PBP2B genes from penicillin-resistant strains of *S. pneumoniae* contain blocks of nucleotides apparently originating from *S. mitis* (Dowson *et al.*, 1993). The observation that oral streptococci, such as *S. mitis*, *S. oralis* and *S. sanguis*, which are increasingly becoming resistant to penicillin, may act as donors of low-affinity PBPs to the closely related species *S. pneumoniae* could have great significance for future studies in this clinically important area of research.

REFERENCES

Beighton, D., Hardie, J.M. and Whiley, R.A. (1991) A scheme for the identification of viridans streptococci. *Journal of Medical Microbiology*, **35**, 367–372.

Beighton, D., Carr, A.D. and Oppenheim, B.A. (1994) Identification of viridans streptococci associated with bacteraemia in neutropenic cancer patients. *Journal of Medical Microbiology*, **40**, 202–204.

Beighton, D., Homer, K.A., Bouvet, A. *et al.* (1995) Analysis of enzymatic activities for differentiation of two species of nutritionally variant streptococci, *Streptococcus defectivus* and *Streptococcus adjacens*. *Journal of Clinical Microbiology*, **33**, 1584–1587.

Bentley, R.W., Leigh, J.A. and Collins, M.D. (1991) Intrageneric structure of *Streptococcus* based on comparative analysis of small-subunit rRNA sequences. *International Journal of Systematic Bacteriology*, **41**, 487–494.

Bouvet, A.F., Grimont, F. and Grimont, P.A.D. (1989) *Streptococcus defectivus* sp. nov. and *Streptococcus adjacens* sp. nov., nutritionally variant streptococci from human clinical specimens. *International Journal of Systematic Bacteriology*, **39**, 290–294.

Bowden, G.H.W. (1991) Which bacteria are cariogenic in humans? In *Risk Markers for Oral Diseases, Volume 1. Dental Caries* (ed. N.W. Johnson), pp. 266–286. Cambridge University Press, Cambridge.

BSAC (1992) Antibiotic prophylaxis of infective endocarditis. *Lancet*, **339**, 1292–1293.

Caufield, P.W., Cutter, G.R. and Dasanayake, A.P. (1993) Initial acquisition of mutans streptococci by infants: evidence for a discrete window of infectivity. *Journal of Dental Research*, **72**, 37–45.

Clarke, J.K. (1924) On the bacterial factor in the aetiology of dental caries. *British Journal of Experimental Pathology*, **5**, 141–147.

Collins, M.D. and Wallbanks, S. (1992) Comparative sequence analyses of the 16S rRNA genes of *Lactobacillus minutus*, *Lactobacillus rimae* and *Streptococcus parvulus*: proposal for the creation of a new genus *Atopobium*. *FEMS Microbiology Letters*, **95**, 235–240.

Colman, G. and Williams, R.E.O. (1972) Taxonomy of some human viridans streptococci. In *Streptococci and Streptococcal Diseases* (ed. L.W. Wannamaker and J.M. Matsen), pp. 281–299. Academic Press, London.

Coykendall, A. (1989) Classification and identification of the viridans streptococci. *Clinical Microbiology Reviews*, **2**, 315–328.

Devriese, L.A. (1991) Streptococcal ecovars associated with different animal species: epidemiological significance of serogroups and biotypes. *Journal of Applied Bacteriology*, **71**, 478–483.

Douglas, C.W.I., Heath, J., Hampton, K.K. *et al.* (1993) Identity of viridans streptococci isolated from cases of infected endocarditis. *Journal of Medical Microbiology*, **39**, 179–182.

Dowson, C.G., Coffey, T.J., Kell, C. and Whiley, R.A. (1993) Evolution of penicillin resistance in *Streptococcus pneumoniae*: the role of *Streptococcus mitis* in the formation of a low affinity PBP2B in *S. pneumoniae*. *Molecular Microbiology*, **9**, 635–643.

Facklam, R.R. (1977). Physiological differentiation of viridans streptococci. *Journal of Clinical Microbiology*, **5**, 184–201.

Facklam, R.R. and Sahm, D.F. (1995) *Enterococcus*. In *Manual of Clinical Microbiology* (ed. P.R. Murray,

E.J. Baron, M.A. Pfaller *et al.*), pp. 308–314. ASM Press, Washington, DC.

Farrow, J.A.E., Kruze, J., Phillips, B.A. *et al.* (1984) Taxonomic studies on *Streptococcus bovis* and *Streptococcus equinus*: description of *Streptococcus alactolyticus* sp. nov., and *Streptococcus saccharolyticus* sp. nov. *Journal of Systematic and Applied Microbiology*, **6**, 467–482.

Fiehn, N.-E., Gutschik, E., Larsen, T. *et al.* (1995) Identity of streptococcal blood isolates and oral isolates from two patients with infective endocarditis. *Journal of Clinical Microbiology*, **33**, 1399–1401.

Freedman, L.R. (1987) The pathogens of infective endocarditis. *Journal of Antimicrobial Chemotherapy*, **20** (Suppl. A), 1–6.

Freney, J., Bland, S., Etienne, J. *et al.* (1992) Description and evaluation of the semiautomated 4-hour Rapid ID 32 Strep method for identification of streptococci and members of related genera. *Journal of Clinical Microbiology*, **30**, 2657–2661.

Hamada, S. and Slade, H.D. (1980) Biology, immunology and cariogenicity of *Streptococcus mutans*. *Microbiological Reviews*, **44**, 331–384.

Hardie, J.M. (1992) Oral microbiology: current concepts in the microbiology of dental caries and periodontal disease. *British Dental Journal*, **172**, 271–278.

Hardie, J.M. and Whiley, R.A. (1992) The genus *Streptococcus* – oral. In *The Prokaryotes*, 2nd edn, Vol. II (ed. A. Balows, H.G. Trüper, M. Dworking *et al.*), pp. 1421–1449. Springer-Verlag, New York.

Hardie, J.M. and Whiley, R.A. (1994) Recent developments in streptococcal taxonomy: their relation to infections. *Reviews in Medical Microbiology*, **5**, 151–162.

Hardie, J.M. and Whiley, R.A. (1995) The genus *Streptococcus*. In *The Genera of Lactic Acid Bacteria. The Lactic Acid Bacteria*, Vol. 2, (ed. B.J.B. Wood and W.H. Holzapfel), pp. 55–124. Blackie Academic and Professional, London.

Kawamura, Y., Hou, X.-G., Sultana, F. *et al.* (1995a) Determination of 16S rRNA sequences of *Streptococcus mitis* and *Streptococcus gordonii* and phylogenetic relationships among members of the genus *Streptococcus*. *International Journal of Systematic Bacteriology*, **45**, 406–408.

Kawamura, Y., Hou, X.-G., Sultana, F. *et al.* (1995b) Transfer of *Streptococcus adjacens* and *Streptococcus defectivus* to *Abiotrophia* gen. nov. as *Abiotrophia adiacens* comb. nov. and *Abiotrophia defectiva* comb. nov. respectively. *International Journal of Systematic Bacteriology*, **45**, 798–803.

Kidd, E.A.M. and Joyston-Bechal, S. (1989) *Essentials of Dental Caries: The Disease and its Management*. Wright, Bristol.

Kikuchi, K., Enari, T., Totsuka, K.-I. *et al.* (1995) Comparison of phenotypic characteristics, DNA–DNA hybridisation results, and results with a commercial rapid biochemical and enzymatic reaction system for identification of viridans group streptococci. *Journal of Clinical Microbiology*, **33**, 1215–1222.

Kilian, M., Mikkelsen, L. and Henrichsen, J. (1989) Taxonomic study of viridans streptococci description of *Streptococcus gordonii* sp. nov. and emended descriptions of *Streptococcus sanguis* (White and Niven 1946), *Streptococcus oralis* (Bridge and Sneath 1982) and *Streptococcus mitis* (Andrews and Horder 1906). *International Journal of Systematic Bacteriology*, **39**, 471–484.

Kilpper-Bälz, R., Wenzig, P. and Schleifer, K.H. (1985) Molecular relationships and classification of some viridans streptococci as *Streptococcus oralis* and emended description of *Streptococcus oralis* (Bridge and Sneath 1982). *International Journal of Systematic Bacteriology*, **35**, 482–488.

Kitada, K., Nagata, K., Yakushiji, T. *et al.* (1992) Serological and biological characteristics of '*Streptococcus milleri*' isolates from systemic purulent infections. *Journal of Medical Microbiology*, **36**, 143–148.

Littler, W. and Shanson, D.C. (1989) Infective endocarditis. In *Septicaemia and Endocarditis: Clinical and Microbiological Aspects* (ed. D.C. Shanson), pp. 143–171. Oxford University Press, Oxford.

Loesche, W.J. (1986) Role of *Streptococcus mutans* in human dental decay. *Microbiological Reviews*, **50**, 353–380.

Longman, L.P., Pearce, P.K., McGowan, P. *et al.* (1991) Antibiotic-resistant oral streptococci in dental patients susceptible to infective endocarditis. *Journal of Medical Microbiology*, **34**, 33–37.

McWhinney, P.H.M., Patel, S., Whiley, R.A. *et al.* (1993) Activities of potential therapeutic and prophylactic antibiotics against blood cultures isolates of viridans group streptococci from neutropenic patients receiving ciprofloxacin. *Antimicrobial Agents and Chemotherapy*, **37**, 2493–2495.

Ohkuni, H., Todome, Y., Mizuse, M. *et al.* (1993) Biologically active extracellular products of oral viridans streptococci and the aetiology of Kawasaki disease. *Journal of Medical Microbiology*, **39**, 352–362.

Phillips, I., Warren, C., Harrison, J.M. *et al.* (1976) Antibiotic susceptibility of streptococci from the mouth and blood of patients treated with penicillin or lincomycin and clindamycin. *Journal of Medical Microbiology*, **9**, 393–404.

Potgieter, E., Carmichael, M., Koornhof, H.J. *et al.* (1992) *In vitro* antimicrobial susceptibility of viridans streptococci isolated from blood cultures. *European Journal of Clinical Microbiology and Infectious Diseases*, **11**, 543–546.

Ross, P.W. (1990) Streptococcal diseases. In *Topley and Wilson's Principles of Bacteriology, Virology and Immunity*, Vol. 3. (Ed. M.T. Parker and L.H. Collier), pp. 239–262. Edward Arnold, London.

Rudney, J.D. and Larson, C.J. (1993) Species identification of oral viridans streptococci by restriction fragment polymorphism analysis of rRNA genes. *Journal of Clinical Microbiology*, **31**, 2467–2473.

Russell, M.W. (1992) Immunization against dental caries. *Current Opinion in Dentistry*, **2**, 72–80.

Russell, R.R.B. (1994) The application of molecular genetics to the microbiology of dental caries. *Caries Research*, **28**, 69–82.

Schleifer, K.H., Kilpper, B. and Bälz, R. (1987) Molecular and chemotaxonomic approaches to the classification of streptococci, enterococci and lactococci: a review. *Journal of Systematic and Applied Microbiology*, **10**, 1–19.

Sherman, J.M. (1937) The streptococci. *Bacteriological Reviews*, **1**, 3–97.

Skinner, F.A. and Quesnel, L.B. (1978) *Streptococci*. Academic Press, London, New York, San Francisco.

van der Meer, J.-T., van Vianen, W., Hu, E. *et al.* (1991) Distribution, antibiotic susceptibility and tolerance of bacterial isolates in culture-positive cases of endocarditis in The Netherlands. *European Journal of Clinical Microbiology and Infectious Diseases*, **10**, 728–734.

Whiley, R.A. and Beighton, D. (1991) Emended descriptions and recognition of *Streptococcus constellatus*, *Streptococcus intermedius*, and *Streptococcus anginosus* as distinct species. *International Journal of Systematic Bacteriology*, **41**, 1–5.

Whiley, R.A., Beighton, D., Winstanley, T.G. *et al.* (1992) *Streptococcus intermedius*, *Streptococcus constellatus*, and *Streptococcus anginosus* (the *Streptococcus milleri* group): association with different body sites and clinical infections. *Journal of Clinical Microbiology*, **30**, 243–244.

Whiley, R.A., Freemantle, L., Beighton, D. *et al.* (1993) Isolation, identification and prevalence of *Streptococcus anginosus*, *S. intermedius* and *S. constellatus* from the human mouth. *Microbial Ecology in Health and Disease*, **6**, 285–291.

Young, S.E.J. (1987) The aetiology and epidemiology of infective endocarditis in England and Wales. *Journal of Antimicrobial Chemotherapy*, **20** (Suppl. A): 7–14.

1b

β-HAEMOLYTIC STREPTOCOCCI

Michael Barnham

HISTORY

Streptococcal illnesses such as scarlet fever, erysipelas and puerperal fever have been familiar problems in medical practice for many centuries. Fehleisen first isolated streptococci from infected patients in 1883 and in the following year Rosenbach gave the name *Streptococcus pyogenes* to cocci that grew in chains in suppurating human wounds. The haemolytic activity of certain streptococci was first noted by Marmorek in 1895 and it was suggested by Schottmuller in 1903 that the forms of haemolysis should be used to classify the organisms.

The system of grouping according to carbohydrate or teichoic acid cell wall antigens devised by Lancefield in the late 1920s ('Lancefield grouping') allowed the first proper division of haemolytic streptococci to be made. The name *S. pyogenes* was retained for the group A streptococci (GAS), the principal human streptococcal pathogens, while the further alphabetical groups (B to U, here termed GBS, GCS, etc.) defined organisms regularly found in man or animals. The agglutination tests developed by Griffiths and others, detecting some of the later-recognized array of T antigen types, proved helpful for subdividing GAS and some GCS and GGS. In the early 1940s Lancefield distinguished the surface protein T and M antigens of *S. pyogenes* and from the mid-1950s a combined T/M typing scheme became widely used to differentiate strains.

Early clinical and epidemiological studies defined the modes of streptococcal transmission and helped to lay the broad foundations of modern hygienic medical and surgical practice. The improvements in social hygiene, housing and nutrition in developed countries during the early twentieth century are thought to have played a major part in bringing about the observed early decline in serious *S. pyogenes* infections, including severe scarlet fever and invasive disease. Following the development of sulphonamides and antibiotics in the 1930s and 1940s there was a further profound reduction in the incidence of rheumatic fever and overt post-streptococcal glomerulonephritis (PSGN).

In more recent years the introduction of Lancefield grouping and rapid streptococcal identification kits for routine use in diagnostic laboratories has led to an increased interest in the role of non-GAS in human and animal infections. Advances in molecular biology, genetics and immunology have greatly enhanced our understanding of streptococcal pathogenicity and host immunity. Interest has been maintained in the

Principles and Practice of Clinical Bacteriology. Edited by A.M. Emmerson, P.M. Hawkey and S.H. Gillespie

clinical and epidemiological aspects of strepto-coccal infection and increasing problems have been noted in haemolytic streptococcal infections of neonates, the immunocompromised and the elderly. Most recently there has been a resurgence of serious streptococcal infection and an increase in rheumatic fever in certain parts of the devel-oped world.

Despite the advances in knowledge and tech-nique and the high levels of infection control achieved in many Western countries, classic streptococcal diseases remain very common in most parts of the developing world. The burden of streptococcal disease continues to pose a challenge to clinicians and research workers.

DESCRIPTION OF THE ORGANISMS

Definition

The haemolytic streptococci are Gram-positive, spherical, aerobic and facultatively anaerobic bacteria arranged in chains, non-sporing, catalase negative, oxidase negative and non-motile. They ferment carbohydrates with the production of lactic acid but no gas, and they fail to reduce nitrate.

The organisms are distinguished from other streptococci by the lytic action of their products (haemolysins) on the red blood cells on blood agar culture, producing clear zones of variable size around each colony after overnight incubation. The appearances depend on the particular strain of *Streptococcus*, the composition of the culture medium, the species of blood employed and the cultural conditions. Non-haemolytic streptococci will occasionally produce β-haemolysis if the culture medium and conditions are suitable, and haemolytic enterococci also occur (now classified separately from the streptococci); these organisms will not be considered further in this chapter.

Classification

Haemolytic streptococci are divided according to the carriage of particular polysaccharide and tei-choic acid Lancefield group antigens in the cell wall. The majority of haemolytic streptococcal isolates carry group-defining polysaccharide anti-gens (such as for groups A, B, C, G, L); cytoplasmic membrane-associated lipoteichoic acid (group D) antigens may be found in *S. suis*. This system of division has proved to be a useful and sufficient practice for many laboratory and clinical purposes, although several of the Lancefield groups of streptococci contain more than one species. Non-haemolytic streptococci may also produce certain Lancefield group antigens. The identification of haemolytic streptococci to species level usually involves extended physiological testing.

Table 1b.1 lists the main haemolytic strep-tococci of medical importance; others which are principally of veterinary importance, such as *S. equi* (group C), *S. canis* (group G) and *S. iniae*, are excluded. GAS, GCS and GGS are frequently associated with purulent infection in man and are often referred to as the pyogenic streptococci. *Streptococcus anginosus* (also widely referred to

TABLE 1b.1 FEATURES OF HAEMOLYTIC STREPTOCOCCI OF MEDICAL IMPORTANCE

Name	Lancefield group antigens carried	Nature of group antigen	Usual form of haemolysis
S. pyogenes	A	P	β
S. agalactiae	B	P	β
S. equisimilis	C	P	β
S. zooepidemicus	C	P	β
Streptococcus spp.	G	P	β
Streptococcus spp.	L	P	β
S. suis, type 2	R (+D)	P (T)	β or non
S. anginosus ('*milleri*')	–, F, G, A or C	P	β or non

P, polysaccharide; T, teichoic acid.

TABLE 1b.2 DIVISION OF SELECTED PYOGENIC STREPTOCOCCI INTO CLUSTERS BY DNA HOMOLOGY

Cluster 1	*S. pyogenes*
	S. dysgalactiae (group C)
	S. equisimilis (group C)
	Large colony group G *Streptococcus*
	Group L *Streptococcus*
	S. equi (group C)
	S. zooepidemicus (group C)
Cluster 2	*S. agalactiae* (group B)
	Group M *Streptococcus*
Cluster 3	Group R *Streptococcus*
	Group S *Streptococcus*
Cluster 4	Group P *Streptococcus*
	Group U *Streptococcus*
	Group V *Streptococcus*
Cluster 5	*S. anginosus* (minute colony group F, G etc.)
	Streptococcus MG, *S. intermedius*)

After Schleifer and Kilpper-Bälz (1987).

as '*S. milleri*' or 'the *S. milleri* group') is an organism which produces minute colonies on blood agar culture and possesses variable haemolytic and Lancefield grouping properties (Ruoff, 1988; Whitworth, 1990) (see p. 7).

Molecular Classification

Recent studies of DNA structure have thrown new light on the genetic relatedness of the various species of haemolytic streptococci (Schleifer and Kilpper-Bälz, 1987). Table 1b.2 shows the clustering of these organisms according to DNA–DNA hybridization values. Within cluster 1 *S. pyogenes* stands distinct from the other pyogenic streptococci; the horse pathogen *S. equi* is closely related to *S. zooepidemicus*, which is found widely in animals and occasionally in man; the group C *S. equisimilis*, large colony group GGS and GLS are closely related to the non-haemolytic group C *S. dysgalactiae*. Distinct clusters contain *S. agalactiae* (group B), *S. suis* (group R and S) and *S. anginosus*.

PATHOGENESIS

The interactions of streptococci with the host depend on 'host factors', such as immunological response (including previous antigenic experience

of the organisms) and general state of health, hygiene and nutrition; these factors may vary according to the individual, community or race. Pathogenic factors in the streptococci can be conveniently divided under the headings of surface structures, soluble products and cross-reacting antigenic constituents; these act in concert in the living organism and the genes that regulate them are known (in some cases) to occur in clusters (regulons) which may be up- or down-regulated according to local conditions.

Cell Surface Structures

The streptococcal cell wall is a complex structure consisting of an inner cell membrane, a tough supporting layer of cross-linked peptidoglycan and an array of projecting surface molecules including M protein, T and R proteins, immunoglobulin-binding proteins and the group carbohydrate antigens. Recent studies have shown that the various molecules in the wall are not distributed as entirely discrete layers but exist as a three-dimensional mosaic, with expression of most components on the inner as well as the outer surface of the wall. The hyaluronic acid capsule which surrounds the cell is produced principally during phases of logarithmic bacterial growth in the host.

Streptococcal M protein

The M protein molecule is the principal virulence factor on the surface of haemolytic streptococci, present and functional on virtually all clinical isolates of GAS and at least some of GCS, GGS and GLS (Fischetti, 1989). It occurs as a double-stranded coiled-coil structure projecting from the cell surface and visible in thin-section electron micrographs of the cell as a fringe of hair-like projections. More than 80 varieties of the molecule have been recognized so far in *S. pyogenes*, currently named M1, M2, M3, and so on. These 'types' reflect differences in the variable and hypervariable domains that occur in the molecule towards its free end. The functional properties of M protein include fibrinogen, fibronectin and

β_2-microglobulin binding, adherence to host cells, interference with complement deposition and the conferring of resistance to phagocytosis. Certain M proteins also act as superantigens, capable of activating a broad range of T lymphocytes. The quantity of M protein expressed on the cell surface appears to be important: freshly isolated strains of GAS, GCS and GGS, particularly those from severe or septicaemic infections, are often rich in this substance and serotypes of *S. pyogenes* such as M1, which express large quantities, are commonly associated with invasive (i.e. locally aggressive or bacteraemic) disease.

The structure of the streptococcal M protein molecule has been analysed in detail and is now one of the best characterized of bacterial virulence factors (Fischetti, 1989). Two classes of M protein (I and II) have been described according to differences in the C-repeat domain of the molecule; the activity of the serum opacity factor (OF) surface structure, which functions as an apoproteinase to render high-density lipoproteins insoluble, is closely associated with class II M proteins. Although there appears to be a fundamental difference in genetic coding for class I and II M proteins, isolates of both classes are found in nasopharyngeal, skin and systemic infections and in association with post-streptococcal glomerulonephritis. However, there appears to be a close correlation of acute rheumatic fever with infection with *S. pyogenes* strains bearing class I M proteins. Anti-M responses are often poor in infection with OF-positive strains but a specific anti-OF immune response may be detected in such cases. Type-specific immunity to M protein following natural infection is thought to confer resistance to challenge with the same type of *Streptococcus*. Certain immunological cross-reactions occur between M protein and mammalian tissues, as noted below.

Other cell surface structures

Other projecting cell surface molecules of haemolytic streptococci include the Lancefield group carbohydrates, lipoteichoic acids, the T, R, X and c protein antigens, C5 peptidase, plasminogen-binding and surface dehydrogenase proteins and immunoglobulin-binding proteins (including those currently designated Sir, Arp and protein H). Many of these substances possess a structure resembling that of M protein. Among the known functions of these surface structures are the destruction of complement C5a, binding and activation of plasminogen, and binding to the Fc portion of IgG and IgA antibodies. Immunoglobulin binding has been found in a high proportion of clinical isolates of *S. pyogenes* but its role in pathogenesis remains unclear; IgG-binding activity is particularly common in pyoderma isolates, while high binding of IgA has been found in a large proportion of deep tissue isolates. In GBS there are at least four varieties of R protein antigen which confer resistance to opsonophagocytic killing; the organisms may also carry X and c protein antigens (the latter occurring in two forms, α and β) which are thought to confer similar protection. The Lancefield group antigens and T antigens are not known to have pathogenic significance.

The non-immunogenic hyaluronic acid capsule of streptococci impedes phagocytosis and favours bacterial survival in the host. Capsular polysaccharide antigens of GBS also confer resistance to complement activity. Streptococcal cell wall fragments contain peptidoglycan which can produce fever and shock when injected into experimental animals. Certain surface components of GAS and GBS can also stimulate macrophages to produce tumour necrosis factor.

Soluble Products

Certain streptococcal enzymes and other soluble products are thought to contribute significantly both to the progress of local infection and to systemic components and sequelae of infection (Ginsburg, 1985).

Streptococcal pyrogenic exotoxins

At least three distinct forms of streptococcal pyrogenic exotoxins (SPE), termed A, B and C and formerly known together as erythrogenic or scarlet fever toxins, may be elaborated singly or in combinations by strains of *S. pyogenes* (Wannamaker, 1983; Bohach *et al.*, 1990) but apparently not by other species of streptococci. SPEs show an affinity for certain dermal cells and are thought to produce the scarlet fever rash by an enhancement of local hypersensitivity reactions to other streptococcal products previously encountered by the host. The varying clinical severity of scarlet fever over the years may relate to the prevalence of streptococcal infection in the community and states of immunity to their products, and to the variable production of the three principal forms of SPE by prevailing streptococci.

In addition to its role in the production of rashes SPE A may cause enhancement of susceptibility to Gram-negative endotoxin shock, stimulation of macrophages to produce tumour necrosis factor, pyrogenicity, cytotoxicity for various tissues including the heart, depression of the clearance function of the reticuloendothelial system, alteration of the blood–brain barrier, non-specific mitogenicity for T cells and suppression of B lymphocyte function. SPE A shows almost 50% structural homology with staphylococcal enterotoxin B, one of the main staphylococcal toxins associated with the toxic shock syndrome. The gene for production of SPE A is located on the temperate bacteriophage T12. SPE C is also associated with bacteriophage and shows structural similarity to SPE A; both SPE A and C are known to function as superantigens. SPE B has a different structure, being secreted as a zymogen and converted to a proteinase with biological functions including mitogenicity and cytotoxicity for cardiac and other tissues; the substance binds to plasmin and may have a role as a cofactor in the pathogenesis of PSGN.

In a recent world collection of clinical isolates of *S. pyogenes,* genes encoding for production of SPE A, B and C were found in 29%, 100% and 50% respectively. Isolates from patients with scarlet fever in the Western world during the last 30–40 years have mainly been producers of SPE B or C, whereas isolates saved from earlier years, when the disease was more severe, were more often producers of SPE A. During the last 10 years

there have been increasing reports from the USA and UK of SPE A-producing *S. pyogenes*, isolated particularly from patients with severe local infections or with marked systemic toxicity resembling the staphylococcal toxic shock syndrome (Hoge *et al.*, 1993). It is likely that the features of infection in these patients are attributable, at least in part, to the effects of SPE. Antibody to SPE is thought to play a protective role against toxin-mediated streptococcal disease in man.

A novel pyrogenic toxin has been identified recently in GBS isolates associated with toxic shock-like clinical conditions. Invasive infections with toxic shock-like symptoms are occasionally seen with GCS and GGS and it is suspected (but not yet shown) that some isolates of these streptococci may also be able to produce pyrogenic toxins.

Streptolysins

The streptolysins (also known as streptococcal haemolysins and streptococcal cytolytic toxins) form a family of toxins with a facility to lyse a wide variety of mammalian cells in addition to the familiar haemolytic effect on red blood cells (Wannamaker, 1983).

The oxygen-stable streptolysin S is largely responsible for the haemolytic effects seen on culture of GAS and large-colony GCS and GGS; only very occasional strains in these Lancefield groups lack haemolysin production and are non-haemolytic. The substance appears to be non-immunogenic; it is lytic for a wide range of cells, able to suppress some T lymphocyte functions and probably responsible for the leukotoxic properties of *S. pyogenes*, whereby polymorphs are killed after ingestion of streptococci.

Streptolysin O is a heat-sensitive and oxygen-labile protein, classed as a thiol-activated cytolysin (see page 77). It is produced by most strains of *S. pyogenes* and human strains of GCS and GGS. Streptolysin O has a special affinity for cell membranes containing cholesterol and is lytic for a wide range of cells including heart muscle; it can also damage platelets, lysosomes and mitochondria. The toxin suppresses chemotaxis and mobility of neutrophils and inhibits phagocytosis by macrophages.

The haemolysins of other streptococci have not yet undergone extensive study. GBS elaborate a haemolysin resembling but not identical to strepto-lysin S.

Streptokinase

Most haemolytic streptococci of groups A and C produce streptokinase enzymes and an antibody response can often be detected after natural infection with these organisms (Ginsburg, 1985). Streptokinases act as plasminogen activators to produce clot lysis and may enhance the spread of streptococci in the tissues.

Streptokinases form a heterogeneous group of enzymes and at least 10 classes have been described in the internal variable domain of the gene that encodes for them. Variant streptokinases with affinity for the glomerular basement membrane – 'nephrostreptokinases' or nephritis-associated protein (NSAP) (Johnston and Zabriskie, 1986) – are strong contenders as pathogenicity determinants in PSGN developing after GAS and occasional GCS and GGS infections. Other proposed pathogenicity determinants include endostreptosin (ESS), thought to be an intracellular precursor of NSAP, and 'pre-absorbing antigen', which may be a breakdown product of NSAP. Binding of nephrostreptokinase–plasmin complexes to the glomerular basement membrane is followed by deposition of complement and antibody, infiltration by inflammatory cells and cellular proliferation in the glomerulus, with consequent disturbance of function. High levels of antibody to NSAP and ESS are found in patients with this condition.

Other streptococcal products

At least four serological varieties of deoxyribonuclease (DNAase) enzymes are elaborated by streptococci, termed A, B, C and D. They liquefy purulent exudates and are thought to act as streptococcal 'spreading factors'. DNAase B is consistently formed by strains of S. pyogenes and may be exclusive to this species. Streptococcal

hyaluronidases digest hyaluronic acid and may also promote the spread of organisms in the tissues. Further products which may be injurious to the host include proteinases, nicotinamide adenine dinucleotide glycohydrolase (NADase), neuraminidases and various hydrolytic enzymes.

Immunological Cross-reactions with the Host

Immunological cross-reactivities have been shown between certain streptococcal components (including protoplast membrane, M protein and capsular materials), and mammalian proteins in heart, kidney, brain, eye and joint tissue (Fischetti, 1985). What significance these structural similarities between organism and host might have remains largely unclear; it is thought that they may provoke the induction of autoimmune damage to various organs in the body following streptococcal infection, particularly in patients of certain histocompatibility (HLA) classes. Such reactions are probably important in the pathogenesis of rheumatic fever, where non-suppurative inflammation of body tissues is the dominant feature; for example, the occurrence of Sydenham's chorea in rheumatic fever patients may relate to the known cross-reactivity between streptococcal membrane antigens and tissue in the relevant nuclei of the brain.

Pathogenic Interactions Between Streptococci and Other Microorganisms

Several forms of microbial interaction may be important in streptococcal epidemiology and pathogenesis. The normal host flora on mucosal surfaces is thought to play an important role in preventing streptococcal attachment, colonization and infection. In skin infection pyogenic streptococci are often mixed with Staphylococcus aureus and significant synergy may occur between them. In animal models of necrotizing streptococcal fasciitis co-injection with S. aureus or staphylolysin is required to initiate the spreading process, and in experimental lesions in mice the presence of β-lactamase enzymes from S. aureus protects streptococci from the effects of penicillin treatment.

Streptococcal and viral infections are likely to occur together by chance in some individuals and the combined effects may produce unusual arrays of symptoms and signs. There may also be potentiation of bacterial infection as a result of temporary immunosuppression and local tissue damage when viral infection occurs in a patient (Barnham, 1989). Invasive streptococcal disease has been associated with acute viral infections including measles, enteroviruses and varicella.

EPIDEMIOLOGY

Carriage

Pyogenic streptococci are commonly carried in the human nasopharynx and carriage rates vary according to the population studied, the age of the patients and from time to time according to the changing prevalence of streptococcal infection in the community; in a recent study of healthy young adults in North Yorkshire nasopharyngeal carriage rates were 1.5% for GAS, 0.5% (GBS), 2% (GCS), 1.3% (GGS) and 1.1% (GFS and non-groupable streptococci), giving a total carriage rate of all streptococcal groups of 6.4%. In closed communities, such as residential schools and detention centres, carriage rates can approach 50%. Patients carrying large numbers of streptococci in the upper respiratory tract (sometimes termed 'dangerous carriers') may disperse organisms liberally, particularly from the nose, leading to widespread contamination of the hands, other parts of the skin and clothes (Hamburger et al., 1945). In patients with streptococcal pyoderma respiratory colonization occurs within two to three weeks of onset of infection in about 25% of cases.

Haemolytic streptococci may sometimes be found on normal healthy skin (such as on the wrist, ankle, back and behind the pinna of the ear) but at non-epidemic times the number of organisms there is usually very low (Ferrieri et al., 1972). In communities where streptococcal pyoderma is common, such as in the Indian reservations of the USA and amongst children in many parts of Africa, skin colonization rates with pyogenic streptococci may approach 40% at epidemic times. There is a greater risk of streptococcal pyoderma developing in those already carrying streptococci on healthy skin. Streptococci may also colonize areas of abnormal skin, such as in eczema, psoriasis, ulcers and wounds, and may be found in the healthy umbilicus of some neonates.

Streptococcus pyogenes has been recovered from the faeces in up to 20% of patients with upper respiratory streptococcal infection but it is otherwise very rarely found in this site. Up to 6% of children with *S. pyogenes* pharyngitis may temporarily carry the organism in the perianal region, usually inoculated there by the fingers. Outbreaks of surgical wound infection have been traced to perianal carriage of *S. pyogenes* amongst members of the staff. GBS, GCS, GGS and *S. anginosus* are regularly found in the faeces, which provide an endogenous source for infection of the peritoneum, perianal structures and abdominal surgical wounds (Barnham, 1983). These streptococci are likely to be found transiently on the hands and in small numbers elsewhere on the skin. From their main habitat in the rectal mucosa GBS are commonly found in the perineum and natal cleft. Two per cent of normal people have been found to carry GGS in substantial numbers in the perineum or in the toe webs.

The urethra and genital tract are colonized with GBS in up to 30% of women and, less commonly, with GCS, GGS and *S. anginosus*. The presence of *S. pyogenes* in the urinary tract is usually associated with signs of infection.

Sources of Infection and Modes of Spread

Acquisition of streptococci from others may occur by contagion, inoculation or inhalation of recently expelled airborne droplets. Direct physical contact provides an efficient means of streptococcal transmission, as shown in studies during the First and Second World Wars, where poor handling and dressing techniques were found to be responsible for much of the observed streptococcal infection in wounded men. Direct inoculation of streptococci through the skin by contaminated penetrating injury is a highly efficient mode of transmission; an example of this form of transmission was shown in pathologists developing severe streptococcal infection after accidental cuts at autopsy. Direct airborne transmission involving contaminated droplets coughed or sneezed out by an index case or carrier is important in the spread of streptococcal respiratory tract infections although other routes of acquisition (such as by ingestion of contaminated food) may also lead to infection at this site. Autogenous infection, involving organisms already carried by the patient, is thought to account for a proportion of wound, puerperal and abdominal infections.

Streptococci are shed in large numbers into the immediate environment from sites of infection or carriage. In outbreaks of respiratory tract or skin infection viable organisms may be readily cultured from sites such as clothing, bedding and furniture but their significance as a source of further infection is doubtful. Strains of S. pyogenes from the throat, in particular, are known to lose their ability to infect others very quickly once away from their human host; this is associated with reduced expression of M protein and other adhesins on the cell surface.

The importance of animals as a source of human streptococcal infection is mainly restricted to a small range of particular zoonotic diseases. *Streptococcus zooepidemicus* infection is usually acquired by close contact with horses or by the consumption of contaminated dairy products or undercooked pork, GLS infection in those in close occupational contact with chickens or pigs, and *S. suis* infection in those in contact with pigs or pork products. Human infection and carriage with GBS, GCS and GGS generally involves non-zoonotic, human strains of the organisms.

Streptococcus pyogenes is highly host specific to man but there are a few reports of infection in animals as a result of exposure to a human source. Bovine mastitis with *S. pyogenes* has led to outbreaks of pharyngeal infection amongst humans consuming the milk in a raw state. Domestic pets occasionally become involved during family outbreaks of infection and may contribute to reinfection and persistence until they have been treated. Occasional reports from tropical areas suggest that contaminated wound-feeding flies, such as *Hippelates* gnats, may play a part in transmitting GAS infection from patient to patient.

Evolution from Colonization to Infection

The evolution of infection in a patient follows stages of exposure to the organism, attachment, multiplication and invasion. In the case of epidemic *S. pyogenes* pyoderma the organisms colonize normal skin for, on average, 10 days before the onset of lesions (Ferrieri *et al.*, 1972). Experimental inoculation of the skin with pyoderma strains often fails to establish colonization, a result that has been ascribed to the bactericidal effects of skin fatty acids. It is not known how large the presented inoculum needs to be to succeed under natural circumstances, but exposure is likely to increase in the setting of an outbreak, where the excretion of streptococci from others is high. The transition from colonization to pyoderma infection usually follows some minor trauma to the skin. The course of events from colonization to infection has not been studied closely with non-GAS and at sites other than the skin.

Endemic and Epidemic Infection

Studies of *S. pyogenes* infection in the community, such as that conducted in Oxfordshire for five years to 1980, show relatively constant isolation of certain endemic T/M types with periodic outbreaks caused by other, epidemic types (Mayon-White and Perks, 1982); more virulent clones within a type may also occur from time to time.

Community-wide outbreaks vary from short, sharp local episodes to persistent outbreaks lasting for years and spreading in variable geographical patterns through city and country areas. Factors affecting the prevalence of clinical infection in a community include season (respiratory streptococcal infections are generally more common in the winter, and skin infections in the summer), geographical location (respiratory infection is generally more common in colder climates with long winters) and levels of hygiene and crowding. Supplementary factors, such as the occurrence of skin injuries or scabies infection, are often relevant in producing or sustaining outbreaks.

National trends

Analysis of data from national reference laboratories shows an ebb and flow of predominant T/M types of *S. pyogenes* submitted over the years. In the UK (Colman *et al.*, 1993) M types 6 and 49 became dominant in the early 1980s to be replaced by types 1 and 12 by mid-decade, and more recently by type 4; in the USA (Schwartz *et al.*, 1990) increases in types 1, 3 and 18 occurred during this period. These changes are likely to be due to chance introductions and opportunities for spread, and are thought to be restricted by the prevailing levels of type-specific immunity in the population. There are insufficient data yet available to know whether infections with particular streptococcal types have a natural periodicity in the human populations. Changes in the prevailing types and clones of streptococci in the community are associated with fluctuations in the prevalence of related complications such as acute rheumatic fever, PSGN, scarlet fever, invasive infection and antibiotic resistance.

Changes comparable to those seen with *S. pyogenes* probably also occur in the types of non-GAS circulating in the community and causing human disease. There appears to have been a significant and sustained increase in serious GBS infection occurring in neonates from the 1960s in many developed countries and recent reports suggest that this organism may also have become more common as a cause of serious community-

TABLE 1b.3 SUMMARY OF REPORTED SETTINGS FOR OUTBREAKS OF HAEMOLYTIC STREPTOCOCCAL INFECTION

Setting	Infection with streptococci of group			
	A	B	C	G
Community				
General	+[a,b]		+[a,b]	+[a]
Family	+	+[b]	+	+
School	+		+	+
Day care centre	+			
Occupations				
Red meat and poultry handlers	+			
Farmers	+			
Carpenters	+			
Gymnastic teams	+			
Football players (rugby, American)	+			
Seamen	+			
Prison	+			
Military camps	+		+[a]	+[a]
Ethnic reservations	+			
Religious communities	+		+	
Police training centre	+			
Hospitals				
Surgical wards	+			
Maternity/baby units	+	+	+	+
Burns unit	+		+	+
Other wards	+	+	+[a]	+
Outpatient clinics	+			+
Nursing/residential homes	+		+	+

Principal route of infection person to person; additionally: [a] food-borne, [b] milk-borne outbreaks described.

acquired infection in adults. Published reports of significant GCS and GGS infections have also increased in recent years (Efstratiou, 1989) but it is not clear whether this represents a true increase in disease, improved case recognition or greater interest amongst researchers.

Outbreaks

The main reported settings for outbreaks of streptococcal infection are summarized in Table 1b.3. Much of the global burden of streptococcal infection occurs amongst children living in poor socioeconomic conditions of overcrowding and poor hygiene, particularly in warm and humid parts of the world. In developed countries there may be relatively closed communities where such conditions still pertain, including certain tightly knit religious groups and isolated ethnic enclaves. Community-based outbreaks of streptococcal infection in industrialized countries are often focused in particular social groupings or occupational activities, as shown in Table 1b.3. Outbreaks of streptococcal tonsillopharyngitis or impetigo occur regularly amongst 'schoolchildren and can spread to affect parents and others in the household at home; school-based outbreaks often persist for more than one term.

Food-borne outbreaks

Food-borne or milk-borne outbreaks of streptococcal infection usually affect a high proportion of those who consume the contaminated items; they usually feature an abrupt, synchronized onset amongst those eating at a particular event (such as at an hotel or wedding) or consuming unpasteurized milk or dairy products from a particular source (Claesson et al., 1992). Food vehicles for outbreaks of GAS and GGS infection have often included cold boiled eggs and other salad items. Faulty food-handling techniques have been identified in many instances, such as the storage of prepared foods at high ambient temperatures for prolonged periods before consumption. Milk-borne outbreaks of S. pyogenes infection have become rare since the widespread introduction of pasteurization; occa-

sional outbreaks of milk-borne S. zooepidemicus infection have been reported in association with clinical or subclinical mastitis in dairy herds.

Skin infections

Wounding of the skin underlies the occurrence of occupational streptococcal pyoderma such as that seen in carpenters and farmers. Trauma to the face and other parts of the skin amongst rugby football and American football players leads to outbreaks of streptococcal 'scrumpox', a condition which may otherwise be caused by Staphylococcus aureus or Herpes simplex virus. Military and police trainees suffer outbreaks of skin infection associated with the cuts and scratches inflicted during outdoor exercises or from the abrasions from coconut matting and burns from rope exercises in gymnasia. Military servicemen under combat conditions, particularly in tropical and subtropical areas of the world, are also subject to high rates of streptococcal pyoderma; in these men insect bites, blisters, thorns and other forms of trauma to the skin are the usual predisposing factors. Infection may also be seen in civilian travellers experiencing such conditions.

The occurrence of outbreaks of streptococcal skin sepsis in red meat and poultry handlers became increasingly recognized in the UK during the late 1970s (Barnham and Kerby, 1984) and has also been reported from Norway and the USA. Injury from knives, saws and sharp bones is a major predisposing factor for infection in these workers. The subsequent skin infection takes various forms including septic cuts and scratches, paronychia, abscess and lymphangitis. Outbreaks of infection are mainly centred in the abattoir and processing plants but they may affect others down the line of the trade, including deliverymen, retail butchers, chefs and housewives.

Respiratory tract infections

Streptococcal respiratory tract infection, sometimes complicated by rheumatic fever, has been a feature amongst young adults grouped closely together in residential schools, detention centres and military training centres. When there is an adequate intake of new susceptible patients to such an institution, outbreaks may become persistent, endemic problems. Scarlet fever, PSGN or both complications together may feature in outbreaks of cutaneous or respiratory tract infection.

Hospital patients

Outbreaks of pyogenic streptococcal infection in elderly patients grouped together in residential and nursing homes have been regularly reported in recent years (Efstratiou, 1989; Schwartz *et al.*, 1992). Infections are often related to chronic lesions of the skin (such as pressure sores) and there may be a high rate of invasive complications including cellulitis, pneumonia and septicaemia, particularly in patients with predisposing medical and surgical conditions. Investigations usually show a substantial rate of carriage of the outbreak organism amongst other patients and staff in the facility.

Localized outbreaks of streptococcal infection in hospital are still regularly reported. These episodes tend to occur when inadequate attention has been given to hygiene, such as during periods of insufficient staffing or when there is a particularly heavy case-load, and they may commence with the inadvertent admission of an infected patient shedding large numbers of streptococci. Outbreaks of postoperative wound infection with *S. pyogenes* have been traced to carriers in the surgical team or other operating room staff. Wound infection or colonization with pyogenic streptococci in burns and plastic surgery units generally results in failure of skin grafts and delays in wound healing, and may progress to serious invasive disease. Haemolytic streptococcal infection in babies may be acquired directly from the mothers or transmitted via the staff in nurseries. Outbreaks of streptococcal puerperal fever involving cross-infection in the hospital setting are now infrequently reported from developed countries.

In the national epidemics of *S. pyogenes* M type 1 infection reported from the USA, UK and Scandinavian countries in the late 1980s, a wide variety of clinical forms were encountered (Stevens, 1992; Bucher *et al.*, 1992), with increased rates of serious infection in otherwise healthy young adults and a high mortality rate in elderly patients (Schwartz *et al.*, 1992).

CLINICAL FEATURES

Skin Infection

The various forms of streptococcal skin infection range from superficial primary or secondary lesions to aggressive, invasive disease. *Streptococcus pyogenes* is the principal pathogen in these infections but other streptococci also play a part. Figure 1b.1 shows the principal sites of infection in streptococcal diseases of the skin and soft tissues.

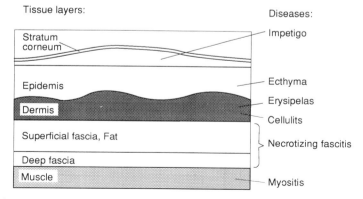

Figure 1b.1. Schematic cross-section of the skin and underlying soft tissues to show the principal location of active infection in various streptococcal diseases. (After Seal, D.V. and Leppard, B. *Transactions of the Royal Society of Tropical Medicine and Hygiene* 1982; **76**: 392–395.)

Pyoderma

Streptococcal pyoderma is a broad term used to describe purulent infections including streptococcal impetigo and localized infections such as otitis externa, paronychia and infections in tattoos and pierced ear lobes. Superficial impetiginous lesions usually develop on traumatized exposed areas of the skin. They start as small erythematous papules and progress to vesicles and pustules, developing thick, honey-coloured crusts on an enlarging erythematous base. The lesions are often associated with moderate tender enlargement of local lymph nodes. Untreated lesions may persist for several weeks, discharging streptococci in large numbers, before healing without a scar; in many cases they are tolerated by the patient without complaint. Figures 1b.2 and 1b.3 show examples of *S. pyogenes* pyoderma lesions.

Ecthyma is a deep and persistent form of ulcerated pyoderma usually showing a raised, oedematous edge and a hard, adherent crust; these lesions are most often found on exposed areas of the lower extremities.

Streptococci and *Staphylococcus aureus* are often found mixed together in pyoderma lesions and there has been controversy over which is the major pathogen in various forms of the disease. Although earlier work suggested that streptococci were the primary pathogens in vesicular impetigo, staphylococci now appear to be the dominant causative organism in this condition in many parts of the USA, Europe and the Middle East. GCS and GGS usually account for only a minority of pyoderma infections but in some parts of West Africa they have been reported as the dominant organisms in this infection. The lesions of angular cheilitis yield haemolytic streptococci, particularly GBS, from about 15% of patients.

Secondary infections with streptococci in other rashes include the 'impetiginization' of scabies, dermatophytosis, eczema and other forms of dermatitis. Streptococcal infection in varicella lesions may lead on to invasive disease.

Infection of superficial wounds such as abrasions and minor burns may produce pyoderma, whereas infection of deeper lesions, including ulcers, surgical incisions, accidental lacerations, the deeper burns and bites, may prove more serious. Wound infection may lead to cellulitis, where there is a rapidly advancing and painful deep inflammation of the skin and subcutaneous

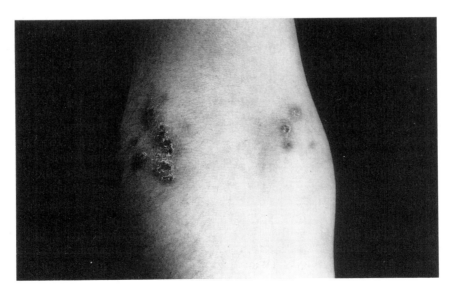

Figure 1b.2. Superficial pyoderma lesions with crusting caused by M-type 80 *S. pyogenes* in the antecubital fossa of a chicken processing factory worker.

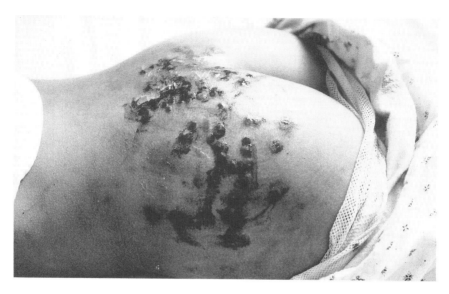

Figure 1b.3. Multiple excoriated and inflamed pyoderma lesions on the buttocks of a schoolboy from Hong Kong. This infection with M-untypable *S. pyogenes* was followed by acute post-streptococcal glomerulonephritis.

tissue with oedema and overlying erythema. The form termed acute perianal cellulitis is largely a disease of childhood, often occurring in association with streptococcal upper respiratory tract infections. In some patients with streptococcal cellulitis or wound infection there is an associated spread of streptococci into the local lymphatic channels to produce ascending lymphangitis (featuring characteristic red streaks in the skin ahead of the focus of infection) and regional lymphadenitis, and a risk that this may lead to suppuration of the nodes or a rapid progression to septicaemia. Subcutaneous abscess is an uncommon local complication of streptococcal infection.

Erysipelas

Erysipelas is an acute, tender, erythematous lesion with an irregular and sharply defined edge associated with streptococcal infection spreading in the dermis; the lesion may in part be due to a hypersensitivity to streptococcal products (Wannamaker, 1983). Lesions occur most commonly on the face in association with upper respiratory tract infection (Figure 1b.4) but they may occur else-where in the body, particularly following wounds and abrasions of the skin. This is an uncommon disease, principally of adults, and now mainly seen in the elderly. In patients with lymphatic or vascular obstruction recurrent forms of erysipelas or streptococcal cellulitis may occur in the dependent area.

Haemolytic streptococci sometimes colonize or infect the umbilicus in neonates or older patients and this can produce a persistent granuloma at the site. Other local forms of streptococcal infection include keratoconjunctivitis, which has been noted in patients of all ages with group A, B and G streptococci, and suppurative hidradenitis in which *S. anginosus* sometimes plays a part, often in conjunction with anaerobic bacteria.

Respiratory Infection

Streptococcal pharyngitis (as a term taken to include superficial infection of the pharynx and/or tonsils) is particularly common in childhood, peaking in incidence between 5 and 14 years of age, and common in adults who live or work at close quarters with children (Wannamaker, 1970;

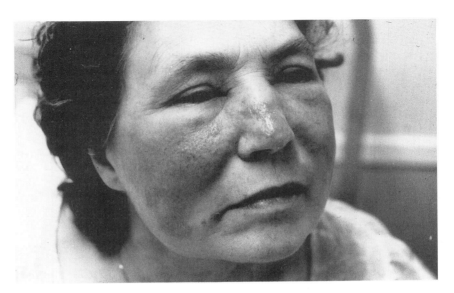

Figure 1b.4. Erysipelas on the face, showing well-defined superficial oedema and typical 'butterfly' distribution across the nose and onto the cheeks.

Peter and Smith, 1977). Pharyngitis probably represents the commonest form of streptococcal infection in the human host (Colman *et al.*, 1993). After an incubation period of one to five days the disease is characterized by a rapid onset of sore throat, malaise and fever, often accompanied by nausea, headache and abdominal pain. Erythema and swelling of the mucosa of the pharynx and tonsils are usually evident, with a purulent exudate and local petechiae in some cases. Enlargement and tenderness of the anterior cervical lymph nodes are particularly common findings. Organisms are excreted in large numbers in the saliva during the first week from onset, when the infection is most easily transmitted to others, but the infectivity falls sharply from 14–21 days after onset despite the persistent carriage of organisms in some patients.

The distinction on clinical signs between streptococcal infection and other common causes of pharyngitis is difficult, as each of the main clinical features seen with streptococcal infection may occur in association with other organisms. The use of score cards and clinical algorithms has been advocated to improve the accuracy of diagnosis (Breese, 1977). The streptococcal aetiology may

be confirmed by bacteriological and serological tests (Kaplan, 1972).

Streptococcal respiratory infection in children below the age of four years often follows a sub-acute, protracted form with only a feeble antibody response. The illness usually shows little or no clinical evidence of infection in the throat but may include rhinorrhoea with nasal excoriation – features that are largely restricted to the disease in infants.

Direct extension of infection may produce otitis media and sinusitis although, presently, GAS account for only a small proportion of the cases seen in clinical practice. Further suppurative complications have been rarely seen in recent years in developed countries; they include local tissue invasion by the infecting streptococci to produce a peritonsillar abscess, suppurative cervical lymphadenitis and extension from the sinuses to produce osteomyelitis in the bones of the skull. These extending forms of the infection may result in streptococcal septicaemia.

Evidence from food-borne, milk-borne and other outbreaks indicates that at least some strains of GCS and GGS have the ability to produce significant pharyngitis in man, although illness is usually relatively mild. Pharyngeal infection with *S. zooepidemicus* has been followed by PSGN in three published outbreaks (Francis *et al.*, 1993). *S. anginosus* may be isolated from oral, dental and sinus abscesses but it does not appear to have the ability to produce pharyngitis.

Genital and Urinary Tract Infections

Specimens collected from patients with a variety of symptoms related to the urethra and lower genital tract commonly yield haemolytic streptococci in pure or mixed culture, but it is often difficult to distinguish carriage from genuine infection. *Streptococcus pyogenes* is clearly associated with a syndrome of vulvovaginitis in young girls during the childhood years (Donald *et al.*, 1991) and similar signs and symptoms are found in a substantial proportion of older women yielding this organism from local swabs. Several centres in the UK reported increasing isolation of *S. pyogenes* from the genital tract during the late 1980s, involving many different T/M types; the reasons for this apparent increase remain unclear. Streptococcal puerperal fever, involving ascending genital tract infection in the postnatal period, is usually associated with poor hygiene and cross-infection within maternity units. Without prompt treatment the infection can produce endometritis, pelvic peritonitis and septicaemia and may be rapidly fatal. In the male genital tract *S. pyogenes* may cause balanitis and anterior urethritis.

GBS colonization may be found in the rectal mucosa or genital tract in up to 30% of women. The importance of this organism as a cause of infection within the tract has been difficult to estimate, especially as there is no widely available serological test to confirm an immune response in the patient. GBS are sometimes isolated in pure, heavy growth from patients with vaginal discharges or Bartholin's gland abscess and are probably a genuine cause of infection in such cases. Maternal endocarditis may result from bacteraemia with GBS at parturition.

Recorded outbreaks of puerperal fever featuring GCS and GGS show that these organisms can cause a spectrum of local and invasive diseases resembling that of *S. pyogenes*, although usually of a lesser severity (Lewis, 1989). *Streptococcus anginosus* is also found as a commensal organism in the perineum and genital tract and may be involved in abscesses in these areas.

Babies born to mothers with high levels of genital colonization with haemolytic streptococci are at high risk of colonization and infection. The risk of neonatal disease is highest in premature babies and in complicated or slow deliveries involving premature rupture of the membranes. GBS have been the leading pathogens in this situation in recent years (Yagupsky *et al.*, 1991; Zangwill *et al.*, 1992; Wessels and Kasper, 1993) but similar infection is sometimes encountered with GAS, GCS, GGS or *S. anginosus*. Urinary tract infection with haemolytic streptococci is uncommon; in pregnancy there is a recognized

TABLE 1b.4 REPORTED SOURCES OF INFECTION IN STREPTOCOCCAL BACTERAEMIA

Source	Percentage of bacteraemic patients with		
	GAS[a] (*n* = 480)	GCS[b] (*n* = 88)	GGS[c] (*n* = 186)
Skin/soft tissues	39	17	43
Respiratory	26[d]	20	9
Gastrointestinal	3	18	3
Genitourinary	4	6	5
Unknown	28	39	40

[a] Compiled from 14 published reports 1987–1992.
[b] Data from review by Bradley *et al.* (1991).
[c] Compiled from nine reports 1983–1989.
[d] Includes primary pneumonia 10%, supra/epiglottitis 1%.

association between GBS urinary tract infection and premature delivery.

Invasive infection

Signs of impending invasion from local sites of streptococcal infection include lymphangitis, cellulitis and endometritis; within a few hours the patient may be critically ill with septicaemia. Reported local sources of infection in patients with streptococcal bacteraemia are summarized in Table 1b.4; in about a quarter of patients with *S. pyogenes* bacteraemia, and up to 40% of those with GCS or GGS, the initial site of infection remains unknown. Haemolytic streptococci account for about 5% of total reports of bacteraemia in man.

The major forms of disease associated with streptococcal invasion are listed in Table 1b.5. These range from local tissue destruction to bacteraemia, which may be associated with secondary focal infections in many different parts of the body (Hoge *et al.*, 1993; Barnham, 1989; Stevens, 1992; Bucher *et al.*, 1992). Underlying conditions in the patient that may predispose to invasion range from the effects of age and acute intercurrent illnesses to chronic debilitating conditions including cardiovascular, metabolic, immunosuppressive and malignant diseases. Infection with virulent strains of streptococci, as in recent national outbreaks with SPE A-producing *S. pyogenes*, may lead to higher than normal rates of invasive disease amongst otherwise healthy children and adults (Stevens, 1992; Bucher, *et al.*, 1992).

Overall mortality rates of 20–50% have been described in recent reports of *S. pyogenes* septicaemia (Hage *et al.*, 1993; Stevens, 1992; Francis and Warren, 1988) with most fatalities occurring within the first 48 hours of clinical presentation. Features associated with a particularly high risk of death include the age of the patient (high risk for neonates and those over 60 years) and the development of respiratory distress syndrome or shock. Aspects of the streptococcal toxic shock syndrome are discussed in the section on scarlet fever below.

Infective endocarditis

Infective endocarditis occurs less commonly with haemolytic than with non-haemolytic streptococci. Recent reports suggest that amongst the pyogenic streptococci endocarditis occurs more commonly with GGS than with GCS or GAS (Bradley *et al.*, 1991; Gaunt and Seal, 1987; Burkert and Watanakunakorn, 1991). This complication is seen also with systemic *S. anginosus* infection and in very occasional patients with *S. suis*. The majority of these patients are over the age of 45 years and many show underlying medical disorders; the infection often follows an acute course with valvular destruction, embolism and signs of streptococcal septicaemia, and reported mortality rates range from 21% to 36%. Streptococcal infection in intravenous drug abusers commonly affects valves on the right side of the heart.

Meningitis

Meningitis is a particular feature of bacteraemic infection with GBS (Yagupsky *et al.*, 1991), the highly capsulated *S. zooepidemicus* (Bradley *et al.*, 1991) and *S. suis* (Arends and Zanen, 1988). The condition is rare with *S. pyogenes* and other

TABLE 1b.5 DISEASES ASSOCIATED WITH INVASIVE STREPTOCOCCAL INFECTION

Bacteraemia/septicaemia
Vascular
   Disseminated intravascular coagulation
   Endocarditis/endarteritis
   Mycotic aneurysm
   Septic thrombophlebitis
   Peripheral gangrene (auto-amputation)
Streptococcal toxic shock syndrome
Abscess/empyema
Cellulitis erysipelas, lymphangitis
Necrotizing fasciitis
Myositis
Septic arthritis
Osteomyelitis
Meningitis
Pericarditis
Peritonitis
Ascending genital tract infection
Cholangitis
Mediastinitis
Pneumonia
Epiglottitis
Ophthalmitis

pyogenic streptococci, occurring with these species mainly by direct spread from adjacent foci of infection in or around the skull, or following head injury or craniospinal surgery.

Respiratory infection

Haemolytlc streptococcal pneumonia is now a rare disease in most parts of the industrialized world. It may occur in association with acute viral infections of the respiratory tract (particularly with influenza and measles) and is sometimes seen in outbreaks of streptococcal infection in the elderly. *Streptococcus pyogenes* is the principal infecting organism but GBS, GCS, GGS and *S. suis* have been noted in occasional cases. Streptococcal pneumonia carries a high risk of empyema; bacteraemia occurs in about 40% of cases. *Streptococcus anginosus* is frequently isolated from lung abscesses.

Septic arthritis and osteomyelitis

Septic arthritis and osteomyelitis occur either by direct extension from a local focus of streptococcal infection or as a complication of bacteraemia. Infec-

tion may develop both in previously healthy bones and joints and in those previously affected by trauma or chronic disease. In a recent compilation of reports from the UK septic arthritis or osteomyelitis was recorded in 10% of patients with systemic GAS, 8% of GCS and 6% GGS infections.

In streptococcal pyomyositis *S. pyogenes* causes a painful, necrotic infection within the muscle, leading to abscess formation. It is frequently seen as part of a multi-focal, septicaemic illness in chronically debilitated patients. In streptococcal necrotizing fasciitis, infection, usually associated with a local injury, spreads in the fascial planes to cause thrombosis of vessels and patchy necrosis of the skin and subcutaneous fat (Barker *et al.*, 1987). The condition features cellulitis, haemorrhagic bullae and areas of deep necrosis, and there is a risk of septicaemia and rapid death (Figure 1b.5); it is most commonly seen in elderly patients, usually in association with serious underlying medical disorders.

Other clinical manifestations

Abdominal pain occurs as a feature of streptococcal respiratory tract infection in childhood,

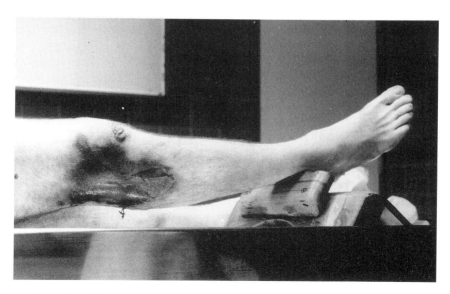

Figure 1b.5. Necrotizing fasciitis on the lateral aspect of the knee showing typical haemorrhagic bullae, bruising and scald-like appearances of early skin necrosis. This patient died of M-type I *S. pyogenes* septicaemia within three days of onset.

possibly related to a tender enlargement of mesenteric nodes. A temporary, palpable enlargement of the spleen has been recorded in children and young adults with *S. pyogenes* pharyngitis.

The presence of haemolytic streptococci in the alimentary tract provides a possible source for abdominal infection (Barnham, 1983). Acute bacteraemic cholangitis has been described in patients with GCS and GGS, and haemolytic streptococci may be cultured from some patients with peritonitis or localized para-intestinal abscesses. *Streptococcus pyogenes* septicaemia can present with signs of gastroenteritis: in a recent series 28% of the patients gave a history of diarrhoea, often with vomiting (Francis and Warren, 1988); in some cases the disturbance has been associated with the presence of pelvic or diffuse peritonitis.

Pyogenic streptococci are a cause of septic bursitis or tenosynovitis around the knee, shoulder, elbow and wrist; they are, however, found less frequently than *S. aureus* in these conditions. It is thought that infection usually arises from direct traumatic inoculation of the organisms.

Group B Streptococcus

GBS were first reported as a cause of occasional serious human infections in the 1930s, soon after their initial characterization by Lancefield. In the 1960s and 1970s these organisms emerged as one of the leading causes of infection in neonates and young infants in many parts of the industrialized world.

Of the two main clinical forms (Yagupsky *et al.*, 1991), early-onset disease, occurring within the first seven days of life and particularly in premature babies following prolonged rupture of the membranes and chorioamnionitis, features pneumonia, septicaemia or meningitis; the organism in this condition may also be cultured from the mother's genital tract. Late-onset disease occurs in otherwise healthy infants, particularly in the first three months of life, following normal delivery, and features septicaemia, meningitis and other focal lesions; the infection is thought to be mainly due to cross-infection. Invasive GBS occurs with an incidence of one in 800–4000 live births in many parts of the world. The fatality rate for serious infantile GBS infection in a recent study in the USA was 5.8%, similar in early- and late-onset disease (Zangwill *et al.*, 1992). Infection with GBS has also been reported as a cause of intrauterine fetal death and miscarriage.

In adults GBS may be the cause of a range of serious infections including septicaemia, pneumonia, arthritis, osteomyelitis, pyelonephritis, endocarditis, meningitis and endophthalmitis (Barnham, 1989). Such disease may be seen in mothers following bacteraemia at parturition or, more commonly, in adults with serious underlying medical disorders, particularly diabetes mellitus and malignancy; the incidence increases with age (Wessels and Kasper, 1993). To date there have been six reports of overwhelming GBS sepsis in splenectomized patients. The case fatality rate amongst adults in the recent study in the USA was 16%, including 57% of those with meningitis (Zangwill *et al.*, 1992). Milder forms of GBS infection in adults include skin, soft tissue and genitourinary tract infections.

Streptococcus anginosus

Streptococcus anginosus is the most commonly found streptococcus in abscesses, particularly those involving internal organs such as the brain, liver, lungs, spleen and peritoneum (Ruoff, 1988; Whitworth, 1990). It is also recorded as an occasional cause of septic arthritis and osteomyelitis; skin and soft tissue infections occur, particularly after human bites. Transient bacteraemia with *S. anginosus* occurs following oral and dental surgery but endocarditis is seen less frequently with this species than with the extracellular polysaccharide-producing 'viridans' streptococci. There is no clear association between haemolysis and pathogenicity in this species but the carriage of the Lancefield group C antigen appears to identify a subgroup of strains that are more commonly found in invasive infection. In general, the presence of *S. anginosus* in blood cultures should raise suspicions of abscess or endocarditis; in about 50% of patients there is underlying disease such as diabetes mellitus or malignancy. The presence of *S. anginosus* in the female genital tract may occasionally lead to ascending infection which, in pregnancy, can result in chorioamnionitis, abortion or serious neonatal infection.

Zoonotic streptococcal infections

Bovine strains of GBS have been found to colonize members of farming families living closely with their animals, and are probably mainly acquired by drinking unpasteurized milk. GBS may also be found in pigs, dogs and certain other large animals encountered by man. There is no clear evidence that these strains are associated with human disease.

The host ranges of the five principal streptococcal species found within Lancefield group C are shown in Table 1b.6. A recent review in the author's laboratory of more than 200 group C streptococci from human infection showed, in superficial lesions, 94%, *S. equisimilis*, 5% *S. anginosus* and 1% *S. zooepidemicus* while from deeper, more aggressive infection the proportions were 67%, 27% and 6.7% respectively. *Streptococcus equisimilis* carriage and infection occur quite commonly in man but this usually involves human strains and there are only a few reported instances of acquisition from an animal source.

Streptococcus zooepidemicus is a relatively rare but important cause of zoonotic infection in man (Francis *et al.*, 1993; Bradley *et al.*, 1991). Table 1b.7 lists the clinical features of 31 cases of infection with this organism detected in the UK in the eight years 1979–1986. Infection is usually seen as sporadic disease in people closely exposed to horses, pigs or other carrier animals or as out-breaks amongst those consuming contaminated milk or dairy products from cattle with *S. zooepidemicus* mastitis. Two principal syndromes of infection occur: one of an acute pharyngitis with cervical lymphadenopathy, complicated in a proportion of cases by PSGN, the other of an acute invasive disease seen particularly in the elderly, the pregnant and the very young with a high risk of focal complications and death. Meningitis and endocarditis are regular features of systemic infection with *S. zooepidemicus* and are probably associated with the high levels of encapsulation and fibrinogen binding shown by this organism.

Streptococcus equi is a highly host-adapted species and there are very few convincing case reports of infection in man; the non-haemolytic *S. dysgalactiae* has also been reported very rarely from humans. There are, as yet, no reports of zoonotic infection with *S. anginosus* in man. The place of *S. canis* (group G) as a potential zoonosis in man has not been clarified.

Wound infections and paronychia caused by GLS have been reported in red meat and poultry handlers (Barnham and Neilson, 1987). The organisms are commonly found in the upper respiratory passages of chickens and pigs and these animals have been the source of most human infections. GLS have also been isolated on rare occasions from the human throat and from endocarditis and septicaemia.

Streptococcus suis is a frequent commensal and opportunistic pathogen in pigs. Strains of this species carry the Lancefield group antigens R, S and T and also react with antisera to group D. Most human disease has been with group R, serotype 2 but infections with types 4 and 14 have

TABLE 1b.6   HOST RANGES OF GROUP C STREPTOCOCCI

S. equisimilis	Man, pig, monkey, dog, cat, poultry, cow, (horse)
S. zooepidemicus	Horse, pig, sheep, goat, cow, fox, poultry, rabbit, guinea-pig, monkey, (man)
S. equi	Horse, mule, donkey
S. dysgalactiae[a]	Cattle, sheep, pig
S. anginosus[b]	Man, pig, monkey, guinea-pig

[a] non-haemolytic;
[b] haemolysis variable;
underlining, principal hosts;
( ), rarely implicated.

TABLE 1b.7 CLINICAL FEATURES OF 31 *S. ZOOEPIDEMICUS* INFECTIONS REPORTED IN ENGLAND 1979–1986

Feature	No. of patients showing feature
Systemic infections	
Meningitis	7
Septicaemia	8
Endocarditis	5
Mycotic aneurysm	1
Pneumonia[a]	2
Cholecystitis	1
Septic arthritis	1
Local infections	
Tonsilopharyngitis, cervical lymphadenopathy[a,b]	8
Asymptomatic throat carriage	1
Otitis externa	1
Infected leg ulcer	1
Infected finger wound	1

[a] Includes one sporadic case of post-streptococcal nephritis in each of these categories.
[b] Also includes five cases of post-streptococcal nephritis in a milk-borne outbreak.
Data from M. Barnham (unpublished compilation).

also been described; both haemolytic and non-haemolytic strains are encountered. Significant human infection with *S. suis* occurs predominantly in pig-breeding countries such as Holland and Denmark or where large quantities of pork are consumed, such as in Hong Kong (Arends and Zanen, 1988). A high proportion of reported cases has occurred in people working in direct contact with pigs or their meat, including farmers, slaughtermen, butchers and housewives, and there is often a history of wounding to the skin which may act as a portal of entry. Infection has also been reported from exposure to wild boar.

The features of systemic infection with *S. suis* in man are listed in Table 1b.8. The organism is most commonly associated with a syndrome of septicaemia and meningitis with a high risk of persistent hearing loss in those who survive, but other localized forms of infection include endocarditis, septic arthritis and pneumonia. A study in New Zealand showed serological evidence of infection with *S. suis* type 2 in 10% of meat inspectors and 21% of pig farmers, suggesting that mild or subclinical forms of infection occur commonly in these occupational groups.

TABLE 1b.8 REPORTED CLINICAL FEATURES IN SYSTEMIC *S. SUIS* INFECTIONS IN MAN

Meningitis
Persistent deafness and vestibular disturbance in convalescence
Uncomplicated septicaemia
Endocarditis
Septic arthritis
Gastroenteritis
Endophthalmitis, uveitis
Pneumonia
Disseminated intravascular coagulation
Peripheral gangrene

Distant Manifestations and 'Non-suppurative Sequelae' of Streptococcal Infection

Scarlet fever and associated conditions

Scarlet fever is most commonly associated with *S. pyogenes* infection in the upper respiratory tract but it may follow infection elsewhere in the body such as in burns, pressure sores and wounds (as in 'surgical scarlet fever'). The disease has not been recorded in association with any other organism.

After a latent period of three to five days from the onset of streptococcal infection there is an abrupt onset of malaise and headache with the appearance of the erythematous rash, which typically shows circumoral pallor, a 'strawberry' tongue and later desquamation of the skin. Historical records show that the severity of scarlet fever fluctuates greatly from time to time and place to place; the disease was one of the commonest causes of death in children in Britain during the second half of the nineteenth century but subsequently there has been a great decline in its associated morbidity and mortality. Throughout much of the developed world the disease has been mild in recent years and there have been difficulties in reliably diagnosing the condition on clinical grounds alone (Perks and Mayon-White, 1983).

The rash of scarlet fever is thought to result from an SPE-enhanced acquired hypersensitivity in the patient to one or more streptococcal products rather than from a primary effect or toxicity of SPE (Wannamaker, 1983). The affinity of SPE for dermal cell may play a part in localizing these interactions. Previous exposure to the relevant antigens by earlier streptococcal infection may be necessary to produce scarlet fever. The disease has been associated over the years with a restricted range of T/M types of *S. pyogenes* including types 1, 3, 4, 6, 12, 18, 22 and 66.

The resurgence of SPE A-producing *S. pyogenes* infections in the USA in the 1980s and early 1990s has been associated with serious clinical disease including cellulitis, necrotizing fasciitis and other invasive forms of infection together with marked systemic toxicity (Hoge *et al.*, 1993; Stevens, 1992); a rash may be present in some patients but it is often atypical of scarlet fever. The main features of this streptococcal toxic shock syndrome are listed in Table 1b.9; this 'new' disease is probably analogous to the serious 'toxic scarlet fever' recorded in earlier years. The clinical resemblance of this disease to the staphylococcal toxic shock syndrome is reflected in the similar molecular structures of SPE A and staphylococcal enterotoxin B. SPE A-producing strains of *S. pyogenes* have been found only rarely in Europe in recent years and the possible involvement of SPE B and/or C in the pathogenesis of toxic shock-like symptoms in patients from this part of the world is currently a matter of debate.

A further 'septic' variety of scarlet fever was once recognized in which the streptococcal infection became locally invasive or disseminated to produce septicaemia and distant foci of infection in

TABLE 1b.9 PRINCIPAL FEATURES OF THE STREPTOCOCCAL TOXIC SHOCK SYNDROME

Physical findings
  Fever >38 °C
  Confusion
  Tachycardia
  Hypotension
  Signs of severe local infection[a] (swelling, erythema, bullae, desquamation)

Complications
  Acute respiratory distress syndrome
  Renal impairment
  Septicaemia[b]
  High fatality rate[c]

After Stevens (1992). In the series reported by that author ($n = 20$) the following percentage of patients showed the feature: [a] 80%, [b] 60%, [c] 30%.

the bones, joints and soft tissues. This form of disease has been seen only rarely in developed countries since the introduction of antibiotics but a few typical cases have been reported during the recent rise in invasive M type 1 *S. pyogenes* in Europe and the USA.

Psoriasis and other rashes

Numerous studies have shown an association between acute streptococcal infection (or local colonization) and the development of acute guttate psoriasis in children and young adults, or exacerbation of pre-existing psoriatic lesions (Colman *et al.*, 1993; Noah, 1990). Many different T/M types of *S. pyogenes* appear to be involved and serological evidence of recent streptococcal infection may be found in up to two-thirds of patients with acute guttate psoriasis; GBS, GCS and GGS have also been isolated with unusually high frequency from various body sites in association with the disease. Both infection and colonization with these organisms appear to act as trigger factors for the production of the psoriasis rash; some have postulated that the extensive exfoliation of psoriasis may represent the body's attempt to rid itself of potentially harmful bacteria detected at the surface (Noah, 1990).

Other cutaneous manifestations of streptococcal infection include urticaria and diffuse erythematous rashes, erythema multiforme, erythema nodosum, and the papular and nodular lesions that occur in patients with rheumatic fever. Petechial haemorrhages in the skin are commonly associated with *S. pyogenes* upper respiratory tract infection in childhood and they may occur in some patients with scarlet fever. More profuse purpuric lesions may be seen in patients with streptococcal septicaemia; gangrene of the extremities can occur in particularly severe cases.

Rheumatic fever and associated conditions

Acute rheumatic fever occurs as a sequel to *S. pyogenes* infections of the tonsils and pharynx, usually affecting less than 3% of patients with untreated infection at that site (Ayoub and Chun, 1990; Bisno, 1991); it is most commonly seen in patients between the ages of five and 15 years. The features of the disease (as shown in Table 1b.10) develop 10–35 days after the start of streptococcal infection. The onset is usually rapid with a painful, flitting, asymmetrical polyarthritis of the major joints, fever, sweating and tachycardia. In some patients the disease may be

TABLE 1b.10   THE REVISED JONES CRITERIA FOR DIAGNOSIS OF RHEUMATIC FEVER[a]

Major manifestations	Minor manifestations
Carditis	Fever
Murmurs (apical systolic, mid-diastolic or basal diastolic)	Arthralgia[b]
	Previous rheumatic fever or rheumatic heart disease
Pericarditis	Increased erythrocyte sedimentation rate or plasma viscosity
Cardiomegaly	raised C-reactive protein
Congestive failure	
Polyarthritis	
Chorea	
Erythema marginatum	
Subcutaneous nodules	Prolonged P–R interval[c]
Evidence of antecedent *S. pyogenes* infection	
Recent scarlet fever	
Positive culture or rapid streptococcal antigen test	
Elevated or rising ASOT (anti-streptolysin O titre) or other anti-streptococcal antibody	

[a] A high probability of rheumatic fever is indicated by two major, or one major and two minor manifestations supported by evidence of antecedent *S. pyogenes* infection.
[b] Not a valid minor manifestation when polyarthritis is counted as a major manifestation.
[c] Not a valid minor manifestation when carditis is counted as a major manifestation.

insidious and present non-specifically with fatigue, malaise and weight loss. In at least one-third of patients there is no history of a preceding overt pharyngitis and the organism may no longer be cultivable from the site.

Sterile, migratory arthritis is the most common manifestation of rheumatic fever, occurring in about 70% of cases. Carditis occurs in about 50% of patients and is a more specific and important characteristic of the disease. The pericardium, myocardium and endocardium may all be affected to produce tachycardia and murmurs during the acute phase of the disease; severe myocarditis may be manifest by dysrhythmias or cardiac failure. In convalescence fibrosis produces thickening and distortion of the valve leaflets and chordae tendineae, affecting the mitral valve disproportionately. Sydenham's chorea affects 5–15% of patients after a latent period of 3–12 months. Erythema marginatum develops on the trunk and limbs of about 5% of patients; painless subcutaneous nodules are found over the extensor surfaces of joints in 2–3% of patients. The minor manifestations shown in Table 1b.10 are relatively non-specific but provide supporting evidence of the disease.

Rheumatic fever is believed to be an autoimmune disorder triggered by streptococcal infection. The disease follows infection with certain strains of *S. pyogenes*, particularly within M types 1, 3, 4, 5, 6, 12, 14, 17, 18, 19 and 24; distinct patterns of superantigenic V-*β* specificity have been found in this group of M proteins. Immunological cross-reactions may also play a role in the disease, such as those found between capsular hyaluronic acid and host connective tissues, the group A polysaccharide and mitral valve glycoprotein, M proteins and cardiac myosin and sarcolemmal membrane proteins, and between the streptococcal protoplast membrane and the subthalamic and caudate nuclei of the brain (Fischetti, 1989; Ayoub and Chun, 1990; Bisno, 1991). Host factors also appear to be important in the aetiology of the disease, with higher than expected attack rates in some families and races (particularly where individuals show the D8/17 antigen on the surface of B lymphocytes) and there is a 50% likelihood of further attacks in susceptible patients.

TABLE 1b.11 PRINCIPAL REACTIONS IN LABORATORY IDENTIFICATION OF HAEMOLYTIC STREPTOCOCCI

Organism (Lancefield group)	Acetoin production (VP)	Hydrolysis of			Production of				Fermentation of				
		Arginine	Aesculin	Hippurate	*β*-Galactosidase	*β*-Glucuronidase	PYR[a]	Alkaline phosphatase	Sorbitol	Lactose	Trehalose	Ribose	Glycogen
S. pyogenes (A)	–	+	–	–	–	V	+	+	–	+	+	–	V
S. agalactiae (B)	+	+	–	+	–	V	–	+	–	V	V	V	–
S. equisimilis (C)	–	+	–	–	–	V	–	+	–	V	+	+	V
S. zooepidemicus (C)	–	+	V	–	–	+	–	+	+	+	–	V	+
S. equi (C)	–	+	–	–	–	+	–	+	–	–	–	–	+
Streptococcus sp., large colony (G)	–	+	–	–	–	V	–	+	–	V	+	+	V
S. canis (G)	–	+	–	–	V	V	–	+	–	V	V	+	–
Streptococcus sp., (L)	–	+	–	V	–	+	–	+	–	V	+	+	+
S. suis (R)	–	+	V	–	V	+	V	–	–	+	+	–	+
S. anginosus ('milleri')	+	+	V	–	V	–	–	+	–	V	+	–	–

–, reaction seen in <10% isolates tested; v, 10–90%; +, >90%.
[a]PYR, pyrrolydonyl arylamidase; VP, Voges–Proskauer test.

Rheumatic fever has declined greatly in incidence in industrialized countries during the twentieth century, probably as a result of improved living standards, better health care for children and the widespread use of antibiotics for respiratory tract infections, but the disease is still the most common cause of acquired heart disease in developing countries. An unexpected resurgence in acute rheumatic fever occurred in the USA in the mid- to late 1980s (Schwartz *et al.*, 1990), associated with infection with highly mucoid strains of *S. pyogenes*.

Some patients feature post-streptococcal reactive arthritis in an illness that falls short of the case definition of rheumatic fever, but a number later have secondary and more characteristic attacks. This form of arthritis is therefore thought to lie within the same spectrum of disease as rheumatic fever and to warrant a similar approach in clinical management and prevention.

Post-streptococcal glomerulonephritis

The symptoms and signs of PSGN develop after a latent period of 10–21 days from the onset of infection and include haematuria, oedema, fever, hypertension and oliguria. Laboratory findings include proteinuria, haematuria, reduced serum complement levels and abnormal renal function tests. PSGN is a disease of variable severity and asymptomatic cases usually outnumber those with overt disease several-fold; attack rates of overt PSGN do not usually exceed 15% even after infection with known nephritogenic strains of streptococci. Second attacks occur only very rarely. Renal biopsy examination of asymptomatic children with decreased serum complement and/or abnormal urinalysis following streptococcal infections of the skin or throat show changes compatible with PSGN in a high proportion of cases. The long-term prognosis is generally good but 7–10% of patients develop chronic glomerulonephritis and may eventually require dialysis or renal transplantation. The incidence of the disease has declined markedly in developed countries in recent decades but it remains a common complication in most parts of the world (Ayoub and Chun, 1990; Ferrieri, 1975).

Nephritis occurs more readily after streptococcal infections of the skin than of the throat (Ferrieri, 1975). There are differences in clinical presentation according to the epidemiology of infection at these two sites: in PSGN after pyoderma patients tend to be younger (often less than six years old), there is a longer latent period (commonly 18–21 days compared with an average 10 days after respiratory infection) and the seasonal peak of disease occurs in the summer and autumn (as compared with the winter and spring after respiratory infections).

Certain T/M types of *S. pyogenes*, the so-called 'nephritogenic types', have been regularly implicated with the occurrence of PSGN, including M1, T25/Imp19M2, M4, T12M12, M49 and T25/Imp19M55; nephritogenicity appears to be associated only with certain strains within these types. Outbreaks and sporadic cases of PSGN have also been described in association with *S. zooepidemicus* (Francis *et al.*, 1993) and with occasional *S. equisimilis* and GGS infections. The responsible organisms in some of these cases have been shown to produce ESS or molecular variants of NSAP. The precise aetiology of PSGN and the parts played by candidate nephritogenic antigens in the initiation and amplification of effects in the glomerulus are not yet clearly understood.

LABORATORY DIAGNOSIS

The major tasks in diagnosis are to distinguish acute streptococcal infection from other causes of disease and from carriage of streptococci at the site in question (Kaplan, 1972). Ideally the diagnosis should result from a clinical interpretation of the patient's history, symptoms and signs supported by microbiological evidence including (1) positive culture or specific antigen detection and (2) evidence of an immune response to the organism from the examination of acute and convalescent sera. Each of these components has its limitations and a comprehensive approach is usually too slow, too costly and impractical for routine clinical purposes; however, it may be desirable in the investigation of severe or unusual streptococcal disease, in the management of suspected outbreaks and in audit or research.

Culture

The careful collection of specimens from the patient and rapid transport to the laboratory are fundamental to achieve good, reliable results. Most strains of haemolytic streptococci can be cultured without difficulty in aerobic or anaerobic atmospheres on conventional laboratory media. Growth in both solid and liquid culture media may be enhanced by the presence of 5–10% blood or horse serum and by an atmosphere containing 5% carbon dioxide. After 18–24 hours incubation at 37 °C isolated colonies of pyogenic streptococci measure up to 1.5 mm diameter, although the size may be much smaller in those who have recently received antibiotics. Colonies of *S. anginosus* are usually minute and culture for 48 hours may be required to reveal them; the cultures give a characteristic caramel odour. The colonies of organisms with pronounced encapsulation, such as *S. zooepidemicus* and certain isolates of *S. pyogenes*, appear large and mucoid. Colonies of streptococci rich in surface M protein usually show a matt appearance. Few strains of *S. pyogenes* will grow on media containing bile but GBS and *S. anginosus* are more tolerant of this substance. The number of streptococcal colonies growing on primary isolation plates has been suggested as a discriminating factor between infection (often yielding a substantial growth) and carriage (often small numbers); however, the distinction is not clear cut and results are easily affected by testing procedures and conditions.

Streptococcal haemolysis varies according to the species of red blood cell employed, but results are generally similar with the horse or sheep blood used in many laboratories. Haemolysis associated with oxygen-labile haemolysins is enhanced by anaerobic culture. The size of zone of haemolysis may be particularly large with GLS but is usually small with GBS and *S. suis*. The recognition of streptococci in specimens where heavy mixed growths are expected may be aided by the use of blood agar rendered selective by the addition of inhibitors such as crystal violet, gentamicin or neomycin. With all species of haemolytic streptococci occasional non-haemolytic isolates occur and these are likely to be overlooked in mixed bacterial cultures; such variants appear to be more common amongst streptococci of animal rather than human origin.

Identification

From the primary culture of suspected haemolytic streptococcal colonies, initial confirmatory tests should include a Gram-stained film (positive cocci in chains) and a catalase test (negative result with streptococci).

Convenient laboratory kits for Lancefield grouping incorporate a two-stage technique involving rapid acid or enzymic antigen extraction followed by specific precipitation, latex particle agglutination or co-agglutination reactions. Tests are usually carried out on one to five colonies picked from the primary isolation plate. In modern kits the group antigens are extracted from the organisms by exposure to nitrous acid at room temperature or by digestion using *Streptomyces*- or *Achromobacter*-derived enzymes at 37 °C for 10 minutes. The older techniques of antigen extraction using hot hydrochloric acid, formamide or autoclaving remain as reference standards but are no longer widely used. In the second stage of the test antigen detection reagents are usually used in combinations (such as groups A, B, C, D, F and G) to identify the majority of haemolytic streptococci found in clinical specimens. These tests have now supplanted the bacitracin identification discs which were formerly used to distinguish *S. pyogenes* (sensitive) from non-GAS (usually resistant).

More detailed identification of streptococci may be achieved by the use of extended biochemical and physiological tests. Standardized laboratory kits for this purpose, such as the API 20STREP and Rapid ID 32STREP tests incorporating multiple test reagents aligned on a strip, are now readily available for routine laboratory use. These tests have the advantages of stability, good reproducibility of results between different laboratories and an extensive database for interpretation of the profile of results. Some laboratories continue to prepare their own media for these purposes and use a shorter series of relevant and discriminating tests. Details of expected test results in the principal tests used to identify haemolytic streptococci are shown in Table 1b.11. Detailed identification of haemolytic streptococcal isolates is advisable in cases of serious invasive disease and, in research, for accurate case description and consistent epidemiological study.

Recent molecular biological techniques, including digested DNA and RNA fragment analysis and gene probing, are currently too complex and costly for routine diagnosis but they may be used for selective subtyping and taxonomic studies; they also hold promise for the future development of rapid tests for the recognition of streptococci in clinical specimens.

Antigen Detection

The commercial development of rapid detection tests for GAS antigen in clinical specimens offers the hope to physicians of near-patient testing with results that could help both with diagnosis and with initial decisions on the use of antibiotic therapy (Pichichero *et al.*, 1992). Studies in patients with pharyngitis have shown a high specificity (>95% with most kits) but variable sensitivity of these tests in comparison with culture, according to the experience and training of the investigator (55–95% in a number of studies). Positive results may be used as a basis for treatment decisions, although a proportion are probably related to simple carriage of substantial numbers of streptococci. A further limitation is that the kits only detect group A antigen, whereas some non-GAS are also relevant in the aetiology of pharyngitis. False negative results with the kits are common in office practice and, where a microbiological result is required, all patients with pharyngitis and a negative antigen result should undergo routine culture for streptococci. In addition, if positive antigen tests are not followed up by culture confirmation there is a loss of potentially useful data for laboratory-based infection surveillance and epidemiology. In view of these limitations, the cost of kits and the extra clinical time involved in carrying out the tests, near-patient antigen testing for rapid diagnosis of streptococcal pharyngitis has not proved popular in most parts of the world.

Antigen detection kits have been employed to test urine and gastric aspirate samples in the rapid investigation of suspected neonatal GBS disease; however, the usefulness of results as a guide in clinical practice is not yet clearly established.

Streptococcal antigen tests have also been used in the laboratory as a rapid preliminary investigation on specimens before culture results are known; a sensitivity of up to 95% compared with culture results has been achieved in experienced hands but some false positives have occurred, particularly with group C reagents.

Typing

A summary of the most frequently used streptococcal typing tests is given in Table 1b.12 and the (relatively limited) indications for such testing are set out in Table 1b.13. The antibiotic susceptibility

TABLE 1b.12 SUMMARY OF TYPING TECHNIQUES APPLIED TO STREPTOCOCCI

Biotyping (from physiological test results used in identification)
T, M, R antigen typing (especially for groups A, C, G)
Opacity factor (OF) and anti-OF (especially for group A)
Polysaccharide antigen typing, proteins R, X (especially for group B)
Bacteriophage typing
Bacteriocin typing (producer – and sensitivity – types)
DNA fingerprinting
Ribotyping
Multi-locus enzyme electrophoresis
Whole cell protein analysis

profiles (antibiograms) and physiological test result profiles of streptococci (biotypes, such as the API 20STREP profile number) are often poorly discriminating and of little use for typing purposes.

The detection of T, M and R protein antigens on the streptococcal surface by agglutination and precipitation tests forms the basis of the principal typing scheme employed for *S. pyogenes* throughout the world. Patterns of T antigens, present in the cell wall either singly or in regular multiples (such as 3/13/B3264 and 8/25/Imp19), are each associated with only one or a short range of possible M antigens. Available T-typing sera usually achieve >90% typability, depending on geographical area (a recent study in England reported 99% T typability) but discrimination of strains is not very high if this test is used alone. There are now more than 80 established M antigen types and a number of provisional M types have also been described; the typability of isolates (97% in the recent English study) depends largely on the quality of antisera, the size of panel employed and on geographical location. Some isolates that give negative results in M typing may be typed according to R protein or specific inhibition of the OF reaction (anti-OF typing). Alternative or complementary typing schemes which have been applied to *S. pyogenes* include bacteriophage susceptibility testing and bacteriocin producer and sensitivity typing.

Some GCS and GGS carry M proteins but these substances have not yet been utilized widely for typing the organisms. *Streptococcus equisimilis* and the large colony GGS carry T antigens that may be used for typing human clinical isolates; in a recent study in the UK this achieved typability rates of 88% and 82% respectively (Efstratiou, 1989). Bacteriophage and bacteriocin typing techniques have also been usefully employed to subdivide streptococci in these groups.

GBS may be divided into a number of serotypes according to the carriage of major and minor polysaccharide antigens and protein antigens (including R, X and c protein in its α and β antigenic forms) and further divided by bacteriophage typing.

The recent application of modern molecular biological methods to the typing of streptococci, including fingerprinting of restriction enzyme digests of DNA or ribosomal RNA, whole cell protein analysis and pyrolysis mass spectrometry, has provided highly detailed profiles of the organisms. DNA fingerprints of *S. pyogenes* appear to be M type specific and minor band differences may be used to distinguish between clones within the types (Cleary *et al.*, 1988); the technique has also been used to investigate clusters of infection with *S. zooepidemicus*, an organism which is poorly typable by conventional techniques. Enzyme electrophoretic typing has been used to analyse clonal diversity in isolates of particular M types of *S. pyogenes* causing invasive or complicated infections.

Certain features of *S. pyogenes* infection appear to be more or less type specific – that is, they are

TABLE 1b.13   INDICATIONS FOR STREPTOCOCCAL TYPING

Epidemiology	Outbreaks (control, research, medicolegal)
	Carrier studies and selective treatment
	Prevalence of types in communities
	Acquisition studies
	Study of type-related features and diseases
Research	Characterization of organisms
	Treatment studies (relapse, reinfection)
	New type-related features
Surveillance	In sentinel districts
	Detect community outbreaks
	Define vaccine requirements
	For cross-infection (hospitals, schools etc.)

mainly restricted to infection with strains within a limited range of T/M types. Such conditions include scarlet fever, PSGN, rheumatic fever, invasive infection and antibiotic resistance. Streptococcal skin infection has been associated traditionally with organisms showing higher-number M types and more complex T types than are seen in throat infection (Wannamaker, 1970). The significance of M type number is purely historical, as the sequence was begun at a time of particular interest in commonly occurring strains from respiratory and systemic infections; the genetic and molecular basis of multiple T-typing patterns in *S. pyogenes* has not yet received detailed attention. An analysis of GAS strains collected recently in the UK appeared to show that these differences in typing between skin and throat strains were becoming less clear cut (Colman, 1993); this may, however, have been due to the increase at that time in infections with particular strains (such as M49) which can cause infection at both sites.

Antibody Responses

The serological responses to streptococcal products may be used either to confirm the clinical significance of isolated streptococci or as an alternative approach to diagnosis for patients in whom cultures are unsuccessful or unobtainable (Kaplan, 1972; Ayoub, 1991). Some serological tests used for routine or special diagnostic purposes are shown in Table 1b.14; those most commonly used include the anti-streptolysin O (ASO), anti-DNAase B (ADB) and anti-hyaluronidase (AH) tests. It is advisable to use more than one of these

tests as a routine in view of the variable host response to different antigens. In particular, skin infection with *S. pyogenes* is associated with an absent or poor ASO response as a result of inactivation of streptolysin O by skin lipids and cholesterol, but it is often accompanied by a brisk response in ADB. In addition, the early treatment of *S. pyogenes* infection with antibiotics has been shown to inhibit serological responses, including the M-specific antibodies which confer immunity to reinfection with the homologous type.

The ideal for confirmation of acute streptococcal infection is to detect a four-fold (or more) rise or fall in specific antibody titre in sera collected in the early and convalescent phases of the illness. Titres in single sera may be interpreted against a notional 'upper limit of normal' which should be established locally and will vary according to the patient's age and the prevalence of streptococcal infections in the community. The ADB response in infected patients usually lasts longer than the rise in ASO titre, and may be used as a serological marker in late convalescence. It has not been determined what proportion of patients with genuine infection show no, or low, serological response to particular antigens.

The serological changes after infection vary with the species of streptococcus involved, as shown in Table 1b.15. Changes in ASO may be found in infection with *S. pyogenes*, *S. equisimilis* and large-colony GGS but not with *S. zooepidemicus*, *S. anginosus* or GBS. Discriminating AH tests may be carried out using antigen derived from group A or from group C/G streptococci. The ADB response is generally considered to be highly specific for infection with *S. pyogenes* but recent

TABLE 1b.14   SEROLOGICAL TESTS IN STREPTOCOCCAL INFECTION

Streptococcal product	Antibody test (common abbreviation)
Streptolysin O	Anti-streptolysin O (ASO)
Hyaluronidase (of group A, or C/G)	Anti-hyaluronidase (AH) against A, C/G
DNAase B	Anti-DNAase B (ADB)
Streptokinase	Anti-streptokinase (ASK)
NADase[a]	Anti-NADase
Lancefield group antigen	Anti-A (or C,G)-carbohydrate (anti-A (C,G)-CHO)

[a] Nicotinamide adenine dinucleotidase.

TABLE 1b.15 EXPECTED SEROLOGICAL CHANGES IN ACUTE STREPTOCOCCAL INFECTION

Organism	ASO	AH(A)	AH(C/G)	ADB
S. pyogenes (group A)	+	+	–	+
Large colony group G streptococcus	+	–	+	–
S. equisimilis (group C)	+	–	+	–
S. zooepidemicus (group C)	–	–	–	+[a]

[a] Preliminary finding, based on small numbers of human cases.

investigations on patients with *S. zooepidemicus* suggest that this infection may also produce a rise in the antibody. Antibodies to the Lancefield group antigens (A, B, C, G, etc.) may be detected after acute infection with the relevant streptococci (Ayoub, 1991) but these tests are not yet widely available. Various other surface antigens of GBS are known to produce antibody responses in man, including the capsule and certain cell wall proteins, but routine diagnostic tests have not yet been developed. There are currently no tests available for the serodiagnosis of infection with *S. anginosus* or *S. suis*.

ANTIMICROBIAL SUSCEPTIBILITY

All isolates of *S. pyogenes* and most other haemolytic streptococci remain highly susceptible to penicillin despite the extensive use of this antibiotic for the last 50 years. Some typical minimal inhibitory concentrations of commonly used *β*-lactam drugs for clinical isolates of *S. pyogenes* are as follows (minimal inhibitory concentration (MIC), mg/l): benzyl penicillin 0.01, ampicillin 0.03, methicillin 0.25, cephradine 0.5, cefotaxime 0.03. In contrast, penicillin resistance may be found in oral non-haemolytic streptococci and in occasional isolates of *S. anginosus*, particularly in patients who have recently received penicillin. A wide discrepancy between penicillin minimum inhibitory and bactericidal concentrations ('tolerance') has been noted in some isolates of pyogenic streptococci; the clinical significance of this is at present uncertain but the phenomenon may be important in serious infections, such as endocarditis, where a highly bactericidal treatment is needed.

Erythromycin resistance was first reported in the UK in 1959; in recent years it has been reported from many parts of the world at a basic prevalence of 2–5% of isolates of *S. pyogenes*, increasing locally (and usually temporarily) to 20–70% of isolates according to the spread in the community of particular clones of streptococci. A recent study in the UK involving large numbers of isolates from 61 diagnostic laboratories recorded erythromycin resistance rates of 3% with GAS, 2.5% with GBS, 4.5% with GCS, 4.3% with GFS and 6.4% with GGS (Spencer *et al.*, 1989). Cross-resistance occurs in these organisms between erythromycin and other macrolides (including clarithromycin and azithromycin), and high-level resistant strains will usually also resist clindamycin and lincomycin.

Tetracycline resistance in haemolytic streptococci was first reported in the UK in 1954 and increased in prevalence significantly during the following decades in most parts of the world. This resistance occurs in many different serotypes of *S. pyogenes*, with higher levels in skin- than in throat-infecting strains. The recent national study in the UK showed tetracycline resistance in 9.5% of GAS, 68% of GBS, 31% of GCS, 25% of GFS and 47% of GGS (Spencer *et al.*, 1989). Strains showing resistance to both tetracycline and erythromycin are uncommon and mainly seen with GCS and GGS.

Haemolytic streptococci are resistant to aminoglycoside antibiotics including gentamicin, neomycin and amikacin (MIC values usually >4 mg/l) and to sodium fusidate. They are, however, susceptible to the topical antibiotic mupirocin (MIC of *S. pyogenes* 0.06–0.5 mg/l) with no reports to date of acquired resistance to this substance. β-Haemolytic streptococci are susceptible to ciprofloxacin and chloramphenicol at MIC values around 0.5 mg/l and 2–4 mg/l respectively, but occasional resistant strains may be encountered.

MANAGEMENT

The management of streptococcal infection in a patient should include (1) an initial clinical diagnosis supported, whenever possible, by specific microbiological confirmation, (2) specific antibiotic therapy given as soon as possible and revised in the light of clinical response and microbiological findings, (3) supportive therapy according to the severity of the case (including control of underlying diseases, surgical drainage of abscess, etc., as required), (4) a consideration of infection control requirements including isolation nursing (particularly in the case of *S. pyogenes* infection in hospital) and a possible search for further cases and (5) the notification of public health authorities of certain forms of streptococcal disease according to local or national requirements. The important supplementary medical, surgical and nursing procedures that may be needed for particular patients will not be considered in further detail here.

A wide variety of active antimicrobial agents is now available for treatment of streptococcal infections and many different regimens have been used with success. This is a field where the familiar, time-tested drugs remain the standard and usually the best choice in clinical practice; further comparative studies of treatment with modern agents are needed to establish what particular advantages they may have. In the sections below the antibiotic treatments of upper respiratory, cutaneous and invasive infections are considered in more detail.

Upper Respiratory Tract Infection

Antibiotic treatment of β-haemolytic streptococcal pharyngitis shortens the illness in the majority of patients and reduces both infectivity and the likelihood of rheumatic fever (Peter and Smith, 1977;

Pichichero *et al.*, 1992; Bass, 1991). Penicillin given orally for 10 days or by a single injection of a long-acting formulation (such as benzathine penicillin) has long been regarded as the treatment of choice for streptococcal infection of the pharynx and associated structures. Alternative drugs for those who are allergic to penicillin include erythromycin and cephalosporins. Oral or injectable cephalosporins (including cephalexin, cephradine and cefuroxime) are as efficacious as penicillin V in the initial treatment of these infections but are more expensive and more likely to disturb the patient's commensal flora. Ampicillin and co-amoxiclav may be appropriate drugs for the treatment of acute otitis media and sinusitis, where the susceptibility of pathogens other than streptococci needs to be considered, but they will produce a rash in those who are suffering from infectious mononucleosis and should therefore be avoided for the treatment of patients with undiagnosed pharyngitis.

Penicillin or erythromycin treatments achieve high rates of clinical improvement in acute streptococcal infection but rather lower rates of bacterial eradication; a meta-analysis of reports showed that 15% of patients give persistent positive cultures. Causes of failure to eradicate the organisms include misdiagnosis of chronic streptococcal carriage, poor patient compliance with the 10 days of treatment and reacquisition of streptococci from immediate contacts (Kaplan *et al.*, 1982). Reinfections or symptomatic relapses of acute infection may warrant a second course of antimicrobial treatment using a different drug. Chronic streptococcal carriers have low infectivity to others and a low risk of rheumatic fever, and they do not usually require antibiotic treatment. For the treatment of pharyngeal carriers clindamycin or the combination of penicillin plus rifampicin have given good results.

Clarithromycin given for 10 days or azithromycin for three days appears to be comparable in efficacy to erythromycin for the treatment of upper respiratory streptococcal infections, giving a low incidence of side effects; however, resistance to macrolides can occur and the drugs are costly.

Skin Infection

Many commonly used topical antibiotic preparations are unsuitable for the treatment of streptococci, including those containing sodium fusidate, polymyxin, neomycin, gentamicin and framycetin to which the organisms are naturally resistant, and they pose is a risk of sensitizing patients to the drugs and promoting bacterial resistance. Tetracycline is often contraindicated because of the high rate of resistance to the agent amongst skin-infecting isolates. Debridement and local disinfection of pyoderma lesions with antiseptics gives little improvement over the spontaneous resolution rate for this infection.

Skin sepsis often involves both *Staphylococcus aureus* and streptococci and, until the bacteriological results are known, it is advisable to choose agents with activity against both organisms, such as flucloxacillin (which has sufficient anti-streptococcal activity to give good results), erythromycin or topical mupirocin. For the treatment of known streptococcal skin infection penicillin and erythromycin both give high rates of success (Peter and Smith, 1977).

Serious and Systemic Infections

In invasive streptococcal infections it is essential to achieve a rapid diagnosis and institute antibiotic therapy without delay (Stevens, 1992); patients are also likely to require urgent access to modern medical and surgical interventive and supportive measures, according to the nature of the infection and its complications.

The mainstay of antibiotic treatment for serious β-haemolytic streptococcal infection is penicillin by injection; adult dosage should be in the region of 1200 mg (2 megaUnits) every 4–6 hours. Those with known penicillin allergy may be treated with intravenous erythromycin (50 mg/kg daily in divided doses every 6 hours). There have been few comparative studies of different antibiotic regimens in these uncommon infections, largely because of the difficulties of patient recruitment. Concern for adequate antimicrobial activity against penicillin-tolerant strains has led to the use of penicillin/aminoglycoside combinations in the treatment of severe disease such as septicaemia and endocarditis; however, it has not been clearly demonstrated that this approach is more successful than monotherapy. Penicillin, ampicillin or chloramphenicol have been used successfully to treat β-haemolytic streptococcal meningitis, including patients infected with GBS, GCS and *S. suis*.

The mortality rate for patients with *S. pyogenes* septicaemia remains high and patients often die within 24–48 hours of hospital admission despite receiving seemingly appropriate therapy with penicillins or cephalosporins. The results of *in vitro* studies and experimental infection in mice suggest that clindamycin may be superior to β-lactam drugs for the treatment of serious (i.e. locally aggressive, bacteraemic and toxigenic) forms of *S. pyogenes* infection (Stevens, 1992). Clinical data on the use of clindamycin in serious human streptococcal infection are few but appear to be promising; the drug may be used in intravenous doses of 600–1200 mg (adult dose) given up to four times per day, singly or in combined treatment with penicillin.

Antibiotic Prophylaxis

Those who have suffered an attack of rheumatic fever are at risk of exacerbations following further streptococcal respiratory infections and should receive regular prophylaxis with penicillin or erythromycin; in children this treatment should be continued until adulthood. There is, however, no indication for prophylaxis in patients who have had a previous attack of nephritis.

Patients liable to recurrent attacks of streptococcal cellulitis or erysipelas, such as those with lymphatic obstruction, often benefit from long-term anti-streptococcal prophylaxis. Intrapartum prophylaxis with ampicillin has been used successfully to reduce the rate of GBS transmission from mothers carrying the organisms in the genital tract to their babies, particularly in the setting of premature delivery or obstetric complications, where there is a risk of serious infection. There has been some concern that antibiotic treatment of the mother in this manner might select and increase infection with other potentially pathogenic organisms, such as *Escherichia coli*, but there is little information on the extent of this possible risk.

INFECTION CONTROL AND PREVENTION

General Aspects of Prevention, Surveillance and Infection Control

Good housing, nutrition and personal hygiene are important for the prevention of pyogenic streptococcal infection in the community. Modern hygienic arrangements in health care premises help to ensure that risks of cross-infection involving patients and staff are kept to a minimum at all times; these include good professional hygiene (including regular and thorough handwashing), the application of aseptic and no-touch techniques in the management of wounds, the use of sterilized equipment and dressings for invasive and other critical procedures, and careful arrangements for prompt disposal of contaminated items. Patients in hospital with *S. pyogenes* infection should be nursed in isolation until at least 48 hours of appropriate antibiotic therapy have been given to minimize the possibility of transmission to others. Patients infected with other species of β-haemolytic streptococci are thought to pose a lesser risk to others.

Routine surveillance for streptococcal infection may include: (1) the reports of infection control nursing staff, (2) clinical reports and statutory notifications on streptococcal diseases (such as scarlet fever) and (3) the analysis of laboratory results for patterns of isolation from the patients. For social groups in which outbreaks of infection have previously occurred (such as in schools, factories or military training centres) more active surveillance may be arranged with the relevant managers, medical officers and nursing staff.

National data on the occurrence of streptococcal diseases may be collected and published by streptococcal reference laboratories and surveillance units (such as, in the UK, the central laboratories of the Public Health Laboratory Service, the Communicable Disease Surveillance Unit and the Office of Population Censuses and Surveys) who receive isolates and information on a voluntary or statutory basis from participating laboratories and clinicians throughout the country. Special surveys may be organized from time to time by professional groups, such as the recent UK study of rheumatic fever undertaken by the British Paediatric Surveillance Unit.

Detection and Control of Outbreaks

The surveillance measures outlined above will often give an early warning of streptococcal outbreaks. The principles used to define and control suspected outbreaks of streptococcal infection are in most respects similar to those required for other microorganisms. Staff should be questioned, case records reviewed and surveillance intensified to improve case ascertainment and help decide whether an outbreak is actually occurring. A programme of appropriate bacteriological testing of suspected cases should be instituted to establish the microbiology, including typing to pinpoint the responsible strains and antibiotic testing to provide a basis for rational treatment. All those found to be infected should be treated without delay; exclusion of cases from work until clinical recovery may sometimes be required. Bacteriological screening tests for carriers, animals, incriminated food or environmental contamination may be indicated where they are thought to be relevant to the infection of patients. Associated issues that may require attention to halt an outbreak include scabies infection, high rates of occupational injury, eddies of infection in household contacts and compliance with suggested therapies.

In the assessment and control of outbreaks good teamwork and rapid dissemination of information are essential between the laboratory, public health authorities, clinicians and managers involved. Where animals are incriminated the discussions and investigations should involve both medical and veterinary specialists. Appropriate treatment guidelines should be prepared according to the susceptibility of the organisms and the nature of the infections and circulated to clinicians at an early stage. Mass treatment of cases and susceptibles with antibiotic is not usually required but it may be considered as a tactic to gain control (1) in outbreaks involving large numbers of patients, where comprehensive bacteriological assessments are difficult to achieve, (2) when outbreak control based on individual case detection and treatment is failing and (3) where serious sequelae such as rheumatic fever are thought likely to occur. In the settings shown in Table 1b.3 outbreaks frequently relapse or recur and at the end of an episode it is good practice to maintain a heightened level of surveillance to detect and treat any further cases that may arise.

Recommended measures for the investigation and control of suspected GBS cross-infection in maternity and neonatal units broadly follow the scheme described above. There is normally a high prevalence of colonization with various types of these streptococci in adults and the routine typing of isolates from serious infection will help to alert staff to the possible occurrence of a common epidemic strain. The main measures for control of outbreaks of this infection include the securing of adequate numbers of staff to ensure that safe working practices are not compromised at busy times, and arranging intensified personal, professional and environmental hygiene, particularly in the delivery suite and nurseries.

Prospects for Streptococcal Vaccines

Despite intensive current research no vaccine is yet available for protection against streptococcal infections in man. Priority in this area is afforded to the development of *S. pyogenes* vaccines to protect against rheumatic fever, and for vaccines to prevent serious GBS infection, particularly in neonates. Difficulties include the heterogeneity of these streptococci, the likely need to produce and maintain both circulating and mucosal immunity to the organisms and the possibility of enhancing pathogenesis in some patients. Current experimental vaccines include hybrid GAS proteins and conjugated GBS capsular polysaccharides (Fischetti, 1989; Wessels and Kasper, 1993). The use of specific immunoglobulins for protection of babies against GBS is also being investigated. Recent progress in the molecular biology and immunology of streptococci holds promise for refinements in these areas, particularly in the study of common surface antigens of streptococci which elicit strong immunity while avoiding cross-reactions with the host.

REFERENCES

Arends, J.P. and Zanen, H.C. (1988) Meningitis caused by *Streptococcus suis* in humans. *Reviews of Infectious Diseases*, **10**, 131–137.

Ayoub, E.M. (1991) Immune response to group A streptococcal infections. *Pediatric Infectious Diseases Journal*, **10**, S15–S19.

Ayoub, E.M. and Chun, C.S.Y. (1990) Nonsuppurative complications of group A streptococcal infection. *Advances in Pediatric Infectious Diseases*, **5**, 69–92.

Barker, F.G., Leppard, B.J. and Seal, D.V. (1987) Streptococcal necrotising fasciitis: comparison between histological and clinical features. *Journal of Clinical Pathology*, **40**, 335–341.

Barnham, M. (1983) The gut as a source of the haemolytic streptococci causing infection in surgery of the intestinal and biliary tracts. *Journal of Infection*, **6**, 129–139.

Barnham, M. (1989) Invasive streptococcal infections in the era before the acquired immune deficiency syndrome: a 10 years' compilation of patients with streptococcal bacteraemia in North Yorkshire. *Journal of Infection*, **18**, 231–248.

Barnham, M. and Kerby, J. (1984) A profile of skin sepsis in meat handlers. *Journal of Infection*, **9**, 43–50.

Barnham, M. and Neilson, D.J. (1987) Group L beta-haemolytic streptococcal infection in meat handlers: another streptococcal zoonosis? *Epidemiology and Infection*, **99**, 257–264.

Bass, J.W. (1991) Antibiotic management of group A streptococal pharyngotonsillitis. *Pediatric Infectious Diseases Journal*, **10**, S43–S49.

Bisno, A.L. (1991) Group A streptococcal infections and acute rheumatic fever. *New England Journal of Medicine*, **325**, 783–793.

Bohach, G.A., Fast, D.J., Nelson, R.D. and Schlievert, P.M. (1990) Staphylococcal and streptococcal toxins involved in toxic shock syndrome and related illnesses. *Critical Reviews in Microbiology*, **17**, 251–272.

Bradley, S.F., Gordon, J.J., Baumgartner, D.D. *et al.* (1991) Group C streptococcal bacteraemia: analysis of 88 cases. *Reviews of Infectious Diseases*, **13**, 270–280.

Breese, B.B. (1977) A simple scorecard for the diagnosis of streptococcal pharyngitis. *American Journal of Diseases of Children*, **131**, 514–517.

Bucher, A., Martin, P.R., Hoiby, E.A. *et al.* (1992) Spectrum of disease in bacteraemic patients during a *Streptococcus pyogenes* serotype M-1 epidemic in Norway in 1988. *European Journal of Clinical Microbiology and Infectious Diseases*, **11**, 416–426.

Burkert, T. and Watanakunakorn, C. (1991) Group A streptococcus endocarditis: report of five cases and review of literature. *Journal of Infection*, **23**, 307–316.

Claesson, B.E.B., Svensson, N.G., Gotthardsson, L. *et al.* (1992) A foodborne outbreak of group A streptococcal disease at a birthday party. *Scandinavian Journal of Infectious Diseases*, **24**, 577–586.

Cleary, P.P., Kaplan, E.L., Livdahl, C. *et al.* (1988) DNA fingerprints of *Streptococcus pyogenes* are M type specific. *Journal of Infectious Diseases*, **158**, 1317–1323.

Colman, G., Tanna, A., Efstratiou, A. *et al.* (1993) The serotypes of *Streptococcus pyogenes* present in Britain during 1980–1990 and their association with disease. *Journal of Medical Microbiology*, **39**, 165–178.

Donald, F.E., Slack, R.C.B. and Colman, G. (1991) *Streptococcus pyogenes* vulvovaginitis in children in Nottingham. *Epidemiology and Infection*, **106**, 459–465.

Efstratiou, A. (1989) Outbreaks of human infection caused by pyogenic streptococci of Lancefield groups C and G. *Journal of Medical Microbiology*, **29**, 207–219.

Ferrieri, P. (1975) Acute post-streptococcal glomerulonephritis and its relation to the epidemiology of streptococcal infections. *Minnesota Medicine*, **58**, 598–602.

Ferrieri, P., Dajani, A.S., Wannamaker, L.W. *et al.* (1972) Natural history of impetigo: 1. Site sequence of acquisition and familial patterns of spread of cutaneous streptococci. *Journal of Clinical Investigation*, **51**, 2851–2862.

Fischetti, V.A. (1989) Streptococcal M protein: molecular design and biological behavior. *Clinical Microbiology Reviews*, **2**, 285–314.

Francis, J. and Warren, R.E. (1988) *Streptococcus pyogenes* bacteraemia in Cambridge: a review of 67 episodes. *Quarterly Journal of Medicine*, new series **68**, 603–613.

Francis, A.J., Nimmo, G.R., Efstratiou, A. *et al.* (1993) Investigation of milk-borne *Streptococcus zooepidemicus* infection associated with glomerulonephritis in Australia. *Journal of Infection*, **27**, 317–323.

Gaunt, P.N. and Seal, D.V. (1987) Group G streptococcal infections. *Journal of Infection*, **15**, 5–20.

Ginsburg, I. (1985) Streptococcal enzymes and virulence. In *Bacterial Enzymes and Virulence* (ed. I.A. Holder), pp. 121–144. CRC Press, Boca Raton, FL.

Hamburger, M., Green, M.J. and Hamburger, V.G. (1945) The problem of the 'dangerous carrier' of hemolytic streptococci: II. Spread of infection by individuals with strongly positive nose cultures who expelled large numbers of hemolytic streptococci. *Journal of Infectious Diseases*, **77**, 96–108.

Hoge, C.W., Schwartz, B., Talkington, D.F. *et al.* (1993) The changing epidemiology of invasive group A streptococcal infections and the emergence of streptococcal toxic shock-like syndrome. *Journal of the American Medical Association*, **269**, 384–389.

Johnston, K.H. and Zabriskie, J.B. (1986) Purification and partial characterization of the nephritis strain-associated protein from *Streptococcus pyogenes*, group A. *Journal of Experimental Medicine*, **163**, 697–712.

Kaplan, E.L. (1972) Unresolved problems in diagnosis and epidemiology of streptococcal infection. In *Streptococci and Streptococcal Diseases* (ed. L.W. Wannamaker and J.M. Matsen), pp. 557–570. Academic Press, New York.

Kaplan, E.L., Gastanaduy, A.S. and Huwe, B.B. (1982) The streptococcal carrier: an explanation for frequent treatment failures with antibiotics. In *Basic Concepts of Streptococci and Streptococcal Diseases* (ed. S.E. Holm and P. Christensen), pp. 165–166. Reedbooks, Chertsey, UK.

Lewis, R.F.M. (1989) Beta-haemolytic streptococci from the female genital tract: clinical correlates and outcome of treatment. *Epidemiology and Infection*, **102**, 391–400.

Mayon-White, R.T. and Perks, E.M. (1982) Why type streptococci? The epidemiology of group A streptococci in Oxfordshire 1976–1980. *Journal of Hygiene (Cambridge)*, **88**, 439–452.

Noah, P.W. (1990) The role of micro-organisms in psoriasis. *Seminars in Dermatology*, **9**, 269–276.

Perks, E.M. and Mayon-White, R.T. (1983) The incidence of scarlet fever. *Journal of Hygiene (Cambridge)*, **91**, 203–209.

Peter, G. and Smith, A.L. (1977) Group A streptococcal infections of the skin and pharynx. *New England Journal of Medicine*, **297**, 311–317, 365–370.

Pichichero, M.E., Disney, F.A., Green, J.L. *et al.* (1992) Comparative reliability of clinical, culture and antigen detection methods for the diagnosis of group A beta-hemolytic streptococcal tonsillopharyngitis. *Pediatric Annals*, **21**, 798–805.

Ruoff, K.L. (1988) *Streptococcus anginosus* ('*Streptococcus milleri*'): the unrecognized pathogen. *Clinical Microbiology Reviews*, **1**, 102–108.

Schleifer, K.H. and Kilpper-Bälz, R. (1987) Molecular and chemotaxonomic approaches to the classification of streptococci, enterococci and lactococci: a review. *Systematic Applied Microbiology*, **10**, 1–19.

Schwartz, B., Facklam, R.R. and Breiman, R.F. (1990) Changing epidemiology of group A streptococcal infection in the USA. *Lancet*, **336**, 1167–1171.

Schwartz, B., Elliott, J.A., Butler, J.C. *et al.* (1992) Clusters of invasive group A streptococcal infections in family, hospital, and nursing home settings. *Clinical Infectious Diseases*, **15**, 277–284.

Spencer, R.C., Wheat, P.F., Magee, J.T. *et al.* (1989) Erythromycin resistance in streptococci. *Lancet*, **i**, 168.

Stevens, D.L. (1992) Invasive group A streptococcus infections. *Clinical Infectious Diseases*, **14**, 2–13.

Wannamaker, L.W. (1970) Differences between streptococcal infections of the throat and of the skin. *New England Journal of Medicine*, **282**, 23–31, 78–85.

Wannamaker, L.W. (1983) Streptococcal toxins. *Reviews of Infectious Diseases*, **5**, S723–S732.

Wessels, M.R. and Kasper, D.L. (1993) The changing spectrum of group B streptococcal disease. *New England Journal of Medicine*, **328**, 1843–1844.

Whitworth, J.M. (1990) Lancefield group F and related streptococci. *Journal of Medical Microbiology*, **33**, 135–151.

Yagupsky, K., Menegus, M.A. and Powell, K.R. (1991) The changing spectrum of group B streptococcal disease in infants: an eleven-year experience in a tertiary care hospital. *Pediatric Infectious Disease Journal*, **10**, 801–880.

Zangwill, K.M., Schuhat, A. and Wenger, J.D. (1992) Group B streptococcal disease in the United States, 1990: report from a multi-state active surveillance system. *Morbidity and Mortality Weekly Report*, **41** (Surveillance Summaries), SS–6, 25–32.

1c

STREPTOCOCCUS PNEUMONIAE (PNEUMOCOCCUS)

James C. Paton

HISTORICAL INTRODUCTION

The organism which we now refer to as *Streptococcus pneumoniae*, or the pneumococcus, remains one of the world's foremost human pathogens. It was first isolated (separately) by Sternberg and Pasteur in 1880; in both cases the source of the organism was the saliva of individuals who were not suffering from pneumococcal disease at the time. The body of information on the biology of the pneumococcus and its importance as a cause of human disease expanded rapidly in the decades following its discovery and these studies have been eloquently reviewed by Austrian (1981a). By 1890, the pneumococcus had been recognized as a causative agent of pneumonia, bacteraemia, otitis media, meningitis, endocarditis and arthritis. Studies carried out during the first half of the twentieth century established that there were numerous serotypes of *S. pneumoniae*, each producing a structurally distinct capsular polysaccharide. These substances were the first non-protein molecules shown to be immunogenic and anti-polysaccharide antibodies were shown to provide type-specific protection against challenge with virulent pneumococci. Perhaps the most important of all, however, were the experiments carried out by Avery and his many collaborators on the capsular transformation phenomenon, which led to the discovery that DNA was the carrier of genetic information (Avery *et al.*, 1944).

MORPHOLOGICAL AND PHYSIOLOGICAL CHARACTERISTICS

Microscopic and Colonial Appearance

Streptococcus pneumoniae is a small, lancet-shaped, Gram-positive coccus, approximately $0.5-1.0 \, \mu m$ in diameter (see Figure 1c.1). Its tendency to form pairs joined along the long axis when grown on solid media accounted for its former name of '*Diplococcus pneumoniae*'. However, in broth cultures it forms short chains, and DNA analysis has confirmed that it is appropriately placed in the genus *Streptococcus*. On blood agar, pneumococci form smooth, glossy colonies $0.5-2$ mm in diameter, which initially are dome shaped. However, after extended incubation the centres of the colonies collapse due to cellular autolysis, resulting in a flattened draughtsman or

Principles and Practice of Clinical Bacteriology. Edited by A.M. Emmerson, P.M. Hawkey and S.H. Gillespie
© 1997 John Wiley & Sons Ltd

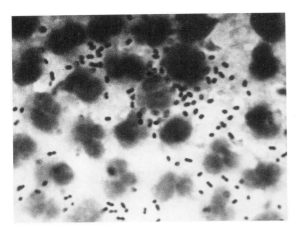

Figure 1c.1. Gram stain of *S. pneumoniae* in CSF.

doughnut-like appearance. Colonies incubated aerobically are surrounded by a greenish hue (α-haemolysis), for which the oxygen-labile haemolytic toxin pneumolysin is not responsible. Pneumolysin is, however, responsible for the β-haemolysis observed when incubation is carried out anaerobically.

Physiological Characteristics

Streptococcus pneumoniae is a facultative anaerobe, which lacks cytochromes and utilizes oxygen via a flavoenzyme system yielding H_2O_2. It is catalase negative and so the presence of an exogenous source of catalase (e.g. erythrocytes) is essential for the survival of the organism *in vitro*. Glucose metabolism is fermentative, via the hexose monophosphate pathway, resulting in the generation of lactic acid. Most pneumococci will grow well in air, but a small percentage require the presence of 5–10% carbon dioxide. Optimal growth occurs at 37 °C at pH 7.0–7.8.

Structure of the Pneumococcal Cell Surface

Peptidoglycan and teichoic acid

Like other Gram-positive bacteria, the pneumococcal cell wall is composed of peptidoglycan and teichoic acid and is approximately 15–25 nm thick (Sorensen *et al.*, 1988). The peptidoglycan is made up of chains of alternating *N*-acetylglucosamine and *N*-acetylmuramic acid residues, with peptide side chains covalently attached to the latter forming cross-links between adjacent glycan chains (Tomasz, 1981). The phosphorylcholine-containing teichoic acid (also referred to as C-polysaccharide) is also covalently attached to the *N*-acetylmuramic acid residues (Tomasz, 1981), and is uniformly distributed on both the inner and outer surfaces of the cell wall (Sorensen *et al.*, 1988) The presence of phosphorylcholine in the cell wall teichoic acid is responsible for two important features. The first of these is the interaction of pneumococci with C-reactive protein (an important human acute-phase serum protein). The second is susceptibility to digestion with the pneumococcal autolysin, an *N*-acetylmuramic acid-L-alanine amidase, located in the cell wall (Tomasz, 1981). In actively growing cells, this enzyme is relatively inactive, possibly a consequence of interaction with the Forssman antigen, located immediately beneath the cell wall. Forssman antigen is a lipoteichoic acid, i.e. C-polysaccharide covalently linked to a lipid moiety, which anchors it firmly to the outer surface of the plasma membrane (Tomasz, 1981). Cessation of growth due to nutrient starvation or treatment with antibiotics such as penicillin, or treatment with detergents such as deoxycholate, somehow disrupts the interaction between the Forssman antigen and autolysin, enabling the enzyme to cleave the amide bond between the peptide cross-links and the glycan chains of peptidoglycan, thereby inducing cellular autolysis (Tomasz, 1981). Detergent-induced autolysis accounts for the characteristic 'bile solubility' of pneumococci.

Capsule

The most important pneumococcal surface structure is the polysaccharide capsule. It is produced by all fresh clinical isolates, is approximately 200–400 nm thick (Sorensen *et al.*, 1988), and is covalently attached to the outer surface of the cell wall. The presence of a capsule was noted by

Pasteur in his original description of the organism, and by 1910 Neufeld had demonstrated the presence of a diversity of capsular serotypes. This made sense of earlier observations of the protective effects of convalescent serum against challenge with a homologous pneumococcal strain, but not necessarily against challenge with a heterologous strain (Austrian, 1981a). The capsular material was first isolated in 1917 by Dochez and Avery, but it was not until 1925 that it was demonstrated that it was composed entirely of polysaccharide (Austrian, 1981a).

To date 84 structurally and serologically distinct polysaccharide types have been recognized. The simplest types are linear polymers with repeat units of one or more monosaccharides. The more complicated structural types are multi-chained polysaccharides with repeat units composed of two to five monosaccharides with additional side chains (Lee *et al.*, 1991). Two nomenclature systems for capsular serotypes have been developed, but the Danish system, which combines antigenically cross-reacting types into groups, is now preferred to the American system, which lists serotypes in chronological order of identification.

Several pneumococcal surface proteins have also been described (Tomasz, 1981) At least some of these protrude through the peptidoglycan–teichoic acid layer of the cell wall and are exposed on the surface of 'rough' pneumococci which have lost the ability to produce a capsule (Sorensen *et al.*, 1988). However, the extent to which they are exposed on the surface of encapsulated strains is not known, and may vary from strain to strain depending on capsule thickness and stage of growth.

NORMAL HABITAT

Pneumococci are frequently isolated from the nasopharynx of healthy people, forming a natural reservoir for infection. Virtually all humans are colonized by pneumococci at some stage, and in certain populations nasopharyngeal carriage rates at any given time may exceed 70% (Riley and Douglas, 1981). Rates of pneumococcal carriage are higher in young children and where people are living in crowded conditions, and the carriage rate in a community is related to the incidence of pneumococcal disease (Riley and Douglas, 1981). There are two possible consequences of nasopharyngeal colonization by *S. pneumoniae*. In a proportion of cases, the pneumococcus is able to invade tissues and cause disease. Alternatively, carriage may result in an immune response capable of eliminating the pneumococcus. This immunity is serotype specific, but may not necessarily prevent recolonization by the same serotype at a later point in time. Duration of carriage is generally longer in children than in adults, because the former have poorer immune responses to pneumococcal polysaccharides. Progression from carriage to invasive disease is more likely in persons who have only recently become colonized. Moreover, pneumococci clearly vary in their invasive capacity. Studies carried out in Papua New Guinea showed that certain serotypes (e.g. 1, 7 and 46) were only occasionally isolated from healthy adult carriers, but were frequent causes of disease, implying a very short lag period between initial colonization and invasion. Conversely, serotypes such as 6, 15, 16 and 17 were frequently carried, but seldom caused disease (Riley and Douglas, 1981). In children, however, pneumococci belonging to serotypes/groups such as 6, 14, 19 and 23, which are frequent causes of paediatric disease in both developed and developing countries, are also the most commonly carried types (Riley and Douglas, 1981; Douglas *et al.*, 1986). Extended carriage is probably a consequence of the poor immunogenicity of these particular polysaccharides in children.

PATHOGENICITY

Polysaccharide Capsule

For many years the polysaccharide capsule has been considered to be the *sine qua non* of pneumococcal virulence. This was based on the observation that all fresh clinical isolates of *S. pneumoniae* were encapsulated and spontaneous non-encapsulated (rough) derivatives of such strains were almost completely avirulent. More-over, Avery and Dubos (1931) demonstrated that enzymic depolymerization of the capsule of a type 3 pneumococcus increased its LD_{50} approximately 10^6-fold. More recently, a similar effect on virulence of type 3 *S. pneumoniae* was achieved by transposon mutagenesis of a gene essential for capsule production (Watson and Musher, 1990). The precise manner in which the pneumococcal capsule contributes to virulence is not fully understood, although it is known to have strong anti-phagocytic properties in non-immune hosts. The majority of capsular polysaccharide serotypes are highly charged at physiological pH and this may directly interfere with cell–cell interactions with phagocytes (Lee *et al.*, 1991). Pneumococcal cell wall teichoic acid is capable of activating the alternative complement pathway. In addition, antibody to cell wall constituents, which is found in most adults, results in activation of the classical complement pathway, as does interaction of the pneumococcal C-polysaccharide with C-reactive protein. However, the capsule forms an inert shield, which appears to prevent interaction of either the Fc region of IgG or iC3b fixed to the bacterial surface from interacting with receptors on phagocytic cells (Winkelstein, 1981; Musher, 1992). Clearly, some polysaccharide serotypes are more effective inhibitors of phagocytosis than others, as certain types are far more commonly associated with human disease. Moreover, within a given serotype, virulence appears to be related to the amount of capsular polysaccharide produced. In the immune host, however, binding of specific antibody to the capsule results in opsonization and rapid clearance of the invading pneumococci (Austrian, 1981b; Lee *et al.*, 1991).

Notwithstanding the importance of the capsule in evading host defences, the various poly-saccharides are completely nontoxic and cannot themselves account for death from pneumococcal infection.

Cell Wall Degradation Products

Both the peptidoglycan and teichoic acid components of the pneumococcal cell wall are potent mediators of host inflammatory responses and as such may play an important role in the patho-genesis of pneumococcal disease (Johnston, 1991; Bruyn *et al.*, 1992). In pneumococcal meningitis, the cell wall components induce a rapid influx of inflammatory cells into the cerebrospinal fluid (CSF), as well as activation of the alternative complement pathway, and production of proinflammatory cyto-kines such as interleukin 1 and tumour necrosis factor α, as well as arachidonic acid metabolites. These in turn may result in altered cerebral blood flow, cerebral oedema and increased intracranial pressure (Tuomanen *et al.*, 1985; Bruyn *et al.*, 1992). Recent studies using a chinchilla model of pneumococcal otitis media have also clearly demonstrated the major contribution of cell wall components to middle ear inflammation (Carlsen *et al.*, 1992).

The major pneumococcal autolysin is largely responsible for solubilization and release of peptidoglycan and teichoic acid fragments from the cell wall. Thus, treatment with antibiotics such as penicillin or other β-lactams, which mediate lysis of pneumococci by activation of autolysin, might further contribute to inflammatory tissue injury and possibly mortal-ity, despite effective sterilization of the site of infection (Tuomanen *et al.*, 1987; Kawana *et al.*, 1992). Studies in both animals and humans have shown that this problem can be attenuated by adjunctive therapy with anti-inflammatory agents (Tuomanen *et al.*, 1987; Kennedy *et al.*, 1991).

Protein Virulence Factors

The involvement of toxins in pneumococcal pathogenesis has long been suspected from the clinical features of disease, in particular the rapid onset of symptoms, the profound toxicity and the fact that death may occur days after the implemen-tation of apparently effective antimicrobial therapy. However, convincing evidence supporting such a role for pneumococcal protein virulence factors has only recently become available, and this has recently been reviewed (Boulnois, 1992; Paton *et al.*, 1993).

Pneumolysin

All pneumococci produce pneumolysin, which is a member of the 'thiol-activated cytolysin' family of toxins. Pneumolysin has a variety of detrimental effects on human cells and tissues *in vitro*, including inhibition of migration and bactericidal activity of polymorphonuclear leucocytes and macrophages, inhibition of proliferative responses and production of lymphokines and immunoglobulins by lymphocytes, and activation of the classical complement pathway in the absence of specific antibody, with concomitant reduction in serum opsonic activity. Pneumolysin has also been shown to slow ciliary beating and disrupt the surface integrity of human respiratory epithelium in organ culture. Thus, the toxin has the capacity directly to interfere with the clearance of invading pneumococci as well as the establishment of a humoral immune response to the infection (Paton *et al.*, 1993). Direct cytotoxicity of pneumolysin for pulmonary epithelial and endothelial cells has also been demonstrated, a property which might contribute to entry of alveolar pneumococci into the blood (Rubins *et al.*, 1992). Injection of purified pneumolysin into the apical lobe bronchus of rat lung *in vivo* also induces all the salient histological features of pneumococcal pneumonia (Feldman *et al.*, 1991). Moreover, immunization of mice with pneumolysin confers a significant degree of protection against challenge with virulent *S. pneumoniae* (Paton *et al.*, 1983).

Derivatives of *S. pneumoniae* in which the pneumolysin gene has been insertionally inactivated are significantly less virulent than the otherwise isogenic wild type. Full virulence can be reconstituted by back-transformation of the pneumolysin-negative pneumococcus with a cloned DNA fragment carrying an intact copy of the pneumolysin gene (Berry *et al.*, 1989a, 1992). Thus, pneumolysin is directly involved in the pathogenesis of pneumococcal infections, but the finding that inactivation of the pneumolysin gene did not completely abolish the capacity of pneumococci to kill their host indicates that other pneumococcal products are also involved. Comparison of the amino acid sequence of pneumolysin and other thiol-activated toxins has identified a conserved 11 amino acid sequence (including a unique cysteine residue) towards the carboxyl terminal. Site-directed mutagenesis of this region resulted in pneumolysin derivatives with markedly reduced cytotoxic activities (Boulnois *et al.*, 1991). The capacity of pneumolysin to activate complement was found to reside in its ability to bind the Fc region of immunoglobulins, and mutations in a region of the pneumolysin coding sequence which has a degree of amino acid sequence homology with human C-reactive protein significantly reduced these properties (Mitchell *et al.*, 1991).

Autolysin

In addition to inflammatory cell wall degradation products referred to above, the pneumococcal autolysin may also be responsible for release of protein toxins from the pneumococcus. Pneumolysin is not actively secreted by *S. pneumoniae* and is located in the cytoplasm, and other potentially deleterious pneumococcal products, such as neuraminidase, may also be strongly cell associated. Thus, autolysin-induced lysis of a proportion of the invading pneumococci could directly harm the host by releasing high local concentrations of potent toxins and hydrolytic enzymes, in addition to inflammatory cell wall degradation products.

The direct contribution of autolysin to pneumococcal virulence has been studied by using the cloned gene to construct defined autolysin-negative encapsulated pneumococci. These mutants did not spontaneously autolyse and did not release pneumolysin or neuraminidase into the culture medium. Moreover, they were significantly less virulent than their otherwise isogenic parental types (Berry *et al.*, 1989b, 1992). Immunization of mice with purified autolysin provides a similar degree of protection against challenge with virulent pneumococci to that achieved by immunization with pneumolysin (Berry *et al.*, 1989b; Paton *et al.*, 1993). However, the relative contribution to pathogenesis of autolysin-mediated release of pneumolysin versus cell wall degradation products is yet to be determined.

Pneumococcal surface protein A

Pneumococcal surface protein A (PspA) is a surface protein produced by all pneumococci, which is highly variable, both immunologically and in molecular size (Crain et al., 1990). Passive immunization with anti-PspA monoclonal antibodies or active immunization with purified antigen protects mice from challenge with virulent pneumococci producing similar types of PspA (McDaniel et al., 1984; Talkington et al., 1991), and pneumococci in which the PspA gene has been insertionally inactivated are significantly less virulent than the respective wild-type strain (McDaniel et al., 1987). The precise function of PspA in virulence, however, is not understood.

Pneumococcal adhesins

The ability of bacteria to adhere to epithelial cells is considered to be an important requirement for colonization, but various studies have produced conflicting data on the capacity of pneumococci to do this (Paton et al., 1993). It has been postulated that host glycolipids containing either GlcNAcβ1-3Gal or GalNAcβ1-4Gal are the targets for pneumococcal adhesion, but the pneumococcal factor mediating this remains largely uncharacterized. It has also been reported recently that pneumococci are capable of binding laminin and type IV collagen. These proteins are components of basement membranes, which might become exposed when respiratory epithelial cells are damaged by virus infection (a known predisposing factor for pneumococcal pneumonia). In this context it is also interesting that S. pneumoniae is known to produce a serine protease capable of degrading these extracellular matrix proteins (Paton et al., 1993).

Other proteins

Pneumococci also produce several other proteins which might function in pathogenesis, particularly neuraminidase, hyaluronidase and IgA1 protease. These three enzymes appear to be produced by the majority of clinical S. pneumoniae isolates.

Neuraminidase has the potential to cause great damage by cleaving terminal sialic acid residues from a wide variety of glycolipids, glycoproteins and oligosaccharides on host cell surfaces or in body fluids, and might also unmask potential cell surface receptors for putative pneumococcal adhesins (Paton et al., 1993). Immunization with purified pneumococcal neuraminidase partially protects mice from challenge with virulent S. pneumoniae. This protection, however, was not as great as that achieved by immunization with pneumolysin, and no additive protective effect could be seen when mice were immunized with both proteins (Lock et al., 1988).

Direct evidence for the involvement of hyaluronidase in pneumococcal pathogenesis is not available, but it could function by allowing greater microbial access to host tissue for colonization. It may also play a role in the migration of the organism between tissues, for example translocation from the lung to the vascular system (Paton et al., 1993).

The pneumococcal IgA1 protease cleaves human IgA1 at a specific point within the hinge region, yielding intact Fab and Fc fragments. Investigation of its involvement in pathogenesis has been frustrated, because the enzyme is highly specific and does not cleave IgA from any animal species commonly used as models for disease. However, the Fab fragments generated by IgA1 proteases retain their specificity for antigen and it has been proposed that such fragments bound to the surface of a bacterium could protect it from the immune system by blocking access to intact immunoglobulins. Also, any mechanism of IgA–immune complex elimination that depends on the Fc fragment would be abolished (Kilian and Reinholdt, 1987).

EPIDEMIOLOGY

High-risk Groups

The rate of nasopharyngeal carriage of S. pneumoniae and the incidence of pneumococcal infection is greatest in young children and the elderly. Inability to mount an effective immune response to the most prevalent capsular polysaccharide serotypes is largely responsible for the increased susceptibility of children, and waning naturally acquired anticapsular antibody levels may also contribute to susceptibility in older individuals. The incidence of pneumococcal disease in healthy young adults is generally low, except in groups such as military recruits or South African mine workers, where individuals are living in crowded, communal accommodation. High rates of both carriage and disease have been reported in such groups, with recent (presumably immunologically naive) arrivals being the most susceptible.

Natural resistance to pneumococcal infection is dependent on intact specific and non-specific host defences. Thus, persons with humoral defects such as hypogammaglobulinaemia and complement deficiencies are at increased risk of serious pneumococcal infection, as are those with AIDS. The spleen and liver are principally responsible for phagocytic clearance of pneumococci and so persons with functional or anatomical hyposplenia (including those with sickle cell anaemia or thalassaemia) are at high risk of overwhelming pneumococcal bacteraemia. Other predisposing factors include perturbation of physical defences (e.g. skull fractures or dural tears in pneumococcal meningitis, and damage to the respiratory epthelium as a consequence of viral infection (particularly influenza in pneumococcal pneumonia), alcoholism, diabetes mellitus, chronic obstructive lung disease and renal failure (Johnston, 1991). Reduced pressure in the middle ear cavity, caused by blockage of the Eustachian tubes (e.g. during viral upper respiratory tract infection) is also a predisposing factor in pneumococcal otitis media.

Serotype Prevalence

The 84 known serotypes of *S. pneumoniae* vary in their capacity to cause disease in humans, and serotypes are therefore not uniformly distributed. Serotype prevalence varies with site of infection, age, time and geographical location (Nielsen and Henrichsen, 1992), which complicates comparison of data from various studies.

Amongst children in Western Europe and North America, 6A + 6B, 7F, 14, 18C, 19F and 23F (not in rank order) are generally the most prevalent serotypes, collectively accounting for about 70% of isolates from blood or CSF (Klein, 1981; Nielsen and Henrichsen, 1992). These same types, with the inclusion of type 3, are also the commonest causes of otitis media. Data for developing countries are scanty, but types 1 and 5 also appear to be important causes of invasive pneumococcal disease in children in these regions (Dagan *et al.*, 1992).

For adults, the position is more complicated. In the first half of this century, types 1, 2 and 3 were most frequently responsible for invasive disease in the USA and Europe, but today type 2 infection is very rare and the most prevalent types are 1, 3, 4, 6A + 6B, 7F, 8 and 14, collectively accounting for about 50% of isolates from blood and CSF (Austrian, 1981b; Nielsen and Henrichsen, 1992). However, type 2 remains an important cause of disease in Africa. The geographical variation in type prevalence is also exemplified by types 5 and 46, which are uncommon in North America, but frequently cause disease in Africa and New Guinea (Austrian, 1981b; Riley and Douglas, 1981).

CLINICAL FEATURES

Pneumonia

Streptococcus pneumoniae is the leading cause of community-acquired pneumonia throughout the world. It most likely develops after inhalation of pneumococci colonizing the nasopharynx. Pneumococci that are not cleared multiply rapidly within the alveolar space, and outpouring of fibrinous fluid into the alveoli aids spread into surrounding regions until the lung segment is completely involved. Thus, most cases present with segmental or lobar consolidation. Estimation of the actual incidence of pneumococcal pneumonia is complicated by the difficulty in unequivocal determination of the aetiological agent in non-bacteraemic cases and attack rates vary greatly in different geographical and socioeconomic settings

(Austrian, 1981b). In North America the overall attack rate has been estimated to range from 68 to 260 cases per 100 000 population per year (Immunization Practices Advisory Committee, 1981). The majority of these cases occur in persons over 55 years of age or with underlying chronic illnesses and for non-bacteraemic cases the fatality rate is about 5% (Immunization Practices Advisory Committee, 1981). In developing countries, the incidence is greatest in children under five years of age and annual attack rates may be as high as 1000 per 100 000. It has been estimated that as many as three million children die from pneumococcal pneumonia each year in developing countries.

Bacteraemic Pneumonia

Approximately 15–30% of cases of pneumococcal pneumonia are bacteraemic, which is a poor prognostic sign. Pneumococci are thought to enter the blood via the lymphatic vessels in the lungs, the hilar lymph nodes and the thoracic duct. The case fatality rate for bacteraemic pneumonia depends on the age of the patient (mortality rates in those over 70 years are more than double those in under 40s), pneumococcal serotype and the presence or absence of underlying disease. The overall case fatality rate in the USA is approximately 20% (Immunization Practices Advisory Committee, 1981), but may be as high as 60% in high-risk groups, even with appropriate antimicrobial therapy.

Meningitis

Except during epidemics of meningococcal disease, *S. pneumoniae* is also the principal cause of bacterial meningitis in adults (Musher, 1992). It is currently the second most common cause of meningitis in children, behind *Haemophilus influenzae* type b (Hib). However, effective Hib conjugate vaccines have been licensed for use in infants and young children, and the widespread utilization of these has resulted in the pneumococcus assuming primacy as a cause of meningitis in this age group as well. Pneumococcal meningitis may arise as a complication of bacteraemic

pneumonia, or untreated otitis media, sinusitis or mastoiditis. Except in cases where trauma, such as skull fracture, disrupts the dura mater and permits direct entry of nasopharyngeal pneumococci into the subarachnoid space, the pathway by which they gain access to the meninges is not understood. Haematogenous spread is likely, but it has only occasionally been demonstrated in animal models. Another possibility suggested by early animal studies in which pneumococci appeared in the subarachnoid space shortly after intranasal challenge, is that pneumococci can enter via perineural spaces surrounding olfactory neurons (Moxon, 1981).

The annual attack rate for pneumococcal meningitis in the USA has been estimated at 1.2–2.8 per 100 000, with an estimated case fatality rate of 30% (Immunization Practices Advisory Committee, 1981), although mortality may be significantly higher than this in infants and the elderly. Morbidity in survivors is high.

Primary Bacteraemia

A major proportion of cases of pneumococcal bacteraemia are associated with pneumonia or meningitis, as discussed above. Primary pneumococcal bacteraemia, on the other hand, may result from invasion from the nasopharynx, via the cervical lymphatics (Austrian, 1981b). It most commonly occurs in children aged 6–24 months (Bratton *et al.*, 1977), although it has been reported in adult South African gold-miners (Austrian, 1981b). It is characterized by fever, and patients may complain of headache and malaise, but there is no other apparent focus of infection. Most patients are only moderately ill, and frequently have recovered (often without antimicrobial therapy) by the time the positive blood culture results become available. However, in some cases, pneumococcal meningitis or pneumonia may subsequently develop (Bratton *et al.*, 1977; Austrian, 1981b).

Otitis Media and Acute Sinusitis

Streptococcus pneumoniae is the single commonest cause of otitis media in children. Although not life threatening in the postantibiotic era, it is a disease of high prevalence throughout the world. Nearly all children suffer at least one attack, and in many cases recurrent attacks, during the first five years of life. Overall morbidity is thus high, and hearing impairment in children suffering recurrent attacks may interfere with learning processes. The portal of entry of pneumococci into the middle ear cavity is the Eustachian tube. Congestion, resulting in reduced middle ear pressure, such as may occur during viral upper respiratory infection, increases susceptibility to otitis media.

Acute sinusitis is another less serious, but nevertheless prevalent infection caused by *S. pneumoniae*. Unlike otitis media, it is more common in adults than in children.

Other Pneumococcal Infections

Pneumococcal mastoiditis is now rare, but in the preantibiotic era was a sequel to otitis media. Untreated mastoiditis may lead to development of meningitis or brain abscess. Similarly, pneumococcal empyema and pericarditis are also much rarer than in the past, and usually occur as complications of pneumonia. Endocarditis is also a possible complication of pneumonia or meningitis. Pneumococcal peritonitis and arthritis are very uncommon and probably develop after transient bacteraemia.

LABORATORY DIAGNOSIS

Culture of *S. pneumoniae*

Culture of *S. pneumoniae* from appropriate clinical specimens is clearly the cardinal diagnostic procedure. Pneumococci are delicate and therefore cultures should be inoculated as soon after collection as possible, and when delay is unavoidable specimens should be refrigerated. Swabs should be placed in an appropriate transport medium. Specimens such as CSF, middle ear or lung aspirates, swabs, or sputum should be cultured on a nutritious blood agar medium (e.g. Columbia agar base + 5% defibrinated horse or sheep blood),

or blood agar + 5 μg/ml gentamicin (to inhibit viridans streptococci) and incubated at 37 °C in 5–10% carbon dioxide. Sputum samples should be rinsed with sterile saline (to reduce contamination with saliva) before culturing and subsequent growth interpreted in accordance with Gram stain findings, as discussed below. Moreover, the presence of significant numbers of viridans streptococci on blood plates without gentamicin may indicate that the sputum sample was contaminated with saliva and therefore not truly representative of lower respiratory secretions. The diagnostic value of sputum culture is entirely dependent on specimen quality; satisfactory samples are not always available, and are very difficult to obtain from children. In such circumstances, although invasive, percutaneous transtracheal aspiration could be considered, particularly in cases of serious disease, where the need to establish an unequivocal diagnosis is greatest. Blood cultures and other liquid specimens requiring enrichment in addition to direct plating, such as CSF, should be inoculated into an appropriate rich medium, such as brain heart infusion, or a suitable commercial blood culture medium.

Presumptive identification of typical colonies as *S. pneumoniae* has traditionally been achieved by subculturing on fresh blood agar and testing for inhibition of growth around a 5 μg optochin disk after further overnight incubation, or by testing for bile solubility. However, optochin-resistant pneumococci have been reported (albeit as a subpopulation of sensitive colonies) and so there is the potential for misidentification of these strains as viridans streptococci (Klugman, 1990). Moreover, optochin zone size is smaller when plates are incubated in 5–10% carbon dioxide rather than in air, and in these circumstances a zone diameter >13 mm is presumptively diagnostic (Klugman, 1990). Faster identification can be achieved by testing colonies on primary culture plates or aliquots of broth cultures by coagglutination or latex agglutination (see below), but these techniques are significantly more expensive. Rapid identification can also be achieved by Quellung reaction using omnivalent antiserum (see below).

Microscopy

Examination of smears for the presence of Gram-positive lancet-shaped cocci (usually as diplococci or short chains) is particularly valuable in the diagnosis of pneumococcal disease.

CSF

In meningitis, CSF may contain up to 10^9 pneumococci per millilitre; in untreated cases 75–90% of culture-positive specimens are Gram stain-positive, although sensitivity diminishes in pretreated cases (Gray and Fedorko, 1992). Acridine orange is also useful for staining CSF smears if a fluorescence microscope is available. Bacteria appear bright red and are easily visible against a black background, with leucocytes staining pale green. The sensitivity limit has been reported to be of the order of 10^4 cfu/ml, whereas for Gram stain the limit is about 10 times this number (Gray and Fedorko, 1992). A Gram stain should be performed on any specimens which are positive.

Sputum

Gram stain is also important for examination of sputum smears from patients with suspected pneumococcal pneumonia. Positive sputum samples should contain Gram-positive cocci and large numbers of polymorphonuclear leucocytes. The presence of epithelial cells is a clear indication of contamination with saliva and such specimens are of little diagnostic value (Musher, 1992).

Capsule swelling reaction (Quellung)

Where Gram stain suggests the presence of pneumococci, rapid confirmation of the identity of the organism can be achieved using the Quellung (capsular swelling) reaction. This involves mixing a drop of CSF (or a drop of broth culture, an aliquot of sputum, or a colony emulsified in saline, as appropriate) with a loopful of omnivalent antiserum (a mixture of antibodies directed against all 84 pneumococcal capsular serotypes, which can be obtained from Statens Seruminstitut,

Copenhagen). Antibody becomes deposited on the outer surface of the pneumococcal capsule within a couple of minutes, and this results in a change in its refractive index; cells appear swollen and are clearly visible under bright field or phase-contrast microscopy. The Quellung reaction can also be used to serotype pneumococci, using a panel of pooled and monospecific antisera. In the preantibiotic era, serotyping was an essential prerequisite for administration of appropriate (monovalent) serum therapy, but these days is usually only carried out in reference laboratories. Nevertheless, it is a simple, rapid and cheap method of confirming pneumococcal aetiology, where organisms are present in sufficient numbers to be visible under the microscope.

Antigen Detection

Direct detection of pneumococcal antigen in clinical samples is based on the fact that soluble capsular polysaccharide is frequently released into body fluids (e.g. serum and CSF) during pneumococcal infection, and also is excreted in the urine. Such methods may be useful in establishing a diagnosis in cases where antimicrobial therapy was commenced before collection of specimens (Kalin and Lindberg, 1983).

Counter-immunoelectrophoresis

Counter-immunoelectrophoresis (CIE) was the first rapid antigen detection technique to be used extensively in clinical laboratories. Patient samples are placed in wells cut in an agarose gel and the negatively charged polysaccharide antigen is electrophoretically accelerated towards wells containing specific antibody. The procedure is highly specific and takes a little over 30 minutes to perform. CIE for rapid detection purposes employs omnivalent antiserum, although monospecific antisera can also be used to determine the serotype of the infecting pneumococcus, where desired. However, the polysaccharides produced by *S. pneumoniae* types 7 and 14, which are important causes of human disease, are not negatively charged, and therefore cannot be detected by CIE without chemical modification.

Latex and co-agglutination

CIE has now been largely replaced by latex particle agglutination (LA) or coagglutination (CA). These techniques employ omnivalent antibody adsorbed onto the surface of polystyrene latex beads, or *Staphylococcus aureus* cells (Cowan's strain), respectively, and high-quality reagents are available commercially. In the presence of specific antigen, visible agglutination occurs. The techniques take less than 15 minutes to perform, and unlike CIE do not require specialized equipment. LA appears to be slightly more sensitive than CA, and both are more sensitive than CIE (Ballard *et al.*, 1987; Gray and Fedorko, 1992). Moreover, neither are affected by charge and so can detect polysaccharide types 7 and 14. Both techniques are susceptible, however, to non-specific agglutinations with interfering substances which may be present in CSF, serum or urine, and so specimens must always be tested in parallel with control particle suspensions. Non-specific reactions can be minimized by appropriate pretreatment of specimens, for example by brief heating.

LA is very effective when used to test CSF in the diagnosis of meningitis, and most studies have shown 90–100% sensitivity with respect to culture. However, it is less sensitive when urine is tested, even when samples are concentrated up to $25 \times$ by ultrafiltration before testing, and <50% of meningitis patients have levels of antigen in urine detectable by LA (Ballard *et al.*, 1987; Gray and Fedorko, 1992). LA is clearly less reliable for the diagnosis of pneumococcal pneumonia, and estimates of sensitivity and specificity vary markedly from study to study. In bacteraemic pneumonia, 24–38% of serum specimens were LA positive, but the positivity rate for urine ranged from 0 to 88% (Cerosaletti *et al.*, 1985; Agello *et al.*, 1987). In non-bacteraemic cases, <8% of sera and 0–38% of urines are LA positive (Cerosaletti *et al.*, 1985; Boersma and Holloway, 1992). O'Niell *et al.* (1989) have reported that the sensitivity of LA for the diagnosis of pneumococcal pneumonia can be improved significantly by the use of panels of latex reagents coated with monospecific antisera. In this study, concentrated urine specimens from 16/21 Gambian children with culture-proven pneumococcal pneumonia were LA positive for the respective serotype, whereas none of the specimens had tested positive using a commercial omnivalent LA reagent.

Antigen detection has also been used in other specimens such as pleural fluid, peritoneal fluid or sputum. In the latter case, samples need to be washed carefully to remove contaminating oropharyngeal flora and also digested with sputolysin before testing. Moreover, a Gram-stained smear should be examined to ensure specimen quality.

C-polysaccharide antigen detection

The cell wall teichoic acid (C-polysaccharide), which is common to all pneumococci, has also been used as a target for antigen detection assays. Yolken *et al.* (1984) described an enzyme immunoassay utilizing immobilized anti-C-polysaccharide and biotinylated antibodies to capsular (type-specific) polysaccharides for the direct detection of pneumococcal antigens in CSF. A quantitative enzyme-linked immunosorbent assay (ELISA) to detect C-polysaccharide in sputum has been described (Gillespie *et al.*, 1994a). However, reliable commercial reagents for detection of C-polysaccharide in body fluids are not currently available.

Molecular Biological Methods

Recently a test system (Accuprobe) based on hybridization of rRNA sequences with a chemiluminescent acridinium ester-labelled DNA probe has become available for rapid identification of *S. pneumoniae* from plate or broth cultures. The test is rapid and highly specific, but again is expensive. Moreover, it is only suitable for culture confirmation and is not sensitive enough for direct detection purposes (Denys and Carey, 1992).

Amplification of specific nucleic acid sequences using the polymerase chain reaction (PCR) has the potential to provide fast and sensitive direct detection of pneumococci in clinical samples, particularly in those such as blood or CSF, which are usually sterile. Interpretation of results obtained using specimens such as sputum, which might be contaminated with oropharyngeal flora, is more complicated, and requires microscopic assessment of specimen quality. The sensitivity of PCR is likely to be greater than alternative rapid methods, as the theoretical detection limit is one copy of the target DNA sequence. Moreover, sensitivity is unlikely to be affected by pretreatment with antibiotics. However, maximum sensitivity is usually only achieved using at least 35–40 amplification cycles, as well as a secondary hybridization step to detect specific PCR product, and this would delay the result often until the next day. Thus, protocols may need to be based on a compromise between speed and maximum sensitivity. PCR is also significantly more labour intensive than alternative rapid methods, although reagent costs are similar. The pneumococcal genes encoding pneumolysin and autolysin have both been used as targets for PCR amplification (Rudolph *et al.*, 1993) with positive results obtained for all 20 serotypes tested. The partial sequence homology between the pneumolysin gene and those encoding related thiol-activated cytolysins produced by other bacteria did not cause problems with specificity. Buffy coat extracts from 6/8 blood samples from culture-proven pneumococcal pneumonia patients and 3/5 culture-negative, CIE-positive blood samples yielded positive PCR results (Rudolph *et al.*, 1993). The autolysin gene has also been successfully used as a PCR amplification target in sputum samples from pneumonia patients and showed 100% specificity and 95% sensitivity (Gillespie *et al.*, 1994b). Comprehensive data on the relative diagnostic efficacy of PCR compared with other direct detection techniques is not yet available.

Serological Diagnosis

Serological techniques based on measurement of immune responses to specific pneumococcal antigens have been of limited clinical value, largely because of the need to test acute and convalescent sera, with concomitant delay in diagnosis. Such techniques are, however, of great epidemiological value, particularly in confirming the aetiology of pneumonia, given the small proportion of such cases which yield positive blood cultures. Such information is important in efficacy trials of candidate pneumococcal vaccines. Radioimmunoassay or ELISAs for measurement of antibodies to capsular polysaccharide, C-polysaccharide and pneumolysin have been developed. However, assessment of anticapsular responses are impractical because of the large number of serotypes, and insensitive because of the poor antibody response to these antigens in children. The problem of multiple serotypes is avoided by testing for C-polysaccharide or pneumolysin antibodies. The former is also poorly immunogenic in children, but an anti-C-polysaccharide ELISA may be of value in establishing a diagnosis of pneumococcal pneumonia in adults (Burman *et al.*, 1991). Measurement of IgG antibodies to pneumolysin by ELISA also appears to be capable of establishing pneumococcal aetiology in cases of adult pneumonia (Jalonen *et al.*, 1989).

ANTIBIOTIC SUSCEPTIBILITY

Disk Diffusion

Laboratory determination of antibiotic susceptibility patterns of pneumococci is generally carried out by disk diffusion, using Mueller–Hinton blood agar, as recommended by the National Committee for Clinical Laboratory Standards (NCCLS, 1990a). Susceptibility using penicillin disks has not been a reliable indicator of penicillin resistance in pneumococci, and the current recommended method uses a 1 μg oxacillin disk at a zone size cut-off of 20 mm (Klugman, 1990; NCCLS, 1990a). This methodology, however, is not capable of distinguishing penicillin-resistant from intermediately resistant strains and so minimal inhibitory concentration (MIC) determination should be carried out on any strains with zone diameters below the cut-off (Jacobs, 1992). The relationship between recommended MIC breakpoints and disk diffusion cut-offs is shown in Table 1c.1.

Agar Dilution

Agar dilution, carried out in accordance with NCCLS recommendations (NCCLS, 1990b), is

TABLE 1c.1 MIC AND DISK DIFFUSION BREAKPOINTS FOR SUSCEPTIBILITY TESTING OF PNEUMOCOCCI[a]

Drug	Susceptible		Intermediate		Resistant	
	MIC (μg/ml)	Disk (mm)	MIC	Disk	MIC (μgml)	Disk (mm)
Penicillin G	≤0.06	≥21[b]	0.12–1 μg/ml	≤20 mm[b]	>1	≤20[b]
Chloramphenicol	≤4	≥22	NA[c]	NA	≥8	≤21
Erythromycin	≤0.5	≥20	NA	NA	≥1	≤19
Tetracycline	≤4	≥20	NA	NA	≥8	≤19
Trimethoprim/ sulphamethoxazole	≤0.5/9.5	–[d]	NA	NA	≥1/19	–

[a] As described by Jacobs (1992).
[b] 1 μg oxacillin disk used, but this does not distinguish resistant from intermediate strains.
[c] NA denotes intermediate category is not applicable.
[d] Disk diffusion breakpoints not available.

the preferred method for MIC determination for pneumococci (Jacobs, 1992). Broth microdilution (NCCLS, 1990b) can also be employed. However, commercial microdilution systems have been reported to be inaccurate for penicillin MICs, falsely classifying a number of resistant or intermediately resistant strains as sensitive. The accuracy of commercial panels can be improved by modifying the protocol, but results should still be interpreted with caution (Jacobs, 1992). A simple MIC procedure known as the E test, which involves application of a calibrated, antibiotic-impregnated plastic strip to the surface of an inoculated plate, can also be used for determining MICs of pneumococci, although it has a tendency to slightly underestimate penicillin G MICs (Jacobs, 1992).

Prevalence and Distribution of Drug-Resistant Pneumococci

Streptococcus pneumoniae was the first organism to demonstrate the capacity to acquire resistance to antimicrobial drugs. During the early part of the twentieth century, optochin (a quinine derivative) was used in the treatment of pneumococcal infections, and acquisition of resistance during therapy in experimentally infected mice and in patients was demonstrated in 1912 and 1917, respectively (Austrian, 1981a; Klugman, 1990). Acquisition by pneumococci of resistance to the sulphonamides

sulphapyridine and sulphadiazine during therapy was documented in 1939 and 1943, respectively (Klugman, 1990). For penicillin, acquisition of resistance was demonstrated in 1943 in a mouse model, and intermediately resistant clinical isolates (MIC 0.1–1 μg/ml) were first reported in the mid-1960s. Pneumococci with high-level resistance to penicillin (MIC > 1.0 μg/ml), as well as to several other antibiotics, were first reported in 1977 (Klugman, 1990).

As might be expected, the prevalence of drug-resistant pneumococci has steadily increased over the past 20 years, although there is significant geographical variation, presumably a consequence of local antibiotic-prescribing practices. There are also significant variations in frequency amongst studies carried out within a given country, perhaps reflecting differences in the source of the isolates tested; very high rates of resistance to a number of antimicrobial drugs have been reported for pneumococcal strains isolated from hospital carriers. High rates of carriage of resistant pneumococci have also been reported in child care centres (Klugman, 1990). Prior exposure to antibiotics appears to be a predisposing factor for both carriage of, and infection with, resistant pneumococci (Klugman, 1990). Recent data (post 1980) for the frequency of resistant pneumococci amongst clinical isolates for various countries are summarized in Table 1c.2. For penicillin, erythromycin, trimethoprim–sulphamethoxazole,

TABLE 1c.2 PREVALENCE OF RESISTANT PNEUMOCOCCI CAUSING DISEASE IN VARIOUS COUNTRIES[a]

Country	Percentage resistant to:				
	Penicillin MIC ≥0.1 μg/ml	Erythromycin MIC ≥1.0 μg/ml	Trimethoprim/ Sulfamethoxazole MIC ≥1/19 μg/ml	Tetracycline MIC ≥8.0 μg/ml	Chloramphenicol MIC ≥8.0 μg/ml
N. and S. America					
United States	5.1	0.3–0.8	4.5–11.5	2.3–2.9	1.2
Canada	1.3	0.4	–	1.7	–
Chile	21.9	–	–	12.4	1.1
Brazil	18.7	6.1	29.2	44.6	7.2
Australasia					
New Zealand	1.3	0.4	6.4	3.9	–
Europe					
Hungary	58.0	48.5	39.7	66.5	25.5
Spain	14.3–52.7	2.5–7.9	37.7–67.0	49.0–72.5	33.7–47.3
France	12	26	24	20	9
England	4.0	–	–	–	0.4
N. Ireland	0.8	–	–	5.1	4.9
Italy	–	0.5	4.5	35.0	15.0
Switzerland	2.3	1.5	1.5	17.3	1.6
Poland	–	2.6	–	12.2	–
Asia					
Malaysia	2.0	0.8	–	18.4	–
Pakistan	8.9	–	32.9	83.5	36.7
Africa					
South Africa	7.0	1.9	–	2.8	0.8
Middle East					
Israel	–	1.3	8.7	–	0.9
Saudi Arabia	–	2.9	64.9	25.0	2.9

[a] Data are for clinical isolates, which were collected since 1980, collated from the data presented by Klugman (1990), except for the figures from Brazil (Sessegolo *et al.*, 1994), France (Geslin *et al.*, 1992) and Hungary (Marton, 1992). Studies involving pneumococci isolated from carriers were excluded. Where data are derived from more than one study, the range is shown; – indicates no recent data is available.

tetracycline and chloramphenicol, the proportion of resistant isolates from a given country ranged from approximately 1% to >50%. Countries with very high prevalence of resistant pneumococci included Hungary, Spain, Brazil and Pakistan. On the other hand, pneumococci isolated from patients in the USA, Canada, New Zealand, South Africa and Switzerland had much lower rates of resistance. Additional foci of high prevalence of penicillin resistance have been reported in the past from a number of other regions, including New Guinea, Israel, Alaska, Mexico, Kenya and parts of South Africa (Klugman, 1990). Recent studies have also shown that the proportion of penicillin-resistant pneumococci with high-level resistance is increasing,

and roughly half of the resistant strains from France or Hungary have an MIC > 1.0 μg/ml (Geslin *et al.*, 1992; Marton, 1992). Penicillin-resistant pneumococci are also more likely to be resistant to non-β-lactam antibiotics than penicillin-sensitive strains (Marton, 1992). For penicillin-resistant pneumococci, increases in the MIC for other β-lactam antibiotics roughly parallel that for penicillin G. Cefotaxime, ceftriaxone and imipenem have the highest *in vitro* activity of the currently available β-lactams against penicillin-resistant pneumococci (Klugman, 1990).

Multi-drug-resistant pneumococci, defined as those with resistance to at least three different classes of antibiotics, have caused considerable concern since their first isolation in Durban in 1977, from a hospitalized child who had previously received therapy with penicillin and cephalothin (Klugman, 1990). The first isolate was resistant to penicillin, tetracycline, clindamycin, chloramphenicol and trimethoprim–sulphamethoxazole (Klugman, 1990). Very high prevalence rates of multiply resistant pneumococci amongst hospital carriers were reported from both Durban and Johannesburg at the time and in subsequent studies, but they represented only 1–2% of blood or CSF isolates (Klugman, 1990). Multiply resistant strains have now been isolated from Britain, Canada, the USA, Eastern and Western Europe, Pakistan and Australia.

The vast majority of pneumococci with high-level penicillin-resistant or multiply resistant phenotypes isolated to date belong to serogroups/types 6, 14, 19 and 23. These same groups/types also dominate the intermediately penicillin-resistant phenotype, although this level of resistance has been now demonstrated in over 30 serotypes (Klugman, 1990).

Mechanisms of Resistance

Penicillin

Penicillin resistance in *S. pneumoniae* is not due to β-lactamase production, but rather to alterations in a family of chromosomally encoded penicillin-binding proteins (PBPs). Six PBPs have been identified by electrophoretic analysis in susceptible pneumococci (PBPla, PBPlb, PBP2x, PBP2a, PBP2b and PBP3), and these are believed to be enzymes catalysing the final stages of murein biosynthesis (Klugman, 1990). These enzymes are inhibited by penicillin and other β-lactams, which bind covalently to the active sites. The affinity of a particular β-lactam drug for the various PBPs is not uniform, and this specificity may be due at least in part to the R1 side chain (see Figure 1c.2) of the particular agent. Capacity to bind PBP2b may be essential for lytic activity of β-lactams. Drugs such as ceftazidime, which cannot bind PBP2b (it binds preferentially to PBP3), cannot induce lysis (Klugman, 1990).

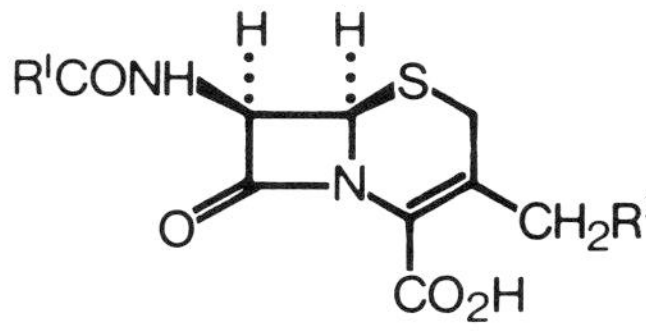

cephalosporin

Figure 1c.2. General structure of cephalosporins, showing location of R1 side chain.

The PBPs of penicillin-resistant pneumococci have reduced affinity for penicillin, and electrophoretic analysis using radiolabelled drug has identified alteration of up to five of the PBPs in such strains. DNA sequence analysis has revealed that there is very little variability in the PBP genes of susceptible pneumococci. However, many resistant strains contain highly variable 'mosaic' PBP2b genes, containing one or more blocks of nucleotides (with up to 21% sequence divergence with respect to that of sensitive pneumococci) which originated from *S. mitis*. In other examples PBP2b genes contained sequences derived from *S. mitis* as well as from at least one other (unidentified) species. Mosaic PBPla and PBP2x genes have also been detected in penicillin-resistant pneumococci. These events have presumably been mediated by direct transformation and homologous recombination, and have resulted in the generation of different families of PBP types (Dowson *et al.*, 1993).

Tolerance

The term 'penicillin tolerant' has been used to describe strains of *S. pneumoniae* which do not lyse and are more slowly killed after exposure to penicillin concentrations in excess of the MIC. Penicillin-induced lysis in susceptible strains is mediated by the pneumococcal autolysin, but the mechanism of autolysin induction is not understood. The majority of penicillin-resistant strains exhibit defective autolysis when the drug concentration exceeds the MIC, and it has been suggested that this may be due to an alteration in the autolytic regulatory mechanism (Klugman, 1990).

Other antibiotics

Tetracycline resistance in *S. pneumoniae* is encoded by the *tetM* gene. The product of this gene is a soluble 7.25 kDa protein, which shares N-terminal sequence homology with translational elongation factors. The TetM protein is thought to bind to the ribosome, thereby blocking the inhibitory action of tetracycline (Klugman, 1990). Pneumococcal erythromycin resistance is encoded by the *ermAM* gene, which also confers resistance to macrolides, lincosamide and streptogramin B. The mechanism of action of the ermAM protein is thought to involve methylation of rRNA, as there is substantial sequence homology with the staphylococcal *ermC* gene, which encodes an enzyme responsible for dimethylation of adenine in the 23S rRNA. A 3'-aminoglycoside phosphotransferase type III enzyme encoded by the *aphA-3* gene is responsible for kanamycin resistance in *S. pneumoniae*, by phosphorylating the 3'-hydroxyl group of aminohexose I of kanamycin, thereby inactivating the drug (Klugman, 1990).

Chloramphenicol-resistant pneumococci produce an inducible chloramphenicol acetyltransferase. Sulphonamide resistance in pneumococci does not appear to be caused by mutation in the gene encoding dihydropteroate synthase, as originally thought, and presumably is due to mutation in one of the other enzymes in the folate synthesis pathway. Information on the mechanism of trimethoprim resistance in pneumococci is not available (Klugman, 1990).

The genes responsible for resistance to a number of antimicrobial drugs in *S. pneumoniae* have been shown to be located on a conjugative transposon Tn*1545*. This element contains the *tetM*, *ermAM* and *aphA-3* genes, and also encodes chloramphenicol resistance. A transposon containing *tetM* has also been shown to be present in a multiply resistant pneumococcus isolated in Minnesota in 1977. Another conjugative element (BM6001) isolated from resistant *S. pneumoniae* has been shown to encode both tetracycline and chloramphenicol resistance. Plasmids encoding antimicrobial drug resistance have not been detected in *S. pneumoniae* (Klugman, 1990).

MANAGEMENT

Penicillin G remains the drug of choice for treatment of serious disease due to susceptible pneumococci. A daily intramuscular dose of 1.2 million units is adequate for treatment of pneumonia, including that caused by pneumococci with intermediate resistance to penicillin. For hospitalized patients, 500 000 units administered intravenously every 4 hours provides optimum therapy. Where oral therapy is appropriate, amoxycillin (500 mg, 8-hourly) is the drug of choice, due to superior absorption (Musher, 1992). Much higher doses (up to 20 million units of aqueous crystalline penicillin, administered intravenously) are required for treatment of meningitis and arthritis, because of poor penetration of drug to the site of infection. Third-generation cephalosporins such as ceftriaxone and cefotaxime are increasingly being used to treat meningitis. Adjunctive therapy with glucocorticoids has also been shown to be beneficial in children with pneumococcal meningitis. In patients with penicillin allergy, erythromycin or chloramphenicol can be used for treatment of pneumonia and meningitis, respectively, provided the organism is susceptible. In view of the high risk of overwhelming pneumococcal infection in patients who have been splenectomized, or have hypogammaglobulinaemia, oral penicillin V or ampicillin may be given prophylactically.

Treatment of infections due to penicillin-resistant pneumococci is problematic, and may be exacerbated by delay in recognition of the fact that the organism is resistant, and the fact that penicillin-resistant strains are frequently resistant to other antibiotics as well. High intravenous doses of penicillin G are appropriate for treatment of pneumonia due to intermediately resistant strains, but for those with MICs > 1 μg/ml ceftriaxone, cefotaxime or imipenem are more effective β-lactam agents; alternatively, vancomycin could be used. Treatment of meningitis due to penicillin-resistant pneumococci is complicated by poor penetration of many antimicrobial agents into CSF. Thus, the response to penicillin therapy has been poor even for intermediately resistant strains, although high doses (500 000 units/kg per day) have been effective in some cases (Viladrich *et al.*, 1988). Failure of chloramphenicol therapy has also been reported in meningitis caused by penicillin-resistant, chloramphenicol-susceptible pneumococci. This was attributed to lower bactericidal activity of chloramphenicol in such strains, compared with penicillin-susceptible pneumococci, perhaps a consequence of defective autolysis. Alternatives for treatment of meningitis due to penicillin-resistant pneumococci include cefotaxime, ceftriaxone or vancomycin (Viladrich *et al.*, 1988; Klugman, 1990; Jacobs, 1992). However, high-level resistance to the former two agents has recently been described (Bradley and Connor, 1991).

VACCINATION AGAINST *S. PNEUMONIAE*

A polyvalent pneumococcal vaccine consisting of purified capsular polysaccharides was first licensed for use in the USA in 1977, after successful efficacy trials in healthy young adults (South African mine workers). However, there were some doubts as to the efficacy of the vaccine in other groups at high risk of pneumococcal infection (such as the elderly, patients with underlying pulmonary, cardiac or renal disease, and immuno-compromised patients), for whom vaccination was specifically recommended. A recent case– controlled study in this target population has indicated that for immunocompetent individuals the vaccine is 61% effective in preventing disease caused by pneumococci belonging to serotypes included in the formulation. However, efficacy was only 21% for immunocompromised patients (Shapiro *et al.*, 1991).

The current vaccine contains purified poly-saccharide from 23 serotypes, namely 1, 2, 3, 4, 5, 6B, 7F, 8, 9N, 9V, 10A, 11A, 12F, 14, 15B, 17F, 18C, 19A, 19F, 20, 22F, 23F and 33F. The protection imparted is type specific and these serotypes account for approximately 85–90% of serious pneumococcal infections in Europe and North America. Thus, the overall efficacy of the vaccine in preventing pneumococcal disease in immunocompetent adults in these regions is of the

order of 55%. Serotype prevalence data is scarce for other parts of the world, but it is known that in several Asian countries the 23 vaccine serotypes account for as little as 63% of infections, and thus overall efficacy may be substantially lower (Lee *et al.*, 1991).

The second shortcoming of the present vaccine is that in children less than two years old antibody responses to most capsular types are generally poor, particularly to types 6A, 6B, 14, 19F and 23F, which are the commonest causes of serious paediatric disease. This has generally correlated with suboptimal clinical efficacy in this age group. Nevertheless, a large vaccination trial in Papua New Guinea children demonstrated that the vaccine was approximately 50% effective in preventing death from pneumococcal disease (Riley *et al.*, 1986). The problem of poor immunogenicity is being addressed by conjugation of the least immuno-genic polysaccharide types to protein carriers, such as tetanus or diphtheria toxoids or meningococcal outer membrane protein complex. Conjugation confers T cell dependence on the polysaccharide antigens, resulting in a booster effect and immun-ological memory (Vella *et al.*, 1992). However, the number of serotypes covered by polyvalent conjugate vaccines is likely to be considerably lower than the current 23, and so variations in serotype prevalence will continue to limit the overall efficacy of such vaccines, notwithstanding their vastly improved immunogenicity in young children.

The vaccine potential of pneumococcal protein antigens such as pneumolysin, pneumococcal surface protein A and a 37 kDa surface antigen is currently being examined. Preliminary data indicate that these antigens are partially protective in animal models of pneumococcal disease (Paton *et al.*, 1993). Moreover, at least in the case of pneumolysin, there is no evidence for antigenic variation between pneumococcal serotypes, and a genetically toxoided derivative has been shown to be a suitable carrier for polysaccharide (Paton *et al.*, 1991, 1993). Thus, pneumococcal protein antigens may become important components of conjugate vaccine formulations to provide protection against non-included serotypes.

REFERENCES

Agello, G.W., Bolan, G.A., Hayes, P.S. *et al.* (1987) Commercial latex agglutination tests for detection of *Haemophilus influenzae* type b and *Streptococcus pneumoniae* antigens in patients with bacteremic pneumonia. *Journal of Clinical Microbiology*, **25**, 1388–1391.

Austrian, R. (1981a) Pneumococcus: the first one hundred years. *Reviews of Infectious Diseases*, **3**, 183–189.

Austrian, R. (1981b) Some observations on the pneumococcus and on the current status of pneumococcal disease and its prevention. *Reviews of Infectious Diseases*, 3 (Suppl.), S1–17.

Avery, O.T. and Dubos, R.(1931) The protective action of a specific enzyme against type III pneumococcus infections in mice. *Journal of Experimental Medicine*, **54**, 73–89.

Avery, O.T., MacLeod, C.M. and McCarty, M. (1944) Studies on the chemical nature of the substance inducing transformation of pneumococcal types: induction of transformation by a desoxyribonucleic acid fraction isolated from pneumococcus type III. *Journal of Experimental Medicine*, **79**, 137–158.

Ballard, T.L., Roe, M.H., Wheeler, R.C. *et al.* (1987) Comparison of three latex agglutination kits and counterimmunoelectrophoresis for the detection of bacterial antigens in a pediatric population. *Pediatric Infectious Disease Journal*, **6**, 630–634.

Berry, A.M., Yother, J., Briles, D.E. *et al.* (1989a) Reduced virulence of a defined pneumolysin-negative mutant of *Streptococcus pneumoniae*. *Infection and Immunity*, **57**, 2037–2042.

Berry, A.M., Lock, R.A., Hansman, D. *et al.* (1989b) Contribution of autolysin to the virulence of *Streptococcus pneumoniae*. *Infection and Immunity*, **57**, 2324–2330.

Berry, A.M., Paton, J.C. and Hansman, D. (1992) Effect of insertional inactivation of the genes encoding pneumolysin and autolysin on the virulence of *Streptococcus pneumoniae* type 3. *Microbial Pathogenesis*, **12**, 87–93.

Boersma, W.G. and Holloway, Y. (1992) Clinical relevance of pneumococcal antigen detection in urine. *Infection*, **20**, 240–241.

Boulnois, G.J. (1992) Pneumococcal proteins and the pathogenesis of disease caused by *Streptococcus pneumoniae*. *Journal of General Microbiology*, **138**, 249–259.

Boulnois, G.J., Paton, J.C., Mitchell, T.J. *et al.* (1991) Structure and function of pneumolysin, the multifunctional, thiol-activated toxin of *Streptococcus pneumoniae*. *Molecular Microbiology*, **5**, 2611–2616.

Bradley, J.S. and Connor, J.D. (1991) Ceftriaxone failure in meningitis caused by *Streptococcus pneumoniae* with reduced susceptibility to beta-lactam antibiotics. *Pediatric Infectious Disease Journal*, **10**, 871–873.

Bratton, L., Teele, D.W. and Klein, J.O. (1977) Outcome of unsuspected pneumococcemia in children not initially admitted to the hospital. *Journal of Pediatrics*, **90**, 703–706.

Bruyn, G.A.W., Zegers, B.J.M. and van Furth, R. (1992) Mechanisms of host defence against infection with *Streptococcus pneumoniae*. *Clinical Infectious Diseases*, **14**, 251–262.

Burman, L.A., Trollfors, B., Andersson, B. *et al.* (1991) Diagnosis of pneumonia by cultures, bacterial and viral antigen detection tests, and serology with special reference to antibodies against pneumococcal antigens. *Journal of Infectious Diseases*, **163**, 1087–1093.

Carlsen, B.D., Kawana, M., Kawana, C. *et al.* (1992) Role of the bacterial cell wall in middle ear inflammation caused by *Streptococcus pneumoniae*. *Infection and Immunity*, **60**, 2850–2854.

Cerosaletti, K.M., Roghmann, M.C. and Bentley, D.W. (1985) Comparison of latex agglutination and counterimmunoelectrophoresis for the detection of pneumococcal antigen in elderly pneumonia patients. *Journal of Clinical Microbiology*, **22**, 553–557.

Crain, M.J., Waltman, W.D. II, Turner, J.S. *et al.* (1990) Pneumococcal surface protein A (PspA) is serologically highly variable and is expressed by all clinically important capsular serotypes of *Streptococcus pneumoniae*. *Infection and Immunity*, **58**, 3293–3299.

Dagan, R., Englehard, D. and Piccard, E. (1992) Epidemiology of invasive childhood pneumococcal infections in Israel. *Journal of the American Medical Association*, **268**, 3328–3332.

Denys, G.A. and Carey, R.B. (1992) Identification of *Streptococcus pneumoniae* with a DNA probe. *Journal of Clinical Microbiology*, **30**, 2725–2727.

Douglas, R.M., Hansman, D., Miles, H.B. and Paton, J.C. (1986) Pneumococcal carriage and type-specific antibody: failure of a 14-valent vaccine to reduce carriage in healthy children. *American Journal of Diseases of Children*, **140**, 1183–1185.

Dowson, C.G., Coffey, T.J., Kell, C. *et al.* (1993) Evolution of penicillin resistance in *Streptococcus pneumoniae*: the role of *Streptococcus mitis* in the formation of a low affinity PBP2b in *S. pneumoniae*. *Molecular Microbiology*, **9**, 635–643.

Feldman, C., Munro, N.C., Jeffery, P.K. *et al.* (1991) Pneumolysin induces the salient histological features of pneumococcal infection in the rat lung in vivo. *American Journal of Respiratory Cell and Molecular Biology*, **5**, 416–423.

Geslin, P., Buu-Hoi, A., Frémaux, A. *et al.* (1992) Antimicrobial resistance in *Streptococcus pneumoniae*: an epidemiological survey in France, 1970–1990. *Clinical Infectious Diseases*, **15**, 95–98.

Gillespie, S.H., Smith, M.D., Dickens, A. *et al.* (1994a) Diagnosis of *Streptococcus pneumoniae* pneumonia by quantitative enzyme linked immunosorbent assay of C-polysaccharide. *Journal of Clinical Pathology*, **47**, 749–751.

Gillespie, S.H., Ullman, C., Smith, M.D. *et al.* (1994b) Detection of *Streptococcus pneumoniae* in sputum samples by PCR. *Journal of Clinical Microbiology*, **32**, 1308–1311.

Gray, L.D. and Fedorko, D.P. (1992) Laboratory diagnosis of bacterial meningitis. *Clinical Microbiology Reviews*, **5**, 130–145.

Immunization Practices Advisory Committee (1981) Pneumococcal polysaccharide vaccine. *Morbidity and Mortality Weekly Reports*, **30**, 410–412, 417–419.

Jacobs, M.R. (1992) Treatment and diagnosis of infections caused by drug-resistant *Streptococcus pneumoniae*. *Clinical Infectious Diseases*, **15**, 119–127.

Jalonen, E., Paton, J.C., Koskela, M. *et al.* (1989) Measurement of antibody responses to pneumolysin: a promising method for the aetiological diagnosis of pneumococcal pneumonia. *Journal of Infection*, **19**, 127–134.

Johnston, R.B., Jr (1991) Pathogenesis of pneumococcal pneumonia. *Reviews of Infectious Diseases*, **13**, (Suppl. 6), S509–517.

Kalin, M. and Lindberg, A.A. (1983) Diagnosis of pneumococcal pneumonia: a comparison between microscopic examination of expectorate, antigen detection and cultural procedures. *Scandinavian Journal of Infectious Diseases*, **15**, 247–255.

Kawana, M., Kawana, C. and Giebink, G.S. (1992) Penicillin treatment accelerates middle ear inflammation in experimental pneumococcal otitis media. *Infection and Immunity*, **60**, 1908–1912.

Kennedy, W.A., Hoyt, M.J. and McCracken, G.H. Jr (1991) The role of corticosteroid therapy in children with pneumococcal meningitis. *American Journal of Diseases of Children*, **145**, 1374–1378.

Kilian, M. and Reinholdt, J. (1987) A hypothetical model for the development of invasive infection due to IgA protease producing bacteria. *Advances in Experimental Medicine and Biology*, **216**B, 1261–1269.

Klein, J.O. (1981) The epidemiology of pneumococcal disease in infants and children. *Reviews of Infectious Diseases*, **3**, 246–253.

Klugman, K.P. (1990) Pneumococcal resistance to antibiotics. *Clinical Microbiology Reviews*, **3**, 171–196.

Lee, C.-J., Banks, S.D. and Li, J.P. (1991) Virulence, immunity and vaccine related to *Streptococcus pneumoniae*. *Critical Reviews in Microbiology*, **18**, 89–114.

Lock, R.A., Paton, J.C. and Hansman, D. (1988) Comparative efficacy of pneumococcal neuraminidase and pneumolysin as immunogens protective against *Streptococcus pneumoniae* infection. *Microbial Pathogenesis*, **5**, 461–467.

Marton, A. (1992) Pneumococcal antimicrobial resistance: the problem in Hungary. *Clinical Infectious Diseases*, **15**, 106–111.

McDaniel, L.S., Scott, G., Kearney, J.F. *et al.* (1984) Monoclonal antibodies against protease-sensitive pneumococcal antigens can protect mice from fatal infection with *Streptococcus pneumoniae*. *Journal of Experimental Medicine*, **160**, 386–397.

McDaniel, L.S., Yother, J., Vijayakumar, M. *et al.* (1987) Use of insertional inactivation to facilitate studies of biological properties of pneumococcal surface protein A (PspA). *Journal of Experimental Medicine*, **165**, 381–394.

Mitchell, T.J., Andrew, P.W., Saunders, F.K. *et al.*, (1991) Complement activation and antibody binding by pneumolysin via a region of the toxin homologous to a human acute phase protein. *Molecular Microbiology*, **5**, 1883–1888.

Moxon, E.R. (1981) Experimental infections of animals in the study of *Streptococcus pneumoniae*. *Reviews of Infectious Diseases*, **3**, 354–357.

Musher, D.M. (1992) Infections caused by *Streptococcus pneumoniae*: clinical spectrum, pathogenesis, immunity and treatment. *Clinical Infectious Diseases*, **14**, 801–807.

National Committee for Clinical Laboratory Standards (1990a) *Performance Standards for Antimicrobial Disk Susceptibility tests*, 4th edn. Approved standard. Document M2-A4, NCCLS, Villanova, PA.

National Committee for Clinical Laboratory Standards (1990b) *Methods for Dilution Antimicrobial Susceptibility Tests for Bacteria that Grow Aerobically*. 2nd edn. Approved standard. Document M7-A2, NCCLS, Villanova, PA.

Nielsen, S.V. and Henrichsen, J. (1992) Capsular types of *Streptococcus pneumoniae* isolated from blood and CSF during 1982–1987. *Clinical Infectious Diseases*, **15**, 794–798.

O'Niell, K.P., Lloyd-Evans, N., Campbell, H. *et al.* (1989) Latex agglutination test for diagnosing pneumococcal pneumonia in children in developing countries. *British Medical Journal*, **298**, 1061–1064.

Paton, J.C., Lock, R.A. and Hansman, D. (1983) Effect of immunization with pneumolysin on survival time of mice challenged with *Streptococcus pneumoniae*. *Infection and Immunity*, **40**, 548–552.

Paton, J.C., Lock, R.A., Lee, C.-J. *et al.* (1991) Purification and immunogenicity of genetically obtained pneumolysin toxoids and their conjugation to *Streptococcus pneumoniae* type 19F polysaccharide. *Infection and Immunity*, **59**, 2297–2303.

Paton, J.C., Andrew, P.W., Boulnois, G.J. *et al.* (1993) Molecular analysis of the pathogenicity of *Streptococcus pneumoniae*: the role of pneumococcal proteins. *Annual Review of Microbiology*, **47**, 89–115.

Riley, I.D. and Douglas, R.M. (1981) An epidemiological approach to pneumococcal disease. *Reviews of Infectious Diseases*, **3**, 233–245.

Riley, I.D., Lehmann, D., Alpers, M.P. *et al.* (1986) Pneumococcal vaccine prevents death from acute lower respiratory tract infections in Papua New Guinea children. *Lancet*, **ii**, 877–881.

Rubins, J.B., Duane, P.G., Charboneau, D. *et al.* (1992) Toxicity of pneumolysin to pulmonary endothelial cells in vitro. *Infection and Immunity*, **60**, 1740–1746.

Rudolph, K.M., Parkinson, A.J., Black, C.M. *et al.* (1993) Evaluation of polymerase chain reaction for diagnosis of pneumococcal pneumonia. *Journal of Clinical Microbiology*, **31**, 2661–2666.

Sessegolo, J.F., Levin, A.S.S., Levy, C.E. *et al.*, (1994) Distribution of serotypes and antimicrobial resistance of *Streptococcus pneumoniae* strains isolated in Brazil from 1988 to 1992. *Journal of Clinical Microbiology*, **32**, 906–911.

Shapiro, E.D., Berg, A.T., Austrian, R. *et al.* (1991) The protective efficacy of polyvalent pneumococcal polysaccharide vaccine. *New England Journal of Medicine*, **325**, 1453–1460.

Sorensen, U.B.S., Blom, J., Birch-Andersen, A. *et al.* (1988) Ultrastructural localization of capsules, cell wall polysaccharide, cell wall proteins, and F antigen in pneumococci. *Infection and Immunity*, **56**, 1890–1896.

Talkington, D.F., Crimmins, D.L., Voellinger, D.C. *et al.* (1991) A 43-kilodalton pneumococcal surface protein, PspA: isolation, protective abilities, and structural analysis of the amino-terminal sequence. *Infection and Immunity*, **59**, 1285–1289.

Tomasz, A. (1981) Surface components of *Streptococcus pneumoniae*. *Reviews of Infectious Diseases*, **3**, 190–211.

Tuomanen, E., Liu, H., Hengstler, B. *et al.* (1985) The induction of meningeal inflammation by components of the pneumococcal cell wall. *Journal of Infectious Diseases*, **151**, 859–868.

Tuomanen, E., Hengstler, B., Rich, R. *et al.* (1987) Nonsteroidal anti-inflammatory agents in the therapy for experimental pneumococcal meningitis. *Journal of Infectious Diseases*, **155**, 985–990.

Vella, P.P., Marburg, S., Staub, J.M. *et al.* (1992) Immunogenicity of conjugate vaccines consisting of pneumococcal capsular polysaccharide types 6B, 14, 19F and 23F and a meningococcal outer membrane protein complex. *Infection and Immunity*, **60**, 4977–4983.

Viladrich, P.F., Gudiol, F., Liñares, J. *et al.* (1988) Characteristics and antibiotic therapy of adult meningitis due to penicillin-resistant pneumococci. *American Journal of Medicine*, **84**, 839–846.

Watson, D.A. and Musher, D.M. (1990) Interruption of capsule production in *Streptococcus pneumoniae* serotype 3 by insertion of transposon Tn916. *Infection and Immunity*, **58**, 3135–3138.

Winkelstein, J.A. (1981) The role of complement in the host's defense against *Streptococcus pneumoniae*. *Reviews of Infectious Diseases*, **3**, 289–298.

Yolken, R.H., Davis, D., Winkelstein, J. *et al.* (1984) Enzyme immunoassay for detection of pneumococcal antigen in cerebrospinal fluid. *Journal of Clinical Microbiology*, **20**, 802–805.

1d

ENTEROCOCCUS

Volkan Korten and Barbara E. Murray

HISTORY

The term 'entérocoque' was first encountered in a French paper published in 1899 emphasizing the intestinal origin of a new Gram-positive coccus (Murray, 1990). Because of its cell shape, staining characteristics and lack of catalase, enterococci were considered to be members of the genus *Streptococcus* during the early 1900s. The name *Streptococcus faecalis*, which came to used for the most common species, emphasized the relationship of these organisms to faeces. In Sherman's classification scheme of streptococci from the 1930s, the term 'enterococcus' was used for those 'streptococci' which had the ability to grow at 10 °C and 45 °C, in 6.5% NaCl and at pH 9.6 and to split aesculin (Sherman, 1937). Using Lancefield's serological classification, enterococci were considered salt-tolerant group D streptococci. Biochemical characteristics that distinguished *Streptococcus faecium* from *S. faecalis* were clarified in the 1940s and the species status of *S. faecium* was formally accepted in the mid-1960s (Murray, 1990). Recent application of modern bacterial taxonomic techniques have divided the genus *Streptococcus* into three genera: *Enterococcus*, *Lactococcus* and *Streptococcus*. Enterococcal strains formerly called *S. faecalis*, *S. faecium*, etc. were designated *Enterococcus faecalis*, *E. faecium*, etc. (Schleifer and Kilpper-Bälz, 1984). A number of new species of the genus *Enterococcus* have also been described in recent years.

DESCRIPTION OF THE GENUS

Biochemical Characteristics

Enterococci are Gram-positive, facultatively anaerobic organisms which are catalase negative, although a weak 'pseudocatalase' is occasionally produced. Most strains have the ability to grow in the presence of 6.5% NaCl at 10 °C and usually at 45 °C at pH 9.6, and can survive at 60 °C for 30 minutes. Enterococci are capable of hydrolysing aesculin in the presence of bile and most strains react with group D antisera; some react also with group Q antisera. Detection of the group D antigen, which is a cell wall-associated glycerol teichoic acid antigen, is not specific for enterococci, but may also be found in other Gram-positive bacteria including *Streptococcus bovis*, *S. equinus*, *S. suis*, *Pediococcus* spp. and *Leuconostoc* spp. Genera of catalase-negative, facultatively anaerobic bacteria whose members may also show some of the other phenotypic characteristics of enterococci include

Principles and Practice of Clinical Bacteriology. Edited by A.M. Emmerson, P.M. Hawkey and S.H. Gillespie
© 1997 John Wiley & Sons Ltd

Aerococcus, *Gemella*, *Streptococcus*, *Lactococcus*, *Pediococcus* and *Leuconostoc* (Table 1d.1). The recent emergence of vancomycin resistance in enterococci has increased the importance and difficulty of differentiation of enterococci from intrinsically vancomycin-resistant Gram-positive cocci, e.g. *Leuconostoc* spp. or *Pediococcus* spp., which also can be isolated from human specimens. Enterococci possess the enzyme pyrrolidonyl arylamidase, and hydrolyse L-pyrrolidonyl-β-naphthylamide (PYR) (Facklam *et al.*, 1989). This reaction is very useful for differentiation of enterococci from most streptococci, *Leuconostoc* spp. and pediococci. Among streptococci, only group A and nutritionally variant streptococci are PYR positive. *Leuconostoc* spp. and pediococci can be group D positive, but they are PYR negative and leuconostocs produce gas from glucose in Mann, Rogosa, Sharpe *Lactobacillus* (MRS) broth (Facklam and Collins, 1989). A DNA probe complementary to enterococcal rRNA may prove useful in the future (Daly *et al.*, 1991). Table 1d.1 shows reactions useful for differentiating selected Gram-positive organisms.

Growth Characteristics

It has been known for decades that enterococci have complex growth requirements. *E. faecalis* has been shown to grow well on Davis minimal medium (consisting of salts, citrate, thiamine, glucose and agar) supplemented with additional vitamins (biotin, calcium pantothenic acid, pyridoxine, nicotinic acid, riboflavin and folic acid) plus 20 amino acids. By deleting individual amino acids from this medium, it was shown that most of 23 *E. faecalis* strains tested were prototrophic for purines and pyrimidines and eight amino acids (Ala, Asn, Asp, Gln, Lys, Pag, Pro and Tyr), and auxotrophic (or almost so) for Arg, Glu, Gly, His, Ile, Leu, Met, Trp and Val. Cys, Ser and Thr were stimulatory for the growth of some *E. faecalis* (Murray *et al.*, 1993). A restriction map has been generated of the chromosome of a widely used strain, OG1, and the location of known genes including genes for purine and pyrimidine biosynthesis are known (Murray *et al.*, 1993).

Habitat

Enterococcus spp. are typically found in the intestinal tracts of warm-blooded animals, and can be found in insects and on plants. In the majority of the studies, *E. faecalis* is more common in human faeces than *E. faecium*, with average counts of 10^5-10^7 and 10^4-10^5 per gram, respectively (Murray, 1990). Enterococci are less frequently found at other sites such as vagina, oral cavity and dental plaque. Enterococci are also found routinely in

TABLE 1d.1 TESTS WHICH ARE USEFUL TO DIFFERENTIATE SELECTED GRAM-POSITIVE ORGANISMS FROM ENTEROCOCCI

Test	Enterococci	Viridans streptococci	Lactococci	Aerococci	Pediococci	Leuconostocs	Lactobacilli
Gas from glucose	−[a]	−	−	−	−	+	V+
Vancomycin resistance	±[b]	−	−	−	+	+	V+
Reaction with group D antiserum	V+	−	−	−	+	V−	V−
Bile aesculin	+	V−	V+	V+	+	V+	V+
Hydrolysis of PYR	+	−[a]	V+	+	−	−	−
Leucine aminopeptidase	+	+	+	−	+	−	
Growth							
in 6.5% NaCl broth	+	−	V+	+	V−	V+	V−
at 45 °C	+	V	V−	−	V+	−	V+
at 10 °C	V+	−[a]	+	−	−	V+	+

+, most (>90%) strains positive; −, most (>90%) strains negative; V+, more than half of the strains positive; V−, more than half of the strains negative; −[a], occasionally positive; ±[b], intrinsic and acquired resistance to vancomycin have been described in some species (see text); PYR, L-pyrrolidonyl-β-naphthylamide.
Adapted from Facklam and Collins (1989) and Facklam and Sahm (1995).

sewage and their presence has been used to monitor faecal contamination. Because of their production of lactic acid, enterococci have been used as starters in the manufacture of cheese and have been isolated from cheese products as well as from certain meats and other foods (Garcia de Fernando, 1991; Andre Gordon and Ahmad, 1991).

PATHOGENICITY

Enterococci are generally not considered as being as virulent as organisms such as *Streptococcus pyogenes* or *Staphylococcus aureus*. Factors augmenting the ability of enterococci to colonize and to cause infections outside the gastrointestinal tract are poorly understood although it has been suggested that the antibiotic resistance may play a major role in their ability to persist in hospitalized patients who are receiving multiple antibiotics. The enterococcal bacteriocin haemolysin, capable of lysing other bacteria and certain eukaryotic cells including erythrocytes, has been shown to enhance virulence of enterococci in some animal studies (Ike *et al.*, 1984). A recent study also suggests an adverse outcome for patients with enterococcal bacteraemia caused by haemolytic strains (Huycke *et al.*, 1991). The aggregation substance produced by pheromone-responsive strains may mediate adhesion of producing organisms to cultured renal tubular cells, suggesting a possible role of this property in enterococcal urinary tract infections (Kreft *et al.*, 1992). The virulence factors which may be important in other severe infections such as endocarditis are still to be defined.

CLINICAL INFECTIONS

Nosocomial Infections

Nosocomial infections due to enterococci have increased considerably in the last two decades. This increase has been attributed to an increase in the use of antimicrobial agents to which enterococci are resistant, an increase in the use of invasive devices, and/or the number of immunocompromised patients (Korten and Murray, 1993; Pallares *et al.*, 1993). Between 1986 and 1989, the

National Nosocomial Infections Surveillance (NNIS) system listed the enterococcus as the second most common cause of nosocomial infections in the USA, isolated from 12% of such infections (Schaberg *et al.*, 1991). During the same years the enterococcus was the second most common cause of urinary tract and wound infections, and the third most common cause of bacteraemia. Many epidemiological studies have documented intra- and/or inter-hospital spread and have indicated that person-to-person transmission via the hands of health care personnel may occur (Korten and Murray, 1993). Inanimate objects can also be a source of nosocomial enterococcal infection. Outbreaks caused by enterococci possessing different antibiotic resistance traits, such as high-level gentamicin resistance, β-lactamase production, high-level penicillin resistance due to mechanisms other than β-lactamase production, glycopeptide resistance and a combination of these, have been described in recent years (Korten and Murray, 1993). *E. faecalis* followed by *E. faecium* are commonly isolated from nosocomial infections, while other enterococcal species are seldom implicated.

Among many methods used for molecular epidemiology studies of enterococci, total plasmid content, plasmid DNA digestion patterns, ribotyping and conventional as well as pulsed-field gel electrophoresis (PFGE) of chromosomal DNA have been used to evaluate nosocomial enterococcal infections. In our hands, PFGE was better at identifying clonality, at least during prolonged outbreaks (Korten and Murray, 1993), and is also reproducible and easy to perform. Results of these analyses have shown both intra-hospital as well as inter-state spread of clones with new resistance properties.

Urinary Tract Infections

Enterococci are common causes of nosocomial UTIs, especially those associated with instrumentation, structural abnormalities and antibiotic use. Enterococci are also among the leading organisms causing UTI in elderly men, including those suffering from prostatitis. In contrast, enterococci cause <5% of uncomplicated UTIs in young women. The prevalence of enterococcal UTIs has increased in recent years probably as a result of increasing use of broad-spectrum antibiotics and of catheterization (Morrison and Wenzel, 1986). In spite of the low morbidity and mortality, enterococcal UTIs have clinical importance because of additional costs of hospitalization and therapy.

Endocarditis

Enterococci are the third most common cause of infective endocarditis following viridans streptococci and *Staphylococcus aureus*, accounting for 5–20% of cases (Megran, 1992). *E. faecalis* is responsible for the majority of these. In men, endocarditis is more common after the fifth decade of life, presumably because of the high prevalence of genitourinary conditions and degenerative valvular disease. In women, enterococcal endocarditis is observed during childbearing years. Enterococci are implicated in 6–7% cases of prosthetic valve endocarditis (Megran, 1992). Enterococcal endocarditis is also seen in 2–13% of intravenous drug abusers (Megran, 1992). Endocarditis often occurs in patients with a previous history of valvular heart disease, but can also affect apparently normal valves, the aortic and mitral valves being most commonly involved. Presentation can be acute or subacute in onset. Right-sided endocarditis is extremely uncommon, even in intravenous drug abusers. The source of infection often appears to be the genitourinary tract, although gastrointestinal diseases, procedures and surgery involving the biliary tract or large bowel are also common as predisposing conditions. In one study, five of 37 cases of enterococcal infective endocarditis were associated with bowel carcinoma or polyps (Herzkein *et al.*, 1984). Dental manipulation and obstetric and gynaecological conditions are less common predisposing factors.

Bacteraemia Without Endocarditis

Enterococcal bacteraemia is much more common than enterococcal endocarditis, accounting for about 9% of positive blood cultures in the USA (Emori and Gaynes, 1993) and enterococci are the most frequently found Gram-positive organisms in polymicrobial bacteraemia. A marked increase in enterococcal bacteraemia was noted after 1975 (Maki and Agger, 1988). These authors also analysed the source of bacteraemia and found 12 cases of enterococcal endocarditis among the 33 patients with community-acquired enterococcal bacteraemias (36%), but only one case in the 120 patients with nosocomial bacteraemia (0.8%). In the same report, 77% of patients with enterococcal bacteraemia had either a urinary or an intravascular catheter. Other possible sources included intra-abdominal, biliary, pelvic and wound infections. Enterococcal bacteraemia, especially if polymicrobial and if Gram-negative organisms are present, is associated with high mortality ranging from 34% to 68% (Graninger and Ragette, 1992). It is not always clear whether the high mortality in patients with enterococcal bacteraemia is due to the organism *per se* or to the underlying conditions, but bacteraemia *per se* does appear to contribute to increased morbidity and mortality.

Neonatal Infections

Enterococci can also cause neonatal sepsis and/or meningitis although *Escherichia coli* and group B streptococci are much more commonly seen. While this can occur in normal term infants, low birth weight and premature infants with severe underlying conditions are a high-risk group for enterococcal infections. A nosocomial outbreak of *E. faecium* in newborns has also been described (Coudron *et al.*, 1984). Use of a non-umbilical central catheter, length of time the central line was in place, gastrointestinal surgery, intubation and umbilical vessel catheterization have been identified as significant risk factors for neonatal enterococcal disease in various studies (Korten and Murray, 1993).

Central Nervous System Infections

Besides neonatal meningitis, enterococci can also cause shunt infections and meningitis in older children and adults. In most of these patients, invasive procedures of the central nervous system, underlying diseases or previous antibiotic therapy were recognized as risk factors.

Intra-abdominal and Pelvic Infections

The role of enterococci in intra-abdominal and pelvic infections remains controversial, particularly in the initial presentation of lower intra-abdominal infections. Animal experiments show that enterococci alone do not cause infections or sepsis when given intraperitoneally but can cause abscess formation by acting synergistically with other organisms (Nichols and Muzik, 1992). Enterococci are an important cause of spontaneous peritonitis in cirrhotic and nephrotic patients and have also been identified as a cause of peritonitis in patients on continuous ambulatory peritoneal dialysis. Enterococcal abscesses and bacteraemia also occur with biliary and other intra-abdominal infections. Enterococci have also been identified as a cause of various pelvic infections, including salpingitis, endometritis and abscess formation after caesarean section.

LABORATORY DIAGNOSIS

Isolation Procedures

Enterococci grow well on blood agar base media containing 5% animal blood, and will also grow on many other media (e.g. Mueller–Hinton, Brain Heart Infusion, dextrose phosphate, chocolate) that are not selective for Gram-negative bacteria. Some strains of *E. faecalis* produce β-haemolysis on media containing rabbit, human or horse blood but not sheep blood. Bile–aesculin azide or other commercially available azide-containing media, Columbia colistin–nalidixic acid agar (CNA), phenylethyl alcohol agar (PEA), SF agar, m-Enterococcus agar, and Enterococcosel agar, among others, can be used to isolate enterococci from mixed samples containing Gram-negative bacteria.

Species Identification

While the majority (85–95%) of clinical enterococcal isolates are *E. faecalis*, approximately 5–10% are *E. faecium*. Some of the other species are encountered only rarely, and some are only isolated from non-human sources. Differentiation of non-*faecalis* enterococci can be helpful in serious infections because of the differences in the susceptibility of some species or for epidemiological purposes within hospitals. The genus *Enterococcus* now contains over a dozen species, some of which have been isolated from plants and animals. The taxonomic status of two proposed species, *E. solitarius* and *E. seriolocida*, is unclear (Williams *et al.*, 1991; Domenech *et al.*, 1993). In addition to the species described in Table 1d.2, four new species have been proposed: *E. sulfureus* (Martinez-Murcia and Collins, 1991), *E. columbae* (Devriese *et al.*, 1990), *E. saccharolyticus* (Rodrigues and Collins, 1990) and *E. cecorum* (Williams *et al.*, 1989). The latter three species do not possess all the phenotypic characteristics of other enterococcal species; e.g. they have a negative PYR reaction, and have less homology as determined by rRNA sequence analysis. The tests listed in Table 1d.2, which were previously described by Facklam and Collins and modified according to recent data, can be used to identify the species (Facklam and Sahm, 1995).

Conventional tests

In their scheme published in 1989, Facklam and Collins separated the species into three groups on the basis of acid formation in conventional tubes of mannitol, sorbitol, and sorbose broths, and hydrolysis of arginine. According to this scheme, group I species, *E. avium*, *E. malodoratus*, *E. raffinosus* and *E. pseudoavium* form acid in mannitol, sorbitol, and sorbose broths, but do not hydrolyse arginine. Group II species (*E. faecalis*, *E. solitarius*, *E. faecium*, *E. casseliflavus*, *E. mundtii*, *E. flavescens* and *E. gallinarum*) produce acid in mannitol broth and hydrolyse arginine but do not produce acid in sorbose broth; variable reactions are seen in sorbitol broth. Group III species (*E. durans*, *E. hirae*, *E. dispar* and *E. faecalis* asaccharolytic variant) hydrolyse arginine but fail to form acid in these three carbohydrate

TABLE 1d.2   TESTS FOR IDENTIFICATION OF *ENTEROCOCCUS* SPECIES

	Test[a]										
	Man	Sorb	Sor	Arg	Arab	Raf	Tel	Mot	Pig	Suc	Pyu
E. avium	+	+*	+	−	+	−	−	−	−	+	+*
E. malodoratus	+	+*	+	−*	−	+	−	−	−	+	+*
E. raffinosus	+	+	+	−*	+	+	−	−	−	+	+*
E. pseudoavium	+	+	+	−	−	−	−	−	−	+	+*
E. faecalis	+	+	−	+	−	−	+	−	−	+	+*
E. faecium	+	−	−	+	+	−	−	−	−	+	−
E. casseliflavus	+	V−	−	+*	+	+	−[b]	+	+	+	−
E. mundtii	+	V−*	−	+	+	+	−[b]	−	+	+	−*
E. flavescens	+	−	−	+	+	+	−	+	+	+	−
E. gallinarum	+	−	−	+*	+	+	−[b]	+	−	+	−
E. durans	−	−	−	+*	−	−	−	−	−	−	−
E. hirae	−	−	−	+	−	V+*	−	−	−	V+*	−
E. dispar	−	−	−	+	−	+	−	−	−	+	+
E. faecalis (var)	−	−	−	+	−	−	+	−	−	−	V+

[a]Man, mannitol; Sorb, sorbitol; Sor, sorbose; Arg, arginine; Arab, arabinose; Raf, raffinose; Tel, tellurite; Mot, motility; Pig, pigmentation; Suc, sucrose; Pyu, pyruvate.
+, most (>90%) strains positive; −, most (>90%) strains negative; V+, more than half of the strains positive; V−, more than half of the strains negative; −[b], occasional strains are tolerant.
* Discrepancies were reported in a recent study (Knudtson and Hartman, 1992) as compared with Facklam and Collins' (1989) results.

broths. The species within each group can be identified by specific reactions shown in Table 1d.2. *Enterococcus faecalis* strains are usually tellurite tolerant when tested on agar medium containing 0.04% potassium tellurite and form black colonies. A few *E. gallinarum*, *E. casseliflavus* and *E. mundtii* strains may also be tellurite tolerant. Tellurite reduction or ribose fermentation is essential for the differentiation of lactose-negative *E. faecalis* and *E. solitarius* (Ruoff *et al.*, 1990). Motility and yellow pigmentation are helpful for the differentiation of three species in the Group II. *E. casseliflavus* is motile and produces yellow pigment; *E. mundtii* produces yellow pigment, but it is not motile; *E. gallinarum* is motile but does not produce yellow pigment. New pigment-producing *Enterococcus* spp. were also described recently: *E. flavescens* and *E. sulfureus*. *E. flavescens*, a motile-pigment producer, is distinguished from *E. casseliflavus* by being unable to ferment ribose; it also lacks α-haemolysis on sheep blood (Pompei *et al.*, 1992). *E. sulfureus*, a non-motile pigment producer, does not possess group D antigen and mannitol, inulin, arabinose and arginine tests are negative (Martinez-Murcia and Collins, 1991). Pigment

production and motility may occasionally be unreliable features on which to base identification of *E. gallinarum* and *E. casseliflavus* (Vincent *et al.*, 1991). Other investigators found discrepancies in conventional tube test results described by Facklam and Collins, particularly in arginine and sorbitol tests (Table 1d.2) (Knudtson and Hartman, 1992).

Commercial identification systems

Commercially available identification systems usually identify *E. faecalis* and *E. faecium* correctly, but other species may be misidentified (Ruoff *et al.*, 1990). Several commercial identification systems also showed discrepancies between each other and conventional tube test results (Knudtson and Hartman, 1992). Test schemes supplemented with motility, pigmentation and sucrose have been described for the API Rapid Strep or the MicroScan system panel (Knudtson and Hartman, 1992). In addition, a number of studies have used a combination of reactions in API 20S and API 50CH to characterize new species (Martinez-Murcia and Collins, 1991; Pompei *et al.*, 1992; Collins *et al.*, 1986).

Susceptibility Testing

Routine testing (Kirby–Bauer)

Since enterococcal susceptibility to antimicrobial agents is unpredictable, the site of infection and/or the significance of a particular isolate determines which antimicrobials should be included in susceptibility testing. Drugs to which enterococci are intrinsically resistant, such as cephalosporins, oxacillin, trimethoprim–sulphamethoxazole (TMP-SMX) (in vivo resistance), clindamycin and aminoglycosides at standard concentrations, should not be tested. Susceptibility to penicillin or ampicillin and vancomycin should be determined routinely. For urine isolates, fluoroquinolones, nitrofurantoin and tetracycline may be added (National Committee for Clinical Laboratory Standards (NCCLS), 1993a). Using the Kirby–Bauer technique, a 16 mm or less zone diameter around ampicillin 10 μg disks and a zone of 14 mm or less around penicillin 10 μg disks are considered resistant. New vancomycin disk diffusion breakpoints for enterococci have been set to improve the accuracy for detecting low-level vancomycin resistance (NCCLS, 1993a). A zone of $\leqslant 14$ mm is considered resistant; 15–16 mm, intermediate; and $\geqslant 17$ mm, susceptible. It is recommended that any haze or colonies within the zone should be taken into account and that an minimal inhibitory concentration (MIC) test be performed for strains with intermediate susceptibility zones if vancomycin is to be used for treatment (Swenson et al., 1992). Alternative methods including breakpoints and Stokes–Ridgeway comparative plates are also used.

Agar incorporation MICs

For agar dilution testing, interpretive criteria for ampicillin and penicillin are MICs of $\leqslant 8$ (susceptible) and $\geqslant 16$ (resistant) μg/ml (NCCLS, 1993b). For vancomycin, MICs of $\leqslant 4$ μg/ml and 8–16 μg/ml are considered susceptible and intermediate, respectively. An MIC of vancomycin of $\geqslant 32$ μg/ml is considered resistant. The NCCLS has recently suggested use of an agar screen using BHI agar plus vancomycin 6 μg/ml and an inoculum of 1–10 μl of a suspension equal to a 0.5 McFarland standard. Growth after 24 hours incubation at 35 °C is interpreted as resistant (NCCLS, 1993b).

Aminoglycoside high-level resistance

For serious infections, particularly for endocarditis, and possibly for meningitis and deep-seated infections in immunocompromised patients, aminoglycoside high-level testing and β-lactamase testing should also be performed. High-level resistance (HLR) to gentamicin also indicates resistance to synergism with all currently available aminoglycosides except streptomycin. High-level aminoglycoside resistance can be detected by agar or single-tube broth screening with 500 μg of gentamicin per millilitre; for streptomycin, 2000 μg/ml is used for agar screening and 1000 μg/ml is used for broth screening. Recent changes in testing recommendations included the use of brain heart infusion agar or broth in place of Mueller Hinton. High-content disks containing 300 μg streptomycin and 120 μg gentamicin can also be used to predict synergy or the lack of synergy (Murray, 1990; NCCLS, 1993b). The E test also demonstrates concordance in the detection of high-level aminoglycoside resistance among enterococci as compared with agar dilution screening (Sanchez et al., 1992). Broth microdilution systems appear reliable for HLR to gentamicin, but they may miss some strains with HLR to streptomycin. Automated and rapid systems have had difficulties in accurately detecting HLR, particularly to streptomycin.

MECHANISMS OF RESISTANCE TO ANTIMICROBIAL AGENTS

Antimicrobial resistance among enterococci can be divided into two types: intrinsic (or inherent) and acquired. Intrinsic resistance refers to chromosomally encoded species characteristics which are encountered in all or almost all of the strains of a particular species. Acquired resistance is caused by acquisition of new DNA or mutations in the existing DNA.

Intrinsic Resistance

Intrinsic resistance of enterococci is exemplified by resistance to cephalosporins, penicillinase-resistant penicillins (e.g. methicillin), mono-bactams, low-level resistance to aminoglycosides, low-level resistance to clindamycin, and only moderate susceptibility to available fluoro-quinolones. Relative resistance of enterococci to β-lactams is a characteristic feature of these organisms. MICs of penicillin for *E. faecalis* are generally between 1 and 4 μg/ml, approximately 10–1000 times greater than these for most strep-tococci. Generally, MICs of ampicillin and the ureidopenicillins are one dilution lower than those of penicillin. *E. faecium* is even more resistant to β-lactams with typical MICs of penicillin of 8–32 μg/ml. *E. raffinosus* has been shown to be more resistant to penicillin in recent years (Grayson *et al.*, 1991a). The intrinsic resistance and relative resistance of enterococci to β-lactam drugs are thought to be due to the presence of low-affinity penicillin-binding proteins (Fontana *et al.*, 1992). *E. faecium* strains with higher MICs of penicillin (64 to >256 μg/ml) are increasingly reported in recent years and will be discussed in the section on acquired resistance. None of the cephalosporins inhibits enterococci sufficiently to be used clinically, and enterococcal superinfec-tions may occur in patients receiving cephalosporins. As with the penicillins, imipenem is more active against *E. faecalis* than *E. faecium*. A nosocomial outbreak of *E. faecium* associated with heavy imipenem use was reported in which the occurrence of non-epidemic resistant strains was 16 times more likely in those who had received imipenem (Boyce *et al.*, 1992). Low-level resistance to clindamycin is another charac-teristic feature of enterococci and acquired HLR also occurs. Another example of intrinsic resist-ance of enterococci is the low-level resistance to aminoglycosides (4–64 μg/ml for gentamicin and 32–500 μg/ml for streptomycin). This resistance may be due to low penetration of aminoglycoside agents through the cell wall, since combining aminoglycoside agents with cell wall active agents, such as penicillins or vancomycin, results

in a synergistic effect (defined as $\geq 2 \log_{10}$ enhanced killing relative to the effect of the cell wall active agent alone when the aminoglycoside effect is subinhibitory). Strains of *E. faecium* normally contain a chromosomally located gene encoding an aminoglycoside-modifying enzyme, 6'-*N*-acetyltransferase (*aac(6')-Ii*), which is specific for this species (Costa *et al.*, 1993). Although the low-level production of this enzyme does not confer HLR to aminoglycosides, MICs are higher than those of *E. faecalis* and synergism between cell wall-active agents and the aminogly-cosides carrying an unprotected amino group at the 6' position (tobramycin, kanamycin, netilmicin and sisomicin) but not gentamicin is abolished. Another apparently intrinsic property of entero-cocci is that of *in vivo* resistance to TMP-SMX; although TMP-SMX may be active *in vitro*, it has been found to be ineffective in both animal and clinical case report studies, probably due to the ability of enterococci to use exogenous folates (Murray *et al.*, 1993).

Acquired Resistance

Enterococci possess several different types of mobile genetic elements that can be transferred from one strain to another. One class consists of broad-host range plasmids which can be trans-ferred between enterococci and to various other Gram-positive bacteria such as staphylococci, streptococci, *Bacillus* spp. and lactobacilli. These plasmids can transfer during filter matings but not usually in broth. Another type of plasmid, referred to as narrow-host range plasmids because they appear to be restricted primarily to *E. faecalis*, respond to sex pheromones produced by recipient cells. There are a number of different known pheromones which act on specific pheromone-responsive plasmids. In response to pheromones, these plasmids initiate the production of aggre-gation substance (clumping factor) which leads to sticking together of donor and recipient cells (Clewell, 1989). The transfer frequency of plasmids is markedly increased by this mechanism and transfer occurs in broth as well as during filter matings (Clewell, 1989). Transposons are also common in enterococci. An erythromycin resistance determinant (*ermB*), which is commonly found in human enterococcal isolates, is often encoded on a transposon, exemplified by the well-studied Tn*917*. Macrolide–lincosamide–streptogramin B (MLS) type resistance also causes HLR to clindamycin. Chloramphenicol resistance, found in 20–42% of enterococci, is mediated by chloramphenicol acetyltransferase (Murray, 1990). Tetracycline resistance, which is found in 60–80% of enterococci, can be mediated by different genes including *tetL*, *M* (by far the most common), *O* and probably *N*. The well-studied conjugative transposon Tn*916* carries the tetracycline resistance gene *tetM*, the same gene found in tetracycline resistant *Neisseria gonorrhoeae*. This and other conjugative transposons differ from ordinary or non-conjugative transposons (e.g. Tn*917*) because they can initiate bacterial mating (conjugation) which allows them to move from one bacterial cell to another.

High-level resistance to aminoglycosides

Besides intrinsic low-level resistance to aminoglycosides, a number of enterococcal strains have acquired HLR (MIC ⩾ 2000 μg/ml) to an aminoglycoside; this resistance causes resistance to the synergism otherwise seen between cell wall-active agents and the involved aminoglycoside. HLR to aminoglycosides is most often due to the production of one or more aminoglycoside-modifying enzymes: aminoglycoside phosphotransferases (APH), nucleotidyltransferases (ANT) and acetyltransferases (AAC). *E. faecalis* strains with HLR to gentamicin were first reported in 1979 and strains highly resistant to all aminoglycosides (including gentamicin and streptomycin) were first reported in 1983 (Murray, 1990; Patterson and Zervos, 1990). Such strains have now been reported around the world and non-faecalis enterococci with this trait have been increasingly reported in recent years. In some centres over 50% of enterococci are resistant to penicillin and gentamicin synergy at present (Patterson and Zervos, 1990). Many enterococci with HLR to gentamicin contain plasmids with a gene coding for a bifunctional enzyme with 2"-phosphotransferase-6'-acetyltransferase (APH(2")-AAC(6')) activity, identical to the gene found in gentamicin-resistant staphylococci (Ferretti *et al.*, 1986). This gene can be located on a transposon probably inherited from *Staphylococcus aureus* (Hodel-Christian and Murray, 1991). This enzyme produces resistance to synergy between cell wall-active agents and all currently available aminoglycosides, except streptomycin; in most instances there is also HLR to the involved aminoglycosides, with amikacin being a notable exception. HLR to streptomycin can coexist with HLR to gentamicin in the same strain and is caused by either mutational ribosomal resistance or enzymatic modification. The strains with ribosomal resistance have very high MICs of streptomycin (>32 000 μg/ml), whereas the ANT(6) enzyme producers have MICs of streptomycin which range from 4000 to 16 000 μg/ml. Strains with the lower levels of streptomycin resistance may be difficult to detect (Weissmann *et al.*, 1991). HLR to kanamycin without HLR to gentamicin is caused by the production of APH(3') or rarely ANT(4'); the latter enzyme also causes HLR to tobramycin. These enzymes also prevent penicillin–amikacin synergy, even though they do not produce HLR to amikacin (Leclercq *et al.*, 1992).

β-Lactamase production and high-level penicillin resistance due to other mechanisms

The first β-lactamase-producing enterococcus was an isolate of *E. faecalis* recovered from a urine culture in 1981. Since then, such strains have been isolated from different geographical locations in the USA and several other countries (Murray, 1992). The gene encoding β-lactamase in enterococci is identical to that of the major β-lactamase found in *Staphylococcus aureus* (Murray, 1992). Enterococcal β-lactamase is often found on conjugative plasmids, although chromosomally located β-lactamase genes have been described. One of these appears to be incorporated into a transposon-like element derived from staphylococci (Rice and Marshall, 1992). Since the amount of the enzyme produced by enterococci is lower than that of *S. aureus*, β-lactamase-producing strains may be missed by routine susceptibility-testing methods unless a high inoculum is used. β-Lactamase-producing enterococci can be detected with the chromogenic cephalosporin nitrocefin as well as other methods. Although such strains are still rare among clinical isolates, they may cause outbreaks and severe infections. For this reason, it is advisable to test enterococci which are isolated from severe infections for β-lactamase production. With few exceptions, β-lactamase-producing enterococci are also highly resistant to gentamicin. A β-lactamase-producing *E. faecium* was isolated in a hospital in which a prolonged outbreak due to β-lactamase-producing *E. faecalis* was described previously, suggesting possible spread of this resistance determinant (Coudron *et al.*, 1992).

Although it has been known for a long time that strains of *E. faecium* are more resistant to β-lactams than *E. faecalis*, there have been a number of reports suggesting that strains of *E. faecium* with much higher penicillin MICs (>64 μg/ml) are increasing (Grayson . *et al.*, 1991b). Since routine laboratories typically have not tested concentrations above 16 μg/ml, it is unclear whether the more highly resistant isolates are actually more common or are being increasingly noticed. Penicillin-resistant *E. raffinosus* isolates have also been reported (Grayson *et al.*, 1991a). Mechanisms that have been implicated in causing high levels of penicillin resistance include overproduction of penicillin-binding protein(s) (i.e. cell wall synthesis enzymes) with low affinity for β-lactams and/or a reduction in the affinity of penicillin-binding protein(s) for β-lactams (Klare *et al.*, 1992).

Glycopeptide resistance

Glycopeptide resistance, the most worrisome acquired resistance in enterococci, was first encountered in England and France, with a rapidly increasing number of reports from the USA and other countries. The majority of vancomycin-resistant isolates are *E. faecium*, but glycopeptide resistance has also been found in *E. faecalis* and in some other enterococcal species. Three phenotypic types of glycopeptide resistance, VanA, VanB and VanC, have been described, and were originally defined based on the level of resistance to vancomycin and teicoplanin, inducibility and transferability of the resistance (Table 1d.3). Many of the genes responsible for glycopeptide resistance have been investigated in detail (Arthur and Courvalin, 1993) and the phenotypic classification has largely been replaced by a genotypic classification.

VanA strains typically have high-level vancomycin and teicoplanin resistance while VanB strains have low- or high-level resistance to vancomycin and are usually susceptible to teicoplanin. VanA strains, after exposure to vancomycin, produce a new 39 kDa cytoplasmic membrane protein which has been identified as a D-alanine-D-alanine-like ligase with altered substrate specificity. VanA ligase produces depsipeptides, that is, D-alanyl-D-2-hydroxy acids instead of the dipeptide, D-alanyl-D-alanine; typically, the D-2-hydroxy acid is D-lactate.

TABLE 1d.3   GLYCOPEPTIDE RESISTANCE IN ENTEROCOCCI

Resistance type and genotype	Phenotype	MIC (μg/ml)		Expression	Transferability	Strains found
		Vancomycin	Teicoplanin			
Acquired						
vanA	VanA	64 to >1000	16–512	Inducible	+	*E. faecium, E. faecalis, E. avium, E. durans, E. mundtii, E. raffinosus*
vanB	VanB	4–1000	≤1[a]	Inducible	+	*E. faecium, E. faecalis*
Intrinsic						
vanC	VanC	2–32	≤1	Constitutive	−	*E. gallinarum*
Other	VanC-like	2–32	≤1	Constitutive	−	*E. casseliflavus, E. flavescens*

[a] Mutants constitutively producing VanB are resistant to teicoplanin.

D-ala-D-ala, when incorporated into cell wall peptidoglycan precursors, is the target for binding by vancomycin, which results in inhibition of cell growth, but D-ala-D-lac-containing precursors have much lower affinity for glycopeptides. Thus, when D-ala-D-lac becomes incorporated into cell wall peptidoglycan precursors, the altered peptidoglycan precursors bind glycopeptides less well, allowing peptidoglycan synthesis to proceed even in the presence of vancomycin. A multi-gene cluster (*vanA*, *vanH*, *vanX*, *vanY*, *vanZ*) and a two-component regulatory system (*vanS* and *vanR*) carried on a transposon designated Tn*1546* has recently been characterized (Arthur and Courvalin, 1993).

VanB strains produce a 39.5 kDa cytoplasmic membrane protein which is inducible by subinhibitory concentrations of vancomycin, but not teicoplanin. Once induced by vancomycin, strains become resistant to teicoplanin. Mutants that are constitutive producers of VanB are teicoplanin resistant, and such mutants arise both *in vivo* and *in vitro*. The structural relatedness of *vanB* and *vanA* suggests that the product of *vanB* is also involved in synthesis of modified peptidoglycan precursors. Partial DNA sequence analysis showed very close similarity between VanB strains with high or low vancomycin MICs, suggesting that regulatory mechanisms or strain differences are involved in different expression.

VanC strains have lower MICs of vancomycin and are susceptible to teicoplanin. The expression of the resistance is constitutive. The *vanC* gene is a characteristic of *E. gallinarum* and is a normal chromosomally located gene in these organisms. VanC-like phenotypes are also found in *E. casseliflavus* and *E. flavescens* but the genes encoding VanC-like ligases are not identical to the VanC ligase gene of *E. gallinarum*.

MANAGEMENT OF ENTEROCOCCAL INFECTIONS

Common Infections

The majority of infections such as urinary tract and soft tissue infections caused by enterococci are typically treated with bacteriostatic agents alone:

either ampicillin, penicillin or vancomycin. Ureidopenicillins which might be used in mixed infections should also be effective. Erythromycin, tetracycline, rifampin and chloramphenicol have had little clinical use against enterococci. Because available quinolones are marginally active against enterococci, they should not be used for treating systemic infections unless no other option exists. For β-lactamase-producing strains of *E. faecalis*, ampicillin–sulbactam, amoxicillin–clavulanic acid, piperacillin–tazobactam, vancomycin or imipenem are active.

Serious Systemic Infections

Therapy of endocarditis and other serious systemic infections has been a challenge to clinicians since the beginning of the antibiotic era. Many patients with enterococcal endocarditis failed even with high doses of penicillin alone, presumably because a bactericidal effect is required in the treatment of such infections, and penicillin is usually not bactericidal for enterococci. With the introduction of streptomycin, successful outcome with penicillin–streptomycin therapy was reported and bactericidal synergism between penicillin and streptomycin could be demonstrated by time-kill techniques. The usual choices for the aminoglycoside component of combined therapy are streptomycin or gentamicin, as discussed earlier. The traditional treatment of enterococcal endocarditis has consisted of penicillin or ampicillin (or vancomycin for patients with β-lactam intolerance) combined with gentamicin or streptomycin administered for four to six weeks. Many authorities recommend low-dose gentamicin (3 mg/kg per day, because of lower toxicity) plus high-dose penicillin (20×10^6 U/day) or ampicillin (12 g/day) for six weeks. Recent data showed that the course of enterococcal prosthetic valve endocarditis resembles that caused by less destructive organisms and can be treated with antibiotics alone (Rice *et al.*, 1991).

High-level aminoglycoside resistance

HLR to either streptomycin or gentamicin abolishes the bactericidal synergism usually seen with these agents. HLR to gentamicin prevents synergistic killing when cell wall-active antibiotics are combined with available aminoglycosides, except streptomycin. For this reason, all high-level gentamicin-resistant isolates should be screened for high-level streptomycin resistance. Because of the normally present chromosomally encoded aminoglycoside modifying enzyme AAC(6') of *E. faecium*, synergism is not observed with the combination of penicillin and tobramycin for this species. Because both speciation and screening for HLR to tobramycin (for detecting APH(2")-AAC(6') or ANT(4')) would need to be performed, most clinicians avoid using tobramycin for enterococci. Amikacin is also generally avoided because of the need to perform screening for HLR to kanamycin, or to perform time-kill synergy studies, which many laboratories are not prepared to do. Optimal therapy for patients with enterococcal endocarditis caused by isolates with HLR to all aminoglycosides is unknown (Eliopoulos, 1993). High-dose ampicillin alone for six to eight weeks has resulted in relapse. Recent work suggests administration of cell wall-active agents by continuous infusion is less likely to cause development of tolerance than repeated pulses (Hodges *et al.*, 1992) and one animal study suggests this approach is preferable to intermittent infusion of ampicillin. Cardiac valve replacement as an adjunct to medical therapy may be considered in patients with inadequate initial response. For β-lactamase-producing strains, ampicillin–sulbactam, vancomycin or imipenem should be used instead of penicillin or ampicillin. The recognition of enterococcal isolates resistant to clinically achievable concentrations of penicillins or glycopeptides or both further complicates the therapy of enterococcal endocarditis. While vancomycin can be used for strains which are highly resistant to penicillins or in penicillin-intolerant patients, there is no established regimen for strains resistant to both. Teicoplanin has been used successfully in the treatment of enterococcal endocarditis caused by vancomycin-susceptible organisms, although high serum concentrations seem to be needed (Schmit, 1992); this agent could be considered for teicoplanin-susceptible,

vancomycin-resistant strains, but resistance might emerge during therapy. For some vancomycin-resistant isolates, favourable interactions between vancomycin and β-lactams have been observed, but an aminoglycoside is still needed for bactericidal therapy. Various combinations of ciprofloxacin, rifampin, cell wall-active agents and/or aminoglycosides in animal models have shown inconsistent results. If such combinations are to be used for multi-resistant enterococcal isolates, *in vitro* documentation of a favourable interaction is desirable.

Enterococcal bacteraemia without endocarditis and with a known extracardiac source generally responds well to 10–14 days of therapy. Maki and Agger recommend four weeks of bactericidal therapy for patients for whom an extracardiac source cannot be identified, especially if the infection is community acquired, and/or if the patient has known valvular heart disease (Maki and Agger, 1988).

Intra-abdominal Infection

Despite the fact that enterococci are frequently isolated from mixed intra-abdominal infections, most clinical trials with antibiotics without specific anti-enterococcal coverage do not show clinical failure or persistent isolation of these organisms. For this reason, many authorities do not recommend specific anti-enterococcal therapy initially (Gorbach, 1993). However, in some cases, enterococci can be important pathogens and patients with persistent positive cultures in the absence of clinical improvement should be treated with specific anti-enterococcal therapy.

INFECTION CONTROL

Prudent use of antimicrobial agents and strict application of infection control practices seem mandatory for prevention and control of nosocomial enterococcal infections. Strict application of handwashing, barrier precautions and cohorting infected or colonized patients is successful in controlling outbreaks of infection. Besides these measures, the removal of chronically colonized health care personnel or inanimate sources has been necessary for controlling some outbreaks (Korten and Murray, 1993). Daily perineal washing with chlorhexidine in patients with groin or rectal colonization and showering with chlorhexidine by colonized personnel have been suggested as useful control measures in a recent outbreak caused by vancomycin-resistant enterococci (Handwerger et al., 1993). Because of the positive selective pressure caused by vancomycin use, the use of this agent as empirical therapy of febrile neutropenic patients and for *Clostridium difficile* infections must be undertaken with caution, in hopes of reversing the recent trends in nosocomial infections due to vancomycin-resistant enterococci. Similarly, the use of multiple antibiotics for selective decontamination of digestive tracts in intensive care units should be limited to the situations where clear benefit has been shown.

REFERENCES

Andre Gordon, C.L. and Ahmad, M.H. (1991) Thermal susceptibility of *Streptococcus faecium* strains isolated from frankfurters. *Canadian Journal of Microbiology*, **37**, 609–612.

Arthur, M. and Courvalin, S.P. (1993) Genetics and mechanisms of glycopeptide resistance in enterococci. *Antimicrobial Agents and Chemotherapy*, **37**, 1563–1571.

Boyce, J.M., Opal, S.M., Potter-Bynoe, G. et al. (1992) Emergence and nosocomial transmission of ampicillin-resistant enterococci. *Antimicrobial Agents and Chemotherapy*, **36**, 1032–1039.

Clewell, D.B. and Weaver, K.E. (1989) Sex pheromones and plasmid transfer in *Enterococcus faecalis*. *Plasmid*, **21**, 175–184.

Collins, M.D., Farrow, J.A. and Jones, D. (1986) *Enterococcus mundtii* sp. nov. *International Journal of Systematic Bacteriology*, **36**, 8–12.

Costa, Y., Galimand, M., Leclercq, R. et al. (1993) Characterization of the chromosomal *aac(6')-Ii* gene specific for *Enterococcus faecium*. *Antimicrobial Agents and Chemotherapy*, **37**, 1896–1903.

Coudron, P.E., Mayhall, C.G., Facklam, R.R. et al. (1984) *Streptococcus faecium* outbreak in a neonatal intensive care unit. *Journal of Clinical Microbiology*, **20**, 1044–1048.

Coudron, P.E., Markowitz, S.M. and Wong, E.S. (1992) Isolation of a β-lactamase-producing, aminoglycoside-resistant strain of *Enterococcus faecium*. *Antimicrobial Agents and Chemotherapy*, **36**, 1125–1126.

Daly, J.A., Clifton, N.L., Seskin, K.C. et al. (1991) Use of rapid, nonradioactive DNA probes in culture confirmation tests to detect *Streptococcus agalactiae*, *Haemophilus influenzae*, and *Enterococcus* spp. from pediatric patients with significant infections. *Journal of Clinical Microbiology*, **29**, 80–82.

Devriese, L.A., Ceyssens, K., Rodrigues, U.M. et al. (1990) *Enterococcus columbae*, a species from pigeon intestines. *FEMS Microbiology Letters*, **71**, 247–252.

Domenech, A., Prieta, J., Fernandez-Garayzabal, J.F. et al. (1993) Phenotypic and phylogenetic evidence for a close relationship between *Lactococcus garvieae* and *Enterococcus seriolicida*. *Microbiologia*, **9**, 63–68.

Eliopoulos, G.M. (1993) Aminoglycoside resistant enterococcal endocarditis. *Infectious Disease Clinics of North America*, **7**, 117–133.

Emori, T.G. and Gaynes, R.P. (1993) An overview of nosocomial infection, including the role of the microbiology laboratory. *Clinical Microbiology Reviews*, **6**, 428–442.

Facklam, R.R. and Collins, M.D. (1989) Identification of *Enterococcus* species isolated from human infections by a conventional test scheme. *Journal of Clinical Microbiology*, **27**, 731–734.

Facklam, R.R. and Sahm, D.A. (1995) The enterococci. In *ASM Manual of Clinical Microbiology*, 6th edn. ASM Press, Washington, DC (in press).

Facklam, R.R., Hollis, D. and Collins, M.D. (1989) Identification of Gram-positive coccal and coccobacillary vancomycin-resistant bacteria. *Journal of Clinical Microbiology*, **27**, 724–730.

Ferretti, J.J., Gilmore, K.S. and Courvalin, P. (1986) Nucleotide sequence analysis of the gene specifying the bifunctional 6'-aminoglycoside acetyltransferase 2"-aminoglycoside phosphotransferase enzyme in *Streptococcus faecalis* and identification and cloning of gene regions specifying the two activities. *Journal of Bacteriology*, **167**, 631–638.

Fontana, R., Amalfitano, G., Rossi, L. et al. (1992) Mechanisms of resistance to growth inhibition and killing by β-lactam antibiotics in enterococci. *Clinical Infectious Diseases*, **15**, 486–489.

Garcia de Fernando, G.D., Hernandez, P.E., Burgos, J. et al. (1991) Extracellular proteinase from *Enterococcus faecalis* subsp. *liquefaciens*. *Folia Microbiologica*, **36**, 423–428.

Gorbach, S.L. (1993) Treatment of intra-abdominal infections. *Journal of Antimicrobial Chemotherapy*, **31** (Suppl A), 67–78.

Graninger, W. and Ragette, R. (1992) Nosocomial bacteremia due to *Enterococcus faecalis* without endocarditis. *Clinical Infectious Diseases*, **15**, 49–57.

Grayson, M.L., Eliopoulos, G.M., Wennersten, C.B. *et al.* (1991a) Comparison of *Enterococcus raffinosus* with *Enterococcus avium* on the basis of penicillin susceptibility, penicillin-binding protein analysis, and high-level aminoglycoside resistance. *Antimicrobial Agents and Chemotherapy*, **35**, 1408–1412.

Grayson, M.L., Eliopoulos, G.M., Wennersten, C.B. *et al.* (1991b) Increasing resistance to β-lactam antibiotics among clinical isolates of *Enterococcus faecium*: a 22-year review at one institution. *Antimicrobial Agents and Chemotherapy*, **35**, 2180–2184.

Handwerger, S., Raucher, B., Altarac, D. *et al.* (1993) Nosocomial outbreak due to *Enterococcus faecium* highly resistant to vancomycin, penicillin and gentamicin. *Clinical Infectious Diseases* **16**, 750–755.

Herztein, J., Ryan, J.L., Mangi, R.J. *et al.* (1984) Optimal therapy for enterococcal endocarditis. *American Journal of Medicine*, **76**, 186–191.

Hodel-Christian, S.L. and Murray, B.E. (1991) Characterization of the gentamicin resistance transposon Tn*5281* from *Enterococcus faecalis* and comparison to staphylococcal transposons Tn*4001* and Tn*4031*. *Antimicrobial Agents and Chemotherapy*, **35**, 1147–1152.

Hodges, T.L., Zighelboim-Daum, S., Eliopoulos, G.M. *et al.* (1992) Antimicrobial susceptibility changes in *Enterococcus faecalis* following various penicillin exposure regimens. *Antimicrobial Agents and Chemotherapy*, **36**, 121–125.

Huycke, M.M., Spiegel, C.A. and Gilmore, M.S. (1991) Bacteremia caused by hemolytic, high-level gentamicin-resistant *Enterococcus faecalis*. *Antimicrobial Agents and Chemotherapy*, **35**, 1626–1634.

Ike, Y., Hashimoto, H. and Clewell, D.B. (1984) Hemolysin of *Streptococcus faecalis* subspecies *zymogenes* contributes to virulence in mice. *Infection and Immunity*, **45**, 528–530.

Klare, I., Rodloff, A.C., Wagner, J. *et al.* (1992) Overproduction of a penicillin-binding protein is not the only mechanism of penicillin resistance in *Enterococcus faecium*. *Antimicrobial Agents and Chemotherapy*, **36**, 783–787.

Knudtson, L.M. and Hartman, P.A. (1992) Routine procedures for isolation and identification of enterococci and fecal streptococci. *Applied and Environmental Microbiology*, **58**, 3027–3031.

Korten, V. and Murray, B.E. (1993) The nosocomial transmission of enterococci. *Current Opinion in Infectious Diseases*, **6**, 498–505.

Kreft, B., Marre, R., Schramm, U. *et al.* (1992) Aggregation substance of *Enterococcus faecalis* mediates adhesions to cultured renal tubular cells. *Infection and Immunity*, **60**, 25–30.

Leclercq, R., Dutka-Malen, S., Brisson-Noel, A. *et al.* (1992) Resistance of enterococci to aminoglycosides and glycopeptides. *Clinical Infectious Diseases*, **15**, 495–501.

Maki, D.G. and Agger, W.A. (198) Enterococcal bacteremia: clinical features, the risk of endocarditis, and management. *Medicine*, **67**, 248–269.

Martinez-Murcia, A.J. and Collins, M.D. (1991) *Enterococcus sulfureus*, a new yellow-pigmented *Enterococcus* species. *FEMS Microbiology Letters*, **80**, 69–74.

Megran, D.W. (1992) Enterococcal endocarditis. *Clinical Infectious Diseases*, **15**, 63–71.

Morrison, A.J., Jr and Wenzel, R.P. (1986) Nosocomial urinary tract infections due to enterococcus: ten years' experience at a university hospital. *Archives of Internal Medicine*, **146**, 1549–1551.

Murray, B.E. (1990) The life and times of the enterococcus. *Clinical Microbiology Reviews*, **3**, 46–65.

Murray, B.E. (1992) β-Lactamase-producing enterococci. *Antimicrobial Agents and Chemotherapy*, **36**, 2355–2359.

Murray, B.E., Singh, K.V., Ross, R.P. *et al.* (1993) Generation of restriction map of *Enterococcus faecalis* OG1 and investigation of growth requirements and regions encoding biosynthetic function. *Journal of Bacteriology*, **175**, 5216–5223.

National Committee for Clinical Laboratory Standards (1993a) Performance standards for antimicrobial disk susceptibility tests. Approved standard M2-A5. National Committee for Clinical Laboratory Standards, Villanova, PA.

National Committee for Clinical Laboratory Standards (1993b) Methods for antimicrobial susceptibility tests for bacteria that grow aerobically. Approved standard M7-A3. National Committee for Clinical Laboratory Standards, Villanova, PA.

Nichols, R.L. and Muzik, A.C. (1992) Enterococcal infections in surgical patients: the mystery continues. *Clinical Infectious Diseases*, **15**, 72–76.

Pallares, R., Pujol, M., Pena, C. *et al.* (1993) Cephalosporins as risk factor for nosocomial *Enterococcus faecalis* bacteremia: a matched case–control study. *Archives of Internal Medicine*, **153**, 1581–1586.

Patterson, J.E. and Zervos, M.J. (1990) High-level gentamicin resistance in *Enterococcus*: microbiology, genetic basis, and epidemiology. *Reviews of Infectious Diseases*, **12**, 644–652.

Pompei, R., Berlutti, F., Thaller, M.C. *et al.* (1992) *Enterococcus flavescens* sp. nov., a new species of enterococci of clinical origin. *International Journal of Systematic Bacteriology*, **42**, 365–369.

Rice, L.B. and Marshall, S.H. (1992) Evidence of incorporation of the chromosomal β-lactamase gene of *Enterococcus faecalis* CH19 into a transposon derivated from staphylococci. *Antimicrobial Agents and Chemotherapy*, **36**, 1843–1846.

Rice, L.B., Calderwood, S.B., Eliopoulos, G.M. *et al.* (1991) Enterococcal endocarditis: a comparison of prosthetic and native valve disease. *Reviews of Infectious Diseases*, **13**, 1–7.

Rodrigues, U. and Collins, M.D. (1990) Phylogenetic analysis of *Streptococcus saccharolyticus* based on 16S rRNA sequencing. *FEMS Microbiology Letters*, **71**, 231–234.

Ruoff, K.L., De La Maza, L., Murtagh, M.J. *et al.* (1990) Species identities of enterococci isolated from clinical specimens. *Journal of Clinical Microbiology*, **28**, 435–437.

Sanchez, M.L., Barrett, M.S. and Jones, R.N. (1992) Use of the E test to predict high-level resistance to aminoglycosides among enterococci. *Journal of Clinical Microbiology*, **30**, 3030–3032.

Schaberg, D.R., Culver, D.H. and Gaynes, R.P. (1991) Major trends in the microbial etiology of nosocomial infection. *American Journal of Medicine*, **91** (Suppl 3B), 72–75.

Schleifer, K.H. and Kilpper-Bälz, R. (1984) Transfer to *Streptococcus faecalis* and *Streptococcus faecium* to the genus *Enterococcus* nom. rev. as *Enterococcus faecalis* comb. nov. and *Enterococcus faecium* comb. nov. *International Journal of Systematic Bacteriology*, **34**, 31–34.

Schmit, J.L. (1992) Efficacy of teicoplanin for enterococcal infections: 63 cases and review. *Clinical Infectious Diseases*, **15**, 302–306.

Sherman, J.M. (1937) The streptococci. *Bacteriology Reviews*, **1**, 3–97.

Swenson, J.M., Ferraro, M.J., Sahm, D.F. *et al.* (1992) New vancomycin disk diffusion breakpoints for enterococci. The National Committee for Clinical Laboratory Standards Working Group on Enterococci. *Journal of Clinical Microbiology*, **30**, 2525–2528.

Vincent, S., Knight, R.G., Green, M. *et al.* (1991) Vancomycin susceptibility and identification of motile enterococci. *Journal of Clinical Microbiology*, **29**, 2335–2337.

Weissmann, D., Spargo, J., Wennersten, C. *et al.* (1991) Detection of enterococcal high-level aminoglycoside resistance with MicroScan freeze-dried panels containing newly modified medium and Vitek gram-positive susceptibility cards. *Journal of Clinical Microbiology*, **29**, 1232–1235.

Williams, A.M., Farrow, J.A.E. and Collins, M.D. (1989) Reverse transcriptase sequencing of 16S ribosomal RNA from *Streptococcus cecorum*. *Letters in Applied Microbiology*, **8**, 185–189.

Williams, A.M., Rodrigues, U.M. and Collins, M.D. (1991) Intrageneric relationships of enterococci as determined by reverse transcriptase sequencing of small-subunit rRNA. *Research in Microbiology*, **142**, 67–74.

2a

STAPHYLOCOCCUS AUREUS

Barry D. Cookson

HISTORICAL INTRODUCTION

The name *Staphylococcus* was first given to the grape-like clusters of cocci seen in abscesses by Sir James Ogston in 1881. However, Rosenbach was officially credited for the name, because although he described the genus four years later, he complied with the subsequent rules of the first bacteriological code in 1948. Rosenbach had pointed out the variable pigment production of staphylococci, but undue importance is still given to this property and that of pathogenic potential. The importance of the coagulase test, although described by Loeb in 1903, was ignored until the 1930s.

The next 60 years saw the gradual emergence of a family, the Micrococcaceae. This now contains four genera (*Planococcus*, *Micrococcus*, *Staphylococcus* and *Aerococcus*) which share little other than their external appearance. Modern methods of taxonomy have confirmed that *S. aureus* is related to the other staphylococci, of which there are now 28 species and many subspecies or ill-described variants, and that they are probably in the *Lactobacillus–Streptococcus–Staphylococcus* group. The reader is referred to Chapter 2b for detailed discussion of the coagulase-negative staphylococci.

Staphylococcus aureus became recognized in the first half of the twentieth century as the major cause of postoperative sepsis. Altemeier *et al.* (1981), for example between 1930 and 1939, observed that 60–65% of postoperative noso-comial surgical infections were due to *S. aureus*. In this review these workers list 56 different septic conditions caused by the bacterium, although endocarditis is omitted. A 90% mortality was observed in staphylococcal septicaemia in the pre-antibiotic era and its epidemic potential was also recognized.

DESCRIPTION OF THE ORGANISM

General Properties

Staphylococcus aureus is an aerobic and faculta-tively anaerobic non-motile Gram-positive coccus with an average diameter of 0.5–1.5 μm. The organism divides in a number of planes producing irregular grape-like clusters. In fluid media the cocci may appear as singletons, pairs and even in chains. Many isolates (particularly from clinical specimens) have a capsule, but in some this is in the form of a microcapsule.

The most useful identifying biochemical fea-tures are extracellular and cell wall-bound protein A, cell-bound clumping factor and extracellular coagulase and heat-stable nuclease. It is catalase

Principles and Practice of Clinical Bacteriology. Edited by A.M. Emmerson, P.M. Hawkey and S.H. Gillespie
© 1997 John Wiley & Sons Ltd

positive, has teichoic acid in the cell wall and glycine as the interpeptide bridge of the peptidoglycan. The G + C content is approximately 35%, it lacks cytochromes c and d, and has MK6–8 as the major menaquinones. The latter properties distinguish all staphylococci from *Micrococcus* spp.

Carbohydrates and/or amino acids are used as carbon and energy sources. A variety of carbohydrates (including glucose) are used aerobically with the production of acetate and carbon dioxide. The requirement for different amino acids can be changed by subculture on minimal media. These requirements and others for various vitamins have been used to biotype *S. aureus* and *S. intermedius*.

Pigment is due to the production of carotenoids in the cell membrane. There are many different types described and this accounts, in part, for the many different colonial colours.

Protein A

This protein is responsible for the agglutination of most strains by all normal human sera and is due to non-specific combination with the Fc portion of some human IgGs, IgAs and IgM.

Free coagulase

Coagulase clots plasma in the absence of calcium, but it does not clot purified fibrinogen unless a coagulase-reacting factor (CRF) is present. CRF varies in type and specificity, and is similar but not identical to prothrombin. Coagulase enables the organism to grow in serum and to resist phagocytosis and produces disseminated intravascular coagulation. However, coagulase-negative mutants are no less virulent than their parent strains.

Bound coagulase (clumping factor)

Provided organisms are easily emulsified, this factor provides a useful, rapid means of identifying *S. aureus*, although up to 12% of strains, including methicillin-resistant *S. aureus* (MRSA), are negative. It can be obscured by large capsules and differs from free coagulase in that it only requires fibrinogen.

Susceptibility to Physical and Chemical Agents

Growth can occur at a wide range of temperatures (10–45 °C) and pH (4–9); it is optimal at 37 °C and pH 7–7.5. The organism is killed at 60 °C in 30 minutes. It is quite resistant to freezing and drying and can survive for six months on sealed agar tubes or threads. It will grow on high concentrations of salt (hence the affinity to the secretions of patients with cystic fibrosis) or sucrose. It is highly susceptible to many disinfectants, such as chlorhexidine, triclosan, iodine and hexachlorophane, as well as aniline dyes. Lysostaphin (but not lysozyme) and fatty acids such as linoleic acid are highly active against *S. aureus*.

PATHOGENICITY OF *S. AUREUS*

The ability to produce disease by different strains of *S. aureus* is, as for other organisms, the result of the interaction between the organism, the patient and numerous factors in the environment. Although certain organism factors are associated with specific conditions (e.g. exfoliative toxins and scalded skin syndrome), despite an enormous number of studies we are still unable to determine the true basis of *S. aureus* virulence. The same can be said for the determinants of *S. aureus* epidemicity. Virulence was certainly never defined convincingly for the phage 80/81 pandemic clone and its descendants, which were generally agreed to be virulent.

Virulence and epidemicity may well be unrelated, in that there are examples of epidemic strains of organisms that have established themselves on certain units and have caused little or no disease (Lacey, 1987).

Studies of isolates from human lesions and others in various animal models have given conflicting information and it is most probable that many factors combine to product a 'shock' environment around the organism. A mouse model, for instance, demonstrated that skin necrosis was related to α-toxin production by certain strains of *S. aureus*. However, other strains that could produce enormous amounts of this toxin were unable to persist or metabolize *in vivo* and were avirulent in this model.

The bacterial inoculum required to produce a pustule in skin is thought to be about 6 million cfu. This perhaps explains why infection is commoner in nasal carriers, who are likely to produce greater contamination of their skin than those who acquire it from other sources. This inoculum can be reduced by 4 logs if a suture is in place and even further if the suture encompasses necrotic tissue. Moisture and the presence of serum exudates encourage a skin lesion to develop. In a skin-stripping model a few hundred organisms can produce a spreading cellulitis, provided the organisms are applied within 24 hours of the procedure. Other experiments in skin models have shown that the presence of leucocytes and competing organisms can reduce the capacity to produce disease.

Some of the virulence factors are listed in Table 2a.1 and will be outlined briefly below.

Resistance to Phagocytosis

Staphylococcal disease is commoner in a number of conditions which inhibit the phagocytic

TABLE 2a.1 VIRULENCE FACTORS OF *S. AUREUS*

Coagulase and other exoenzymes such as DNAase, hyaluronidase, lipases, phosphatase, proteases, staphylokinase

Toxins
α, β, γ and δ leucocidin, exfoliatin, toxic shock protein (TSST-1), exfoliative toxins A and B, enterotoxin, pyrogenic exotoxins

Cellular surface proteins such as lipoteichoic acid, clumping factor, protein A, capsule (serotypes 5 and 8 in particular)

Receptors for binding, e.g. fibronectin, fibrinogen, thrombospondin, tissue-binding receptors to, for example, endothelial cells

Superantigens (e.g. TSST-1, enterotoxin)

Catalase

Hydrophobicity

Resistance to desiccation

response (e.g. Job's syndrome, chronic granulomatous disease, diabetes mellitus) and this is clearly an important factor. A number of *S. aureus* factors (cell-free coagulase, cell wall-associated aggressins, capsule and protein A) are said to assist in the resistance to phagoctosis but the evidence for some of these is conflicting.

Lipase Production

Almost all organisms that are isolated from boils produce lipases that are active on Tween 80 and egg yolk agar (produce opacity). It is thought that the conversion of the 80/81 clone to non-virulence was related to the loss of lipase activity. However, other factors are also thought to be important, in that some lipase producers from postoperative infected patients have not caused boils. Lipase, like hyaluronidase, might enable the organism or other toxic products to spread in tissues.

General Extracellular Toxins

Staphylococcus aureus produces several general toxic substances that may contribute to pathogenesis of local or general disease.

Haemolytic Toxins

Four such toxins are produced; they differ in their ability to damage different species of animal blood cells.

α-Lysin

This lyses rabbit, human and sheep erythrocytes, produces necrosis upon intradermal injection and, when injected intravenously in certain animals, produces many profound effects (abnormal EEG changes, damage to blood vessels, paralysis of muscles, liberation of catecholamines, renal damage and death). It is also lethal to some species' white blood cells. Almost all human *S. aureus* and fewer animal isolates produce it, although serological responses are not always seen following deep human sepsis. Animal models would support a role for the toxin being important in producing necrosis and facilitating invasiveness.

β-Lysin

This is a phospholipase C which acts on sphingomyelin and lysolecithin. It acts on a variety of blood cells such as sheep, but not rabbit or human erythrocytes. It produces 'hot–cold' haemolysis, i.e. damage is only observed when the exposed cells are cooled, potentiated by pH or osmotic pressure, or exposure to toxins produced by group B streptococci (the CAMP test). A minority of human (approximately 10%) and many animal strains produce this lysin. It can be switched off by phage insertion, as can lipase production along with the gaining of enterotoxin A and staphylokinase production (Coleman et al., 1989).

γ-Lysin

This is inactive against horse erythrocytes but active against those of human, rabbit and sheep. It is a leucocidin and can be lethal when injected into animals. Serological response to it may be useful in diagnosis.

δ-Haemolysin

This is produced by most human strains of S. aureus (approximately 99%). It has the widest lytic spectrum for erythrocytes, it is a leucocidin, a dermonecrotic agent and appears to regulate other haemolysin production.

Leucocidin (Panton Valentine toxin)

This also produces dermonecrosis and comprises two factors.

Specific Toxins

Epidermolytic toxins

There are two such toxins (ETA and ETB), both high-molecular-weight proteins. ETA is heat stable and chromosomal in origin; ETB is probably plasmid controlled (a bacteriocin plasmid which is also evident in ETA isolates) and is heat labile. Phage group II organisms are usually implicated and both or either toxins can be carried. Both toxins cause separation of cells in the stratum granulosum of the skin.

Enterotoxins

Staphylococcus aureus can produce seven antigenically distinct enterotoxins (A to E, including C1, C2 and C3). About 40% of strains produce one or more of these toxins. They produce emesis by stimulating the vomiting centre via the vagus nerve. In addition, the toxins are pyrogenic, mitogenic, produce hypotension and thrombocytopenia and can also damage tissue culture cells. Enterotoxin B is also associated with lethal staphylococcal disease (see below) and as such is more often found in organisms of phage group V. Recently, Arbuthnott and co-workers found that enterotoxin and TSST-1 production were more frequent than expected in septicaemia cases compared with strains from healthy carriers (Arbuthnott et al., 1990).

Toxic shock toxin (TSST-1)

Formally named enterotoxin F, this toxin is a protein of molecular weight approximately 2200. Production is decreased in anaerobic conditions. It is a pyrogen, releases interleukin 1 (IL-1) and is a superantigen. Most producers are of phage group I and lysed by phages 29 or 52. Numerous animal models for development of TSST-1 have suggested mechanisms of toxin action, though the exact molecular action is not known. Other toxins are also associated with toxic shock (see below) and have similar modes of action in that they are all potent pyrogens, induce T lymphocyte proliferation, require IL-1 release from macrophages, suppress immunoglobulin production, enhance endotoxin shock, and produce hypersensitivity skin reactions.

Superantigens

Superantigens (e.g. TSST-1, enterotoxin) are restricted to Gram-positive organisms and are polyclonal stimulators of T cells that are independent of antigen processing, class II major histocompatibility restriction or specific T cell receptors. They cause massive lymphokine release (IL-1, interferon and tumour necrosis factor). In severe invasive infection and non-menstrual and menstrual toxic shock, this activity manifests itself in multi-organ failure.

Antibiotic Resistance and Virulence

Another highly disputed area is that of the virulence of antibiotic-resistant strains. Workers have shown increases and decreases phenotypically in a number of the above factors in such strains. In addition, there is often no correlation with pathogenicity in animal models or changes in other properties such as formation of soluble products, or alterations in survival on glass or membrane polypeptides. MRSA has been examined by many workers and, although certain trends are described, e.g. to produce low levels of protein A and high levels of coagulase, there are always exceptions that prove the rule. The generally accepted view is that MRSA, although not a primary pathogen, can be as virulent as susceptible *S. aureus* (MSSA), but there is a wide spectrum of virulence in both (Cookson and Phillips, 1990).

NORMAL HABITAT

Staphylococcus aureus is a human commensal and pathogen, although biovars of it are found in cattle and chickens. Other coagulase-positive staphylococci are described; *S. intermedius*, a commensal and pathogen of dogs but also isolated from pet owners, *S. hyicus* a skin commensal of cattle and pigs (causing disease in piglets) and, most recently described, *S. delphini* has been recovered in pus from dolphin cutaneous lesions. The coagulase and heat-stable nucleases from these organisms are serologically distinct. There are also differences in protein A, biochemistry, location and in the proportion of positive strains.

The major habitat for *S. aureus* in humans is the anterior nares; carriage rates vary between 10% and 40%. Carriage is lower in primitive people.

Identical/non-identical twin and human leucocyte antigen (HLA) studies would indicate that there are genetic factors which can affect carriage (Noble, 1993). Carriage varies with age; it is high in the first two weeks (60–90%), declining to 20% at the end of the first year, rising again to reach the adult level by five to eight years of age and then declining again in old age to about 20%.

Carriage increases with increasing lengths of hospital stay and is also higher in hospital staff. Other parts of the body have lower carriage rates (<10%, e.g. throat, perineum, groin and axilla). However, there are large discrepancies in such studies. Throat carriage has varied between 4% and 64%; it is probably an important source of relapse following attempts to eradicate nasal carriage with topical antibiotics. Faecal carriage is related to nasal carriage. Perhaps 20% of patients carry small numbers of organisms; carriage can be detected very intermittently. Sampling of the perineum must be performed thoroughly as 'hot spots' of carriage are described. Hair and finger carriage is said to reflect dispersion of the organism. Skin disease, such as eczema, psoriasis and dermatitis, results in increased skin carriage.

Carriage can be intermittent (30–70%) or permanent (10–40%) for the organism or a strain. In some cases intermittent nasal acquisition has been shown from another site on the same subject or from a close contact. Interference with the non-staphylococcal flora by antibiotics appears to increase the likelihood of acquisition of *S. aureus*.

The incidence of carriage may vary in different studies for a variety of methodological reasons. The usual sampling method is to rub a moistened swab over the surface to be examined and then to smear it over a Petri dish with blood agar, serum agar, or media containing salt, e.g. salt mannitol. Some advocate the use of carbon-containing swabs or transport media if there is to be a delay of several hours before culture. Many broth enrichment methods have been used in the food industry; the medium of Baird Parker is the most popular but, although it does contain pyruvate which stimulates the recuperation of stressed bacterial cells exposed to high or low temperatures, it is only slightly selective for *S. aureus*.

Most investigators in medical microbiology have chosen a salt-containing medium for *S. aureus* detection. The choice would appear logical for unstressed bacteria from human sites, although not perhaps for sampling the environment. Broth methods will increase detection of *S. aureus* carriage but also the detection of transient carriers; it can be particularly cost effective in outbreak situations as more than one swab can be processed in the same broth (Cookson, 1990).

Sources and Routes of Transmission

Most *S. aureus* infection is endogenous. However, particularly in hospitals and perhaps some institutions, acquisition occurs after direct contact with hands of staff transiently or otherwise carrying the organism (Cookson *et al.*, 1989). In some recent studies MRSA acquisition occurred in the wounds of some (but not all) patients before the nose was colonized.

A more contentious issue is the role of the environment and airborne transmission. The survival of the organism in the environment is better than for Gram-negative rods, but the weight of evidence points to organisms becoming non-infectious after 24 hours. Some investigators have found the immediate environment to be heavily contaminated and that, in such circumstances, certain articles such as sphygmomanometers and bed mattresses may act as fomites.

Airborne spread from exudates or skin scales is thought to be important in certain settings, such as dermatology or burns wards. The median diameter of particles carrying the organism is 12 μm (range 4–24 μm). This was perhaps more important, historically, when the ventilation in operating theatres was suboptimal. The dispersion of *S. aureus* by normal people occurs rarely, and is a very variable and unpredictable phenomenon. Males disseminate more often than females and the lower half of the body is more important than the upper. The number of organisms isolated from a person or any one site is a poor predictor of the ability to disperse (Blowers *et al.*, 1973).

Most of the recent data on *S. aureus* acquisition relates to studies of MRSA infection and colonization. There are many risk factors that have been described for such spread (see Table 2a.2 and we still do not know why certain MRSA strains appear to have a greater epidemic potential than others. The introduction of MRSA to a hospital (and presumably on occasion susceptible *S. aureus*) is now known to occur after international transfer of patients and, less often, hospital staff. Such spread more often occurs between hospitals in the same country or city. More recently in the UK, but for several years in the USA, elderly care and nursing homes have been implicated as reservoirs and sources of outbreaks in hospitals. Spread within a hospital is facilitated if there are frequent transfers of patients and, on occasion, staff between wards.

TABLE 2a.2 FACTORS THAT AFFECT THE SPREAD OF AN MRSA

Patient factors
Case mix, e.g. severity of illness, pressure sores, catheter use, antibiotics

Intensity of patient care and length of hospital stay

Staff
Numbers, morale, skills, attitudes, workloads, agency staff usage

Wards implicated
Intensive care units, neonatal intensive care units, burns units, elderly care, surgical, mixed medical and surgical

Other hospital factors
Size and whether a teaching hospital

Availability of isolation facilities

Patient referral patterns; transfers intra- and inter-hospital, inter-country and readmissions

Infection control
Resources, policies (including antibiotic prescribing), practice, surveillance and audit activities

Nursing or elderly care homes
Whether affected, numbers of transfers and their standards of infection control

CLINICAL FEATURES

Predisposing Conditions

All *S. aureus* infections occur more frequently in males than in females, with the exception of mastitis. There are several conditions that predispose to infection and these are outlined where relevant below.

Diseases of the Skin and Subcutaneous Tissues

Impetigo

This is characterized by blisters or golden crusts and is commoner in patients in the first two decades of life. In many parts of the world it is now a commoner cause than the group A *Streptococcus*, although the two do occur together in mixed infections in about a third of cases. The condition can be particularly aggressive in AIDS patients, with extensive intertriginous bullous lesions.

Exacerbations and colonization of skin conditions

The skin of many patients with a variety of skin conditions such as atopic eczema, dermatitis and, to a lesser extent, psoriasis is heavily colonized with *S. aureus*. This may be due to lipases in exudates destroying the protective action of skin lipids or these being deficient *per se*. Colonization is usually asymptomatic but exacerbations (exudative or impetiginous lesions) can be associated with an increase in the *S. aureus* numbers, and topical antiseptics appear to help the condition.

Boils and carbuncles

Diabetes mellitus predisposes to boils and especially carbuncles. Sties occur particularly in stressed individuals, and sycosis barbae is commoner in individuals with curly hair. Pressure and minor trauma result in an increased risk of boils. *Staphylococcus aureus* can also cause paronychia and sometimes deeper abscesses, e.g. in the breast or axilla.

Boils occur more frequently under the age of 40, with peaks in the first decade and the third decade, perhaps due to transmission from infected children. In general practice the same organisms are found in the nose and boils, particularly of the head and neck. In the 1950s and 1960s organisms of phage 52, 52A, 80, 81 complex caused boils in patients and staff. Whereas family infection was commoner following patients discharged from hospital in the 1950s, this is now uncommon. Recent MRSA studies have shown that familial spread, although unusual, may be commoner for certain strains.

Wound, burns and device-related infections

Colonization of traumatic lesions, burns or surgical infection is often as common as infection. Colonization may not result in delayed healing or even the rejection of grafts, although many surgeons prefer to see it eliminated before attempting such procedures. Traumatic, thermal or surgical wounds (see associated risk factors under 'Prevention', below) can be infected with *S. aureus*. Indeed, in most studies *S. aureus* is the commonest single agent causing surgical wound infection and accounts for between 33% and 50% of such infections, depending on the type of surgery and other factors. Haemodialysis and peritoneal dialysis patients have significantly more shunt or exit site infection if they are nasal carriers. Some authorities have advocated the continuous prophylactic use of nasal antiseptics such as mupirocin, although resistance is emerging in some centres.

Scalded skin syndrome

This has to be distinguished from another cause of 'toxic epidermal necrolysis' due to drug reactions. The organisms which cause this condition are usually of phage group II and carry either or both ETA or ETB toxins (see above). These toxins cause the separation of cells in the stratum granulosum of the skin and result in the splitting of the upper layers of the skin and the pathognomonic Nikolsky's sign, where the skin can be rubbed away by gentle pressure with the finger. Abscess formation is rare. The condition is often seen in infants or neonates and also in children between one and two years of age. Perhaps the remaining 20% of cases are adult patients, a few of whom are immunosuppressed. The condition was described by Ritter and Lyell and is a dermatological emergency. Acute toxaemia and death will ensue unless the correct antibiotic therapy is commenced (see below). Interestingly, large numbers of staphylococci may not be seen in the lesions as the toxin can act at some distance from their site of multiplication.

Necrotizing fasciitis

Staphylococcus aureus can, like group A β-haemolytic streptococci, occasionally cause this condition. It can follow superficial lesions and trauma, including surgery. There is widespread destruction of subcutaneous tissues and ulceration of the skin. Toxaemia is evident and rapid death can follow. Treatment is with surgery and antibiotics (see below).

Urinary Tract Infections

Cystitis and pyelonephritis are rare and nosocomially rather than community acquired. They follow catheterization or other manipulations or surgery of the urological tract. Although uncommon, they often result in septicaemia and renal or perinephric abscesses. The asymptomatic isolation of the organism from the urine during septicaemia is a common but unexplained finding.

Osteomyelitis

Staphylococcus aureus is the commonest cause of acute and chronic osteomyelitis. The condition often follows rather minor trauma, and transient bacteraemia is thought to result in localization of the organism, causing pain, tenderness, fever, malaise and subsequent infection (anachoresis).

Once established, bacteraemia is usually evident. Although mainly a disease of children it can occur at all ages. It sometimes affects the vertebrae, more often in adults, where it may present as pain and little else.

Septic Arthritis

Infection can occur at all ages and in previously normal joints. However, it more commonly occurs in chronic arthritis treated with steroids. It is often mistaken as an acute flare-up of the underlying inflammatory condition. Gram stain and culture of the aspirate are usually required to establish the proper diagnosis.

Respiratory Infection

Invasion of the lungs can occur in various groups of patients:

(1) Young infants. Immediate mortality is high, as are complications such as empyaema, lung abscess and pneumocystocoeles evident upon X-ray. Respiratory viruses or measle infection predisposes to pneumonia in young children.
(2) Post influenza. This seems to occur in healthy adults, although the pneumococcus is probably a commoner pathogen overall in this situation. Data are scarce. The condition follows extensive damage of the lower tract by the virus. Massive invasion with *S. aureus* ensues, resulting in rapid onset of profuse watery and blood-stained sputum; death can occur within two days and even in a matter of hours.
(3) As an opportunist in patients suffering from other disease. In recent years it has become evident that *S. aureus* is a far commoner cause of ventilator-associated pneumonia than many had suspected.

Another condition that has been recently recognized in young children and perhaps adults is that of *S. aureus* tracheitis. It is said to mimic the viral condition and is very difficult to diagnose with certainty.

Clinical Significance of *S. aureus* in Cystic Fibrosis

Staphylococcus aureus is usually the initial bacterial pathogen detected in the respiratory secretions of cystic fibrosis patients. It is probable that colonization follows the initial damage by viral infection of the respiratory epithelial cells. Affinity of staphylococci for salt-enriched cystic fibrosis mucus, mucociliary abnormalities and other factors contribute to persistent colonization, causing progressive pulmonary damage. It may possibly influence subsequent *Pseudomonas aeruginosa* infection. Most of the evidence indicates that aggressive antibiotic management directed against *S. aureus* is essential in all stages of broncho-pulmonary infection. Other strategies are being researched at present, including vaccines, anti-toxins, anti-inflammatory agents, immunomodulators and antibiotic regimens.

Generalized Infections

Infection may spread from superficial lesions, particularly in babies, resulting in lymphangitis and regional lymphadenopathy, subsequent bacteraemia and, on occasion, septicaemia. Transient bacteraemia following perhaps minor lesions is commoner than is thought, as evidenced by osteomyelitis (see above). Abscesses localized to the renal cortex, and others in the spleen and liver, may follow bloodstream invasion.

Septicaemia

Staphylococcus aureus septicaemia probably comprises about 20% of all septicaemias (Gransden *et al.*, 1984). It may occur as a complication of sepsis anywhere in the body or as a primary condition. Underlying conditions include neoplasia, hepatic disease and some extensive skin diseases (see above). It can also follow interventions such as surgery, intravenous or other vascular catheterization. Indeed vascular access site infection accounts for about 20–37% of cases. Infection at the access site may not be apparent, despite the usually severe consequences of the infection. The device has usually been *in situ* for six or more days but for as little as two on occasion. Rheumatoid arthritis, if severe, can result in septicaemia with pyoarthrosis. There is some disagreement as to whether the incidence of septicaemia is higher in diabetes mellitus, although most agree that when sepsis does occur it tends to be more severe and/or prolonged.

Septicaemia can be associated with disseminated intravascular coagulation, thrombocytopenia, glomerulonephritis and peripheral gangrene, and may also result in positive urinary culture (with or without renal involvement) and even meningitis. Mortality varies in different series from 21% to 46%. Mortality is related to the underlying diagnosis and delay in starting appropriate therapy.

Endocarditis

The organism perhaps accounts for a third of all native valve endocarditis, affecting normal or abnormal valves. A toxic middle- or old-aged patient (no age is exempt), often without heart murmurs is initially seen by the physician, who may elicit a history of a mild flu-like illness with or without sterile meningitis and gastrointestinal upset. Valvular destruction can be very rapid, and commensurate with this is the appearance of the more classical features such as a new or changing murmur and a major embolic event. About 10% of cases are nosocomial and follow intravascular cannulation; they are usually right sided. The organism can of course also affect prosthetic valves; early prosthetic valve endocarditis (usually caused by *S. aureus*) appears to have decreased in certain centres.

The condition can follow any septicaemia but is particularly common in intravenous drug addicts. In these it is usually right sided and tricuspid, and has a lower mortality than left-sided endocarditis. In the USA, MRSA community-acquired infections are described in such patients.

Toxic Shock Syndrome

Toxic shock syndrome (TSS) is an acute-onset, multi-organ illness which resembles severe scarlet fever. The syndrome has certain features; all patients have a scarlatiniform rash with fine desquamation of the hands and feet during convalescence, high fever, headache, myalgia, confusion, subcutaneous oedema, vomiting, diarrhoea and profound hypotensive shock. In more severe or undiagnosed cases it may go on to acute renal and or hepatic failure, disseminated intravascular coagulation, peripheral gangrene and death in between 5% and 10% of cases. Microbiological investigations yield positive cultures from a variety of sites but without positive blood cultures. The Centres for Disease Control (CDC) revised the criteria for the clinical classification of staphylococcal bacteraemia as follows:

(1) Confirmed TSS; satisfying all the criteria outlined above.
(2) Probable TSS; where one criterion is missing.
(3) Possible TSS; where two criteria are missing.
(4) Unconfirmed; three criteria missing.
(5) Not TSS; an alternative diagnosis seemed appropriate.
(6) No data; so unclassifiable.
(7) Sudden infant death syndrome (SIDS).

A proportion of cases occurs in menstruating women and is associated with the use of high-absorbency tampons, particularly when these are used continuously or left unchanged for long periods. In Wisconsin in 1980 the incidence was calculated to be 6/10 000 menstruating women per year, but lower rates are thought to have occurred outside the USA. Increasing recognition of the condition has resulted in more non-menstrual cases being described. It is now known that they can follow almost any staphylococcal infection (Bohach et al., 1990).

Staphylococcus aureus strains from cases of toxic shock contain TSST-1, enterotoxin B or enterotoxin C. TSST-1 is associated with menstrual TSS and approximately one-half of non-menstrual cases; the other two toxins cause non-menstrual cases, approximately 40% and <5%, respectively. The three toxins are expressed in culture media under similar environmental conditions and may explain the association of certain tampons with menstrual TSS.

In a recent analysis of seven years of toxic shock cases referred to the Laboratory of Hospital Infection (LHI) (Marples and Wieneke, 1993) it was possible to classify 128 (73 menstrual) as confirmed or probable and 199 (45 menstrual) as possible or unconfirmed. Phage group I strains were associated with the menstrual cases, many of whom (49%) were aged less than 20 and were using non-introducer tampons. It was thought that lack of education and poor hygiene had been contributing factors. The course of the disease was swift and occasionally fatal within a few hours of the first alarm.

There were interesting relationships with phage and toxin type. TSST-1 production was associated with phage group I strains, enterotoxin B with group V and enterotoxin C with phage type 95. Enterotoxin A without TSST-1 was associated with phage group III strains and septicaemia without toxic shock. TSST-1 together with enterotoxin A production was evident in confirmed and possible toxic shock cases. Enterotoxin B was associated with non-menstrual toxic shock missing two of the criteria (perhaps milder forms) and were of local or pneumonic origin (others have associated this with toxic shock from burn infections).

Food Poisoning

Vomiting following ingestion of food in which S. aureus has multiplied with the formation of enterotoxin was described in the late nineteenth century. Enterotoxin A is the commonest toxin implicated in such incidents. The food in 70% of cases is meat or poultry, but many other foods are also implicated, such as trifle and cream cakes. It is usually contaminated by an infected or colonized handler. In some countries the source of the outbreak is produce from cow's milk from a cow with subclinical or clinical mastitis.

Enterotoxin production is optimal at 35–40 °C. The main clinical signs are projectile effortless vomiting, abdominal pain and diarrhoea some two to six hours after ingestion. In severe cases dehydration and collapse can occur.

Severe choleraic diarrhoea was described in the 1950s following the administration of tetracyclines and other antibiotics such as neomycin and chloramphenicol. The faecal flora had been super-colonized with strains resistant to the antibiotic and often producing enterotoxin A or B, although the significance of this is disputed. Dehydration and death often occurred but the condition was curable with the appropriate antibiotic to which the strain was susceptible.

There is little doubt that post-antibiotic colitis is mainly due to *Clostridium difficile*. However, cases (particularly in Japan) have been documented following *S. aureus* infection, where *C. difficile* appears to have been ruled out as the cause. There is some dispute as to whether necrosis of the bowel occurs, as in the clostridial disease.

DIAGNOSIS OF INFECTIONS

Microscopy

Microscopic examination of specimens for Gram-positive cocci in clumps (or on occasion in chains in fluids) may be a useful diagnostic method. Some laboratories are using polymerase chain reaction (PCR) with primers for various genes (e.g. *mec*, staphylococcal nuclease, coagulase or protein A) directly on screening or clinical specimens. Antigen detection in the blood has been attempted, with varying results. In the future, PCR of buffy coat layers of blood samples might be fruitful.

Growth Conditions and Colonial Appearance

Staphylococus aureus grows well on plain nutrient media and forms smooth circular, opaque and often yellow pigmented colonies, about 1–2 mm in diameter after 16–24 hours incubation at 37 °C. Pigment is not formed in fluid culture, and on solid culture it can vary with incubation conditions such as exposure to an anaerobic environment and light, age of culture, storage at low temperatures and number of subcultures. It is thought that non-pigmented strains are more susceptible to drying and survive less well at colonized sites. If heavily capsulated they will appear mucoid. In general the colonies are easy to emulsify. On MacConkey's agar, the colonies are small and pale pink at 24 hours and deep pink at 48 hours. Other media such as phenolphthalein phosphate agar is recommended for use in environmental studies, as it aids the recovery of physically damaged organisms.

Cell wall-deficient and other variants

These are occasionally isolated from primary lesions or more often from patients receiving antibiotic therapy. They produce small colonies on ordinary media, which are often defective in the production of coagulase or other characteristic staphylococcal proteins. Thymidine-dependent strains have been isolated from antibiotic-treated patients with cystic fibrosis.

Interpretation

Interpretation of culture results is more difficult when swabs or specimens arrive from sites where carriage can also occur. Differentiation from coagulase-negative staphylococci is essential and can be achieved with tube coagulase (the gold standard method) or with the less sensitive and/or specific but faster methods such as slide coagulase or latex particles coated with coagulase and/or protein A. Newer methods are undergoing evaluation, such as a rapid method to detect staphylo-coagulase within two hours by a fluorescence test. Because some European MRSA have fewer target sites or thick capsules which may obscure these sites others have advocated the use of latex particles coated with a monoclonal antibody to capsular serotype 5, the commonest serotype found in MRSA (Adams and Van Enk, 1994).

A variety of indicator media have been suggested (e.g. mannitol salt, milk agar, phenolphthalein phosphate agar). Such media can have added appropriate antibiotics (such as methicillin) to facilitate the identification of antibiotic-resistant *S. aureus*.

Serological Diagnosis

Some clinicians use serology to assist in the diagnosis of deep-seated infections or to chart the response to therapy of certain long-standing conditions such as cystic fibrosis, bone or joint infections. α-Haemolysin response is said to be poor in half of some series of osteomyelitis. Nuclease antibodies may be helpful in such cases. Teichoic acid antibodies have been used more recently, particularly by several Swedish workers, who found it of value in detecting complications of septicaemia such as metastatic abscesses. However, others have had problems with standardization of the method, specificity and the choice of cut-off values to distinguish between normal and abnormal values.

Susceptibility Testing

Staphylococcus aureus is relatively easy to test for susceptibility to antimicrobial agents, although methods for testing against disinfectants are much debated. Disk testing if performed in a standardized manner is satisfactory for most antibiotics. Some laboratories may use breakpoint methods, automated methods or the E-test.

Testing against methicillin requires a lower temperature (30 or 35 °C) or incubation with salt in the medium. In this way any heteroresistant subpopulation can be detected. Isolates producing large quantities of β-lactamase may appear to be resistant to methicillin and so testing against clavulanic acid and a penicillin is recommended. There are still problematic isolates that exhibit intermediate resistance to methicillin; testing against other agents, such as oxacillin, may clarify the situation for these, as may probing with *mec*. Dissociated resistance to clindamycin is usually assumed for all erythromycin-resistant organisms. Mupirocin requires testing against low- and then high-content disks and it might be cost effective to test in future with an E-test or breakpoints.

Phage typing

Fisk first described a set of bacteriophages that could be used to type epidemiologically related strains of *S. aureus* in 1942. The concept was then introduced of a routine test dilution (RTD) in typing, defined as the concentration of phage that produced semi-confluent lysis on the propagating strain. This had to be defined for every phage and every propagation. Williams and Rippon (1952) developed the concept of the two strong difference rule, whereby there was less than a 5% likelihood that two isolates were of common origin if they differed by two strong (>50 plaques) reactions. These workers also introduced 1000 × RTD typing because 40% of their strains were untypeable at RTD. However, this higher concentration produced many inhibition reactions and, although these were occasionally useful in strain identification, they were too susceptible to variations of the initial inoculum of *S. aureus* on the typing plate.

The International Subcommittee on Phage Typing, formed in 1955 to supervise the development of the method and to select a basic set of phages for international use, agreed that the current phage-typing set should consist of 23 phages. The LHI at the Central Public Health Laboratory in Colindale, London, became the WHO Centre in 1961 and since that time has maintained and distributed the phages of the International Basic Set and their propagating strains to national centres. It is generally advised that someone from each centre is trained by the LHI to ensure accurate transfer of the method to new laboratories.

Phage typing is more helpful in the short-term circumscribed outbreak, because in long-continued outbreaks new phage patterns can evolve in a strain, probably because of phage modification, addition or loss. Where a strain has widely disseminated then extensive fieldwork is needed to establish sources, reservoirs and possible routes of *S. aureus* transmission.

Phages that lyse human strains may be divided into serogroups with sera that neutralize the phage activity, and lytic groups in which the phages commonly react together. Eleven serogroups (A to L) have been described: only A (the most stable), B and F are represented in the international human phage set. Six lytic groups of phages have been described and each set may contain phages of different serogroups.

In the present international phage set for human strains, five phages (29, 52, 52A, 79 and 80) belong to lytic group I, four (3A, 3C, 55 and 71) to group II, 10 (6, 42E, 47, 53, 75, 77, 83A, 84, 85) to group III, and two (94 and 96) to group V. Phages 81 and 95 belong to a miscellaneous group and 42D, no longer in the current set, to group IV. The restricted lytic spectrum of strains that react with phages of groups II and V are known to be, in part, dependent on their own restriction/ modification systems; only group II, for instance, produces an enzyme with *Sau*AI endonuclease activity.

Additional phage-typing techniques

There are a number of additional techniques which have been used on occasion for poorly typeable organisms. These include reverse phage typing, where the spectrum of phage found in the organism is determined; cross-spotting, where the derived phage is tested against other encountered strains; and heat 'shock' phage typing, where it is thought that exposure to a variety of heat treatments inactivates restriction endonucleases in some strains and that they thus become more phage typeable.

Probably the most useful additional technique is the use of experimental phages. There are a number of such phages around the world that have been used. There are plans to collect these together and select about 20 for distribution internationally.

Serotyping of S. aureus

Serotyping of *S. aureus* is less popular than phage typing and few countries have access to it. There are several systems, including capsular and coagulase serotyping. However, they suffer from various problems, such as poor reproducibility and discrimination.

Determination of antibiotic and chemical susceptibility patterns

This can also be used to type the organism, although with increasing knowledge of the genetics of resistance it is now realized that many of the agents tested are conveyed on plasmids or

transposons and thus can be evanescent, or spuriously distinguish otherwise identical isolates. However, if enough epidemiological background of the isolates is known, the method may be useful in exploring outbreak dynamics, or even subtyping of strains.

Analysis of proteins

High-resolution polyacrylamide gel electrophoresis (PAGE) of proteins has been used increasingly in bacterial systematics both at and below the species level and more recently for typing. Several workers have found that the techniques may be of some use for typing *S. aureus*, especially MRSA (Costas *et al.*, 1989). Whole cell or exported proteins have been examined. In addition, others have also Western blotted the proteins with various types of antisera and found the method useful, although it is not a true typing but a fingerprinting or tentative typing technique. Criteria for distinguishing strains have not been agreed.

Multi-locus enzyme electrophoresis is a useful tool to explore clonal hypotheses but rather expensive and time consuming as a typing tool.

Genotypic methods

There are a whole host of methods that have now been used for typing *S. aureus*, especially MRSA.

Plasmid analysis Analysis of plasmid DNA has been used in many studies. Techniques include determination of size, number, copy number, restriction enzyme analysis and determining the nature of the carried genes by transfer, cure or specific probing. The ability to transfer is also of epidemiological importance and can include conjugative transfer, mixed cell culture transfer, transduction and transformation.

Some plasmids which are readily lost from certain strains do not provide reliable epidemiological markers, although this has been documented more often in coagulase-negative staphylococci. A single plasmid may be present in multiple molecular forms and will require further examination with the above techniques.

Chromosomal genotyping techniques These techniques are now widely used, but many suffer from poor reproducibility or discrimination.

Approaches include ribotyping, use of the PCR to amplify a variety of sequences such as those for coagulase, protein A, random or repetitive sequences (e.g. ERIC or REP). Digestion of the chromosome with rare cutting restriction enzymes and various types of pulsed-field gel electrophoresis (PFGE) is generally thought to be the 'gold standard' for these techniques. There are difficulties in deciding criteria for distinguishing strains as insertions of phage or plasmids, deletions, transpositions, inversions and point mutations can generate band differences. Increasingly investigators are combining PFGE with Southern blotting and trying to identify certain bands, e.g. with IS256, protein A, *mec* or ribotyping probes.

In a recent study of many of these techniques no one technique was superior. All had a place and the general feeling was that the methods had to be used hierarchically (Tenover *et al.*, 1994).

MANAGEMENT

General Principles

Clinical acumen will decide what therapeutic approach to use for *S. aureus* infections. Purulent lesions, particularly if 'closed', will require drainage. Septicaemia following intravascular cannulation can respond rapidly to the removal of the device, and short courses of therapy are usually satisfactory unless there has been splenic or cardiac involvement or other metastatic spread. In the treatment of burn infection subcutaneous blood flow appears to be critical and histamine administration, heating, pain relief and optimization of blood volume are all advocated (Benhaim and Hunt, 1992). Chronic (or poorly responding acute) osteomyelitis will require sequestrectomy.

Severe sepsis, e.g. endocarditis, pneumonia, TSS, osteomyelitis and severe wound infection, will require antibiotic therapy. Where there is a clear focus of infection, a susceptible organism and a rapid response, a short course with one antibiotic is sufficient. Where this is not the case, combined therapy, e.g. flucloxacillin with oral fusidic acid and/or intravenous gentamicin, for several weeks (two to four) will be required. In endocarditis, large doses of a bactericidal (preferably intravenous) combination of antibiotics should be given. Laboratory tests should be performed to confirm this, many also perform serum back-titrations. Treatment will be required for several weeks; opinions differ but at least two weeks intravenously and another two weeks orally are sufficient, provided the response has been adequate.

Development of Resistance

The Second World War, with its commensurate cases of *S. aureus* sepsis, provided a good testing ground for sulphonamides and a spur to the development of penicillin, which in the 1940s reversed the appalling prognosis of *S. aureus* infections. However, resistance to sulphonamides and then penicillin soon followed. Indeed, by 1948 about 60% of *S. aureus* in the UK were resistant to penicillin, and penicillinase-producing *S. aureus* strains of phage group I were the cause of worldwide nosocomial infection in maternity and special care baby units, and similar strains of phage group III were the cause of infection in non-maternity areas. This pattern was repeated when the versatile *Staphylococcus* developed, in turn, resistance to streptomycin, tetracycline, chloramphenicol and erythromycin.

Multiple drug-resistant *S. aureus* became a world-wide problem in the 1950s. At this same time a new virulent strain of penicillin-resistant *S. aureus* appeared, first in Australia, where it reacted with phage 80, and then in Canada, where it reacted with phage 81. In 1959 the organism was still amongst the strains associated with boils and wound infection, in both healthy people and patients (particularly on obstetric wards). Although much of the early history of nosocomial infection control is anecdotal, it seems fairly clear that this staphylococcal pandemic was the major stimulus to an organized infection control effort, although throughout the 1960s and 1970s many clinicians were blissfully unaware of the magnitude of nosocomial infection in their hospitals.

After 1960 the 'hospital *Staphylococcus*', as the 80/81 strain had become known, was much less common. The isolation of 6-aminopenicillinic acid in 1959 resulted in the subsequent synthesis of a large number of compounds with different radicals on the side-chain of the penicillinic acid nucleus. Methicillin was one such compound, and it proved of value in the treatment of penicillin-resistant staphylococci because of the molecule's stability to staphylococcal penicillinase.

Barber (1961) reported artificially induced methicillin-resistant strains in 1960, but it was Jevons (1961) who first described naturally occurring methicillin-resistant *S. aureus*, shortly after the therapeutic agent had been introduced in the UK in 1960. In 1963 the first nosocomial MRSA outbreak was described; over a 14-month period 37 children were affected on eight wards. In this same year 102 MRSA were found amongst 27 000 *S. aureus* sent to the UK PHLS. All these strains showed a similar antibiotic and mercurial salt resistogram, and most belonged to phage group III. MRSA was also described in countries such as Poland and Turkey before the introduction of methicillin (see Cookson and Phillips, 1990).

The early MRSA strains were heterogeneously resistant to methicillin, although it is clear that even then, as now, this property varied from one strain to another. The small resistant proportion could be increased by changing the physical conditions of the test, e.g. with added 5% (w/v) sodium chloride or 7.5% (w/v) ammonium sulphate, lower temperatures of incubation, low pH, chelating agents, trace metals and β-lactam antibiotics themselves.

One of the features of MRSA has been the different experiences described between and within countries, cities and even hospital wards. However, one could make the following generalizations. A gradual increase in the incidence of methicillin resistance was seen throughout the 1960s in the UK and Europe. In the UK, for instance, the incidence of 1% in 1965 increased to 5% in 1969. During the early half of the 1970s many centres in the UK experienced a decrease in MRSA. In Switzerland it fell from 20% in 1971 to 3% in 1975 and in Denmark the incidence fell from 19% in 1969 to 6% in 1974, probably as a result of intensive antibiotic control policies. The geographical differences in experience with MRSA were also evident in the USA. In the late 1960s, MRSA comprised less than 1% of *S. aureus* isolates. However, problems did arise in the 1970s and these have since continued. The number of Veterans Administration Medical Centers, for instance, with MRSA increased from three in 1975 to 11 in 1984.

In the late 1970s, after a decade of use of the agent, there emerged in Europe outbreaks of gentamicin-resistant *S. aureus*. The overall incidence was low, about 1% in 1976 in the USA and probably about the same in London. However, by the late 1970s and early 1980s most parts of the world were experiencing problems with patient colonization and infection with MRSA strains also resistant to many other antibiotics, including aminoglycosides. This trend has continued and in the 1990s, with the exception of certain countries such as Holland and Scandinavia, most of the world has problems with endemic MRSA. As before, there were hospitals with a very low incidence amidst others with a high incidence.

Choice of Agent

Few organisms in hospital today are susceptible to penicillin. Penicillinase-stable antibiotics (flucloxacillin, cloxacillin) are the first therapeutic choices. In serious sepsis they may be combined with oral (to lower the risk of jaundice) fusidic acid or parenteral aminoglycoside (carefully monitored to avoid nephrotoxicity). Cephalosporins are also used (first and second generation, preferably). In those allergic to β-lactams, erythromycin or alternatives such as clarithromycin can be used, vancomycin (or teicoplanin) if the infection is severe. Fusidic acid, quinolones and clindamycin penetrate bone well; several months treatment is required for osteomyelitis. Chloramphenicol may also be useful, particularly in cases of meningitis or resistant isolates. Vancomycin and teicoplanin may be the only agents available for some MRSA infections. If necrotic tissue is present this should be removed. Clindamycin appears to be the antibiotic of choice in life-threatening necrotizing infections. Much of the evidence for this is anecdotal although based on good theory (the agent is active against anaerobes and streptococci which may also be present, it penetrates well and is not inactivated by pus or necrotic tissue).

The susceptibility of MRSA varies with time and location, depending on the prevalence of various strains in different parts of the world, a country or even within a city or hospital. It is important that clinicians are aware of these changes and local prevalence, so that any empiric therapy is as safe and effective as possible. Probably the best data on variation in antibiotic susceptibility patterns in epidemic MRSA (EMRSA) comes from the UK. EMRSA-15 and 16 are always resistant to the quinolones and EMRSA-3 is becoming so. On the east coast of Australia and the USA and parts of the Mediterranean, MRSA is also resistant to quinolones, and many strains are also resistant to rifampicin and trimethoprim, popular systemic agents used in eradication strategies. In many countries in northern Europe (Spain, Portugal, France, Belgium, northern Germany) a phage 77 strain and its clonal derivatives are widely disseminated and are all resistant to quinolones. Resistance to erythromycin and clindamycin is common, as is that to tetracycline, but less so to minocycline. Aminoglycoside resistance is extremely common throughout the world, although some of these agents are of value, depending on the nature of the resistance mechanism (see below).

Topical Therapy

Topical agents to treat cutaneous infection and/or eradicate carriage of *S. aureus* include mupirocin, which seems far more effective than topical agents used previously (e.g. neomycin). However, resistance has become a significant problem in certain parts of the world. Alternative topical agents are under consideration, e.g. azelaic acid and tea tree oil, and antiseptic-containing agents such as chlorhexidine, triclosan, povidone iodine, silver sulphadiazine and hexachlorophane.

Some authorities advocate the use of topical antibiotics to treat infection of certain sites with poor vasculature, e.g. bone in osteitis, cartilage in chondritis and the avascular burn eschar. Antibiotics have included mupirocin and also gentamicin beads, which also serve to provide some structure in areas that would otherwise collapse following surgery. Once again the problems of resistance are ever present.

Mechanism of Resistance Development

Staphylococcus aureus is not only a versatile pathogen but also exhibits an unfortunate ability for developing or acquiring resistant mechanisms to numerous antimicrobial agents, sometimes quite shortly after a new therapeutic agent has been introduced into clinical practice. The history of the emergence of some of these resistances is described above. The reader is also referred to the extensive literature on the nature of the resistance mechanisms, their mechanisms of transfer and genetic location (Foster 1983; Lyon and Skurray, 1987; Brumfitt and Hamilton-Miller, 1989).

Initially, the origin of the resistance in *S. aureus* was thought to be similar to that found in the laboratory, where point mutations could be induced at a frequency of 10^{-6} to 10^{-8} per cell. This is true for several resistances (e.g. rifampicin, fusidic acid, quinolones). However, at least in the laboratory, these mutations could result in crippled organisms, and alternative mechanisms evolved to increase the repertoire of resistance mechanisms without reducing the organism's competitive abilities. These mechanisms include plasmids, transposons (Tn) and insertion sequences (IS).

The IS are found on plasmids or the chromosome and enable other resistance genes carried on plasmids or transposons or transduced into the organism to become inserted without disturbing other gene functions. One IS (IS257) is associated with the *mec*, and mercury and tetracycline resistance genes. At least 11 transposons have been described in *S. aureus* (Lyon and Skurray, 1987) and there is certainly evidence for the existence of others such as that encoding mupirocin resistance.

Plasmids are found in many strains of *S. aureus* and on almost all MRSA. There exist at least 13 incompatibility groups of plasmids; in some instances a plasmid has probably become inserted into the chromosome so that another plasmid of the same incompatibility group could be acquired (e.g. EMRSA-1; Cookson and Phillips, 1990).

The various resistance mechanisms are outlined in Table 2a.3. In certain instances, the same mechanism is able to confer resistance to more than one agent. The efflux mechanism that confers resistance to ethidium bromide and propamidine isethionate is also thought to confer low-level resistance to chlorhexidine and some other disinfectants, although the significance of this resistance is uncertain (Cookson *et al.*, 1991).

TABLE 2a.3 MECHANISMS AND EXAMPLES OF RESISTANCE TO ANTIMICROBIAL AGENTS

Efflux mechanisms
Arsenate, cadmium, streptomycin, quaternary ammonium and nucleic acid binding compounds and perhaps tetracycline and quinolone resistances

Enzymatic destruction or alteration
Aminoglycosides (acetylation, adenylation or phosphorylation; see text), chloramphenicol (acetyltransferase), penicillin (β-lactamase), mercury (mercuric reductase), organomercurials (organomercurial lyase), streptogramin A (an *o*-acetyltransferase), streptogramin B (a hydrolase)

Binding of agent
Cadmium (ion binding)

Reduced affinity
Erythromycin (23S rRNA methylation), mupirocin (isoleucyl tRNA-transferase), novobiocin (DNA gyrase), quinolones (altered DNA gyrase A and occasionally B), rifampicin (RNA polymerase?), sulphonamides (dihydropteroate synthetase), high-level trimethoprim (dihydrofolate reductase)

Decreased permeability
Perhaps for fusidic acid

Multi-factorial
Methicillin resistance (see text)

Unknown
Arsenite, antimony, bismuth, lead

There are at least five genes that confer resistance to various aminoglycosides. Probably the commonest aminoglycoside resistance genes are *aacA-aphD* which encode the acetylating (AAC) and phosphorylating (APH) enzymes AAC(6') and APH(2") and confer resistance to gentamicin, tobramycin and kanamycin. Others comprise *aadE* encoding an adenylating enzyme AAD(6) and resistance to streptomycin; *aadA* encoding AAD(3")(9) and resistance to streptomycin and spectinomycin; *aadD* for AAD(4')(4") and resistance to neomycin, kanamycin, pristinamycin, tobramycin and amikacin; *aphA* for APH(3')III and neomycin and kanamycin resistance.

Transfer of resistance

The methods of acquisition of these resistance genes include conjugation, mixed cell culture transfer (phage-mediated conjugation), transformation, and transduction. The importance in nature of the rather unnatural process of transformation is uncertain. Transduction results in a rather low transfer rate and requires the recipient to be protected by lysogeny. It is thus thought that the other two mechanisms are probably more important *in vivo*. Various conjugative plasmids have been described, and the conjugative genes have been sequenced in certain instances. Most encode aminoglycoside resistance, but some have also been described which encode other antibiotic resistances, e.g. mupirocin and erythromycin resistance. Conjugative plasmids are able to mobilize other non-conjugative plasmids on occasion. Phage-mediated conjugation does not require the donor to be lysogenic; the exact role of phage in the process is unclear, but chromosomal or plasmid resistance genes can be transferred in this process (Lyon and Skurray, 1987).

There is good evidence that many identical *S. aureus* genes may be found in *S. epidermidis* and that these may be transferred to and between *S. aureus* strains by a process resembling conjugation (Archer and Mayhall, 1983). This process is, to an extent, governed by plasmid incompatibility (Townsend *et al.*, 1985). There is also evidence that other species may act as a reservoir for resistance genes; identical aminoglycoside, tetracycline and chloramphenicol resistance genes are found in *Streptococcus* spp., for instance. It remains to be seen whether vancomycin resistance will transfer from *Enterococcus* spp. as has occurred, albeit unstably, *in vitro* (Noble *et al.*, 1992).

Methicillin Resistance

Methicillin resistance is probably the most complex of the resistance mechanisms found in *Staphylococcus* spp. *MecA*, the structural gene for an additional penicillin-binding protein (PBP2' or PBP2a), has been located on the chromosomal map of *S. aureus* close to the novobiocin resistance gene *nov* and is additional DNA not present in isogenic-sensitive strains (Beck *et al.*, 1986), and is probably transposable (Trees and Iandolo, 1988); it is also found in coagulase-negative methicillin-resistant staphylococci.

PBP2' has low affinity for methicillin and is probably a transpeptidase that produces poorly cross-linked cell wall structures. However, the situation is far more complex than this and there are at least 20 additional loci that have been identified and are thought to be involved in cell wall growth and expression of methicillin resistance (Berger-Bächi, 1989; Murakami and Tomasz, 1989; de Lancastre *et al.*, 1994). They probably account for the heterogeneity of expression of methicillin resistance. Some strains contain *mecR1-mecI*, which encode elements regulating *mecA* transcription (Tesch *et al.*, 1990). Penicillinase determinants may also have a similar but smaller effect on this transcription. The various *fem* loci (*A*, *B* and *C*) are native to staphylococci and participate in normal cell wall production. Mutations destroying these enzymes lower the methicillin minimal inhibitory concentrations (MICs) in MRSA despite normal PBP2' content.

PREVENTION

Infection Control Measures

Staphylococcus aureus infections were the stimulus in the 1950s to improve many aspects of infection control in the UK and many other countries. The re-emergence of MRSA as a significant problem in the 1980s and 1990s resulted in our relearning many of the lessons from that time. However, there have also been many other changes in health services which have added to this challenge, and new ways of monitoring and controlling the problem will have to be considered.

The main elements of a control programme to prevent *S. aureus* infections are as follows:

(1) To reduce the number of organisms gaining access to the wound by auto-infection with the appropriate use of antiseptics and prophylactic antibiotics. If there is infection elsewhere this should be treated before operation. Eradication of nasal carriage with neomycin or mupirocin creams is considered in certain types of surgery, e.g. cardiothoracic surgery, where the consequences of infection are particularly dire.

(2) To minimize the number of organisms entering the wound during operation: well-designed theatres, theatre procedures and ventilation, careful aseptic technique, use of gloves and handwashing.

(3) To minimize spread of organisms to patients from other patients or staff, particularly when performing close-contact procedures such as wound dressings or drainage care: handwashing and gloves, consideration of identification of dispersers, particularly on dermatology or burns units, and the implementation of different isolation measures, targeted or cohort nursing.

(4) To maximize the resistance of the host to infection by encouraging surgeons to consider their surgical technique. This is often done by feeding back their rates of infection to them. It is unclear what it is that the surgeons do to lower their rates of infection. Cruse and Foord (1980) suggest that they should consider whether they are operating as quickly as is safe, in that the infection risk increases with operative time, whether cautery is used judiciously, the avoidance of the use of drainage through the wound and depilatory creams or shaving patients just before the operation.

They also advocate special care with patients identified as at particular risk of infection. Many such 'risk factors' have been suggested, but these often include the obese, patients over 60 years of age, those with malignancy or diabetes mellitus, and the malnourished.

(5) To minimize the risks of colonization or infection from the environment. There should be effective decontamination policies, procedures, audit, and an efficient hospital decontamination and sterilization department.

The increasing antibiotic resistance that is being seen in MRSA throughout the world is a great cause for concern; infections are difficult and expensive to treat. Control policies are described in many countries, states and hospitals (Ayliffe *et al.*, 1990). They vary depending on many factors: the type of unit involved, the virulence of the organism and its endemicity and transmissibility and last, but not least, the facilities and resources available. It should be emphasized that it is not sufficient merely to record the number of cases seen in a hospital but also how the organism was acquired. In some tertiary care centres the majority of their cases will be transferred to them and new case acquisition may be low.

Some authorities have suggested grading the response to MRSA depending on the resources and the size of the problem. If there are few clinical infections and resources then it may be sufficient to emphasize the use of appropriate hygienic measures. Isolation or cohort nursing and MRSA screening would be the next tier of measures. A maximal response would be indicated if resources were sufficient and, for instance, the unit was a high-risk area, or there were few recent MRSA problems. Measures would include the screening or means to identify early on the international or other inter-hospital transfer of patients or staff, readmitted patients and patients admitted from affected nursing or elderly care homes. There should be screening of other patients if more than one case occurs on a ward or if it is thought to be an epidemic strain (EMRSA). MRSA isolates should be sent early on to the reference laboratory for identification and a view sought if it is similar or identical to current EMRSA. There should be consideration (and policies for) the eradication or reduction in the numbers of MRSA on colonized or infected patients. This will include the use of disinfectants, antiseptics (in particular mupirocin) and systemic antibiotics if there is wound or perhaps throat carriage. Faecal carriage should also be considered. The quality of patient care and implications for staff numbers and workloads should be considered when deciding isolation and/ or cohort or targeted nursing. Some centres have established a dedicated ward/area for MRSA patients, although this need not necessarily be physically separate from other wards. Inter-ward transfer of patients and staff should be minimized and other hospitals or nursing homes informed as to the MRSA status of transferred patients. In a significant outbreak (say more than four patients) the use of disinfectants for all patients on the ward should be considered.

There are several new threats to UK MRSA control in that the length of hospital stay is reducing the denominator of alert organism surveillance. There is increasing inter-ward transfers, resulting in problems in tracking patients and exposure of large numbers of staff and patients to the organism. In addition, there is an emerging problem of misuse of mupirocin and resistance to this valuable agent (Marples *et al.*, 1995). Sometimes, it has been used on staff without establishing if the carriage is transient. Others have not assessed the full extent of carriage and considered whether the agent should be used with systemic agents. It has also been used prophylactically, in situations where it is impossible to prevent MRSA recolonization and 'blanket use' after initial MRSA screening of all patients and staff. Control of its use is imperative and alternative effective agents are required urgently.

Immunization

There have been various attempts to develop a vaccine. Target groups would include those particularly prone to infection, e.g. diabetes mellitus and cystic fibrosis patients, or others suffering from chronic infection, e.g. osteomyelitis or recurrent skin sepsis. The emergence of certain strains that are resistant to almost all antibiotics and the possibility that vancomycin resistance might transfer from enterococci to *S. aureus* may result in renewed efforts to develop an effective vaccine.

Formalin-treated toxoid preparations have not affected the course of chronic or recurrent infections despite high antibody responses to α-toxin and Panton Valentine leucocidin toxin. However, there is some evidence that such preparations may lower the incidence of infection acquisition at least in neonates born to immunized mothers and for mastitis in the mothers. Surface polysaccharides and proteins from *S. aureus* which could serve as components of a future subunit vaccine against staphylococcal disease in man and animals have recently been characterized and other workers in the USA are also exploring capsular polysaccharide vaccines (see Foster, 1991).

Bacterial Interference

An alternative strategy to immunization is that of bacterial interference. Shinefield and co-workers successfully lowered the incidence of sepsis in nurseries in the 1960s by colonizing the neonates with a strain of lowered virulence (502A strain). However, the practice fell into disrepute with the subsequent descriptions of mild purulent lesions and fatal septicaemia with the strain. The use of other organisms might also be considered, e.g. coagulase-negative staphylococci.

REFERENCES

Adams, J. and Van Enk, R. (1994) Use of commercial particle agglutination systems for the rapid identification of methicillin-susceptible and methicillin-resistant *Staphylococcus aureus*. *European Journal of Clinical Microbiology and Infectious Diseases*, **13**, 86–89.

Altemeier, W.A., Lewis, S. and Brackett, K. (1981) The versatile *Staphylococcus*. In *The Staphylococci: Proceedings of the Alexander Ogston Centennial Conference* (ed. A. Macdonald and G. Smith), pp. 125–148. Aberdeen University Press, Aberdeen.

Arbuthnott, J.P., Coleman, D.C. and de Azavedo, J.S. (1990) Staphylococcal toxins in human disease. *Journal of Applied Bacteriology, Symposium Supplement*, 101S–107S.

Archer, G.L. and Mayhall, C.G. (1983). Comparison of epidemiological markers used in the investigation of an outbreak of methicillin-resistant *Staphylococcus aureus* infections. *Journal of Clinical Microbiology*, **18**, 395–399.

Ayliffe, G.A.J., Brumfitt, W., Casewell, M.W.C. *et al.* (1991) Revised guidelines for the control of epidemic methicillin-resistant *Staphylococcus aureus*. Report of a combined working party of the Hospital Infection Society and the British Society of Antimicrobial Chemotherapy. *Journal of Hospital Infection*, **16**, 351–377.

Barber, M. (1961) Methicillin-reistant staphylococci. *Journal of Clinical Pathology*, **14**, 385–393.

Beck, W.F., Berger-Bächi, B. and Kayser, F.H. (1986) Additional DNA in methicillin-resistant *Staphylococcus aureus* and molecular cloning of mec-specific DNA. *Journal of Bacteriology*, **165**, 373–378.

Benhaim, P. and Hunt, T.K. (1992) Natural resistance to infection: leukocyte functions *Journal of Burn Care and Rehabilitation*, **13**, 287–297.

Berger-Bächi, B. (1989) Genetics of methicillin-resistance in *Staphylococcus aureus*. *Journal of Antimicrobial Chemotherapy*, **23**, 671–680.

Blowers, R., Hill, J. and Howell, A. (1973) Shedding of *Staphylococcus aureus* by human carriers. In *Airborne Transmission and Airborne Infection* (ed. J.F.P. Hers and K.C. Winkler), pp. 432–434. Oosthoek, Utrecht.

Bohach, G.A., Fast, D.J. Nelson, R.D. *et al.* (1990) Staphylococcal and streptococcal pyrogenic toxins involved in toxic shock syndrome and related illnesses. *Critical Reviews in Microbiology*, **17**, 251–272.

Brumfitt, W. and Hamilton-Miller, J. (1989) Methicillin-resistant *Staphylococcus aureus*. *New England Journal of Medicine*, **320**, 1188–1196.

Coleman, D.C., Sullivan, D.J., Russell, R.J. *et al.* (1989) *Staphylococcus aureus* bacteriophages mediating the simultaneous lysogenic conversion of β-lysin, staphylokinase and enterotoxin A: molecular mechanism of triple conversion. *Journal of General Microbiology*, **135**, 1679–1697.

Cookson, B.D. (1990) Selective staphylococcal broth. *Journal of Clinical Microbiology*, **28**, 2380–2381.

Cookson, B.D. and Phillips, I. (1990) Methicillin-resistant staphylococci. *Journal of Applied Bacteriology*, **69** (Suppl. 19), 55–70.

Cookson, B.D., Peters, B., Webster, M. *et al.* (1989) Staff carriage of epidemic methicillin-resistant *Staphylococcus aureus*. *Journal of Clinical Microbiology*, **27**, 1471–1476.

Cookson, B.D., Bolton, M.C. and Platt, J.H. (1991) Chlorhexidine resistance in methicillin-resistant *Staphylococcus aureus* or just an elevated MIC? An in vitro and in vivo assessment. *Antimicrobial Agents and Chemotherapy*, **35**, 1997–2002.

Costas, M., Cookson, B.D., Talsania, H. *et al.* (1989) Numerical analysis of SDS–PAGE protein electrophoretic patterns of MRSA. *Journal of Clinical Microbiology*, **27**, 2574–2581.

Cox, R.A., Conquest, C., Mallaghan, C. *et al.* (1995) A major outbreak of methicillin-resistant *Staphylococcus aureus* caused by a new phage type. *Journal of Hospital Infection*, **29**, 87–106.

Cruse, P.J.E. and Foord, R. (1980) The epidemiology of wound infection. Symposium on Surgical Infection. *Surgical Clinics of North America*, **60**, 27–40.

de Lancastre, H., de Jonge, B.L.M., Mathews, P.R. *et al.* (1994) Molecular aspects of methicillin resistance in *Staphylococcus aureus*. *Journal of Antimicrobial Chemotherapy*, **33**, 7–24.

Foster, T.J. (1983) Plasmid determined resistance to antimicrobial drugs and toxic metal ions in bacteria. *Microbiological Reviews*, **47**, 361–409.

Foster, T.J. (1991) Potential for vaccination against infections caused by *Staphylococcus aureus*. *Vaccine*, **9**, 221–227.

Gransden, W.R., Eykyn, S. and Phillips I. (1984) *Staphylococcus aureus* bacteraemia: 400 episodes in St Thomas' hospital. *British Medical Journal*, **288**, 300–303.

Jevons, M.P. (1961) 'Celbenin'-resistant staphylococci. *British Medical Journal*, **i**, 124–125.

Lacey R.W. (1987) Multi-resistant *Staphylococcus aureus*: a suitable case for inactivity? *Journal of Hospital Infection*, **9**, 103–105.

Lyon, B.R. and Skurray, R. (1987) Antimicrobial resistance of *Staphylococcus aureus*: genetic basis. *Microbiological Reviews*, **51**, 88–134.

Marples, R.R. and Wieneke, A.A. (1993) Enterotoxins and toxic-shock syndrome toxin-1 in non-enteric staphylococcal disease. *Epidemiology and Infection*, **110**, 477–488.

Marples, R.R., Speller, D.C.E. and Cookson, B.D. (1995) Prevalence of mupirocin resistance in *Staphylococcus aureus*. *Journal of Hospital Infection*, **25**, 153–155.

Murakami, K. and Tomasz, A. (1989) Involvement of multiple genetic determinants in high-level methicillin resistance in *Staphylococcus aureus*. *Journal of Bacteriology*, **171**, 874–879.

Noble W.C. (1993) Staphylococci on the skin. In *The Skin Microflora and Microbial Skin Disease* (ed. W.C. Noble), pp. 153–172. Cambridge University Press, Cambridge.

Noble, W.C., Virani, Z. and Cree, R.G.A. (1992) Co-transfer of vancomycin and other resistance genes from *Enterococcus faecalis* NCTC 12201 to *Staphylococcus aureus*. FEMS *Microbiological Letters*, **72**, 195–198.

Tenover, F.C., Arbeit, R., Archer, G. *et al.* (1994) Comparison of traditional and molecular methods of typing isolates of *Staphylococcus aureus*. *Journal of Clinical Microbiology*, **32**, 407–415.

Tesch, W., Ryffel C., Strassle, A. *et al.* (1990) Evidence of a novel staphylococcal *mec*-encoded element (mecR) controlling expression of penicillin-binding protein 2'. *Antimicrobial Agents and Chemotherapy*, **34**, 1703–1706.

Townsend, C., Ashdown, N. and Grubb, W.B. (1985) Evolution of Australian isolates of methicillin-resistant *Staphylococcus aureus*: a problem of plasmid incompatibility. *Journal of Medical Microbiology*, **20**, 49–61.

Trees, D.L. and Iandolo, J.J. (1988) Identification of a *Staphylococcus aureus* transposon (Tn4291) that carries the methicillin resistance gene(s). *Journal of Bacteriology*, **170**, 149–154.

Williams, R.E. and Rippon, J.E. (1952) Bacteriophage typing of *Staphylococcus aureus*. *Journal of Hygiene (Cambridge)*, **50**, 320–353.

2b

COAGULASE-NEGATIVE STAPHYLOCOCCI

Roger G. Finch

INTRODUCTION

Coagulase-negative staphylococci (CONS) comprise an ever-expanding group of bacteria whose medical importance has largely emerged in the past two decades. They now count among the most frequent of nosocomial pathogens featuring prominently among blood culture isolates, often in association with intravascular devices, and as a cause of infection of more deep-seated prosthetic implants. Clinically, infection may be silent, overt and occasionally fulminant, and reflects the diverse pathogenic profile of this group of organisms. CONS are also characterized by an unpredictable pattern of susceptibility to commonly used antibiotics. Multiple drug resistance is common and adds to the difficulties of treating infections caused by this group of microorganisms.

HISTORICAL ASPECTS

Staphylococcus aureus was first described by Rosenbech in 1884. Its pathogenic profile includes local invasion, systemic spread and toxin-mediated disease. It was included among the group of pyogenic cocci and hence its former description, *S. pyogenes*. In contrast, CONS were considered for many years to be non-pathogenic commensal organisms of the skin. *Staphylococcus albus* was widely used to describe all CONS as distinct from the colonial appearance of the golden pigmented *S. aureus*. The first widely accepted pathogenic role of CONS was the association of *S. saprophyticus* (novobiocin-resistant coagulase-negative staphylococci) with urinary tract infections in women (Pereira, 1962).

The widely held view that CONS were largely commensals and indeed 'contaminants' of clinical specimens frustrated recognition of the pathogenic potential of this group of organisms for many years. However, by the 1980s CONS had clearly been identified with a wide variety of clinical problems such as bacteraemia, endocarditis of both prosthetic and native heart valves, septic arthritis, peritonitis complicating continuous ambulatory peritoneal dialysis (CAPD), mediastinitis, pacemaker associated infections, cerebrospinal fluid (CSF) shunt device infections, prosthetic joint and other orthopaedic device infections, osteomyelitis, urinary tract infection and prostatitis (Kloos and Bennerman, 1994). While *S. saprophyticus* was clearly associated with the urinary tract, the predominant species among the remaining infections was *S. epidermidis*. However, many hospital diagnostic laboratories have used the species *S. epidermidis* description loosely to

Principles and Practice of Clinical Bacteriology. Edited by A.M. Emmerson, P.M. Hawkey and S.H. Gillespie
© 1997 John Wiley & Sons Ltd

encompass all CONS, further frustrating recognition of the diverse microbial nature of CONS infections. This has changed in recent years largely as a result of increased awareness of the importance of CONS infections, together with the availability of commercial identification systems.

DESCRIPTION OF THE ORGANISM

CONS, together with *S. aureus*, are members of the family Micrococcaceae. They are Gram-positive facultative anaerobes which appear in clusters, are non-motile, non-spore forming and catalase positive, and in general do not produce the enzyme coagulase. A thin capsule may be detected in some strains.

CONS are divided into more than 30 species (Table 2b.1), of which approximately half have been associated with man (Kloos and Bennerman, 1994). The remainder are associated with domestic and other species of mammals. The relatedness of these species has been confirmed by guanine + cytosine ratios. DNA sequence homology of >50% has been used to group the species, although a number of species are too distantly related to fit into this arrangement.

Coagulase production is generally absent among CONS although some strains of *S. intermedius* and *S. hyicus* are weak producers. Thermonuclease is produced by *S. intermedius*, *S. hyicus*, *S. schleiferi* and some strains of *S. carnosus*, *S. epidermidis* and *S. simulans*.

Classification

CONS have been divided into various species based on a variety of characteristics including

TABLE 2b.1 COAGULASE-NEGATIVE STAPHYLOCOCCI ASSOCIATED WITH MAN

S. epidermidis	*S. pasteurii*
S. auricularis	*S. saccharolyticus*
S. capitis	*S. saprophyticus*
S. caprae	*S. schleiferi*
S. cohnii	*S. simulans*
S. haemolyticus	*S. warneri*
S. hominis	*S. xylosus*
S. lugdunensis	

colonial morphology, coagulase and phosphatase production, acid formation from maltose, sucrose, D-mannitol, D-trehalose and D-xylose as well as susceptibility to novobiocin using a 5 μg disc (Pfaller and Herwald, 1988). More extensive biochemical testing is necessary to speciate less common strains such as *S. warneri*, *S. capitis*, *S. simulans* and *S. hominis*, although little call is made for this outside reference or research laboratories (Kloor *et al.*, 1991). Table 2b.2 summarizes the major differentiating biochemical features (see Barrow and Feltham, 1993).

PATHOGENICITY

CONS should not be considered biologically inactive despite the fact that relatively few virulence factors have been defined to date. A number of proteins and exoenzymes are expressed to varying degrees among the various species of CONS (Gemmell, 1986). These include haemolysins, phosphatases, lipase, galactosidase and various decarboxylases.

The process of bacterial attachment to cells and inanimate surfaces has been subject to much investigation (Tenney *et al.*, 1986). In the case of CONS, it is quite clear that the mechanism is complex, strain variable and affected by the nature of the solid surface and the environment in which attachment occurs.

Biomaterials are largely synthetic polymers but may occasionally be natural substances. Physicochemical factors affecting attachment include electrostatic forces and hydrophobicity. While more hydrophobic strains in general attach more readily to these surfaces there is considerable variation which may be further affected by nutrient limitation, pH and variation in carbon dioxide tension (pCO_2) (Denyer *et al.*, 1990).

Adhesins

Implanted medical devices readily become coated with host substances such as collagen, fibrinogen, fibronectin, vitronectin and laminin. Variation in binding affinities to these proteins can be demonstrated; *S. haemolyticus* binds more strongly than

TABLE 2b.2 LABORATORY CHARACTERISTICS OF THE GENUS *STAPHYLOCOCCUS*

	1	2	3	4	5	6	7	8	9	10	11	12	13	14	15	16	17	18	19	20	21	22	23	24	25	26
Growth anaerobically	+	+	+	+	+	w	w	+[a]	+	w	+	+	w	w	w	+	+	w	–	–	w	–	–	w	+	+
Oxidase	–	–	–	–	+	–	–	–	+	–	+	–	–	–	–	–	–	+	–	–	–	–	w	+	–	–
*VP	+	–	–	–	+	+	d	?	+	+	+	–	+	+	–	+	+	–	–	–	–	d	–	–	+	+
*Coagulase	+	+	d	–	–	–	–	–	–	–	–	–	–	–	–	–	–	–	–	–	–	–	–	–	–	–
Acid from																										
Lactose	+	+	+	+	D	–	–	–	D	+	–	+	+	–	+	+	d	+	+	+	d	d	+	–	–	–
*Maltose	+	+	–	d	+	–	d	–	+[b]	+	d	–	+	+	+	d	–	+	+	+	+	+	d	+	+	–
Mannitol	+	+	–	d	+	+	–	–	d	–	d	–	+	+	+	–	+	–	+	+	+	+	+	+	+	+
Fructose	+	+	+	+	+	+	+	+	+	+	+	+	+	+	+	+	+	+	+	+	+	+	+	+	+	+
Sucrose	+	+	+	+	+	+	d	–	d	+	+	+	+	–	+	+	d	d	+	+	+	+	+	+	+	+
*Trehalose	+	+	+	+	+	–	+	–	+	+	+	–	–	+	+	+	+	d	+	+	–	+	+	+	+	d
Xylose	–	–	–	–	–	–	–	?	–	–	–	–	–	–	+	–	–	–	–	–	d	–	–	–	–	–
Cellobiose	–	–	–	–	–	–	–	?	d	–	–	d	–	–	–	–	?	?	d	–	?	+	–	d	–	–
Raffinose	–	–	–	–	–	–	–	–	–	–	–	w	–	–	–	–	–	?	+	–	+	+	–	–	–	–
Mannose	+	+	+	+	+	+	+	+	–	+	+	+	+	+	+	+	+	+	+	+	+	+	+	+	+	+
*Phosphatase	+	+	+	+	+	+	–	?	d	–	–	d	–	–	–	–	+	?	d	+	?	–	+	d	+	+
Nitrate	+	+	+	+	+	+	d	+	+	+	+	+	+	+	+	+	+	+	+	+	+	+	+	+	+	+
*Arginine	+	+	+	+	+	–	–	+	+[d]	+[d]	+[d]	+	–	–	–	+	+	+	–	–	–	–	–	+	+	+
Urea	d	+	+	+	+	w	–	?	–	+	–	–	d	d	+	+	–	?	–	–	+	–	d	–	–	–
Protease	+	D	+	+	w	w	–	–	–	+	–	–	+	–	–	+	–	+	–	+	–	–	w	w	–[c]	?
*Novobiocin	s	s	s	s	s	s	s	s	s	s	s	s	r	r	r	s	s	s	r	r	r	r	r	r	s	s

1 *Staph. aureus*
2 *Staph. intermedius*
3 *Staph. hyicus*
4 *Staph. chromogenes*
5 *Staph. epidermidis*
6 *Staph. capitis*

7 *Staph. auricularis*
8 *Staph. saccharolyticus*
9 *Staph. haemolyticus*
10 *Staph. hominis*
11 *Staph. warneri*

12 *Staph. simulans*
13 *Staph. saprophyticus*
14 *Staph. cohnii*
15 *Staph. xylosus*
16 *Staph. caprae*

17 *Staph. carnosus*
18 *Staph. caseolyticus*
19 *Staph. arlettae*
20 *Staph. equorum*
21 *Staph. gallinarum*

22 *Staph. kloosii*
23 *Staph. lentus*
24 *Staph. sciuri*
25 *Staph. lugdunensis*
26 *Staph. schleiferi*

s = sensitive
r = resistant

[a] = No growth anaerobically.
[b] = Usual reaction.
[c] = Ornithine decarboxylated.
[d] = Inferred reaction.
* = These tests are usually sufficient to identify the species that may infect man.

Reproduced from Barrow and Feltham (1993) by permission of Cambridge University Press.

strains of *S. epidermidis* (Paulsson *et al.*, 1992). The binding of *S. epidermidis* to fibronectin may be linked to their ability to colonize damaged tissues (Wadström, 1989). In contrast, strains of *Staph. saprophyticus* associated with urine infections have a higher capacity to adhere to laminin.

Polysaccharide adhesin

The search for a specific adhesin continues. A capsular immunodominant polysaccharide adhesin (PSA) with a molecular weight of >500 000 has been described (Tojo *et al.*, 1988). Antibodies to PSA have been shown to block adherence of *S. epidermidis* (strain RP-62A) to silastic catheter surfaces. The same adhesin has been demonstrated in other species such as *S. capitis*, subsp. *ureolyticus*. Anti-adhesin antibodies have also been shown to enhance opsonophagocytosis by polymorphonuclear leucocytes (PMNs). Another protein that may be associated with attachment is a 220 kDa surface antigen of *S. epidermidis* which immunogold electron microscopy suggests could be fimbrial in nature (Timmerman *et al.*, 1991).

Slime

Staphylococci, including CONS, produce variable amounts of capsular material. External to this is extracellular slime material produced under certain circumstances of growth (Bayston and Rodgers, 1990). The term glycocalyx encompasses both capsular and extracellular slime material within which the microorganisms grow to produce a biofilm. The importance of extracellular slime material and biofilm formation lies in the relationship of CONS to medical device-associated infections and colonization of the uroepithelium. Extracellular slime production appears to occur more readily with certain strains of *S. epidermidis* associated with foreign bodies and in particular indwelling medical devices. The function of slime has been much debated but it is believed to act as an ion-exchange resin for nutritional purposes. Bacterial growth within a biofilm differs markedly from the planktonic state and has been intensively studied in recent years. Biofilm-associated CONS appear to be protected from a number of control mechanisms. Slime from CONS interferes with various aspects of phagocytosis (Johnson *et al.*, 1986). Leucocyte migration is inhibited, as is degranulation. Oxygen-dependent intracellular killing, as measured by chemiluminescence, is also impaired. In addition, complement and/or IgG opsonic phagocytosis and killing have also been shown to be inhibited (Noble *et al.*, 1990). It is thought that surface-exposed proteins may be important in this regard (Shiro *et al.*, 1994). Human T cell lymphocyte proliferation is inhibited (Gray *et al.*, 1984). This may be a direct inhibitory effect or may be mediated by enhanced production of prostaglandin E_2 (Stout *et al.*, 1992). In addition, slime production has been associated with increased production of interleukin 1 and tumour necrosis factor α (Beutler and Cerami, 1989; Dinarello, 1989), as have changes in immunoglobulin production as a result of impaired B cell blastogenesis. Whilst these phenomena are of interest, they do not clarify the exact molecular and genetic nature whereby slime production is inhibitory to host defences.

Chemical analysis of slime indicates that it is a glycoconjugate composed of glycerol phosphate, D-alanine, *N*-acetylglucosamine and usually glucose (Hussain *et al.*, 1991; Kotilainen *et al.*, 1990). Slime production is strain variable and affected by circumstances of growth (Hussain *et al.*, 1992a). Class I and class II phenotypes have been described (Barker *et al.*, 1990). The former demonstrate good slime production under aerobic conditions but not in anaerobic states, whereas class II produce little or no slime under either condition. Slime production has been measured qualitatively and quantitatively. The Congo Red agar test has been widely used for individual colony testing, while radiochemical analyses have also been described (Hussain *et al.*, 1992b).

Most reports have focused on *S. epidermidis* and have generally, but not universally, shown slime production to be linked with pathogenic potential in relation to device-associated infections. *Staphylococcus saprophyticus* can also produce slime; urea appears to be an essential nutrient and is associated with biofilm production and the formation of urinary struvite and apatite stones (McLean *et al.*, 1985).

Iron-Scavenging Systems

Many bacteria have developed sophisticated iron-scavenging systems since this element is essential for survival. They have been well characterized for Gram-negative bacteria; however, their significance among Gram-positive pathogens is just emerging. Coagulase-negative staphylococci exemplify the process of microbial adaptation. For example, *S. epidermidis*-associated CAPD catheter-associated infections express two iron-regulated proteins in the cytoplasmic membrane when grown in used dialysate (Williams *et al.*, 1988). These have been shown to be antigenic and in a rat chamber model are immunodominant (Modun *et al.*, 1992). Furthermore, using lectin-binding studies human transferrin but not transferrin of other species has been shown to bind to a 42 kDa transferrin receptor protein (Modun *et al.*, 1994). This suggests that *S. epidermidis* has developed sophisticated iron-scavenging systems which include not only siderophores but also receptor and transportation systems to internalize this essential element.

EPIDEMIOLOGY

Normal Habitat

The distribution and concentration of CONS on the human skin and surface mucosae varies. The density of organisms ranges from 10^3 to 10^6 cfu/cm^2, with the lowest counts in the dry areas of the skin. They are particularly concentrated in the perineum, inguinal region, axillae and anterior nares. The distribution pattern is reflected in the relative frequency with which the various species are isolated from pathological specimens. For example, *S. capitis* generally prefers the scalp and face. *Staphylococcus epidermidis* is the most widely distributed species on the skin and achieves the highest concentrations in moist skin areas. *Staphylococcus haemolyticus* and *S. hominis* are most numerous in the perineum, axillae and inguinal regions in association with apocrine glands. *Staphylococcus auricularis* is largely confined to the external auditory meatus. *Staphylococcus warneri* and *S. lugdunensis* are less frequent commensals than are other species, but when present are widely distributed (Kloos and Bennerman, 1994).

The increasing importance of CONS as human pathogens has been recognized over the past two decades. Prior to this, *S. epidermidis* was an uncommon pathogen and *S. saprophyticus* was recognized as an occasional cause of community-acquired urinary tract infection in sexually active young women. However, community-acquired CONS infections are rare, and although they may arise in patients who have been discharged from hospital following the insertion of prosthetic implants such as joints, heart valves and intracardiac patches, infection by these organisms is generally a delayed expression of hospital-acquired infection. However, the recent growth in CAPD and interest in home intravenous drug therapy suggest that CONS infections will increase within the community.

Hospital

It is in the hospital setting that CONS infections have made their greatest impact. Many studies confirm the rising frequency of CONS infections (Sehaberg *et al.*, 1991). This is demonstrated in surveys of nosocomial bacteraemia; rates of 5–10% in the early 1980s are now of the order of 25–30% for all nosocomial bacteraemias a decade

TABLE 2b.3 NOTIFIED TOTAL OF STAPHYLOCOCCAL BACTERAEMIAS – ENGLAND AND WALES

Year	Total	*S. aureus*	*S. epidermidis*
1984	18405	2724	906
1985	20845	2984	906
1986	22338	3318	962
1987	23937	3525	998
1988	26253	3758	1094
1989	30872	4436	1376
1990	33365	4911	1408
1991	33834	4925	1347
1992	35159	5090	1425
1993	36318	5660	1460

Acknowledgement: Central Public Health Laboratory, London

later (Bannerjee *et al.*, 1991). CONS are now the leading cause of hospital-acquired bacteraemia as demonstrated in the National Nosocomial Infection Survey in the USA (Sehaberg *et al.*, 1991). These surveys suggest infection rates of 5.2–38.6 cases per 10 000 admissions in one institution (Martin *et al.*, 1989). This increase is greatest in patients within critical care areas such as the intensive care unit (ICU), haematology and oncology facilities, dialysis and other high-dependency units, although no service is entirely free of this problem. CNS bacteraemia among neonatal intensive care units has increased and is more common in the low birth weight infant of <1000 g (Freeman *et al.*, 1987). The impact of nosocomial CONS bacteraemia is an overall mortality of 30.5% and an attributable mortality of 13.6%, with a relative risk ratio for dying of 1.8 in comparison with controls and prolonged hospitalization (Martin *et al.*, 1989).

One population of patients in whom CONS infections have figured prominently are those with malignant disease undergoing cytotoxic chemotherapy. Gram-positive infections are an increasing cause of neutropenic febrile episodes, among which CONS predominate (EORTC, 1990). This not only reflects the use of intravascular devices such as Hickman lines (Quinn *et al.*, 1986), but also an absolute reduction in Gram-negative bacteraemia as a result of improved chemoprophylactic regimens. More aggressive cytotoxic regimens also increase the risks of infection as a result of their effects on skin and mucous membranes.

Whilst most nosocomial CONS infections are device associated, others have been clearly linked to infections at other sites such as skin and soft tissue, septic arthritis, mediastinitis, pneumonia and meningitis (Kloos and Bennerman, 1994). In many situations CONS infection has been linked to surgical wound infection or mechanical ventilation. Although the possibility of contamination is high, it is important not to dismiss the isolation of CONS from a range of non-device-associated situations without assessing the full aspects of a case carefully.

Although most CONS infections arise from the host's normal flora, there is increasing evidence to suggest that some are the result of nosocomial transmission. Studies have indicated transmission from staff to patients, whilst in other reports epidemic strains have been found circulating within high dependency units such as a neonatal ICU (Huebner *et al.*, 1994). Part of the difficulty in defining the epidemiology of nosocomial CONS infections accurately is the lack of good data concerning normal carriage rates of the various CONS species, and the factors that affect these. Furthermore, inexpensive yet reliable discriminative typing systems have been lacking. However, with the increased availability of various molecular typing systems, improved epidemiological data is likely to be forthcoming (Bingen *et al.*, 1994).

CLINICAL FEATURES

Infection with CONS does not usually exhibit characteristic clinical symptoms or signs. Patients may have a fever which is usually low grade. Other signs are those of infection at the site and are described below.

Bacteraemia and Endocarditis

CONS are now among the most frequent of blood culture isolates, especially in hospitalized patients. However, the risk of contamination with commensal CONS, either during collection or as a result of laboratory manipulations, cannot be entirely eliminated despite the use of automated blood culture systems. As a result it is generally considered desirable to have evidence that a similar isolate be present in at least two sets of blood cultures collected from different sites at different times. In routine diagnostic laboratories evidence of similarity is often restricted to colonial morphology, coagulase activity, and antibiogram with or without biochemical testing.

The microbiological diagnosis of infective endocarditis affecting a prosthetic valve or implant, or indeed a native valve, presents a particular challenge. Here repeated isolation of a similar strain from samples collected from different venepuncture sites over a period of time and viewed in the context of the overall clinical picture provides the best evidence for active infection (Caputo *et al.*, 1987). Among CONS causing endocarditis *S. epidermidis*, *S. capitis*, *S. warneri* and more recently *S. lugdunensis* predominate (Herchline and Ayers, 1991).

Intravascular Line Infections

CONS are the commonest cause of intravascular line infections (Goldman and Pier, 1993). Clinical evidence for sepsis includes inflammation, with or without a purulent discharge at the insertion site. Evidence of systemic infection and occasionally metastatic sepsis at other sites may be present. Endocarditis is always a concern with regard to infected centrally placed vascular catheters.

Peripheral blood cultures are often collected simultaneously with cultures collected through the catheter and compared in an attempt to define a pathogenic role. Since peripheral devices are more readily removed they have been sampled in various ways.

Some recommend quantitative blood cultures in this situation, although this can only increase the risk of contamination. Semi-quantitative cultures of the distal (intravascular) section of peripheral venous catheters, cultured by rolling the cut off tip across an agar plate, have provided guidance in differentiating between contamination and true colonization; counts of >15 cfu have been used to indicate catheter-related sepsis (Maki *et al.*, 1977). However, this approach is not usually of great practical value in the clinical management of such patients. Alternative approaches have included flushing of removed catheter systems, a section of which is then incubated in broth media; the ability to distinguish infection from contamination is poor and may therefore lead to confusion in the management of such patients.

Soft Tissue and Deep Wound Samples

In the case of soft tissue and wound infections, aspirated material for culture on solid media is preferred. Surface swabs will almost certainly be contaminated by normal flora. Gram stain of

infected material is valuable as a means of initial assessment and as an aid to interpretation of subsequent culture findings. In the case of infected medical implants such as joint prostheses, arthrocentesis and, when appropriate, surgical exploration allow sampling of synovial fluid, the surrounding soft tissue as well as the bone cement interface. This permits a full range of cultures including tissue homogenates to be set up. When infected prosthetic valves are removed, vegetations and infected valve rings should be processed carefully to avoid laboratory contamination. Culturing tissue homogenates may improve the yield. Likewise, an infected joint prosthesis should also be subject to microbiological sampling and culture in order to provide the best information for eradicating deep-seated infection.

Urine

Midstream specimens of urine (MSU) are generally adequate for the diagnosis of urinary tract infection (UTI). CONS count for approximately 10% of UTIs in young women. *Staphylococcus saprophyticus* and *S. epidermidis* are the most frequent CONS isolates (Latham *et al.*, 1983). The risk of contamination of the sample can present difficulties when interpreting culture findings, particularly in the absence of pyuria. Standard quantitative microbiological techniques are satis-

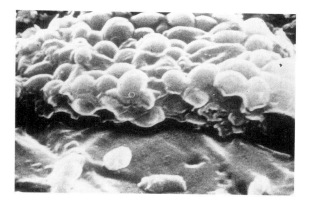

Figure 2b.1. Microcolony of coagulase-negative staphylococci growing within a biofilm on the internal surface of a central venous catheter.

factory in indicating levels of significance. Counts of 10^5 cfu/ml are considered significant but in patients with dysuria and frequency counts as low as 10^3 cfu/ml can also be found. CONS grows satisfactorily on standard laboratory media used in the diagnosis of UTI such as cysteine lactose electrolyte deficient (CLED) and MacConkey agar. Colonial morphology, coagulase negativity and resistance to a 5 μg novobiocin disk is generally satisfactory for the routine identification of *S. saprophyticus*. Isolation in pure culture is usual, although repeat mixed cultures may occur. It is rarely necessary to resort to suprapubic aspiration of urine.

Dialysis Infections

CONS are the most common cause of dialysis-associated infections and together with *S. aureus* comprise the leading bacteria responsible for infection of either short-term or chronic dialysis catheter devices (Cheesbrough *et al.*, 1986). The temporary use of double-lumen catheters for haemodialysis is often complicated by infection, usually with microorganisms of skin origin including CONS. These infections may be clinically evident but are often covert and are only recognized once the catheter is removed and cultured. Microbial attachment, colonization and biofilm production are common and are particularly associated with CONS (Baddour *et al.*, 1986). The diagnosis is usually made clinically and supported by positive blood cultures which may be collected from a peripheral vein as well as through the device.

Arteriovenous fistulae created for haemodialysis are prone to infection during needle insertion. Staphylococci are the leading pathogens; *S. aureus* predominates but CONS may also occur. The risks from both these dialysis catheter-associated infections are recurrence and metastatic spread of infection. Diagnosis is largely based on clinical evidence of sepsis and positive blood cultures. Local evidence of inflammation with exudate formation may be present. Removal of dialysis catheters provides an opportunity to culture the endovascular and subcutaneous portions through techniques such as catheter rolling and flushing (Maki *et al.*, 1977). Examination by scanning electron microscopy to visualize microcolony formation has been described within the research environment.

CONS are the most frequent cause of peritonitis in patients managed by CAPD (Working Party of the BSAC, 1987). The microbiological diagnosis is partly hampered by the low colony counts present in spent dialysate, which may be as few as <1 cfu/ml. Furthermore, the risk of contaminating samples at the time of collection or during processing, often with skin microorganisms, presents an added problem. The diagnosis is therefore based on clinical and microbiological evidence of peritonitis. The latter should include evidence of a minimum of 100 white blood cells per microlitre. The cellular effluent is made up of polymorphonuclear cells and peritoneal macrophages (Verbrugh *et al.*, 1983). Direct Gram staining of spun dialysate yields a positive result in only about 15% of instances and thus lacks sensitivity. Because of the low bacterial counts, techniques aimed at improving the yield have been adopted. Centrifuged deposits and millipore filtered samples are used in some diagnostic laboratories. However, broth enrichment culture is now widely adopted as the simplest diagnostic approach, often using conventional blood culture systems (Working Party of the BSAC, 1987). Isolation, identification and antibiotic susceptibility should follow. Recurrent infections are not uncommon and reflect either persistence of the original infection, usually from continued colonization of the implanted Tenkhoff catheter, or reinfection with a different microorganism. An interval of six weeks between two episodes of infection is often used to distinguish recurrence from reinfection. However, this is an arbitrary separation which does not always stand up to close microbiological scrutiny. Hence it is important to retain isolates in case more detailed microbiological analysis becomes necessary.

CSF Shunts/Valves

CSF-shunting systems include valves and ventriculoatrial and ventriculoperitoneal systems used in the management of hydrocephalus. Ventriculoperitoneal shunts are currently preferred. Unfortunately these are subject to microbial contamination, often at the time of insertion or subsequent manipulations, and cause considerable difficulties with regard to early diagnosis and management. Those inserted in the first few months of life are at greatest risk of infection with rates of 10–20%, of which CONS accounts for approximately three-quarters of the infecting organisms (Bayston, 1994). Shunt infections may be internal when they affect the lumen of the shunt, or less commonly external when the surgical insertion site and surrounding tissues become infected. Ventriculitis is common and requires examination of CSF for its diagnosis. Aspiration of CSF from the valve chamber of the shunt must be carried out carefully to avoid introducing infection; adequate skin disinfection is essential. Ventriculoperitoneal shunts may be associated with low-grade peritonitis. Bacteraemia is a rare complication of ventriculoarterial shunts.

LABORATORY DIAGNOSIS

Specimens

CONS may be isolated from a wide range of laboratory specimens submitted for bacteriological analysis. However, difficulties in defining their pathogenic role are common. Repeated isolation from a normally sterile body site presents few problems when ascribing aetiology. However, the fact that CONS are ubiquitous members of the normal flora of the skin and surface mucosae inevitably leads to concerns with regard to contamination of samples collected from these sites or from regions contiguous or deep to such areas. Furthermore, the association of CONS with deeply situated medical device implants presents difficulties with sampling, processing and interpretation of cultures, should these become infected. In many clinical situations the risks associated with the removal of implanted medical devices, such as prosthetic hip joints and heart valves or CSF shunting systems, present a major clinical dilemma in which the risks of removal must be carefully weighed against the failure to control the

infectious process. Various procedures have been developed, aimed at increasing the sensitivity and specificity of laboratory diagnosis.

Media

CONS can be isolated using a variety of laboratory media such as blood agar, nutrient agar, tryptic soya agar, brain heart infusion agar and their broth equivalents. Colonies vary in diameter from 1 to 3 mm following overnight incubation in air. Morphological variation provides some assistance in identification and to some extent speciation. Colonies of CONS tend to be smaller than those of *S. aureus*, usually lack pigment and were formerly called '*S. albus*' because of their white appearance. *S. lugdunensis* often appears creamy or yellow in colour. Occasional strains are sticky, reflecting slime production. In general, the colonies are entire, complex and smooth. Colonial variation occurs; for example, those of *S. haemolyticus* are usually larger than *S. epidermidis*.

Speciation

Another laboratory dilemma includes the desirability of speciating CONS isolates accurately for diagnostic and epidemiological purposes. The lack of widely available, sensitive, reliable and economical typing systems creates difficulties in recognizing outbreaks of CONS infections.

A number of commercial miniaturized rapid identification systems have been produced. The API-STAPH is widely used and has permitted ready speciation by routine diagnostic laboratories. These diagnostic kits, in conjunction with novobiocin susceptibility testing, provide speciation accuracy of 70% to >90% (Kloos and Bennerman, 1994). Occasional difficulties arise in speciating *S. warneri* and *S. haemolyticus*. However, for routine diagnostic purposes such systems are generally unnecessary and relatively expensive, especially those combined with automated reading systems. Speciation still has limitations in establishing the epidemiology of clusters of CONS infections. However, they are useful in defining the nature of repeat isolates from blood, implanted medical devices and other sites when distinguishing contaminant from pathogen.

Finally, the increasing problem of multi-drug resistance among CONS has implications for the range of susceptibility tests that should be provided. In turn the necessity for therapeutic drug monitoring of vancomycin adds an additional complexity to management.

Antibiotic Susceptibility

The growing importance of CONS as a cause of human infection has been matched by an increasing problem of drug resistance. Multiply antibiotic resistant strains of CONS are now commonly recognized either as colonizers or as pathogens. Evidence for cross-infection between patients and staff is accumulating and CONS, as part of the normal human flora, provide a reservoir in which antibiotic resistance can be spread to other CONS, and other potentially pathogenic bacteria.

The majority of CONS are able to elaborate an inducible β-lactamase and hence are resistant to penicillin, while the production of a low-affinity penicillin-binding protein, PB2a, is responsible for resistance to methicillin and related anti-staphylococcal drugs (Chambers, 1987). The *mecA* gene is common to all staphylococci exhibiting methicillin resistance and is expressed heterotypically among a variable minority of isolates within a bacterial population. Recognition is sometimes difficult to detect, requiring a higher inoculum and prolonged incubation; 2% NaCl and prolonged incubation often improves detection although *mecA* gene probe is probably the most sensitive method (Archer and Pennell, 1990). Up to 60% of CONS are methicillin resistant and of these more than half will be resistant to other agents such as gentamicin, trimethoprim, erythromycin and clindamycin. Tetracycline, chloramphenicol and quinolone resistance is more variable. Methicillin-resistant CONS should be considered to be multi-resistant unless there is *in vitro* evidence to the contrary (Archer and Climo, 1994).

Gentamicin resistance among CONS is usually enzymatic as a result of either acetylation (AAC (6')) or phosphorylation (APH (2")) (Thomas and Archer, 1989). Such resistance may be plasmid or chromosomally mediated and is common to most aminoglycosides. This is of particular concern when treating infections such as infective endocarditis for which a β-lactam–aminoglycoside regimen is widely used.

Quinolone resistance was recognized shortly after the introduction of agents such as ciprofloxacin and ofloxacin (Kotilainen *et al.*, 1990). The widespread use of these agents within hospital populations led to a rapid decline in the susceptibility of CONS as a result of DNA gyrase (*gyrA*) mutation (Piddock, 1994). More recently, alterations to the *norA* gene have been linked to increased efflux of quinolones and other antibiotics (Piddock, 1994). Resistance rates vary throughout the world but are of the order of 7–22%. Cross-resistance to other quinolones is common and includes the more recently developed agents active against Gram-positive cocci.

Tetracycline resistance has declined owing to less frequent use in hospitals. Resistance rates of about 25–35% (Archer and Scott, 1991) occur and are related to either reflux or ribosomal resistance; while the *tet* (K) gene is responsible for plasmid-mediated resistance (Bismuth *et al.*, 1990), the *tet* M gene is chromosomally carried and is responsible for resistance in minocycline, tetracycline and doxycycline, although minocycline often retains activity against other tetracycline-resistant strains.

Macrolide resistance is often linked to clindamycin and streptogramin resistance since they share a similar target on the 50S ribosomal subunit, which is important in translocation and transpeptidation. The majority of methicillin-resistant CONS and even some methicillin-sensitive strains will be resistant to erythromycin and related compounds (Archer and Climo, 1994). Dissociated resistance between erythromycin and clindamycin is the result of differential induction of the *erm* gene (Jenssen *et al.*, 1987), although mutational resistance can occur during treatment with clindamycin. New macrolides—clarithromycin and azithromycin—appear to offer no advantage with regard to CONS since *in vitro* activity is comparable and cross-resistance occurs (Hamilton-Miller, 1992).

Rifampicin is increasingly used to treat deep-seated CONS infection in combination with other antibiotics. CONS are usually highly sensitive but rifampicin-resistant mutants occur spontaneously at a rate of approximately 1 in 10^6 as a result of genetic mutation in coding for the subunit of DNA-dependent RNA polymerase. It is therefore important that use of this agent be limited and should be based on *in vitro* evidence of susceptibility.

Vancomycin is currently the glycopeptide of choice for the treatment of most serious CONS infections. To date most CONS remain susceptible to 4 mg/l vancomycin or less, although occasional strains of *S. haemolyticus* are resistant (Schwalbe *et al.*, 1987). Vancomycin resistance among *S. epidermidis* isolates is even more uncommon.

Teicoplanin is being increasingly used as an alternative to vancomycin in the treatment of a wide range of staphylococcal infections. However, CONS of reduced susceptibility (minimal inhibitory concentration > 8 mg/l) among *S. epidermidis* and *S. haemolyticus* are now recognized (Bannerman *et al.*, 1991). Resistance to *S. haemolyticus* can be readily reduced *in vitro* and among *S. epidermidis* by stepwise exposure (Biavasco *et al.*, 1991). However, such strains are currently uncommon.

MANAGEMENT OF INFECTION

The clinical presentations of CONS infection vary widely according to the circumstances in which they express disease. In patients with deep-seated infections, such as those complicating a prosthetic hip implant, clinical features are usually localized to the joint with progressive pain, and eventually instability; constitutional symptoms are often absent. This contrasts with the patient in an ICU with multiple endovascular lines, in whom fever and persistent bacteraemia should rapidly raise the suspicion of line-associated sepsis. Peritonitis complicating CAPD is usually accompanied by a cloudy effluent dialysate and may precede clinical symptoms of peritonitis.

The diagnostic and management problems of CONS-associated infections are accentuated by the difficulties in establishing a microbiological diagnosis, particularly in situations associated with deep-seated infection. Removal of an infected prosthetic device presents specific and individual problems; an implanted heart valve is less easily dealt with than an endovascular catheter which may be readily removed. The diagnostic problems are compounded by the occasional difficulties in confidently ascribing pathogenicity to organisms which are the most common laboratory or sampling contaminant. Furthermore, antibiotic choice is restricted owing to the frequency of multi-drug resistance. Finally, there may be uncertainty with regard to duration of therapy, and the likelihood of success if prescribed in the continued presence of an infected medical device.

Urinary Tract Infection

Staphylococcus saprophyticus, and less commonly *S. epidermidis* and other species of CONS, are a cause of UTI. Although most commonly associated with acute cystitis in young women, the upper urinary tract or prostate may occasionally be involved. Acute cystitis can usually be treated with an appropriate antibiotic, although susceptibility guidance is desirable. Trimethoprim, nitrofurantoin or a quinolone such as norfloxacin are all appropriate choices provided the organism is sensitive. Short-course therapy is now widely practised using a three-day regimen with arrangements for checking MSU six weeks after treatment, or earlier should symptoms fail to resolve.

Intravascular Line Infection

The range and complexity of intravascular lines in current medical use are reflected in the diverse nature of the infectious complications. One of the most widely used devices is the intravenous cannula of the 'Venflon' variety. These may or may not have an integral injection port. Most are sited in peripheral veins for short-term vascular access. The complications include phlebitis and infection which are often interrelated and vary with the type of plastic, the length of the device and the site of insertion (Cheesbrough and Finch, 1985). Evidence of infection at the exit site is usually managed by device removal with spontaneous resolution. Occasionally cellulitis or septic phlebitis may occur, with the necessity for antibiotic therapy. Most respond to an anti-staphylococcal penicillin, such as flucloxacillin, although occasionally metastatic infection may arise with positive blood cultures. Antibiotic selection should then be governed by sensitivity testing but will usually include either a penicillase-stable penicillin or a glycopeptide such as vancomycin.

Central venous catheters are used for a variety of purposes including pressure monitoring, infusion of fluids, blood or drugs and parenteral nutrition. Infectious complications are much more frequent, usually because of the multiple uses these systems are put to. Hickman, Broviac, Swan–Ganz and haemodialysis catheters are particularly subject to infectious complications from skin microorganisms (Cheesbrough et al., 1986; Goldman and Pier, 1993). Staphylococci including CONS predominate (Mermel et al., 1991). There should be a low threshold for suspecting such an infection in any patient running a fever with a central line in place. Blood cultures should be obtained and the exit site inspected and sampled (Linares et al., 1985). It is occasionally helpful to draw blood cultures through the catheter (Moyer et al., 1983).

The principles of treatment are the same as for peripheral devices. However, these devices are often essential to patient management, particularly those patients in a high-dependency unit, so that a trial of antibiotic therapy is often conducted before a decision to remove the device is made; ideally the catheter should be removed and resited. Antibiotic choice should again be guided by laboratory susceptibility testing. In the case of CONS infections greatest reliance is now placed on vancomycin, with teicoplanin as an alternative choice. This strategy will occasionally prove successful, but as stated, line removal is often necessary to eradicate infection. There is the risk of developing metastatic infection or endovascular infection such as right-sided endocarditis when the catheter tip is sited within the heart.

Infective Endocarditis

Staphylococci are the most frequent cause of prosthetic valve endocarditis (PVE) and less commonly native valve endocarditis (Caputo et al., 1987). Although predominantly arising within two months following valve insertion, it has become increasingly apparent that endocarditis beyond this period may also be staphylococcal in nature. CONS figure prominently in both situations (Karchmer et al., 1983). The key clinical features of endocarditis include low-grade fever, a murmur and systemic embolization. There should be a low threshold for suspecting infective endocarditis in patients with prosthetic heart valves, intracardiac patches or ventricular support systems. The diagnosis is normally confirmed microbiologically by evidence of persistent bacteraemia on blood culture.

The management of PVE includes prolonged high-dose intravenous bactericidal antibiotic, and careful monitoring of clinical response supported by investigations such as echocardiography. Failure to control bacteraemia, a changing murmur, conduction abnormalities suggesting a septal abscess, progressive heart failure and major embolic phenomena are all indications for urgent valve replacement.

The antibiotic regimen should be guided by laboratory information on the nature and susceptibility of the infecting organism. In the case of CONS endocarditis an anti-staphylococcal penicillin such as flucloxacillin in combination with gentamicin, with or without the addition of rifampicin, is commonly prescribed (Massanari and Donta, 1978). In those allergic to penicillin an appropriate cephalosporin or vancomycin is widely used, again in association with gentamicin. Teicoplanin provides an alternative to vancomycin (Galetto et al., 1986). The latter will require careful monitoring of blood levels to avoid drug toxicity, especially to the kidney. Treatment of PVE requires a minimum of six weeks therapy with careful follow-up to detect relapse. PVE complicates approximately 2–3% of procedures. Prevention requires careful surgical technique with practices similar to those adopted for prosthetic joint insertion (q.v.). Perioperative antibiotic prophylaxis regimens vary but a broad-spectrum cephalosporin such as cefuroxime is generally suitable. If surgery is prolonged, a second dose may need to be administered.

CAPD Peritonitis

Peritonitis is the commonest complication of CAPD. The infecting organisms often arise from the skin of the patient and gain access to the Tenkhoff catheter during bag changes. Less commonly the catheter exit site becomes infected. There is considerable individual variation in the frequency of such infections. Patients need to be educated in the practice of sterile technique and observed to ensure good practices, since repeated episodes of peritonitis can alter the efficiency of the peritoneal surface as a dialysis membrane.

The principles of management have evolved over the past decade or so. Systemic antibiotics are less able to achieve sufficiently high therapeutic concentrations within the infected peritoneal cavity than those administered directly with the dialysate. The latter is the preferred route of administration although in patients with systemic features of sepsis one or two doses of antibiotic are given intravenously at the start of therapy (Report of BSAC, 1987).

The choice of agent should be guided by microbiological information. However, the initial empirical regimen takes account of the importance of skin staphylococci and in particular CONS. Vancomycin plus gentamicin is the most widely adopted combination. Alternatives have included cefuroxime, quinolones, other cephalosporins and carbapenems. Whilst the drug has frequently been given into each dialysate bag it is now recognized that alternate bag therapy, or even the overnight dwell bag, may be adequate for the control of such infections (Ad Hoc Advisory Committee, 1993). However, before varying the regimen it is important to monitor response to treatment clinically by observing the clearing of the dialysate bag. Microbiological information may permit subsequent simplification of the regimen to a single drug. Treatment is usually continued for a period of 7–10 days when managing CONS infections, but longer periods for infections caused by yeasts or Gram-negatives such as *Pseudomonas aeruginosa* will be required (Report of BSAC, 1987).

Patients should be monitored to detect early relapse. Should this occur within a six-week period then careful consideration should be given to whether the Tenkhoff catheter is heavily colonized with bacteria within a biofilm. This makes eradication of infection extremely difficult and catheter change is often necessary for its clearance. Traditionally this required a period of haemodialysis following peritoneal catheter removal and the subsequent insertion of a new Tenkhoff device. However, removal and insertion of a new catheter as a single procedure has proved successful under cover of appropriate antibiotic therapy, and has the advantage of avoiding unnecessary haemodialysis and a further surgical procedure to insert a new catheter as a delayed procedure (Ad Hoc Advisory Committee, 1993).

CSF Shunt Infections

The management of CSF shunt infections is a specialized problem requiring close collaboration between experienced neurosurgical and microbiological services and an individualized decision as to whether this should be managed surgically or non-surgically (Bayston, 1994). Surgical treatment requires shunt removal and reshunting, with or without a period of external ventricular CSF drainage. An alternative approach includes shunt removal and regular ventricular taps in selected patients. However, both approaches run the risk of either ventriculitis from retrograde spread of organisms through the external ventricular drainage system or from direct puncture, which of itself may result in porencephalic cysts (Mayhall *et al.*, 1984). Another approach has been to remove the infected shunt and replace it immediately with a fresh system. However, this can be technically difficult and the risk of infecting the new shunt, despite appropriate antibiotic cover, may occur.

The antibiotic management of CSF shunt infections depends upon the causative microorganisms, their known susceptibility to antibiotics and the ability to deliver the antibiotic in sufficient concentrations to the site of the infection (Bayston *et al.*, 1995). Furthermore, the ability of many microorganisms to form microcolonies and exist within a biofilm presents further difficulties with regard to eradicating these infections.

Various antibiotics have been used, such as flucloxacillin, cephalosporins such as cefuroxime, fusidic acid, erythromycin, and to a lesser extent clindamycin. The modest inflammatory response in the CSF produced by infections such as CONS presents further difficulties in achieving adequate concentrations of β-lactam agents within the CSF. Furthermore, these drugs are only active against dividing cells, and within an infected CSF shunt cells are often dividing extremely slowly. Greatest reliance is therefore currently placed on the use of vancomycin, with or without rifampicin (Bayston *et al.*, 1995). It is important that the infecting organism be identified carefully, and in the case of CONS the laboratory evidence should suggest a true infection rather than the presence of a contaminating organism.

Intraventricular administration of antibiotics is usually essential to achieve sufficient bactericidal concentrations to sterilize an infected shunt and the ventricular CSF. In the case of ventriculoperitoneal shunts infection is also present within the peritoneal cavity (although often clinically inapparent) and systemic antibiotics should also be given.

Vancomycin has achieved greater importance in the management of multiply antibiotic resistant staphylococcal shunt infection. A daily dose of 20 mg vancomycin administered intraventricularly has proved effective and safe (Bayston *et al.*, 1987). CSF fluid concentrations of between 200 and 300 mg/l are achieved. Systemic antibiotic is also given and oral rifampicin is preferred when dealing with staphylococccal infections. The response to treatment is measured clinically and by repeated CSF fluid examination. CONS infections generally disappear within four to five days. CSF fluid levels of antibiotic should be measured preferably to ensure adequate bactericidal concentrations. A decision whether to attempt medical eradication of infection or to reshunt requires assessment of all factors relevant to the case.

Prosthetic Joint Infections

Many thousands of total hip arthroplasties and total knee procedures are performed annually. The majority give rise to few complications. However, the development of a wound infection, and more seriously infection of the prosthesis, can result in failure of the prosthetic implant (Fitzgerald *et al.*, 1977). Infection rates for total hip replacements vary between 0.6% and 2%. The rate for total knee arthroplasties is approximately two-fold higher. Underlying problems such as diabetes mellitus, rheumatoid arthritis, advanced age and infection remote from the operation site are all recognized risk factors for infection which may arise by direct implantation through the open wound, or as a result of haematogenous spread, or less commonly as a result of the reactivation of latent infection in a previously infected operative site. Infections are reduced in frequency by the use of prophylactic antibiotics in the perioperative period and by high-efficiency particulate air (HEPA) exhaust ventilation systems in the operating theatre suite (Salvati *et al.*, 1982). The use of exhausted suits for the operating team are an additional refinement, but have not been widely adopted.

The diagnosis of joint infection can be difficult and may be delayed since local symptoms often occur late (Inman *et al.*, 1984). Loosening of the prosthesis is a late sign. Systemic signs of infection are often lacking in the early stages. Monitoring the erythrocyte sedimentation rate (ESR) can be valuable. Early acute infections are more likely to be caused by *S. aureus* and associated with poor wound healing and local evidence of infection. Infections delayed beyond a three-month period are more usually associated with low-grade pathogens such as CONS and other skin bacteria such as *Propionibacterium* spp. Infection should be suspected if there is persistent joint pain and a raised ESR.

The management of prosthetic joint infections needs to be individualized and is a balance between medical and surgical treatment. Prolonged antibiotic therapy for periods ranging from 1 to 12 months according to response is widely practised. The choice of agent should be guided by microbiological data, but should be directed at Gram-positive cocci including CONS in the absence of any laboratory information. Drugs such as flucloxacillin, co-amoxiclav or a cephalosporin are commonly used. These may be given parenterally for the first few weeks until there is clinical evidence of response, including a falling ESR. Surgical drainage of any infected material should be part of the early management, whilst early resection of an obviously infected arthroplasty should not be delayed. A replacement implant should only be considered once all evidence of local infection has disappeared.

Prevention of prosthetic joint infections requires careful consideration of the operative environment, which should include a satisfactory ventilation system, preferably with a HEPA air filtration arrangement (Lidwell et al., 1984). Meticulous preparation of the operative site and observance of all aspects of sterile technique are essential. Double glove techniques and operator isolator systems have their devotees. Patients should be free of infection at other sites and in particular the skin.

The use of antibiotic prophylaxis is now well established and in general when given as a short perioperative course is effective in encouraging a sterile operative site. The combined benefits of clean air within the operating room and short-course perioperative antibiotic prophylaxis have been associated with the lowest complication rates of <1%. Among the agents selected cloxacillin, flucloxacillin and the cephalosporins have proved the most popular (Pollard et al., 1979; Hill et al., 1981). Cefuroxime, cephradine and cefazolin possess antistaphylococcal activity, which is a primary consideration although the increasing frequency of antibiotic resistance has led to alternative choices such as co-amoxiclav (Nelson, 1987). Other techniques such as joint irrigation and antibiotic-impregnated bone cement have been used by some but have not been widely adopted.

REFERENCES

Ad Hoc Advisory Committee on Peritonitis Management (1993) Peritoneal dialysis-related peritonitis treatment recommendations: 1993 update. *Peritoneal Dialysis International*, **13**, 14–28.

Archer, G.L. and Climo, M.W. (1994) Antimicrobial susceptibility of coagulase-negative staphylococci. *Antimicrobial Agents and Chemotherapy*, **38**, 2231–2235.

Archer, G.L. and Pennell, E. (1990) Detection of methicillin resistance in staphylococci by using a DNA probe. *Antimicrobial Agents and Chemotherapy*, **34**, 1720–1724.

Archer, G.L. and Scott, J. (1991) Conjugative transfer genes in staphylococcal isolates from the United States. *Antimicrobial Agents and Chemotherapy*, **35**, 2500–2504.

Baddour, L.M., Smalley, D.L., Kraus, A.P., Jr et al. (1986) Comparison of microbiologic characteristics of pathogenic and saprophytic coagulase-negative staphylococci from patients on continuous ambulatory peritoneal dialysis. *Diagnostic Microbiology and Infectious Diseases*, **5**, 197–205.

Bannerjee, S.N., Emori, T.G., Culver, D.H. et al. (1991) Secular trends in nosocomial primary bloodstream infections in the United States, 1980–1989. *American Journal of Medicine*, **91** (Suppl. 3B), 86S–89S.

Bannerman, T.L., Wadiak, D.L. and Kloos, W.E. (1991) Susceptibility of staphylococcus species and subspecies to teicoplanin. *Antimicrobial Agents and Chemotherapy*, **35**, 1919–1922.

Barker, L.P., Simpson, W.A. and Christensen, G.D. (1990) Differential production of slime under aerobic and anaerobic conditions. *Journal of Clinical Microbiology*, **28**, 2578–2579.

Barrow, G.I., and Feltham, R.K.A. (1993) *Cowan and Steel's Manual for the Identification of Medical Bacteria*. Cambridge University Press, Cambridge.

Bayston, R. (1994) Hydrocephalus shunt infections. *Journal of Antimicrobial Chemotherapy*, Suppl. A, 75–84.

Bayston, R. and Rodgers, J. (1990) Production of extracellular slime by *Staphylococcus epidermis*, during stationary phase of growth: its association with adherence to implantable devices. *Journal of Clinical Pathology*, **43**, 866–870.

Bayston, R., Hart, C.A. and Barniecoat, N. (1987) Intraventricular vancomycin in the treament of ventriculitis associated with cerebrospinal shunting and draining. *Journal of Neurology, Neurosurgery Psychiatry*, **50**, 1419–1423.

Bayston, R., de Louvois, J., Brown, E.M. et al. (1995) Treatment of infections associated with shunting for hydrocephalus. *British Journal of Hospital Medicine*, **53**, 368–373.

Beutler, B. and Cerami, A. (1989) The biology of cachectic/TNFα: a primary mediator of the host response. *Annual Review of Immunology*, **7**, 625–656.

Biavasco, F., Giovanetti, E., Montanari, M.P. et al. (1991) Development of in-vitro resistance to glycopeptide antibiotics: assessment in staphylococci of different species. *Antimicrobial Chemotherapy*, **27**, 71–79.

Bingen, E.H., Denamur, E. and Elion, J. (1994) Use of ribotyping in epidemiological surveillance of nosocomial outbreaks. *Clinical Microbiology Reviews*, **7**, 311–327.

Bismuth, R., Zilhao, R., Sakamoto, H. *et al.* (1990) Gene heterogeneity for tetracycline resistance in *Staphylococcus* spp. *Antimicrobial Agents and Chemotherapy*, **34**, 1611–1614.

Caputo, G.M., Archer, G., Calderwood, S.B. *et al.* (1987) Native valve endocarditis due to coagulase-negative staphylococci: clinical and microbiologic features. *American Journal of Medicine*, **83**, 619–625.

Chamber, H.F. (1987) Coagulase-negative staphylococci resistant to β-lactam antibiotics in vivo produce penicillin-binding protein 2a. *Antimicrobial Agents and Chemotherapy*, **31**, 1919–1924.

Cheesbrough, J.S. and Finch, R.G. (1985) Studies on the microbiological safety of the valved side-port of the 'Venflon' cannula. *Journal of Hospital Infection*, **2**, 201–208.

Cheesbrough, J.S., Finch, R.G. and Burden, R.P. (1986) A prospective study of the mechanisms of infection associated with hemodialysis catheters. *Journal of Infectious Diseases*, **154**, 579–589.

Denyer, S.P., Davies, M.C., Evans, J.A. *et al.* (1990) Influence of carbon dioxide on the surface characteristics and adherence potential of coagulase-negative staphylococci. *Journal of Clinical Microbiology*, **28**, 1813–1817.

Dinarello, C.A. (1989) Interleukin 1 and its biologically related cytokines. *Advances in Immunology*, **44**, 153–206.

EORTC International Antimicrobial Therapy Cooperative Group (1990) Gram-positive bacteremia in granulocytopenic cancer patients: results of a prospective randomized therapeutic trial. *European Journal of Cancer and Clinical Oncology*, **26**(5), 569–574.

Fitzgerald, R.H., Nolan, D.R., Illstrup, D.M. *et al.* (1977) Deep wound sepsis following total hip arthroplasty. *Journal of Bone and Joint Surgery*, **59A**, 847–855.

Freeman, J., Platt, R., Sidebottom, D.G. *et al.* (1987) Coagulase-negative staphylococcal bacteremia in the changing neonatal intensive care population. *Journal of the American Medical Association*, **258**, 2548–2552.

Galetto, D.W., Boscia, J.A., Kobasa, W.D. and Kaye, D. (1986) Teicoplanin compared with vancomycin for treatment of experimental endocarditis due to methicillin-resistant *Staphylococcus epidermidis*. *Journal of Infectious Diseases*, **154**, 69–75.

Gemmell, C.G. (1986) Virulence characteristics of *Staphylococcus epidermidis*. *Journal of Medical Microbiology*, **22**, 287–289.

Goldman, D.A. and Pier, G.B. (1993) Pathogenesis of infections related to intravascular catheterization. *Clinical Microbiology Reviews*, **6**, 176–192.

Gray, E.D., Peters, G., Verstegen, M. *et al.* (1984) Effects of extracellular slime substance from *Staphylococcus epidermidis* on the cellular immune response. *Lancet*, **i**, 365–367.

Hamilton-Miller, J. (1992) In-vitro activities of 14-, 15- and 16-membered macrolides against Gram-positive cocci. *Journal of Antimicrobial Chemotherapy*, **29**, 141–147.

Herchline, T.E. and Ayers, L.W. (1991) Occurrence of *Staphylococcus lugdunensis* in consecutive clinical cultures and relationship of isolation to infection. *Journal of Clinical Microbiology*, **29**, 419–421.

Hill, C., Flamant, R., Mazas, F. *et al.* (1981) Prophylactic cefazolin versus placebo in total hip replacement. *Lancet*, **i**, 795–797.

Huebner, J., Pier, G.B., Maslow, J.N. *et al.* (1994) Endemic nosocomial transmission of *Staphylococcus epidermidis* bacteraemia isolates in a neonatal intensive care unit over 10 years. *Journal of Investigative Dermatology*, **169**, 526–531.

Hussain, M., Hastings, J.G.M. and White, P.J. (1991) Isolation and composition of the extracellular slime made by coagulase-negative staphylococci in a chemically defined medium. *Journal of Infectious Diseases*, **163**, 534–541.

Hussain, M.A., Wilcox, M.H., White, P.J. *et al.* (1992a) Importance of medium and atmosphere type to both slime production and adherence by coagulase-negative staphylococci. *Journal of Hospital Infection*, **20**, 173–184.

Hussain, M., Collins, C., Hastings, J.G.M. *et al.* (1992b) Radiochemical assay to measure the biofilm produced by coagulase-negative staphylococci on solid surfaces and its use to quantitate the effects of various antibacterial compounds on the formation of the biofilm. *Journal of Medical Microbiology*, **37**, 62–69.

Inman, R.D., Gallegos, K.V., Brause, B.D. *et al.* (1984) Clinical and microbial features of prosthetic joint infection. *American Journal of Medicine*, **77**, 47–53.

Jenssen, W.D., Thakker-Varia, S., Dublin, D.T. *et al.* (1987) Prevalence of macrolide–licosamides–streptogramin B resistance and *erm* gene classes among clinical strains of staphylococci and streptococci. *Antimicrobial Agents and Chemotherapy*, **31**, 883–888.

Johnson, G.M., Lee, D.A., Regelmann, W.E. *et al.* (1986) Interference with granulocyte function by *Staphylococcus epidermidis* slime. *Infection and Immunity*, **54**, 13–20.

Karchmer, A.W., Archer, G.L. and Dismukes, W.E. (1983) *Staphylococcus epidermidis* causing prosthetic valve endocarditis: microbiologic and clinical observations as guides to therapy. *Annals of Internal Medicine*, **98**, 447–455.

Kloos, W.E. and Bennerman, T.L. (1994) Update on clinical significance of coagulase-negative staphylococci. *Clinical Microbiology Reviews*, **7**, 117–140.

Kloos, W.E., Schleifer, K.H. and Götz, F. (1991) The genus *Staphylococcus*. In *The Prokaryotes* (ed. A. Balows, H.G. Trüper, M. Dworkin *et al.*), pp. 1369–1420. Springer-Verlag, New York.

Kotilainen, P., Maki, J., Oksman, P. *et al.* (1990) Immunochemical analysis of the extracellular slime substance of *Staphylococcus epidermidis*. *European Journal of Clinical Microbiology and Infectious Diseases*, **9**, 262–270.

Kotilaninen, P., Nikoskelainen, J. and Huovinen, P. (1990) Emergence of ciprofloxacin-resistant coagulase-negative staphylococcal skin flora in immunocompromised patients receiving ciprofloxacin. *Journal of Infectious Diseases*, **161**, 41–44.

Latham, R.H., Running, K. and Stamm, W.E. (1983) Urinary tract infections in young adult women caused by *Staphylococcus saprophyticus*. *Journal of the American Medical Association*, **250**, 3063–3066.

Lidwell, O.M., Lowbury, E.J.L., Whyte, W. *et al.* (1984) Infection and sepsis after operations for total hip or knee-joint replacement: influence of ultra-clean air, prophylactic antibiotics and other factors. *Journal of Hygiene (Cambridge)*, **93**, 505–529.

Linares, J., Sitges-Serra, A., Garau, J. *et al.* (1985) Pathogenesis of catheter sepsis: a prospective study with quantitative and semiquantitative cultures of catheter hub and segments. *Journal of Clinical Microbiology*, **25**, 357–360.

Maki, G.D., Weise, C.E. and Sarafin, H.W. (1977) A semiquantitative culture method for identifying intravenous catheter-related infection. *New England Journal of Medicine*, **296**, 1305–1309.

Martin, M.A., Pfaller, M.A. and Wenzel, R.P. (1989) Coagulase-negative staphylococcal bacteraemia. *Annals of Internal Medicine*, **110**, 9–16.

Massanari, R.M. and Donta, S.T. (1978) The efficacy of rifampicin as adjunctive therapy in selected cases of staphylococcal endocarditis. *Chest*, **73**, 371–375.

Mayhall, C.G., Archer, N.H., Lamb, A. *et al.* (1984) Ventriculostomy-related infections: a prospective epidemiologic study. *New England Journal of Medicine*, **310**, 553–559.

McLean, R., Nicket, J.C., Noakes, V. *et al.* (1985) An in vitro ultrastructural study of infectious kidney stone genesis. *Infectional and Immunity*, **49**, 805–811.

Mermel, L.A., McCormick, R.D., Springman, S.R. *et al.* (1991) The pathogenesis and epidemiology of catheter-related infection with pulmonary artery Swan–Ganz catheters: a prospective study utilizing molecular subtyping. *American Journal of Medicine*, **91**, S197–205.

Modun, B., Williams, P., Pike, W.J. *et al.* (1992) Cell envelope proteins of *Staphylococcus epidermidis* grown in vivo in a peritoneal chamber implant. *Infection and Immunity*, **60**, 2551–2553.

Modun, B., Kendall, D. and Williams, P. (1994) Staphylococci express a receptor for human transferrin: identification of a 42-kilodalton cell wall transferrin-binding protein. *Infection and Immunity*, **62**, 3850–3958.

Moyer, M.A., Edwards, L.D. and Farley, L. (1983) Comparative culture methods on 101 intravenous catheters: routine, semiquantitative and blood cultures. *Archives of Internal Medicine*, **143**, 66–69.

Nelson, C.L. (1987) The prevention of infection in total joint replacement surgery. *Reviews of Infectious Diseases*, **9**, 613–618.

Noble, M.A., Grant, S.K. and Hajen, E. (1990) Characterization of a neutrophil-inhibitory factor from clinically significant *Staphylococcus epidermidis*. *Journal of Infectious Diseases*, **162**, 909–913.

Paulsson, M., Ljungh, A. and Wadström, T. (1992) Rapid identification of fibronectin, vitronectin, laminin, and collagen cell surface binding proteins on coagulase-negative staphylococci by particle agglutination assays. *Journal of Clinical Microbiology*, **30**, 2006–2112.

Pereira, A.T. (1962) Coagulase-negative strains of *Staphylococcus* possessing antigen 51 as agents of urinary infections. *Journal of Clinical Pathology*, **15**, 252–259.

Pfaller, M.A. and Herwald, L.A. (1968) Laboratory, clinical and epidemiological aspects of coagulase-negative staphylococci. *Clinical Microbiology Reviews*, **1**, 281–299.

Piddock, L. (1994) New quinolones and Gram-positive bacteria., *Antimicrobial Agents and Chemotherapy*, **38**, 163–169.

Pollard, J.P., Hughes, S.P.F., Scott, J.E. *et al.* (1979) Antibiotic prophylaxis in total hip replacement. *British Medical Journal*, **i**, 707–709.

Quinn, J.P., Counts, G.W. and Meyers, J.D. (1986) Intracardiac infections due to coagulase-negative staphylococcus associated with Hickman catheters. *Cancer*, **57**, 1079–1082.

Report of a Working Party of the British Society for Antimicrobial Chemotherapy (1987) Peritonitis complicating continuous peritoneal dialysis: recommendations for its diagnosis and management. *Lancet*, **i**, 845–849.

Salvati, E.A., Robinson, R.P., Zeno, S.M. *et al.* (1982) Infection rates after 3175 total hip and total knee replacements performed with and without a horizontal unidirectional filtered air-flow system. *Journal of Bone and Joint Surgery*, **64A**, 525–535.

Schwalbe, R.S., Stapleton, J.T. and Gilligan, P.H. (1987) Emergence of vancomycin resistance in coagulase-negative staphylococci. *New England Journal of Medicine*, **316**, 927–931.

Sehaberg, D.R., Culver, D.H. and Gaynes, R.P. (1991) Major trends in the microbial etiology of nosocomial infection. *American Journal of Medicine*, **91** (S3B), 72–75.

Shiro, H., Muller, E., Gutierrez, N. *et al.* (1994) Transposon mutants of *Staphylococcus epidermidis* deficient in elaboration of capsular polysaccharide/adhesin and slime are avirulent in a rabbit model of endocarditis. *Journal of Infectious Diseases*, **169**, 1042–1049.

Stout, R.D., Ferguson, K.P., Li, Y. *et al.* (1992) Staphylococcal exopolysaccharides inhibit lymphocyte proliferative responses by activation of monocyte prostaglandin production. *Infection and Immunity*, **60**, 922–927.

Tenney, J.H., Moody, M.R., Newman, K.A. *et al.* (1986) Adherent microorganisms on luminal surfaces of long-term intravenous catheters. *Archives of Internal Medicine*, **146**, 1949–1954.

Thomas, W.D., Jr and Archer, G.L. (1989) Mobility of gentamicin resistance genes from staphylococci isolated in the United States: identification of Tn*4031*, a gentamicin resistance transposon from *Staphylococcus epidermidis*. *Antimicrobial Agents and Chemotherapy*, **33**, 1335–1341.

Timmerman, C.P., Fleer, A., Besnier, J.M. *et al.* (1991) Characterization of a proteinaceous adhesin of *Staphylococcus epidermidis* which mediates attachment to polystyrene. *Infection and Immunity*, **59**, 4187–4192.

Tojo, M., Yamashita, N., Goldman, D.A. *et al.* (1988) Isolation and characterization of a capsular polysaccharide/adhesin from *Staphylococcus epidermidis*. *Journal of Infectious Diseases*, **157**, 713–722.

Verbrugh, H.A., Keane, W.F., Hoidal, J.R. *et al.* (1983) Peritoneal macrophages and opsonins: antibacterial defense in patients undergoing chronic peritoneal dialysis. *Journal of Infectious Diseases*, **147**, 1018–1029.

Wadström, T. (1989) Molecular aspects of bacterial adhesion, colonization, and development of infections associated with biomaterials. *Journal of Investigative Surgery*, **2**, 353–360.

Williams, P., Denyer, S.P. and Finch, R.G. (1988) Protein antigens of *Staphylococcus epidermidis* grown under iron-restricted conditions of human peritoneal dialysate. FEMS *Microbiology Letters*, **50**, 29–33.

Working Party of the British Society for Antimicrobial Chemotherapy (1987) Diagnosis and management of peritonitis in continuous ambulatory peritoneal dialysis. *Lancet*, **i**, 845–849.

3

CORYNEBACTERIUM

Philip G. Murphy

INTRODUCTION

History

The *Corynebacterium* genus was first proposed by Lehmann and Neumann in 1896 to include the diphtheria bacillus and other morphologically similar organisms. Klebs first observed *Corynebacterium diphtheriae* in 1883 and Loeffler in 1884 first cultured the species. The genus name emphasizes the tendency towards club-like formation in culture (Greek: *koryne* = club) which is characteristic of the diphtheria bacillus and several other species within the coryneform group, particularly in old cultures. The generic name was accepted by the committee appointed by the Society of American Bacteriologists (Winslow *et al.*, 1920). The genus encompasses other morphologically similar organisms derived from plant, water, air and soil to give a large and heterogeneous collection. These organisms are often referred to as diphtheroids but a more correct term would be coryneforms, as the term diphtheroid implies close resemblance to *C. diphtheriae*, while the term coryneform simply refers to a morphologic appearance.

Classification

Neither the term diphtheroid nor coryneform is of any specific taxonomic meaning. The coryneforms can be defined as 'pleomorphic Gram-positive rods occurring in angular arrangements and developing a varied proportion of coccoid cells in stationary cultures. Rudimentary branching may occur but definite mycelia are not formed. These organisms do not produce endospores, are not acid fast, and may be motile (Coyle *et al.*, 1985). There may be up to 21 genera within the coryneform group, 60% of which can be identified to genus level. These include *Corynebacterium*, *Brevibacterium*, *Arthrobacter*, *Cellulomonas*, *Curtobacterium*, *Microbacterium*, *Caseobacter*, *Rhodococcus*, *Oerskovia*, and arguably *Propionibacterium* as many strains of *P. granulosum*, *P. avidum*, and occasionally *P. acnes* are facultative anaerobes and resemble the coryneform group (Goodfellow and Minikin, 1981; Keddie and Jones, 1981).

Within this coryneform group are the diphtheroids; these are pleomorphic Gram-positive bacilli which stain irregularly and may contain metachromatic (polyphosphate) granules. A collection of aerobic coryneforms isolated from human skin

Principles and Practice of Clinical Bacteriology. Edited by A.M. Emmerson, P.M. Hawkey and S.H. Gillespie
© 1997 John Wiley & Sons Ltd

characterized on the basis of cell wall amino acids and sugars proved to be *Corynebacterium* spp., in 60%, another 20% were related to *Brevibacterium* spp., 5% resembled aerobic *Propionibacterium* spp., and 15% appeared to be environmental isolates from a variety of other unnamed genera (Noble, 1984; Pitcher, 1977). The *Corynebacterium* genus is the genus of greatest medical importance but even here the taxonomy is complex and changing, e.g. *C. ulcerans* has not been properly accepted into the genus and *C. aquaticum* and *C. bovis* may not be appropriately placed in the genus.

An upsurge in the isolation of coryneforms, particularly the *Corynebacterium* spp., has been seen in recent years, due in part to the combination of advanced medical and surgical procedures. Immunosuppression therapies and transplant procedures lead to an increased use of multiple courses of broad-spectrum antimicrobial agents and prolonged use of intravascular devices which breach skin defences. The ensuing opportunistic infections arising from skin sources have included most skin residents and transients and among the corynebacteria the following have been reported: *C. xerosis*, *C. pseudodiphtheriticum* (*C. hofmannii*), *Rhodococcus equi* (*C. equi*), *Bacterionema matruchotti* (*C. matruchotti*), *C. striatum*, *C. aquaticum*, *Actinomyces pyogenes* (*C. pyogenes*), *C. genitalium*, '*C. pseudogenitalium*', and in non-compromised individuals *C. ulcerans*, *C. bovis*, *Arcanobacterium haemolyticum* (*C. haemolyticum*), *C. pseudotuberculosis* (*C. ovis*), *C. minutissimum* and of course *C. diphtheriae* (Lipsky *et al.*, 1982). The Special Pathogens Section of the Centers for Disease Control (CDC) in Atlanta, Georgia, USA, have described the G-2, A-3, A-4, A-5, I-2, D-2 (now *Corynebacterium urealyticum*) and JK (now *Corynebacterium jeikeium*) groups of organisms in immunocompromised patients (Hollis and Weaver, 1981). Although these last two opportunistic pathogens are the commonest infectious aetiology presented by the corynebacteria in modern clinical practice, owing to their broad antimicrobial resistance, nevertheless the most important species from the pathogenesis and clinical priority viewpoint remains *C. diphtheriae* (and to a lesser extent the other toxin producers *C. ulcerans* and *C. pseudotuberculosis*), which is historically the major pathogen and even today can be a significant problem particularly in an unimmunized population.

The Multiply Resistant Corynebacteria

Corynebacterium jeikeium and *C. urealyticum* are the two major species of emerging prominence. The *C. jeikeium* species was probably first recognized from isolated reports of non-toxigenic diphtheria-like organisms, e.g. causing endocarditis (Howard, 1893; Roosen-Runge, 1903; Sutherland and Willis, 1936), which were first reported in 1893 and later in 1963 (Davis *et al.*, 1963) and were opportunistic infections caused by coryneforms which were resistant to a broad range of antimicrobial agents. This report was of four cases of endocarditis following open heart surgery, three of whom were treated with various penicillins and died and one who was treated with vancomycin and survived. However, the first large detailed review was reported by Johnson and Kaye (1970), who reviewed 52 cases of infections caused by corynebacteria other than *C. diphtheriae*. Thirty-one of the 52 patients had bacterial endocarditis and it was noted that most of the strains were characteristically resistant to a wide range of antimicrobials and often only sensitive to vancomycin. A new species was first proposed in 1976 (Hande *et al.*, 1976) of organisms resistant to penicillins and aminoglycosides. A CDC group JK (named after Johnson and Kaye) was proposed in 1979 (Riley *et al.*, 1979) based on morphological and biochemical characteristics of a collection of 95 strains which had been referred to them over the previous 15 years. They were all human clinical isolates, 53 of them from blood. It has been suggested that the CDC group JK corynebacteria are biotypes of either *C. genitalium* or *C. pseudogenitalium* (Evangelista *et al.*, 1984). However, this suggestion has been based on the phenotypic biochemical reactions and antimicrobial susceptibilities and not on any more definitive investigations. In 1987, a proposal was made on the basis of biochemical tests – polyacrylamide electrophoresis of proteins, DNA base composition, mycolic acid composition and DNA–DNA homology of a new species *C. jeikeium* – for the group JK taxon and the name has been widely adopted (Jackmann *et al.*, 1987).

The *C. urealyticum* taxon has emerged more recently with a similar historical background to *C. jeikeium*; however, it differs in being urea positive and has a particular trophism for the urinary tract. It was first reported in 1979 as a cause of pneumonia and in 1985 as a cause of cystitis (Soriano *et al.*, 1985). Eighty-two cases were reviewed in 1990 (Sorriano *et al.*, 1990) and the taxon was proposed as a species in 1992 (Pitcher *et al.*, 1992).

GENERAL DESCRIPTION

Corynebacteria are pleomorphic Gram-positive bacilli, often showing an irregular expansion at one end and are described as club shaped. They are characteristically arranged in palisades and V-forms or described as having a Chinese lettering arrangement, which is due to the nature of their cell division. They are non-motile, non-capsulate and non-sporing. Using Albert's stain, characteristic metachromatic phosphate volutin granules can be demonstrated in *C. diphtheriae* and *C. xerosis* (see Figure 3.1). These are staining artefacts arising from the heat fixation process. The cell walls are composed of a characteristic peptidoglycan and ester-linked fatty acids, which they share with the other genera *Nocardia* and *Mycobacterium*, the three genera being collectively known as the CMN group.

Cultural Characteristics

They will grow on ordinary blood agar, with varying degrees of preference for carbon dioxide. For example *C. diphtheriae* prefers 10% carbon dioxide but with *C. jeikeium*, although enrichment with 5% carbon dioxide does not affect growth (Ersgaard and Justesen, 1984), nevertheless there is no growth under strictly anaerobic conditions (Jackmann *et al.*, 1987).

Corynebacterium diphtheriae is usually cultured from clinical specimens on selective media such as tellurite-containing medium (e.g. Hoyle's), which produces black colonies due to the reduced tellurite, or on Loeffler's serum medium, which

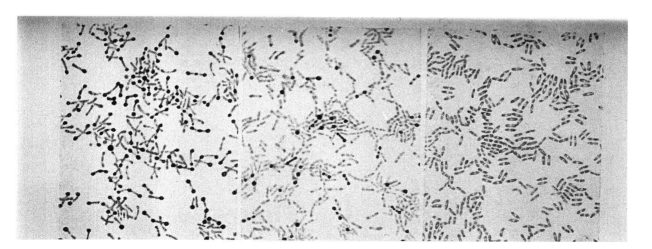

Figure 3.1. Staining reactions using Albert's stain of (left) *C. diphtheriae*, (middle) *C. xerosis* and (right) *C. pseudodiphtheriticum* (*C. hofmannii*). The presence of many volutin granules is characteristic of *C. diphtheriae* although their presence also in *C. xerosis* demands that they must be differentiated by further tests. *Corynebacterium pseudodiphtheriticum* shows a characteristic clear unstained central bar and no volutin granules (×100). (Reproduced by permission of *Bacteriology Illustrated*.)

allows them to grow rapidly in 12–18 hours while suppressing other commensal flora. The three classical colonial variants of *C. diphtheriae* var. *gravis*, *intermedius* and *mitis* may be distinguished on tellurite medium, particularly using sheep rather than horse blood. The *gravis* variant is a semi-rough domed colony and is the only one to ferment starch; although the least common, it is associated with the most serious clinical presentation. The *intermedius* variant is a smooth, domed, dwarf colony of intermediate occurrence and pathogenicity, while the *mitis* variants are smooth, convex, translucent colonies and, although the most prevalent, are the least pathogenic. Haemolytic reactions can also distinguish the three colonial variants.

Other species of clinical significance are not usually selectively sought in the routine laboratory but are easily cultured and are usually suspected as being clinically significant due to predominance, or pure growths, or due to their broad antimicrobial resistance such as with *C. jeikeium* or *C. urealyticum*. All species grow more luxuriantly on subculture compared with initial isolation. Although there may be a requirement for lipid there is always sufficient lipid present in blood agar, and any additional lipid is of little value. Similar colonial morphological differences have been described for *C. jeikeium* (Bayston and Higgins, 1986) on Columbia blood agar at 48 hours and five types are described ranging from 0.5–1.0 mm up to 2.0–3.0 mm, entire, rough or dry, flat or domed, and white or grey in appearance. Strict requirements for lipid are controversial. It has been shown that there is a strict nutritional requirement using 0.5% Tween 80 as a lipid source (McGinley *et al.*, 1985a). This is a large molecule containing small amounts of available oleic acid, and growth of *C. jeikeium* is supported by concentrations as low as 0.01% Tween 80. This suggests that lipid is not used as a carbon source but probably as a cofactor. The fact that most agar preparations, especially blood agar, support growth and are not specifically known to have lipid is explained by the fact that trace amounts of lipid are usually present and are usually sufficient for growth. If lipid is extracted

from these media growth is not supported. Growth enhancement was reported optimal using 1% Tween 80 (Bayston and Higgins, 1986), although Tween 60 has been reported to hydrolyse more completely (Riley *et al.*, 1979). Growth on brain heart infusion agar was superior to that on Columbia agar, nutrient agar, and tryptone soy agar (Bayston and Higgins, 1986). Growth was also supported on 0.03% tellurite agar and bile salt agar (Bayston and Higgins, 1986) but Riley *et al.* (1979) state that there was no growth on MacConkey agar. A differential medium called Tween purple agar (Coppola and Furness, 1985) with 1% fructose differentiates *C. genitalium* from *C. pseudogenitalium*, although these taxa are in dispute. Various antimicrobial agents have been incorporated in culture media particularly when used for clinical or environmental studies, but this has the disadvantage of repressing sensitive strains.

Biochemical reactions are the main method of routine speciation when required but variations can exist in the materials and methods used in each reaction. Commercial kits, e.g. API CORYNE (Biomerieux, France) are available which can standardize reactions between laboratories (see 'Diagnostic methods', below). Otherwise, use could be made of reference laboratories such as the Diphtheria Reference Unit in Colindale, London, or the Special Bacteriology Section at the CDC, Atlanta, Georgia, USA.

PATHOGENICITY

Diphtheria

Lysogenic phage

The type strain *C. diphtheriae* has the greatest potential for serious pathogenicity, due to its propensity to express toxin production. The exotoxin is coded for by a gene which is carried in a lysogenic (tox$^+$) β phage. During lysogeny the phage DNA integrates into the bacterial DNA, which then expresses the toxin. The amount of toxin produced also depends on the amount of iron available to the organism. Later the bacterial cell may undergo lysis, releasing new β phage.

Restriction enzyme electrophoresis has shown that indistinguishable strains *in vivo* may be toxigenic (tox [+]) or non-toxigenic (tox [−]) (Papenheimer, 1983). Those strains not susceptible to lysogenic phage do not produce toxin. There are three suggested routes by which virulence may arise: person-to-person spread of toxigenic bacilli; phage spread to previously non-toxigenic bacilli; and incomplete phages from non-toxigenic bacilli may recombine in a susceptible strain to allow expression of the tox [+] gene and produce toxin. Degrees of invasiveness among strains independent of toxin production are other determinants of pathogenicity. *Corynebacterium ulcerans* and *C. pseudotuberculosis* (*C. ovis*) are also able to express the toxin and it seems more common for *C. diphtheriae* phages to infect the other species than the reverse (Groman, 1984).

Diphtheria toxin

The toxin is a polypeptide of 535 amino acids containing two disulphide bridges. The first of these is easily broken by serine proteases and reduction after binding to the eukaryotic cell membrane to release two dissimilar fragments, A active and B binding fragment. A hydrophobic domain of fragment B forms ion-conducting channels in the phospholipid membrane which are large enough to allow passage of fragment A. The A fragment is now enzymically active and catalyses a reaction of ADP ribosylation of active elongation factor 2 (EF2), which is essential for ribosomal transfer of code from mRNA to tRNA (see Figure 3.2). This inactivation of EF2 stops the building of polypeptide chains, which is the primary event leading to necrotic lesions in all cells of the body, particularly the cardiac, nervous and renal systems. A single molecule of fragment A is lethal within a few hours to any mammalian cell, even if from a toxin-resistant species.

Non-toxin-producing Species

The non-toxin-producing species are predominantly opportunists, causing less dramatic pathology in the immunocompromised, although in this setting a wide spectrum of infections are seen, the most significant being the life-threatening conditions of bacteraemia, meningitis and endocarditis. The antimicrobial-resistant species present major therapeutic problems. *Corynebacterium urealyti-*

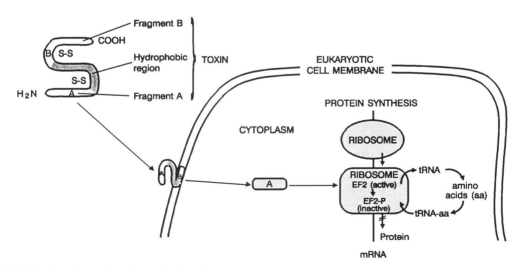

Figure 3.2. Mechanism of action of diphtheria toxin. Toxin fragment B binds to the cell membrane and after S–S cleavage fragment A enters the cell. As ribosomes move along the mRNA during protein synthesis, the interaction with tRNA is interrupted by the inactivation (ADP-ribosylation) of elongation factor 2 (EF2). Toxin fragment A catalyses this inactivation and prevents protein synthesis.

cum also has a pathogenic niche in urinary tract infection due to its urease activity, causing it to act as a cofactor in the development of struvite (ammonium magnesium phosphate) stones and an encrusted cystitis. Other cofactors are pre-existing urinary tract infection, immunosuppression, urological instrumentation and pathology such as neoplasm (see below). Infection with *Corynebacterium jeikeium* requires predisposing factors before colonization. The epidemiological risk factors of long-term or recurrent short-term hospitalization, multiple courses of broad-spectrum antimicrobial agents, chronic intravascular catheterization and chemotherapeutic immune-suppressing agents are important. Also important are the skin colonization mechanisms. It would seem highly likely that colonization is a prerequisite for infection in most cases, regardless of the true significance of gastrointestinal carriage as discussed above. The opportunistic nature of the pathology reported, in particular endocarditis following cardiac surgery and other invasive infection associated with skin penetration by intravascular catheterization, suggests that invasion from a skin source is the commonest route of infection. Factors which influence the occurrence and the degree of skin colonization can reasonably be expected to be the same as for other skin residents or transients. However, several special circumstances for *C. jeikeium* are beginning to be elucidated.

Firstly, the strict nutritional requirement for low concentrations of lipid, also shared by *C. bovis*, may provide an environmental advantage as the sebum production (lipids and free fatty acids) of human skin provides a niche for lipophilic organisms. Although levels of colonization are lower in lipid-rich sebaceous regions, as with many bacteria, this is not inconsistent as only very low levels of lipid are required.

Secondly, ultrastructural differences exist between sensitive and resistant strains of *C. jeikeium* (see below), which may account for permeability to antibiotics (Blom and Heltberg, 1986). The fatty acid composition of the cell wall of corynebacteria as shown by gas−liquid chromatography is modified by different cultural conditions and can be particularly influenced by Tween 80 (Chevalier *et al.*, 1987). It might be hypothesized that the nature of the lipids or quantity available may play a role in the survival, resistance to therapy, or even the pathogenicity of *C. jeikeium*.

A third colonization factor, which is probably of greatest significance, at least in terms of survival and quantity of organisms, is the amount of water on the skin surface. Most of the water is derived from eccrine sweat and in the axillary region a contribution from apocrine sweat. A very small amount of water is contributed by transpiration through the stratum corneum (Schuplein and Blank, 1971). Cutaneous lipophilic diphtheroids are more prevalent in the moist areas (nose, axilla, groin and toe web) and very few in the dry (arm and leg) or oily (forehead and scalp) regions (McGinley *et al.*, 1985b). Corroborating evidence of this was shown when a dry region was covered with occlusive dressings and a great increase of the lipophilic diphtheroid population was observed within 48 hours (Leyden *et al.*, 1983). Since one of the major effects of occlusion is an increase in the amount of water on the skin surface these findings taken together suggest that moisture is an important ecological determinant for lipophilic diphtheroids.

A fine balance of many features exists on the skin, as in any ecosystem. Other examples may be bacteriostatic and bactericidal components, e.g. bacterial lipases hydrolysing lipids to form free fatty acids, pH effects, etc. A plasmid-associated bacteriocin produced by a 'JK-type coryneform' has been reported (Kerry-Williams and Noble, 1984). This showed antibacterial activity against some strains of other JK coryneforms, *C. bovis*, *Rhodococcus equi*, *C. hoagii*, *C. pseudodiphtheriticum*, *C. renale* and *Micrococcus* spp. In a follow-up study, 39 isolates of JK-type coryneforms, 23 of which contained plasmids, were investigated. Using restriction endonuclease analysis, plasmids were allocated into six groups and four of these produced a similar bacteriocin-like substance. Skin flora studies of volunteers on tetracycline therapy have shown an inverse relationship between lipophilic diphtheroids and coagulase-negative staphylococci (Marples and Williamson, 1969). When the diphtheroid population density fell, as a result of treatment, the staphylococci were able to multiply, and as the lipophilic diphtheroids returned the staphylococcal population density fell without loss of resistance. The interpretation of this data was that lipophilic diphtheroids are able to suppress the growth of staphylococci and are the main group controlling the composition of the flora of the axilla.

The opposite effect, satellitism, i.e. growth enhancement of one organism by another, has also been demonstrated *in vitro* by the enhanced growth of skin coagulase-negative staphylococci by several skin organisms (Selwyn and Ellis, 1972). However, the role of these co-action phenomena in specific relation to *C. jeikeium* has yet to be determined.

EPIDEMIOLOGY

Habitat

The coryneform bacteria are widely distributed in soil and plants in nature, and have been isolated in air, water and milk. They are common inhabitants of the mucous membranes and skin of animals and man, and this is the most probable site from which infection could arise. Man is the only known reservoir for *C. diphtheriae*. The other species also recognized as human skin pathogens and human opportunists have only been reported in human studies and the animal and plant pathogens in their respective habitats. The reservoirs for the other rarer species such as some of the CDC groups are unknown.

Diphtheria

Corynebacterium diphtheriae is rarely isolated in immunized communities although recently non-toxigenic strains were reported in homosexual men attending genitourinary clinics (Wilson *et al.*, 1992). In non-immunized communities carrier rates are higher, at 3–5% throat carriage (Kalapothaki *et al.*, 1984). In Russia, where vaccination rates are high among children (96%) and low among adults, 80–90% of diphtheria occurs among adults

(Korzenkova *et al.*, 1991). In addition to this throat carriage, the skin is another source of *C. diphtheriae* among the homeless of developed countries or among travellers to tropical areas with high incidences of cutaneous diphtheria, and it is suggested that person-to-person spread is more efficient than respiratory spread in this environment (Koopman and Campbell, 1975).

There has been a dramatic decrease in the incidence of diphtheria from 75 years ago, when it was a leading cause of childhood deaths, to the current rarity it is today (Figure 3.3a). However, the WHO reference unit in the UK have recorded a five-fold increase in isolates of non-toxigenic *C. diphtheriae* between 1990 and 1992, most of which were *gravis* subtype (Efstratiou *et al.*, 1993). More dramatically in Eastern Europe, a slow increase in the 1980s was

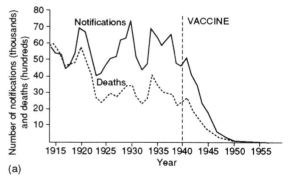

(a)

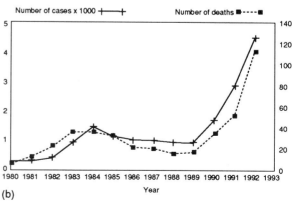

(b)

Figure 3.3. (a) Diphtheria: notifications and deaths, England and Wales, 1914–1959. (b) Diphtheria cases and deaths in the Russian Federation (WHO).

noted in the Soviet Union which first peaked in 1983–1985 with 1400–1600 cases per annum, and a second wave has occurred since 1990 with 1896 cases in 1991 and 4685 cases in the first seven months of 1993 (Figure 3.3b). The Ukraine has experienced a similar incidence and it seems to be spreading to the neighbouring countries of Azerbaijan, Belorussia, Kazakhstan and Uzbekistan (World Health Organization, 1993). The resurgence is thought to be due to (a) low and decreasing childhood immunity, (b) the weakening of adult immunity, and (c) a large demographic shift in these countries facilitating the spread of virulent forms.

Hospital corynebacteria

Among the non-diphtheria species the skin is the most relevant habitat. *Corynebacterium jeikeium* has been extensively studied in the hospital environment because of its increasingly recognized pathology particularly in immunocompromised patients and its broad antimicrobial resistance, so it will be described in detail as a representative species. One of the earliest epidemiological studies, which refers to 'antibiotic-resistant *Corynebacterium* species', reported 11% of bone marrow transplant patients being bacteraemic with these isolates, 17/42 patients colonized, 13% of adults in a general hospital, and only 1% of non-hospitalized healthy adults (Stamm *et al.*, 1979). There was also evidence of nosocomial acquisition and lower bacteraemic rates in patients in laminar air-flow rooms. A marked age–sex predilection was shown, i.e. colonization and infection were rare under 16 years of age, and in patients over 16 years of age the colonization and infection rates were much higher in males than females. This may relate to differing levels of androgenic and oestrogenic hormones in these groups. A strict nutritional requirement for lipid and similar components of cell wall fatty acids gives the species a predilection for human skin, particularly the more moist areas. As sebum concentration is related to these hormones and increased sebum results in more lipid, particularly free fatty acids, this could promote the lipophilic diphtheroids. Another explanation for the male predominance might be the male urethra colonization as opposed

to the female urethra, although other studies have failed to show this colonization of the urethra (Stamm *et al.*, 1979; Holmes *et al.*, 1975).

Another study of healthy adults and hospitalized patients looked separately for antibiotic-resistant and antibiotic-sensitive coryneforms (Larson *et al.*, 1986). Among healthy adults ($n = 80$) prevalence rates of resistant organisms were greatest in the perineum, quite scanty in the toe webs and absent in the nose and axilla. However, in leukaemia patients ($n = 28$) they were present in all four sites, although more so in the perineum and toe webs than in the nose and axilla. Other hospitalized patients were also examined ($n = 15$) and prevalence rates were in between the two former groups. Overall the resistant lipophilic diphtheroids were more prevalent in patients than controls, and in the skin of adult controls with poor hygiene than those with good hygiene. There were no significant differences in types or numbers of organisms by age (greater or less than 40 years) or race. There was also no significant difference in the prevalence of resistant lipophilic diphtheroids among those who had or had not received antimicrobial therapy in the previous 30 days. However, there was a significant inverse correlation between the proportion of resistant and sensitive lipophilic diphtheroids, and the suggestion has been made that the resistant strains were normal lipophilic diphtheroids that had acquired resistance. This has also been suggested based on the fact that no differences in resistant group JK or other lipophilic diphtheroids were noted when cellular fatty acids and mycolates, cell wall peptidoglycan composition, nutritional requirements and biochemical reactions were examined (McGinley *et al.*, 1985a). Resistance was found to be long lasting and was unlike Gram-negative resistance, which decreases when the antimicrobial pressure is removed (Gill *et al.*, 1981). Crossed immunoelectrophoresis assay and fatty acid isomer patterns have shown that simple mutation of a sensitive strain to a resistant clone does not occur (Heltberg *et al.*, 1986), although a single point mutation in quinolone susceptibility of repeated isolates from one patient has been reported (Murphy and Ferguson, 1987).

It has been suggested that since the perineum is the most frequent and usually the first site of colonization antimicrobial resistance is acquired in the gastrointestinal tract and subsequently spreads to skin (Larson *et al.*), and colonization in three patients after initial rectal colonization and subsequent persistence after three, six and nine months has been shown (Khabbaz *et al.*, 1988). These follow-up strains were indistinguishable by typing with restriction endonuclease analysis of chromosomal DNA.

A four-year period review of *C. jeikeium* in one hospital found 30–35% of patients colonized, with the most prevalent sites being inguinal, rectal and axillae (Gill *et al.*, 1981). It was also found that the urine, umbilicus, nose, hands, ears and throat sites were colonized with various prevalence rates. Colonization persisted in some patients for up to six months. New patients may have been already colonized on admission although this could still have been nosocomial as some were admitted from other hospitals. Males were found to be colonized more frequently or to a greater degree than females.

Another study of *C. jeikeium* also found males to be colonized significantly more than females and oncology patients were colonized more often (51%) than haemodialysis patients (33%) or hospital staff (36%) (Wichmann *et al.*, 1985).

A cluster of four cases of *C. jeikeium* bacteraemia and one line infection was reported to have occurred over a four-week period in a haematology ward from which the organism had not been isolated during the previous year (Quinn *et al.*, 1984). Isolates were also identified from the environment in 10/17 air samples and 9/13 surfaces in patient rooms. Results also showed patient colonization after the outbreak (44%) and by way of comparison colonization of patients on an oncology ward of the same hospital (12%). Hand colonization of ward staff showed 4/13 positive at the end of the outbreak and 0/9 positive two weeks later after infection control measures had been instituted. The staff of the oncology ward which had no outbreak had a prevalence rate of 0/4 hand colonization. Although the numbers are too small for statistical

significance, the outbreak seems to have been related to increased colonization of patients, staff and the ward environment. The bacteraemic strains were subsequently typed by multilocus enzyme electrophoresis and found to be a single clone (Murphy, 1990).

Another large outbreak of 26 cases of septicaemia over an 18-month period, 24 of which occurred in patients with haematological malignancies, was reported (Lange *et al.*, 1980). However, no infection or even colonization occurred in any patient in the marrow transplant unit of the hospital at this time. The authors suggest that this was due to the housing of the transplant unit, which was a special infection control-orientated facility. The role of good infection control practices was further emphasized in their study by the dramatic fall in the incidence of bacteraemia from 2.7 per month to 1.6 per month following their cluster or outbreak. In addition, following this period the rate fell to zero over a further seven-month period coincident with an organized nursing audit of patient hygiene.

The environment has also been strongly implicated using surface swabs (Telander *et al.*, 1988). Two isolation rooms occupied by colonized patients in a haematology ward were implicated. This contamination decreased after cleaning with disinfectant. In two other rooms contaminated to a lesser extent the patients were not colonized.

In another study 59 isolates of *C. jeikeium* from 25 patients in intensive care and oncology wards over a 15-month period were reported in which, using clinical and microbiological criteria, seven of the patients were regarded as infected (Finger *et al.*, 1983).

Colonization is clearly widespread on human skin and prevalence rates vary, with maximum colonization seen in long-term hospitalized male patients receiving multiple courses of broad-spectrum antimicrobial agents. Infection, on the other hand, is not as widespread and is usually seen as an opportunistic event although probably related to the same factors, i.e. gender, neutropenia, antimicrobial therapy, duration of hospitalization and intravascular catheterization. Although most clinical isolates are contaminants, up to 20% have been reported to be associated with serious nosocomial infection (Riebel *et al.*, 1986). However, the mode of acquisition is still controversial. Patient-to-patient and environment-to-patient transmission would seem to occur with this nosocomial pathogen, and by using plasmid-associated bacteriocin production and multilocus enzyme electrophoresis as markers these modes of transmission have been confirmed (Murphy, 1990; Kerry-Williams and Noble, 1986). On the other hand, studies using restriction endonuclease analysis of chromosomal DNA have suggested that patient-to-patient transmission did not occur when 18 epidemiologically related isolates were investigated, which included strains from two apparent clusters (Khabbaz *et al.*, 1986).

Other corynebacteria

Among the other *Corynebacterium* spp., *C. pseudo-diphtheriticum* (*C. hofmannii*), *C. xerosis*, *C. urealyticum* (CDC group D2), *C. minutissimum*, *C. striatum*, and the *Arcanobacterium haemolyticum* (*C. haemolyticum*) and some of the CDC groups can be predominantly found as residents of human skin, while *Actinomyces pyogenes* (*C. pyogenes*), *C. ovis*, *C. pseudotuberculosis*, *C. ulcerans* and *Rhodococcus equi* (*C. equi*) are predominantly found in animal sources from which man becomes infected. The tendency towards broad antimicrobial resistance among *C. jeikeium* and *C. urealyticum* is probably aided by their high prevalence among hospitalized patients exposed to antimicrobial pressures.

CLINICAL FEATURES

Diphtheria

The symptoms and signs of *C. diphtheriae* infection are due to local inflammation in the respiratory tract and skin, and to toxin-mediated effects in the cardiac, nervous and renal systems. Both the incidence and severity of symptoms are inversely related to the degree of immunity and consequently mortality is rare in a fully immunized person. Mortality rates are consistently less than 10% in a predominantly immunized population and 50% of cases are mild. Most deaths occur in the first few days from respiratory or cardiac effects. Also the frequency of cardiac or neurological signs is related to both the size of initial infective lesion and the time between onset and the administration of antitoxin. The incubation period is one to four days, with most cases presenting at two days. Initial symptoms will depend on the initial site of infection, usually tonsillar or faucial, although other sites of initial infection less commonly seen are cutaneous, nasopharyngeal, anterior nasal, laryngeal/tracheal/bronchial/bronchopneumonic, aural, conjunctival, genital and gastrointestinal. In tonsillar infection, the onset is insidous with no initial complaint. A sore throat is surprisingly not a characteristic, nor is a very raised temperature. The child is quiet and non-interactive with food and toys. The face is pale and muscle tone is weak. There may be vomiting but nausea is more common. The pulse is fast but of low volume and easily compressible. The tonsillar surface at first shows white specks of exudate which later coalesce and darken, becoming more adherent to the tissue and leaving a bleeding surface if removed. In severe presentation the membranes extend from the entire tonsil to the hard palate, which is oedematous and often into the postnasal space (Figure 3.4). There is a

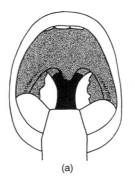 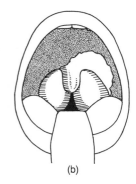

(a)   (b)

Figure 3.4. (a) Faucial diphtheria, demonstrating the membrane on the opposed surfaces of the tonsils. (b) Hypertoxic diphtheria has an extensive membrane covering the tonsils and extending on to the palate and uvula, which are swollen and oedematous.

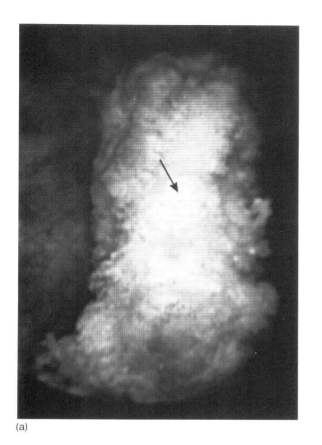

(a)

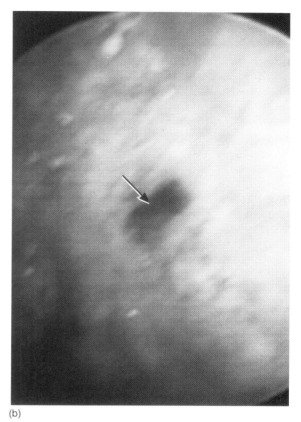

(b)

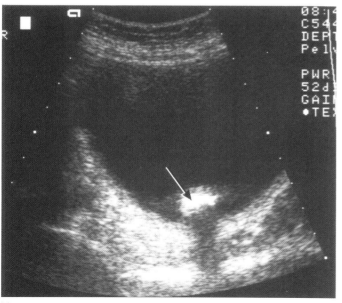

(c)

Figure 3.5. A bleeding ulcer on the bladder wall (a) seen in an 85-year-old patient with persistent *C. urealyticum* urinary tract infection, (b) left after removal of an ammonium magnesium phosphate calculus. On ultrasound examination of the bladder (c) the calculus appears as a mass with an echogenic area behind suspicions of a bladder tumour.

remarkable oral fetor which can pervade the room or even a patient's house. Cervical gland enlargement and local oedema produce the 'bull neck' appearance.

The toxin effects are mainly seen in cardiac and renal systems. Cardiac toxicity is seen in up to 70% of cases, often one to two weeks into the illness. It may be an acute myocarditis with failure and cardiovascular collapse or insidious with dyspnoea and weakness. Dysrhythmias can present as first-degree heart block or progress to atrioventricular block, left bundle branch block and other dysrhythmias which have a four-fold increase in mortality compared with patients with normal electrocardiograms. The neurological toxicity is due to toxin-mediated demyelination and can present initially with pharyngeal and laryngeal paralysis leading to aspiration. Later a proximal muscle motor neuropathy may develop and other peripheral sensory or motor nerves can be affected. The neuronal damage is usually slowly reversible.

Cutaneous diphtheria is seen in the homeless with poor hygiene or in tropical countries, and presents as a slow healing ulcer with a membrane. The culture is often mixed with other pathogens and the significance of *C. diphtheriae* might be queried as toxin effects are rarely seen.

Non-diphtheria Coryneforms

Among the other species of the *Corynebacterium* genus, *C. ulcerans* may produce a pharyngitis, but although it may produce the toxin it rarely gives rise to classical diphtheria. *Corynebacterium pseudotuberculosis* rarely produces human infection but can cause a suppurative granulomatous lymphadenitis.

Most reports of *C. jeikeium* infection are of bacteraemia and endocarditis but in practice it is most commonly isolated from skin infections at the site of catheter insertions, usually in immunocompromised patients (Johnson and Efstratiou, 1993). However, a very wide range of pathology has been reported (Murphy, 1990).

The other species can rarely cause a wide range of infections as seen with *C. jeikeium* and are also usually opportunists in the immunocompromised.

Rhodococcus equi, formerly *C. equi*, has also become increasingly recognized in recent years as a cause of pneumonic cavitation in patients with deficient T cell immunity such as in AIDS.

Corynebacterium minutissimum is the cause of erythrasma, the skin infection seen in intertriginous areas. *Corynebacterium urealyticum*, formerly CDC group D2, has recently been recognized (over 200 cases reported since 1985) in association with alkaline encrusted cystitis in immunocompromised patients in general and with encrusted pyelitis in renal transplant patients in particular (Soriano *et al.*, 1990). The bladder wall has one or more encrusted stones of ammonium magnesium phosphate (Figure 3.5a) which can be readily seen during cystoscopy and which leave a bleeding ulcer (Figure 3.5b) on removal by the cystoscope. These lesions may be suspected on ultrasound (Figure 3.5c) by a bladder wall mass beneath which is an echogenic area suggestive of a bladder tumour.

DIAGNOSTIC METHODS

Diphtheria

The priority is the rapid diagnosis of tonsillar diphtheria caused by a toxigenic strain of *C. diphtheriae*. This is usually made clinically in endemic populations which have low immunization and high endemicity of diphtheria. However, in the developed countries with high immunization levels and low levels of clinical diphtheria it is generally only those laboratories in the larger urban areas with substantial migration of people from countries with lower levels of immunization who specifically look for *C. diphtheriae* in all throat swabs submitted. A case can be made for screening all throat swabs as even the non-toxigenic strains may cause a pharyngitis in children and young adults and the incidence seems to be rising in the UK (Efstratiou *et al.*, 1993). The herd immunity effect seen in immunized populations seems to protect by reducing carriage of toxigenic strains as protection occurs even though non-toxigenic carriage is unaffected (Karzon and Edwards, 1988).

Microscopy

Provisional diagnosis on microscopy using a methylene blue stain from a throat swab is diagnostically unreliable and must be confirmed with culture and toxin testing, although Albert's stain demonstrates characteristics as seen in Figure 3.1. Immunofluorescent techniques offer improved specificity and sensitivity when performed on smears made from swabs preincubated in glucose broths for 3–4 hours (McCracken and Mauney, 1971).

Culture

Swabs should be taken from nose and throat including the pharyngeal wall and inoculated without delay or transported in Amies medium. A tellurite-containing medium will both suppress other nasopharyngeal flora and provide prominence to corynebacteria by the black pigment produced by the reduction of tellurite. Suspicious colonies can be screened further for potential toxin production by culture on Tinsdale's medium for the detection of cysteinase, as only *C. diphtheriae*, *C. ulcerans* and *C. pseudotuberculosis* produce black colonies with a brown halo. Another useful screen of suspicious colonies is pyrazinamidase activity and toxin detection by the Elek test. This three-test procedure is recommended by the WHO Reference Unit at Colindale, UK. Although these tests have been difficult to perform and control in the routine laboratory recent modifications have improved their performance and ease of use (Coleman *et al.*, 1992). Nevertheless the performance of the Elek test is difficult and many laboratories would appropriately refer cultures to a reference laboratory. The biochemical identification has been greatly facilitated by the commercial development of the API CORYNE kit (Biomerieux) using 20 biochemical tests to distinguish 33 related taxa. Although the *intermedius* biotype is not specifically recognized such kits have the advantage of international quality control, are easy to perform in most routine laboratories and are reliable (Freney *et al.*, 1991). Another kit called the Minitek System (BBL

Microbiology Systems, Cockeysville, MD, USA) has been investigated using 44 strains of group JK corynebacteria and a number of other *Corynebacterium* spp. (Slifkin *et al.*, 1986). When compared with conventional tests as described by Riley *et al.* (1979) complete agreement was found and results were readable at 12–18 hours for most reactions, with only maltose fermentation taking up to three days.

In vivo tests such as guinea-pig inoculation are confined to reference laboratories with animal facilities. The newer molecular methods such as polymerase chain reaction (PCR) have also been developed as screening procedures for toxin detection. A 246 bp fragment of the toxin gene has been used successfully and a 910 bp fragment has also been used and verified with an ADP-ribosylation activity test (Pallen, 1991). These are good rapid toxin tests and particularly useful for screening negative strains, although false positive results may occur if the toxin gene is present but not expressed. Immunoassays are also being developed and may be applicable using an immunoblotting technique (Efstratiou, 1993).

Non-diphtheria Species

The non-diphtheria species are normally easier and of less clinical priority in laboratory isolation and identification. The two species which show broad antimicrobial resistance are conspicuous by their antibiograms although identification to species level, if required, can be problematic. The API CORYNE kit can differentiate many strains conveniently, including many related CDC group taxa, *Rhodococcus equi* and other taxa not in the *Corynebacterium* genus. However, taxonomic developments continue and using the presence of mycolic acids as a prerequisite for membership of the *Corynebacterium* genus it has been shown that 26 of 42 isolates which the API CORYNE kit had speciated as *C. minutissimum*, *C. striatum* and CDC group I did not contain mycolic acids and therefore could not be placed in the genus (Barreau *et al.*, 1993). Furthermore, a recent study using 21 biochemical tests found that only 60% of coryneform clinical isolates could be assigned to any species or

CDC group (Slifkin *et al.*, 1986). Another example of the lack of agreement is the recent proposal that 10 commercially available reference strains of *C. xerosis* represent six different new species (Coyle *et al.*, 1993a). Also the stability of the biotypes of *C. diphtheriae* has been questioned (Coyle *et al.*, 1993b). The CDC manual *Gram Positive Organisms: A Guide to Identification* is a useful reference (Hollis and Weaver, 1981).

MANAGEMENT OF INFECTION

Antitoxin

Antitoxin is the treatment priority in clinical diphtheria. This is a hyperimmune antiserum produced in horses which can neutralize the toxin before cell entry. A human antiserum has been prepared but has insufficient potency for therapy (Hartman, 1979). Administration is of extreme urgency as the prognosis is dependent on the time from onset of illness to administration. A test dose should be given to exclude hypersensitivity and it may be administered intramuscularly or intravenously in doses dependent on the clinical condition (20 000–100 000 units). Unimmunized close case contacts should be followed up by screening and given antimicrobial prophylaxis and vaccination.

Antimicrobial Therapy

In the management of diphtheria, antimicrobial therapy augments antitoxin therapy and may reduce the bacterial load and thereby reduce the further production of toxin. It should also improve the initial inflammatory site and may also reduce the risk of further spread. Erythromycin has been the traditional drug of choice although there is usually a wide range of agents with sufficient activity such as penicillin, tetracyclines, rifampicin, clindamycin, imipenem, the glycopeptides vancomycin and teicoplanin, the quinolones ciprofloxacin and ofloxacin and the newer macrolides clarithromycin and azithromycin. Initial prescribing must be empirical, and susceptibility testing should be performed for support of efficacy as *in vitro* resistance can occur. Some

strains of *mitis* and *intermedius* do not grow on Mueller–Hinton agar so 5% blood should be added to solid agar or 10% fetal calf serum to an appropriate broth such as Trypticase Soy or brain heart infusion broths for broth dilution tests.

In severe cases parenteral penicillin or erythromycin should be administered and oral administration for milder cases when the patient can swallow. A single intramuscular dose of benzathine penicillin is appropriate for patients suspected of having poor compliance. A tracheostomy may be required in severe cases and other multisystem complications should be detected by close clinical monitoring and with serial echocardiograms and liver function tests.

Eradication of Carriage

Several regimens have been shown to be effective for clearance of carrier status. Seven-day oral courses of erythromycin or clindamycin gave 93% and 92% eradication but a single injection of benzathine penicillin only cleared 84% in a study of 294 carriers (McCloskey *et al.*, 1974). Relapse of the cleared carrier state is not uncommon and may not be associated with antimicrobial resistance. Cultures should therefore be repeated two and three weeks after treatment.

Non-diphtheria Corynebacteria

The non-diphtheria species, being less virulent, rarely present the same degree of clinical urgency. Although *C. jeikeium* is commonly a cause of bacteraemia and occasionally of endocarditis or meningitis the priority here is to prescribe antimicrobial agents based on susceptibility tests. If treatment is to be commenced in advance of susceptibilities becoming known the glycopeptides vancomycin and teicoplanin can be wholly depended upon for activity. Rifampicin, fusidic acid and the new quinolones are also usually active and have better tissue-penetrative properties so are appropriate as second agents if required. The nature of resistance is not definitely known but using transmission electron microscopy on sections of *C. jeikeium* cells, and comparing two antibiotic-susceptible strains with two multiply resistant strains, the cells of all four strains had a typical Gram-positive cell wall with an extra surface layer (Blom and Heltberg, 1986). Although such extra surface layers have been observed in other *Corynebacterium* spp., the interesting feature was that this layer was significantly thicker in the resistant strains than in the sensitive strains. Such a structural difference on the exterior of the cell wall, if real and not arte-factual may affect the cell permeability to antimicrobial agents. This layer is 7–9 nm thick and is enhanced in density by ruthenium red treatment, which indicates that acidic mucopoly-saccharides are constituents of this layer.

Examination of penicillin-binding proteins (PBPs) has shown six PBPs in a sensitive *Coryne-bacterium* and five in a resistant *C. jeikeium* (Quinn *et al.*, 1986). PBPs 4 and 5 of *C. jeikeium* had a much lower affinity for penicillin than those of the sensitive *Corynebacterium* and this was proposed as the mechanism of resistance to peni-cillin. No plasmids were detected in either isolate and both were β-lactamase negative.

It has been shown, using crossed immuno-electrophoresis with *C. jeikeium*, that there are antigenic differences between two strains, one sensitive and one resistant, both from the same patient (Heltberg *et al.*, 1986). It would appear therefore that surface structures may influence cell permeability to antibiotics, and such resistance might be considered a virulence factor, or at least provide an environmental advantage in a hospital-ized patient on antimicrobial therapy.

Another hypothesis which may explain the difficulty in treatment is that of adhesion of cells. Electron microscopy and histochemical methods have been used to study adhesion of coryne-bacteria to axillary hairs (Shelley and Millar, 1984). A thready extracellular surface layer was seen to 'glue' the cells to the hair shaft. In addi-tion this surface layer was only revealed by treatment with ruthenium red. Although it is only speculative at this stage nevertheless such adhe-sion factors would fit well the clinical observation of pathology associated with intravascular catheterization.

Similar factors may apply to *C. urealyticum* although it appears less invasive. As these infec-tions are commonly seen in immunocompromised patients the underlying factors should be addressed, such as removal of intravascular or urinary catheters and intensive use of multiple courses of broad spectrum antimicrobials. *C. minutissimum* skin infection – erythrasma – responds to topical treatment with antibacterials. The cavitating pneumonia seen in *Rhodococcus equi* infection is prone to relapse after short courses of antimicrobial therapy, so several weeks of therapy may be required and surgery may ultimately be needed. Similarly the uncommon lymphadenitis due to *C. pseudotuberculosis* also requires several weeks' therapy and occasionally surgery. The other species are associated less commonly with a wide range of pathology and treatment must be pathogen directed with regard to the penetrative properties of active antimicrobial agents.

PREVENTION AND CONTROL

Diphtheria

The management of a clinical case of diphtheria should be strict isolation until antimicrobial therapy is complete; contacts must be followed up, including obligatory notification in most countries. Cutaneous diphtheria cases should be isolated also as they are a potential source of infection. However, the crucial factor in the prevention of *C. diphtheriae* infection is the population herd immunity, which when sufficiently high will break the chain of transmission of toxigenic carrier strains even though non-toxigenic carrier rates are unaffected. Active immunization has been shown to achieve this but high vaccine uptake must be maintained as natural immunity from sub-clinical infection is then unlikely. The immunogen is a formaldehyde-treated toxoid which is adsorbed onto an aluminium adjuvant. *Bordetella pertussis* is also an effective adjuvant and is usually combined with the adsorbed diphtheria and tetanus toxoid. Immuniz-ation schedules vary but the current UK schedule is a primary course of three intramuscular or deep sub-cutaneous injections starting at two months of age with an interval of one month between each dose. A booster dose is given at school entry (four to five years). This schedule now closely approximates the WHO recommendations and reduces the potential for low vaccine uptake due to young families with high geographic mobility. If primary immunization is commenced over the age of 10 years a special low-dose vaccine is used in a similar time schedule. The WHO have recently recommended a booster dose of tetanus–diphtheria toxoid for any traveller whose last dose of vaccine was more than 10 years ago and who intends to travel to the Russian Federation or the neighbouring countries where a diphtheria epidemic is in progress (World Health Organization, 1993). Contacts of a diphtheria case or carriers of a toxigenic strain should be swabbed and receive booster doses of vaccine according to their vaccine history and age and a prophylactic course of erythromycin or a single intramuscular injection of benzathine penicillin. Health care workers and others who may be exposed in their work should have their immune state checked by the Schick test, which is an intradermal injection of toxin in a test forearm and a similar injection of inactivated toxin in a control forearm. These are examined at one to two days and again at seven days for an erythematous reaction. A negative Schick test shows no skin reaction and indicates immunity whereas a positive Schick test shows a reaction in the test arm which lasts several days, while the control is negative. This positive test indicates lack of immunity and a requirement for vaccination. About 2% of healthy adults may fail to achieve sufficient protection after immunization (Edsall *et al.*, 1954). Fully immunized persons may rarely become infected but outbreaks may even occur among immunized groups. Patients who have suffered clinical diphtheria are not always immune and should be screened and immunized. However, it may now be difficult to obtain Schick toxin.

Non-diphtheria Corynebacterium

Infection control for the other non-diphtheria species is not generally as strict and prevention is more difficult. Transmission of skin infection such as *C. minutissimum* can be minimized by using antimicrobial soap in intertriginous skin areas.

Patients infected with those species with broad antimicrobial resistance, *C. jeikeium* and *C. urealyticum*, if occurring in a hospital area in which other immunocompromised patients are in close proximity should be isolated because clusters of infection have been described with a predominant outbreak clone and they may present a therapeutic problem (Murphy, 1990). The main preventative measures which will help are strict infection control procedures, careful hand hygiene, and minimization of the main risk factors of multiple courses of broad spectrum antimicrobials, breakage in skin defences such as catheterization, and prolonged periods of immunosuppression.

REFERENCES

Barreau, C., Bimet, F., Kiredjian, M. *et al.* (1993) Comparative chemotaxonomic studies of mycolic acid-free coryneform bacteria of human origin. *Journal of Clinical Microbiology*, **31**(8), 2085–2090.

Bayston, R. and Higgins, J. (1986) Biochemical and cultural characteristics of 'JK' coryneforms. *Journal of Clinical Pathology*, **39**, 654–660.

Blom, J. and Heltberg, O. (1986) The ultrastructure of antibiotic-susceptible and multi-resistant strains of group JK diphtheroid rods isolated from clinical specimens. *Acta Pathologica Microbiologica et Immunologica Scandinavica*, Section B, **94**, 301–308.

Chevalier, J., Pommier, M.T. and Crémieux, A. (1987) Rôle du Tween-80 utilisé dans la culture des corynébactéries cutanées (Group JK) sur la composition en acides gras cellulaires. *Annals of the Institue of Pasteur*, **138**, 427–437.

Coleman, G., Weaver, E. and Efstratiou, A. (1992) Screening tests for pathogenic corynebacteria. *Journal of Clinical Pathology*, **45**, 46–48.

Coppola, K.M. and Furness, G. (1985) Evaluation of differential media for the identification of *C. genitalium* and *C. pseudogenitalium* (group JK Corynebacteria). *Canadian Journal of Microbiology*, **31**, 32–34.

Coyle, M.B., Hollis, D.G. and Groman, N.B. (1985) *Corynebacterium* spp. and other coryneform organisms. In *Manual of Clinical Microbiology* (ed. E.H. Lennette, A. Balows, W.J. Hausler *et al.*), Ch. 18, pp. 193–204. 4th edn, American Society of Microbiology, Washington, DC.

Coyle, M.B., Leonard, R.B., Nowowiejski, D.J. *et al.* (1993a) Evidence of multiple taxa within commercially available reference strains of *C. xerosis. Journal of Clinical Microbiology*, **31**(7), 1778–1793.

Coyle, M.B., Nowowiejski, D.J., Russell, J.Q. *et al.* (1993b) Laboratory review of reference strains of *C. diphtheriae* indicates mistyped *intermedius* strains. *Journal of Clinical Microbiology*, **31**(11), 3060–3062.

Davis, A., Maxwell, J.B., Burroughs, J.T. *et al.* (1963) Diphtheroid endocarditis after cardiopulmonary bypass surgery for the repair of cardiac valvular defects. *Antimicrobial Agents and Chemotherapy*, **3**, 643–656.

Edsall, G., Altman, J.S. and Gaspar, A.J. (1954) Combined tetanus–diphtheria immunisation of adults: use of small doses of diphtheria toxoid. *American Journal of Public Health*, **44**, 1537.

Efstratiou, A. (1993) The laboratory diagnosis of diphtheria. *British Society for Microbial Technology Newsletter*, **15**, 3–11.

Efstratiou, A., George, R.C. and Begg, N.T. (1993) Non-toxigenic *Corynebacterium diphtheriae* var *gravis* in England. *Lancet*, **341**, 1592–1593.

Ersgaard, H. and Justesen, T. (1984) Multiresistant lipophilic corynebacteria from clinical specimens. *Acta Pathologica Microbiologica et Immunologica Scandinavica*, Section B, **92**, 39–43.

Evangelista, A.T., Coppola, K.M. and Furness, G. (1984) Relationship between group JK corynebacteria and the biotypes of *Corynebacterium genitalium* and *Corynebacterium pseudogenitalium*. *Canadian Journal of Microbiology*, **30**, 1052–1057.

Finger, H., Wirsing von Koenig, C.H., Wichmann, S. *et al.* (1983) Clinical significance of resistant corynebacteria group JK. *Lancet*, **i**, 538.

Freney, J., Duperron, M.T., Courtier, C. *et al.* (1991) Evaluation of API Coryne in comparison with conventional methods for identifying coryneform bacteria. *Journal of Clinical Microbiology*, **29**, 38–41.

Gill, V.J., Manning, C., Lamson, M. *et al.* (1981) Antibiotic-resistant group JK bacteria in hospitals. *Journal of Clinical Microbiology*, **13**, 472–477.

Goodfellow, M. and Minikin, D.E. (1981) Introduction to the coryneform bacteria. In *The Prokaryotes: A Handbook on Habitats, Isolation and Identification of Bacteria* (ed. M.P. Starr, M. Stolp, A. Truper *et al.*), Ch. 140, pp. 1811–1826.

Groman, N.B. (1984) Conversion by corynephages and its role in the natural history of diphtheria. *Journal of Hygiene*, **93**(3), 405–417.

Hande, K.R., Witebsky, F.G., Brown, M.S. *et al.* (1976) Sepsis with a new species of *Corynebacterium*. *Annals of Internal Medicine*, **85**, 423–426.

Hartman, L.J. (1979) Bioavailability study of diphtheria immunoglobulin (human). *Pathology*, **11**(3), 385–387.

Heltberg, O., Friis-Moller, A. and Ersgaard, H. (1986) Group JK diphtheroid bacteremia. *Acta Pathologica et Microbiologica et Immunologica Scandinavica*, Section B, **94**(4), 285–289.

Hollis, D.G. and Weaver, R.E. (1981) *Gram Positive Organisms: A Guide to Identification*. Special Bacteriology Laboratory, Centers for Disease Control, Atlanta, GA.

Holmes, K.K., Handsfield, H.H., Wang, S.P. *et al.* (1975) Etiology of nongonococcal urethritis. *New England Journal of Medicine*, **292**, 1199–1205.

Howard, W.T. (1893) Acute ulcerative endocarditis due to the *Bacillus diphtheriae*. *Bulletin of the Johns Hopkins Hospital*, **4**, 32–33.

Jackmann, P.J.H., Pitcher, D.G., Pelczynska, S. *et al.* (1987) Classification of corynebacteria associated with endocarditis (group JK) as *Corynebacterium jeikeium* sp. nov. *Systematic and Applied Microbiology*, **9**, 83–90.

Jacobs, D. (1990) *S.A.S./Graph and Numerical Taxonomy*. S.A.S. Users Group International Conference, Nashville, TN, April 1–4, 1990.

Johnson, A.P. and Efstratiou, A. (1993) *Corynebacterium jeikeium*: a multiresistant nosocomial pathogen. *Reviews in Medical Microbiology*, **4**, 242–248.

Johnson, W.D. and Kaye, D. (1970) Serious infections caused by diphtheroids. *Annals of the New York Academy of sciences*, **174**, 569–576.

Kalapothaki, V., Sapounas, T., Xirouchaki, E. *et al.* (1984) Prevalence of diphtheria carriers in a population with disappearing clinical diphtheria. *Infection*, **12**(6), 387–389.

Karzon, D.T. and Edwards, K.M. (1988) Diphtheria outbreaks in immunised populations. *New England Journal of Medicine*, **318**(1), 41–43.

Keddie, R.M. and Jones, D. (1981) Saprophytic, aerobic coryneform bacteria. In *The Prokaryotes: A Handbook on Habitats, Isolation, and Identification of Bacteria* (ed. M.P. Starr, M. Stolp, A. Truper *et al.*), Ch. 142, pp. 1838–1878. Springer-Verlag, New York.

Kerry-Williams, S.M. and Noble, W.C. (1984) Plasmid-associated bacteriocin production in a JK-type coryneform bacterium. *FEMS Microbiology Letters*, **25**, 179–182.

Kerry-Williams, S.M. and Noble, W.C. (1986) Plasmids in group JK coryneform bacteria isolated in a single hospital. *Journal of Hygiene*, **97**(2), 255–263.

Khabbaz, R.F., Kaper, J.B., Moody, M.R. *et al.* (1986) Molecular epidemiology of group JK *Corynebacterium* on a cancer ward: lack of evidence for patient-to-patient transmission. *Journal of Infectious Diseases*, **154**, 95–99.

Koopman, J.S. and Campbell, J. (1975) The role of cutaneous diphtheria infections in a diphtheria epidemic. *Journal of Infectious Diseases*, **131**, 239–244.

Korzenkova, M.P., Ivanov, U.A., Platonova, T.V. *et al.* (1991) Routine screening for *Corynebacterium diphtheriae*. *Lancet*, **338**, 577–578.

Lange, M., Sobeck, K., Blevin, A. *et al.* (1980) *Corynebacterium* species (CDC-JK) in a cancer hospital. *2nd International Conference on Nosocomial Infection*, Atlanta, GA, August 5–8, 1980.

Larson, E.L., McGinley, K.J., Leyden, J.J. *et al.* (1986) Skin colonisation with antibiotic resistant (JK group) and antibiotic sensitive lipophilic diphtheroids in hospitalised and normal adults. *Journal of Infectious Diseases*, **153**(4), 701–706.

Lehmann, K.B. and Neumann, R.O. (1886) *Atlas und Grundiss der Bakteriologie und Lehrbuch der Speciellen Bakteriologischen Diagnostik*, 1st edn. Munich.

Leyden, J.J., McGinley, K.J. and Webster, G.F. (1983) Cutaneous microbiology. In *Biochemistry and Physiology of the Skin* (ed. L.A. Goldsmith), pp. 1153–1165. Oxford University Press, New York.

Lipsky, B.A., Goldberger, A.C., Tompkins, L.S. *et al.* (1982) Infections caused by nondiphtheria corynebacteria. *Review of Infectious Diseases*, **4**, 1220–1235.

Marples, R.R. and Williamson, P. (1969) Effects of systemic demethylchlortetracycline on human cutaneous microflora. *Applied Microbiology*, **18**, 228–234.

McCloskey, R.V., Green, M.J., Eller, J. *et al.* (1974) Treatment of diphtheria carriers: benzathine penicillin, erythromycin and clindamycin. *Annals of Internal Medicine*, **81**(6), 788–791.

McCracken, A.W. and Mauney, C.U. (1971) Identification of *Corynebacterium diphtheriae* by immunofluorescence during a diphtheria epidemic. *Journal of Clinical Pathology*, **24**, 641–644.

McGinley, K.J., Labows, J.N., Zeckman, J.M. *et al.* (1985a) Pathogenic JK group Corynebacteria and their similarity to human cutaneous lipophilic diphtheroids. *Journal of Infectious Diseases*, **152**(4), 801–806.

McGinley, K.J., Labows, J.N., Zechmann, J.M. *et al.* (1985b) Analysis of cellular components biochemical reactions and habitat of human cutaneous lipophilic diphtheroids. *Journal of Investigative Dermatology*, **85**, 374–377.

Murphy, P.G. (1990) *Corynebacterium jeikeium* infection and the development of a multilocus enzyme electrophoresis typing system. MD thesis, Faculty of Medicine, University College, Dublin.

Murphy, P.G. and Ferguson, W.P. (1987) *Corynebacterium jeikeium* (Group JK) resistance to ciprofloxacin emerging during therapy. *Journal of Antimicrobial Chemotherapy*, **20**(6), 922–923.

Noble, N.C. (1984) Skin microbiology: coming of age. *Journal of Medical Microbiology*, **17**, 1–12.

Pallen, M.J. (1991) Rapid screening for toxigenic *Corynebacterium diphtheriae* by the polymerase chain reaction. *Journal of Clinical Pathology*, **44**, 1025–1026.

Papenheimer, A.M. and Murphy, J.R. (1983) Studies on the molecular epidemiology of diphtheria. *Lancet*, **ii**, 923–926.

Pitcher, D.G. (1977) Rapid identification of cell wall components as a guide to the classification of aerobic coryneform bacteria from human skin. *Journal of Medical Microbiology*, **10**, 439–445.

Pitcher, D., Soro, A., Soriano, F. *et al.* (1992) Urinary tract infection (group D2) as *Corynebacterium urealyticum* sp. nov. *International Journal of Systematic Bacteriology*, **42**(1), 178–181.

Quinn, J.P., Arnow, P.M., Weil, D. *et al.* (1984) Outbreak of JK diphtheroid infections associated with environmental contamination. *Journal of Clinical Microbiology*, **19**, 668–671.

Quinn, J.P., Lucks, D.A. and Divencenzo, C.A. (1986) A comparison of penicillin binding proteins in group JK bacteria and penicillin-susceptible *Corynebacteria*. *Abstracts of the Annual Meeting of the American Society of Microbiology*, Washington, A-112, 19.

Riebel, W., Frantz, N., Adelstein, D. *et al.* (1986) *Corynebacterium* JK: a cause of nosocomial device-related infection. *Reviews of Infectious Diseases*, **8**(1), 42–49.

Riley, P.S., Hollis, D.G., Utter, G.B. *et al.* (1979) Characterisation and identification of 95 diphtheroid (group JK) cultures isolated from clinical specimens. *Journal of Clinical Microbiology*, **9**, 418–424.

Roosen-Runge, (1903) Ein Fall von Diphtherienbazillen Sepsin. *Meunchen Medische Wocheschrift*, **50**, 1253.

Scheuplein, R.J. and Blank, I.H. (1971) Permeability of the skin. *Physiological Reviews*, **51**, 702.

Selwyn, S. and Ellis, H. (1972) Skin bacteria and skin disinfection reconsidered. *British Medical Journal*, **i**, 136–140.

Shelley, W.B. and Millar, M.A. (1984) Electron microscopy, histochemistry, and microbiology of bacterial adhesion in trichomycosis axillaris. *Journal of the American Academy of Dermatology*, **10**, 1005–1014.

Slifkin, M., Gil, G.M. and Engwall, C. (1986) Rapid identification of Group JK and other Corynebacteria with the Minitek system. *Journal of Clinical Microbiology*, **24**(2), 177–180.

Soriano, F., Ponte, C., Santa Maria, M. *et al.* (1985) *Corynebacterium* D2 as a cause of alkaline encrusted cystitis: report of 4 cases and characterisation of the organisms. *Journal of Clinical Microbiology*, **21**(5), 788–792.

Soriano, F., Agnado, J.M., Ponte, C. *et al.* (1990) Urinary tract infection caused by *Corynebacterium* group D2: report of 82 cases and review. *Reviews of Infectious Diseases*, **12**(6), 1019–1034.

Stamm, W.E., Tompkins, L.S., Wagner, K.F. *et al.* (1979) Infection due to *Corynebacterium* species in marrow transplant patients. *Annals of Internal Medicine*, **91**, 167–173.

Sutherland, J. and Willis, R.A. (1936) A case of endocarditis due to a diphtheroid bacillus structurally resembling the diphtheria bacillus. *Journal of Pathology and Bacteriology*, **43**, 127–135.

Telander, B., Lerner, R., Palmblad, J. *et al.* (1988) *Corynebacterium* group JK in a hematological ward: infections, colonization, and environmental contamination. *Scandinavian Journal of Infectious Diseases*, **20**(1), 55–61.

Wichmann, S., Wirsing von Köenig, C.H., Becker-Boost, E. *et al.* (1985) Group JK corynebacteria in skin flora of healthy persons and patients. *European Journal of Clinical Microbiology*, **4**, 502–504.

Wilson, A.P.R., Efstratiou, A., Weaver, E. *et al.* (1992) Unusual non-toxigenic *Corynebacterium diphtheriae* in homosexual men. *Lancet*, **339**, 998.

Winslow, C.-E.A., Broadhurst, J., Buchanan, R.E. *et al.* (1920) *Journal of Bacteriology*, **5**, 191.

World Health Organization (1993) Outbreak of diphtheria, update. Expanded Programme on immunisation. *Weekly Epidemiological Record*, No. 19 (7 May 1993), **68**, 134–138.

4

LISTERIA AND ERYSIPELOTHRIX

Kevin G. Kerr

HISTORICAL BACKGROUND

In 1911 a Swedish veterinary microbiologist isolated a bacterium from necrotic lesions in the liver of a rabbit. From his description, this could well have been the earliest example of the isolation of *Listeria monocytogenes*, but unfortunately the culture was not preserved. Seven years later, a bacterium resembling *Erysipelothrix rhusiopathiae* was isolated from the cerebrospinal fluid of a soldier serving in France. This isolate was deposited in the Institut Pasteur, Paris, but it was to be many years before this bacterium was recognized as *L. monocytogenes*.

In 1924 Murray and colleagues, during the investigation of an epizootic among experimental animals, isolated a bacterium from the enlarged mesenteric glands of affected animals. When injected into healthy animals the bacillus induced a monocytosis and was accordingly given the name *Bacillus monocytogenes*. Three years later in South Africa, Pirie during an investigation of carriage of *Yersinia pestis* by rodents isolated a bacterium from the livers of gerbils, which he named *Listerella hepatolytica*. This bacillus was found to be indistinguishable from *B. monocytogenes* and Pirie later proposed the name *Listeria monocytogenes*.

In 1929 Nyfeldt isolated *L. monocytogenes* from blood cultures of a patient with glandular fever and was convinced he had isolated the causative agent of infectious mononucleosis. Not surprisingly, other investigators were unable to substantiate his claim. Over the ensuing years, anecdotal reports of human listeriosis in both neonates and adults continued to appear in the literature but the consensus, however, was that listeriosis was an extremely rare zoonotic pathogen. The pioneering work of Reiss and his colleagues, and of Heinz Seeliger in the 1950s, established the first truly systematic studies of human listeriosis, but it was not until three decades later, following a series of well-publicized outbreaks, that *L. monocytogenes* was catapulted from relative obscurity into the microbiological limelight.

THE GENUS *LISTERIA*

Taxonomy and General Description of the Genus

The intra- and intergeneric relatedness of the genus *Listeria* has been the subject of much debate. At first considered as a member of the family Corynebacteriaceae, primarily because of morphological characteristics, later chemotaxonomic studies demonstrated that *Listeria* spp. are quite distinct from the corynebacteria. It was not until 1984, however, that partial sequencing of 16S rRNA unambiguously confirmed the phylogenetic place of the genus *Listeria* in the *Clostridium–Bacillus–Lactobacillus* group, with *Brochothrix thermosphacta* as its nearest neighbour.

The genus *Listeria* as originally described was monotypic, with *L. monocytogenes* the sole member. In the ensuing years a further seven species were recognized: *L. ivanovii* (previously *L. monocytogenes* serovar 5), *L. innocua*, *L. welshimeri*, *L. seeligeri*, *L. murrayi*, *L. grayi* and *L. denitrificans*. *Listeria denitrificans* has been since reclassified as *Jonesia denitrificans*. *Listeria murrayi* and *L. grayi* were once considered sufficiently distinct from other *Listeria* spp. to warrant the creation of a new genus, *Murraya*, but have now been assigned to a single species *L. grayi*. Most recently, *L. ivanovii* has been divided into two subspecies: subsp. *ivanovii* and subsp. *londoniensis*. Of the non-monocytogenes species, only *L. ivanovii* is recognized as a human pathogen (Cummins *et al.*, 1994).

The mol% G&C content of *L. monocytogenes* is 37–39 and, for other species, 36–38 (except for *L. grayi*: 41–42.5). Between 0 and 20% of isolates of *L. monocytogenes* carry plasmids. Although most of these are cryptic, a 37 kb plasmid which specifies antimicrobial resistance has been reported (Poyart-Salmeron *et al.*, 1990).

Listeria spp. are short (0.4–0.5 μm × 0.5–2.0 μm) Gram-positive rods. They are non-acid fast and do not produce spores. At 20 °C they are motile by means of peritrichous flagella, but motility is not observed in cultures incubated at 37 °C. They are facultatively anaerobic and grow over a wide temperature range of 0–45 °C (optimum 30–36 °C). Growth over a wide pH range occurs, with some strains growing at pH 9.6, but is optimal at neutral to slightly alkaline pH. Key biochemical and other characteristics are listed in Tables 4.2 and 4.3.

The major antigenic determinants of *Listeria* spp. are the somatic (O) and flagellar (H) antigens.

The current serotyping scheme, based on 14 somatic and four flagellar antigens, distinguishes five serogroups (1/2, 3, 4, 5 and 6) divided into 19 serovars for all species except *L. grayi*. Whilst *L. innocua*, *L. ivanovii* and *L. welshimeri* can be readily differentiated from *L. monocytogenes*, some strains of *L. seeligeri* may be antigenically indistinguishable from serogroup 1/2 of *L. monocytogenes*. It should also be noted that in excess of 90% of clinical isolates of *L. monocytogenes* belong to only three serovars – 1/2a, 1/2b and 4b – thereby limiting the value of this technique in epidemiological studies.

PATHOGENESIS OF LISTERIOSIS

Apart from the very rare exception of direct inoculation via skin or conjunctiva, it is most likely that the bacteria in the adult gain access to the host via the gastrointestinal tract. In the case of the fetus, infection in the majority of cases arises from haematogenous seeding of the placenta and only a few cases are thought to be acquired intra partum as the neonate exits the birth canal. Late-onset neonatal listeriosis is acquired through direct or indirect person-to-person transmission.

Although it has been suggested that co-infection with another gastrointestinal pathogen may predispose to invasion of the gut by *L. monocytogenes*, it is now known that the bacterium can specify its own uptake by mammalian cells, including those which are non-professional phagocytes. The expression of an 80 kDa protein – internalin – whose carboxy terminal amino acid sequence is similar to the membrane attachment proteins of Gram-positive cocci, such as *Streptococcus pyogenes* M protein, is of key importance in this process. Another protein (p60), the product of the *iap* gene, may also play a role in this context.

Following internalization by the host cell, the bacterium escapes from the phagosomal vacuole to enter the cytoplasm, whereupon rapid growth ensues. Lysis of the vacuole is due to the production of listeriolysin O, a haemolysin which shows sequence homology with other thiol-activated cytolysins, such as streptolysin O.

After escaping from the phagosomes, the bacteria mediate the nucleation of host actin filaments, which then rearrange to form a 'tail' consisting of these filaments and actin binding proteins, allowing them to move through the cell at a rate of up to 1.5 μm/s. Some bacteria move to the edge of the host cell and are extruded from it in pseudopod-like structures, which are apparently recognized by an adjacent cell and phagocytosed. The bacterium is now in a double membrane vacuole, which is then lysed by a phospholipase C (lecithinase), thus allowing it free access to its new host cell. The expression of these and other virulence factors is regulated by the *prf*A gene, whose product is a site-specific binding protein, which acts as a transcriptional activator of these genes. Mutants of *L. monocytogenes* lacking a functional PrfA protein are avirulent.

There is little consensus on either the infective dose of *L. monocytogenes* or the possibility that some strains are more virulent than others. Despite reports using experimental animals, the wide range of assay systems and lack of standardized protocols make it extremely difficult to draw firm conclusions. However, quantitative bacterial counts from implicated foodstuffs in some clinical cases of listeriosis have allowed estimates of minimum infectious doses to be made. In some instances, the counts were in excess of 10^6 cfu/g and in one case, involving unpasteurized goats' milk cheese, an infective dose of 4×10^9 was calculated (Azadian *et al.*, 1989).

EPIDEMIOLOGY

Ecology of *Listeria monocytogenes*

The environment

Listeria monocytogenes has been isolated from a wide range of environmental sources, including vegetation, dust, soil and sewage. Although it is often considered that *L. monocytogenes* in soil and vegetation results from faecal contamination by animals, Weiss and Seeliger (1976) noted that the bacterium was isolated in greatest numbers from plants and soil from uncultivated areas, whereas

the lowest numbers were obtained from samples taken in agricultural environments.

Listeria monocytogenes can survive for extended periods in the environment. It can survive for up to 1500 days in certain types of soil and has also been shown to survive and multiply in water. It has been isolated from surface water in canals and lakes and from estuarine environments. The bacterium has also been isolated from raw and treated sewage. When sprayed on agricultural land, numbers of *L. monocytogenes* did not significantly decrease over an eight-week period (Watkins and Sleath, 1981). Of particular concern is that crops grown in soil treated with sewage sludge may become contaminated with *L. monocytogenes*. Similarly, aquatic environments may become contaminated by the addition of animal manure or human soil to water, as occurs in several countries.

Listeria monocytogenes can be found in environmental samples taken from food production facilities and at retail outlets. Contamination of the domestic environment with *L. monocytogenes*, although not widely investigated, appears to be rare.

Food

Following the recognition that listeriosis is often food-borne (see below), there have been few foods which have not escaped the attention of the microbiologist seeking *L. monocytogenes*. Studies to determine the extent of listerial contamination for a given food product often yield markedly different results. The reasons for this are complex, and whilst geographic, seasonal and other differences must be acknowledged, wide variations in protocols for isolation are also important. Differences in experimental technique also account for the discrepancies in the results of investigations into the growth, survival and heat tolerance of *L. monocytogenes* in foods.

To date, *L. monocytogenes* has been associated with a variety of food products, particularly raw milk and dairy products, principally surface-ripened (soft) cheese. Hard cheese, because of the decrease in pH and a_w which occur during ripening, is much less likely to become contaminated. Soft cheeses made from pasteurized milk are equally as likely to be contaminated as those made from raw milk (Bind, 1989).

Listeriosis has been associated with the consumption of contaminated poultry (Kerr *et al.*, 1988), and up to 66% of fresh chickens and 17% of cooked birds may harbour *L. monocytogenes* (Art and Andre, 1991). Other meat products, both raw and cooked, may also be contaminated with the bacterium (Farber *et al.*, 1989). As with poultry, it is uncertain as to whether bacteria present in cooked items are organisms which have survived the cooking process or merely represent post-cooking contaminants.

Other foods in which *L. monocytogenes* has been detected include pâté, vegetables (including pre-packed salads), seafood and both commercial and institutional cook-chill products.

Animal and human carriers

At least 42 species of wild, zoo and domestic animals and birds have been shown to harbour *L. monocytogenes*. Rates of faecal carriage in cattle, sheep and goats vary widely, but may be extremely high, even in listeriosis-free herds.

Early studies investigating faecal carriage in humans suggested that up to 70% of selected populations may excrete *L. monocytogenes* for short periods, but these reports must be viewed with caution, as many of the isolates, given contemporary identification criteria, would not now be recognized as *L. monocytogenes*. More recent reports suggest that faecal carriage is, in fact, rare, with rates ranging from 0.1% to 2.7% (Oakley *et al.*, 1992; Lamont and Postlethwaite, 1986).

Carriage of *Listeria* spp. in the vagina has been investigated, but does not seem to occur outside the context of recent maternofetal listeriosis.

Human Infection

For many years *L. monocytogenes* was considered a rare zoonotic pathogen. The first case of food-borne listeriosis was reported by Potel as long ago as 1951 during a *Listeria* epidemic in which raw milk was suspected as the source of infection. Similar reports continued to appear in the ensuing two decades, but were largely ignored, presumably because the East German and Czechoslovak researchers had little contact with fellow investigators in the West. It was not until the large outbreaks of listeriosis in the 1980s that systematic studies of the epidemiology of *L. monocytogenes*-associated infection were initiated.

In many countries human listeriosis has been perceived for many years to be on the increase. The question as to whether this represents a true increase in frequency or merely greater awareness amongst clinicians and bacteriologists has long been the subject of debate. Whilst there can be no doubt that diagnostic techniques and reporting systems have improved, most authorities now believe that there has indeed been a 'real' increase in the number of cases of listeriosis. This is probably because of the growing number of individuals with conditions which render them vulnerable to *L. monocytogenes* infection; but changes in food production and retailing practices, such as the introduction of refrigerated products with extended 'shelf lives', and altered dietary habits, may be additional factors.

Data on the incidence of listeriosis is influenced by methods used for ascertainment. In 1986, in the USA, an active surveillance system established in six areas with a total population of 33.5 million reported an annual rate of seven cases per 10^6 population; this compares with rates of 0.5–3.6 cases per 10^6 in previous studies using passive surveillance techniques (Gellin *et al.*, 1991). Marked year-to-year variations can occur, even in the apparent absence of epidemics. Most studies report a peak during the summer, although others have failed to identify any seasonal differences. More recently, in several countries such as the UK, the incidence of listeriosis has fallen sharply. This may have been due to increased microbiological monitoring and surveillance by public health agencies, improved food production practices and changes in consumer awareness relating to 'high-risk' foods.

Listeria monocytogenes as a Food-borne Pathogen

Evidence that contaminated food is the principal route of transmission of *L. monocytogenes* comes from three main sources: investigation of outbreaks (Table 4.1), case–control studies of sporadic listeriosis and individual case reports.

Even before the well-publicized outbreaks in North America and Europe in the 1980s, epidemics of listeriosis were well recognized. Several of these involved large numbers of individuals (in the 1966 outbreak in Halle, Germany, there were 279 cases) but insufficient data were collected to allow the precise identification of the source of these outbreaks. In practice, identification of an outbreak may be difficult and it is likely that some go unnoticed. For example, in their retrospective study, Ciesielski *et al.* (1988) observed three clusters which had, at that time, gone undetected. In addition, several outbreaks may have only come to light because of fortuitous circumstances. The Los Angeles outbreak, which mainly involved the City's Hispanic community, was recognized because women in this particular population favoured a single hospital for obstetric care (Linnan *et al.*, 1988).

Further evidence supporting *L. monocytogenes* as a food-borne pathogen has come from a number of case–control studies. Schuchat *et al.* (1992) compared 165 sporadic cases with 376 carefully matched controls. The former were significantly more likely to have eaten soft cheeses, undercooked chicken or food purchased from delicatessen counters. In a parallel investigation, the bacterium was isolated in at least one food specimen in 79 of 123 (64%) cases and of these 26 (33%) contained an

isolate of *L. monocytogenes* indistinguishable by multilocus enzyme electrophoresis typing.

A limited number of anecdotal reports have incriminated a variety of contaminated foodstuffs, particularly soft cheese and undercooked poultry, in cases of sporadic listeriosis. The investigation of such cases is often difficult, particularly as the incubation period may be very long, compared with that of other food-borne pathogens. The mean incubation period, as determined by the investigators of the Los Angeles outbreak, was 31 days (range 11–70 days). As a result, accurate food histories may be impossible to obtain and, additionally, left-over food items may have been eaten or discarded in the interim.

Other Routes of Transmission of Listeria monocytogenes

Person-to-person transmission outside the hospital setting has never been convincingly demonstrated, but nosocomial spread of *L. monocytogenes* is well recognized, particularly on neonatal units, typically following the introduction of a case of early-onset sepsis onto the ward, resulting in late-onset cases several days later. Routes of transmission include contaminated resuscitation equipment, rectal thermometers, tape measures and mineral oil which was applied to the skin of newborns after delivery. In other outbreaks, transmission of the bacterium by health care personnel or mothers appears to have occurred.

Zoonotic cases of listeriosis are very uncommon and have presentations which differ from the more commonly recognized syndromes, and include cutaneous lesions, conjunctivitis and pneumonia. Some authors have suggested that *L.*

TABLE 4.1 EXAMPLES OF OUTBREAKS OF LISTERIOSIS WITH A FOOD-BORNE VECTOR

Location	Date	No. cases	No. deaths/still-births/abortions	Foodstuff	Reference
Maritime Provinces, Canada	1980–81	41	17	Coleslaw	Schlech *et al.* (1983)
Los Angeles, USA	1985	142	48	Soft cheese	Linnan *et al.* (1988)
Canton de Vaud, Switzerland	1983–87	122	31	Soft cheese	Bille (1990)
France	1992	279	95	Pork tongue in aspic	Jacquet *et al.* (1995)
France	1995	20	4	Soft cheese	Goulet *et al.* (1995)

monocytogenes may be transmitted by sexual intercourse, or by ticks and tabanid flies, but there is no convincing evidence for this. Transmission via blood transfusion, although theoretically possible given the psychrotrophic nature of the bacterium, has never been reported.

Molecular Epidemiology of *Listeria monocytogenes*

Conventional typing systems such as serotyping are poorly discriminative, and bacteriophage typing, for many years the 'gold standard', is available only at a few centres and is limited by the non-typeability of many strains. The application of genotypic techniques has contributed much to the understanding of the epidemiology of *L. monocytogenes* infections: these include DNA macrorestriction analysis (Moore and Datta, 1994) and polymerase chain reaction (PCR)-based methods, such as a multiple arbitrary amplicon profiling (Kerr *et al.*, 1995). Currently, a WHO-sponsored international multicentre study is attempting to standardize typing systems.

CLINICAL MANIFESTATIONS OF *L. MONOCYTOGENES* INFECTION

Listeriosis in Pregnancy

This syndrome accounts for approximately one-third of all cases of listeriosis, although the proportion may be much higher in epidemics. Although most frequently documented in the third trimester, listeriosis in the early stages of pregnancy has also been reported. However, as early fetal loss is very often incompletely investigated, the number of cases occurring in the first trimester of pregnancy may be underestimated.

Bacteraemia is the most common manifestation of listeriosis in pregnancy and is classically accompanied by an episode of 'flu-like' illness with fever, headache and myalgia. Associated low back pain may suggest a urinary tract infection. Gastrointestinal symptoms, including abdominal pain and diarrhoea, are less common. In up to 45% of cases, however, the pregnant woman may be asymptomatic with the first indication of infection being the abortion or stillbirth of the fetus, or neonatal listeriosis in a live-born child.

In contrast to adult listerial infections, complications in pregnant women are very rare and are usually seen in the context of underlying illness, such as systemic lupus erythematosis or AIDS and, in the overwhelming majority of women, the infection is self-limiting, even in the absence of antimicrobial therapy.

There is evidence that untreated *L. monocytogenes* bacteraemia in the gravid female does not inevitably lead to transmission of the infection to the fetus; in the Los Angeles outbreak, for example, 10% of maternal cases did not lead to fetal sepsis (Linnan *et al.*, 1988).

The hypothesis that maternal 'genital listeriosis' is a cause of repeated abortion was first proposed over 30 years ago, but there is no compelling evidence to uphold it.

Neonatal Listeriosis

Somewhat analogous to neonatal sepsis with group B β-haemolytic streptococci, neonatal listeriosis can be divided into early- and late-onset groups. Early-onset disease is defined as sepsis manifesting within five days of birth but typically presents within 48 hours post partum. Late-onset disease develops five or more days after birth and several investigators have reported a mean age of onset of 14 days. Overall mortality rates for both types vary widely but can be as high as 50%.

Early-onset listeriosis results, in most cases, from *in utero* transmission of *L. monocytogenes* from a bacteraemic mother. Ascending vaginal infection is uncommon. The classical manifestation of early-onset disease is granulomatosis infantisepticum characterized at autopsy by widely disseminated granulomas in several organs, most frequently in the liver and placenta. Although frequently noted in early reports, it has been less commonly observed by later investigators.

In practice, it is difficult to distinguish early-onset listeriosis from other forms of neonatal sepsis. Respiratory distress, occasionally associated with interstitial chest infiltrates, poor perfusion of the extremities and hypotonia, are common features. Petechial or pustular rashes are seen less frequently.

In contrast to early-onset disease, infants who manifest the late-onset form of listeriosis are usually healthy at birth. It has been suggested that affected infants are colonized at birth but, as a result of hitherto unexplained factors, the onset of infection is delayed. Much more likely, however, particularly in the light of numerous reports of clusters of late-onset listeriosis, is that nosocomial transmission has occurred. As many as 95% of infants with late-onset infection present with meningitis or meningoencephalitis. Onset is more insidious than the early form of the infection, with poor feeding, irritability and fever common presenting symptoms.

Listeriosis in Adults

Listeriosis in adults is often seen against a background of immune suppression, particularly where cell-mediated immunity is affected, e.g. lymphoreticular neoplasms, corticosteroid therapy and anti-rejection regimens in organ transplantation. Early in the AIDS epidemic, *L. monocytogenes* was not considered to be a significant pathogen in HIV-infected individuals and several plausible explanations for this, including the anti-*Listeria* activity of cotrimoxazole used as *Pneumocystis carinii* prophylaxis, were advanced. Later studies, however, have demonstrated that listeriosis is 150–350 times more common in HIV-positive patients than matched control groups from the general population. Other chronic diseases, such as diabetes and alcoholism, predispose to *L. monocytogenes* infection. Age has also been suggested as a predisposing factor, but as many elderly patients have other underlying conditions it is difficult to determine the exact contribution which age, per se, makes to the development of listeriosis in this population.

The fact that listeriosis can develop in previously apparently healthy individuals is often overlooked. Indeed, in several published series, approximately one-third of cases had apparently no obvious predisposing factor (e.g., Skogberg *et al.*, 1992).

Reported mortality rates vary widely according to age, sex, and underlying illness, thus making it extremely difficult to make useful comparisons between published studies, but overall mortality rates of 35–45% are typical. More recently, several investigators have reported decreasing case:fatality ratios, perhaps because of more vigorous bacteriological investigation and antimicrobial therapy in immunosuppressed patients.

Adult listeriosis can be categorized according to clinical manifestations into three groups: central nervous system disease, primary bacteraemia and a miscellaneous group which embraces a wide spectrum of localized infections.

Meningitis, with or without focal neurological signs, is the commonest form of central nervous system (CNS) listeriosis. As with other pyogenic meningitides, listerial meningitis is usually acute in onset with high fever, nuchal rigidity and photophobia, but there are often other additional features, such as movement disorders, including tremor and/or ataxia. Seizures also appear to be more common than in other types of meningitis.

The most common non-meningitic form of CNS listeriosis is encephalitis, most frequently affecting the rhombencephalon. This has a characteristic biphasic course: a non-specific prodrome of headache, nausea, vomiting and fever, followed by progressive asymmetrical cranial nerve palsies, cerebellar signs or hemiparesis and impairment of consciousness. Prognosis is poor, with significant rates of neurological sequelae in survivors. Given the frequency of CNS involvement in listeriosis, it is, perhaps, surprising to note that listerial brain abscesses are rare. All cases reported thus far appear to be haematogenous in origin, with no evidence of spread from infected contiguous sites.

Primary bacteraemia is the second most common manifestation of listeriosis in non-pregnant adults, occurring in 25–43% of cases. There are no distinguishing clinical features associated with this form of listeriosis. Patients may be profoundly hypotensive, with an overall clinical picture which mimics Gram-negative endotoxic shock which may be accompanied by the adult respiratory distress syndrome (Blot *et al.*, 1994).

A variety of other clinical syndromes are associated with adult listeriosis. Listeria infections of the locomotor system include osteomyelitis and septic arthritis, with the latter occurring in both native and prosthetic joints. Pulmonary infection, in contradistinction to neonatal listeriosis, is rare, but cases of pneumonia and/or empyaema have occasionally been reported. Hepatic involvement in listeriosis is also comparatively rare, but hepatic abscesses, both single and multiple, are recognized, the former almost exclusively occurring in insulin-dependent diabetic subjects. Hepatitis in a liver transplant patient has also been described (Bourgeois *et al.*, 1993). Spontaneous bacterial peritonitis caused by *L. monocytogenes* has been reported in both cirrhotic and non-cirrhotic patients, as has peritonitis in individuals undergoing continuous ambulatory peritonitis (Polanco *et al.*, 1992).

Listerial endocarditis occurs on both native and prosthetic valves and has also been reported as a complication of coronary artery bypass surgery (Baddour, 1989). Infections of arteriovenous shunts, intravenous cannulae and prosthetic grafts have also been recorded (Gauto *et al.*, 1992).

Ocular infections, although rare, have been described by several investigators. These infections are difficult to manage and are often sight threatening (Eliott *et al.*, 1992). Primary cutaneous listeriosis is an infrequently observed manifestation of *L. monocytogenes* sepsis and is usually seen in veterinarians and farm workers after accidental inoculation of the skin following exposure to animals.

Other clinical forms of listeriosis, frequently described in earlier reviews, such as the 'oculoglandular syndrome' and 'typhoid-like pneumonia', do not feature in studies published by contemporary observers.

LABORATORY DIAGNOSIS OF *LISTERIA* INFECTION

Diagnosis of listeriosis on clinical grounds is problematic, partly because there are few, if any, pathognomic signs, and partly because it is a rare infection and is often not considered in the differential diagnosis.

Direct Detection of *L. monocytogenes* in Clinical Material

Gram staining of specimens from normally sterile sites may suggest the diagnosis of listeriosis. Short Gram-positive rods may be seen in both extra- and intracellular locations, but it should be remembered that the bacteria may appear filamentous, coccoid or even Gram negative, especially in cerebrospinal fluid (CSF) from patients with partially treated meningitis. It should also be noted that analysis of CSF specimens may not yield a typical pyogenic picture; in up to 30% of cases, there is no hypoglycorrhachia and there may be no predominance, or even an absence, of polymorphs (Niemann and Lorber, 1980).

A number of different antigen detection techniques have been reported for the rapid detection of *L. monocytogenes* in clinical material, e.g. chemiluminescent enzyme-linked immunoassay (ELISA), but these are not available for routine use. There are several commercially available systems which rely on DNA hybridization, PCR-based DNA amplification and antigen detection by ELISA, but these have been developed for the identification of *Listeria* spp. in foodstuffs, and there is little experience of these techniques in the clinical laboratory.

Isolation of *L. monocytogenes*

Listeria monocytogenes is easily isolated from specimens obtained from normally sterile sites and the bacterium will grow on most commonly used non-selective media after 24–48 hours incubation. Where the number of organisms may be low, specimens may be enriched by incubation on broth media, such as brain heart infusion, at 37 °C. Isolation of *L. monocytogenes* from clinical or food samples which are likely to be contaminated requires the use of selective/differential media, such as modified Oxford or PALCAM agars (van Netten *et al.*, 1989). On both of these media, aesculin-hydrolysing colonies, such as *Listeria* spp., are surrounded by a black halo of aesculin (which diffuses widely throughout the medium on prolonged incubation, making it difficult to identify individual aesculin-hydrolysing colonies). With the exception of the uncommonly encountered *L. grayi*, *Listeria* spp. do not ferment mannitol and this property is made use of in PALCAM agar, which contains a mannitol/phenol red indicator system. Additionally, food or contaminated clinical material may be incubated for 48 hours at 30 °C in an enrichment broth, such as L-PALCAMY (van Netten *et al.*, 1989) before subculture onto a selective agar. Cold enrichment by incubation at 4 °C is a lengthy process and may lead to significant delays in the isolation and identification of *Listeria* spp.

Identification of *Listeria monocytogenes*

There are several reasons why *L. monocytogenes* may be misidentified in the diagnostic laboratory, other than the well-recognized tendency to appear as a 'diphtheroid', which occasionally leads to an isolate being discarded as a contaminant. Zones of β-haemolysis may not be obvious and may require removal of a colony from the plate for this to become apparent. In addition, *L. monocytogenes* may cross-react with reagents in some, but not all (MacGowan *et al.*, 1988; Farrington *et al.*, 1991), commercially available streptococcal grouping

kits. Furthermore, tests for motility are sometimes carried out at 20 °C only without simultaneously testing for absence of motility at 37 °C. It should be noted that only a minority of the motile population may exhibit the so-called characteristic 'tumbling leaf' motility when viewed in a hanging drop preparation. Very rarely, tests for catalase may be negative (Swartz *et al.*, 1991).

Although biochemical identification of *Listeria* spp. using traditional biochemical and other techniques, as outlined in Tables 4.2 and 4.3, should not be beyond the capability of most clinical laboratories, a number of commercially produced identification systems can be used (Kerr *et al.*, 1991; Bille *et al.*, 1992). These are, however, primarily designed for food microbiology facilities and it is unlikely, given the infrequency of isolation of *Listeria* in the clinical setting, that the routine diagnostic laboratory would find it cost effective to employ these methods. The API CORYNE system (Kerr *et al.*, 1993) includes the genus *Listeria* in its database, but requires additional tests to distinguish *L. monocytogenes* from *L. innocua* (β-haemolysis, CAMP reaction with *Staphylococcus aureus*). The API 20S kit also contains tests useful in the identification of *Listeria* to the genus level.

TABLE 4.2   DIFFERENTIATION OF *LISTERIA* SPECIES

Test	L. monocytogenes	L. innocua	L. seeligeri	L. ivanovii	L. welshimeri	L. grayi subsp. grayi	L. grayi subsp. murrayi
β-Haemolysis on blood agar	+	–	+	+	–	–	–
CAMP test							
S. aureus	+	–	w	–	–	–	–
R. equi	–	–	–	+	–	–	–
Nitrate reduction	–	–	–	–	–	–	+
Acid from:							
D-Mannitol	–	–	–	–	–	+	+
L-Rhamnose	+	v	–	–	–	–	v
D-Xylose	–	–	+	+	+	–	–
α-Methyl-D-glucoside	+	+	+	+	+	v	v
α-Methyl-D-mannoside	+	+	–	+	+	v	v
D-Ribose	–	–	–	v	–	+	+
D-Tagatose	–	–	–	–	v	–	–

+, ≥90% strains positive; –, ≤10% strains positive; w, weakly positive; v, 11–89% strains positive.
L. ivanovii subsp. *ivanovii* +; subsp *londoniensis* –.

TABLE 4.3 DIFFERENTIATION OF *LISTERIA* SPECIES AND *ERYSIPELOTHRIX RHUSIOPATHIAE*

Test	*Listeria* spp.	*Erysipelothrix rhusiopathiae*
Catalase	+	−
Oxidase	−	−
Motility		
20 °C	+	−
37 °C	−	−
Growth at 4 °C	+	−
Haemolysis on blood agar	*β*/non-haemolytic	*α*/non-haemolytic
H₂S production	−	+
Aesculin hydrolysis	+	−
Indole production	−	−
VP	+	−
Urease	−	−
Vancomycin susceptibility	S	R

VP, Voges–Proskauer test; S, susceptible; R, resistant.

The CAMP test, originally employed in the identification of *Streptococcus agalactiae*, has been modified for use in the characterization of *Listeria* spp. The test relies upon synergism of haemolysis between cultures of *L. monocytogenes* and *S. aureus*, and *Rhodococcus equi* and *L. ivanovii* (*L. seeligeri* may also give a weak positive CAMP test with *S. aureus*). In this test *S. aureus* or *R. equi* is streaked across in a 5% (v/v) sheep blood agar plate and the *β*-haemolytic *Listeria* isolate is streaked at 90° to the *S. aureus* or *R. equi*. Plates are incubated in air overnight at 37 °C. With *R. equi* and *L. ivanovii* an easily identifiable 'arrow-head' zone of haemolysis is observed. With *L. monocytogenes* and *S. aureus* synergistic haemolysis also occurs, but this is less obvious and a more 'blunt' zone of haemolysis is seen (Figure 4.1). It must be emphasized that for the test to be successful only sheep blood cells should be used and these must be washed (twice) in phosphate-buffered saline prior to media preparation as some lots of cells contain inhibitors of haemolysis. Not all strains of *S. aureus* and *R. equi* are suitable for use and strains NCTC 1803 and NCTC 1621, respectively, have been recommended (McLauchlin, 1988).

Commercial antisera are available for agglutination of isolates belonging to serogroups 1 and 4 although, as discussed earlier, this is of limited epidemiological value. In addition, antigenic cross-reactions between *Listeria* and other genera, including *Staphylococcus* and *Streptococcus*, may yield misleading results. Antigenic cross-reactivity is also responsible for the poor specificity of serodiagnostic techniques and these cannot be recommended for use in the investigation of listeriosis.

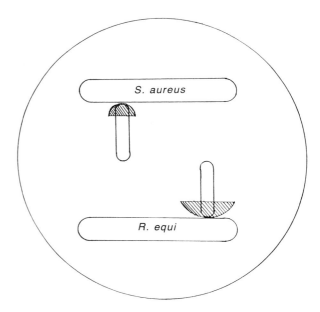

Figure 4.1. CAMP test with *L. monocytogenes* (top) and *L. ivanovii* (bottom). Hatched areas represent zone of haemolysis.

CHEMOTHERAPY OF LISTERIOSIS

Despite *in vitro* susceptibility to a wide range of agents (except the cephalosporins) the outcome of therapy in listeriosis is often disappointing – mainly as a result of delays in the initiation of appropriate therapy because of failure to consider listeriosis in the differential diagnosis and also because many patients have predisposing conditions, such as immune deficiency or debilitating disease, including malignancy. Moreover, *L. monocytogenes* is a facultative intracellular parasite and many agents have poor intracellular penetration. Even if penetration does occur, compounds may be unstable or exhibit reduced activity in this milieu. Information on the most effective agents for listeriosis are derived from *in vitro* data, animal models and clinical reports, but methodologies vary greatly between studies and results are often conflicting. There have been no controlled trials in this field.

Despite poor intracellular penetration and a widely held belief that it is only bacteriostatic against *L. monocytogenes*, ampicillin is regarded as the drug of choice in listeriosis, albeit at higher than usual doses of 8–12 g per day in divided doses. The need to add an aminoglycoside to this regimen remains controversial. *In vitro* data suggest that this is a synergistic combination, but experimental animal studies and clinical experience have produced varying outcomes. The addition of gentamicin (2.5 mg/kg per day) has been suggested if poor prognostic indicators are identified (Jones and MacGowan, 1995). These are defined as age >50 years, organ transplant patients and the need for cardiovascular, renal or ventilatory support. More recently, animal models using liposomal or nanoparticle bound ampicillin have yielded encouraging results, but these have yet to be employed in the clinical context. There are insufficient data at present to recommend the use of carbapenem agents in listeriosis.

The optimal duration of therapy has still to be determined, but a general recommendation is at least two weeks for primary bacteraemia and listeriosis in pregnancy and at least three weeks for meningitis. Shorter courses are often associated with relapsing infection. Extended courses are necessary for less frequently occurring manifestations of listeriosis, such as endocarditis and brain abscesses. Recommendations for the management of these, and other syndromes associated with *L. monocytogenes* infection, are given by Jones and MacGowan (1995).

For patients unable to tolerate an ampicillin ± aminoglycoside regimen, cotrimoxazole is considered optimal second-line therapy, both on account of *in vitro* synergy of the combination at concentrations readily achievable in serum and CSF and also because of favourable clinical outcome. There are insufficient data, however, to recommend trimethoprim monotherapy in this context. In pregnancy, where cotrimoxazole cannot be used, there is limited evidence to suggest that a macrolide may be a reasonable alternative in the penicillin-allergic patient. Another alternative to ampicillin, except in CNS listeriosis, is vancomycin alone, or in combination with, gentamicin. Despite good tissue and intracellular penetration, and evidence from animal models, there is little experience on the use of quinolones in the clinical setting.

Antibiotic resistance in clinical isolates of *L. monocytogenes* is fortunately rare, but an isolate from a patient with meningoencephalitis was found to be resistant to chloramphenicol, erythromycin, streptomycin and tetracycline (Poyart-Salmeron *et al.*, 1990). Sequence homology studies suggested that the conjugative plasmid specifying these determinants had been acquired from enterococci or other streptococci.

ERYSIPELOTHRIX RHUSIOPATHIAE

Historical Background

Although Koch cultured a bacterium, *Erysipelothrix muriseptica*, from the blood of septicaemic mice in 1880, it was not until eight years later that Löffler published the first accurate description of *E. rhusiopathiae*, which he isolated from the vasculature of a pig which had died from swine erysipelas. In the intervening period Pasteur and Dumas (and later Thuillier) used a strain of the bacterium which had been passaged through rabbits to immunize swine against erysipelas – the first time active immunization by a live attenuated vaccine had been demonstrated. The bacterium was first identified as a human pathogen in 1909 when Rosenbach reported its isolation from a patient with localized cutaneous lesions to which he gave the name 'erysipeloid' to distinguish them from those of human erysipelas.

Taxonomy and Description of the Genus

Erysipelothrix spp. are facultative anaerobes which grow over a wide temperature range with an optimum of 30–37 °C. They are non-motile, asporogenous, non-acid-fast, short Gram-positive rods (0.2–0.4 μm in diameter, 0.8–2.5 μm in length). They usually occur singly but, according to growth conditions, may be observed as chains, clusters or filamentous forms. Growth is favoured under alkaline conditions (range pH 6.7–9.2; optimum pH 7.2–7.6). Biochemical characteristics are discussed below and in Table 4.3.

Until recently the genus *Erysipelothrix* contained only one species, *E. rhusiopathiae*, but DNA–DNA homology studies have identified a distinct subgroup of strains which have been named as *E. tonsillarum*.

Heat-stable antigens extracted from the cell wall of *E. rhusiopathiae* form the basis of a serotyping system, in which serotypes 1 and 2 are most frequently associated with sepsis in both human and veterinary settings; however, some strains – 'type N' – are untypeable by this method. More recently, multi-locus enzyme electrophoresis has been utilized to examine the genetic diversity of *Erysipelothrix* spp. (Chooromoney *et al.*, 1994).

PATHOGENESIS OF ERYSIPELOTHRIX RHUSIOPATHIAE INFECTION

Virulence factors of *E. rhusiopathiae* remain ill defined, particularly with regard to human infection. It has been reported that production of neuraminidase and hyaluronidase and *in vitro* adherence to porcine kidney cells is more common in virulent strains. More recently, it has been suggested that the presence of an antiphagocytic capsule is an important virulence determinant (Shimoji *et al.*, 1994).

EPIDEMIOLOGY

Ecology of *Erysipelothrix rhusiopathiae*

Erysipelothrix rhusiopathiae is distributed widely and has been identified in a number of environmental samples, including soil. The primary reservoir for this bacterium is, however, mammals and birds, in which it can behave as a commensal or pathogen. Particularly important in this respect are pigs, in which *E. rhusiopathiae* infection is associated with a number of syndromes including swine erysipelas, septicaemia and polyarthritis which resembles rheumatoid arthritis in humans. In addition, lambs, calves, poultry and, more recently, farmed emu, are also susceptible to this infection, which has a major economic impact on the farming industry. *Erysipelothrix tonsillarum*, isolated from the tonsils of healthy pigs, has not been shown to cause veterinary or human infection. *Erysipelothrix rhusiopathiae* can be isolated from the mucoid slime covering finned fish and also from shellfish but has not been associated with disease in this setting.

Human Infection

There is no carrier state in humans. Although infection associated with *E. rhusiopathiae* in humans is apparently rare, difficulties in the microbiological diagnosis of erysipeloid (see below) and the rapid response of this condition to many antibiotics, coupled with the fact that the disease is not notifiable, may lead to an underestimation of the true number of cases.

Given the reservoirs of the bacterium, it is not surprising that individuals who have frequent contact with animals, poultry, fish and their associated products are most at risk for *Erysipelothrix* infection. These include abattoir workers, butchers, fishermen, farmers etc., and these occupational factors presumably explain why these infections are more common in males. In most instances it is likely that the bacterium is acquired via cutaneous inoculation.

In some cases, no history of animal or fish contact can be elicited, whilst in others consumption of raw fish, shellfish or undercooked pork has been associated with subsequent systemic infection. There is no evidence that person-to-person transmission occurs.

CLINICAL MANIFESTATIONS OF *ERYSIPELOTHRIX RHUSIOPATHIAE* INFECTION

The commonest form of *E. rhusiopathiae* infection in man, accounting for 90% of cases reported in the literature, is the cellulitis which is also known as erysipeloid. Most cases are occupationally related and follow puncture wounds or inoculation of cuts and abrasions. Very uncommonly, infection may follow dog bites. There is no convincing evidence that the bacterium is able to penetrate intact skin. After an incubation period of two to seven days the lesions, which are usually located on the hands or forearms, are noted to have a sharply defined edge with a blue or purplish coloration. Lesions are painful and are often described as burning or intensely itchy. The lesion may spread proximally with central clearing. Systemic symptoms are rare and although there may be swelling and complaints of stiffness in adjacent joints, aspirates are sterile on culture. The differential diagnosis includes erysipelas caused by *Streptococcus pyogenes* and staphylococcal cellulitis; although in these syndromes the incubation time is shorter, constitutional symptoms are more frequent and pitting oedema is common. In addition, lymphangitis and regional lymphadenopathy are infrequently observed in erysipeloid.

A more severe form of cutaneous infection in which the cellulitis spreads more widely, often in conjunction with the appearance of additional lesions at other sites, occurs much less commonly. Although systemic symptoms may be pronounced, blood cultures are negative. The most serious manifestation of *E. rhusiopathiae* is endocarditis. Approximately 40% of patients give a history of preceding, or coexisting, skin lesions. Very rarely consumption of raw or undercooked seafood has anteceded endocarditis. All but two reported cases have involved native valves (Hayek, 1993) and in as many as 60% of cases infection occurs in individuals without a history of valvular heart disease. In their review of 49 cases of *Erysipelothrix* endocarditis Gorby and Peacock (1988) note that in comparison with other bacterial endocarditides the former have a longer mean duration of symptoms to diagnosis (6.6 weeks), a higher male : female ratio (probably reflecting occupational factors) and a predilection for the aortic valve. Despite the more insidious onset of *Erysipelothrix* endocarditis, it is often associated with significant valve destruction (30% of cases require valve replacement) which accounts, in part, for the higher mortality rate when compared to endocarditis caused by other bacteria.

Bacteraemia without endocarditis also occurs usually, but not always, in immunocompromised individuals, particularly those with chronic liver disease and in patients receiving glucocorticosteroids (Fakoya *et al.*, 1995).

DIAGNOSIS OF *ERYSIPELOTHRIX RHUSIOPATHIAE* INFECTION

A PCR-based detection system has been reported, but its use outside the veterinary setting has not been evaluated (Makino *et al.*, 1994). Serological tests have been used for sero-epidemiological studies but have, at present, no place in the routine diagnosis of *Erysipelothrix* infections. Diagnosis of *E. rhusiopathiae* infection remains dependent on the isolation and identification of the bacterium from clinical material.

The bacterium is not fastidious and will grow in standard blood culture media in cases of septicaemia or endocarditis. Swabs are unsuitable for the diagnosis of erysipeloid and aspirates, or preferably, skin biopsies from the edge of the lesion should be obtained. As the number of bacteria in these specimens may be small, enrichment for up to two weeks in glucose serum broth is recommended, with frequent subcultures to blood agar. Primary cultures and subcultures should be incubated aerobically at 37 °C in 5–10% carbon dioxide. For isolation from heavily contaminated samples, e.g. foodstuffs, selective media are available (Bratberg, 1981).

After 24 hours incubation colonies are pinpoint, but extended incubation permits the observation of two colonial types. 'Smooth' colonies are 0.5–1.5 mm in diameter, are convex and have a bluish transparent appearance. These are more likely to be seen in isolates from acute infections. Rough colonies are classically associated with more chronic conditions and are larger, flatter, opaque and have a rough irregular edge. Intermediate forms also occur. On blood agar a narrow zone of α-haemolysis is seen on prolonged incubation and which may, occasionally, lead to misidentification of *E. rhusiopathiae* as a viridans group streptococcus. In addition, granules in the bacilli may resemble those of diphtheroids and smears made from older colonies may appear Gram negative.

Erysipelothrix rhusiopathiae can be identified using commercially available systems, e.g. the API CORYNE kit, but the biochemical and other tests outlined in Table 4.3 and below should suffice to identify the bacterium in the clinical laboratory.

When identifying *E. rhusiopathiae* and *Listeria* spp. in foodstuffs it is important to distinguish the bacterium from the Gram-positive genera *Brochothrix* and *Kurthia*. In practice this is not difficult as *Brochothrix* does not grow above 30 °C, and *Kurthia* spp. are obligate aerobes and oxidase positive.

In clinical material, *E. rhusiopathiae* can be distinguished from *Lactobacillus* spp. by hydrogen sulphide production and from *Corynebacterium* spp. by failure to produce catalase and resistance to vancomycin. *Listeria* spp. can be distinguished from the former on the grounds of motility and catalase test and from the latter on testing for motility. (*C. aquaticum*, however, is motile but unlike *Listeria* spp. is negative in the Voges–Proskauer test).

MANAGEMENT OF *ERYSIPELOTHRIX* INFECTION

Although the lesions of erysipeloid may resolve spontaneously, resolution may be prolonged and relapses may occur, and antimicrobial chemotherapy is recommended. Additionally, this may prevent progression to bacteraemia and/or endocarditis.

There have been no controlled clinical trials to determine optimal antimicrobial therapy of *E. rhusiopathiae* infections. Although there are several reports on the *in vitro* susceptibility of the bacterium to a variety of antimicrobials these have involved the testing of very small numbers of strains and there is a paucity of information regarding the clinical relevance of these data. The bacterium remains exquisitely susceptible to penicillin (minimal inhibitory dose (MIC) ≤0.01 μg/ml) and this agent has been agent of choice for 50 years. Of the other β-lactams, imipenem appears the most active (Venditti *et al.*, 1990). *In vitro* susceptibility to erythromycin, tetracycline and chloramphenicol is variable. Although generally regarded as resistant to gentamicin and other aminoglycosides Schuster *et al.* (1993) report an isolate with an MIC to gentamicin of 1 μg/ml. Of particular interest is the resistance of *E. rhusiopathiae* to vancomycin, as this agent may be employed as empirical therapy in prosthetic valve endocarditis. Teicoplanin susceptibility, however, has been observed in some strains (Jensen *et al.*, 1992).

Although penicillin is regarded as the agent of choice, there is very little reported experience of the management of penicillin-allergic patients. Ciprofloxacin appears highly active *in vitro* (MIC range ≤0.01–0.06 μg/ml) and has been used in the management of *E. rhusiopathiae* endocarditis in a patient who could not tolerate penicillin therapy (MacGowan *et al.*, 1991).

Optimal dosing regimens and duration of therapy remain ill defined. Benzylpenicillin in doses of up to 12 g per day in six divided doses for four to six weeks has been recommended for the therapy of serious *E. rhusiopathiae* infections, although shorter courses of two weeks' intravenous therapy followed by two–four weeks' oral therapy have been used with success (Reboli and Farrar, 1989).

REFERENCES

Art, D. and Andre, P. (1991) Clinical and epidemiological aspects of listeriosis in Belgium, 1985–1990. *International Journal of Medical Microbiology*, **275**, 549–556.

Azadian, B.S., Finnerty, G.T. and Pearson, A.D. (1989). Cheese-borne *Listeria* meningitis in immunocompetent patients. *Lancet*, **i**, 322–323.

Baddour, L.M. (1989) Listerial endocarditis following coronary artery bypass surgery. *Reviews of Infectious Diseases*, **4**, 669–670.

Bille, J. (1990) Epidemiology of human listeriosis in Europe, with special reference to the Swiss outbreak. In: *Foodborne Listeriosis* (ed. A.J. Miller, J.L. Smith and G.A. Somkuti). Elsevier, Amsterdam.

Bille, J., Catimel, B., Bannerman, E. *et al.* (1992) API *Listeria*, a new and promising one-day system to identify *Listeria* isolates. *Applied and Environmental Microbiology*, **58**, 1857–1860.

Bind, J.L. (1989) International aspects of the control of animal listeriosis. *Acta Microbiologica Hungarica*, **30**, 91–94.

Blot, F., Hermann, J.L., Brunengo, P. *et al.* (1994) Septic shock and adult respiratory distress syndrome due to *Listeria monocytogenes*. *Intensive Care Medicine*, **20**, 83–84.

Bourgeois, N., Jacobs, F., Tavares, M.L. *et al.* (1993) *Listeria monocytogenes*, hepatitis in a liver transplant recipient: a case report and review of the literature. *Journal of Hepatology*, **18**, 284–289.

Bratberg, A.M. (1981) Observations on the utilisation of a selective medium for the isolation of *Erysipelothrix rhusiopathiae*. *Acta Veterinaria Scandinavica*, **22**, 55–59.

Chooromoney, K.N., Hampson, D.J., Eamens, G.J. and Turner, M.J. (1994). Analysis of *Erysipelothrix rhusiopathiae* and *Erysipelothrix tonsillarum* by multilocus enzyme electrophoresis. *Journal of Clinical Microbiology*, **32**, 371–376.

Ciesielski, C.A., Hightower, A.W., Parsons, S.K. and Broome, C.V. (1988) Listeriosis in the United States, 1980–1982. *Archives of Internal Medicine*, **148**, 1416–1419.

Cummins, A.J., Fielding, A.K. and McGlauchlin, J. (1994) *Listeria ivanovii* infection in a patient with AIDS. *Journal of Infection*, **28**, 89–91.

Eliott, D., O'Brien, T.P., Green, W.R. *et al.* (1992) Elevated intraocular pressure, pigment dispersion and dark hypopyon in endogenous endophthalmitis from *Listeria monocytogenes*. *Survey of Ophthalmology*, **37**, 117–124.

Fakoya, A., Bendall, R.P., Churchill, D.R. *et al.* (1995) *Erysipelothrix rhusiopathiae* bacteraemia in a patient without endocarditis. *Journal of Infection*, **30**, 180–181.

Farber, J.M., Sanders, G.W. and Johnston, M.A. (1989) A survey of various foods for the presence of *Listeria monocytogenes*. *Journal of Food Protection*, **52**, 456–458.

Farrington, M., Winters, S.M., Rubenstein, D. *et al.* (1991) Streptococci from primary isolation plates grouped by reverse passive haemagglutination. *Journal of Clinical Pathology*, **44**, 670–675.

Gauto, A.R., Cone, L.R., Woodard, D.R. *et al.* (1992). Arterial infections due to *Listeria monocytogenes*: report of four cases and review of world literature. *Clinical Infectious Diseases*, **14**, 23–28.

Gellin, B.G., Broome, C.V., Bibb, W.F. *et al.* (1991) The epidemiology of listeriosis in the United States, 1986. *American Journal of Epidemiology*, **133**, 392–401.

Gorby, G.L. and Peacock, J.E. (1988) *Erysipelothrix rhusiopathiae* endocarditis: microbiologic, epidemiologic, and clinical features of an occupational disease. *Reviews of Infectious Diseases*, **10**, 317–325.

Goulet, V., Jacquet, C., Vaillant, V. *et al.* (1995) Listeriosis from consumption of raw milk cheese. *Lancet*, **345**, 1581–1582.

Hayek, L.J.H.E. (1993) Erysipelothrix endocarditis affecting a porcine xerograft heart valve. *Journal of Infection*, **27**, 203–204.

Jacquet, C., Catimel, B., Brosch, R. *et al.* (1995) Investigations related to the epidemic strain involved in the French listeriosis outbreak in 1992. *Applied and Environmental Microbiology*, **61**, 2242–2246.

Jensen, K.T., Schonheyder, H., Pers, C. and Thomsen, V.F. (1992) *In vitro* activity of teicoplanin and vancomycin against gram-positive bacteria from human clinical and veterinary sciences. *Acta Pathologica Microbiologica et Immunologica Scandinavica*, **100**, 542–543.

Jones, E.M. and MacGowan, A.P. (1995) Antimicrobial chemotherapy of human infection due to *Listeria monocytogenes*. *European Journal of Clinical Microbiology and Infectious Diseases*, **14**, 165–175.

Kerr, K.G., Dealler, S.F. and Lacey, R.W. (1988) Materno-fetal listeriosis from cook-chill and refrigerated food. *Lancet*, **ii**, 1133.

Kerr, K.G., Rotowa, N.A., Hawkey, P.M. and Lacey, R.W. (1991) Evaluation of the Rosco system for the identification of *Listeria* species. *Journal of Medical Microbiology*, **35**, 193–196.

Kerr, K.G., Hawkey, P.M. and Lacey, R.W. (1993) Evaluation of the API CORYNE system for the identification of *Listeria* spp. *Journal of Clinical Microbiology*, **31**, 749–750.

Kerr, K.G., Kite, P., Heritage, J. and Hawkey, P.M. (1995) Typing of epidemiologically associated environmental and clinical strains of *Listeria monocytogenes* by random amplification of polymorphic DNA. *Journal of Food Protection*, **58**, 609–613.

Lamont, R.J. and Postlethwaite, R. (1986) Carriage of *Listeria monocytogenes* and related species in pregnant and non-pregnant women in Aberdeen, Scotland. *Journal of Infection*, **13**, 187–193.

Linnan, M.J., Mascola, L., Lou, X.D. *et al.* (1988) Epidemic listeriosis associated with Mexican-style cheese. *New England Journal of Medicine*, **319**, 823–828.

MacGowan, A.P., Marshall, R. and Reeves, D. (1988) False positive reactions with *Listeria monocytogenes* using a commercial test for Lancefield grouping of beta haemolytic streptococci. *European Journal of Clinical Microbiology and Infectious Diseases*, **7**, 208–210.

MacGowan, A.P., Reeves, D.S., Wright, C. and Glover, S.C. (1991) Tricuspid valve infective endocarditis and pulmonary sepsis due to *Erysipelothrix rhusiopathiae* successfully treated with high doses of ciprofloxacin but complicated by gynaecomastia. *Journal of Infection*, **22**, 100–101.

Makino, S., Okada, Y., Maruyama, T. *et al.* (1994) Direct and rapid detection of *Erysipelothrix rhusiopathiae* DNA in animals by PCR. *Journal of Clinical Microbiology*, **32**, 1526–1531.

McLauchlin, J. (1988) The identification of *Listeria* species. *DMRQC Newsletter*, **3**, 1–3.

Moore, M.A. and Datta, A.R. (1994) DNA fingerprinting of *Listeria monocytogenes* by pulsed-field gel electrophoresis. *Food Microbiology*, **11**, 31–38.

Niemann, R.E. and Lorber, B. (1980) Listeriosis in adults: a changing pattern. Report of eight cases and a review of the literature. *Reviews of Infectious Diseases*, **2**, 207–227.

Oakley, W., MacVicar, J., Jones, D. and Andrews, P. (1992) Vaginal and faecal carriage of listeria during pregnancy. *Health Trends*, **24**, 117–119.

Polanco, A., Giner, C., Cantón, R. *et al.* (1992) Spontaneous bacterial peritonitis caused by *Listeria monocytogenes*: two case reports and literature review. *European Journal of Clinical Microbiology*, **11**, 346–349.

Poyart-Salmeron, C., Carlier, C., Trieu-Cuot, P. *et al.* (1990) Transferable plasmid-mediated antibiotic resistance in *Listeria monocytogenes*. *Lancet*, **i**, 1422–1426.

Reboli, A.C. and Farrar, W.E. (1989) *Erysipelothrix rhusiopathiae*: an occupational pathogen. *Clinical Microbiology Reviews*, **2**, 354–359.

Schlech, W.F., Lavigne, P.M., Bortolussi, R.A. *et al.* (1983) Epidemic listeriosis: evidence for transmission by food. *New England Journal of Medicine*, **308**, 203–206.

Schuchat, A., Deaver, K.A., Wenger, J.D. *et al.* (1992) Role of foods in sporadic listeriosis: case control study of diet risk factors. *Journal of the American Medical Association*, **267**, 2041–2045.

Schuster, M.G., Brennan, P.J. and Edelstein, P. (1993) Persistent bacteremia with *Erysipelothrix rhusiopathiae* in a hospitalised patient. *Clinical Infectious Diseases*, **17**, 783–784.

Shimoji, Y., Yokomizo, Y., Sekizaki, T. *et al.* (1994) Presence of a capsule in *Erysipelothrix rhusiopathiae* and its relationship to virulence for mice. *Infection and Immunity*, **67**, 2806–2810.

Skogberg, K., Syrjänen, J., Jakhola, M. *et al.* (1992) Clinical presentation and outcome of listeriosis in patients with and without immunosuppressive therapy. *Clinical Infectious Diseases*, **14**, 815–821.

Swartz, M.A., Welch, D.F., Narayanan, R.D. and Greenfield, R.A. (1991) Catalase negative *Listeria monocytogenes* causing meningitis in an adult. *American Journal of Clinical Pathology*, **96**, 130–133.

van Netten, P., Perales, I., van de Moosdijk, A. *et al.* (1989) Liquid and solid selective differential media for the detection and enumeration of *Listeria monocytogenes* and other *Listeria* species. *International Journal of Food Microbiology*, **8**, 299–316.

Venditti, M., Gelfusa, V., Tarasi, A. *et al.* (1990) Antimicrobial susceptibilities of *Erysipelothrix rhusiopathiae*. *Antimicrobial Agents and Chemotherapy*, **24**, 2038–2040.

Watkins, J. and Sleath, K.P. (1981) Isolation and enumeration of *Listeria monocytogenes* from sewage, sewage sludge, and river water. *Journal of Applied Bacteriology*, **50**, 1–9.

Weis, J. and Seeliger, H.P.R. (1976) Incidence of *Listeria monocytogenes* in nature. *Applied Microbiology*, **30**, 29–32.

5

BACILLUS, *ALICYCLOBACILLUS* AND *PAENIBACILLUS*

Roger C.W. Berkeley and Niall A. Logan

HISTORICAL INTRODUCTION

The organism now known as *Bacillus subtilis* was first described as '*Vibrio subtilis*' by Christian Ehrenberg in 1835. Nearly 30 years later Casimir Davaine (1864) gave the name '*Bacteridium*' to the organism associated with anthrax infection – *la maladie charbonneuse* – but the name *Bacillus* was first applied to these organisms by Ferdinand Cohn in 1872, who, five years later, observed and illustrated spores, although he was not aware of their importance as resistant forms and did not use sporulation as a generic character in his classifications. In the next 40 years at least 30 keys for the classification of bacteria were produced, many of which used the presence of spores as a character but there were many which did not. The last scheme not to do so was constructed in 1912 and since then there has been general acceptance that endospore formation is an important character in classification and identification of members of the genus *Bacillus*.

The first major study of *Bacillus*, by Ford and his colleagues (Laubach *et al.*, 1916; Lawrence and Ford, 1916) who allocated 1700 strains to 27 species, produced an incomplete classification, particularly because of the absence of adequate differential tests. The next was 30 years later when Smith *et al.* (1946) published a monograph on aerobic mesophilic spore-formers dealing with 625 strains. Subsequently this work was expanded to include 1134 strains and to cover all known aerobic spore-formers (Smith *et al.*, 1952). The work of these authors was thorough. They collected all possible strains and studied rod, spore and sporangium morphology as well as many physiological characters. This approach contrasted with the tendency at that time to describe new species on the basis of a single strain differing from the description of an existing taxon by a single character. The organisms were placed in three groups according to their spore shape and size relative to the sporangia in which they were produced. Organisms with ellipsoidal to cylindrical spores and unswollen sporangia, which accounted for 65% of cultures studied, were allocated to group 1; those with ellipsoidal spores and swollen sporangia (30% of cultures) to group 2; and those with spherical spores and swollen sporangia (5% of cultures) to group 3. The soundness of this work was established when the scheme was successfully applied to 246 strains isolated by Knight

Principles and Practice of Clinical Bacteriology. Edited by A.M. Emmerson, P.M. Hawkey and S.H. Gillespie
© 1997 John Wiley & Sons Ltd

and Proom (1950) from soil and to 400 obtained from spinal fluid, tissue, other human sources, laboratory dust and soil (Burdon, 1956). An updated and expanded version of the scheme has been published (Gordon *et al.*, 1973) and, despite attempts to split the genus (Gibson and Gordon, 1974), was widely followed from 1952 to 1992.

During this period the number of recognized species in the genus declined from its peak number of 146, in the 1939 (fifth) edition of *Bergey's Manual of Determinative Bacteriology*, to 22, with 26 of uncertain status in the 1974 (eighth) edition and to only 31 species in the ICSB Approved Lists of Bacterial Names (Skerman *et al.*, 1980). In spite of this relatively small number of species, however, it was generally agreed that the genus *Bacillus* was heterogeneous. The range of DNA base composition in a homogeneous genus is agreed to be no more than 10% (Bull *et al.*, 1992) whereas that found in *Bacillus* was over 30% (Claus and Berkeley, 1986). This gives confirmation of heterogeneity, and numerical studies such as that by Logan and Berkeley (1981) have also indicated that the genus should be divided into five or six genera.

Consistent with this, studies of rRNA sequences of single representatives of 51 *Bacillus* spp. suggest the existence of at least five phylogenetically distinct clusters (Ash *et al.*, 1991b). Division of the genus has started with the separation of a few strains isolated from hot, acid environments into the new genus *Alicyclobacillus* (Wisotzkey *et al.*, 1992) and the reclassification of *B. polymyxa* and its relatives, comprising the rRNA group 3 of Ash and her colleagues (1991a), which form sporangia swollen by ellipsoidal spores, as the new genus *Paenibacillus* (Ash *et al.*, 1993).

Alicyclobacillus strains growing at 45 °C and pH 3.0 are unlikely to be encountered in the clinical context and are not considered further. Those *Paenibacillus* spp. which have been identified with clinical problems are described below, with members of the genus *Bacillus*, using the designation *Bacillus* (now *Paenibacillus*) spp.

At the same time as rearrangement at the generic level, the number of species has been rising rapidly; in mid-1995 there were over 70 recogn-

ized species. The habitats and physiologies of most of these organisms are such that only in extraordinary circumstances would they be of clinical interest, but several of the remainder, in addition to the well-recognized pathogens *B. anthracis* and *B. cereus*, must be considered because they do occasionally cause clinical problems and the frequency of recognition of these problems is increasing.

DESCRIPTIONS OF ORGANISMS

The genus *Bacillus* comprises aerobic or facultative organisms which are rod shaped, Gram positive, Gram variable or, in some instances, Gram negative. The cells may be motile by means of peritrichous flagella. The defining feature for the genus (and those derived from it) is the production of one endospore per cell (Figure 5.1) in the presence of air (oxygen). Endospores are very resistant to many adverse conditions. Asporogenous organisms, otherwise phenotypically similar to sporulating strains, do exist in laboratory collections, but apparently do not survive long in nature.

Bacillus is a physiologically heterogeneous genus, containing some species which do not sporulate readily, but all the clinically significant isolates reported to date are of species that grow, and often sporulate, on routine laboratory media such as blood agar or nutrient agar, at 37 °C. It is unlikely that clinically important, but more fastidious, strains of *Bacillus* are being missed for want of appropriate growth conditions. Occasional isolates are sent to reference laboratories as *Bacillus* spp. because they are large Gram-positive rods, even though spores have not been seen or, sometimes because poly-β-hydroxybutyrate granules or other inclusion bodies have been mistaken for spores.

Although many *Bacillus* spp. are strict aerobes, the genus contains facultative anaerobes as well. This can be a valuable character in identification – for example, the two large-celled species *B. cereus* and *B. megaterium* are, respectively, facultative and strictly aerobic as are *B. licheniformis* and *B. subtilis*, which are colonially and microscopically (Figure 5.1a) very similar.

Bacillus anthracis and *B. cereus*

These are the two *Bacillus* spp. of greatest medical and veterinary importance, and with *B. mycoides* and *B. thuringiensis* they form the *B. cereus* group.

The colonies of this group are very variable, but usually recognizable nonetheless. They are characteristically large (2–7 mm in diameter, and usually near the top end of this range) and vary in shape from circular to irregular, with entire to undulate, crenate or fimbriate ('medusa head') edges; they have matt or granular textures and have been likened to little heaps of ground glass. Smooth and moist colonies are not uncommon, however.

Colonies of *B. anthracis* and *B. cereus* are similar in appearance, but those of the former are non-haemolytic, may show spiking or tailing along lines of inoculation streaks, and may have a more tenacious, rather than a butyrous, consistency, so that they may be pulled into standing peaks with a loop. The edges of *B. anthracis* colonies are often described as 'medusa head', but this is a character to be found throughout the *B. cereus* group. *Bacillus cereus* itself has colonies which are butyrous and cream to whitish in colour. The white colonies often contain spores. On blood agar, which is usually vigorously haemolysed, the colonies may be tinged with pigments derived from haemoglobin degradation. Fresh cultures characteristically smell mousy. *Bacillus mycoides* colonies are characteristically rhizoid or hairy looking, adherent and readily cover the whole surface of an agar plate.

Bacillus anthracis cells are Gram-positive, non-motile rods, 1.0–1.2 μm × 3.0–5.0 μm. They commonly appear as long, entangled chains, but some strains of *B. cereus* and *B. mycoides* (which is non-motile) may look similar. Fresh isolates of *B. anthracis*, and laboratory strains grown on serum-containing agar in the presence of carbon dioxide, produce a poly-D-glutamic acid capsule. Spores are ellipsoidal, central, or nearly so, and do not cause the sporangium to swell. This organism is a chemoorganotroph and grows above 15–20 °C and below 40 °C; its optimum is about 37 °C.

Bacillus cereus cells are Gram-positive and similar in size to those of *B. anthracis* but are usually motile, and single organisms, pairs and short chains are more common than in *B. anthracis* cultures. Capsules are not formed, but spore and sporangial morphology are similar to those of *B. anthracis* (Figure 5.1c). *Bacillus cereus* is chemoorganotrophic and grows above 10–20 °C and below 35–45 °C with an optimum of about 37 °C.

Bacillus thuringiensis can be distinguished from *B. cereus* by the production of parasporal crystals (Figure 5.1d), which are toxic for insects. Spores may lie obliquely in the sporangium, as may happen in *B. cereus*.

Vegetative cells of all members of the *B. cereus* group may, when grown on a carbohydrate medium, accumulate poly-β-hydroxybutyrate and their cytoplasm appear vacuolate or foamy.

Figure 5.1. (*overleaf*) Photomicrographs of *Bacillus* spp. viewed by phase-contrast microscopy. Bar markers represent 2 μm. (a) *B. subtilis*, ellipsoidal, central and subterminal spores, not swelling the sporangia; (b) *B. pumilus*, slender cells with cylindrical, subterminal spores not swelling the sporangia; (c) *B. cereus*, broad cells with ellipsoidal, subterminal spores, not swelling the sporangia; (d) *B. thuringiensis*, broad cells with ellipsoidal, subterminal spores, not swelling the sporangia, and showing parasporal crystals of insecticidal toxin (arrowed); (e) *B. megaterium*, broad cells with ellipsoidal and spherical, subterminal and terminal spores, not swelling the sporangia and showing poly-β-hydroxybutyrate inclusions (arrowed); (f) *B.* (now *Paenibacillus*) *alvei*, cells with tapered ends, ellipsoidal, paracentral to subterminal spores, not swelling the sporangium; (g) *B. brevis*, ellipsoidal subterminal spores, one swelling its sporangium slightly; (h) *B.* (now *Paenibacillus*) *polymyxa*, ellipsoidal, paracentral to subterminal spores, slightly swelling the sporangia; (i) *B. circulans*, ellipsoidal, subterminal spores, swelling the sporangia; (j) *B. coagulans*, ellipsoidal, subterminal spores, swelling the sporangia; (k) *B. laterosporus*, ellipsoidal, central spores with thickened rims on one side (arrowed), swelling the sporangia; (l) *B. sphaericus*, spherical, terminal spores, swelling the sporangia.

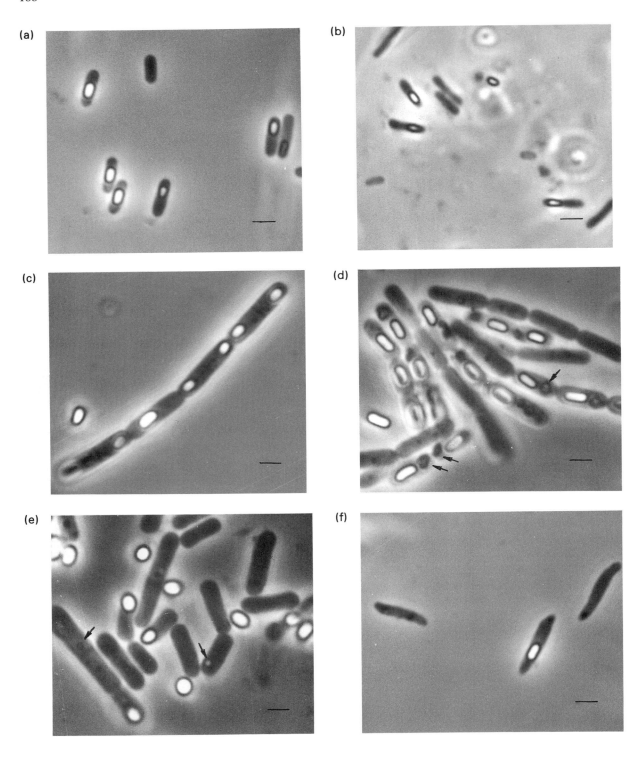

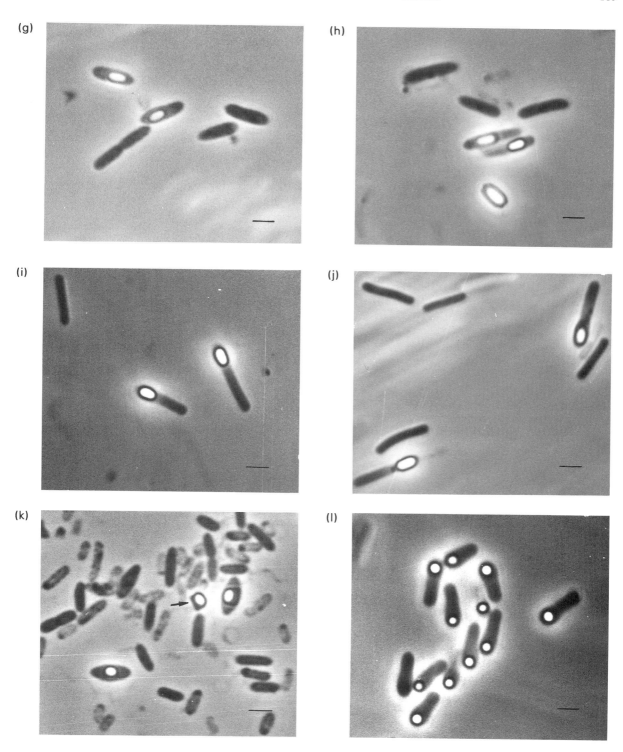

Other *Bacillus* species

Other species show a very wide range of colonial morphologies, both within and between species, and this has been extensively illustrated by Parry *et al.* (1983). Colonial appearance varies from moist and glossy, through granular, to wrinkled; shape varies from round to irregular, sometimes spreading, with entire, through undulate or crenate, to fimbriate edges; sizes range from 1 to 5 mm; colour commonly ranges from buff or creamy-grey to off-white in colour, and strains of some species may produce orange pigment; haemolysis may be absent, slight or marked, partial or complete; elevations range from effuse, through raised, to convex; consistency is usually butyrous, but mucoid and dry, adherent colonies are not uncommon. Despite this diversity, *Bacillus* colonies are not generally difficult to recognize, and some species have characteristic, yet seemingly infinitely variable, colonial morphologies, as with the *B. cereus* group.

Bacillus subtilis and *B. licheniformis* produce similar colonies which are exceptionally variable in appearance and often appear to be mixed cultures; colonies are irregular in shape and of moderate (2–4 mm) diameter, and range from moist and butyrous or mucoid, with margins varying from undulate to fimbriate, through membranous with an underlying mucoid matrix, with or without mucoid beading at the surface, to rough and crusted as they dry. The 'licheniform' colonies of *B. licheniformis* tend to be quite adherent.

Bacillus circulans was so named because a protoplasm-like, circular motion of the interior of its colonies was observable by low-power microscopy. Rotating and migrating microcolonies, which may show spreading growth, have been observed macroscopically in about 13% of strains received as *B. circulans* (Logan *et al.*, 1985b), but the species is exceptionally heterogeneous and its taxonomy is undergoing radical revision. Motile microcolonies with spreading growth are more characteristic of *Bacillus* (now *Paenibacillus*) *alvei* (Figure 5.1f); plate cultures of this species will readily grow across the entire agar surface and commonly have an unpleasant smell.

Other species that have been encountered in the clinical laboratory include *B. brevis* (Figure 5.1g), *B. circulans* (Figure 5.1i), *B. coagulans* (Figure 5.1j), *B. laterosporus* (Figure 5.1k), *B.* (now *Paenibacillus*) *macerans*, *B. megaterium* (Figure 5.1e), *B.* (now *Paenibacillus*) *polymyxa* (Figure 5.1h), *B. pumilus* (Figure 5.1b) and *B. sphaericus* (Figure 5.1l); and they do not produce particularly distinctive growth. Illustrations can be seen in Parry *et al.* (1983), but it must be appreciated that few species have colonies sufficiently characteristic or invariant to allow tentative identification, even by the experienced worker.

Microscopic morphologies, particularly of sporangia (Figure 5.1), are much more helpful than colonial characters in distinguishing between all these non-*B. cereus* group species. Vegetative cells are usually round ended, but cells of *B.* (now *Paenibacillus*) *alvei* may have tapered ends (Figure 5.1f). The large cells of *B. megaterium* (Figure 5.1e) may accumulate poly-β-hydroxybutyrate and appear vacuolate or foamy when grown on glucose nutrient agar. Overall, cell widths vary from about 0.5 to 1.5 μm, and lengths from 1.5 to 5 μm. Most strains of these species are motile. Spore shapes vary from cylindrical, through ellipsoidal, to round, and bean or kidney-shaped, curved-cylindrical, and pear-shaped spores are occasionally seen. Spores may be terminally, subterminally, or centrally positioned within sporangia and may distend it. Although there is some within-species and within-strain variation, spore shape, position and size tend to be characteristic of species (Figure 5.1), and may allow tentative identification by the experienced worker. One species, *B. laterosporus*, produces very distinctive ellipsoidal spores which have thickened rims on one side, so that they appear to be laterally displaced in the sporangia (Figure 5.1k).

All these species are mesophilic, and will grow well between 30 and 37 °C; minimum temperatures for growth lie mostly between 5 and 20 °C, maxima mostly between 35 and 50 °C. For more information on growth temperatures, see Claus and Berkeley (1986).

NORMAL HABITATS

Bacillus anthracis

Long before this organism was recognized as the cause of anthrax it was understood that putting animals to graze in certain places was likely to lead to an outbreak of the disease. At one time this was attributed to the persistence of spores in the soil, introduced from infected animals. This does not, however, explain the regular, seasonal outbreaks in some areas (anthrax districts) and the long intervals between infections in others. Bacillus anthracis is now regarded as part of the normal soil flora, usually present in small numbers. In areas with nitrogen/organic matter-rich soils with sufficient calcium, a pH above 6.0 and temperature above 15.5 °C, and given a major change such as a drought or heavy rain, B. anthracis numbers rapidly increase until they reach a level leading to infection of grazing animals (Kaufmann, 1990). Bacillus anthracis may also occur in unsterilized animal products such as carcasses, wool, hair, bristle, hides, bones and bone meal.

Bacillus cereus

Typically this organism is found in soil and the bottom deposits of fresh and sea waters. From the former it becomes distributed to foods of all sorts, including milk.

Other species

Strains of other Bacillus spp. are very common in soils of all types: from those with acid pH to those which are alkaline; from those in very cold regions to those which are very hot; and from fertile types to deserts. Very often, isolation from soils of aerobic, mesophilic, chemoorganotrophic bacteria at about neutral pH will result in a great preponderance of Bacillus strains amongst the organisms obtained, but this does not necessarily mean that they are the numerically dominant type in the soil sampled. Furthermore, neutral soils from temperate regions may yield strains capable of growth under more extreme conditions.

These organisms are also common in water of all types. In sea water it has been estimated that up to a fifth of the total heterotrophic population is accounted for by Bacillus strains; however, the numbers vary greatly, declining as the coast is distanced but increasing with temperature and depth. Where there is pollution, large quantitative and qualitative changes in the population may occur.

Similarly, unpolluted marine sediments contain a different population of Bacillus spp. from those of polluted areas. Bacillus strains which are often orange or yellow pigmented – features perhaps associated with salt tolerance – are easily isolated from estuarine deposits and salt marsh muds, where evaporation causes higher than normal salt concentrations.

Bacillus strains in fresh water are derived mainly from adjacent soils, their numbers reflecting weather conditions. They are frequently found in water treatment plant such as cation exchangers and sand filters, and distilled and demineralized water can also contain these organisms.

Airborne dispersal from soil results in Bacillus strains occurring in dust as well as on the surfaces of animals and plants. The use of B. thuringiensis as a highly selective, hence environmentally friendly, insecticide results in very high numbers on plants and in soils, where it has been applied. Bacillus strains also occur in faeces. Foodstuffs such as bread, cocoa, rice, sugar, spices and milk, as well as those preserved by freezing and canning, are also sources of these organisms.

In short, these organisms are ubiquitous contaminants of man, other animals, their foodstuffs, water and environments, natural, domestic and hospital. This distribution is at least partly due to the extraordinary longevity of their endospores which are, relative to vegetative cells, very resistant to cold, heat, dehydration and toxic chemicals but only slightly more resistant to radiation damage. When protected from radiation, spores can survive for several thousand years and there is evidence that they can lie dormant for between 25 million and 40 million years. Given this spore longevity it would be surprising if the distribution of these organism was not ubiquitous (Logan,

1988). More detailed information about environments in which particular species may be found are given in Claus and Berkeley (1986), Norris *et al.* (1981) and Priest (1989).

PATHOGENICITY

Bacillus anthracis

Once in the host tissue, there are two main requirements for the virulence of this organism: a toxin consisting of an 85 kDa protective antigen (PA), an 83 kDa lethal factor (LF) and 89 kDa oedema factor (EF), all coded for by the 110 MDa plasmid pX01, and a poly-D-glutamic acid capsule, which interferes with phagocytosis, coded for by the 60 MDa plasmid pX02 (Robertson *et al.*, 1990). Absence of either plasmid, as in the vaccine strains, results in loss of virulence.

None of the three toxin components alone apparently has any effect on the host. Injection of PA and EF into the skin of experimental animals causes localized oedema and injection of PA and LF causes death in about an hour. The role of PA, injection of which leads to protective immunity, is to allow the passage of LF and EF across the membrane of animal cells. Following initial binding to a membrane receptor, a 20 kDa fragment is cleaved from PA by host proteolysis and the remaining 63 kDa membrane-bound fragment, with high affinity for LF and EF, mediates their entry into the host cell. When in the cell EF, an adenylate cyclase, associates with calmodulin and causes increased cyclic AMP levels and, in turn, the oedema characteristic of anthrax (Leppla, 1982, 1984). LF is assumed to be an enzyme but its action is not understood (Leppla *et al.*, 1990).

The genes of the toxin components have been cloned and pure PA, LF and EF are available in quantity. This will allow re-examination of the several suggestions for the cause of death (Smith, 1990).

Bacillus cereus

The cause of intoxications by this organism leading to vomiting, nausea and abdominal cramps, which become evident from one to six hours after eating contaminated food (usually cooked rice that has been improperly stored) is a heat-stable enterotoxin. This emetic toxin is specific to primates but little is known about it as, until recently, its activity could only be tested using monkeys; now, however, a cell test has been developed (Shinagawa *et al.*, 1992). The toxin is very stable to heat, proteolysis and a pH range of 2–11, and it has a molecular weight of 5–7 kDa. It is not a protein, and it has been suggested that it might be a lipid (Shinagawa *et al.*, 1992), but its production, structure and mode of action remain unknown (Granum, 1994).

The diarrhoeal form of the illness, which occurs 8–16 hours after contaminated food is eaten, leading to diarrhoea, nausea and abdominal cramps, is caused by a heat-labile enterotoxin. This is a single cytotoxic, non-haemolytic protein of molecular weight about 40 kDa. It is degraded by proteolytic enzymes and is unstable below pH 4, and so it has been suggested that the ingestion of preformed toxin plays no part in the illness, but that toxin is formed in the small intestine (Granum, 1994). Levels of enterotoxin produced by different strains vary widely, but the *B. cereus* enterotoxin may be considerably more toxic than that of *Clostridium perfringens*, causing membrane disruption and leakage (Granum, 1994).

Bacillus cereus also produces a variety of extracellular enzymes and toxins which may be involved in infections of tissue. These include phospholipase C, haemolysin, necrotizing toxin and lethal toxin (Farrar and Reboli, 1992).

EPIDEMIOLOGY

Bacillus anthracis

Anthrax infections in man normally occur as a result of transmission from animals or their products. The distribution of the disease in animals is therefore of importance in public health but, due to variations in practice and standards in different countries, this is not easy to establish. In the world as a whole there is under-reporting. In some places anthrax in sheep and goats is not counted and from others there is no information. Scandinavia is essentially free of the disease and it is at low levels in many European countries, although increasing in parts of the south and east. Countries in northern and southern Africa are better placed than those in the tropical region where anthrax is enzootic, as it is in many, but not all, countries in the Middle East and Southeast Asia. Elsewhere in Asia the situation is not clear. The last case in New Zealand was in 1954 and many of the world's smaller islands had their last case long ago or have never had an outbreak. It is commoner on larger islands. In North America there are few cases and in parts South America there is fair control (Hugh-Jones, 1990).

Nearly all (95%) human infections result from inoculation of spores through cuts and abrasions, usually from animal products such as carcasses, wool, hair, bristle, hides, bones or bone meal, but the source may also be soil, leading to a cutaneous infection. Sometimes inoculation is caused by the animal product itself, particularly by bristles and long bone fragments, and possibly by bites from flies. Rarely (5%), infection occurs as a result of inhalation. Once more common, and known as wool-sorter's disease, it follows from inhalation of spore-contaminated dust produced when handling wool and hair. Both cutaneous and inhalation anthrax may lead, following bacteraemia, to anthrax meningitis (Farrar and Reboli, 1992).

Intestinal anthrax is very rare in humans and results from eating insufficiently cooked, infected meat. It has never been recorded in the USA but there are reports of two fairly recent outbreaks in Africa (Logan, 1988). Oropharyngeal anthrax is also very rare. An outbreak in Thailand resulted from eating infected, imported meat (Logan, 1988).

Bacillus cereus

After *B. anthracis*, amongst *Bacillus* spp., *B. cereus* is undoubtedly next in importance as a pathogen of man. Its ubiquity ensures that many foods are contaminated and this may lead to diarrhoeal illness involving meat, vegetables, sauces and puddings. Intoxications leading to vomiting due to this organism are largely associated with rice. These occur, as would be expected, as they are caused by improper food handling, at any time of year and without any particular distribution pattern within a country. Between countries, however, there are differences in the proportions of all outbreaks of foodborne disease due to *B. cereus*. In Japan and Scotland, it accounts for less than 1%, in contrast to more than 22% in the Netherlands (Kramer and Gilbert, 1989). In Norway too, the incidence of *B. cereus* foodborne illnesses is high relative to those by other organisms (Granum, 1994). It is probable that underestimation of the frequency occurs widely.

The universal distribution of *B. cereus* ensures that infections due to it are not uncommon, particularly in immunocompromised patients, following surgical procedures or where there are other predisposing factors. As with *B. cereus* food poisoning, there is no particular temporal or geographical pattern.

Other *Bacillus* Species

Opportunistic infections with *Bacillus* spp. have been reported since the late nineteenth century. A common feature of such reports, right up to the present, has been emphasis on the importance of interpreting isolates of *Bacillus* in the light of any other species cultured and the clinical context, and the danger of dismissing them as mere contaminants. The fact that individual case histories of infections with these organisms continue to warrant published reports indicates that incidents are rare and that authors feel that awareness needs to be improved. Only cases reported since 1950 are mentioned here; the earlier literature was reviewed by Norris *et al.* (1981).

The factors contributing to the increasing frequency with which opportunistic infections are encountered are well known: host predisposition by suppressed or compromised immunity; malignant disease or metabolic disorder; exposure by accidental trauma, and clinical and surgical procedures; drug abuse; and advances in bacteriological technique, interpretation and awareness. It seems unlikely that these organisms have changed in virulence over the last century.

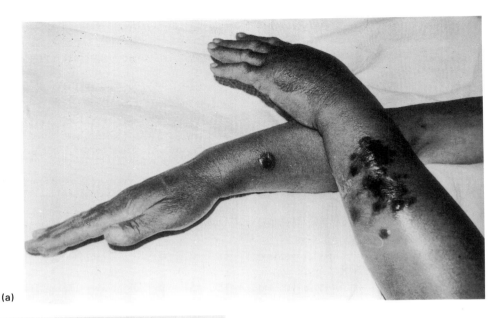

(a)

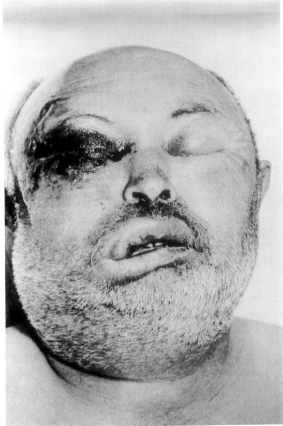

(b)

Figure 5.2. (a) Anthrax infection of the forearms. (Photograph kindly supplied by Professor Mehmet Doganay, Erciyes Universitesi, Kaysari, Turkey.) (b) Anthrax infection of the eye. The characteristic black eschar on the upper lid, particularly, is evident. The eye itself is usually not damaged. Oedema of the right side of the face can also be seen. (Photograph kindly supplied by Professor Mehmet Doganay, Erciyes Universitesi, Kaysari, Turkey.)

Given the ubiquity of *Bacillus* spp., infections with them might be commonplace were it not for their low invasiveness and virulence. It is certain that many clinically significant isolates of *Bacillus* were disregarded in the past, and the perceived difficulties of identification may have contributed to this. Although awareness is now better than ever, the problem remains one of recognizing what is a contaminant and what is not.

CLINICAL FEATURES

Bacillus anthracis

Results from a study of cutaneous anthrax cases in Turkey indicate that these occur in decreasing order of frequency on hands and fingers, eyelids and face, wrists and arms, feet and legs, and neck (Doganay, 1990). Following spore germination and multiplication of the vegetative organisms in the host tissue, a papule appears at the inoculation site. This develops into an ulcer and then to a necrotic, black eschar (Figure 5.2a) often with surrounding oedema (Figure 5.2b). The disease derives its name from the black eschar; *anthrakitis* is the Greek word for a kind of coal. If diagnosed early it is easy to treat – indeed a very high proportion of infections heal spontaneously. In untreated cases airway obstruction, meningitis and bacteraemia are all possible causes of death, with a mortality of about 20%. Prompt diagnosis and antibiotic treatment reduces this to about 1%.

Inhalation anthrax is rare and the most difficult form to diagnose. Initially the symptoms are those of a respiratory virus illness. There is no local lesion and spores are generally thought to be carried by alveolar macrophages via the lymphatic system to the mediastinal lymph nodes, where they germinate and multiply. There is, however, evidence that in guinea-pigs the spores germinate before macrophage uptake. After the initial phase of the disease, lasting two to three days, acute pulmonary disease develops, with death within 24 hours. Deaths from respiratory obstruction due to oedema of the soft tissue of the neck may sometimes be wrongly attributed to pulmonary anthrax

(Pugh and Davies, 1990). Mortality is high (up to 90%), even when treated, because correct diagnosis is usually late in the course of the disease.

In oropharyngeal anthrax the primary lesion is on the tongue, tonsil or wall of the pharynx. As with the cutaneous form, ulceration, necrosis and oedema are features of the lesion, with marked swelling of the neck. Mortality even with penicillin treatment may be up to 50%.

Intestinal anthrax results from eating undercooked, heavily infected meat; so few cases have been reported that no typical picture of the clinical features can be given but the mortality seems to be quite high (Farrar and Reboli, 1992).

Bacillus cereus

The diarrhoeal, or long-incubation, form of *B. cereus* food poisoning has an onset period of 8–16 hours, followed by abdominal cramps, profuse watery diarrhoea and rectal tenesmus. Occasionally there is fever and vomiting. Thus the symptoms are similar to those of *Clostridium perfringens* food poisoning. Recovery is usually complete in 24 hours, although there have been two reports of death (Logan, 1988).

Emetic food poisoning due to *B. cereus* is characterized by a shorter onset period of one to six hours and the symptoms resemble those of *Staphylococcus aureus* food poisoning. Nausea, vomiting and malaise, occasionally with diarrhoea, characterize the disease. There are rarely complications and recovery within 24 hours is usual (Logan, 1988).

Infections by *B. cereus* (Figure 5.1c) are often severe. For example, this organism is one of the most virulent and destructive ocular pathogens. The most serious of these conditions is panophthalmitis, a rapidly developing infection which may follow penetrating trauma of the eye (commonly by a metal fragment in an environment such as a farm or a garage), or haematogenous dissemination of the organism from another site (typically in intravenous drug abusers). Either way, the condition usually evolves so rapidly that irreversible damage occurs before effective treatment can be started; vision is therefore lost, and loss of the eye is normal.

Bacillus cereus can also cause a range of respiratory tract infections, including pneumonia, empyaema, pleurisy, lung abscess, and mild infections of neonates. Most of the cases have been associated with predisposing conditions such as leukaemia, alcoholism, chronic hepatitis and cirrhosis, steroid-dependent asthma and, possibly, heart disease. However, two cases, both fatal, occurred in normal hosts. Overall, fatality has been about 50%.

Infections of the central nervous system have also been associated with particularly vulnerable individuals, including infants, both full term and premature, surgical patients following treatment for adenoma or insertion of shunts to treat hydrocephalus, a drug and alcohol abuser, and a leukaemic patient undergoing chemotherapy.

Bacteraemias, in addition to those occurring with pneumonia and meningitis, have been associated with a variety of underlying conditions. In each case the organism probably gained access through direct openings into the veins, from haemodialysis, intravenous infusion, hepatic perfusion, other surgical procedures, accidental trauma and intravenous drug addiction. Despite the compromised condition of the patients, most recovered. Wound infections and gangrenous conditions involving this organism are probably common, but the clinical significance of *B. cereus* isolates can be difficult to determine, as many such infections yield mixed cultures. In the opinion of Barnham and White (1980), however, moderate or heavy growths of *Bacillus* spp. from wounds are usually of clinical significance.

Miscellaneous infections with *B. cereus* have included osteomyelitis, salpingitis, prosthetic infusions, abscesses of the brain and lung, and dissemination in a maternity unit with umbilical stump colonization.

Bacillus thuringiensis

The insect pathogen *B. thuringiensis* is a close relative of *B. cereus*, and preparations of this organism are widely used as insecticides. Splash-ing of one such commercial preparation has led to an eye infection in a healthy person (Samples and Buettner, 1983). This species has also been implicated in a fatal bovine mastitis and in a severe inflammation of the finger web of a laboratory worker following accidental inoculation (see Claus and Berkeley, 1986), and in a gastroenteritis outbreak. Following this outbreak, further *B. thuringiensis* isolates from other sources showed cytotoxic effects characteristic of enterotoxin production (Jackson *et al.*, 1995).

Bacillus licheniformis

Reports of infections with *B. licheniformis* include ventriculitis following the removal of an intraventricular meningioma, cerebral abscess following a penetrating orbital injury (Jones *et al.*, 1992), septicaemia following arteriography, bacteraemia in a pregnant woman who was suffering from eclampsia and acute fibrinolysis, peritonitis with bacteraemia in an immunologically normal person with volvulus and small-bowel perforation, a case of ophthalmitis, and corneal ulcer after trauma (Logan, 1988).

There have been reports of L-form organisms, occurring in blood and other body fluids, which reverted to small acid-fast diphtheroids and then to non-acid-fast, Gram-positive, endospore-forming rods on subculture or greatly prolonged (up to two years) primary culture, especially when exposed to agents known to induce reversion of other L-forms. These organisms produced licheniform colonies and were phenotypically similar to *B. licheniformis*. Claims of a positive relationship between these organisms and certain diseases which are believed to have immunological involvement, such as arthritis and cancer, remain unproven (Logan, 1988).

There have been many isolations of apparently typical strains of *B. licheniformis* in association with bovine and ovine abortion. Pathogenesis is unclear, but the organism's association with distinct placental and fetal lesions is strongly suggestive of a primary aetiological role (Mitchell and Barton, 1986; Logan, 1988). It has also been isolated in association with bovine mastitis, from areas of local disruption of bovine gut mucosa, and in mixed culture from areas of congestion, ulceration and oedema of the bovine gut mucosa (Al-Mashat and Taylor, 1983).

There is strong circumstantial evidence that *B. licheniformis* can cause food poisoning which manifests as diarrhoea, sometimes with vomiting, after 4–15 h incubation. Cooked-meat dishes were the foods mainly implicated, and these had *B. licheniformis* counts of 10^5–10^9 cfu/g (Kramer *et al.*, 1982).

Bacillus subtilis

Early reports of infection ascribed to *B. subtilis* (Figure 5.1a) often used the name to mean any aerobic, endospore-forming organism, but since 1970 there have been several reports of infection with *B. subtilis* in which accurate identification of the species appears to have been made. They include cases of bacteraemia, septicaemia and pneumonia associated with neoplastic disease and infection of a necrotic tumour. Cases associated with implants include two ventriculo-atrial shunt infections (Tuazon *et al.*, 1979) and an isolation from a breast prosthesis. There have also been a case of endocarditis in a drug abuser and isolations from a pleural effusion contiguous to a subphrenic abscess, and from several surgical wound-drainage sites (Logan, 1988). Also, *B. subtilis* derivatives containing proteolytic enzymes for use in laundry products have given rise to respiratory ailments and dermatitis (Norris *et al.*, 1981). *Bacillus subtilis* is, however, widely used in biotechnology and is Generally Regarded as Safe (GRAS) for these purposes. *Bacillus subtilis* may also cause bovine mastitis (Fossum *et al.*, 1986).

Like *B. licheniformis*, *B. subtilis* has been implicated in several incidents of food poisoning. Symptoms of vomiting, with diarrhoea in more than half of the cases, followed incubation periods ranging from 15 minutes to 10 hours. High counts of the organism ($>10^6$ cfu/g) were found in the implicated foods, which included wholemeal bread, pizza, stuffed poultry, sausage rolls and meat pasties (Kramer *et al.*, 1982).

Other Species

Bacillus (now *Paenibacillus*) *alvei* has been isolated from two cases of meningitis (one isolate, from a neonate, was an atypical strain) (Weidermann, 1987), a prosthetic hip infection in a patient with sickle cell anaemia (Reboli *et al.*, 1989), a wound infection and, in association with *Clostridium perfringens*, a case of gas gangrene.

Bacillus brevis has been isolated from corneal infection and bacteraemia and has been implicated in several incidents of food poisoning (Gilbert *et al.*, 1981).

Bacillus circulans has been isolated from the cerebrospinal fluid of a neonate with fatal meningitis, and from a wound infection, following surgery in an elderly patient with ovarian carcinoma (Logan *et al.*, 1985b), and from septicaemia and abscesses.

Bacillus coagulans has been isolated from corneal infection, bacteraemia and bovine abortion (Logan, 1988).

Bacillus laterosporus has been reported from a case of endophthalmitis which resulted in loss of the eye.

Bacillus (now *Paenibacillus*) *macerans* has been isolated from a wound infection following surgical removal of a large malignant melanoma, and from bovine abortion (Logan, 1988).

Bacillus (now *Paenibacillus*) *polymyxa* was isolated from a case of ovine abortion in Scotland.

Bacillus pumilus has been found in cases of pustule and rectal fistula infection (Gilbert *et al.*, 1981), in association with bovine mastitis and has been implicated in foodborne illness (Turnbull and Kramer, 1995).

Bacillus sphaericus has been implicated in several serious infections: a fatal pseudotumour of the lung in a chronic asthmatic who was receiving steroid therapy (Isaacson *et al.*, 1976), and two cases of meningitis in which the portal of entry could not be determined – a rapidly fatal case with generalized Schwartzmann reaction in a normal subject, and a case associated with bacteraemia and endocarditis in an alcoholic; the latter was successfully treated with penicillin (Logan, 1988). It has also been implicated in foodborne illness (Turnbull and Kramer, 1995).

LABORATORY DIAGNOSIS

Specimens, Transport and Culture

Bacillus anthracis

Although anthrax is not highly contagious, special precautions are required in the collection and handling of specimens, when it is suspected. Surgical gloves, disposable overalls, apron and disinfectable boots should be worn, and where large numbers of spores are thought to be present in dry, dusty material, headwear and a dust mask are appropriate.

Exudate from early lesions may be collected with a dry swab. Where the eschar is well developed, its edge should be lifted and fluid obtained using a capillary tube. Faeces and blood may also be collected as appropriate for culture if intestinal anthrax is suspected, and blood for smear and culture in the case of pulmonary patients. Post mortem, fluid may be swabbed from nose, mouth or anus and, in the case of animals, samples of soil under the nose and anus. Blood may also be collected for smear and culture, as it does not clot at death from anthrax. If these are negative, peritoneal fluid, spleen and lymph node specimens should be collected by aspiration, to avoid fluid spillage, for smear and culture. All specimens should be placed in secure containers for transport.

Bacillus anthracis must be handled at Laboratory Containment Level 3 as it is a Hazard Group 3 biological agent (Advisory Committee on Dangerous Pathogens, 1995). Smears should be fixed chemically as heat from a flame may not kill all spores; 10% formalin for 10 minutes is one suitable method. In the case of cultures likely to be mixed, from soil, for example, plating on polymyxin–lysozyme–EDTA–thallous acetate (PLET) medium (Knisely, 1966) will help to select for *B. anthracis*.

Disposable items should be discarded into a container, autoclaved and incinerated. Other equipment should be placed in 10–40% formalin, depending on the degree of contamination, and surfaces disinfected with 10% formalin or 1% hypochlorite in 50:50 v/v methanol:water (Turnbull and Kramer, 1995).

Bacillus cereus *and other species*

Clinical specimens for isolation of other species of *Bacillus* need no special precautions and can be collected, transported and cultivated in the normal way.

Culture Maintenance

Maintenance of all species is simple if spores can be obtained, but it is a mistake to assume that a primary culture or subculture on blood agar will automatically yield spores if stored on the bench or in the incubator. It is best to grow the organism on nutrient agar containing 5 mg/l manganese sulphate for a few days, check for spores by microscopy (see below), and refrigerate when most cells appear to have sporulated. For most species, sporulated cultures on slopes of this medium, sealed after incubation, can survive in a refrigerator for years. Alternatively, slopes can be frozen at $-70\,°C$, or cultures can be freeze-dried.

Identification

In addition to *Bacillus* and the two genera derived from it, *Alicyclobacillus* and *Paenibacillus*, dealt within this chapter, and *Clostridium* (see Chapter 19a), there are a number of other validly described genera of endospore-forming bacteria. Very few of these, if any, are likely to encountered by clinicians but information enabling them to be identified to the generic level is available in Berkeley and Ali (1994), if needed.

Bacillus anthracis *and* Bacillus cereus

Bacillus anthracis, *B. cereus* and *B. thuringiensis* have only very small differences in their rRNA sequences (Ash *et al.*, 1991a; Ash and Collins, 1992). This is entirely consistent with the difficulty commonly experienced of distinguishing *B. anthracis* from *B. cereus*. It is, however, usually not difficult to identify *B. anthracis* from clinical material associated with a case of human or animal anthrax, or virulent strains from other sources. The distinction of avirulent strains, which have lost either or both of the pX01 and pX02 plasmids (see Pathogenicity, above), from *B. cereus* is less simple.

Identification as *B. anthracis* of organisms from humans or animals with symptoms of anthrax depends on them producing a capsule, being susceptible to γ-phage and to penicillin, being non-motile and non-haemolytic. The methods for carrying out these tests are described by Logan and his colleagues (1985a). No one test is diagnostic, however, as not all strains are obviously susceptible to phage, some strains are penicillin resistant, if the physiological conditions are not right the McFadyean test will be negative, and some *B. cereus* strains are non-motile and some are weakly or non-haemolytic. Thus the pattern of results must be considered rather than the result of a single test.

The polymerase chain reaction (PCR) has been used to detect *B. anthracis* strains from the environment carrying plasmids pX01 and pX02 (Titball *et al.*, 1991; Carl *et al.*, 1992). For epidemiological purposes, and to monitor vaccine seed cultures, it is also desirable to be able to identify avirulent strains lacking one or both these plasmids and reliably to distinguish them from other members of the *B. cereus* group. PCR fingerprinting of isolated total DNA enables this to be done and, using the sequence-specific coliphage M13-based primer, *B. anthracis* strains could be assigned to three groups (Henderson *et al.*, 1994).

Pyrolysis mass spectrometry also enables the clear separation of *B. anthracis* from *B. cereus*, the discrimination between some strains of *B. anthracis*, and grouping of others (Helyer *et al.*, in press).

Other Bacillus *species*

As pointed out by Logan (1988), *Bacillus* isolates from clinical material, other than *B. anthracis*, were not identified beyond the generic level until quite recently. This was because they were believed to be of no clinical significance and difficult to identify (Logan and Berkeley, 1984). The identification system established by these authors based on morphological observation and API tests allows recognition of all those species likely to be encountered by the clinician. Kämpfer

(1991) has established a probability matrix for the identification of 36 *Bacillus* spp. based on miniaturized biochemical tests, as an alternative to the perceived high cost of commercial systems.

Information about alternative, traditional approaches to identification at the species level may be found in the reviews by Berkeley and colleagues (1984) and by Priest (1989). A colour atlas to aid this process is available (Parry *et al.*, 1983).

Another approach is to use pyrolysis mass spectrometry. The instrumentation needed is expensive, but the method has the advantages of accuracy, rapidity, transferability, universal applicability and, despite the initial capital expenditure, cost-effectiveness (Berkeley *et al.*, 1992).

As was indicated earlier, before attempting to identify to species level it is important to establish that any suspect isolate really is an aerobic endospore-former, and that other kinds of inclusions are not being mistaken for spores. With phase-contrast microscopy or spore staining of cultures that appear 'moth eaten' when Gram stained, such errors are entirely avoidable. A Gram film showing Gram-positive cells with unstained areas suggestive of spores can, at a pinch, be stripped of any immersion oil with acetone/alcohol, washed, and then spore stained in the usual way. Phase contrast (at $1000\times$ magnification) should be used if it is available, however, because it is greatly superior to staining and much more convenient. Spores are larger, more phase-bright, and more regular in shape, size and position than other kinds of inclusion such as poly-β-hydroxybutyrate granules (see Figure 5.1). Members of the *B. cereus* group and *B. megaterium* will produce large numbers of storage granules when grown on carbohydrate media, so that the cytoplasm may appear vacuolate or foamy when viewed by phase-contrast microscopy, but on routine media this phenomenon is rarely sufficiently pronounced to cause confusion.

ANTIMICROBIAL SENSITIVITY

Bacillus anthracis

Information relating to the sensitivity of this organism is sparse. In two separate studies – both using agar dilution, one on 70 *B. anthracis* isolates (Lightfoot *et al.*, 1990), the other on 22 organisms (Doganay and Aydin, 1991) – most strains were sensitive to penicillins, with minimal inhibitory concentrations (MICs) of 0.03 mg/l or less. In the first study two strains, both from the same fatal case of pulmonary anthrax, were found to be resistant, with MICs in excess of 0.25 mg/l. MICs for erythromycin, tetracycline and chloramphenicol are, respectively 0.25–1.0, 0.06–1.0 and 2.0–4.0 mg/l. Ofloxacin and ciprofloxacin showed very good activities and had MIC values of 0.03–0.06 mg/l.

Bacillus cereus

Microdilution sensitivity tests of 54 *B. cereus* strains showed that they were susceptible to imipenem, vancomycin, chloramphenicol, gentamicin and ciprofloxacin, with MICs of 0.25–4.0, 0.25–2.0, 2.0–4.0, 0.25–2.0 and 0.25–1.0 mg/l, respectively (Weber *et al.*, 1988).

Other *Bacillus* Species

A study of seven other *Bacillus* species: *B. megaterium* (five strains), *B.* (now *Paenibacillus*) *polymyxa* (five strains), *B. pumilus* (four strains), *B. subtilis* (four strains), *B. circulans* (three strains), *B. amyloliquefaciens* (two strains) and *B. licheniformis* (one strain) by Weber *et al.* (1988) showed that in microdilution sensitivity tests more than 95% of these organisms were susceptible to imipenem, vancomycin and ciprofloxacin, with MICs of 0.25–16, 0.25–4 and 0.25–1.0 mg/l, respectively. Other work has been summarized by Claus and Berkeley (1986).

MANAGEMENT OF INFECTION

B. anthracis

This organism is normally penicillin and cephalosporin sensitive, and β-lactams remain the drugs of choice, although four penicillin-resistant strains have been isolated. Where alternative treatment is indicated, erythromycin, tetracycline and chloramphenicol may be used (Dogany and Aydin, 1991).

B. cereus

In contrast to *B. anthracis*, *B. cereus* is resistant to antibiotics such as penicillin and cephalosporin because it produces an extracellular, broad-spectrum β-lactamase. Clindamycin or vancomycin, in combination with an aminoglycoside, such as gentamicin, are usually effective.

Other *Bacillus* Species

Strains of a number of other species have been shown to be susceptible to imipenem, vancomycin and ciprofloxacin (Weber *et al.*, 1988). Farrar and Reboli (1992), however, advocated further studies before imipenem and ciprofloxacin are used for treatment of *Bacillus* infections and suggested that the drug of choice is vancomycin.

PREVENTION AND CONTROL

Bacillus anthracis

Cross-infection is not a problem with this organism as person-to-person transmission is very rare and direct infections from soil are few. Soil is, however, a main reservoir from which animals and hence man are infected. *Bacillus anthracis* is known to persist in soil, and the period of persistence will vary from site to site and according to the conditions in any one place. It is not possible to generalize about the longevity of organisms introduced into the soil but the view has been expressed that it will not normally be for more than a few years. It was shown in South Africa that *B. anthracis* was not present in naturally contaminated soil some five years after its introduction, due, it was suggested, to its inability to compete successfully with the indigenous soil microflora (Brachman, 1990). In contrast, on Gruinard Island in Scotland, some of the spores artificially introduced in large quantity could be recovered after 45 years, and then limited data available on the rate of decline of the population suggested that spores would remain viable for more than twice this period (Manchee et al., 1990). Given the extreme longevity of spores it would be unwise to assume relatively short persistence in environments in which B. anthracis spores may not germinate, and so avoid competition with other organisms.

Anthrax could be prevented if B. anthracis could be eliminated from soil, and although this has been essentially achieved on Gruinard Island (Manchee et al., 1990) the process was expensive and is not generally applicable. Thus prevention of the disease depends essentially on its eradication from animal populations. This can be achieved by vaccination programmes; anthrax has been more or less eradicated in South Africa and effectively controlled in a number of other countries in this way. Complementary measures such as incineration of carcasses, disinfection of water supplies and burning contaminated vegetation have also helped.

In countries free of the disease, disinfection of animal products imported from epizootic areas of the world is necessary to prevent its reintroduction. Hair and wool can effectively be treated with formaldehyde, as can hides and bone meal by heat (Brachman, 1990).

The vaccines most widely used for animals are derived from the Sterne live spore vaccine and are made with organisms descended from his original 34F2 strain. Such vaccines are considered unsuitable for human use in the West, and cell-free products containing high levels of PA and relatively little LF and EF from the Sterne strain and strain V770 have been produced in the UK and USA, respectively (Turnbull, 1991). Information on the performance in humans of the former USSR live spore vaccine has recently been presented. It is recorded that in 30 years no adverse effects occurred using the vaccine based on the two avirulent, non-capsulate B. anthracis strains STI-1 and 3, which were derived from virulent parents at the Sanitary-Technical Institute (STI), Kirov (now Viatka), and reconsideration of the suitability of live spore vaccines for human use was therefore suggested (Shlyakhov and Rubinstein, 1994).

Bacillus cereus

Diarrhoeal and vomiting intoxications by this organism are readily preventable by appropriate food-handling procedures. Meat and vegetables should not be held at temperatures between 10 °C and 45 °C for long periods, and rice held overnight after cooking should be refrigerated and not held at room temperature. Prevention of infection by this organism, and by other Bacillus species, in patients following surgery or in those who are immunocompromised or who are otherwise predisposed to infection, depends on good practice.

ACKNOWLEDGEMENTS

We are most grateful to Dr Peter Turnbull and to Professor Mehmet Doganay for assistance during the preparation of this chapter.

REFERENCES

Advisory Committee on Dangerous Pathogens (1995) Categorisation of Biological Agents According to Hazard and Categories of Containment, 4th edn. HSE Books, HMSO, London.

Al-Mashat, R.R. and Taylor, D.J. (1983) Bacteria in enteric lesions of cattle. Veterinary Record, 112, 5–10.

Ash, C. and Collins, M.D. (1992) Comparative analysis of 23S ribosomal RNA gene sequences of B. anthracis and emetic B. cereus determined by PCR-direct sequencing. FEMS Microbiology Letters, 94, 75–80.

Ash, C., Farrow, J.A.E., Dorsch, M. et al. (1991a) Comparative analysis of B. anthracis, B. cereus, and related species on the basis of reverse transcriptase sequencing of 16S rRNA. International Journal of Systematic Microbiology, 41, 343–346.

Ash, C., Farrow, J.A.E., Wallbanks, S. and Collins, M.D. (1991b) Phylogenetic heterogeneity of the genus Bacillus revealed by comparative analysis of small-subunit-ribosomal RNA sequences. Letters in Applied Microbiology, 13, 202–206.

Ash, C., Priest, F.G. and Collins, M.D. (1993) Molecular identification of rRNA group 3 bacilli (Ash, Farrow, Wallbanks and Collins) using a PCR probe test: proposal for the creation of a new genus Paenibacillus. Antonie van Leeuenhoek, 64, 253–260.

Barnham, M. and White, D.H. (1980) B. cereus infections. Journal of Clinical Pathology, 33, 314–315.

Berkeley, R.C.W. and Ali, N. (1994) Classification and identification of the endospore-forming bacteria. *Journal of Applied Bacteriology Symposium Supplement*, **76**, 1S–8S.

Berkeley, R.C.W., Goodacre, R., Helyer, R.J. and Kelley, T. (1992) Pyrolysis mass spectrometry in the identification of *Bacillus* species. In *Identification Methods in Applied and Environmental Microbiology* (ed. R.G. Board, D. Jones and F.A. Skinner), pp. 292–328. Blackwell, London.

Berkeley, R.C.W., Logan, N.A., Shute, L.A. and Capey, A.G. (1984) Identification of *Bacillus* species. In *Methods in Microbiology*, Vol. 16 (ed. T. Bergan), pp. 291–328. Academic Press, London.

Brachman, P.S. (1990) Introductory comments on prophylaxis, therapy and control in relation to anthrax. *Salisbury Medical Bulletin*, **60** (Special Suppl.), 84–85.

Bull, A.T., Goodfellow, M. and Slater, J.H. (1992) Biotechnology as a source of innovation in biotechnology. *Annual Review of Microbiology*, **46**, 219–252.

Burdon, K.L. (1956) Useful criteria for the identification of *Bacillus anthracis* and related species. *Journal of Bacteriology*, **71**, 25–42.

Carl, M.R., Hawkins, N., Coulson, J. *et al.* (1992) Detection of spores of *B. anthracis* using polymerase chain reaction. *Journal of Infectious Diseases*, **165**, 1145–1148.

Claus, D. and Berkeley, R.C.W. (1986) Genus *Bacillus* Cohn 1872, 174[AL]. In *Bergey's Manual of Systematic Bacteriology*, Vol. 2 (ed. P.H.A. Sneath, N.S. Mair, M.E. Sharpe and J.G. Holt), pp. 1105–1139. Williams & Wilkins, Baltimore.

Cohn, F. (1872) Untersuchungen über Bakterien. *Beitrage zur Biologie der Pflanzen*, **1**(2), 127–224.

Davaine, M.C. (1864) Nouvelles recherches sur la nature de la maladie charbonneuse connue sous le nom de sang de rate. *Comptes Rendues de l'Academie des Sciences, Paris*, **59**, 393–396.

Doganay, M. (1990) Human anthrax in Sivas, Turkey. *Salisbury Medical Bulletin*, **60** (Special Suppl.), 13.

Doganay, M. and Aydin, N. (1991) Antimicrobial susceptibility of *B. anthracis*. *Scandinavian Journal of Infectious Diseases*, **23**, 333–335.

Ehrenberg, C.G. (1835) Dritter Beitrag zur Erkenntnis grosser Organisation in der Richtung des kleinsten Raumes. *Abhandlungen der Königlichen Akademie der Wissenschaften zu Berlin aus die Jahre 1833–1835*, 145–336.

Farrar, W.E. and Reboli, A.C. (1992) The genus *Bacillus*: medical. In *The Prokaryotes: A Handbook of Bacteria, Ecophysiology, Isolation, Identification, Applications*, Vol. 2 (ed. A. Balows, H.G. Trüper, M. Dworkin *et al.*), pp. 1746–1768. Springer-Verlag, New York.

Fossum, K., Kerikstad, H., Binde, M. and Pettersen, K.-E. (1986) Isolation of *Bacillus subtilis* in connection with bovine mastitis. *Nordisk Veterinaermedicin*, **38**, 233–236.

Gibson, T. and Gordon, R.E. (1974) Genus *Bacillus* Cohn. In *Bergey's Manual of Determinative Bacteriology*, 8th edn (ed. R.E. Buchanan and N.E. Gibbons), pp. 529–550. Williams & Wilkins, Baltimore.

Gilbert, R.J., Turnbull, P.C.B., Parry, J.M. and Kramer, J.M. (1981) *Bacillus cereus* and other *Bacillus* species: their part in food poisoning and other clinical infections. In *The Aerobic Endospore-forming Bacteria: Classification and Identification* (ed. R.C.W. Berkeley and M. Goodfellow), pp. 297–314. Academic Press, London.

Gordon R.E., Haynes, W.C. and Hor-Nay Pang, C. (1973) The Genus *Bacillus*: *Agriculture Handbook No. 427*. US Department of Agriculture, Washington, DC.

Granum, P.E. (1994) *Bacillus cereus* and its toxins. *Journal of Applied Bacteriology (Symposium Supplement)*, **76**, 61S–66S.

Helyer, R.J., Kelley, T. and Berkeley, R.C.W. (1996) Pyrolysis mass spectrometry studies on *B. anthracis*, *B. cereus* and their close relatives. *Zentralblatt für Bakteriologie*, in press.

Henderson, I., Duggleby, C.J. and Turnbull, P.C.B. (1994) Differentiation of *Bacillus anthracis* from other *Bacillus cereus* group bacteria with the PCR. *International Journal of Systematic Bacteriology*, **44**, 99–105.

Hugh-Jones, M.E. (1990) Global trends in the incidence of anthrax in livestock. *Salisbury Medical Bulletin*, **60** (Special Suppl.), 2–4.

Isaacson, P., Jacobs, P.H., Mackenzie, A.R. and Mathews, A.W. (1976) Pseudotumour of the lung caused by infection with *Bacillus sphaericus*. *Journal of Clinical Pathology*, **29**, 806–811.

Jackson, S.G., Goodbrand, R.B., Ahmed, R. and Kasatiya, S. (1995) *Bacillus cereus* and *Bacillus thuringiensis* isolated in a gasteroenteritis outbreak investigation. *Letters in Applied Microbiology*, **21**, 103–105.

Jones, B.L., Hanson, M.F. and Logan, N.A. (1992) Isolation of *Bacillus licheniformis* from a brain abscess following a penetrating orbital injury. *Journal of Infection*, **24**, 103–105.

Kampfer, P. (1991) Application of miniaturised physiological tests in numerical classification and identification of some bacilli. *Journal of General and Applied Microbiology*, **37**, 225–247.

Kaufmann, A.F. (1990) Observations on the occurrence of anthrax as related to soil type and rainfall. *Salisbury Medical Bulletin*, **60** (Special Suppl.), 16–17.

Knight, B.C.J. and Proom, H. (1950) A comparative survey of the nutrition and physiology of mesophilic species in the genus *Bacillus*. *Journal of General Microbiology*, **4**, 508–538.

Kramer, J.M. and Gilbert, R.J. (1989) *Bacillus cereus* and other *Bacillus* species. In *Foodborne Bacterial Pathogens* (ed. M.P. Doyle), pp. 21–70. Marcel Dekker, New York.

Kramer, J.M., Turnbull, P.C.B., Munshi, G. and Gilbert, R.J. (1982) Identification and characterisation of *Bacillus cereus* and other *Bacillus* species associated with foods and food poisoning. In *Isolation and Identification Methods for Food Poisoning Organisms* (ed. J.E.L. Corry, D. Roberts and F.A. Skinner), pp. 261–286. Academic Press, London.

Knisely, R.F. (1966) Differential media for *B. anthracis*. *Journal of Bacteriology*, **90**, 784–786.

Laubach, C.A., Rice, J.L. and Ford, W.W. (1916) Studies on aerobic spore-bearing non-pathogenic bacteria. Part II. *Journal of Bacteriology*, **1**, 493–533.

Lawrence, J.S. and Ford, W.W. (1916) Studies on aerobic spore-bearing non-pathogenic bacteria. Part I. *Journal of Bacteriology*, **1**, 273–320.

Leppla, S.H. (1982) Anthrax toxin edema factor: a bacterial adenylate cyclase that increases cyclic AMP concentrations in eukaryotic cells. *Proceedings of the National Academy of Sciences USA*, **79**, 3162–3164.

Leppla, S.H. (1984) *Bacillus anthracis* calmodulin-dependent adenylate cyclase: chemical and enzymatic properties and interactions with eukaryotic cells. *Advances in Cyclic Nucleotide Protein Phosphorylation Research*, **17**, 189–198.

Leppla, S.H., Friedlander, A.M., Singh, Y. *et al.* (1990) A model for anthrax toxic action at the cellular level. *Salisbury Medical Bulletin*, **60** (Special Suppl.), 41–43.

Lightfoot, N.F., Scott, R.J.D. and Turnbull, P.C.B. (1990) Antimicrobial susceptibility of *B. anthracis*. *Salisbury Medical Bulletin*, **60** (Special Suppl.), 95–98.

Logan N.A. (1988) *Bacillus* species of medical and veterinary importance. *Journal of Medical Microbiology*, **25**, 157–165.

Logan, N.A. and Berkeley, R.C.W. (1981) Classification and identification of members of the genus *Bacillus* using API tests. In *The Aerobic Endospore-forming Bacteria* (ed. R.C.W. Berkeley and M. Goodfellow), pp. 105–140. Academic Press, London.

Logan, N.A. and Berkeley, R.C.W. (1984) Identification of *Bacillus* strains using the API system. *Journal of General Microbiology*, **130**, 1871–1882.

Logan, N.A., Carman, J.A., Melling, J. and Berkeley, R.C.W. (1985a) Identification of *B. anthracis* by API tests. *Journal of Medical Microbiology*, **20**, 75–85.

Logan, N.A., Old, D.C. and Dick, H.M. (1985b) Isolation of *Bacillus circulans* from a wound infection. *Journal of Clinical Pathology*, **38**, 838–839.

Manchee, R.J., Broster, M.G., Stagg, A.J. *et al.* (1990) Out of Gruinard island. *Salisbury Medical Bulletin*, **60** (Special Suppl.), 17–18.

Mitchell, G. and Barton, M.G. (1986) Bovine abortion associated with *Bacillus licheniformis*. *Australian Veterinary Journal*, **63**, 160–161.

Norris, J.R., Berkeley, R.C.W., Logan, N.A. and O'Donnell, A.G. (1981) The genera *Bacillus* and *Sporolactobacillus*. In *The Prokaryotes: A Handbook on Habitats, Isolation and Identification of Bacteria*, Vol. 2 (ed. M.P. Starr, H. Stolp, H.G. Trüper *et al.*), pp. 1711–1742. Springer-Verlag, Berlin.

Parry, J.M., Turnbull, P.C.B. and Gibson, J.R. (1983) *A Colour Atlas of Bacillus Species*. Wolfe Medical Publications, London.

Priest, F.G. (1989) Isolation and identification of aerobic endospore-forming bacteria. In *Bacillus* (ed. C.R. Harwood), pp. 27–56. Plenum Press, New York.

Pugh, A.O. and Davies, J.C.A. (1990) Human anthrax in Zimbabwe. *Salisbury Medical Bulletin*, **60** (Special Suppl.), 32–33.

Reboli, A.C., Bryan, C.S. and Farrar, W.E. (1989) Bacteremia and infection of a hip prosthesis caused by *Bacillus alvei*. *Journal of Clinical Microbiology*, **27**, 1395–1396.

Robertson, D.L., Bragg, T.S., Simpson, S. *et al.* (1990) Mapping and characterisation of the *Bacillus anthracis* plasmids pX01 and pX02. *Salisbury Medical Bulletin*, **60** (Special Suppl.), 55–58.

Samples, J.R. and Buettner, H. (1983) Ocular infection caused by a biological insecticide. *Journal of Infectious Diseases*, **148**, 614.

Shinagawa, K., Otake, S., Matsusaka, N. and Sugii, S. (1992) Production of the vacuolation factor of *Bacillus cereus* isolated from vomiting-type food poisoning. *Journal of Veterinary Medical Science*, **54**, 443–446.

Shlyakhov, E.N. and Rubinstein, E. (1994) Human live anthrax vaccine in the former USSR. *Vaccine*, **12**, 727–730.

Skerman, V.B.D., McGowen, V. and Sneath, P.H.A. (1980) Approved lists of bacterial names. *International Journal of Systematic Bacteriology*, **30**, 225–420.

Smith, H. (1990) Anthrax, clinical manifestations and pathogenesis: much unknown and much just forgotten. *Salisbury Medical Bulletin*, **60** (Special Suppl.), 31.

Smith, N.R., Gordon, R.E. and Clark, F.E. (1946) *Aerobic Mesophilic Sporeforming Bacteria: Miscellaneous Publication No. 559*. US Department of Agriculture, Washington, DC.

Smith, N.R., Gordon, R.E. and Clark, F.E. (1952) *Aerobic Endosporeforming Bacteria: Agriculture Monograph No. 16.* US Department of Agriculture, Washington, DC.

Titball, R.W., Turnbull, P.C.B. and Hutson, R.A. (1991) The monitoring and detection of *B. anthracis* in the environment. *Journal of Applied Bacteriology (Symposium Supplement)*, **70**, 9S–18S.

Tuazon, C.E., Murray, H.W., Levy, C. *et al.* (1979) Serious infections from *Bacillus* sp. *Journal of the American Medical Association*, **241**, 1137–1140.

Turnbull, P.C.B. (1991) Anthrax vaccines: past, present and future. *Vaccine*, **9**, 533–539.

Turnbull, P.C.B. and Kramer, J.M. (1995) *Bacillus*. In *Manual of Clinical Microbiology*, 6th edn (ed. P.R. Murray, E.J. Barron, M.A. Pfaller *et al.*), pp. 349–350. ASM Press, Washington, DC.

Weber, D.J., Saviteer, S.M., Rutala, W.A. and Thomann, C.A. (1988) In vitro susceptibility of *Bacillus* spp. to antimicrobial agents. *Antimicrobial Agents and Chemotherapy*, **32**, 642–645.

Weidermann, B.L. (1987) Non-anthrax *Bacillus* infections in children. *Paediatric Infectious Disease Journal*, **6**, 218–219.

Wisotzkey, J.D., Jurtshuk Jr, P., Fox, G.E. *et al.* (1992) Comparative analyses on the 16S rRNA (rDNA) of *B. acidocaldarius*, *B. acidoterrestris* and *B. cycloheptanicus* and proposal for creation of a new genus, *Alicyclobacillus* gen. nov. *International Journal of Systematic Microbiology*, **42**, 263–269.

6a

THE GENUS *MYCOBACTERIUM*

Stephen H. Gillespie and Timothy D. McHugh

INTRODUCTION

The genus *Mycobacterium* contains more than 55 recognized species. Although the genus contains two of the most important human pathogens *M. tuberculosis* and *M. leprae*, and several species which commonly cause infection in compromised hosts the majority of mycobacteria are environmental saprophytic organisms being found in water (fresh and salt) and soil. They also act as commensals in man and animals.

Description of the Genus

Phylogeny

Mycobacteria, together with other mycolic acid-containing organisms, form part of the order Actinomycetales. They are related, therefore, to *Rhodococcus*, *Nocardia*, *Corynebacterium*, *Gordona* and *Tsukamurella*. Species within the genus fall into two broad groups which broadly correspond with the slow and rapid growers (see below). Sequencing of 16S ribosomal DNA has confirmed the division in the genus between rapid and slow growers, and in evolutionary terms this has occurred recently (Pitulle *et al.*, 1995). A summary of the phylogenetic relationships within the genus are illustrated in Figure 6a.1.

Definition

Organisms of the genus *Mycobacterium* are acid fast, contain mycolic acids and have a G + C ratio of 61–71% (Levy-Frebault and Portaels, 1992). Some other closely related genera (e.g. *Corynebacterium* and *Rhodococcus*, may exhibit acid fastness when grown on lipid-rich medium but usually decolorize when acid–alcohol (e.g. Kinyoun method) is applied (Levy-Frebault and Portaels, 1992). Mycolic acids are found in several related genera, but mycobacteria are unique because they synthesize long-chained mycolic acids containing between 60 and 90 carbon atoms. In addition oxygenated mycolic acids are synthesized (methoxy-keto-). When mycolic acids are cleaved by pyrolysis to C_{22}–C_{26} derivatives may be distinguished from mycolic acids of related genera which are characteristically C_{12}–C_{22} and may be monosaturated. The G + C content of 61–71% encompasses related genera, and one species, *M. leprae*, differs from other mycobacteria in that its G + C content is 54–57% and has been shown to be remotely genetically related

Principles and Practice of Clinical Bacteriology. Edited by A.M. Emmerson, P.M. Hawkey and S.H. Gillespie

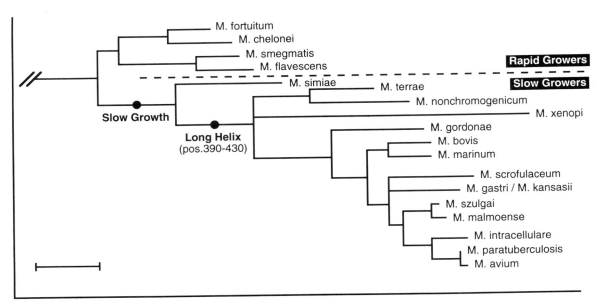

Figure 6a.1. Phylogenetic tree showing the relationships of species belonging to the genus *Mycobacterium*. This tree was constructed by using 16S rRNA sequence and the neighbourliness method The tree was rooted by using *Nocardia asteroides* as an outgroup. Bar = 10 nucleotide differences; pos., positions.

to other mycobacteria by DNA hybridization (Grosskinsky *et al.*, 1989).

Classification

Our understanding of the taxonomy of the genus *Mycobacterium* is expanding rapidly through the application of molecular techniques. The upsurge in interest in mycobacterial disease has resulted in the discovery of several new species. The majority of species are not implicated in clinical disease and any classification should take this into account. Several clusters of organisms are well-recognized pathogens and have similar pathological behaviour and these are detailed below. Table 6a.1 summarizes the main species isolated in clinical practice and the main disease associations.

M. tuberculosis *complex*

The 'tuberculosis' complex consists of several species which are probably variants of a single species which may be differentiated by small but

consistent biochemical differences. It includes *M. tuberculosis*, and a variant often isolated in Africa and given the name '*M. africanum*'. '*Mycobacterium africanum*' is divided into two variants by some authors. The bovine tubercle bacillus *M. bovis* is also closely related to *M. tuberculosis*, differing in only a few biochemical tests.

M. avium–intracellulare–scrofulaceum *complex*

This group of organisms has come to prominence as a result of the HIV epidemic (see below) and includes the following species: *M. avium*, *M. intracellulare*, *M. avium* subsp. *silvaticum* and *M. paratuberculosis*. The results of DNA hybridization indicate that *M. avium* is a distinct species from *M. intracellulare* and this corresponds with some of the distinctions made with species-specific group IV antigen agglutination. Serovars 1–6 and 8–11 are ascribed to *M. avium*, serovar 7 and 12–20 to *M. intracellulare*. The ascription of

TABLE 6a.1   COMMON DISEASE ASSOCIATIONS OF *MYCOBACTERIUM* SPP.

Species	Main disease association	Other syndromes
M. tuberculosis	Chronic pulmonary infection	See Chapter 6b
M. bovis	Bovine tuberculosis	Human tuberculosis
BCG	Human vaccine	Injection abscess
M. leprae	Leprosy	
M. avium–intracellulare	Disseminated infection in AIDS	Chronic pulmonary infection
		Lymphadenitis
		Osteomyelitis
M. scrofulaceum	Lymphadenitis in children	
M. paratuberculosis		
M. kansasii	Chronic pulmonary infection	Cervical lymphadenitis
M. xenopi	Chronic pulmonary infection	Disseminated infection rare
M. malmoense	Chronic pulmonary disease	
M. szlugai	Chronic pulmonary disease	
M. marinum	Chronic cutaneous infection	Spread to deep tissues
M. ulcerans	Penetrating ulcer at the site of trauma 'Buruli' ulcer	
M. fortuitum } *M. chelonei* } *M. abscessus* }	Soft tissue infections, disseminated infections in the immunocompromised, otitis media, chronic pulmonary disease	
M. genevense	Disseminated infection in AIDS patients	
M. haemophilum	Cutaneous and disseminated infection in the immunocompromised	Cervical lymphadenopathy

higher serovar numbers is more controversial although 26 and 27 are probably *M. scrofulaceum* (Wayne *et al.*, 1993). The mycobactin-dependent species *M. paratuberculosis* has been shown to belong to a single species by DNA–DNA hybridization. *Mycobacterium scrofulaceum* is a species closely related to *M. avium*, differing serologically, on DNA hybridization, mycolic acid profile and thermoresistant catalase activity. The species *M. avium* has been shown to be very closely related to the mycobactin-dependent species *M. paratuberculosis* and the wood pigeon strain and these are probably subspecies. They have been given the names of *M. avium* subsp. *paratuberculosis*, and *M. avium* subsp. *sylvaticum* respectively (Thorel *et al.*, 1990).

Rapid growers

The rapidly growing mycobacteria are phylogenetically older than the slow-growing species (Pitulle *et al.*, 1995). All of the species are closely related to each other, and there is good agreement between numerical phenotypic, chemotaxonomic and DNA hybridization and 16S rRNA studies, although the intrageneric relationship of these species is less clear and sometimes contradictory (Pitulle *et al.*, 1995). They may be divided into seven clusters on the basis of 16S rRNA sequencing. Rapidly growing species found in routine clinical practice include *M. fortuitum*, *M. chelonei*, *M. chelonei* subsp. *abscessus*, *M. smegmatis* and *M. phlei*.

Slow growers

The relationships between other slow-growing organisms is slowly emerging (Pitulle *et al.*, 1995). A useful clinical classification might place the organisms responsible for chronic pulmonary infection together, including *M. kansasii*, *M. xenopi*, *M. szlugai* and *M. malmoense*. An example of the taxonomic refinement which can be expected is to be found in *M. kansasii*, within which a genetically distinct subspecies has recently been identified (Ross *et al.*, 1992). The other clinically useful grouping of organisms is the skin pathogens, which include *M. marinum* and *M. ulcerans*. New species which have recently been recognized include *M. geneveuse*, *M. hiberniae*, *M. cookiae* and have not yet found their place in the phylogeny of the genus.

M. leprae

Mycobacterium leprae has traditionally been classified in the genus *Mycobacterium*. Studies by different methodologies have differed about its relationship to the rest of the genus. The G + C% of flanking DNA of immunodominant epitopes and rRNA analysis suggest a close relationship whereas hybridization studies of 16S rRNA oligonucleotide sequences failed to show relationships with other mycobacteria (Grosskinsky *et al.*, 1989). Endonuclease digestion of 16S rRNA showed that *M. leprae* had a unique pattern. The cell wall contains glycine, in comparison to lysine found in other mycobacteria. Some authors suggest that *M. leprae* should be classified with members of the genera *Rhodococcus* and *Nocardia*.

PATHOGENESIS OF MYCOBACTERIAL DISEASE

The precise mechanisms of pathogenesis in mycobacterial disease are the subject of much debate. The survival success of the mycobacteria relates to their ability to survive in hostile environments and the intracellular location of these bacteria is critical in their pathogenesis. In terms of the pathogenic mycobacteria, e.g. *M. tuberculosis* or *M. leprae*, the persistence of a few viable organisms and their ability to reactivate after years of dormancy are important in understanding the pathology of these infections. A delayed-type hypersensitivity reaction (DTH) may be associated with killing of intracellular mycobacteria; this cell-mediated response is dependent on prior activation of macrophages. In the case of non-activated macrophages containing replicating bacteria the cell is killed and tissue damage results. This manifests as a caseous necrosis with cavity formation that does not eradicate the bacilli but does provide an unfavourable environment that inhibits multiplication (Danneburg and Rook, 1994). Activated macrophages secrete tumour necrosis factor (TNF), which initiates granuloma formation. The granuloma becomes encapsulated with a fibrotic wall and necrotic centre; this localizes and retains the mycobacteria but does not eradicate them (Chan and Kaufmann, 1994) (Figure 6a.2). Central to these events is the

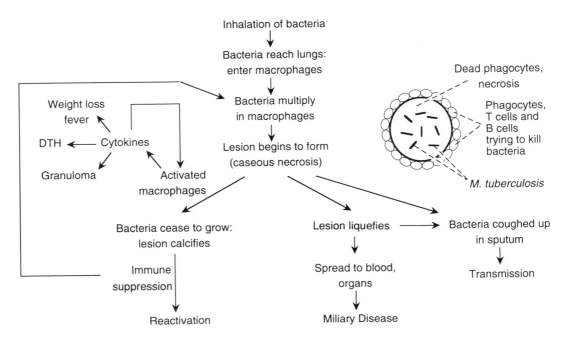

Figure 6a.2. The pathogenesis of tuberculosis.

role of the pathogen surface and its interaction with both macrophages and T cells. The pathology induced appears to be associated with the inappropriate activation of the host immune system rather than specific mycobacterial toxins. As a consequence, the emphasis of the studies of the mechanisms of mycobacterial pathogenesis has been placed in the dissection of the pathogenic and protective components of the host immune response to infective bacilli.

Bacterial Cell Wall

The mycobacterial cell wall is an organized structure comprising soluble proteins, lipids, carbohydrates and an insoluble matrix composed of three covalently linked macromolecules: peptidoglycan, arabinogalactan and mycolic acid (McNeil and Brennan, 1991). Mycobacteria are unusual amongst the bacteria in that they contain as much as 40% of their total lipid in the cell wall (Rastogi, 1991). The precise relationship between the various components of the cell wall and their alignment with respect to each other is not yet resolved: there are anomalies in both electron microscope and biochemical observations. In most of the pathogenic mycobacteria a further capsule-like structure has been noted on invasion of macrophages (Rastogi, 1991). The evidence suggests that this mycobacterial capsule is not a true hydrophilic capsule, as demonstrated by *Escherichia coli* or *Streptococcus pneumoniae*, but a matrix of polymethylated saccharide moieties of lipopolysaccharide anchored in the mycobacterial electron transparent layer (ETL) (Figure 6a.3). The importance of the interaction between the mycobacterium surface and macrophages is demonstrated by the phenolic glycolipids, for example PGL-1. This molecule is an oligoglycosylphenolic phthiocerol diester with a species-specific trisaccharide moiety. Although PGL-1 is universal in *M. leprae* it has restricted expression in *M. tuberculosis*; thus a role in pathogenesis has been postulated for this molecule. *In vitro* macrophage studies have demonstrated that PGL-1 downregulates reactive oxygen intermediates (ROI) and in cell-free systems PGL-1 scavenges oxygen radicles (Besra and Chatterjee, 1994).

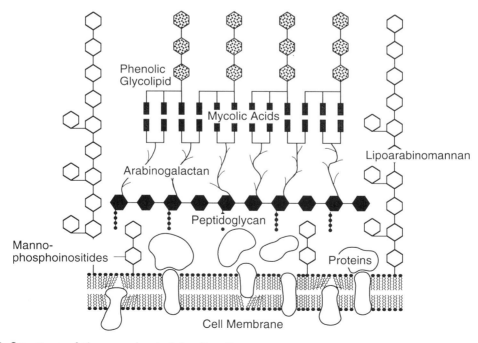

Figure 6a.3. Structure of the mycobacterial cell wall.

Studies of the *M. leprae* capsule indicate that this structure contains both species-specific antigens and antigens common to most mycobacteria (Rastogi, 1991). These cell wall structures are implicated in a number of mechanisms that are related to the development of mycobacterial disease. Processing and presentation of cell wall components to the host immune system, promotion of adhesion to macrophages, inhibition of host antimicrobial activity and drug resistance are all features of the pathogenesis of mycobacterial disease in which the bacterial cell wall has a role. Interaction of the wall lipids with host membranes has received particular attention. Lanéelle & Daffé (1991) hypothesized that protection against host defences and most damage to host cells are the result of the effect of mycobacterial cell wall lipids on host membranes. Indeed, there is considerable data indicating that mycobacterial cell wall lipids contribute to the inappropriate activation of the host immune response associated with mycobacterial pathogenicity. Release of lipoarabinomannan (LAM) (Figure 6a.4) from phagocytosed *M. tuberculosis* cell wall results in activation of the macrophage and the release of a range of cytokines. Amongst these the role of TNF has been defined in the transformation of invasive monocytes to epithelioid cells and Lan-

gerhans giant cells; this process may be involved in the formation of the granuloma characteristic of mycobacterial disease (Rook, 1990).

Mycobacterial Molecules Associated with Pathogenesis

A comprehensive review of the defined proteins identified as targets of humoral and cell-mediated immune responses in patients and animal models was recently published (Young *et al.*, 1992). A large number of mycobacterial proteins do induce an immune response; the value of each moiety as a diagnostic reagent or vaccine target represents the major thrust of much antigen-based research.

Only a small proportion of mycobacterial antigens identified have had specific functions assigned to them. Proteins associated with bacterial responses to stress (e.g. heat, pH or ROI) are particularly prominent and appear to be implicated in mycobacterial pathogenesis. The stress or heat shock proteins (HSPs) include the family of molecular chaperonins: molecules that are concerned with protein folding and assembly as well as membrane translocation. Analogous proteins exist in both prokaryotes and eukaryotes (Murray and Young, 1992). In the mycobacteria, hsp65 is the most fully studied, following the observation that

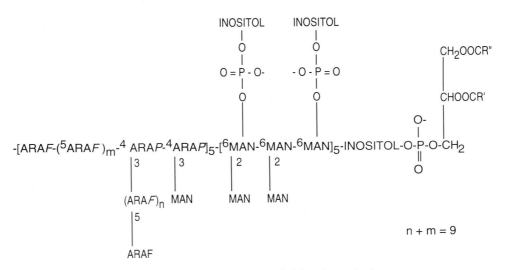

Figure 6a.4. Structure of the native lipoarabinomannan of *M. tuberculosis*.

20% of the T cell response of mice immunized with *M. tuberculosis* is directed against this protein (Lamb *et al.*, 1989). The induction of inappropriate immune responses to self proteins, by mycobacteria, has been proposed as the pathogenic mechanism of some autoimmune diseases, e.g. rheumatoid arthritis. The role of the heat shock proteins in the pathogenesis of infectious disease is not unique to the mycobacteria; a role for T cell responses to hsp60 in chlamydial infections has also been identified (See Chapter 24).

As has already been suggested, the pathology of mycobacterial disease is not associated with the release of exotoxins, however, mycobacteria do secrete a number of highly immunogenic proteins. Indeed, in animal models of BCG vaccination it has been demonstrated that only a live vaccine generates specific protection (Andersen and Brennan, 1994). A further moiety released into the external milieu, by *M. tuberculosis*, is the enzyme superoxide dismutase (SOD). This molecule disarms the macrophage's defensive mechanisms by inactivating superoxide radicles (Fridovich, 1978). SOD makes a further contribution to the pathogenic potential of *M. tuberculosis* as a mutation on the SOD gene correlates with resistance to isoniazid (INH).

The role of the phosphorylated lipopolysaccharides (LPS) as antigens and as virulence factors has recently received attention. Analysis of the role of LAM (Figure 6a.3), a potent downregulator of host cell immunity related functions, has revealed significant differences in activity of LAM purified from the virulent strain of *M. tuberculosis* H37Rv as compared with the avirulent strain H37Ra (Adams *et al.*, 1993). The latter strain was significantly more potent in inducing secretion of TNF-α; this correlated to structural differences between the molecules. Furthermore, LAMs from both *M. tuberculosis* and *M. leprae* block the activation of macrophages. This contributes to the survival of the bacterium within the macrophage as macrophage-mediated killing follows macrophage activation by T cell-derived interferon γ (INF-γ). The downregulation of INF-γ-inducible genes, by LAM, results in the impaired activity of antigen-presenting cells and a consequent non-specific inhibitory effect on proliferating T cells (Britton *et al.*, 1994). Further inhibition of the antimicrobial mechanisms of the macrophage by LAM results from its activity as a reactive oxygen intermediate scavenger and downegulation of the oxidative burst by inhibition of protein kinase C (Britton *et al.*, 1994).

T Cells

The T cell response to mycobacterial infection is complex; the role of the individual populations of T cells is not fully elucidated but the principal groups are CD4$^+$, CD8$^+$ and $\gamma\delta$ cells ($\gamma\delta$ cells represent less than 5% of the resting human T cell population).

CD4$^+$ T cells appear to play the dominant role in the immune response to mycobacteria. These cells provide both protective and memory immunity in adoptive transfer experiments and secrete large amounts of IFN-γ in *in vitro* culture with mycobacterial antigens. Current opinion suggests that the CD4$^+$ response is adequate to eliminate mycobacterial infections, provided that MHC class II presenting cells are present (Orme, 1993). The ability of mycobacteria to downregulate the host response, via the effects of LAM, discussed above, reflects the inadequacy of the CD4$^+$ response and the intricacy of the bacteria–host interaction. Beyond the role of CD4$^+$ T cells as mediators of bactericidal activity through macrophage activation and cytokine production, a further function is in the direct cytolysis of infected host cells; this activity is greatly enhanced at the site of disease as compared· with the peripheral circulation (Barnes *et al.*, 1994). The importance of the CD4$^+$ T cell control of macrophage activation is emphasized when we consider reactivation of tuberculosis; an equilibrium is established between low numbers of viable mycobacteria at the site of infection and circulating memory CD4$^+$ T cells. A reduction in the specific CD4$^+$ cells tips this balance in favour of active infection. Of the wide range of infections established as being associated with reactivation of tuberculosis, co-infection with HIV is the greatest single risk factor (Britton *et al.*, 1994).

Although there is strong evidence of a role for CD8$^+$ T cells in anti-mycobacterial activity in the mouse model of tuberculosis, and that this function is complementary to that of CD4$^+$ cells, the evidence is not so clear and indeed is conflicting in humans. Murine CD8$^+$ cells directly lyse *M. tuberculosis*-infected cells *in vitro* and either depletion or lack of CD8$^+$ cells results in severe manifestations of tuberculosis (Flynn *et al.*, 1992). However, in humans CD8$^+$ cells do not selectively concentrate at the site of disease in tuberculosis, CD8$^+$ cell count does not affect the severity of tuberculosis in HIV patients and the specific cytolytic T cells identified to date are not CD8$^+$ cells. It may be that as the CD4$^+$ cell response fails and the mycobacteriosis disseminates then the CD8$^+$ cell response becomes more important.

Macrophages

Invasion of macrophages by the mycobacteria is via several specific receptors, but no triggering of an oxidative burst occurs as Fc receptors are not involved. Complement receptor types 1 and 3 as well as fibronectin and vitronectin receptors have all been demonstrated to have a function in invasion. Macrophages perform three important defensive functions; firstly, release of antimycobacterial metabolites; secondly, release of cytokines; and thirdly, processing and presentation of mycobacterial antigens to T cells. The released cytokines play specific roles in the disease process as well as anti-mycobacterial activities. For example, a synergistic reaction between TNF and INF-γ results in production of nitric oxide metabolites and contributes to granuloma formation. Conversely, TNF is known to induce fever, weight loss and tissue necrosis – all symptoms typical of tuberculosis (Barnes *et al.*, 1994).

The normal route for macrophage killing of bacteria is the fusion of the phagosome with lysosomes. However, phagolysosomal fusion is inhibited by virulent strains of *M. tuberculosis*, *M. leprae* and *M. avium*. Virulent *M. tuberculosis* is found free in the macrophage cytoplasm, as well as in membrane-bound extrusions of the phago-

lysosome in which replication continues. Avirulent *M. tuberculosis* also form these extra-phagolysosomal vesicles but do not undergo replication. *M. bovis* BCG does not escape the phagolysosome. The presence of mycobacteria in the macrophage cytoplasm makes mycobacterial antigens available for processing via the MHC class I pathway, leading to CD8$^+$ T cell activation. As has been already discussed, components of the mycobacterial cell wall, e.g. LAM and PGL-1, specifically interfere with the normal protective responses of the macrophage, blocking macrophage activation and inhibiting release of reactive metabolites. This facilitates the survival of the bacterium.

Idiopathic Diseases and Autoimmune Disease

The aetiology of a range of autoimmune or idiopathic diseases suggests a role for the mycobacteria, although the evidence for a direct involvement for mycobacteriosis remains equivocal. These infections are characterized by a spectrum of pathology that relates to the balance between T cell-mediated and antibody-mediated responses. They are characteristically diseases of the lung, gut or skin and are accompanied by arthritis, autoantibodies and raised levels of agalactosyl IgG. A clear example of this pattern is Takayasu's arteritis. This granulomatous arteritis has a demonstrated association with tuberculosis but bacteria are often not demonstrable. Other conditions in which mycobacteria have been implicated are rheumatoid arthritis, Crohn's disease, ulcerative colitis, sarcoidosis and psoriasis; all these diseases have the characteristics described (Rook and Stanford, 1992).

Particular attention has been paid to the role of mycobacterioses in Crohn's disease as the clinically similar disease of ruminants, Johne's disease, has been demonstrated to result from the colonization of the intestinal mucosa by *M. paratuberculosis* (Thompson, 1994). Both diseases are chronic granulomatous diseases of the gut affecting nutrient adsorption. There are three strands of evidence for a mycobacterial role in Crohn's disease: the isolation of mycobacteria from

Crohn's disease tissue; development of a granulomatous disease when *M. avium* or *M. paratuberculosis* is administered to neonatal animals; and *M. avium* and *M. paratuberculosis* DNA detected by polymerase chain reaction (PCR) in some though not all studies of cultured Crohn's disease tissues. However, despite the wealth of data seeking a role for the mycobacteria in Crohn's disease the case remains neither proved nor disproved (Thompson, 1994).

The pathology of these autoimmune diseases may be associated with the continued presence of low numbers of viable organisms that drive an inappropriate T cell response. Candidate antigens for this process have been identified amongst the HSPs following the observation that T cells from susceptible rats with Freund's adjuvant-induced arthritis not only are capable of transferring the arthritis but also recognize mycobacterial hsp65 (van Eden *et al.*, 1988). The significance of mycobacterial HSPs in the development of autoimmune disease may be explained by one of three hypotheses, each of which has some degree of supporting evidence. The first case may be simple cross-reactivity between host and mycobacterial HSPs resulting in autoimmune responses. The second hypothesis depends on the specific recognition of HSPs due to their protective role on exposure of the bacterium to the stress associated with the inflammatory response. These highly conserved proteins thus indicate the presence of a stressed pathogen to the host immune response; autoimmunity is an accidental consequence. The final hypothesis relates to the possibility that self-derived HSPs may be adopted as targets for cytotoxic cells, enabling the identification and elimination of stressed host cells indicating the presence of infection.

The evidence for the role of mycobacterioses in development of autoimmune disease is accumulating and in the context of the pathology of tuberculosis and leprosy perhaps is unsurprising; however, there are still considerable anomalies in the data available which need to be addressed before we have a full understanding of this disease process.

LABORATORY DIAGNOSIS

Organization of Laboratories for Diagnosis of Mycobacterial Infection

In countries where the incidence of tuberculosis declined isolation of *M. tuberculosis* became a relatively rare occurrence. This led to a general fall in standards and a rationalization of *Mycobacterium* diagnostic services. To combat this most countries adopt a three-level structure; in the UK, for example, most laboratories will examine smears and culture specimens, sending positive isolates to a regional reference laboratory for identification and first-line sensitivity testing. The national Mycobacterial Reference Laboratory provides a full sensitivity and identification service and organizes a quality control programme (Marks, 1975; Collins *et al.*, 1985). In the USA 'Level I' laboratories collect specimens, may examine smears and forward specimens to a Level II laboratory which cultures specimens, identifies tubercle bacilli and may perform susceptibility testing. Level III laboratories provide a comprehensive diagnostic service and do research (American Thoracic Society, 1983). In developing countries simple smear examination should be provided at district hospitals. A proportion of all specimens and all specimens from patients failing or relapsing on therapy should be sent to a regional or national reference laboratory for culture, identification and sensitivity testing.

Specimens

It is true to say that almost any specimen is suitable for mycobacterial examination but the investigation of each disease requires a different protocol. When pulmonary infection is suspected the principal specimen is sputum but not all patients are capable of producing satisfactory specimens. This may be due to physical weakness or failure to coordinate the effort required for effective specimen production, and some patients have a non-productive cough. Children are very rarely capable of producing sputum. When sputum is not available an early-morning gastric lavage is an alternative. Fluid is aspirated from the gastric contents, which will contain respiratory secretions coughed up and swallowed during the night. Bronchial alveolar lavage, however, provides a better specimen and should be obtained wherever facilities for its collection exist. In this technique individual bronchopulmonary segments are lavaged with saline and the washings collected. The lavage is concentrated by centrifugation and used for direct microscopic examination and culture.

Specimens must be subdivided into those which are sterile or contaminated: those that are normally sterile are particularly suitable for mycobacterial culture as they do not require decontamination (see below); this includes cerebrospinal fluid (CSF), blood, bone marrow, pleural, pericardial, peritoneal and joint fluid. In addition aspirated pus from abscesses may be examined, as may tissue biopsies from any tissue. Contaminated specimens include sputum and faeces. Specimens of urine are required for diagnosis of renal tuberculosis. Twenty-four-hour collections are very likely to become contaminated so early-morning specimens (usually three) are preferred. In the diagnosis of disseminated *M. avium–intracellulare* infection in HIV-infected people faeces can be examined by microscopy and culture.

Sputum specimens should be collected into wide-mouth glass or plastic pots; 2–5 ml should be collected, preferably of early-morning sputum. A minimum of three specimens should be examined.

Aspirated fluids and pus specimens should be collected in sterile universal containers. Containers for pleural, peritoneal or joint fluids should contain an anticoagulant. Tissue specimens should be placed dry in a sterile universal container. Specimens should be transported to the laboratory with the minimum of delay and, whenever possible, processed immediately. If this is not possible they should be stored at 4 °C. Specimens can be transported through the post if appropriate postal regulations are adhered to (Marks, 1975).

Microscopy

Sputum

Microscopy of sputum is one of the most important investigations in mycobacteriology, not only providing a rapid result but also identifying the patients thought to be most important in transmission of disease. A smear may be made directly from sputum or following digestion and centrification. It is difficult to make a consistent, even preparation using undigested sputum. Portions of the slide which are too thick will prevent organisms being seen and may float off during the staining process, causing a biological hazard. Digestion and centrifugation are favoured as the deposit is aqueous and makes a better film. The slides are easier to examine, with less background debris.

Fluid specimens

Specimens of CSF are very valuable and should be processed with great care. A circle should be drawn on the glass slide with a diamond marker, and a drop should be placed within the mark and allowed to dry before subsequent drops are added, thus concentrating the specimen. Aspirated fluid should be concentrated by centrifugation before being placed on a slide. Smears of pus and thick aspirates must be made carefully to provide thin, even preparations. Urine and gastric washings should not be examined microscopically as commensal mycobacteria and acid-fast bacilli in food may result in a false positive diagnosis.

Staining

There are two principal methods for staining mycobacteria. These are: variants on the traditional Ziehl–Neelsen method, and auramine–phenol staining followed by fluorescence microscopy. Ziehl–Neelsen stain is the preferred technique when small numbers of specimens are to be examined. However, when the throughput of specimens is high, the auramine–phenol method should be adopted as it facilitates screening of large numbers of specimens. Although sensitive, this latter technique is less specific and strict criteria for positivity must be laid down (i.e. three fluorescent bacilli) and it is prudent for all fluorescent-positive specimens to be over-stained by the Ziehl–Neelsen method, to confirm the morphology of acid-fast objects.

Ziehl–Neelsen stain The principles of this method were laid down originally by Robert Koch in 1882, and modified in the subsequent year by Ziehl, Erlich and Neelsen. Carbol–fuchsin is driven into the bacterial cell wall by heating the specimen, decolorized with acid–alcohol and counterstained with methylene blue. Organisms which are truly acid fast will retain the carbol–fuchsin in the face of decolorization with acid–alcohol solution. In specimens where *M. leprae* or *Nocardia* spp. are suspected, a weaker acid solution must be used. Cold staining methods (e.g. Kinyouin) can be used where the stain is taken into the bacteria using dimethylsulphoxide or Tween 80. Approximately 6.9×10^3 cfu/ml are required for a 50% chance of a positive result (Cruickshank, 1952).

When very large numbers must be processed automated machines may be used and some studies have shown that these do not result in cross-contamination. They have rarely gained acceptance in routine microbiology laboratories.

The number of bacilli present in the patient's sputum may reflect the severity of the disease. It is traditional to quantify the number of acid-fast bacilli present in the patient's sputum. The fact that organisms may in fact be dead or that individual specimens may represent significant sampling errors means that any quantitative results should be viewed with a degree of caution. However, overall trends in smear positivity when viewed over a number of weeks may be useful. Quantitation is performed on the basis of the number of positive bacilli present in each field, as set out in Table 6a.2 (Collins *et al.*, 1985).

Decontamination

Mycobacterial culture requires long incubation periods and mycobacteria would be readily overgrown if they were not decontaminated before inoculation onto selective media (see below). The

TABLE 6a.2 EXAMPLE OF A SIMPLE METHOD FOR QUANTIFYING MYCOBACTERIA IN ZIEHL–NEELSEN STAINED SPUTUM SMEARS

No. of acid-fast organisms seen	Report
None[a]	–
1–10 in 100 fields	+
1–10 in 10 fields	+ +
1–10 per fields	+ + +
>10 per field	+ + + +

[a] At least 300 high-power fields should be examined.

process of decontamination is one which reduces the number of viable bacterial organisms and may be divided into stringent and non-stringent methods depending on whether they inhibit conventional bacteria only (non-stringent), or also inhibit mycobacteria (stringent). The standard technique for many laboratories is to treat sputum with 4% sodium hydroxide by shaking at room temperature for 15 minutes; *N*-acetylcysteine, a mucolytic, can also be added. The sodium hydroxide method is stringent and therefore must be strictly controlled. If digestion periods are extended for more than 15 minutes, there will be significant loss of mycobacteria and consequent false negative results. An even more stringent method uses oxalic acid. Astringent methods inhibit only normal non-mycobacterial species and are suitable for specimens which are not likely to be heavily contaminated. Sputum is digested with trisodium phosphate with or without the addition of benzalkonium chloride.

Some specimens such as urine are not always contaminated, so rather than decontaminate all specimens a Gram stain can be performed and if no organisms are seen the specimen can be inoculated directly onto mycobacterial medium; otherwise an astringent method can be applied.

An alternative approach to physical decontamination is the use of liquid antibiotic containing medium such as Kirschners (see below) (Mitchison *et al.*, 1972, 1983).

Culture

Where resources are available it is essential to culture all specimens. This is required not only to confirm the identity of organisms seen on direct microscopy and confirm the sensitivity of wild-type strains but also, more importantly, because culture is more sensitive than direct microscopy. Approximately 10^4 organisms per millilitre are required for positive microscopy whereas as few as 10 will result in a positive culture (Cruickshank, 1952). In addition modern typing methods can now distinguish between strains of *M. tuberculosis* (see below) and this enables epidemiological relationships between organisms to be determined (e.g. cross-infection in the hospital environment) (van Embden *et al.*, 1993).

Media

There are three main groups of media used for the culture of mycobacteria: egg-based media, agar-based media and fluid media. Egg-based media are used for primary isolation in most laboratories. A number of variants have been described, including Lowenstein–Jensen, Stonebrink and International Union Against Tuberculosis. Each of these contains inspissated egg to form a solid surface. Contaminating organisms are inhibited by use of varying concentrations of malachite green and the growth of *M. bovis* is encouraged by the incorporation of pyruvate in the medium and the growth of the human strain *M. tuberculosis* is enhanced by glycerol.

Middlebrooks media (7H10, 7H11 and comb) are not usually used for primary isolation: their role is usually confined to identification and sensitivity testing. These media do not contain eggs so an alternative source of lipid must be provided, usually oleic acid. Antibiotics may be added and the medium is supplemented by albumin, dextrose and catalase (Collins *et al.*, 1985). Some of the media used in cultivation of mycobacteria are listed in Table 6a.3.

Fluid media Several fluid media have been described and they have an important role in culture of precious specimens. A larger inoculum is possible and up to 0.5 ml can be inoculated in a fluid medium. One of the most popular media is that of Kirschner, which is made selective by the

TABLE 6a.3 EXAMPLES OF MEDIA USED FOR ISOLATION AND IDENTIFICATION OF MYCOBACTERIA

Egg-based media using malachite green for selection
Lowenstein–Jensen
International Union Against Tuberculosis medium
American Thoracic Society medium
Stonebrink medium

Synthetic media
Kirchner
Kirchner Selective
Acid egg medium
Middlebrook (7Hg broth, 7H10 agar)
Middlebrook OADC enrichment

addition of antibiotics: polymyxin B, carbenicillin, trimethoprim and ampicillin (Mitchison *et al.*, 1983). A combination of two slopes of an egg-based medium such as Lowenstein–Jenssen, one each with pyruvate and glycerol, plus a fluid medium such as Kirschner's is probably the optimal combination for the isolation of mycobacteria. Cultures should be incubated at 37 °C and a duplicate set should be incubated at 30–32 °C when the presence of *M. marinum* is suspected. The slopes should be inspected two to three days after inoculation to detect the presence of rapid growth or contaminants. After this they should be inspected weekly for a minimum of eight weeks. Some larger laboratories will also examine specimens for up to 12 weeks. When colonies are seen on the slopes or the fluid medium becomes cloudy a Ziehl–Neelsen preparation should be made to confirm the identity of the organism isolated. The morphology of colonies on Ziehl–Neelsen staining may be a useful identification criterion (see below).

The radiometric automated blood culture system 'BACTEC 400' has been adapted for mycobacterial culture (Vincke *et al.*, 1982). Mycobacteria are detected by incorporating radioactive ^{14}C-labelled palmitate which is taken up by the organism and metabolized with production of radiolabelled carbon dioxide. The main advantage of this system is that positive cultures are detected much more quickly. When a positive culture is indicated a sample is taken so that the growth can be confirmed by Ziehl–Neelsen and subcultured for identification and sensitivity testing by conventional or adapted radiometric techniques.

Identification

Methods to identify positive isolates can now be divided into two main types: conventional and molecular. Conventional identification is divided into two phases: screening examination and definitive identification. The clinical microbiologist's first priority is to define isolates which belong to the tuberculosis complex. Simple screening tests have been devised which select out these groups of organisms and enable a rapid presumptive identification to be made. These use a range of simple characteristics enabling a result to be given within 10 days, as follows. *Mycobacterium tuberculosis* on Ziehl–Neelsen staining shows characteristic cording (see Figure 6a.5), and is sensitive to paranitrobenzoic acid, whereas other mycobacteria are resistant. Classical human tuberculosis is resistant to thiophen-2-carboxylic acid hydrazine (TCH) but other Asian, African and bovine strains are sensitive. The isolate should also be inoculated onto Lowenstein–Jensen glycerol broth (LJG) and incubated at 37 °C in the dark, in the light and also at 25 °C. Using this combination of tests, strains of the tuberculosis group can be reliably identified using Table 6a.4 (Collins *et al.*,

1985). A BACTEC method uses the ability of *p*-nitro-α-acetylamino-β-hydroxypropiophenone (NAP) to inhibit *M. tuberculosis* complex but not other mycobacterial species.

The identification of other species of mycobacteria requires a wide range of identification tests and this is usually beyond the scope of any single routine laboratory. These tests include a study of pigmentation production and photoreactivity. Some mycobacteria synthesize carotenoid pigments which give the colonies a yellow or red pigmentation. Some organisms exhibit this characteristic when grown in the absence of light and are therefore known as scotochromogens. Photochromogens, in contrast, require light for carotenogenesis to take place. Many mycobacteria do not produce pigment under any circumstances and are known as non-chromogens. This phenomenon was once the basis of a simple classification system by Runyon which has now been superseded.

Mycobacteria have different temperature growth optima; this characteristic reflects differences in their natural environment and can be used for identification. Strains are tested for their ability to grow at 25, 30, 33, 37, 42 and 45 °C. Resistance to anti-tuberculosis agents is, for many species, a stable characteristic; thus resistance testing can be used to separate species. *Mycobacterium kansasii* is naturally resistant to isoniazid, and most mycobacteria other than tuberculosis with the exception of *M. kansasii* are resistant to thiacetazone. TCH and other antibiotics which may be used to speciate mycobacteria include streptomycin, ethambutol, ethionamide, cycloserine and pyrazinamide. Resistance to oleate is tested by the same method.

The presence of various biochemical activities is also a useful identification characteristic and the following enzymes are tested: catalase, a lipase which hydrolyses Tween 80, urease, nitrate reductase, acid phosphatase, aryl sulphatase, pyrazinamidase α-esterase and has the ability to reduce tellurite. Some mycobacteria have a block in the nicotinamide adenine dinucleotide (NAD) scavenging pathway and accumulate extracellular niacin. This is a characteristic of *M. tuberculosis*, *M. simiae* and some *M. avium* spp.

By collating the results of all of these test results

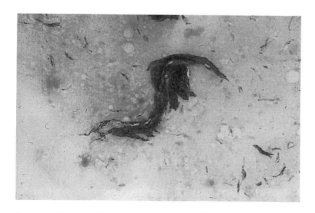

Figure 6a.5. Ziehl–Neelsen stain of colony isolated on Lowenstein–Jensen medium demonstrating the typical cording of *Mycobacterium tuberculosis*.

TABLE 6a.4 RESULTS OF TESTS AND USED IN SEPARATING *M. TUBERCULOSIS* COMPLEX FROM OTHER MYCOBACTERIA

Test	*M. tuberculosis* complex	Mycobacteria other than tuberculosis
Microscopy	Cording	No cording
Growth at 37 °C	+	+
Growth at 25 °C	−	+
Pigment	−	±
Growth on pNB	−	±
Growth on NAP (BACTEC)	−	+

most species of mycobacteria can be identified; examples of some of the more commonly isolated species are recorded in Table 6a.5.

Mycolic acid profile

The pattern of mycolic acids is species specific and may be examined for speciation. The mycolic acid profile is constant in the species and also varies between different genera, such as *Corynebacterium, Gordona, Nocardia, Rhodococcus* and *Tsukamurella* (McNeil and Brennan, 1991). The mycolic acid profile can be determined by thin-layer, high-pressure liquid and gas–liquid chromatographic methods. These methods are more suitable for research than routine diagnosis (Jenkins, 1981; Luquin *et al.*, 1991; Kolk *et al.*, 1994). Pyrolysis–mass spectroscopy has also been used successfully (Sisson *et al.*, 1992).

Molecular identification

As an alternative a molecular approach to speciation can be employed and this approach is likely to become more common in the future. A species-specific molecular technique can be applied to colonies or positive broth cultures enabling a rapid identification of clinically important species, e.g. *M. tuberculosis* and *M. avium–intracellulare*, to be made (Gonzalez and Hanna, 1987; Bull and Shanson, 1992). The techniques which may be employed in this way are Southern hybridization with specific probes, or the PCR (see below). Obviating the need for culture over prolonged periods, this latter approach shortens the time to

definitive species diagnosis. It is, however, limited to those species for which probes or PCR primers have been described. At the moment, for practical purposes this limits it largely to isolates of *M. tuberculosis* and *M. avium–intracellulare* in routine laboratories. Considerable care must be taken in evaluating these techniques to prevent false positive reactions.

DNA probes

DNA probes can be used for the identification of several species of *Mycobacterium*, including *M. tuberculosis*, *M. avium–intracellulare*, *M. kansasii* and *M. gordonae* (Evans *et al.*, 1992, Gonzalez and Hanna, 1987; Bull and Shanson, 1992). Labelled complementary DNA binds to bacterial DNA or RNA to form a stable hybrid. The formation of the hybrid, and thus a positive identification, is made usually by chemo-luminescent detection systems. These probes are commercially available and they may be used to identify isolates cultured conventionally in the BACTEC system. Current DNA probes seem to lack the sensitivity for reliable direct diagnosis from patients' specimens without amplification.

The transcription-mediated amplification system is an isothermal process which provides a 10^9 amplification of the rRNA target of the DNA probe. It can be applied to decontaminated sputum specimens, providing positive results in less than 6 hours. In comparison to conventional culture methods a sensitivity of 97.2% and a specificity of 96.1% have been obtained (Telenti *et al.*, 1994).

TABLE 6a.5 EXAMPLES OF CHARACTERISTICS OF COMMONLY ISOLATED *MYCOBACTERIA*

Species	Pigment	Growth at (°C)					Nitratase	Sulphatase (21 days)	Catalase	Tellurite reduction	Tween hydrolysis	Thiacetazone
		20	25	33	42	44						
M. kansasii	P	−	+	+	v	−	+	+	+++		+	s
M. marinum	P	+	+	+	−	−	−	++	++		+	r
M. avium−intracellulare	−/S	v	+	+	+	v	−	v	−	+	−	v
M. xenopi	−/S	−	−	−	+	+	−	+++	−	−	−	r
M. ulcerans	−/S	−	−	+	−	−	−	−	−	−	−	r
M. fortuitum	−	+	+	+	v	−	+	+++	v	+	−	r
M. chelonei	−	+	+	+	−	−	−	+++	v	+	−	r
M. malmoense	−	−	+	+	−	−	+	−	−	−	+	r

s, sensitive; r, resistant; v, variable; P, photochromogen; S, scotochromogen.
Based on Collins *et al.* (1985).

Polymerase chain reaction

PCR is particularly suitable for the diagnosis of organisms which cannot be cultivated or are slow to grow, and where susceptibilities are predictable or initial treatment is by a standard protocol. The competing conventional methods – culture, Lowenstein–Jensen medium or radiometric broth (BACTEC) – are slow by comparison and initial therapy is an agreed regimen. Consequently the PCR result provides a significant clinical advantage. A wide range of different targets have been selected for amplification, including genes which code for immunologically characterized antigens. The first *M. tuberulosis* PCR used the insertion sequence IS6110, which was originally defined in an *M. fortuitum* plasmid. This is present in almost every isolate of *M. tuberculosis*, usually in multiple copies; this gives the PCR system added sensitivity (Brisson-Noel *et al.*, 1991). A small number of strains contain fewer than five copies and *M. bovis* contains only one copy. Genes coding for the 65, 38 and 32 kDa antigens and superoxide dismutase have been used. This subject has recently been reviewed (Hawkey, 1994). One of the PCR methods directed against the 16S ribosomal RNA is commercially available (Larocco *et al.*, 1994). Several trials of PCR diagnosis have been reported indicating that PCR diagnosis may have superior or equivalent sensitivity as microscopy. Only a few blinded trials have been completed to date, one study suggesting a superiority for IS6110 sequences over 65 kDa

sequences (Noordhoek *et al.*, 1994; deLassence *et al.*, 1992; Walker *et al.*, 1992). PCR has usually been applied to diagnosis in sputum, but also has an application to sterile fluids such as CSF or peritoneal fluid. *Mycobacterium*-specific DNA can also be found in the lymphocyte fraction of peripheral blood (Kolk *et al.*, 1994). Like culture and microscopy, PCR has been shown to be valuable in the early detection of relapse. In this circumstance PCR has much to offer although it might have slightly inferior performance to culture. The results are available almost immediately, enabling patients who are relapsing to be treated quickly (Kennedy *et al.*, 1994).

Susceptibility Testing

The concept of susceptibility as usually applied in microbiological investigation cannot be so readily applied to testing of mycobacteria. The long incubation periods mean that conventional disk susceptibility and broth minimal inhibitory concentration (MIC) methods are not suitable. In any population of mycobacteria, organisms which are spontaneously resistant to anti-tuberculosis drugs will be found.

Methods

There are three main methods in common use: the proportion method, which is very popular in the USA but is also used in Europe; the resistance ratio method, mainly used in the UK and anglophone Africa and India; and a radiometric method which utilizes the BACTEC system.

Proportion method In this method Felson quadrant plates are used. One quadrant contains drug-free medium, usually Middlebrook 7H10, and the other three contain different concentrations of the anti-tuberculosis agent being tested against the isolate. Each quadrant is inoculated with three drops of a suspension of organisms and the plates are sealed and incubated for up to three weeks. The culture rates are examined without opening the plate by looking through the base. The number of colonies on each quadrant is counted and an organism is defined as resistant if the number of colonies in the drug-containing medium is 1% or more of the number found on the drug-free medium (Heifets, 1988).

Resistance ratio method In the resistance ratio method Lowenstein–Jensen medium is used. Test organisms are inoculated onto medium containing different concentrations of antibiotics and a set of non-drug containing slopes. A battery of 'wild-type' strains which are sensitive to the test antibiotics are inoculated in parallel with the test strains. The MIC of individual strains is divided by the modal resistance of the control 'wild-type' strains to define a resistance ratio. Strains giving a resistance ratio of 1 or 2 are reported as sensitive, those giving a resistance ratio of 4 are defined as resistant, and those giving a resistance ratio of 8 as highly resistant. Due to the need to inoculate a battery of control strains, this method is not suitable for laboratories only examining a few isolates per week. As this method uses Lowenstein-Jensen, an egg-containing medium, there is a possibility that antibiotic binding to the albumin will interfere with the results of the test. However, as the results are defined as a ratio this means that effects on the test strain are cancelled out by similar effects on the control strains and it is the simplicity of this technique and robustness for which it is favoured (Collins *et al.*, 1985).

The radiometric BACTEC method The radiometric BACTEC method has been developed for susceptibility testing using a variant of the proportion method. A standard suspension is made and inoculated into a vial containing antibiotic at an appropriate 'breakpoint' concentration. A 1:100 dilution is inoculated into a non-drug-containing vial. The growth index is checked daily and if growth in the drug containing and 1:100 non-drug-containing vial are equal, resistance is implied. Radiometric sensitivity testing is especially valuable in the context of increasing multi-drug resistance where rapid assessment of susceptibility is of critical importance, or for testing of mycobacteria other than tuberculosis where sensitivity patterns are less predictable (Laszlo *et al.*, 1983; Roberts *et al.*, 1983).

Chemiluminescence A method similar in concept to the radiometric method has recently been reported which utilizes chemiluminescence. All living bacteria contain ATP and this substance is used as the energy source in the 'fire-fly' luciferin/luciferase light reaction. The chemical reaction which gives fire-flies their brightly lit tails depends on the enzyme luciferase acting on luciferin with the release of light. In this reaction the amount of light generated is directly proportional to the amount of ATP present in a specimen and therefore proportional to the number of viable organisms. As in the BACTEC method, mycobacterial test strains are incubated for five days and the concentration of ATP or light, or organisms, is detected using a luminometer. Suppression of growth in a 1:100 dilution in comparison to drug-free growth indicates sensitivity.

New methods With the threat of multi-drug-resistant strains, several new attempts have been made for even more rapid detection of resistance. Most novel of these is the mycobacterial 'reporter' phage method described by Jacobs and colleagues (Cooksey *et al.*, 1993). A mycobacterial phage into which the luciperase gene has been cloned is incubated with organisms which have been grown in the presence or absence of antibiotics. Light production is dependent on phage infection, which can only occur in viable organisms. Those strains susceptible to the antibiotic will be killed and the phage will be unable to infect and thus there will be no light production in the luciferin/lucipherase reaction. In contrast, resistant strains will be infected and will glow brightly. Considerable development of this technique is required before it becomes available for routine use.

Molecular methods   Until recently the molecular mechanisms of mycobacterial drug resistance were obscure (see below). For some, resistance arises as a result of a deletion of critical genes, e.g. *katG*, the gene which encodes for the catalase enzyme and is essential for isoniazid susceptibility (Zhang *et al.*, 1992). Other isoniazid resistance is due to point mutation with the *inhA* gene (Zhang and Young, 1993). For other drugs such as rifampicin, resistance is due to point mutations in the RNA polymerase gene *rpoB*, most of which occur in a 'hot spot' (Telenti *et al.*, 1993). The mutated genes result in a RNA polymerase which has lower affinity for the rifampicin molecule. The molecular basis for resistance to other anti-tuberculosis agents has been elucidated, including streptomycin, ethambutol and 4-fluoroquinolones (see Table 6a.6) (Zhang and Young, 1994). This opens the possibility of rapid resistance testing using molecular methods. The presence or absence of these genes can be detected by the PCR. Point mutations can be differentiated by using the single-strand confirmation polymorphism method (Telenti *et al.*, 1993). The two strands of the products are separated by heating and then run on an acrylamide gel. Point mutation results in changes in the confirmation of the single-stranded DNA, which means that the mutated DNA runs at a different speed from native DNA, allowing these differences to be detected.

Typing   There has been a long-standing need for effective typing methods for *M. tuberculosis*. Previously reported methods included serology but this was difficult to use as a large number of strains auto-agglutinate. Phage-typing methods have been described but have not been widely applied.

The restriction fragment length polymorphism (RFLP) method has been applied to typing of *M. tuberculosis*. Genomic DNA is isolated and

TABLE 6a.6 MOLECULAR MECHANISMS OF ANTI-TUBERCULOSIS DRUG RESISTANCE

Anti-tuberculosis agent	Gene
Isoniazid	*KatG inhA*
Rifampicin	*rpoB*
Ciprofloxacin	*gyrA*
Streptomycin	*rpsL*

digested with *Pvu* II, run on an agarose gel, and blotted onto nitrocellulose. A probe to the insertion sequence IS6110 is hybridized with it, giving a ladder-like pattern (Van Soolingen *et al.*, 1991). This insertion sequence is present in almost all *M. tuberculosis* isolates from one to more than 20 copies. Comparison between patterns can be used to determine epidemiological relationships between isolates. The methodology has been standardized to enable comparisons to be made between laboratories and countries. It has proved valuable in determining cross-infection in the hospital environment, identifying routes of transmission for multi-drug-resistant strains or contamination of equipment, and it has been used to detect cross-contamination within the laboratory. Studies in Australia and Switzerland in alcoholics and intravenous drug abusers showed that strains which were circulating in these closed communities were being transmitted to the general population. When sophisticated scanning and computer analysis is applied to this method, relationships between strains, which were not identical, can be derived using a similarity coefficient. This has the potential to be applied to the study of transmission with much larger communities (Gillespie *et al.*, 1995). New alternative probes using repetitive epitopes are becoming available to type strains where IS6110 is not appropriate, notably low-copy number strains.

Serology   Serology has never proved valuable in the routine diagnosis of mycobacterial infection and a large number of methods have been described (Krambovitis, 1986). Most recently a peptide from a 38 kDa protein has been evaluated with some success in patients with smear-negative tuberculosis.

REFERENCES

Adams, L.B., Fukutomi, Y. and Krahenbuhl, J.L. (1993) Regulation of murine macrophage effector functions by lipoarabinomannan from mycobacterial strains with different degrees of virulence. *Infection and Immunity*, **61**, 4173–4181.

American Thoracic Society (1983) Levels of laboratory services for mycobacterial diseases. *American Review of Respiratory Diseases*, **128**, 213.

Andersen, A.B. and Brennan, P. (1994) Proteins and antigens of *Mycobacterium tuberculosis*. In *Tuberculosis: Pathogenesis, Protection, and Control* (ed. B.R. Bloom), pp. 307–332. American Society for Microbiology, Washington, DC.

Barnes, P.F., Modlin, R.L. and Ellner, J.J. (1994) T-cell responses and cytokines. In *Tuberculosis: Pathogenesis, Protection, and Control* (ed. B.R. Bloom), pp. 415–417. American Society for Microbiology, Washington, DC.

Besra, G.S. and Chatterjee, D. (1994) Lipids and carbohydrates of *Mycobacterium tuberculosis*. In *Tuberculosis: Pathogenesis, Protection, and Control* (ed. B.R. Bloom), pp. 285–306. American Society for Microbiology, Washington, DC.

Brisson-Noel, A., Aznar, C., Chureau, C. *et al.* (1991) Diagnosis of tuberculosis by DNA amplification in clinical practice evaluation. *Lancet*, **338**, 364–366.

Britton, W.J., Roche, P.W. and Winter, N. (1994) Mechanisms of persistence of mycobacteria. *Trends in Microbiology*, **2**, 284–288.

Bull, T.J. and Shanson, D.C. (1992) Evaluation of a commercial chemiluminescent gene probe system 'AccuProbe' for the rapid differentiation of mycobacteria, including 'MAIC X', isolated from blood and other sites, from patients with AIDS. *Journal of Hospital Infection*, **21**, 143–149.

Chan, J. and Kaufmann, S.H.E. (1994) Immune mechanisms of protection. In *Tuberculosis: Pathogenesis, Protection, and Control* (ed. B.R. Bloom), pp. 389–415. American Society for Microbiology, Washington, DC.

Collins, C.H., Grange, J.M. and Yates, M.D. (1985) *Organization and Practice in Tuberculosis Bacteriology*. Butterworth, London.

Cooksey, R.C., Crawford, J.T., Jacobs, W.R. and Shinnick, T.M. (1993) A rapid method for screening antimicrobial agents for activities against a strain of *Mycobacterium tuberculosis* expressing firefly luciferase. *Antimicrobial Agents and Chemotherapy*, **37**, 1348–1352.

Cruickshank, D.B. (1952) Bacteriology. In *Modern Practice in Tuberculosis* (ed. T.H. Sellors and J.L. Livingstone), p. 53. Butterworth, London.

Danneburg, A.M. and Rook, G.A.W. (1994) Pathogenesis of pulmonary tuberculosis: an interplay of tissue-damaging and macrophage-activating immune responses: dual mechanisms that control bacillary multiplication. In *Tuberculosis: Pathogenesis, Protection and Control* (ed. B.R. Bloom), pp. 459–483. American Society for Microbiology, Washington, DC.

deLassence, A., Lecossier, D., Pierre, C. *et al.* (1992) Detection of mycobacterial DNA in pleural fluid from patients with tuberculous pleurisy by means of the polymerase chain reaction: comparison of two protocols. *Thorax*, **47**, 265–269.

Evans, K.D., Nakasone, A.S., Sutherland, P.A. *et al.* (1992) Identification of *Mycobacterium tuberculosis* and *Mycobacterium avium–intracellulare* directly from primary BACTEC cultures by using acridinium-ester-labeled DNA probes. *Journal of Clinical Microbiology*, **30**, 2427–2431.

Flynn, J.L., Goldstein, M.M., Triebold, K.J. *et al.* (1992) Major histocompatibility complex class I-restricted T cells are required for resistance to *Mycobacterium tuberculosis* infection. *Proceedings of the National Academy of Sciences of the USA*, **89**, 12013–12017.

Fridovich, I. (1978) The biology of oxygen radicals. *Science*, **201**, 875–880.

Gillespie S.H., Kennedy N., Ngowi F.I. *et al.* (1995) Restriction fragment length polymorphism (RFLP) analysis of *Mycobacterium tuberculosis* isolated from patients with pulmonary tuberculosis in Northern Tanzania. *Transactions of the Royal Society of Tropical Medicine and Hygiene*, **89**, 335–339.

Gonzalez, R. and Hanna, B.A. (1987) Evaluation of Gen-Probe DNA hybridization systems for the identification of *Mycobacterium tuberculosis* and *Mycobacterium avium–intracellulare*. *Diagnostic Microbiology and Infectious Disease*, **8**, 69–77.

Grosskinsky, C.M., Jacobs, W.R., Jr, Clark-Curtiss, J.E. *et al.* (1989) Genetic relationships among *Mycobacterium leprae*, *Mycobacterium tuberculosis*, and candidate leprosy vaccine strains determined by DNA hybridization: identification of an *M. leprae*-specific repetitive sequence. *Infection and Immunity*, **57**, 1535–1541.

Hawkey, P.M. (1994) The role of polymerase chain reaction in the diagnosis of mycobacterial infections. *Reviews in Medical Microbiology*, **5**, 21–32.

Heifets, L. (1988) Qualitative and quantitative drug-susceptibility tests in mycobacteriology. *American Review of Respiratory Disease*, **137**, 1217–1222.

Hermans, P.W., Schuitema, A.R., Van Soolingen, D. *et al.* (1990) Specific detection of *Mycobacterium tuberculosis* complex strains by polymerase chain reaction. *Journal of Clinical Microbiology*, **28**, 1204–1213.

Jenkins, P.A. (1981) Lipid analysis for the identification

of mycobacteria: a reappraisal. *Reviews of Infectious Diseases*, **3**, 862–866.

Kennedy, N., Gillespie, S.H., Saruni, A.O. *et al.* (1994) Polymerase chain reaction for assessing treatment response in patients with pulmonary tuberculosis. *Journal of Infectious Diseases* **170**, 713–716.

Kolk, A.H.J., Kox, L.F.F., Kuijper, S. *et al.* (1994) Detection of *Mycobacterium tuberculosis* in peripheral blood. *Lancet*, **344**, 694.

Krambovitis, E. (1986) Detection of antibodies to *Mycobacterium tuberculosis* plasma membrane antigen by enzyme linked immunosorbent assay. *Journal of Medical Microbiology*, **21**, 257–264.

Lamb, J.R., Lathigra, R., Rothbard, J.B. *et al.* (1989) Identification of mycobacterial antigens recognised by T lymphocytes. *Reviews of Infectious Diseases*, **II** (S2), S443–S447.

Lanéelle, G. and Daffé, M. (1991) Mycobacterial cell wall and pathogenicity: a lipodologist's view. *Research in Microbiology*, **142**, 433–437.

Larocco, M.T., Wanger, A., Ocera, H. and Macias, E. (1994) Evaluation of a commercial rRNA amplification assay for direct detection of *Mycobacterium tuberculosis* in processed sputum. *European Journal of Clinical Microbiology and Infectious Diseases*, **13**, 726–731.

Laszlo, A., Gill, P., Handzel, V. *et al.* (1983) Conventional and radiometric drug susceptibility testing of *Mycobacterium tuberculosis* complex. *Journal of Clinical Microbiology*, **18**, 1335–1339.

Levy-Frebault, V.V. and Portaels, F. (1992) Proposed minimal standards for the genus *Mycobacterium* and the description of new slowly growing *Mycobacterium* species. *International Journal of Systematic Bacteriology*, **42**, 315–323.

Luquin, M., Ausina, V. and Lopez-Calahorra, F. (1991) Evaluation of practical chromatographic procedures for identification of clinical isolates of mycobacteria. *Journal of Clinical Microbiology*, **29**, 120–130.

Marks, J. (1975) Notes on the organization of tuberculosis bacteriology and its quality control. *Tubercle*, **56**, 219–226.

McNeil, M.R. and Brennan, P.J. (1991) Structure, function and biogenesis of the cell envelope of mycobacteria in relation to bacterial physiology, pathogenesis and drug resistance: some thoughts and possibilities arising from recent structural information. *Research in Microbiology*, **142**, 451–463.

Mitchison, D.A., Allen, B.W., Carrol, L. *et al.* (1972) A selective oleic acid albumin agar medium for tubercle bacilli. *Journal of Medical Microbiology*, **5**, 165–175.

Mitchison, D.A., Allen, B.W. and Manickavasagar, D. (1983) Selective Kirchner medium in the culture of specimens other than sputum for mycobacterium. *Journal of Clinical Pathology*, **36**, 1357–1361.

Murray, P.J. and Young, R.A. (1992) Stress and immunological recognition in host–pathogen interactions. *Journal of Bacteriology*, **174**, 4193–4196.

Noordhoek, G.T., Kolk, A.H., Bjune, G. *et al.* (1994) Sensitivity and specificity of PCR for detection of *Mycobacterium tuberculosis*: a blind comparison study among seven laboratories. *Journal of Clinical Microbiology*, **32**, 277–284.

Orme, I.M. (1993) The role of CD8+ T cells in immunity to tuberculosis infection. *Trends in Microbiology*, **1**, 77–78.

Pitulle, C., Dorsch, M., Kazda, J. *et al.* (1995) Phylogeny of rapidly growing members of the genus *Mycobacterium*. *International Journal of Systemic Bacteriology*, **42**, 337–343.

Rastogi, N. (1991) Recent observations concerning structure and function relationships in the mycobacterial cell envelope: elaboration of a model in terms of mycobacterial pathogenicity, virulence and drug-resistance. *Research in Microbiology*, **142**, 464–476.

Roberts, G.D., Goodman, N.L., Heifets, L. *et al.* (1983) Evaluation of the BACTEC radiometric method for recovery of mycobacteria and drug susceptibility testing of *Mycobacterium tuberculosis* from acid-fast smear-positive specimens. *Journal of Clinical Microbiology*, **18**, 689–696.

Rook, G.A.W. (1990) Mechanisms of immunologically mediated tissue damage during infection. In *Recent Advances in Dermatology* (ed. R.H. Champion and R.J. Pye), pp. 193–210. Churchill Livingstone, Edinburgh.

Rook, G.A. and Stanford, J.L. (1992) Slow bacterial infections or autoimmunity? *Immunology Today*, **13**, 160–164.

Ross, B.C., Jackson, K., Yang, M. *et al.* (1992) Identification of a genetically distinct subspecies of *Mycobacterium kansasii*. *Journal of Clinical Microbiology*, **30**, 2930–2933.

Sisson, P.R., Freeman, R., Magee, J.G. *et al.* (1992) Rapid differentiation of *Mycobacterium xenopi* from mycobacteria of the *Mycobacterium avium–intracellulare* complex by pyrolysis mass spectroscopy. *Journal of Clinical Pathology*, **45**, 355–357.

Telenti, A., Imboden, P., Marchesi, F. *et al.* (1993) Detection of rifampicin-resistance mutations in *Mycobacterium tuberculosis*. *Lancet*, **341**, 647–650.

Telenti, M., de Quiros, J.F., Alvarez, M. *et al.* (1994) The diagnostic usefulness of a DNA probe for *Mycobacterium tuberculosis* complex (Gen-Probe) in Bactec cultures versus other diagnostic methods. *Infection*, **22**, 18–23.

Thompson, D.E. (1994) The role of mycobacteria in Crohn's disease. *Journal of Medical Microbiology*, **41**, 74–94.

Thorel, M., Krichevsky, M. and Levy-Frebault, V.V.

(1990) Numerical taxonomy of mycobactin dependent mycobacteria, emended description of *Mycobacterium avium* subsp., *avium* nov., *Mycobacterium avium* subsp., *paratuberculosis* subsp., nov., and *Mycobacterium avium* subsp., *sylvaticum*. *International Journal of Systematic Bacteriology*, **40**, 254–260.

van Eden, W., Thole, J.E., van der Zee, R. *et al.* (1988) Cloning of the mycobacterial epitope recognized by T lymphocytes in adjuvant arthritis. *Nature*, **331**, 171–173.

van Embden, J.D.A., Cave, M.D., Crawford, J.T. *et al.* (1993) Strain identification of *Mycobacterium tuberculosis* by DNA fingerprinting: recommendations for a standardized methodology. *Journal of Clinical Microbiology*, **31**, 406–409.

van Soolingen, D., Hermans, P.W., de Haas, P.E. *et al.* (1991) Occurrence and stability of insertion sequences in *Mycobacterium tuberculosis* complex strains: evaluation of an insertion sequence-dependent DNA polymorphism as a tool in the epidemiology of tuberculosis. *Journal of Clinical Microbiology*, **29**, 2578–2586.

Vincke, G., Yegers, O., Vanachter, H. *et al.* (1982) Rapid susceptibility testing of *Mycobacterium tuberculosis* by a radiometric technique. *Journal of Antimicrobial Chemotherapy*, **10**, 351–354.

Walker, D.A., Taylor, I.K., Mitchell, D.M. *et al.* (1992) Comparison of polymerase chain reaction amplification of two mycobacterial DNA sequences, IS6110 and the 65Kda antigen gene, in the diagnosis of tuberculosis. *Thorax* **47**, 690–694.

Wayne, L.G., Good, R.C., Tsang, A. *et al.* (1993) Serovar determination and molecular taxonomic correlation in *Mycobacterium avium*, *Mycobacterium intracellulare*, and *Mycobacterium scrofulaceum*: a cooperative study of the international working group on mycobacterial taxonomy. *International Journal of Systematic Bacteriology*, **43**, 482–489.

Young, D.B., Kaufmann, S.H., Hermans, P.W. *et al.* (1992) Mycobacterial protein antigens: a compilation. *Molecular Microbiology*, **6**, 133–145.

Zhang, Y. and Young, D.B. (1993) Molecular mechanisms of isoniazid: a drug at the front line of tuberculosis control. *Trends in Microbiology*, **1**, 109–113.

Zhang, Y. and Young, D. (1994) Molecular genetics of drug resistance in *Mycobacterium tuberculosis*. *Journal of Antimicrobial Chemotherapy*, **34**, 313–319.

Zhang, Y., Heym, B., Allen, B. *et al.* (1992) The catalase peroxidase gene and isoniazid resistance of *Mycobacterium tuberculosis*. *Nature* **358**, 591–593.

6b

MYCOBACTERIUM TUBERCULOSIS

Stephen H. Gillespie

HISTORY

Described by Bunyan as the Captain of the men of death and by Oliver Wendell Holmes as the White Plague, tuberculosis has been and remains a major threat to human health. Many of the famous suffered from tuberculosis, including Purcell, the Brontë sisters, George Orwell and Keats.

Tuberculosis is a disease of great antiquity thought to have evolved during the neolithic period and its rise has been associated with the change from a hunter-gatherer lifestyle to pastoralism and farming. Skeletons from the neolithic period, and Egyptian mummies, have evidence of spinal tuberculosis. Ancient Chinese writing more than 4500 years old describes a lung fever with cough and wasting suggestive of tuberculosis. The disease was recognized by Hippocrates, who made an accurate clinical description and probably gave it the name phthisis, which recognized the characteristic wasting. Aristotle and Galen recognized that the disorder was contagious.

It is clear that tuberculosis was a major cause of death; in the seventeenth century 'bills of mortality' from England indicated that approximately 20% of deaths in 11 areas were caused by tuberculosis (1650). In Massachusetts during 1768–1773 pulmonary tuberculosis accounted for 18% of deaths, rising to 25% at the turn of the century. In Europe the peak of the tuberculosis epidemic was reached in the late eighteenth and early nineteenth centuries, while in Eastern Europe this peak was delayed several decades and only occurred in Asia in the late nineteenth and early twentieth centuries (Dubos and Dubos, 1952). In industrialized countries the impact of social improvement brought about a steady fall in the incidence of tuberculosis but was confounded by a steep rise during and after each of the two world wars. Tuberculosis is a disease of overcrowding and poor nutrition. Modern-day rates of tuberculosis correlate closely to economic indicators such as per capita income and unemployment (Enarson and Dirks, 1989).

NATURAL HISTORY OF TUBERCULOSIS INFECTION

When the host first encounters *M. tuberculosis* it is thought that neutrophils are the first phagocytes to come in contact with the organisms. Later macrophages are recruited and although the majority of organisms are probably killed, a number will survive. They are able to multiply inside macrophages and are transported to the regional lymphatics. In this site typical epithelioid cell

Principles and Practice of Clinical Bacteriology. Edited by A.M. Emmerson, P.M. Hawkey and S.H. Gillespie

granulomata develop and central necrosis typical of delayed type hypersensitivity develops associated with tuberculin conversion. As the epithelioid cells are activated and able to kill mycobacteria, most of the remaining organisms are found in an extracellular environment. Bacterial numbers may be very scanty. This initial lesion, a tuberculous bronchopneumonia, is known as the Gohn focus and this together with hilar lymphadenopathy is known as the primary complex of Ranke (Dannenberg, 1989). The bacteria spread via the lymphatics and the bloodstream to other parts of the body, including the brain, kidneys, bone, lungs and heart. In the majority of patients (more than 90%) infection does not progress to clinical disease but bacilli are able to survive at the original pulmonary focus of infection or any of the other organs. Long-term survival of the bacteria in these sites is responsible for persisting infection and relapse, which occurs as a result of failing immunity from many sources, including malnutrition, malignant disease, alcoholism, diabetes and acquired immunodeficiency syndrome, among others. Relapsing infection is also known as post-primary infection and there is an approximately 10% lifetime risk of this complication (Enarson and Rouillon, 1994). Clearly the acquisition of a disease which reduces the host's cell-mediated immunity makes recrudescence of tuberculosis more likely and this is now a common problem in patients dually infected with tuberculosis and HIV (Hawken *et al.*, 1993; Comstock, 1994). Post-primary infection can also arise as a result of exogenous reinfection; although once thought to be rare, it is now recognized that new infections are more common especially in immunocompromised hosts (Nardell *et al.*, 1986).

The main focus of pulmonary infection is in the lung but all other organs of the body can be involved, including the bones, kidney meninges, peritoneum and brain. In each of these sites tuberculous infection can be responsible for localized inflammation expanding space-occupying lesions, which may be followed by fibrosis and result in obstruction of a hollow viscus. Tuberculosis is therefore capable of mimicking almost any other clinical disease. The most common clinical manifestations of tuberculosis are reviewed below (see page 227).

EPIDEMIOLOGY OF TUBERCULOSIS

Mycobacterium tuberculosis is transmitted from person to person via the airborne route. It is spread on droplet nuclei 1–5 μm in diameter which remain suspended in the air for prolonged periods; transmission is consequently favoured when large numbers of organisms are expectorated and overcrowded poorly ventilated conditions exist. The likelihood of acquiring *M. tuberculosis* infection from a contact is a function of the duration and intensity of that contact. Children and patients with deficient cell-mediated immunity are more susceptible to infection (Enarson and Rouillon, 1994). On average approximately one in six people will become infected after contact with a single infectious case. In looking at the transmission dynamics there are three groups to consider: the susceptible individuals, latently infected individuals and active infective tuberculosis cases. Disease develops by one of two mechanisms: by direct progression soon after infection, or reactivation many years after infection. The risk of developing clinical disease is highest immediately after infection and declines exponentially. The incidence of disease is 1–5% in the first year and between 5% and 10% for the first five years with an approximate lifetime risk of 10% (Enarson and Rouillon, 1994).

In communities where tuberculosis is common, the majority are first infected in childhood and the peak of clinical disease is in the group aged between 20 and 25. When tuberculosis is introduced into a community for the first time the incidence of active tuberculosis rises to a peak, rarely more than 1%, and then only when overcrowding, poor nutrition or reduced immunity facilitates it. Thereafter tuberculosis rates decline at approximately 4% per year. A mathematical model of the transmission dynamics of tuberculosis indicates that tuberculosis epidemics take several hundred years to rise, fall and reach a stable endemic level (Blower *et al.*, 1995). This suggests that the current decline in tuberculosis noted in this century is the natural behaviour of a tuberculosis epidemic. The recent rises noted in many cities have a trend which indicates a 'young' epidemic superimposed on a declining curve (Blower *et al.*, 1995). In this situation the proportion of cases due to primary progression should increase and the age distribution should shift to younger individuals, and this is borne out by molecular studies in New York and San Francisco (Shafer *et al.*, 1995; Small *et al.*, 1994). If chemotherapy is used effectively this decline is accelerated. As tuberculosis declines, infection in the young becomes progressively less common and the peak age for disease increases. In addition high-risk groups emerge where rates are up to 60 times higher than in the general population (Comstock, 1994). These groups usually include immigrants from countries with high rates of tuberculosis, and HIV-positive patients. Among the former group the risk of developing active disease is greatest in the first five years after immigration and is thought to be around 10% (Comstock, 1994).

The HIV epidemic has had a major impact on the epidemiology of tuberculosis. In Africa more than half of patients with tuberculosis are also infected with HIV (Elliott *et al.*, 1995). The risk of progression to active disease is increased at least 10-fold. Multiple-drug resistant strains have also emerged among HIV-infected individuals in the USA and have resulted in a very high mortality (Comstock, 1994; Pearson *et al.*, 1992).

Tuberculosis is a potential hazard in the hospital environment, especially when there is a substantial population of immunocompromised patients. Spread has occurred as a result of inadequate sterilization of equipment such as bronchoscopes. Outbreaks of multiple-drug resistant tuberculosis have occurred when an infected patient is managed in accommodation unable to contain aerosol transmission.

CLINICAL FEATURES

Pulmonary Disease

Tuberculous infection of the lung causes a characteristic bronchopneumonia with a predilection for the posterior segments of the upper lobe or the apical segments of the lower lobes. However, almost any pattern of infection can be associated with the disease. The infection is usually patchy or nodular and cavities may develop. This can be complicated by pleurisy, pleural effusion or empyema. Fibrosis is common, leading to shifts in the neighbouring structures; calcification of long-standing disease may be present (Figure 6b.1) (Ormerod, 1994).

The symptoms may be divided into two groups: non-specific constitutional symptoms, and localized respiratory symptoms. The constitutional symptoms are a result of the release of cytokines and consequences of serious disease and include fever, night sweats, weight loss and anorexia (see page 208). Among the respiratory symptoms cough is the most prominent and sputum is usually mucoid or purulent. It may be accompanied by haemoptysis which, when it occurs, is usually light with the sputum mildly blood stained. Catastrophic haemoptysis may occur as a terminal event when a

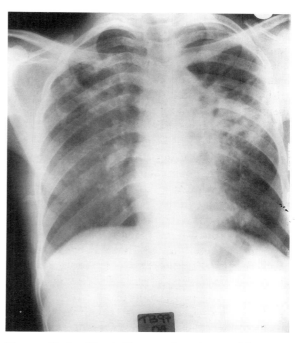

Figure 6b.1 Chest X-ray of patient with acute pulmonary tuberculosis demonstrating consolidation in the left mid-zone

bronchial artery ruptures into a tuberculous cavity. Pulmonary tuberculosis characteristically presents insidiously with progressive constitutional symptoms, fever and weight loss, associated with a cough. It may also present as an acute infection and tuberculosis should be suspected in any patient in whom a pneumonia fails to respond satisfactorily to appropriate antibiotic therapy (Ormerod, 1994).

The signs of tuberculosis are similarly divided into constitutional and respiratory. The patient is often pallid and has signs of weight loss, and a fever may be present with sweats, especially at night. The respiratory signs are those associated with bronchopneumonia and include fine crepitations or signs of consolidation or pleural effusion. The signs of pulmonary cavities or empyema may be found in patients with more advanced disease. Clubbing may be present if the patient presents late in the course of the disease.

Extrapulmonary Tuberculosis

Extrapulmonary tuberculosis is present in a third to a half of all patients with tuberculous infection. There is an increasing trend in extrapulmonary tuberculosis worldwide. This is only partly explained by the rise in HIV infection, in which extrapulmonary tuberculosis is more common (Hopewell, 1992; Stead, 1995).

Lymph Node Infection

Tuberculosis infection of lymph nodes is one of the commonest forms of extrapulmonary tuberculosis. In the past it was frequently caused by *M. bovis* but (*M. tuberculosis*) is now the commonest isolate (Yates and Grange, 1992). Other mycobacteria such as *M. avium–intracellulare* and *M. scrofulaceum* can also be isolated from immunocompetent children (Yates and Grange, 1992; Grange *et al.*, 1995). Tuberculous lymphadenitis commonly occurs in children in areas of high endemicity and in adults between the ages of 25 and 50 in countries where tuberculosis is rare. More than two-thirds of cases are localized to the cervical nodes, and tuberculous infections at other sites are found in half of the patients. Tuberculous

lymphadenitis has an insidious onset and lymph nodes are matted, swollen and usually painless. The overlying skin may break down and discharging sinuses may develop. Up to half of patients may have no constitutional symptoms associated with this infection. Other sites for tuberculous lymphadenitis are hilar and paratracheal glands and the mediastinum.

Spinal Tuberculosis

Spinal tuberculosis is the commonest bony form of extrapulmonary disease and is uncommon in the indigenous populations of industrialized countries. It is more common in patients who acquire their disease in countries of a high endemicity (Girling *et al.*, 1988). This condition gains its importance because of the serious deformities which may result from untreated infection. Patients present with chronic back pain which has been present for months or years and constitutional symptoms may be present (Figure 6b.2). Other signs arise as a result of the neurological consequences of bony disease, resulting in cord transection, radiculitis, lower limb symptoms or sphincter disturbances. Associated psoas abscess may result in pus formation and a 'cold' abscess found in the groin.

Meningitis

Tuberculous meningitis has a high mortality and even when successfully treated may be associated with chronic neurological damage. Infection is often localized in the basal meninges and may be associated with hydrocephalus or cranial nerve palsy. Focal neurological signs may be caused by tuberculomata, which are localized tuberculosis infections in the substance of the brain.

The onset of tuberculous meningitis is slower and more insidious than pyogenic meningitis, ranging from two days to several months (median 10 days) (Kent *et al.*, 1993). It is associated with fever, weight loss, headache, nausea, and vomiting; children may present with irritability or behavioural changes. Coma may be present on admission and is an important indicator; the prognosis is directly

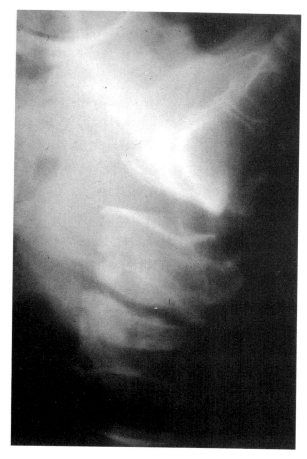

Figure 6b.2 X-ray of lumbar spine of patient with back pain demonstrating lucency in the lumbar vertebrae characteristic of spinal tuberculosis

related to the degree of impairment of the level of consciousness. The severity of the disease can be defined clinically using the BMRC (British Medical Research Council) classification and this is useful in defining the prognosis (Streptomycin in Tuberculosis Trials Committee, 1948):

- *Stage I*: Consciousness normal and no focal neurological signs.
- *Stage II*: Consciousness disturbed but not comatose or delirious; there may be focal neurological signs and cranial nerve palsies.

- *Stage III*: Patient extremely ill, deeply stuporous or comatose, with or without associated neurological signs.

Cranial nerve palsies, especially oculomotor palsies, signs of raised intracranial pressure (e.g. papilloedema) although more common than in other forms of meningitis, are not diagnostic. Epileptic seizures may develop at any stage and hyponatraemia due to inappropriate antidiuretic hormone (ADH) secretion may occur. Choroidal tubercles are rare. Tuberculous meningitis can involve the spinal meninges, also known as spinal tuberculosis, characterized by sciatica associated with flaccid or spastic limb paresis with loss of bladder and anal sphincter control which is usually permanent (Kent *et al.*, 1993; Kilpatrick *et al.*, 1986).

The cerebrospinal fluid (CSF) white cell count is moderately increased ($0.5-2 \times 10^9$/l and is usually lymphocytic, although a polymorph predominance is sometimes found. The glucose is low (<2 mmol/l) and the protein elevated. The CSF abnormalities resolve only slowly on treatment over many months. The peripheral white cell count may be elevated. Less than half of the patients will have any radiographic evidence of tuberculosis in the chest, and only 75 % may have a positive tuberculin reaction; magnetic resonance imaging and computed tomography (CT) scanning contribute to the diagnosis. Direct smear is positive in less than half of the patients, and culture is positive in up to 80%. The sensitivity of both procedures is dependent on volume of CSF studied (Leonard and Des Prez, 1990). Tuberculomas are now rare. They are frequently multiple and give rise to symptoms similar to brain abscess.

Abdominal Tuberculosis

Tuberculous infection may infect any part of the gut but is more commonly localized in the ileocaecal region or the oesophagus. Abdominal tuberculosis has few characteristic clinical signs and is consequently a difficult diagnosis to make; without a high index of suspicion the diagnosis may be missed. Patients present with fever, anorexia, abdominal pain, nausea and weight loss. Constipation and diarrhoea are rare; a small bowel perforation or malabsorption may develop. There are no characteristic signs but fever is common and examination may reveal either localized tuberculous masses in the abdomen or signs of tuberculosis in other organs.

Tuberculous peritonitis usually arises due to rupture of a caseous abdominal lymph node, or more rarely spread from another adjacent site such as a psoas abscess or fallopian abscess. It usually presents in younger patients and the majority have signs of tuberculosis in other organs. It has an insidious onset and may present with tender abdominal masses or with ascites and signs of peritonitis.

Genitourinary Tuberculosis

Tuberculous infection of the kidney is usually asymptomatic early in the course of the disease. Dysuria, haematuria and, in advanced cases, flank pain may be present. Asymptomatic disease is common, but infection of the renal tract may be complicated by fibrosis and renal obstruction which may lead to renal failure. In almost all cases the intravenous pyelogram (IVP) is abnormal, with early signs of pyelonephritis followed by features similar to papillary necrosis, with ureteric strictures and hydronephrosis.

Infection of the epididymis is the commonest form of genitourinary tuberculosis in men and is often associated with renal infection. Infection is spread to the site haematogenously or by local extension (Gorse and Belshe, 1985). In the female genital tract tuberculous infection may result in infertility, pelvic pain, menorrhagia and amenorrhoea.

Skin Tuberculosis

Cutaneous manifestations of tuberculosis arise as a result of direct infection of the skin or the immunological consequences of tuberculosis. There are numerous forms of disease. Primary infection of the skin occurs as the result of a localized inoculation which may take a chronic form or a verrucosa cutis or the more acute verruca necrogenica. A post-primary form of the disease is lupus vulgaris, a dullish red lesion which appears on the head, face and limbs. It is a chronic, mutilating, destructive process of the skin and may also destroy the cartilage of the ears and nose, giving the patient a 'wolf-like' facies – hence its name (Lugt, 1965). Disseminated cutaneous forms of infection may occur in HIV-positive patients (Bassiri et al., 1993).

The immune response to tuberculosis infection may result in cutaneous manifestations. These manifestations are known as tuberculides and include erythema nodosa and Bazin's erythema induratum.

TREATMENT

The clear association between tuberculosis, poverty and overcrowding led indirectly to the development of the sanatorium movement. This provided patients with bed-rest, good food and fresh air, and isolated them from other contacts. The mortality from pulmonary tuberculosis treated in this way, in the absence of chemotherapy, was just under 50%. Alternative surgical approaches were used adjunctively: where tuberculosis was limited to a single lobe, lobectomy was performed. Alternatively phrenic nerve crushing, artificial pneumothorax and artificial pneumoperitoneum and thoracoplasty were practised (Enarson and Rouillon, 1994).

The real revolution occurred with the discovery of streptomycin, which was the first drug active against tuberculosis (Waksman, 1964). It brought about clinical and radiological improvement in patients who relapsed after initial improvement due to the development of drug resistance (Mitchison, 1950). Help was on hand with the development of para-aminosalicylic acid (PAS), which was developed by Leiman in Denmark. Combination therapy of streptomycin and PAS prevented the development of resistance. The introduction of isoniazid in 1952 made available a potent bactericidal agent for the treatment of M.

tuberculosis. Using these drugs in combination for 18 months to two years brought about a high rate of cure. Other agents developed at this time included ethambutol and thiacetazone, which could be substituted for the standard drugs. This was often required as adverse events were common. Pyrazinamide was also introduced for use at this time but a high incidence of side effects due to high dosing meant that it soon fell into disuse. With the introduction of rifampicin and the rediscovery of the role of pyrazinamide, a series of clinical trials showed that it was possible to treat pulmonary tuberculosis effectively with short-course regimens, i.e. six months (see below) (Fox and Mitchison, 1975).

The main drugs currently used in the treatment of tuberculosis can be divided into two broad groups: first- and second-line agents. The first-line agents are those which have been established in regimens of chemotherapy as a result of a series of clinical trials (Mitchison, 1992). These include rifampicin, isoniazid, ethambutol, pyrazinamide and streptomycin. The second-line agents are used for the treatment of patients with multiple-drug resistance or who are unable to tolerate first-line agents as a result of adverse events. These include ethionamide or prothionamide, cycloserine, capreomycin, kanamycin and amikacin and the 4-fluoroquinolones: ofloxacin and ciprofloxacin. PAS and clofazamine can also be used.

Practical Problems of Anti-tuberculosis Chemotherapy

Development of resistance

The piecemeal introduction of anti-tuberculosis agents highlighted the importance of preventing the development of drug resistance during chemotherapy. In any population of MTB spontaneously resistant mutants will exist. The number of tubercle bacilli in a pulmonary tuberculosis cavity is estimated to be about 10^8 organisms. If the probability of resistance is 10^{-6} the pulmonary cavity is likely to contain 100 resistant organisms. However, if two drugs are combined, both of which have a probability of resistance of 10^{-6}, the overall probability

of resistance becomes 10^{-12} and the chance of a drug-resistant mutant being present is 10^{-4}, thus drug-resistant cases are very unlikely to develop. The relationship of probability of resistance to the number of tubercle bacilli in the lesion is expressed by the formula $P = 1 - (1 - R)^N$, where P is the probability of incidence of drug-resistant cases, R is the probability of incidence of drug-resistant mutants, and N is the number of tubercle bacilli in the lesion (Shimao, 1987).

With the availability of a wide range of anti-tuberculosis agents, emphasis is shifted towards bactericidal activity and sterilizing activity. These terms appear to be identical but represent two different concepts applicable to tuberculosis chemotherapy. They arise because of the wide variation in the sites at which tubercle bacilli are found inside the body. This is summarized by the special populations hypothesis evolved by Mitchison (1985). The majority of tubercle bacilli in lesions at the start of treatment are growing and metabolizing quickly. They are located extracellularly in pulmonary cavities. Two other populations of semi-dormant organisms exist: the organisms located at the edge of caseous foci, an environment characterized by low pH and low oxygen tension, and macrophages. The bactericidal activity of a drug measures the ability to kill organisms which are metabolizing rapidly. As these organisms are extracellular and found in the sputum, a bactericidal effect at this site will rapidly render sputum culture negative. This characteristic is of great importance in the control of tuberculosis spread in the community. In practice it can be measured by determining sputum viable count in patients during the first week of therapy (Jindani *et al.*, 1980; Kennedy *et al.*, 1993). Sterilizing activity measures the ability of the drug to kill the slow-growing, slow-metabolizing populations of the organism. Pyrazinamide, which is converted to its active form at low pH, is probably active against organisms inside caseous foci and within the low pH of phagolysosomes. Rifampicin is also active against organisms during spurts of metabolism and it is this characteristic which is thought to be responsible for its sterilizing activity. Sterilizing activity can be determined by measuring the percentage of patient's sputum culture negative at two months and by the rate of relapse.

Early bactericidal activity can be defined as the ability to render sputum culture negative.

Standardized treatment regimens are laid down by national and international bodies. The characteristics of the most successful regimens incorporate an early intensive phase usually incorporating isoniazid, rifampicin and pyrazinamide. When primary drug resistance is common a fourth drug – ethambutol or streptomycin – may be added. This is followed by a consolidation phase usually consisting of isoniazid and rifampicin, although other second-line agents may be used. Trials have demonstrated that pyrazinamide adds little to therapeutic efficacy after the first two months (Mitchison, 1992). It has also been shown that it is not necessary for all the drugs to be given daily and that intermittent treatment two and three times a week are just as effective. Rifampicin given once a week in high dosage is associated with severe adverse reactions. In countries with a low incidence of primary drug resistance six months intermittent therapy is adequate treatment of uncomplicated pulmonary tuberculosis (Fox and Mitchison, 1992). It was also shown early in the course of developing these protocols that sanatorium-based treatment was no more effective than home-based treatment, and the number of secondary cases which arose was similar (Tuberculosis Chemotherapy Centre, 1959). This has clear implications for the cost of delivering treatment regimens in developing countries. The other main distinction in antituberculosis regimens whether they are oral or partly parenteral. Many control programmes have favoured the retention of streptomycin in the programme as investigators consider it is less likely that patients will default if they have to attend hospital for injection. There are in addition to this many other considerations in the effectiveness of a regimen. These include the cost of the drugs to the patient, whether the treatment is supervised or unsupervised, and the toxicity of the regimen.

In countries where patients are required to pay for their drugs, the poorest members of the community most likely to suffer from tuberculosis are likely to stop treatment before bacteriological cure

is to be expected. This has serious consequences for the individual as relapse is likely to occur and the relapse may be with the drug-resistant strain.

Unsupervised treatment has had its problems as patients in the poorest sectors of society may be tempted to sell their drugs for ready cash or for drugs of addiction. Patients who are intravenous drug abusers, homeless or alcoholics are less likely to be sufficiently disciplined to keep a long-term drug regimen and thus incomplete treatment will occur, with the risk of relapse with drug-resistant strains. Against this general background we have seen the emergence of epidemics of multiple-drug resistant tuberculosis in New York and within the American prison system. The recent epidemics of MDRT (multidrug resistant tuberculosis) in the USA and other countries arose as a result of inadequate regimens and poor compliance. Directly observed therapy, where patient compliance is guaranteed, prevents the development of such multiple-drug resistant strains (Anonymous, 1993).

Drug toxicity

The toxicity of anti-tuberculosis agents is now rarely a problem, although when chemotherapy was first begun patients often were unable to complete a course of treatment. The exceptions to the generally favourable position are those with acquired immunodeficiency syndrome, in whom reactions to antituberculosis and other drugs are common.

Treatment of Drug-resistant Tuberculosis

Studies performed on patients treated with streptomycin, isoniazid and PAS demonstrated a small advantage for rapid determination for susceptibility in choosing antituberculosis regimens. It can be seen that six month regimens containing isoniazid, rifampicin and pyrazinamide which may include streptomycin or ethambutol in the initial phase, together with a consolidation phase of isoniazid and rifampicin, are very effective in the treatment of pulmonary tuberculosis even when strains are initially resistant to isoniazid. Where primary rifampicin resistance occurs (usually coupled with isoniazid resistance), these regimens are likely to fail (Anonymous, 1993). When primary rifampicin resistance is present, treatment regimens should be designed to prevent the development of resistance. When treating patients known to be infected with multiple-drug resistant tuberculosis a number of guidelines can be suggested. All patients with tuberculosis should be managed according to the following rules: (1) *in vitro* drugs susceptibility testing should be performed on all initial isolates; (2) all initial treatments should include four anti-tuberculosis drugs to ensure that patients with unsuspected drug resistance are adequately treated until susceptibility test results are available; (3) directly observed therapy should be used to confirm adequate therapeutic levels of antituberculosis agents. Drug-resistant tuberculosis has much higher mortality (approximately 45–56%) and a drug regimen should be evolved that includes three drugs to which the patient's organism is susceptible. When the patient fails to respond it is essential to add two new agents known to be active. The piecemeal addition of individual agents to a failing regimen is likely to result in the development of further drug resistance. As the likelihood of relapse is high in these patients, regimens for the treatment of multi-drug resistance should be prolonged for up to two years. In practice this advice must be modified in the light of drug toxicity or tolerance (Iseman, 1993).

Treatment of Smear-negative Tuberculosis

Attempts have been made to treat smear-negative pulmonary tuberculosis with regimens shorter than the standard six months. A study in Hong Kong of daily treatment with isoniazid, rifampicin, pyrazinamide and streptomycin for two or three months was not adequate because relapse rates of 32% and 13% respectively were found during five years of follow-up (Hong Kong Chest Service *et al.*, 1989). A later study of four months treatment with an initial four-drug regimen for two months followed by consolidation for two months, isoniazid and rifampicin was successful. Consequently a regimen of HRZ (isoniazid, rifampicin, pyrazinamide) for two months followed by HR (insoniazid, rifampicin) for a further two months is recommended by the WHO for treating smear-negative pulmonary tuberculosis (Dutt *et al.*, 1990).

Treatment of Extra-pulmonary Tuberculosis

Tuberculous lymphadenitis is successfully treated with chemotherapy using isoniazid, rifampicin and pyrazinamide for between six and nine months.

Short-course chemotherapy including isoniazid and rifampicin for six to nine months is effective in the treatment of tuberculosis of the spine. Trials have shown that ambulatory therapy is effective and is the treatment of choice. For the majority of patients operative procedures are unnecessary unless spinal instability requires correction. Another exception is acute cord compression, which must be operated on as an emergency.

Tuberculous meningitis is an important life-threatening complication of tuberculosis. Treatment is complicated by the difficulty of ensuring adequate concentrations in the CSF. Isoniazid, pyrazinamide and rifampicin cross the blood–brain barrier in therapeutically useful concentrations, but only very low levels of aminoglycosides do so. Streptomycin may still be valuable early in the course of infection where inflamed meninges permit this drug to penetrate the CSF. Larger doses of antituberculosis agents are used for meningitis than are employed in pulmonary disease. Isoniazid is given at a dose of 10 mg/kg to a maximum of 600 mg per day, although other studies show that 5 mg/kg is adequate. Rifampicin is given at 10 mg/kg per day and pyrazinamide is employed at between 30 and 40 mg/kg per day. The duration of treatment required is uncertain. Those patients presenting with mild disease may be treated for 9–12 months, although for those with more severe disease treatment for at least 12 months is recommended. The presence of an intracranial tuberculoma is an indication for prolonged treatment of between 18 and 24 months. The use of corticosteroids is controversial but they are probably beneficial in patients with medium or severe disease. Other indications are tuberculous encephalopathy and tuberculous meningitis complicated by spinal block or arachnoiditis (Watson *et al.*, 1993).

TUBERCULOSIS CONTROL

There have been many different attempts to control tuberculosis. Shortly after his initial description of the tubercle bacillus, Koch described what he thought was effective immunotherapy. His injection of tuberculin was not protective and the tuberculin skin reaction was in fact damaging. It continues, however, as the intradermal skin test developed by Mantoux.

Efforts to control tuberculosis were focused around the sanatorium movement which identified patients with tuberculosis and transferred them to sanatoria in the countryside, where they could receive improved nutrition and could rest fully. This segregation may have helped to interrupt the cycle of transmission in tuberculosis. Other control measures included the eradication of tuberculosis in cattle by tuberculin skin testing and slaughter of those cattle found to be infected. The universal application of pasteurization of milk also helped to control spread to man from bovine tuberculosis. In the middle of the twentieth century chemotherapy became available, enabling cases to be made rapidly non-infectious, and this was coupled with national case-finding campaigns using mass miniaturized radiography.

In the USA recommendations for management of patients suffering from MDR-tuberculosis have been reported. These focus around early diagnosis, isolation and treatment. This includes the provision of rapid diagnostic methods which allow high-risk patients to be managed in side wards with negative pressure ventilation. Personal protective measures are to be taken when entering the patient's room or performing procedures likely to generate an aerosol (e.g. bronchoscopy). Therapy should be with a four-drug regimen using 'directly observed therapy'. Health care workers themselves, at risk of being immunosuppressed, should be educated as to their risks and be able to exclude themselves from contact with such patients without prejudice (Anonymous, 1992).

Vaccination

Many attempts have been made to control tuberculosis by vaccination; Koch with the Koch reaction was the first unsuccessful attempt. A strain of *M. bovis* was attenuated by Calmette and Guérin by passaging it 231 times through medium containing glycerol and ox bile. Bacille Calmette–Guérin (BCG) was found to be safe and gained wide acceptance throughout Europe. There have been several reports over the years of patients suffering from acute disease with vaccine that was not satisfactorily attenuated.

Many control studies of the efficacy of BCG have been conducted (Bloom and Fine, 1994). These show wide variation in the protective efficacy calculated, ranging from 0 to 70%. It is clear that these differences are real and must be explained. Several theories have been developed to explain these phenomena. These include variation in the vaccine strains, as different strains of BCG vary in their ability to protect laboratory animals and similar effects are likely to occur in the human population. The dosing regimen and means of administration may vary and vaccine potency may also vary depending on the handling of the vaccine before administration.

Others have suggested that sensitization to environmental mycobacteria may modify the immune response to BCG (Palmer and Long, 1966), implying that infection with certain kinds of environmental mycobacteria stimulate immunosuppressive effects and thus the effect of BCG would be determined by, the environmental mycobacteria present in the community. Where 'immunosuppressive' environmental mycobacteria predominate BCG efficacy will be low (Stanford *et al.*, 1981). The possibility that host genetic factors and nutritional factors are in part responsible cannot be ruled out.

The consequence of this debate is uncertainty as to the efficacy of BCG in the prevention of tuberculosis. In some countries, such as the UK, it is recommended for use, whereas in the USA BCG is not given.

Antimicrobial Prophylaxis

A large number of placebo-controlled trials have shown that daily administration of isoniazid to individuals at risk of tuberculosis for 6–12 months reduces the likelihood of developing open disease. Various guidelines have been evolved and the patients at risk are defined by the American Thoracic Society (Ad hoc committee of the Scientific Assembly of Microbiology, 1994). The IUATLD (International Union Against Tuberculosis and Lung Diseases) and the WHO recommend isoniazid preventive therapy for childhood contacts of infectious cases. Studies of prophylactic therapy in patients dually infected with *M. tuberculosis* and HIV show efficacy (Pape *et al.*, 1993). As there are concerns that tuberculosis may accelerate the progression, isoniazid prophylaxis of HIV-infected individuals is now recommended by several agencies (Anonymous, 1994).

Immunotherapy

In recent years injection of a preparation of *M. vaccae* has been used as adjunctive therapy in multiple-drug resistant disease (Stanford *et al.*, 1990). Although initial results are encouraging, the results of further trials are awaited.

REFERENCES

Ad hoc committee of the Scientific Assembly of Microbiology (1994) Treatment of tuberculosis and tuberculosis infection in adults and children. *Journals of Respiratory and Critical Care Medicine*, **149**, 1359–1374.

Anonymous (1992) Transmission of multidrug-resistant tuberculosis among immunocompromised persons in a correctional system: New York, 1991. *Morbidity and Mortality Weekly Report*, **41**, 507–509.

Anonymous (1993) Initial therapy for tuberculosis in the era of multidrug resistance: recommendations of the Advisory Council for the Elimination of Tuberculosis [published erratum appears in *MMWR*

(1993), **42**(27), 536]. *Morbidity and Mortality Weekly Report*, **42**, 1–8.

Anonymous (1994) Tuberculosis preventive therapy in HIV-infected individuals: a joint statement of the International Union against Tuberculosis and Lung Diseases and the Global Programme on AIDS and the Tuberculosis Programme of the World Health Organization. *Tuberculosis and Lung Diseases*, **75**, 96–98.

Bassiri, A., Chan, N.B., Mcleod, A., Rossi, S. *et al.* (1993) Disseminated cutaneous infection due to *Mycobacterium tuberculosis* in a person with AIDS. *Canadian Medical Association Journal*, **148**, 577–578.

Bloom, B.R. and Fine, P.E.M. (1994) The BCG experience: implications for future vaccines against tuberculosis. In *Tuberculosis: Pathogenesis, Protection and Control* (ed. B.R. Bloom), pp. 531–557. American Society of Microbiology, Washington.

Blower, S.M., McLean, A.R., Porco, T.C. *et al.* (1995) Intrinsic transmission dynamics of tuberculosis epidemics. *Nature Medicine*, **1**, 815–821.

Comstock, G.W. (1994) Variability of tuberculosis trends in a time of resurgence. *Clinical Infectious Diseases*, **19**, 1015–1022.

Dannenberg, A.M.J. (1989) Immune mechanisms in the pathogenesis of pulmonary tuberculosis. *Reviews of Infectious Diseases*, **11**(Suppl. 2), S369–S378.

Dubos, R. and Dubos, J. (1952) *The White Plague: Tuberculosis, Man and Society*. Little Brown, Boston, MA.

Dutt, A.K., Moers, D. and Stead, W.W. (1990) Smear-negative, culture-positive pulmonary tuberculosis: six-month chemotherapy with isoniazid and rifampin. *American Review of Respiratory Disease*, **141**, 1232–1235.

Elliott, A.M., Halwiindi, B., Hayes, R.J. *et al.* (1995) The impact of human immunodeficiency virus on mortality of patients treated for tuberculosis in a cohort study in Zambia. *Transactions of the Royal Society of Tropical Medicine and Hygiene*, **89**, 78–82.

Enarson, D.A. and Dirks, J.M. (1989) The incidence of tuberculosis in a large urban area in Canada. *American Journal of Epidemiology*, **129**, 1268–1276.

Enarson, D.A. and Rouillon, A. (1994) The epidemiological basis of tuberculosis control. In *Clinical Tuberculosis* (ed. P.D.O. Davies), pp. 19–32. Chapman and Hall, London.

Fox, W. and Mitchison, D.A. (1975) Short-course chemotherapy for pulmonary tuberculosis. *American Review of Respiratory Disease*, **111**, 325–353.

Fox, W. and Mitchison, D.A. (1992) Community-based short-course treatment of pulmonary tuberculosis in a developing nation. *American Review of Respiratory Disease*, **146**, 536.

Girling, D.J., Darbyshire, J.H., Humphries, M.J. *et al.* (1988) Extra-pulmonary tuberculosis. *British Medical Bulletin*, **44**, 738–756.

Gorse, G.J. and Belshe, R.B. (1985) Male genital tuberculosis: a review of the literature with instructive case reports. *Reviews of Infectious Diseases*, **7**, 511–524.

Grange, J.M., Yates, M.D. and Pozniak, A. (1995) Bacteriologically confirmed non-tuberculous mycobacterial lymphadenitis in south east England: a recent increase in the number of cases. *Archives of Disease in Childhood*, **72**, 516–517.

Hawken, M., Nunn, P., Gathua, S. *et al.* (1993) Increased recurrence of tuberculosis in HIV-I-infected patients in Kenya. *Lancet*, **342**, 332–337.

Hong Kong Chest Service, Tuberculosis Research Centre, and British Medical Research Council (1989) A controlled trial of 3-month, 4-month, and 6-month regimens for sputum smear negative pulmonary tuberculosis. *American Review of Respiratory Disease*, **139**, 871.

Hopewell, P.C. (1992) Impact of human immunodeficiency virus infection on the epidemiology, clinical features, management, and control of tuberculosis. *Clinical Infectious Diseases*, **15**, 540–547.

Iseman, M.D. (1993) Treatment of multidrug-resistant tuberculosis [published erratum appears in *N. Engl. J. Med.* (1993), **329**(19), 1435]. (Review.) *New England Journal of Medicine*, **329**, 784–791.

Jindani, A., Aber, V.R., Edwards, E.A. *et al.* (1980) The early bactericidal activity of drugs in patients with pulmonary tuberculosis. *American Review of Respiratory Disease*, **121**, 939–949.

Kennedy, N., Fox, R., Kisyombe, G.M. *et al.* (1993) Early bactericidal and sterilizing activity of ciprofloxacin in pulmonary tuberculosis. *American Review of Respiratory Disease*, **148**, 1547–1551.

Kent, S.J., Crowe, S.M., Yung, A. *et al.* (1993) Tuberculous meningitis: a 30-year review. *Clinical Infectious Diseases*, **17**, 987–994.

Kilpatrick, M.E., Girgis, N.I., Yassin, M.W. *et al.* (1986) Tuberculous meningitis: clinical and laboratory review of 100 patients. *Journal of Hygiene*, **96**, 231–238.

Leonard, J.M. and Des Prez, R.M. (1990) Tuberculous meningitis. *Infectious Disease Clinics of North America*, **4**, 769–787.

Lugt, L., van der (1965) Some remarks about tuberculosis of the skin and tuberculids. *Dermatologica*, **131**, 266–275.

Mitchison, D.A. (1950) Development of streptomycin resistant strains of tubercle bacilli in pulmonary tuberculosis. *Thorax*, **5**, 144–161.

Mitchison, D.A. (1985) The action of antituberculosis drugs in short-course chemotherapy. *Tubercle*, **66**, 219–225.

Mitchison, D.A. (1992) Understanding the chemotherapy of tuberculosis: current problems. *Journal of Antimicrobial Chemotherapy*, **29**, 477–493.

Nardell, E., McInnis, B., Thomas, B. *et al.* (1986) Exogenous reinfection with tuberculosis in a shelter for the homeless. *New England Journal of Medicine*, **315**, 1570–1575.

Ormerod, L.P. (1994) Respiratory tuberculosis. In *Clinical Tuberculosis* (ed. P.D.O. Davies), pp. 73–91. Chapman and Hall, London.

Palmer, C.E. and Long, M.W. (1966) Effects of infection with atypical mycobacteria on BCG vaccination and tuberculosis. *American Review of Respiratory Disease*, **94**, 553–568.

Pape, J.W., Jean, S.S., Ho, J.L *et al.* (1993) Effect of isoniazid prophylaxis on incidence of active tuberculosis and progression of HIV infection. *Lancet*, **342**, 268–272.

Pearson, M.L., Jereb, J.A., Frieden, T.R. *et al.* (1992) Nosocomial transmission of multidrug-resistant *Mycobacterium tuberculosis*: a risk to patients and health care workers. *Annals of Internal Medicine*, **117**, 191–196.

Shafer, R.W., Small, P.M., Larkin, C. *et al.* (1995) Temporal trends and transmission patterns during the emergence of multidrug-resistant tuberculosis in New York city: a molecular epidemiologic assessment. *Journal of Infectious Diseases*, **171**, 170–176.

Shimao, T. (1987) Drug resistance in tuberculosis control. *Tubercle*, **68**, 5–18.

Small, P.M., Hopewell, P.C., Singh, S.P. *et al.* (1994) The epidemiology of tuberculosis in San Francisco: a population-based study using conventional and molecular methods. *New England Journal of Medicine*, **330**, 1703–1709.

Stanford, J.L., Shields, M.J. and Rook, G.A. (1981) How environmental mycobacteria may predetermine the protective efficacy of BCG. *Tubercle*, **62**, 55–62.

Stanford, J.L., Bahr, G.M., Rook, G.A. *et al.* (1990) Immunotherapy with *Myobacterium vaccae* as an adjunct to chemotherapy in the treatment of pulmonary tuberculosis. *Tubercle*, **71**, 87–93.

Stead, W.W. (1995) Management of health care workers after inadvertent exposure to tuberculosis: a guide for the use of preventive therapy. *Annals of Internal Medicine*, **122**, 906–912.

Streptomycin in Tuberculosis Trials Committee (1948) Streptomycin treatment of tuberculous meningitis. *Lancet*, **i**, 582–597.

Tuberculosis Chemotherapy Centre (1959) A concurrent comparison of home and sanitorium treatment of pulmonary tuberculosis in South India. *Bulletin of the World Health Organization*, **21**, 51.

Waksman, S.A. (1964) *The Conquest of Tuberculosis*. University of California Press, San Francisco.

Watson, J.D.G., Shnier, R.C. and Seale, J.P. (1993) Central nervous system tuberculosis in Australia: a report of 22 cases. *Medical Journal of Australia*, **158**, 408.

Yates, M.D. and Grange, J.M. (1992) Bacteriological survey of tuberculous lymphadenitis in southeast England, 1981–1989. *Journal of Epidemiology and Community Health*, **46**, 332–335.

6c

NON-TUBERCULOSIS MYCOBACTERIA

Stephen H. Gillespie

INTRODUCTION

Non-tuberculosis mycobacteria are increasingly recognized as human pathogens. They were once classified as 'atypical' to differentiate them from the organisms of tuberculosis. They are for the most part environmental organisms, and are more typical of the genus as a whole. The epidemiology, clinical features and management of these infections are set out below.

MYCOBACTERIUM AVIUM–INTRACELLULARE

The *Mycobacterium* responsible for disease induction isolated in 1890 was given the name *M. avium*. A related organism caused an outbreak of pulmonary infection in a state hospital in Georgia, USA, and was for some time known as the 'Battey' bacillus. It was assigned the name *M. intracellulare*. The detailed classification of these two species can be found on page 206.

Epidemiology

Organisms of the *M. avium–intracellulare* complex (MAC) are widely distributed in nature. Recent studies have shown a strong association with acid, brown water swamps in the southern USA. *Mycobacterium avium–intracellulare* occurs worldwide, so we may suppose that the conditions of the swamps are favourable to *M. avium–intracellulare* growth: warm temperatures, low pH, low dissolved oxygen, high soluble zinc, high humic acid and high fulvic acid (Kirschner *et al.*, 1992). This may be the reason for the geographical variation in incidence of infection (Hoover *et al.*, 1995; Horsburgh *et al.*, 1994a). The organisms can also be isolated from soil, dust, animals and tap water (Kirschner *et al.*, 1992). The latter may be an important source of infection for immunocompromised patients in the hospital environment (Peters *et al.*, 1995). *Mycobacterium avium–intracellulare* can be isolated from environmental water samples in Zaire and Kenya where infection in AIDS patients is uncommon (von Reyn *et al.*, 1993).

Before the HIV epidemic pulmonary manifestations of *M. avium–intracellulare* infection were most common. Recent reports are bringing increasing recognition of pulmonary *M. avium–intracellulare* infection in elderly patients with no apparent predisposition.

A chronic lymphadenitis usually in the cervical or facial region is the most common presentation in children between one and 10 years and this

Principles and Practice of Clinical Bacteriology. Edited by A.M. Emmerson, P.M. Hawkey and S.H. Gillespie
© 1997 John Wiley & Sons Ltd

organism is now responsible for the majority of mycobacterial lymphadenitis in the developed world (O'Brien *et al.*, 1987).

Disseminated infection may occur in patients without AIDS, usually associated with malignancy, inherited or iatrogenic immunodeficiency. The HIV epidemic has brought about a massive increase in the number of MAC infections reported. The main portal of infection is thought to be the respiratory and gastrointestinal tracts. Initially the patient may be colonized but later disseminated disease with bacteraemia may develop. Pulmonary infection or invasion of other organs, including the bone, may take place (Benson, 1994). Dissemination does not usually take place under the CD4 count has fallen well below $100/mm^3$ (Benson, 1994). Colonization and infection with *M. avium–intracellulare* are associated with a worse prognosis compared with uninfected patients. The outcome can be improved with effective treatment (Horsburgh *et al.*, 1994b; Chin *et al.*, 1994).

In areas where *M. tuberculosis* is endemic HIV-infected individuals are rarely infected with MAC. The reasons for this dichotomy are not yet elucidated.

Most infections in AIDS patients are thought to be due to *M. avium* serovars, while infections in non-HIV-infected individuals are mainly due to *M. intracellulare* serovars. A relatively small number of serovars are responsible for the majority of *M. avium* infection in AIDS patients (Benson, 1994).

Clinical Features

Lymphadenitis

The submandibular, pre-auricular, submaxillary and rarely intraparotid lymph nodes are involved. The infection follows a chronic course with discharge and sinus formation, and must be differentiated from cat-scratch disease, tuberculosis and lymphoma.

Respiratory infection

There are four main syndromes recognized: solitary pulmonary nodules, chronic bronchitis or bronchiectasis mainly in older patients, a tuberculosis-like syndrome and diffuse pulmonary infiltrates in immunocompromised individuals. A wide range of clinical and radiological features have been described in HIV-positive patients (see below) but bacteraemia usually predominates.

Disseminated disease

The usual symptoms are fever and night sweats, diarrhoea, abdominal pain and weight loss. On examination patients are found to be wasted and febrile. Localized disease is less common but pulmonary nodules or infiltrates, or cavitation may be present. Additionally intra-abdominal abscess, skin infection, osteomyelitis and cervical lymphadenitis have been described (O'Brien *et al.*, 1987). At post-mortem many patients have, often unsuspected, evidence of disseminated MAC infection. On clinical examination patients are wasted and have hepatosplenomegaly. Patients are anaemic with reduced platelets and elevated alkaline phosphatase (Horsburgh *et al.*, 1994b). Intra-abdominal lymphadenopathy can be detected by ultrasound or computed tomography (CT) scanning.

Antimicrobial susceptibility

Mycobacterium avium–intracellulare is naturally resistant to many of the drugs used to treat *M. tuberculosis* and this causes considerable therapeutic difficulties. Resistance to isoniazid, rifampicin, pyrazinamide and streptomycin is common, but many strains are susceptible to clarithromycin, azithromycin, rifabutin, clofazamine, ciprofloxacin, amikacin and ethambutol.

Prophylaxis

Rifabutin has been shown to be effective in reducing the incidence of *M. avium–intracellulare* bacteraemia and, when dissemination did take place, it reduced the frequency of associated symptoms (Nightingale *et al.*, 1993). It is likely that other agents such as the newer macrolides will be effective in a similar situation (Heifets, 1994).

Treatment

Clear guidelines for the management of invasive *M. avium–intracellulare* infection cannot be given in view of the unpredictable susceptibility of this organism. Because of the likelihood of multiple-drug resistance, each of the isolates must be sent for full susceptibility testing. Many clinical trials are underway at present and efficacy has been shown for regimens which include rifabutin, clofazamine, ethambutol and the newer macrolides. Empirical therapy is likely to commence with a combination of ciprofloxacin, ethambutol, clarithromycin or azithromycin and rifabutin. The regimen will then be adjusted in the light of the susceptibility tests and tolerance of the drugs.

As infection occurs late in the course of HIV disease, little immune response can be expected and therapy must be lifelong. As 'cure' is imposs-ible: the clinician must use patient well-being and quality of life as the main therapeutic endpoints. This may mean a careful balance between pre-scription, adverse events and clinical improvement (Chin *et al.*, 1994).

Lymphadenitis

Antimicrobial therapy should be prescribed and benefit has been reported for regimens which include the newer macrolides. Where possible surgery should be considered as this improves the outcome.

MYCOBACTERIUM MARINUM

Epidemiology

Mycobacterium marinum was first recognized as a pathogen of fish. Human infection, when it occurs, usually arises as a result of water contact. Initially most cases were associated with poorly maintained contaminated swimming pools – 'swimming pool granuloma' – but this has now almost disappeared due to improved construction and water chlorination. Most cases seen now arise in association with maintenance of fish tanks (Edelstein, 1994; Collins *et al.*, 1985).

Clinical Features

Infection with *M. marinum* causes a chronic granulomatous infiltration of the skin. Nodular or pustular lesions are most common, and erythema-tous swelling, crusting or swelling may occur. The upper limb, especially the hand, is the most common site of infection. The lesion spreads locally in the majority of cases after four to six weeks.

Mycobacterium marinum infection must be differentiated from other chronic granulomatous skin infections such as tuberculosis, nocardiasis, coccidioidomycosis, histoplasmosis, leishmaniasis, leprosy and syphilis.

Treatment

The organism is often resistant to isoniazid but susceptible to rifampicin, ethambutol and pyrazin-amide. Minocycline and other tetracyclines have been used in treatment but rifampicin and ethambutol appear to be more successful (Edelstein, 1994).

MYCOBACTERIUM XENOPI

Mycobacterium xenopi is a slow-growing non-chromogenic mycobacterium which is frequently isolated from human specimens as a colonizer or infecting organism.

Epidemiology

Mycobacterium xenopi was first isolated from a skin granuloma of a toad (*Xenopus laevis*) kept in a laboratory for pregnancy testing (Schwabacher, 1959). It is regularly recovered from human respiratory specimens, where its significance must be carefully determined. In Western Europe it is the most common non-tuberculosis *Mycobacter-ium* isolated in laboratories, but less commonly isolated in the USA (Miller *et al.*, 1994). It may be isolated from hot-water supplies in hospitals and nosocomial outbreaks have been reported (McSwiggen and Collins, 1974; Costrini *et al.*, 1981). Person-to-person spread is thought not to occur, but in nosocomial outbreaks clusters of cases occur and person-to-person spread cannot be excluded. In this situation the true nature of transmission cannot be determined for certain as the patients and staff also share the same environment and exposure to the hospital water supplies (Costrini *et al.*, 1981) The reservoir of *M. xenopi* in the environment is uncertain, but the clustering of cases in coastal areas has suggested a link with the sea, although the organism has not been isolated in naturally occurring fresh or sea water. Birds are highly susceptible to *M. xenopi* and sea birds have been proposed as a reservoir of infection.

Infection is more common in men after middle age (McSwiggen and Collins, 1974), often with a long history of previous lung problems including obstructive airways disease, emphysema and healed tuberculosis (Simor *et al.*, 1984).

Clinical Features

Isolation of *M. xenopi* is not always associated with disease. Retrospective reviews differ in the proportion of clinical cases attributable to the organism but approximately half of the isolates are considered significant (McSwiggen and Collins, 1974; Simor *et al.*, 1984). An underlying chest abnormality is usual in the patient, making it even more difficult to define the significance of a positive isolation. Repeated isolation from respiratory sites or from bronchiolar lavage may indicate infection. Isolation of the organism from sterile sites such as synovium, peritoneum, bone and lymph nodes indicates invasive disease (Anonymous, 1990).

The presentation of pulmonary infection is subacute in the majority of patients. It is almost always associated with cough but fever is not a prominent sign. Haemoptysis and weight loss may be presenting symptoms. Solitary or multiple nodules or cavitation may be found on radiological examination of the chest (Costrini *et al.*, 1981; Smith and Citron, 1983; Simor *et al.*, 1984). A syndrome indistinguishable from tuberculosis may also develop. Extrapulmonary disease is rare. Disseminated disease has been reported in AIDS patients but is much less common than *M. kansasii* or *M. avium–intracellulare*.

Antimicrobial Susceptibility

Mycobacterium xenopi is usually susceptible to aminoglycosides but susceptibility to other agents is variable. Initial therapy should be with isoniazid, rifampicin and ethambutol, with the possible addition of streptomycin (Costrini *et al.*, 1981; Smith and Citron, 1983; Simor *et al.*, 1984; Anonymous, 1990). Therapy can be adjusted in the light of susceptibility tests. Surgical therapy of localized lesions may be beneficial (Simor *et al.*, 1984; Anonymous, 1990; Miller *et al.*, 1994).

MYCOBACTERIUM KANSASII

Mycobacterium kansasii is a photochromogenic organism which may be isolated from the environment; it causes chronic pulmonary infection and more rarely extrapulmonary lesions.

Epidemiology

Mycobacterium kansasii is a regular but uncommon cause of infection, making up less than 5% of significant mycobacterial isolates (Lillo *et al.*, 1990). Infection is acquired from the environment and person-to-person spread is not thought to be important in the epidemiology of the disease. *Mycobacterium kansasii* may be isolated from swimming pools, hot and cold water supplies and storage tanks and this may be a source of infection in hospitals (McSwiggen and Collins, 1974). Areas of high and low incidence emphasize the sporadic nature of this disease and the deficits in our understanding of routes of transmission of *M. kansasii*. Unlike other non-tuberculosis species the number of *M. kansasii* infections does not appear to be rising (Breathnach *et al.*, 1995; Lillo *et al.*, 1990).

Infection is typically found in older patients and there is a strong male preponderance. A history of cigarette smoking is strongly associated with infection. Chronic lung conditions, including pneumoconiosis, treated tuberculosis, chronic obstructive airways disease and bronchiectasis, all predispose to *M. kansasii* infection (Lillo *et al.*, 1990; Pang, 1991).

Clinical Features

The characteristic clinical association is with a chronically progressive pulmonary infection which follows a rather indolent course (Lillo *et al.*, 1990; Pang, 1991). Clinically the presentation resembles tuberculosis and is frequently mistaken for it. Cough, sputum production, haemoptysis and the constitutional effects of infection are commonly seen. Infection is acquired from the environment and person-to-person spread is not thought to be important in the epidemiology of the disease.

Localized infections are reported but are much less common than in other mycobacterioses. Lymphadenitis, cutaneous and bone infection have all been reported (Breathnach *et al.*, 1995). Cutaneous infection is usually associated with immunosuppression whereas pulmonary infection arises in immunocompetent individuals with a compromised respiratory tract (Breathnach *et al.*, 1995). Disseminated infection may develop in patients with severe immunocompromise who often have a pulmonary predisposition and some are also infected by HIV (Lillo *et al.*, 1990).

The radiological appearances resemble tuberculosis and are characterized by apical cavitation or fibrosis. Hilar lymphadenopathy and pleural effusions are rare (Lillo *et al.*, 1990; Pang, 1991).

Pathology

The histopathological appearances of *M. kansasii* are indistinguishable from those of tuberculosis, with an inflammatory infiltrate of lymphocytes, histiocytes and a few giant cells. Acid-fast bacteria may be scanty.

Treatment

Antituberculosis drugs are less active against *M. kansasii*. Almost all isolates are susceptible to rifampicin. Isoniazid inhibits less than 50% of isolates at the standard breakpoint of 1 mg, but approximately 90% will be susceptible at a breakpoint of 5 mg, perhaps explaining the clinical success of isoniazid-containing regimens. *Mycobacterium kansasii* is also usually susceptible to ethambutol, streptomycin, ethionamide and cycloserine (Lillo *et al.*, 1990). All isolates are resistant to pyrazinamide. Patients should be treated with rifampicin, isoniazid and ethambutol daily for 18 months (Harris *et al.*, 1975; Anonymous, 1990). Shorter regimens including streptomycin in the first three months appear to achieve similarly high cure rates. A recent study suggests that isoniazid is not necessary as part of the regimen (Anonymous, 1994). The addition of another agent such as an aminoglycoside or 4-fluoroquinolone may be required in patients unable to tolerate the standard therapy. Treatment duration must often be extended for 12–24 months. In patients who relapse after treatment, resistance to first-line agents may develop.

MYCOBACTERIUM MALMOENSE

Mycobacterium malmoense is closely related to *M. avium–intracellulare*. It is now the second commonest non-tuberculosis mycobacterium after the latter organism in HIV-infected individuals in some countries (Zaugg *et al.*, 1993). It is a non-chromogenic organism which is very slow growing, with the result that some infections are not detected. *M. malmoense* was first isolated from four patients with pulmonary disease present in Malmo in Sweden (Schroder and Juhlin, 1977).

Epidemiology

Unlike other non-tuberculosis mycobacteria *M. malmoense* has no known environmental reservoir. It has only been isolated from human and animal sources. Most cases have been reported from Northern Europe including the UK, but cases have been reported in the Americas. The number of cases is increasing and this is thought to be a real rise and not the result of improved identification, as a review of the UK Mycobacterial Reference Laboratory records only found a few strains where a misidentification was possible (Jenkins, 1985).

Mycobacterium malmoense has an affinity for the respiratory tract and the majority of infections are pulmonary. Patients are predisposed to pulmonary infection by previous pulmonary disease, notably treated tuberculosis. Other associated conditions include lung carcinoma, chronic obstructive airways disease and pneumoconiosis (Henriques *et al.*, 1994). In one study 80% of patients were current or former smokers (France *et al.*, 1987). Immunosuppression by leukaemia or other malignancy can predispose to infection but *M. malmoense* is rarely isolated in association with HIV (Zaugg *et al.*, 1993). Infection can arise in previously healthy individuals and may progress in a manner analogous to tuberculosis.

The commonest extrapulmonary manifestation is cervical lymphadenitis, which occurs most often in children. Disseminated infection is reported in patients with severe immunocompromise including patients with HIV infection or leukaemia. Colonization of the respiratory tract in otherwise healthy individuals has been reported, as has colonization of the gastrointestinal tract. Despite this the majority of patients – more than 90% in some studies – from whom *M. malmoense* is isolated have clinical disease.

Clinical Features

The presentation may take place after a year of symptoms but some report an illness of only a few weeks' duration. Cough, weight loss and haemoptysis are the most prominent symptoms and the overall picture closely resembles tuberculosis. Radiological examination reveals the presence of cavitation in the majority of patients (Zaugg *et al.*, 1993; France *et al.*, 1987; Alberts *et al.*, 1987).

Antimicrobial Susceptibility

Mycobacterium malmoense has variable susceptibility to anti-tuberculosis agents. All strains are resistant to pyrazinamide and *para-aminosalicyclic* acid though most are susceptible to rifampicin and ethambutol and some strains are resistant to isoniazid (Zaugg *et al.*, 1993; Anonymous, 1990; France *et al.*, 1987). The correlation between outcome and *in vitro* susceptibility testing is poor. In a large study regimens containing rifampicin, isoniazid and ethambutol given for more than 18 months was associated with a favourable outcome

(Banks *et al.*, 1985). Surgery has been used as adjunctive therapy.

MYCOBACTERIUM ULCERANS

Epidemiology

Mycobacterium ulcerans was first isolated from patients in Bairnsdale, Australia, with necrotizing skin ulcers. Buruli ulcer, the lesion caused by this organism, is described in many tropical and subtropical countries in Africa, Central and South America and Southeast Asia (Marston *et al.*, 1995; Amofah *et al.*, 1993; Hayman, 1991).

An environmental source for *M. ulcerans* has not been identified but epidemiological studies indicate that it is to be found near slow-flowing or stagnant water (Marston *et al.*, 1995). Infection is most common in individuals under 15 years of age, and males and females are affected equally. The prevalence of infection is highest in villages close to rivers where farming activities occur. Infection appears to occur by direct inoculation into the skin, as wearing protective clothing such as long trousers makes infection less likely (Marston *et al.*, 1995). The incidence of infection is rising in some countries but this may relate to increasing farming activity and does not appear to be related to HIV co-infection (Marston *et al.*, 1995).

Clinical Features

The disease begins as a small subcutaneous swelling increasing in size until the skin is raised. At first it is attached to the skin but not the deep fascia, but as the lesion progresses it extends to involve this layer. The skin over the lesion is at first darker but then loses its pigmentation before becoming necrotic and ulcerating. Some cases have a small central vesicle. Rarely, the disease may present in an oedematous form mimicking cellulitis. Occasionally the necrosis spreads through the deep fascia involving muscle and bone (Hayman, 1993). Ulcers are typically painless, usually found on the lower limbs, but may more rarely occur on the face or trunk, especially in children. Buruli ulcer should be differentiated from foreign body granuloma, phycomycosis, fibroma or fibrosarcoma (Hayman, 1993).

Pathology

The ulcer usually has a straight or undermined edge with subcutaneous spread, producing nodules and a gelatinous material which is readily removed. An oedematous form of the disease has also been described (Hayman, 1993). Microscopically, necrotic tissue lines the ulcer and multiple acid-fast bacilli can be seen. The bacteria form tangled masses and 'globular' forms where many bacteria are found within macrophages have been described, but this latter term should be avoided as it may give rise to confusion with leprosy.

Caseation is not a characteristic of buruli ulceration. Necrosis is present in the lesion, including fat necrosis due to infarction of the arterioles serving the fat lobules. Mycobacteria can be found in lipid lacunae. The necrosis is characterized by calcification, especially in chronic lesions, although this feature is rarely described in Australian cases. In studies of cases biopsied sequentially three stages are described: necrosis and tissue destruction, an organizing stage and a healing stage.

Treatment

Surgical treatment, including excision and local debridement, may be necessary. Antimicrobial treatment with isoniazid and streptomycin, or oxytetracycline and dapsone, and a combination of rifampicin, minocycline and cotrimoxazole, may be beneficial. A significant number of patients are left with residual disability (Goutzamanis and Gilbert, 1995).

Control

BCG vaccination appears to provide some protection against infection (Amofah et al., 1993). Wearing long trousers may be beneficial by preventing the initial inoculation injury (Marston et al., 1995).

MYCOBACTERIUM FORTUITUM AND M. CHELONEI

These rapid-growing organisms are more closely related to *Nocardia* spp. (see Chapter 27). *Mycobacterium fortuitum* was first isolated from a frog and *M. chelonei* was first isolated from a turtle. These organisms were previously thought to be non-pathogenic but more recently their full potential for infection of many body systems has been recognized.

Epidemiology

Mycobacterium fortuitum and *M. chelonei* are environmental saprophytes. They may also be found in human specimens without evidence of disease. *Mycobacterium fortuitum* and *M. chelonei* are principally pathogens of the skin and soft tissue. Local abscesses following injection which are contaminated before administration. Surgical wounds may be infected postoperatively and infection following augmentation breast surgery with silicon implants has been reported (Wallace et al., 1983). Catheters, both intravenous and chronic ambulatory peritoneal dialysis, can become colonized. Keratitis and lymphadenitis have been reported (Raad et al., 1991). Disseminated infection can develop in immunocompromised patients, particularly those undergoing remission induction in leukaemia in whom neutropenia has developed (McWhinney et al., 1992). Pneumonia and disseminated skin infection can also occur in immunocompromised patients.

Pathology

Infection with rapidly growing mycobacteria is characterized histologically by the presence of an acute inflammatory response with polymorphonuclear leucocytes (PMNs) in microabscesses. Necrosis is almost invariably present and granulomatous change with Langerhan's giant cells is found in 80%. Caseation necrosis is rarely reported (Wallace et al., 1983). Acid-fast bacilli are scanty and may not be seen in as many as two-thirds of patients. When organisms are present they are usually found in clumps lying extracellulary, associated with microabscess.

Clinical Features

A primary source for infection is not usually apparent. Non-surgical skin infection is often described in children or young adults. It usually takes the form of cellulitis, often with abscess formation (Wallace *et al.*, 1983). The infection follows an indolent path with the patient only seeking medical attention after several weeks. The lesions are red and only mildly tender. The organisms are inoculated into the skin as a result of penetrating trauma, foreign body or pre-existing skin disease. Postoperative infections are often associated with implantation of prostheses, including cardiac valves and silicon prostheses used in augmentation mammoplasty. A series of sternotomy wound infections has been reported (Wallace *et al.*, 1983).

Pulmonary infection is associated with underlying pulmonary disease less often than for other non-tuberculosis mycobacteria and may pursue a progressive course to death.

Different clinical patterns of disseminated infection have been associated with renal transplantation, renal failure and collagen vascular disease where skin lesions predominate over organ involvement (Ingram *et al.*, 1993). In patients with malignancy or defects in cell-mediated immunity, disease is more widespread alongside skin involvement. In this latter situation the mortality is high.

Lymphadenitis with rapidly growing mycobacteria has been described in children and has been associated with dental extraction in some cases.

The outcome of infection with rapidly growing mycobacteria is in large part dependent on the nature of any underlying disease. Where there is a severe underlying immune deficit which cannot be reversed, the mortality rate is high.

Antimicrobial Susceptibility

Antimicrobial susceptibility is not predictable and these organisms are often resistant to first-line agents. Antimicrobial susceptibility tests should be performed using disc methods. First-line antituberculosis agents have no place in the management of infection due to rapidly growing mycobacteria. Aminoglycosides are useful and some authors recommend the use of amikacin together with cefoxitin in the initial therapy of infection. Many strains are susceptible to macrolides and some of the new agents look promising as therapeutic agents. Many isolates are susceptible to 4-fluoroquinolones which may be used in treatment (Anonymous, 1990; Ingram *et al.*, 1993).

Wherever possible underlying immune deficits should be reversed. Infected prostheses should also be removed. Surgical removal of infected tissue when this is possible, is beneficial.

MYCOBACTERIUM HAEMOPHILUM

Mycobacterium haemophilum is a fastidious member of the genus which grows more slowly than other species and requires iron-supplemented medium and a lower temperature of incubation (Dawson and Jennis, 1988). It was first identified in an ulcerating skin lesion of a woman with Hodgkin's disease. Since then a small number of cases have been reported in patients with severe defects in cell-mediated immunity.

Epidemiology

Infection with *M. haemophilum* have been reported worldwide. Lymphadenitis has been reported in immunocompetent children but most other reports are from patients who are severely immunocompromised. Before the appearance of the HIV epidemic most patients had been treated with immunosuppressive therapy after organ transplantation, or were patients with lymphoma. *Mycobacterium haemophilum* is now a recognized pathogen in patients with HIV infection (Kiehn and White, 1994). The true extent of *M. haemophilum* infection cannot be judged as there is probably considerable under-reporting due to failure to use appropriate media and conditions to isolate the organism. A recent survey reported 13 cases in 20 months, equivalent to one-third of the number of cases reported in the world literature (Straus *et al.*, 1994).

Little is known of the mode of transmission and cases appear to arise spontaneously. There is no evidence of person-to-person spread.

Clinical Features

Several syndromes have been associated with infection with *M. haemophilum*, including lymphadenitis in immunocompetent children, cutaneous ulceration, bacteraemia, and infection of the joints, bones and lungs in severely immunocompromised patients.

Lymphadenitis may arise in the cervical or perihilar region in children, producing a clinical picture similar to infection with *M. avium–intracellulare*. Cutaneous lesions are the commonest manifestation of *M. haemophilum* infection. The lesions tend to cluster on the extremities, often over joints, and this suggests that this distribution is related to the lower temperatures in these areas. Lesions are typically raised, violaceous and fluctuant, ranging in size from 0.5 to 2 cm. Later the lesions enlarge and become pustular and may be painful. The appearances must be distinguished from Kaposi's sarcoma. The majority of patients report joint symptoms including tenderness and swelling. A small proportion of patients have pulmonary lesions which may be cavitatory in nature.

Laboratory Diagnosis

Mycobacterium haemophilum is fastidious, requiring an egg-based chocolate agar medium supplemented with ferric ammonium citrate haemoglobin and haemin for optimum growth (Dawson and Jennis, 1988). The optimum incubation temperature for isolation is 32 °C. As the organism grows slowly incubation periods should be extended beyond 8 weeks.

Antimicrobial Susceptibility

Strains of *M. haemophilum* have been reported to be susceptible to rifabutin, ciprofloxacin, cycloserine and kanamycin. Approximately half are susceptible to rifampicin, most are resistant to isoniazid and none to pyrazinamide and ethambutol. There are currently no standard methods for determining susceptibility and no recommendations for empirical therapy (Straus *et al.*, 1994).

OTHER MYCOBACTERIA

A wide range of organisms which would once have been dismissed as contaminants have been isolated from patients and shown to be the cause of invasive infections. These include *M. shimoidei*, *M. celatum*, *M. gordonae*, and *M. simiae* (Tsukamura, 1982; Weinberger *et al.*, 1992; Tortoli *et al.*, 1995; Torres *et al.*, 1991). Some of these organisms are found in tap-water supplies in hospitals. This may act as a source of infection for immunocompromised patients or a source of contamination for specimens, microbiological stains and media in the laboratory. Consequently each individual isolate of a mycobacterium should be judged on the clinical features of the case. In most instances a positive diagnosis of infection cannot be made unless the organisms are isolated on more than one occasion. Isolation from a normally sterile site or from bronchoalveolar lavage may indicate invasion.

MYCOBACTERIUM LEPRAE

Although an important cause of disease worldwide leprosy is not usually found in the province of the clinical microbiology laboratory as the organism cannot be cultivated and there are no reliable serological tests (Hastings, 1994).

Epidemiology

Leprosy was once endemic throughout the world, but is now confined to low and middle income countries emphasizing poverty as an important cofactor in maintaining the disease in the community predominantly in Southeast Asia. The prevalence of leprosy has been falling in recent years and WHO estimates that there are between three and five million cases worldwide in comparison to the ten million estimated ten years ago. This difference has been brought about by the application of effective bactericidal chemotherapy.

The mode of transmission of leprosy is uncertain but it is thought that nasal shedding by lepromatous cases has an important role to play.

Clinical Features

Leprosy attacks the skin and the nerves. The presentation of the disease can be subtle or florid, the clinical signs depending on the immunological response to infection (see Chapter 6a). Patients with some cell mediated immunity have 'tuberculoid disease' which is localized to individual nerves and skin patches. Clinical symptoms and signs of thickened nerves, pallid skin patches and anaesthesia are similarly localized. As immunity to *M. leprae* falls, tuberculoid disease gives way to lepromatous disease where there is little immune response and the infection is more generalized as are involvement of nerves and skin. Anaesthesia results in loss of digits. A more detailed account is found in Hastings (1994).

Treatment

The treatment of leprosy has been transformed by the introduction of multidrug therapy which includes rifampicin which rapidly renders the patient non infectious. The regimen for multibacillary disease consists of rifampicin 600 mg once monthly, clofazamine 300 mg once monthly and 50 mg daily together with dapsone 100 mg daily. All medications are continued for two years and preferably to negativity on skin smears. For paucibacillary disease rifampicin 600 mg once monthly and dapsone 100 mg daily for six months. It also includes management of reversal reactions and erythema nodosum leprosum which arise during therapy. Leprosy treatment involves much more than chemotherapy and must encompass restorative plastic surgery tranplanting tendons to restore function to denervated hands and feet. It must also include physiotherapy, and occupational therapy to enable patients to return to their communities and earn again (Hastings, 1994).

Prevention and Control

Prevention must be directed to rendering lepromatous patients non-infectious as speedily as possible. This is achieved by offering open access free services which strive to remove the stigma associated with leprosy and which are capable of providing chemotherapy coupled with effective case finding. Leprosy is a disease of poverty, and will only finally come under control with improvement in living standards.

REFERENCES

Alberts, W.M., Chandler, K.W., Soloman, D.A. and Goldman, A.L. (1987) Pulmonary disease caused by *Mycobacterium malmoense*. *American Review of Respiratory Disease*, **135**, 1375–1378.

Amofah, G.K, Sagoe-Moses, C., Adjei-Acquah, C. and Frimpong, E.H. (1993) Epidemiology of Buruli ulcer in Amansie West district, Ghana. *Transactions of The Royal Society of Tropical Medicine and Hygiene*, **87**, 644–645.

Anonymous (1990) Diagnosis and treatment of diseases caused by non-tuberculosis mycobacteria. *American Review of Respiratory Disease*, **142**, 940–953.

Anonymous (1994) *Mycobacterium kansasii* pulmonary infection: a prospective study of the results of nine months of treatment with rifampicin and ethambutol. Research Committee, British Thoracic Society. *Thorax*, **49**, 442–445.

Banks, J., Jenkins, P.A. and Smith, A.P. (1985) Pulmonary infection with *Mycobacterium malmoense*: a review of treatment and response. *Tubercle*, **66**, 197–203.

Benson, C.A. (1994) Disease due to *Mycobacterium avium* complex in patients with AIDS: epidemiology and clinical syndrome. *Clinical Infectious Diseases*, **18**(Suppl. 3), S218–S222.

Breathnach, A., Levell, N., Munro, C. *et al.* (1995) Cutaneous *Mycobacterium kansasii* infection: case report and review. *Clinical Infectious Diseases*, **20**, 812–817.

Chin, D.P., Reingold, A.L., Stone, E.N. *et al.* (1994) The impact of *Mycobacterium avium* complex bacteremia and its treatment on survival of AIDS patients. *Journal of Infectious Diseases*, **170**, 578–584.

Collins, C.H., Grange, J.M., Noble, W.C. and Yates, M.D. (1985) *Mycobacterium marinum* infections in man. *Journal of Hygiene (Cambridge)*, **94**, 135–149.

Costrini, A.M., Mahler, D.A., Gross, W.M. *et al.*

(1981) Clinical and roentgenographic features of nosocomial pulmonary disease due to *Mycobacterium xenopi*. *American Review of Respiratory Disease*, **123**, 104–109.

Dawson, D.J. and Jennis, F. (1988) Mycobacteria with growth requirement for ferric ammonium citrate, identified as *Mycobacterium haemophilum*. *Journal of Clinical Microbiology*, **11**, 190–192.

Edelstein, H. (1994) *Mycobacterium marinum* skin infections: report of 31 cases and review of the literature. *Archives of Internal Medicine*, **154**, 1359–1364.

France, A.J., McLeod, D.T., Calder, M.A. and Seaton, A. (1987) *Mycobacterium malmoense* infections in Scotland: an increasing problem. *Thorax*, **42**, 593–595.

Goutzamanis, J.J. and Gilbert, G.L. (1995) *Mycobacterium ulcerans* infection in Australian children: report of eight cases and review. *Clinical Infectious Diseases*, **21**, 1186–1192.

Harris, G.D., Johanson, W.G. and Nicholson, D.P. (1975) Response to chemotherapy of pulmonary infection due to *Mycobacterium kansasii*. *American Review of Respiratory Disease*, **112**, 31–36.

Hastings, R.C. (1994) *Leprosy*, 2nd edn. Churchill Livingstone, Edinburgh.

Hayman, J. (1991) Postulated epidemiology of *Mycobacterium ulcerans* infection. *International Journal of Epidemiology*, **20**, 1093–1098.

Hayman, J. (1993) Out of Africa: observations on the histopathology of *Mycobacterium ulcerans* infection. *Journal of Clinical Pathology*, **46**, 5–9.

Heifets, L.B. (1994) Quantitative cultures and drug susceptibility testing of *Mycobacterium avium* clinical isolates before and during antimicrobial therapy. *Research in Microbiology*, **145**, 188–196.

Henriques, B., Hoffner, S.E., Petrini, B. *et al.* (1994) Infection with *Mycobacterium malmoense* in Sweden: report of 221 cases. *Clinical Infectious Diseases*, **18**, 596–600.

Hoover, D.R., Graham, N.M.H., Bacellar, H. *et al.* (1995) An epidemiologic analysis of *Mycobacterium avium* complex disease in homosexual men infected with human immunodeficiency virus type 1. *Clinical Infectious Diseases*, **20**, 1250–1258.

Horsburgh, C.R., Chin, D.P., Yajko, D.M. *et al.* (1994a) Environmental risk factors of acquisition of *Mycobacterium avium* complex in persons with human immunodeficiency virus infection. *Journal of Infectious Diseases*, **170**, 362–367.

Horsburgh, C.R., Metchock, B., Gordon, S.M. *et al.* (1994b) Predictors of survival in patients with AIDS and disseminated *Mycobacterium avium* complex disease. *Journal of Infectious Diseases*, **170**, 573–577.

Ingram, C.W., Tanner, D.C., Durack, D.T. *et al.*

(1993) Disseminated infection with rapidly growing mycobacteria. *Clinical Infectious Diseases*, **16**, 463–471.

Jenkins, P.A. (1985) *Mycobacterium malmoense*. *Tubercle*, **66**, 193–195.

Kiehn, T.E. and White, M. (1994) *Mycobacterium haemophilum*: an emerging pathogen. *European Journal of Clinical Microbiology and Infectious Diseases*, **13**, 925–931.

Kirschner Jr, R.A., Parker, B.C. and Falkinham III, J.O. (1992) Epidemiology of infection by nontuberculous mycobacteria: *Mycobacterium avium*, *Mycobacterium intracellulare*, and *Mycobacterium scrofulaceum* in acid, brown-water swamps of the southeastern United States and their association with environmental variables. *American Review of Respiratory Disease*, **145**, 271–275.

Lillo, M., Orengo, S., Cernoch, P. and Harris, R.L. (1990) Pulmonary and disseminated infections due to *Mycobacterium kansasii*: a decade of experience. *Reviews of Infectious Diseases*, **12**, 760–767.

Marston, B.J., Diallo, M.O., Horsburgh Jr, C.R. *et al.* (1995) Emergence of Buruli ulcer disease in the Daloa region of Cote d'Ivoire. *American Journal of Tropical Medicine and Hygiene*, **52**, 219–224.

McSwiggen, D.A. and Collins, C.H. (1974) The isolation of *M. kansasii* and *M. xenopi* from water systems. *Tubercle*, **55**, 291–297.

McWhinney, P.H., Yates, M., Prentice, H.G. *et al.* (1992) Infection caused by *Mycobacterium chelonae*: a diagnostic and therapeutic problem in the neutropenic patient. *Clinical Infectious Diseases*, **14**, 1208–1212.

Miller, W.C., Perkins, M.D., Richardson, W.J. and Sexton, D.J. (1994) Pott's disease caused by *Mycobacterium xenopi*: case report and review. *Clinical Infectious Diseases*, **19**, 1024–1028.

Nightingale, S.D., Cameron, D.W. and Gordin, F.M. (1993) Two controlled trials of rifabutin prophylaxis against *Mycobacterium avium* complex infection in AIDS. *New England Journal of Medicine*, **329**, 828–833.

O'Brien, R.J., Geiter, L.J. and Snider, D.E. (1987) The epidemiology of nontuberculous mycobacterial diseases in the United States. *American Review of Respiratory Disease*, **135**, 1007–1014.

Pang, S.C. (1991) *Mycobacterium kansasii* infections in Western Australia (1962–1987). *Respiratory Medicine*, **85**, 213–218.

Peters, M., Muller, C., Rusch-Gerdes, S. *et al.* (1995) Isolation of atypical mycobacteria from tap water in hospitals and homes: is this a possible source of disseminated MAC infection in AIDS patients? *Journal of Infection*, **31**, 39–44.

Raad, I.I., Vartivarian, S., Khan, A. and Bodey, G.P. (1991) Catheter-related infections caused by the

Mycobacterium fortuitum complex: 15 cases and review. *Reviews of Infectious Diseases*, **13**, 1120–1125.

Schroder, K.H. and Juhlin, I. (1977) *Mycobacterium malmoense* sp. nov. *International Journal of Systematic Bacteriology*, **27**, 241–246.

Schwabacher, H. (1959) A strain of mycobacterium from skin lesions of a cold-blooded animal. *Journal of Hygiene (London)*, **57**, 57.

Simor, A.E., Salit, I.E. and Vellend, H. (1984) The role of *Mycobacterium xenopi* in human disease. *American Review of Respiratory Disease*, **129**, 435–438.

Smith, M.J. and Citron, K.M. (1983) Clinical review of pulmonary disease caused by *Mycobacterium xenopi*. *Thorax*, **38**, 373–377.

Straus, W.L., Ostroff, S.M., Jernigan, D.B. *et al.* (1994) Clinical and epidemiologic characteristics of *Mycobacterium haemophilum*, an emerging pathogen in immunocompromised patients. *Annals of Internal Medicine*, **120**, 118–125.

Torres, R.A., Nord, J., Feldman, R. *et al.* (1991) Disseminated mixed *Mycobacterium simiae–Mycobacterium avium* complex infection in acquired immunodeficiency syndrome. *Journal of Infectious Diseases*, **164**, 432–433.

Tortoli, E., Piersimoni, C., Bacosi, D. *et al.* (1995) Isolation of the newly described species *Mycobacterium celatum* from AIDS patients. *Journal of Clinical Microbiology*, **33**, 137–140.

Tsukamura, M. (1982) *Mycobacterium shimoidei* sp. nov. rev., a lung pathogen. *International Journal of Systematic Bacteriology*, **32**, 67–69.

von Reyn, C.F., Waddell, R.D., Eaton, T. *et al.* (1993) Isolation of *Mycobacterium avium* complex from water in the United States, Finland, Zaire, and Kenya. *Journal of Clinical Microbiology*, **31**, 3227–3230.

Wallace, R.J., Swenson, J.M., Silcox, V.A. *et al.* (1983) Spectrum of disease due to rapidly growing mycobacteria. *Review of Infectious Diseases*, **5**, 657–679.

Weinberger, M., Berg, S.L., Fuerstein, I.M. *et al.* (1992) Disseminated infection with *Mycobacterium gordonae*: report of a case and review of the literature. *Clinical Infectious Diseases*, **14**, 1229–1239.

Zaugg, M., Salfinger, M., Opravil, M. and Luthy, R. (1993) Extrapulmonary and disseminated infections due to *Mycobacterium malmoense*: case report and review. *Clinical Infectious Diseases*, **16**, 540–549.

7a

BRANHAMELLA, MORAXELLA, KINGELLA

B.I. Davies

INTRODUCTION

The members of the genera *Neisseria*, *Branhamella*, *Moraxella* and *Kingella* have been embroiled in a confusion of nomenclature and taxonomy over the last two decades. Although the true neisseriae have been well described for many years (see Chapters 7b and 7c), the organism originally described in 1896 as *Mikrokokkus catarrhalis* and changed in 1920 to *Neisseria catarrhalis* (Riou, 1986) was renamed *Branhamella catarrhalis* in 1970 in honour of Dr Sara E. Branham and is now proposed as a subgenus of the genus *Moraxella* within the family Neisseriaceae (Bøvre, 1984). Its correct nomenclature would therefore have to be *Moraxella (Branhamella) catarrhalis*. Although this unhandy name was reached on good scientific grounds based on G + C percentages of 40–45% in the DNA, like those of the true moraxellae (also 40–45%), but different from those of the neisseriae (47–52%), the proposal has not received universal acceptance. One of the pioneer workers has reviewed these organisms (Catlin, 1990) and has explained clearly why he still continues to use the nomenclature *Branhamella catarrhalis*. Many authoritative modern reference books (e.g. 5th edition of the *Manual of Clinical Microbiology* (Pickett *et al.*,

1991) and the third edition of *Cowan and Steel's Manual for the Identification of Medical Bacteria* (Barrow and Feltham, 1993)) still prefer to use this nomenclature and we shall do so too. Further controversy arises because *Branhamella catarrhalis* and the 'false neisseriae' (*N. caviae*, from guinea-pigs, *N. ovis* from sheep, and *N. cuniculi* from rabbits) are, almost without exception, Gram-negative cocci and fit poorly in the genus *Moraxella*.

The true *Moraxella* spp. also have a long history extending back to the publications of V. Morax and T. Axenfeld in 1896 and 1897, respectively (reviewed by Wilson and Wilkinson, 1983). For many years the conjunctivitis-causing organism now known as *Moraxella lacunata* was called the Morax–Axenfeld bacillus. Most of the true moraxellae are Gram-negative coccobacilli or obvious rods. *Moraxella urethralis*, a further species, is also composed of coccoid rods but has recently been moved to a different genus because of its DNA composition and its motility. It has been renamed *Oligella urethralis*.

The *Kingella* group started off in 1968 with the Gram-negative rod first known as *Moraxella kingii* (sic), which was then temporarily renamed *Kingella kingii*. Its name was changed again in 1974 to *Kingella kingae* because of the female gender of

Elizabeth O. King. The composition of this group may change again in the future. Despite the prolific literature on the taxonomy and nomenclature of these organisms, *Moraxella* and *Kingella* are seldom encountered in a diagnostic microbiology laboratory, and there is considerable geographical variation in the occurrence of *Branhamella catarrhalis* (Davies and Maesen, 1986).

DESCRIPTION OF THE ORGANISMS

Morphology

Branhamella catarrhalis strains show a typical kidney-bean Gram-negative diplococcal shaped form in Gram-stained smears of tissue exudates, pus, purulent sputum, etc., in which they are often not distinguishable from neisseriae. They may sometimes lie intracellularly (Figure 7a.1). Stained smears made from cultures generally reveal a more spherical form. Sometimes the bacterial cells show a degree of resistance to decolorization during Gram staining.

- *Moraxella bovis* is usually rod-like in shape, with some variation between plump and slender forms.
- *Moraxella lacunata* strains are usually plump bacilli, with a tendency to form pairs end to end: some chain forming is also possible.
- *Moraxella nonliquefaciens* is generally seen in a cocco-bacillary form but thin filaments are also possible.
- *Moraxella osloensis* is usually cocco-bacillary.
- *Moraxella phenylpyruvica* is morphologically similar to *M. nonliquefaciens*.
- All moraxellae are Gram negative.

The three species in the *Kingella* group at present are all short Gram-negative rods 1 μm broad and approximately 2–3 μm in length (Figure 7a.2). There is a tendency towards the formation of end-to-end pairs and short chains.

From these descriptions it is clear that *Branhamella catarrhalis* differs morphologically from the moraxellae and the kingellae but it is also apparent that the members of the two latter groups

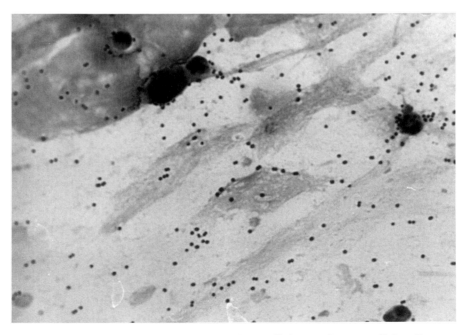

Figure 7a.1. Gram-stained smear of sputum with intracellular and extracellular Gram-negative cocci (*Branhamella catarrhalis*).

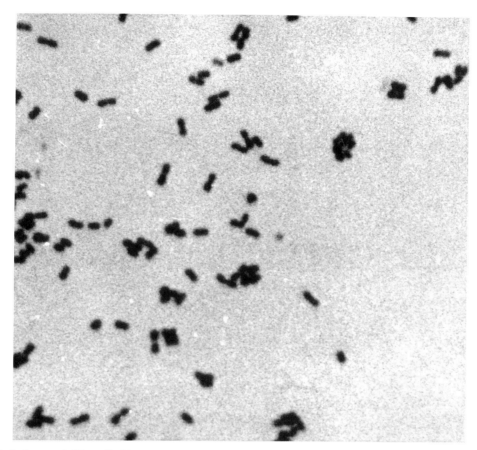

Figure 7a.2. Culture of *Kingella kingae* stained by methylene blue.

cannot always be reliably differentiated on morphological appearances alone.

Cultural Characteristics, Identification

All strains of *Branhamella catarrhalis*, *Moraxella* spp. and *Kingella* spp. grow reasonably well on standard laboratory culture media when enriched with either blood or (especially) serum. Additional carbon dioxide in the atmosphere does not improve growth. Unlike the true haemophilic bacteria, there is no known requirement for specific growth factors, although *B. catarrhalis* will not grow in the absence of arginine and *M. lacunata* requires animal protein. Most species fail to grow on MacConkey medium, exceptions being *M. osloensis*, *M.*

phenylpyruvica and occasional strains of *K. kingae*. Unlike the branhamellae and moraxellae which are strict aerobes, *Kingella* spp. are said to be facultatively anaerobic (Pickett *et al.*, 1991), although growth is comparatively poor. Colonies of *B. catarrhalis* are fairly small after overnight incubation in air (1–2 mm diameter) but grow in size with extended incubation. They are matt and greyish white in appearance and can be easily moved over the culture plate by touching with a bacteriological wire loop (the so-called 'ice-hockey puck' phenomenon). Growth range of *B. catarrhalis* is between 22 and 38 °C, unlike most *Moraxella* and *Kingella* spp. which grow poorly under 30 °C. However, *M. phenylpyruvica* is said to be able to grow at 5 °C. Colonial appearances of *Moraxella* and *Kingella* species are not distinctive except that *M. bovis*, *M. lacunata* and *K. kingae* may cause pitting in the agar surface. Prolonged subculturing of all *Branhamella*, *Moraxella* and *Kingella* strains may lead to unexpected death of the organism, particularly if humidity is inadequate. Freeze-drying of strains for collection purposes is thus recommended. Culture of *Kingella* spp. from joint fluids may be improved by using modern systems such as the BACTEC blood culture system (Yagupsky *et al.*, 1992), in which the clinical material is diluted in the fluid culture medium.

All individual species within the genera *Branhamella* and *Moraxella* are oxidase positive, produce catalase and fail to break down any carbohydrates to form acid. They are all non-motile but a 'twitching' movement has been described. In contrast, *Kingella* spp. do not produce catalase and their oxidase reaction may be feeble, especially if the dimethyl-*p*-phenylenediamine reagent is used in place of the tetramethyl compound. If sufficiently rich media are employed to promote bacterial growth (10–20% ascitic fluid agar, for example) *Kingella* spp. all break down glucose, and some species can also break down maltose and sucrose. However, conventional 'sugar fermentation tests' may well prove negative.

Reduction of nitrate to nitrite is rapid with *B. catarrhalis*, but somewhat slower with the *Moraxella* spp. Some strains of *M. bovis* and *M. osloensis* yield negative nitrate reduction test results. Among the kingellae, only *K. denitrificans* reduces nitrate to nitrite and then further to nitrogen, a property shared with *B. catarrhalis*. The above characteristics are summarized in Table 7a.1.

Because *B. catarrhalis* is so obviously a Gram-negative coccus, it needs to be differentiated from the various neisseriae which have been described earlier. In fact, the colonial appearances are completely different, and no difficulties are encountered in daily laboratory practice. However, the failure to break down any carbohydrates may be shared with atypical meningococci and extra tests for *B. catarrhalis* may be required. In our own experience all *B. catarrhalis* strains were found to hydrolyse tributyrin rapidly in the 4-hour tablet test (Rosco Diagnostica, Denmark), whereas all of a variety of pathogenic and non-pathogenic neisseriae yielded negative results. It appears that among other bacteria only the 'false neisseriae' yield positive results, although the reactions are less strong than those with *B. catarrhalis* (Riou, 1986). A further test, only positive for *B. catarrhalis* (and possibly '*Neisseria*' *caviae*), is the

TABLE 7a.1   FIRST-STAGE TABLE FOR *BRANHAMELLA, MORAXELLA, KINGELLA*

	Branhamella	Moraxella	Kingella
Morphology (all are Gram negative)	Cocci	Coccobacilli, rods, sometimes in pairs	Short rods, sometimes in short chains
Aerobic growth on:			
nutrient agar	+	+	+
serum agar	+ +	+ +	+ +
MacConkey agar	–	Variable	Variable
Anaerobic growth	–	–	Scanty
Catalase production	+	+	–
Oxidase test	+	+	+[a]
Reduction of:			
nitrate to nitrite	+ +	+	+[b]
nitrite to nitrogen	+	–	+[b]
Breakdown of carbohydrate	–	–	+[c]
Hydrolysis of tributyrin	+ + +	–	–
Production of DNAase	+ + +	–	–

[a] Results often only positive when tetramethyl-*p*-phenylenediamine is used for test.
[b] *K. denitrificans* strains positive, other *Kingella* spp. negative.
[c] Carbohydrate breakdown tests may be negative with some conventional methods.

TABLE 7a.2 SECOND-STAGE TABLE FOR *MORAXELLA* AND *KINGELLA*

	Moraxella group					*Kingella* group		
	M. bovis	*M. lacunata*	*M. nonliquefaciens*	*M. osloensis*	*M. phenylpyruvica*	*K. denitrificans*	*K. indologenes*	*K. kingae*
Growth on:								
MacConkey agar	–	–	–	+	+	–	–	Variable[a]
Pitting of agar surface	+	+	–	–	–	+	–	Occasionally
Breakdown of:								
glucose	–	–	–	–	–	+[b]	+[b]	+[b]
maltose	–	–	–	–	–	–	+[b]	+[b]
sucrose	–	–	–	–	–	–	+[b]	–
Reduction of:								
nitrate to nitrite	Variable[a]	+	+	Variable[a]	+	+	–	–
nitrite to nitrogen	–	–	–	–	–	+	–	–
Gelatin liquefaction	+	+	–	–	–	+	–	–
Deamination of phenylalanine	–	31%[c]	–	14%[c]	97%[c]	...[d]	...[d]	...[d]
Production of indole	–	–	–	–	–	–	+	–

[a] Strains yielding 'variable' results are positive in 20–80% of instances.
[b] Carbohydrate breakdown tests may be negative with some conventional methods.
[c] Percentage of strains able to deaminate phenylalanine.
[d] Information not available.

DNAase test which we have also found to yield clear-cut results although requiring incubation for two to four days.

Table 7a.2 therefore only deals with the genera *Moraxella* and *Kingella* and may assist with the identification of the individual species. It must be emphasized, however, that this identification procedure is, at the present time and in our present state of knowledge, far from ideal.

CLINICAL FEATURES AND EPIDEMIOLOGY

Branhamella catarrhalis

We have recently reviewed the clinical significance of *B. catarrhalis* and the therapeutic problems associated with this species (Davies, 1991). Despite the long history of these organisms, it is only in the last 15–20 years that their importance has become accepted. First and foremost, they are associated in many areas with acute purulent exacerbations of chronic bronchitis or chronic obstructive lung disease (COLD). In the De Wever Hospital, 185 of 500 such episodes (37%) yielded *B. catarrhalis* in the sputum cultures and in 127 instances it was the only pathogen demonstrated. Well-documented cases of pneumonia associated with *B. catarrhalis* have been described (Hager *et al.*, 1987) but they are rare, even in immuno-compromised patients or in those with immuno-globulin abnormalities. We have recently seen one single patient with acute community-acquired pneumonia in whom both the sputum and a pro-tected bronchial brush yielded 5×10^6 colony-forming units (cfu) of *B. catarrhalis* per millilitre. In many districts these organisms are also associated with upper respiratory tract infections, particularly paranasal sinusitis and acute otitis media (Shurin *et al.*, 1983) and these have been reviewed (O'Grady and Nord, 1986). Sporadic cases of bacteraemia, meningitis, keratitis and endocarditis have been described, mostly in immunocompromised patients, but these must all be considered rare.

Most of the *B. catarrhalis* lower respiratory tract infections occur in fairly well-defined geo-graphical areas, mainly those associated with heavy industry such as the coal, iron, steel and chemical industries (Davies and Maesen, 1990). However, these infections occur also in large and small cities, in Europe, America and New Zealand (Slevin *et al.*, 1984). Nasopharyngeal carriage rates in normal adults in a variety of cities have varied from zero to 7% in recent years, although rates in children may be age dependent and can range from 24% (under two years of age) to zero rates in older children. Selective culture media containing, amongst other substances, vancomycin and trimethoprim have been developed (Catlin, 1990; Vaneechoutte *et al.*, 1990b).

Moraxella spp., *Kingella* spp.

Cultures yielding true moraxellae are rare in most laboratories and even the reference laboratory at the Centers for Disease Control (CDC) only received 933 isolates over a period of 27 years (Graham *et al.*, 1990). Analysis of our own laboratory results in 1993 showed that, of the 16 420 bacterial isolates, there were 506 isolates of *B. catarrhalis* but only 13 of the various *Moraxella* spp. none of which was *M. lacunata*. Most of the *Moraxella* spp. were oxidase and catalase positive, but failed to produce indole or to liquefy gelatin. This would seem to agree with the CDC data showing that more than a third of the strains there were *M. nonliquefaciens*. Out of the 933 *Moraxella*-like organisms at the CDC, only 79 were identified as *K. kingae*. The single strain of *K. kingae* seen in our laboratory in recent years came from the Dutch microbiology quality assur-ance scheme, and 37 of the 65 participating laboratories identified it correctly! Most of the misidentifications were described as *Eikenella corrodens* (five times), and *Cardiobacterium hominis* or *Moraxella* spp. (each four times). It does seem that sporadic isolates of *Moraxella* and *Kingella* spp. from eye infections (Mollee *et al.*, 1992) in man and animals and from blood or cerebrospinal fluid (CSF) cultures in man (Nam-nyak *et al.*, 1991) will be recorded, but the *K. kingae* association with bone and joint infections in both children (Yagupsky *et al.*, 1992; Chiquito

TABLE 7a.3 CLINICAL INFECTIONS ASSOCIATED WITH *MORAXELLA* AND *KINGELLA* SPECIES

(a) *Moraxella* species	
M. bovis	Conjunctivitis in cattle and horses
M. lacunata	Conjunctivitis and keratitis in humans, now becoming much rarer. Sporadically in blood cultures, more often in nasopharynx
M. nonliquefaciens	Upper respiratory tract (nasopharynx) of humans. Occasionally in eye and blood cultures
M. osloensis	Human upper respiratory tract (nasopharynx), urine. Only occasionally in eye and blood cultures, but becoming more common
M. phenylpyruvica	Positive blood cultures, sometimes unexplained. Sometimes repeatedly positive
(b) *Kingella* species	
K. denitrificans	Endocarditis, prosthetic valve infections, chronic granulomatous disease in AIDS patients
K. indologenes	Eye infections (very rare)
K. kingae	Bone, joint and eye infections, especially in children. Bacteraemia, endocarditis, meningitis

et al., 1991) and adults (Meis *et al.*, 1992) suggests that existing laboratory procedures on materials from patients with such infections may not always be optimal. Table 7a.3 presents the known data on the clinical presentations of infections caused by *Moraxella* and *Kingella*.

LABORATORY DIAGNOSIS

Specimens Required

Eye infections

Obtaining correct specimen materials for the bacteriological diagnosis of eye infection is seldom simple, and it is not sufficient to rub a swab over the eye, place the swab in the transport medium and send it to a distant laboratory. Especially when there is corneal ulceration, the specimens need to be collected by a skilled ophthalmologist who may also wish to take corneal scrapings. Frankly purulent material presents fewer problems, although even then the necessary materials for the diagnosis of underlying viral infection (adenovirus, herpes simplex) or chlamydial infection also need to be

submitted. It is important to ensure that no fluids containing antiseptics or antibiotics have been instilled prior to specimen collection!

Respiratory tract infections

Spontaneously produced purulent sputum is usually sufficient for a reliable bacteriological diagnosis. However, if the patient is not producing frankly purulent material or has unproductive pneumonia, then invasive methods of specimen collection (such as sputum induction with nebulized salt solution, bronchoscopy, bronchoalveolar lavage and protected bronchial brushing) may be used, although our experience is that cultures from these materials are often negative in patients with little or no sputum. Quantitation of these cultures is necessary (a short dilution series) in order to distinguish endobronchial infection from contamination, even though the cut-off points (10^3 or 10^4 organisms per millilitre) have not been definitively agreed. Screening surveys for upper respiratory tract colonization may employ nose, throat or nasopharyngeal swabs (Vaneechoutte *et al.*, 1990b) but pernasal swabs may also be used.

Bone and joint infections

Purulent material obtained directly by surgery or by puncture from patients with bone and joint infections may indicate from the cultures which form of antimicrobial therapy is advisable. Here again, representative material is less adequately obtained by swabbing than by direct sampling. In any case, delicate organisms should not be allowed to die out from excessive drying or exposure to oxygen, and a closed needle and syringe is often useful. Biopsies should be processed without any delay.

Joint aspirates should perhaps be injected on the ward or in the theatre into blood culture bottles and processed further as blood (preferably by means of one of the modern automatic systems).

Endocarditis, bacteraemia, meningitis

Blood cultures will normally be taken from patients suspected of endocarditis, whether or not associated with the presence of prosthetic valves. CSF is usually obtained by careful lumbar puncture of patients suspected of meningitis. Whatever method is used for culture of these normally sterile materials, it should be such that the most demanding bacterial pathogens (e.g. *Haemophilus influenzae*, *N. gonorrhoeae* and *N. meningitidis*) can grow, ensuring that the less demanding *Branhamella*, *Moraxella* and *Kingella* spp. will be cultured if present.

Culture Techniques

Standard culture techniques in many diagnostic microbiology laboratories include a rich basic medium such as blood agar (two plates if one is to be incubated in air and one in a carbon dioxide incubator, and a third if the specimen requires anaerobic incubation). Respiratory and bone and joint materials will usually also be cultured on heated blood agar (chocolate agar) in the carbon dioxide incubator, as will CSF specimens. Most laboratories also include MacConkey medium plates and selective media for anaerobic cocci and bacilli in their routine cultures of pus specimens where anaerobes can be expected. In the routine laboratory, special selective media for

Branhamella, *Moraxella* and *Kingella* species are not employed, although for screening surveys (see above) such media have a certain function, especially if the cultures are deliberately not incubated in a carbon dioxide incubator. This improves the selectivity (Vaneechoutte *et al.*, 1990b).

Minimal Requirements for Identification

It is probably sufficient for *B. catarrhalis* isolates that the following characteristics be determined (Stratton, 1990):

- Gram negative cocci of human origin;
- grow with greyish-white matt colonies on standard media (but not on MacConkey);
- carbohydrates not broken down;
- tributyrin hydrolysed rapidly and/or DNAase produced.

For the members of the genus *Moraxella*, the following may be required:

- Gram-negative coccobacilli, rods or filaments, especially if present as end-to-end pairs or chains in material of human origin;
- oxidase and catalase tests positive;
- carbohydrates not broken down;
- pitting of the agar surface and/or liquefaction of gelatin by some species;
- deamination of phenylalanine by some species.

It is not yet possible to clarify the minimum identification requirements for *Kingella* spp. and the reader is referred to Tables 7a.1 and 7a.2.

IN VITRO ANTIMICROBIAL SUSCEPTIBILITY PATTERNS

Branhamella catarrhalis

There is no shortage of information on the susceptibility patterns of *B. catarrhalis*, reflecting this organism's role as a common respiratory tract pathogen. There is general agreement in the modern literature that the majority of strains now produce β-lactamases, resulting in direct or indirect pathogenicity (Percival *et al.*, 1977), but the actual percentage varies from district to district. In our own laboratory, 81% of strains are currently producers. We have followed the same line as other investigators in claiming that β-lactamase production must automatically lead to interpretation of susceptibility test results for β-lactamase-labile antibiotics as resistant (Davies and Maesen, 1990) even though a large zone of inhibition of growth may be seen in disk diffusion tests or an apparently low ampicillin minimal inhibitory concentration (MIC) value of 0.5 mg/l, or less, may be noted (Fung *et al.*, 1992). Table 7a.4 shows our own MIC results in recent years, from which it is clear that many β-lactamase-producing strains may appear to be highly susceptible to ampicillin and penicillin at first sight. The effect of β-lactamase inhibitors such as clavulanate is, nevertheless, dramatic and all isolates are normally susceptible to the combination co-amoxiclav. As little as 0.5 mg/l clavulanate can reduce the amoxycillin MICs from 1 mg/l or more to 0.25 mg/l, or less (Maesen *et al.*, 1987).

The position with regard to cephalosporins is much less clear cut than the literature would have us believe. Although most countries have agree-ments on breakpoint concentrations for antibiotics (the definition of what is 'susceptible'), these are not always in accordance with clinical practice and therapeutic experience. For example, the MIC value below which strains are to be considered as susceptible to (e.g. cefotaxime) is 0.25 mg/l in Britain (Working Party, 1988) and Germany, but 4 mg/l in The Netherlands, and 8 mg/l in the USA (Baqueiro, 1990). Table 7a.4 also shows our own MIC results from clinical studies with a wide variety of cephalosporins, some not yet registered in the UK, from which one may conclude that MICs of most non-producers lie well below 0.25 mg/l, although there is a considerable spread of results among the β-lactamase-producing strains, some yielding MICs of the order of 1 or 2 mg/l. The differences between the β-lactamase producers and the non-producers are particularly obvious for the new antibiotics cefodizime (Davies *et al.*, 1992) and cefepime. Our own studies with various new cephalosporins have only seemed to reinforce the view that the definition of 'susceptible' for strains of *B. catarrhalis* causing endobronchial infections should preferably lie in

TABLE 7a.4 *B. CATARRHALIS*: ANTIMICROBIAL SUSCEPTIBILITY PATTERNS FOR β-LACTAM ANTIBIOTICS

	No. of strains with these MICs (mg/l)									
	≤0.03	0.06	0.125	0.25	0.5	1	2	4	8	>8
Ampicillin										
β-Lactamase pos. ($n=282$)	2	20	49	66	46	34	29	34	–	2
β-Lactamase neg. ($n=86$)	6	19	45	6	5	5	–	–	–	–
Penicillin										
β-Lactamase pos. ($n=401$)	16	6	2	10	43	102	55	61	40	66
β-Lactamase neg. ($n=132$)	80	17	4	6	15	10	–	–	–	–
Cefepime										
β-Lactamase pos. ($n=36$)	–	–	9	12	5	–	3	7	–	–
β-Lactamase neg. ($n=12$)	1	–	8	3	–	–	–	–	–	–
Cefodizime										
β-Lactamase pos. ($n=142$)	24	47	12	1	11	23	22	2	–	–
β-Lactamase neg. ($n=54$)	34	18	2	–	–	–	–	–	–	–
Cefotaxime										
β-Lactamase pos. ($n=171$)	23	66	27	11	24	19	1	–	–	–
β-Lactamase neg. ($n=100$)	41	51	7	–	–	1	–	–	–	–
Ceftriaxone										
β-Lactamase pos. ($n=126$)	56	2	4	15	35	10	3	–	–	1
β-Lactamase neg. ($n=22$)	20	–	1	1	–	–	–	–	–	–

the region of 0.25–0.5 mg/l for the injectable cephalosporins, and 0.125 mg/l for the oral compounds. Although the cephalosporin MIC results presented in the table only refer to the parenterally administered drugs, the newer oral cephalosporins (often irregularly absorbed even though only given in low dosage) present even greater diversity of activity against *B. catarrhalis*, especially the β-lactamase-producing isolates (Fung *et al.*, 1992; Eliasson *et al.*, 1992). Unrealistically high breakpoints (far above the attainable tissue or sputum concentrations) may yield apparent susceptibility rates of 100%, and only clinical studies including failure analyses will indicate the lability of a drug to the β-lactamases of *B. catarrhalis*.

Apart from problems associated with β-lactamase production, most strains of *B. catarrhalis* yield highly predictable susceptibility patterns which have not changed recently (Doern and Tubert, 1988). Table 7a.5 shows the percentage of strains currently susceptible in our own region (data from the 1993 laboratory records). Although almost all strains are intrinsically resistant to trimethoprim, they are usually susceptible to sulphonamides and thus to the combination, cotrimoxazole. Most strains are highly resistant to vancomycin although occasional hyper-susceptible strains may be noted.

TABLE 7a.5   ANTIMICROBIAL SUSCEPTIBILITY PATTERNS FOR NON-β-LACTAM ANTIBIOTICS

	B. catarrhalis[a]	*Moraxella* spp.[b,c]
Amikacin	100	S
Ciprofloxacin	100	S
Clindamycin	(NT)	R
Cotrimoxazole	97	S
Erythromycin	99	S
Gentamicin	100	S
Ofloxacin	100	S
Tetracycline	99	S/I
Trimethoprim	0	I/R
Vancomycin	0	R

[a] Based on 502 laboratory isolates in the year 1993 (percentage of strains fully susceptible); NT, not tested routinely.
[b] Based on isolates received at CDC, Atlanta (Graham *et al.*, 1990), together with results from the literature.
[c] S, fully susceptible; I, moderately susceptible; R, resistant.
[d] No data in the literature.

Moraxella and *Kingella* Species

There is remarkably little literature on the antibiotic susceptibility patterns of the various species within the genus *Moraxella*. Graham *et al.* (1990) presented the general results of 933 human isolates of *Moraxella* spp. (of which 356 were *M. nonliquefaciens* and 199 *M. osloensis*) which had been submitted to the CDC (Atlanta) over 27 years. In the same period 79 isolates of *K. kingae* were received. Most strains were moderately sensitive to penicillin and ampicillin, with MIC_{90} values of 0.5 and 0.25 mg/l, respectively, and all were sensitive to gentamicin (MIC ≤ 1 mg/l) but resistant to clindamycin. There is some evidence from other reports that β-lactamase production among *Moraxella* spp. may be widespread, especially in *M. nonliquefaciens* (Eliasson *et al.*, 1992) and in *M. lacunata*. Furthermore, it seems that the majority of the true moraxellae are resistant to trimethoprim, but data are lacking on sulphonamides and cotrimoxazole. Tables 7a.4 and 7a.5 attempt to show the general patterns of susceptibility.

Susceptibility data on *Kingella* spp. are even more scarce, most case reports presenting only individual patient details. Data from various sources show that most *K. kingae* isolates are still fully susceptible to the β-lactam antibiotics, the aminoglycosides, the fluoroquinolones, erythromycin and cotrimoxazole, although they are usually resistant to the older quinolones and to clindamycin, trimethoprim and vancomycin (Amir and Shockelford, 1991). *Kingella denitrificans* infections have also been recently reviewed and β-lactamase production has been documented (Minamoto and Sordillo, 1992). It is clear that susceptibility testing of isolates of *Moraxella* and *Kingella* spp. is always necessary, especially if the use of β-lactam antibiotics is envisaged.

Typing Systems for *Branhamella catarrhalis*

Until recently it has not been possible to provide any sort of typing for individual isolates of *B. catarrhalis*, other than noting any unusual resistance patterns (e.g. resistance to erythromycin) and recording the isolation of apparently similar strains during outbreaks. However, it has long been possible to use the sensitive nitrocefin test (Barreiro *et al.*, 1992) to distinguish between producers and non-producers of β-lactamase, but because most strains now produce these enzymes this property is no longer useful for typing purposes.

Many years ago, we attempted to use the API-ZYM system (Humble *et al.*, 1977), testing for 20 specific enzymes (results unpublished). With very few exceptions, nearly all isolates produced the same three enzymes and there was an extensive overlap with *N. meningitidis* and (in particular) with *N. gonorrhoeae*. We did not proceed further. Peiris and Heald (1992) have found the API-ZYM research kit (containing 89 enzyme substrates) to be more useful, and 17 different enzyme patterns were found among 49 *B. catarrhalis* isolates. These authors felt that 20 of the tests gave sufficient discrimination to be useful in a prototype panel.

Catlin (1990) reviewed the biochemical and molecular methods for strain differentiation. Various techniques have been described for analysing the profiles of the soluble proteins or performing electrophoretic analysis of the esterase zymotypes. An inhibition–enzyme-linked immunosorbent assay (ELISA) technique has been developed at the University of Ghent (Vaneechoutte *et al.*, 1990a), allowing separation into four different groups (A, B, C and untypable), but 60% of strains fell into group A and 30% into group B.

More recent investigations have employed molecular methods for characterizing strains of *B. catarrhalis* suspected of causing hospital cross-infections (McKenzie *et al.*, 1992; Morgan *et al.*, 1992). Typically, whole-cell protein extracts were studied by sodium dodecyl sulphate-polyacrylamide gel electrophoresis (SDS-PAGE) and the resultant profiles stained and analysed. Immunoblot studies were also carried out. Other methods involved extraction of bacterial DNA, followed by restriction endonuclease analysis. The results showed evidence of similarity of some of the strains clinically associated with episodes of cross-infection, especially within the individual hospital ward units.

Serological Studies

There are only a limited number of reports on serological studies on patients with proven *B. catarrhalis* infections (Chapman *et al.*, 1985; Eliasson, 1986), but these suggest the active production of bactericidal and complement-fixing antibodies. Furthermore, various ELISA methods have been attempted and seem to confirm active antibody production. However, use of paired (or single) serum specimens for serological studies has not yet become available other than for pure research purposes.

MANAGEMENT OF INFECTIONS

In all patients with infections who require treatment with antimicrobial agents, it is necessary to decide which agent, which method of drug administration, which dosage, and what length of treatment course are needed. As far as lower respiratory tract infections associated with *B. catarrhalis* are concerned, these decisions are vital and relate to the drug concentration which can be brought about at the site of infection, in relation to the concentration required to inhibit the growth of the infecting organisms (in other words, in relation to the MIC value).

Most infections with *B. catarrhalis* in adults are noted in elderly patients with chronic obstructive lung disease (chronic bronchitis) in whom several purulent exacerbations may occur in each year. In these patients, for whom the MIC values for individual antimicrobial agents can readily be measured in the laboratory, the controversy over the method for measuring the drug concentration at the site of infection remains as yet unsettled. Should the concentration in coughed-up sputum be taken into account, or that in bronchial biopsies or in mucus removed at bronchoscopy? We have evidence that extensive penetration of an antimicrobial agent from blood to sputum is of the greatest importance in the treatment of surface (endobronchial) infections, leading to high antibiotic concentrations in the sputum and in the endobronchial tissues. In contrast, in parenchymatous lung infections such as pneumonia, it is the concentration of the antimicrobial agent in the blood which seems to be the most important factor in relation to the drug MIC for the infecting organisms. Table 7a.4 has already shown the various MIC values for β-lactam agents against *B. catarrhalis*, but these must be balanced against the achievable concentration in sputum (generally not higher than approximately 5% of the peak concentration in the blood). With oral ampicillin or amoxicillin, sputum concentrations are seldom higher than 0.5–1 mg/l. Even though the parenteral cephalosporins may reach concentrations of 50–100 mg/l in the blood, the sputum levels seldom exceed 2 mg/l. Failure analysis studies in clinical trials on patients with purulent exacerbations of chronic bronchitis (because of persistent infection) suggest that these concentrations may not be high enough to eradicate β-lactamase-producing *B. catarrhalis* strains, and persistence or recurrence of infection may be the result (Davies *et al.*, 1992). There is usually no difficulty with the non-producing strains. Erythromycin (and the other macrolides) and the new fluoroquinolones are nearly always successful with *B. catarrhalis* infections, mainly due to the extraordinarily high degree of tissue penetration with these drugs, leading to high concentrations in lung tissue and in sputum.

At the present time, there are insufficient study results in the literature to permit similar comments to be made on infections associated with *Moraxella* or *Kingella* spp. although failure of a patient with an intervertebral joint infection to respond to clindamycin or vancomycin may suggest infection with *K. kingae* (Amir and Shockelford, 1991).

PREVENTION AND CONTROL

There are numerous accounts of clusters of *B. catarrhalis* infections, particularly on wards containing patients suffering from COLD serious enough to warrant admission to hospital (Richards *et al.*, 1993). Moreover, such patients are often elderly and generally have bronchospasm, bronchiectasis and emphysema in addition. Superimposition of an acute viral or chlamydial infection in a chronic upper respiratory tract carrier of *B. catarrhalis* with pre-existing chronic bronchitis may lead to colonization with *B. catarrhalis*, followed by an acute purulent exacerbation of the chronic lung disease. Such patients cough freely (sometimes quite unrestrainedly), and the air in the nursing ward or room may become heavily loaded with various respiratory pathogens, certainly including the 'big three': *Haemophilus influenzae*, *Streptococcus pneumoniae* and *B. catarrhalis*. It would seem prudent, therefore, to admit bronchitis and pneumonia patients with uncontrolled cough to single rooms with adequate air input and exhaust systems. Strict isolation is not necessary because the organisms are present in the upper respiratory tract flora of many normal persons.

There is no information at the moment to suggest that *Moraxella* spp. easily cause cross-infection, provided that a normal degree of hygiene is observed and regulations for the disposal of contaminated materials and instruments (e.g. from patients with eye infections) are strictly followed. *Kingella* spp. infections have not (as yet) been seen to cause cross-infection problems.

REFERENCES

Amir, J. and Shockelford, P.G. (1991) *Kingella kingae* intervertebral disk infection. *Journal of Clinical Microbiology*, **9**, 1083–1086.

Baqueiro, F. (1990) European standards for antibiotic susceptibility testing: towards a theoretical consensus. *European Journal of Microbiology and Infectious Diseases*, **9**, 492–495.

Barreiro, B., Esteban, L., Prats, E. *et al.* (1992) *Branhamella catarrhalis* respiratory infections. *European Respiratory Journal*, **5**, 675–679.

Barrow, G.I. and Feltham, R.K.A. (1993) *Cowan and Steel's Manual for the Identification of Medical Bacteria*, pp. 98–105. Cambridge University Press, Cambridge, UK.

Bøvre, K. (1984) Family VIII: Neisseriaceae. In *Bergey's Manual of Systematic Bacteriology* (ed. N.R. Krieg and J.G. Holt), pp. 289–310. Williams & Wilkins, Baltimore.

Catlin, B.W. (1990) *Branhamella catarrhalis*: an organism gaining respect as a pathogen. *Clinical Microbiology Reviews*, **3**, 293–320.

Chapman, A.J., Musher, D.M., Jonsson, S. *et al.*

(1985) Development of bacterial antibody during *Branhamella catarrhalis* infection. *Journal of Infectious Diseases*, **151**, 878–882.

Chiquito, P.E., Elliott, J. and Namnyak, S.S. (1991) *Kingella kingae* dactylitis in an infant. *Journal of Infection*, **22**, 102–103.

Davies, B.I. (1991) *Moraxella catarrhalis*: clinical significance and therapeutic problems. *Infectious Diseases Newsletter*, **10**, 73–77.

Davies, B.I. and Maesen, F.P.V. (1986) Epidemiological and bacteriological findings on *Branhamella catarrhalis* respiratory infections in The Netherlands. *Drugs*, **31** (Suppl. 3), 28–33.

Davies, B.I. and Maesen, F.P.V. (1990) Treatment of *Branhamella catarrhalis* infections. *Journal of Antimicrobial Chemotherapy*, **25**, 1–7.

Davies, B.I., Maesen, F.P.V., van den Bergh, J.J.A.M. *et al.* (1992) Clinical and bacteriological experience with cefodizime in acute purulent exacerbations of chronic bronchitis. *Infection*, **20** (Suppl. 1), S22–S25.

Doern, G.V. and Tubert, T.A. (1988) In vitro activities of 39 antimicrobial agents for *Branhamella catarrhalis* and comparison of results with different quantitative susceptibility test methods. *Antimicrobial Agents and Chemotherapy*, **32**, 259–261.

Eliasson, I. (1986) Serological identification of *Branhamella catarrhalis*. Serological evidence for infection. *Drugs*, **31** (Suppl. 3), 7–10.

Eliasson, I., Kamme, C., Vang, M. *et al.* (1992) Characterization of cell-bound papain-soluble β-lactamases in BRO-1 and BRO-2 producing strains of *Moraxella* (*Branhamella*) *catarrhalis* and *Moraxella nonliquefaciens*. *European Journal of Clinical Microbiology and Infectious Diseases*, **11**, 313–321.

Fung, C.P., Powell, M., Seymour, A. *et al.* (1992) The antimicrobial susceptibility of *Moraxella catarrhalis* isolated in England and Scotland in 1991. *Journal of Antimicrobial Chemotherapy*, **30**, 47–55.

Graham, D.R., Band, J.D., Thornsberry, C. *et al.* (1990) Infections caused by *Moraxella*, *Moraxella urethralis*, *Moraxella*-like groups M-5 and M-6, and *Kingella kingae* in the United States, 1953–1980. *Reviews in Infectious Diseases*, **12**, 423–431.

Hager, H,, Verghese, A., Alvarez, S. *et al.* (1987) *Branhamella catarrhalis* respiratory infections. *Reviews in Infectious Diseases*, **9**, 1140–1149.

Humble, M.W., King, A. and Philips, I. (1977) API-ZYM: a simple rapid system for the detection of bacterial enzymes. *Journal of Clinical Pathology*, **30**, 275–277.

Maesen, F.P.V., Davies, B.I. and Baur, C. (1987) Amoxycillin/clavulanate in acute purulent exacerbations of chronic bronchitis. *Journal of Antimicrobial Chemotherapy*, **19**, 373–383.

McKenzie, H., Morgan, M.G., Jordens, J.Z. *et al.* (1992) Characterisation of hospital isolates of *Moraxella* (*Branhamella*) *catarrhalis* by SDS-PAGE of whole-cell proteins, immunoblotting and restriction-endonuclease analysis. *Journal of Medical Microbiology*, **37**, 70–76.

Meis, J.F., Sauerwein, R.W., Gijssens, I.C. *et al.* (1992) *Kingella kingae* intervertebral diskitis in an adult. *Clinical Infectious Diseases*, **15**, 530–532.

Minamoto, G.Y. and Sordillo, E.M. (1992) *Kingella denitrificans* as a cause of granulomatous disease in a patient with AIDS. *Clinical Infectious Diseases*, **15**, 1052–1053.

Mollee, T., Kelly, P. and Tilse, M. (1992) Isolation of *Kingella kingae* from a corneal ulcer. *Journal of Clinical Microbiology*, **30**, 2516–2517.

Morgan, M.G., McKenzie, H., Enright, M.C. *et al.* (1992) Use of molecular methods to characterize *Moraxella catarrhalis* strains in a suspected outbreak of nosocomial infection. *European Journal of Clinical Microbiology and Infectious Diseases*, **11**, 305–312.

Namnyak, S.S., Quinn, R.J.M. and Fergusson, J.D.M. (1991) *Kingella kingae* meningitis in an infant. *Journal of Infection*, **23**, 104–106.

O'Grady, F. and Nord, C.E. (eds) (1986) Symposium on *Branhamella catarrhalis*. *Drugs*, **31** (Suppl. 3), 1–142.

Peiris, V. and Heald, J. (1992) Rapid method for differentiating strains of *Branhamella catarrhalis*. *Journal of Clinical Pathology*, **45**, 532–533.

Percival, A., Corkill, J.E., Rowlands, J. *et al.* (1977) Pathogenicity of and β-lactamase production by, *Branhamella* (*Neisseria*) *catarrhalis*. *Lancet*, **ii**, 1175.

Pickett, M.I., Hollis, D.G. and Bottone, E.J. (1991) Miscellaneous Gram-negative bacteria. In *Manual of Clinical Microbiology*, 5th edn (ed. A. Balows), pp. 410–428. American Society for Microbiology, Washington, DC.

Richards, S.J., Greening, A.P., Enright, M.C. *et al.* (1993) Outbreak of *Moraxella catarrhalis* in a respiratory unit. *Thorax*, **48**, 91–92.

Riou, J.Y. and Guibourdenche, M. (1986) *Branhamella catarrhalis*: new methods of bacterial diagnosis. *Drugs*, **31** (Suppl. 3), 1–6.

Shurin, P.A., Marchant, C.D., Kim, C.H. *et al.* (1983) Emergence of beta-lactamase-producing strains of *Branhamella catarrhalis* as important agents of acute otitis media. *Pediatric Infectious Diseases Journal*, **2**, 34–38.

Slevin, N.J., Aitken, J. and Thornley, P.E. (1984) Clinical and microbiological features of *Branhamella catarrhalis* bronchopulmonary infections. *Lancet*, **i**, 782–783.

Stratton, C.W. (1990) *Moraxella catarrhalis*: a new name for a new (?) pathogen. *Infectious Diseases Newsletter*, **9**, 4–6.

Vaneechoutte, M., Verschraegen, G., Clays, G. *et al.*

(1990a) Serological typing of *Branhamella catarrhalis* strains on the basis of lipopolysaccharide antigens. *Journal of Clinical Microbiology*, **28**, 182–187.

Vaneechoutte, M., Verschraegen, G., Clays, G. *et al.* (1990b) Respiratory tract carrier rates of *Moraxella* (*Branhamella*) *catarrhalis* in adults and children and interpretation of the isolation of *M. catarrhalis* from sputum. *Journal of Clinical Microbiology*, **28**, 2674–2680.

Wilson, G. and Wilkinson, A.E. (1983) *Neisseria, Branhamella* and *Moraxella*. In *Topley and Wilson's Principles of Bacteriology, Virology and Immunology*, 7th edn, Vol. 2 (ed. G. Wilson, A. Miles and M.T. Parker), pp. 156–172. Edward Arnold, London.

Working Party, British Society for Antimicrobial Chemotherapy (1988) Breakpoints in in-vitro antibiotic sensitivity testing. *Journal of Antimicrobial Chemotherapy*, **21**, 701–710.

Yagupsky, P., Dagan, R., Howard, C.W. *et al.* (1992) High prevalence of *Kingella kingae* in joint fluid from children with septic arthritis revealed by the BACTEC blood culture system. *Journal of Clinical Microbiology*, **30**, 1278–1281.

7b

NEISSERIA GONORRHOEAE

Catherine Ison

DESCRIPTION OF THE GENUS

The genus *Neisseria* belongs to the family Neisseriaceae, which consists of 12 species. Only two species of the genus, *Neisseria gonorrhoeae* and *Neisseria meningitidis*, are considered as primary pathogens in man. *N. gonorrhoeae* causes a sexually transmitted infection and is always considered as a pathogen. *Neisseria meningitidis* colonizes the upper respiratory tract as a commensal and in a small proportion of individuals invades to cause systemic disease. *Neisseria lactamica*, *Neisseria*

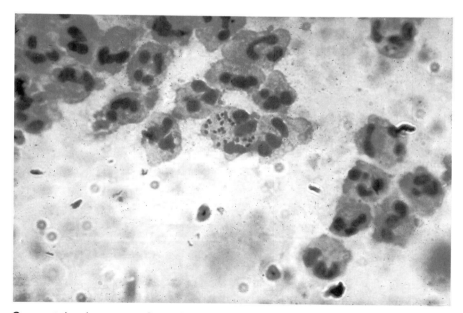

Figure 7b.1. Gram-stained smear of urethral pus showing typical Gram-negative diplococci within neurophils.

Principles and Practice of Clinical Bacteriology. Edited by A.M. Emmerson, P.M. Hawkey and S.H. Gillespie
© 1997 John Wiley & Sons Ltd

TABLE 7b.1   CELL ENVELOPE ANTIGENS OF *NEISSERIA GONORRHOEAE* AND THEIR EQUIVALENT IN *NEISSERIA MENINGITIDIS*

N. gonorrhoeae	N. meningitidis	Description	Function
Por	Class 1 (Por A)	Major OMP	Porin
	Class 2/3 (Por B)	Major OMP	Porin
Rmp	Class 4	Reduction-modified protein	Site for blocking antibody
Opa	Class 5	Heat-modifiable protein	Enhances attachment/ phagocytosis/serum resistance
Pilin	Class I pilin	Pilin	Attachment
LOS	LOS	Lipooligosaccharide	Toxic to epithelial cells
Fbp/Frp	Fbp/Frp	Iron binding/ restricted protein	Iron binding
Tbp	Tbp	Transferrin-binding protein	Iron acquisition

cinerea and *Moraxella catarrhalis* have also been implicated as causes of infection (Johnson, 1983). The remaining species are generally regarded as commensals.

Neisseria spp. are oxidase-positive, Gram-negative cocci. It is relatively simple to distinguish the clinically important species, *N. gonorrhoeae*, *N. meningitidis*, *N. lactamica*, *N. cinerea* and *Moraxella catarrhalis*, from the non-pathogenic *Neisseria*. However, differentiation between the non-pathogenic species has proved difficult and as a consequence the taxonomy has been controversial. Biochemical characteristics that can differentiate between *Neisseria* include production of acid from carbohydrates, production of superoxol, production of hydroxyprolyl- or glutamyl-aminopeptidase, ability to reduce nitrate, deoxyribonuclease production and susceptibility to colistin (Knapp, 1988).

Neisseria have a typical Gram-negative cell envelope which consists of a cytoplasmic membrane, a thin peptidoglycan layer and an outer membrane. The outer membrane acts as a barrier and also interacts with the host. Many of the major antigens of the cell envelope are shared between *N. gonorrhoeae* and *N. meningitidis* and are shown in Table 7b.1.

PATHOGENESIS

Neisseria gonorrhoeae is the causative agent of gonorrhoea, and colonizes mucosal surfaces of humans and has no other known reservoir. It primarily colonizes the mucosa of the lower genital tract and occasionally will ascend to the upper genital tract or invade and colonize the blood. For infection to occur, the organism must adhere to the epithelium, enter or invade the host cells, acquire sufficient nutrients from the host to survive and evade the host's defences. To maintain the infection in the population an efficient mode of transmission is also required.

Attachment

If *N. gonorrhoeae* is successfully to attach to the epithelium, it must avoid being swept away by cervical secretions in women and urine in men. In addition, both the bacterial and epithelial cell are negatively charged and, therefore, would naturally repel. The electrostatic forces between the two cells are believed to be overcome by pili, which are hydrophobic surface appendages, and non-specific factors such as pH and surface charge. Attachment is then mediated by specific receptors on both pili and the Opa proteins. *N. gonorrhoeae* has been shown, in human fallopian tube tissue culture, to adhere preferentially to non-ciliated compared with ciliated cells. However, it is the ciliated cells that are damaged during colonization (McGee *et al.*, 1981). This is thought to result from the toxic effect of lipooligosaccharide (LOS) and peptidoglycan that is found in blebs shed from the bacterial cell envelope.

When the organism has attached to the epithelial cell surface, it is taken into the cell and passes through to the lamina propria, where the infection is established. This transmission is believed to be mediated by the major outer membrane protein, Por. However, it is not known whether the organism is taken into the epithelial cell or remains in a vacuole. It is also possible that at least some of the organisms may pass through the junctions of the epithelial cells by secreting proteases.

Iron Acquisition

Once colonization has been established, *N. gonorrhoeae* need to acquire iron to survive. Unlike other organisms which produce siderophores to chelate iron from the environment, *N. gonorrhoeae* has evolved mechanisms to acquire iron directly from human transferrin and lactoferrin (Alcorn and Cohen, 1994; Van Putten, 1990). It is postulated that in the absence of sufficient iron, transcription of transferrin and lactoferrin receptors and transferrin-binding proteins is induced in the organism. These receptors interact with human transferrin and lactoferrin and iron is removed and transported across the bacterial cell membrane into the periplasmic space. During this process there is a transient association with iron-binding proteins and then iron is transported across the cytoplasmic membrane. Other essential nutrients are transported through the porin, which is a polymer of the outer membrane proteins Por and Rmp.

Intracellular Survival

On successful colonization, the organism will elicit an inflammatory and antibody response in the host (Brooks and Lammel, 1989). *N. gonorrhoeae* is known to be ingested by macrophages and this may be a primary mechanism by which the host eradicates infection. However, evidence that the phagocytosed organisms are killed is inconclusive. Sialylation of LOS and the expression of the Opa proteins has been shown *in vitro* to enhance the ability of the organism to resist phagocytic killing. Antibody to *N. gonorrhoeae*, both IgG and IgA, is produced in response to infection, both in serum and in local secretions. There is little evidence that this antibody affords protection against subsequent colonization and repeated infections in the same patient are common.

Cell Envelope Antigens

The major antigens of the cell envelope of *N. gonorrhoeae* that are exposed to the immune response include pili, LOS and the three outer membrane proteins, Por, Opa and Rmp. Of these antigens, pili, LOS and the Opa proteins exhibit antigenic variation. This process enables the organism to express immunologically distinct proteins which are not recognized by the host's immune system and hence each episode of infection appears as novel (Robertson and Meyer, 1992; Siefert, 1992). Por is a more conserved protein with variable exposed regions and there is some evidence that antibody directed at different serotypes of Por may be protective. Women with repeated episodes of gonococcal pelvic inflammatory disease do not appear to be colonized with strains of the same Por serotype.

The function of antibody produced to *N. gonorrhoeae* is not known (Brooks and Lammel, 1989). Systemic antibody may activate the complement pathway and play a role in limiting disseminated infection. However, it is not known whether complement-mediated lysis occurs in mucosal secretions. Antibody in secretions may inhibit attachment or enhance phagocytosis. The activity of mucosal antibody is likely to be short lived and, therefore, play little role in protection against infection.

EPIDEMIOLOGY

The epidemiology of gonorrhoea has been influenced in recent years by two factors: the advent of acquired immunodeficiency syndrome (AIDS) and the development of resistance to treatment with penicillin and tetracycline.

The advent of AIDS has been linked with a decline in the number of cases of gonorrhoea in Europe and the USA in the last decade. For instance, in the USA the number of reported cases has fallen from 1 million in 1977 to 439 000 in 1993 and in England and Wales reported cases have fallen from approximately 50 000 prior to 1984 to 11 300 in 1993–1994. Changes in sexual practices since the advent of AIDS, either as the result of education or fear of a fatal sexually transmitted disease, is one of many factors which may have influenced this decline. The availability of effective therapies and improved contact tracing have also contributed and may have initiated a fall in the number of cases before any effect resulting from AIDS. Although the incidence of gonorrhoea has fallen in heterosexual men and women the reduction was most marked in homosexual men. Unfortunately while total cases of gonorrhoea continue to fall, infection in homosexual men has shown an increase since 1989. The reasons for this are unclear.

In common with many other sexually transmitted diseases, gonorrhoea is not evenly distributed amongst the population. It is usually restricted to large towns or cities, to ethnic minorities or socioeconomically deprived communities and is more predominant in young sexually active people. A greater number of men than women are diagnosed with gonorrhoea. The male : female ratio of cases of gonorrhoea in England during 1993–1994 was 1.6 : 1.0. The ability of the organism to cause infection on a single sexual contact (transmission rate) is unknown but thought to be greater from infected male to uninfected female (50–60%) than from infected female to uninfected male (35%). The majority of cases of uncomplicated infection in men are symptomatic, in contrast to gonococcal infection in women which is predominantly asymptomatic.

In developing countries, the incidence of gonorrhoea is largely unknown but is considerably higher than in industrial countries. Large cities in Africa are estimated to have an annual incidence rate for gonorrhoea of 3000 per 100 000 inhabitants. This results from high numbers of antibiotic-resistant strains in the population and the lack of effective antibiotics. Inadequate or nonexistent contact tracing facilities and differences in social behaviour also influence incidence rates (Meheus and de Schryver, 1991).

CLINICAL FEATURES AND TREATMENT

Neisseria gonorrhoeae is primarily an infection of mucosal surfaces. Uncomplicated gonococcal infection (UGI) occurs when *N. gonorrhoeae* colonizes the columnar epithelium of the cervix, urethra, rectum and pharynx. The cervix is the primary site of colonization in women and the urethra in men. Colonization of the mucosa often stimulates a polymorph response, resulting in a purulent discharge. In a minority of cases, infection spreads from the lower genital tract to the upper genital tract, causing complicated gonococcal infection which presents as pelvic inflammatory disease (PID) or salpingitis in women and prostatitis or epididymitis in men. Disseminated gonococcal infection (DGI) where *N. gonorrhoeae* invades and colonizes the blood after a primary mucosal infection is only rarely encountered. Unlike complicated infection, DGI does not result from untreated or multiple infections but is a distinct entity.

Uncomplicated infection in men usually presents as urethritis, often with dysuria. The discharge is the most common symptom and can range from scant to copious and purulent. In women, endocervical infection is predominant, resulting in increased secretions manifesting as a vaginal discharge. Asymptomatic infection does occur in a minority of men but is more common in women. Over 50% of cases of gonorrhoea in women can be asymptomatic and are usually detected by tracing contacts of infected men. Rectal gonorrhoea occurs in homosexual men practising anal intercourse and can result in symptoms which range from mild discomfort to discharge and bleeding. In women, urethral and rectal infection are often the result of contamination with vaginal discharge and only occasionally the result of true colonization. Pharyngeal infection occurs in patients practising oral intercourse and there is no evidence that colonization relates to the presence of a sore throat or tonsillitis (Brooks and Donegan, 1985).

Complicated gonococcal infection in men is rare because most mucosal infection is symptomatic and therefore receives adequate therapy. In women, where infection is often asymptomatic, the organisms ascend from the cervical canal to the fallopian tubes and subsequently to the pelvic cavity, causing pelvic pain and tenderness. These symptoms can also be caused by other sexually transmitted diseases, such as chlamydiae, as well as organisms found as part of the normal vaginal flora. PID caused by *N. gonorrhoeae* is uncommon in industrialized countries but is often found in developing countries where treatment and health care are often inadequate. Infertility can result from PID and the incidence increases with sequential episodes of infection.

DGI can present as a low-grade fever followed by a rash and arthritis. DGI is more common in women and in patients with a deficiency in the late components of the complement pathway. It has also been linked to certain nutritional variants of *N. gonorrhoeae* which exhibit hypersusceptibility to penicillin. The interplay between the host and the organism that leads to dissemination of the infection is not understood. In the 1970s a number of cases were reported particularly from Sweden and the west coast of the USA. However, in recent years it has become increasingly less common (Brooks, 1985).

LABORATORY DIAGNOSIS

Rapid Diagnosis

The rapid and accurate detection of any sexually transmitted infection is crucial to allow suitable therapy to be given and for transmission to be prevented. In an ideal situation this will be achieved at the patient's initial visit. Historically, the presence of intracellular Gram-negative cocci has been used for the presumptive diagnosis of gonorrhoea (Ison, 1990). In symptomatic men this has a sensitivity of >95% as compared with culture for *N. gonorrhoeae*. In asymptomatic men and women and for use with rectal smears, the sensitivity is lower: 30–50%. This is probably due to reduced numbers of organisms in asymptomatic infection, and to the presence of many other Gram-negative bacteria in rectal specimens. This is a quick and inexpensive test which can be easily performed in the clinic and has a high specificity when used by experienced personnel.

Alternative approaches to the rapid detection of gonococcal antigen have used immunological and DNA-based techniques.

Enzyme-linked immunosorbent assay (ELISA)

An ELISA using polyvalent antibodies (Gonozyme, Abbott Laboratories) has been the most widely evaluated method. Gonococcal antigen in the specimen is adsorbed onto a solid phase and detected using antibodies specific to *N. gonorrhoeae*. Any antigen/antibody complexes are detected using an antiglobulin linked to an enzyme. The addition of a chromogenic substrate allows a quantitative assessment of the amount of antigen present. When used in high-risk populations of symptomatic men this test has a sensitivity of 87–100% and a specificity of 99.4–100% as compared with culture for *N. gonorrhoeae*. In women the sensitivity and specificity are lower: 60–100% and 70–100%, respectively (Ison, 1990). This test cannot be used as a test of cure because it will detect non-viable organisms and is also not suitable for use with rectal or pharyngeal specimens that may contain a large number of bacteria with cross-reactive epitopes. The performance of such immunologically-based tests is dependent on the antibodies used. The polyvalent antiserum used in this test has the advantage that it will cross-react with many strains of *N. gonorrhoeae* but has the disadvantage that it may also react with other species of *Neisseria*, particularly *N. meningitidis*.

DNA-based tests

DNA-based tests using probes for the detection of gonorrhoea have largely been unsuccessful because of the complexity and expense of the technique. A chemiluminescent acridinium ester-labelled DNA probe that is specific for the rRNA of *N. gonorrhoeae*, Gen-Probe Pace-2, is the latest of the probes to be evaluated. This test has shown a high sensitivity and specificity when used for the diagnosis of gonorrhoea in both men and women (Panke *et al.*, 1991; Hale *et al.*, 1993).

In men neither of these approaches have any advantage over the Gram stain for the presumptive diagnosis of gonorrhoea because the sensitivity is high and it is quick and inexpensive. In women there is the potential to replace the Gram stain with a test that is more sensitive and will provide a rapid and sensitive diagnosis of gonorrhoea. However, such a test will need to be highly specific (Schachter *et al.*, 1984) because of the psychological, social and medicolegal problems associated with false positive results for a sexually transmitted infection.

Isolation

Isolation of *N. gonorrhoeae* is still considered the 'gold standard' for the diagnosis of gonorrhoea and can have a sensitivity approaching 100%. However, successful isolation requires good specimen collection, rapid transport to the laboratory and a suitable culture medium.

Specimens

Specimens for the diagnosis of UGI may be collected from the urethra, cervix, rectum and oropharynx. In heterosexual men it is usual to take specimens only from the urethra, whereas for homosexual men rectal and pharyngeal specimens should also be taken. In women it is essential to sample the cervix but it may also be helpful to take specimens from the urethra and rectum and the pharynx where appropriate.

Specimens can be collected with disposable plastic loops or with swabs that are made of material that is non-inhibitory to *N. gonorrhoeae*. The highest isolation rates for *N. gonorrhoeae* are obtained when the specimen is inoculated directly onto the isolation medium and incubated in 7% carbon dioxide at 36 °C until it is transported to the laboratory. If this is not feasible then the swab should be immersed into a transport medium such as Stuart's or Amies, stored at 4 °C and sent to the laboratory as soon as possible.

Neisseria gonorrhoeae is a fastidious organism which inhabits sites that, in some instances, are colonized by many other bacteria as part of the normal flora. An enriched medium is required that can supply nutrients such as essential amino acids, glucose and iron. Chocolated horse blood agar was used for many years but it is now more common to use a medium containing GC agar base which is supplemented with lysed horse blood or a growth supplement such as Kellogg's or IsoVitaleX. These are modifications of a medium originally described by Thayer and Martin (1966) that contained GC agar base supplemented with haemoglobin. Antibiotics are often added to the primary isolation medium to suppress the growth of other organisms. The cocktail that is most often preferred consists of vancomycin, which inhibits Gram-positive organisms, colistin and trimethoprim, which inhibit Gram-negative organisms, and nystatin or amphotericin to prevent the growth of yeasts. Antibiotics added to culture media to aid the selection of *N. gonorrhoeae* may also retard the growth or inhibit certain gonococcal strains. The use of a combination of non-selective and selective media is favoured by some clinics and laboratories and can overcome this problem.

Identification

Identification of *N. gonorrhoeae* can be achieved by using specific reagents that eliminate other species of *Neisseria* or by using a battery of tests that will allow speciation into the individual members of the genus. In both instances the presence of Gram-negative cocci that are oxidase positive (produce cytochrome oxidase) is used as presumptive identification of *Neisseria* spp. Historically, carbohydrate utilization tests have been used for identification of *N. gonorrhoeae* which allows both differentiation from other species and speciation of other *Neisseria*. *N. gonorrhoeae* produces acid from glucose only whereas *N. meningitidis* also produces acid from maltose and *N. lactamica* from maltose and lactose. Conventional carbohydrate utilization tests use an agar base that supports the growth of *Neisseria* with added carbohydrate. These media require a heavy inoculum of a pure culture and further incubation for 24 hours at 36 °C before a result can be obtained. Interpretation of the colour change can also be difficult. The prolonged incubation time has been overcome by the use of liquid media or commercially available kits which require between 1 and 4 hours incubation for a result. However, all these tests should be inoculated with a heavy growth of a pure culture, which normally requires at least one subculture from the primary isolation plate. Despite these disadvantages, carbohydrate utilization has been considered the definitive means of identifying *N. gonorrhoeae*, particularly for medicolegal purposes.

In an attempt to provide a more rapid identification of *N. gonorrhoeae* that can be obtained direct from the primary isolation medium, specific antibodies to *N. gonorrhoeae* have been utilized. Monoclonal antibodies raised to specific epitopes on the two types of the major outer membrane protein, PIA and PIB (Tam *et al.*, 1982), have been used linked either to a fluorochrome (*Neisseria gonorrhoeae* Culture Confirmation, Syva Company) or to staphylococcal protein A (Phadebact Monoclonal GC Test, Boule Diagnostics AB, Sweden). The immunofluorescent reagent has the advantage of requiring very little growth but the disadvantage that the smears must be examined using a fluorescence microscope. The coagglutination reagent does not need any expensive equipment but requires sufficient growth to provide a cloudy suspension which must then be boiled before use. Both reagents have the advantage that they can be performed on non-viable organisms collected direct from the primary isolation medium. These reagents contain a mixture of specific antibodies to give a reagent that will react with all strains of *N. gonorrhoeae* but that does

not react with other species of *Neisseria*. When mixtures of antibodies are used in this manner, rather than a single antibody to a conserved epitope, there will always be the possibility that some strains will not react. Both of these reagents have been shown to be highly sensitive and specific and any unexpected negatives can be resolved by using biochemical methods. In the laboratories requiring only confirmation of *N. gonorrhoeae*, without identification of the other *Neisseria*, these immunological approaches to identification have largely replaced conventional carbohydrate utilization tests.

Many laboratories prefer to use commercially available kits which are a combination of both carbohydrate utilization tests and tests to detect preformed enzymes, particularly the aminopeptidases. These are useful for laboratories that only isolate *N. gonorrhoeae* occasionally and have little experience with alternative methods. However, these kits are designed to differentiate between the species of *Neisseria* and are most accurate for the clinically important species.

Typing Methods

Typing of *N. gonorrhoeae* can be a useful epidemiological tool to study reinfection versus treatment failure, tracing of contacts particularly in cases of sexual or child abuse and for monitoring trends over time (Sarafian and Knapp, 1989). Methods that have been used include antimicrobial susceptibility patterns, plasmid profiles, auxotyping and serotyping.

Antimicrobial susceptibility patterns and plasmid profiles are limited in their ability to differentiate between strains but give useful information on the development and type of resistance.

Auxotyping

Auxotyping is differentiation between strains by their nutritional requirements (Catlin, 1973). A large number of auxotypes have been identified but four types – non-requiring (prototrophic or wild type), proline requiring (pro⁻), arginine requiring (arg⁻) and arginine, hypoxanthine and uracil requiring (AHU⁻) – predominate in most populations. AHU-requiring strains have been associated with susceptibility to penicillin, disseminated infection and heterosexual gonorrhoea. Non-requiring and proline-requiring strains are more resistant to antibiotics. Initial isolates of PPNG were also differentiated by auxotype. PPNG from Africa carrying the 3.2 MDa plasmid were arginine requiring and Asian PPNG carrying the 4.4 MDa plasmid were proline requiring. This association has largely been lost as the penicillinase plasmids have spread through the gonococcal population worldwide. Although auxotyping revealed some interesting associations, it lacks sufficient discrimination for most purposes.

Serotyping

The use of antibodies to differentiate between strains of *N. gonorrhoeae* has made major advances in the last 15 years. Initially polyvalent antibodies were used, but it was the development of monoclonal antibodies (Tam *et al.*, 1982) that has enabled this technique to be used more widely. Antibodies to specific epitopes on the major outer membrane protein, Por, are used in a coagglutination system. Two panels of antibodies exist – GS (Genetic Systems) and Ph (Pharmacia) – and two nomenclatures (Sarafian and Knapp, 1989). The GS panel has been used most often in recent years and consists of 12 antibodies: six directed to the IA type of Por and six to the IB type. The pattern of reactivity with this panel denotes the serovar, with an arbitary number using the nomenclature of Knapp *et al.* (1984). *N. gonorrhoeae* express either a IA or IB type of Por and it is unusual to encounter hybrids which express epitopes of both types (Gill *et al.*, 1994).

The use of monoclonal antibodies for the serological classification of *N. gonorrhoeae* has greatly increased the ability to differentiate between strains. Discrimination is also enhanced when auxotyping and serotyping – two independent characters – are used in combination to produce auxotype/serovar (A/S) classes. This technique has now been used extensively to study gonococcal populations in different geographical locations and for studying temporal changes.

Certain serovars have also been associated with antibiotic resistance and colonization at particular sites such as the rectum (Gill, 1991).

The development of serotyping has allowed a more detailed study of the epidemiology of gonorrhoea than was possible with any of the previous techniques. It is a phenotypic method and has a subjective endpoint but is easy to perform and inexpensive. It may be possible in future years to use genotypic methods for *N. gonorrhoeae* that may be more reproducible and more discriminatory. However, it is probable that such methods will be used selectively and that serotyping will remain the method of choice in many situations.

Susceptibility Testing

In vitro susceptibility testing is used to the predict the outcome of therapy. This can be achieved by using disk diffusion, breakpoint agar dilution technique or determination of the minimal inhibitory concentration (MIC). All these methods are dependent on type of medium used, inoculum and concentration of antibiotic tested. *Neisseria gonorrhoeae* are fastidious organisms which vary in their growth patterns and this can make interpretation of the results difficult. In North America, susceptibility testing is performed to NCCLS guidelines (National Committee for Clinical Laboratory Standards, 1990), which attempts to standardize methods between laboratories. There are also recommended methods from the World Health Organization (1989) but in most countries outside North America the methodology has not been standardized for testing *N. gonorrhoeae*. The medium used varies from GC agar base to sensitivity test agars such as Diagnostic Sensitivity Test (DST) agar and Isosensitest. A range of supplements has also been employed, including IsoVitaleX, Kellogg's supplement, haemoglobin or lysed horse blood. A major difference between the methods used for disk susceptibility is the use of high-content disks according to NCCLS and lower-content disks in Europe and Australia.

The choice of method is made by individual laboratories and disk diffusion is used most often. An alternative method is the breakpoint agar dilution technique (Ison *et al.*, 1991), where a few concentrations of antibiotic are used to categorize strains into susceptible, reduced susceptibility and resistant. This has the advantage of giving a predicted range for the MIC and can be used with a multi-point inoculator so that up to 20 strains can be tested at one time.

Determination of the full MIC is not required by most laboratories and if necessary should be performed by reference laboratories. However, for those who wish to perform an MIC occasionally the recently developed E-test (AB Biodisk, Solna, Sweden) may be of value. This method uses a plastic carrier strip with a predefined continuous exponential antibiotic gradient on one side which is applied to the surface of a previously seeded agar plate. The MIC is recorded at the point when the zone interacts with the strip. Recent evaluations of the E-test with MICs have shown the test to be accurate and an attractive alternative which may be particularly appropriate for use in developing countries (Dyck *et al.*, 1994; Yeung *et al.*, 1993).

Plasmid-mediated resistance is simpler to detect. Penicillinase production in *N. gonorrhoeae* is most commonly detected using the chromogenic cephalosporin (Nitrocefin, Unipath Laboratories) test (O'Callaghan *et al.*, 1972). The action of the penicillinase changes the colour of the reagent from yellow to pink/red in a few seconds. The starch—iodine method for detection of penicillinase is more time consuming to perform but is efficient and less expensive than the Nitrocefin reagent. Plasmid-mediated resistance to tetracycline can be detected using screening methods of either no zone of inhibition around a 10 μg disk or growth on GC agar containing 10 mg/l tetracycline. Confirmation of the presence of the *tetM* determinant is achieved using hybridization with a suitable probe. However, this is not possible in most laboratories and the screening tests have been shown to be good predictors of the presence of the *tetM* determinant (Ison *et al.*, 1993). For laboratories with appropriate facilities, TRNG can be detected using the polymerase chain reaction (PCR).

Management of Infection

Penicillin has been the antibiotic of choice for the treatment of gonorrhoea for many years because it has been very effective and inexpensive. Until recent years resistance to penicillin was largely overcome by increasing the dosage. However, isolates of *N. gonorrhoeae* that exhibit plasmid or chromosomal resistance to penicillin have now disseminated worldwide and present a therapeutic problem. For these reasons the World Health Organization has recommended that penicillin should not be used as first-line therapy for gonorrhoea unless the strain population is known to be susceptible. Alternative recommended therapies are ciprofloxacin, 500 mg orally; ceftriaxone 250 mg i.m. and spectinomycin 4 g i.m. (World Health Organization, 1989).

Antimicrobial Resistance

Neisseria gonorrhoeae is inherently susceptible to most antibiotics but through increased usage both chromosomally mediated and plasmid-mediated resistance has developed. Chromosomal resistance to penicillin is low level and the result of the additive effect of mutations at multiple loci, including *penA*, *mtr* and *penB*. *penA* encodes for penicillin-binding protein 2 (PBP2), and a mutation which results in a single amino acid change confers decreased affinity for penicillin (Spratt, 1988). The *mtr* locus consists of an operon, *mtrRCDE*, which controls susceptibility to a range of hydrophobic antibiotics and detergents by an efflux system (Pan and Spratt, 1994; Hagman *et al.*, 1995). The function of the locus *penB* is unknown but is either very closely linked or part of the *por* gene that encodes for the major porin of *N. gonorrhoeae*. It is likely that mutations occur within this gene that alter cell wall permeability to penicillin. The additive effect of these mutations can increase the MIC from ≤0.06 mg/l in a susceptible strain to ≥1 mg/l with an increased chance of therapeutic failure. Low-level resistance to antibiotics such as tetracycline and erythromycin that have been used for the therapy of gonorrhoea is also the result of chromosomal mutations.

In contrast, chromosomal resistance to spectinomycin in *N. gonorrhoeae* occurs in a single step and results in an increase in MIC from 8–16 mg/l to ≥256 mg/l which is invariably resistant to therapy. It is the result of mutations on the chromosome affecting binding of the antibiotic to the ribosome (Maness *et al.*, 1974). There have been several documented episodes of spectinomycin-resistant *N. gonorrhoeae* (Ashford *et al.*, 1981; Easmon *et al.*, 1984) but unlike penicillin resistance it has not spread or limited the use of the antibiotic. Spectinomycin is not a widely used treatment for gonorrhoea but will be particularly useful if resistance develops to the newer alternatives such as ceftriaxone and ciprofloxacin.

Therapeutic resistance to ceftriaxone has not been documented. However, the loci that encode for chromosomal resistance to penicillin also confer reduced susceptibility to the cephalosporins (Ison *et al.*, 1990). Indiscriminate use of penicillin or inadequate dosage of ceftriaxone could lead to selection of resistant strains.

Ciprofloxacin, a fluoroquinolone, is an alternative treatment for gonorrhoea. It is highly active against *N. gonorrhoeae*, is given orally, rather than intramuscularly as spectinomycin and ceftriaxone are, and it is effective in a single dose of 250 mg or 500 mg (Echols *et al.*, 1994). There have been only a few reports of therapeutic failure which has occurred in isolates with MICs of $\geqslant 0.12$ mg/l after treatment with a single 250 mg dose (Gransden *et al.*, 1991). The mechanism of resistance or reduced susceptibility in clinical isolates of *N. gonorrhoeae* is unknown. In other bacteria this results from mutations in the DNA gyrase genes or changes in cell wall permeability. There is recent evidence that in spontaneous mutants of *N. gonorrhoeae* with increasing MICs to ciprofloxacin, moderate levels of resistance result from amino acid changes in *gyrA* whereas mutants with high levels of resistance had changes in both *gyrA* and the topoisomerase IV gene, *parC* (Belland *et al.*, 1994).

Resistance to penicillin and tetracycline in *N. gonorrhoeae* can also be plasmid mediated. High-level penicillin resistance was first documented in 1976 in two isolates which originated from Africa (Ashford *et al.*, 1976) and the Far East (Phillips, 1976). The two strains carried plasmids of 3.2 megadaltons (MDa) (African) and 4.4 MDa (Asian) respectively and both encoded for a TEM-1 type β-lactamase, the smaller plasmid having a

deletion in a non-functional region of the plasmid (Elwell *et al.*, 1977). Transfer of penicillinase plasmids can occur between strains of *N. gonorrhoeae* by conjugation but requires the presence of a plasmid of 24.5 MDa in the donor to mobilize the transfer (Roberts and Falkow, 1977). Isolates of *N. gonorrhoeae* carrying these plasmids have been disseminated worldwide. Penicillinase-producing *N. gonorrhoeae* carrying plasmids of differing size have also been reported in recent years (Embden *et al.*, 1985; Gouby *et al.*, 1986; Yeung *et al.*, 1986; Brett, 1989). They are all related to the original plasmids and encode for the TEM-1 β-lactamase but, as yet, have not spread so widely. The prevalence of PPNG has presented a therapeutic problem in many parts of the world. However, it is currently a greater problem in developing countries where alternative therapies are not available or are too expensive.

High-level plasmid-mediated resistance to tetracycline in *N. gonorrhoeae* was not reported until 1985 (Morse *et al.*, 1986). It is due to the acquisition of the *tetM* determinant by the conjugative plasmid (24.5 MDa) of *N. gonorrhoeae*, resulting in a plasmid of 25.2 MDa. This plasmid is self-mobilizable and can move between strains of *N. gonorrhoeae* and other genera. Tetracycline-resistant *N. gonorrhoeae* (TRNG) were initially isolated in the USA and the Netherlands. The DNA sequence of the *tetM* determinant from TRNG appears to vary and can be subdivided into two types which correlate with the location of the original isolates (Gascoyne-Binzi *et al.*, 1993). TRNG have now spread to many countries, including those in the developing world where tetracycline is often used for the treatment of gonorrhoea because it is inexpensive and readily available.

PREVENTION AND CONTROL OF INFECTION

Control of gonococcal infection depends on ready access to confidential diagnostic and treatment facilities. This must be allied to an efficient system to follow up and treat sexual contacts. The impact of health education can be seen following the fall in gonorrhoea incidence associated with the publicity surrounding the HIV epidemic.

Attempts to induce protection by vaccination have been largely unsuccessful. This is mostly due to the heterogeneity of the antigens chosen as vaccine candidates such as pili. The first pilus vaccine used whole pili from a single strain which produced antibody that was specific only for the homologous strain. The use of Por as a vaccine candidate is more hopeful and may give protection against complicated infection particularly in women. In addition there is little information known on the host response required to induce protection and this has hampered the search for a suitable vaccine.

REFERENCES

Alcorn, T.M. and Cohen, M.S. (1994) Gonococcal pathogenesis: adapation and immune evasion in the human host. *Current Opinion on Infectious Diseases*, 7, 310–316.

Ashford, W.A., Golash, R.G. and Hemming, V.G. (1976) Penicillinase-producing *Neisseria gonorrhoeae*. *Lancet*, ii, 657–658.

Ashford, W.A., Potts, D.W., Adams, H.H.J.U. *et al.* (1981) Spectinomycin-resistant penicillinase-producing *Neisseria gonorrhoeae*. *Lancet*, ii, 1035–1037.

Belland, R.J., Morrison, S.G., Ison, C. *et al.* (1994) *Neisseria gonorrhoeae* acquires mutations in analogous regions of *gyrA* and *parC* in fluoroquinolone-resistant isolates. *Molecular Microbiology*, 14, 371–380.

Brett, M. (1989) A novel gonococcal beta-lactamase plasmid. *Journal of Antimicrobial Chemotherapy*, 23, 653–654.

Brooks, G.F. (1985) Disseminated gonococcal infection. In *Gonococcal Infection* (ed. G.F. Brooks and E.A. Donegan), pp. 121–131 (Current Topics of Infection Series.) Edward Arnold, London.

Brooks, G.F. and Donegan, E.A. (1985) Clinical manifestations of gonococcal infection. In *Gonococcal Infection* (ed. G.F. Brooks and E.A. Donegan), pp. 85–138 (Current Topics of Infection Series). Edward Arnold, London.

Brooks, G.F. and Lammel, C.J. (1989) Humoral immune response to gonococcal infections. *Clinical Microbiology Reviews*, 2, S5–10.

Catlin, B.W. (1973) Nutritional profiles of *Neisseria gonorrhoeae*, *Neisseria meningitidis* and *Neisseria lactamica* in chemically defined media and the use of growth requirements for gonococcal typing. *Journal of Infectious Diseases*, 128, 178–194.

Dyck, E. van, Smet, H. and Piot, P. (1994) Comparison of E-test with agar dilution for antimicrobial susceptibility testing of *Neisseria gonorrhoeae*. *Journal of Clinical Microbiology*, 32, 1586–1588.

Easmon, C.S.F., Forster, G.E., Walker, G.D. *et al.* (1984) Spectinomycin as initial treatment for gonorrhoea. *British Medical Journal*, 289, 1032–1034.

Echols, R.M., Heyd, A., O'Keeffe, B.J. *et al.* (1994) Single-dose ciprofloxacin for the treatment of uncomplicated gonorrhoea: a worldwide summary. *Sexually Transmitted Diseases*, 21, 345–352.

Elwell, L.P., Roberts, M., Mayer, L.W. *et al.* (1977) Plasmid-mediated beta-lactamase production in *Neisseria gonorrhoeae*. *Antimicrobial Agents and Chemotherapy*, 11, 528–533.

Embden, J.D.A. van, Dessens-Kroons, M. and Klingeren, B. van (1985) A new beta-lactamase plasmid in *Neisseria gonorrhoeae*. *Journal of Antimicrobial Chemotherapy*, 15, 247–250.

Gascoyne-Binzi, D.M., Heritage, J. and Hawkey, P.M. (1993) Nucleotide sequences of the *tet(M)* genes from the American and Dutch type tetracycline resistance plasmid of *Neisseria gonorrhoeae*. *Journal of Antimicrobial Chemotherapy*, 32, 667–676.

Gill, M.J. (1991) Serotyping *Neisseria gonorrhoeae*: a report of the Fourth International Workshop. *Genitourinary Medicine*, 67, 53–57.

Gill, M.J., Jayamohan, J., Lessing, M.P.A. *et al.* (1994) Naturally occurring PIA/PIB hybrids of *N. gonorrhoeae*. *FEMS Microbiology Letters*, 119, 161–166.

Gouby, A., Bourg, G. and Raamuz, M. (1986) Previously undescribed 6.6 kilobase R plasmid in penicillinase-producing *Neisseria gonorrhoeae*. *Antimicrobial Agents and Chemotherapy*, 29, 1095–1097.

Gransden, W.R., Warren, C. and Phillips, I. (1991) 4-Quinolone-resistant *Neisseria gonorrhoeae* in the United Kingdom. *Journal of Medical Microbiology*, 34, 23–27.

Hagman, K.E., Pan, W., Spratt, B.G. *et al.* (1995) Resistance of *Neisseria gonorrhoeae* to antimicrobial hydrophobic agents is modulated by the *mtrRCDE* efflux system. *Microbiology*, 141, 611–622.

Hale, Y.M., Melton, M.E., Lewis, J.S. *et al.* (1993) Evaluation of the PACE 2 *Neisseria gonorrhoeae* assay by three public laboratories. *Journal of Clinical Microbiology*, 31, 451–453.

Ison, C.A. (1990) Methods of diagnosing gonorrhoea. *Genitourinary Medicine*, 66, 453–459.

Ison, C.A., Bindayna, K.M., Woodford, N. *et al.* (1990) Penicillin and cephalosporin resistance in gonococci. *Genitourinary Medicine*, 66, 351–356.

Ison, C.A., Branley, N.S., Kirtland, K. *et al.* (1991) Surveillance of antibiotic resistance in clinical isolates of *Neisseria gonorrhoeae*. *British Medical Journal*, **303**, 1307.

Ison, C.A., Tekki, N. and Gill, M.J. (1993) Detection of the *tetM* determinant in *Neisseria gonorrhoeae*. *Sexually Transmitted Diseases*, **20**, 329–333.

Johnson, A.P. (1983) The potential of commensal species of *Neisseria*. *Journal of Clinical Pathology*, **36**, 213–223.

Knapp, J.S. (1988) Historical perspectives and identification of *Neisseria* and related species. *Clinical Microbiology Reviews*, **1**, 415–431.

Knapp, J.S., Tam, M.R., Nowinski, R.C. *et al.* (1984) Serological classification of *Neisseria gonorrhoeae* with use of monoclonal antibodies to gonococcal outer membrane protein I. *Journal of Infectious Diseases*, **150**, 44–48.

Maness, M.J., Foster, G.C. and Sparling, P.F. (1974) Ribosomal resistance to streptomycin and spectinomycin in *Neisseria gonorrhoeae*. *Journal of Bacteriology*, **120**, 1293–1299.

McGee, Z.A., Johnson, A.P. and Taylor-Robinson, D. (1981) Pathogenic mechanisms of *Neisseria gonorrhoeae*: observations on damage to human fallopian tubes in organ culture by gonococci of colony type 1 or type 4. *Journal of Infectious Diseases*, **143**, 413–422.

Meheus, A. and de Schryver, A. (1991) Sexually transmitted diseases in the Third World. In *Sexually Transmitted Diseases and AIDS* (ed. J.R.W. Harris and S.M. Forster), pp. 201–217. Churchill Livingstone, Edinburgh.

Morse, S.A., Johnson, S.R., Biddle, J.W. *et al.* (1986) High-level tetracycline resistance in *Neisseria gonorrhoeae* is result of acquisition of streptococcal *tetM* determinant. *Antimicrobial Agents and Chemotherapy*, **30**, 664–670.

National Committee for Clinical Laboratory Standards (1990) Methods for dilution antimicrobial susceptibility tests for bacteria that grow aerobically. NCCLS Document M7-A2, Vol. 10, No. 8. NCCLS, Villanova, PA.

O'Callaghan, C.H., Morris, A., Kirby, S.M. *et al.* (1972) Novel method for the detection of beta-lactamases by using a chromogenic cephalosporin substrate. *Antimicrobial Agents and Chemotherapy*, **1**, 283–288.

Pan, W. and Spratt, B.G. (1994) Regulation of the permeability of the gonococcal cell envelope by the *mtr* system. *Molecular Microbiology*, **11**, 769–775.

Panke, E.S., Yang, L.I., Leist, P.A. *et al.* (1991) Comparison of Gen-Probe DNA probe test and culture for the detection of *Neisseria gonorrhoeae* in endocervical specimens. *Journal of Clinical Microbiology*, **29**, 883–888.

Phillips, I. (1976) Beta-lactamase-producing, penicillin-resistant gonococcus. *Lancet*, **ii**, 656–657.

Roberts, M.C. and Falkow, S. (1977) Conjugal transfer of R plasmids in *Neisseria gonorrhoeae*. *Nature*, **266**, 630–631.

Robertson, B.D. and Meyer, T.F. (1992) Genetic variation in pathogenic bacteria. *Trends in Genetics*, **8**, 422–427.

Sarafian, S.K. and Knapp, J.S. (1989) Molecular epidemiology. *Clinical Microbiology Reviews*, **2**, S49–55.

Schachter, J., McCormack, W.M., Smith, R.F. *et al.* (1984) Enzyme immunoassay for diagnosis of gonorrhoea. *Journal of Clinical Microbiology*, **19**, 57–59.

Siefert, H.S. (1992) Molecular mechanisms of antigenic variation in *Neisseria gonorrhoeae*. In *Molecular and Cell Biology of Sexually Transmitted Diseases* (ed. D. Wright and L. Archard), pp. 1–22. Chapman & Hall, London.

Spratt, B.G. (1988) Hybrid penicillin-binding proteins in penicillin-resistant strains of *Neisseria gonorrhoeae*. *Nature*, **332**, 173–176.

Tam, M.R., Buchanan, T.M., Sandstrom, E.G. *et al.* (1982) Serological classification of *Neisseria gonorrhoeae* with monoclonal antibodies. *Infection and Immunity*, **36**, 1042–1053.

Thayer, J.D. and Martin, J.E. (1966) Improved medium selective for cultivation of *Neisseria gonorrhoeae* and *Neisseria meningitidis*. *Health Laboratory Reports*, **81**, 559–562.

Van Putten, J.P.M. (1990) Iron acquisition and the pathogenesis of meningococcal and gonococcal disease. *Medical Microbiology and Immunology*, **179**, 289–295.

World Health Organizational (1989) Bench-level manual for sexually transmitted diseases. WHO/VDT/89.443.

World Health Organization (1989) *STD Treatment Strategies*, p. 447, WHO/VDT.

Yeung, K.-H., Dillon, J.R., Pauze, M. *et al.* (1986) A novel 4.9 kilobase plasmid associated with an outbreak of penicillinase-producing *Neisseria gonorrhoeae*. *Journal of Infectious Diseases*, **153**, 1162–1165.

Yeung, K.-H., Ng, L.-K. and Dillon, J.R. (1993) Evaluation of E test for testing antimicrobial susceptibilities of *Neisseria gonorrhoeae* isolates with different growth media. *Journal of Clinical Microbiology*, **31**, 3053–3055.

7c

NEISSERIA MENINGITIDIS

Dlawer A.A. Ala'Aldeen

INTRODUCTION

Neisseria meningitidis and *N. gonorrhoeae* are the only two recognized obligate human pathogens of the genus *Neisseria*, family Neisseriaceae. *Neisseria meningitidis* (meningococcus) is the commonest overall cause of pyogenic meningitis worldwide and is the only bacterium that is capable of generating epidemic outbreaks of meningitis. Vieusseaux (1805) was the first to describe an outbreak of an apparently new disease, a cerebrospinal fever, which spread rapidly in and around Geneva in the spring of 1805. Several other outbreaks of similar nature were also recorded over the subsequent decades but the organism was first isolated in Vienna in 1887 by Anton Weichselbaum. He found the causative organism in the meningeal exudate of six cases of cerebrospinal fever and gave it the descriptive name of '*Diplococcus intercellularis meningitidis*', which was later changed to *Neisseria meningitidis*.

DESCRIPTION OF THE ORGANISM

Cultural Characteristics and Biochemical Reactions

Neisseria meningitidis is a Gram-negative, non-sporing, non-motile aerobic diplococcus of approximately 0.8 μm in diameter. On solid media, *N. meningitidis* grows as a transparent, non-haemolytic, non-pigmented (grey) convex colony, approximately 0.5–5 mm in diameter, depending on the length of incubation. The organism is relatively fastidious in its growth requirements and optimal growth conditions are achieved at 35–37 °C, at pH 7.0–7.4 in a moist environment with 5–10% carbon dioxide. It grows poorly on unenriched media but grows reasonably well on blood, chocolate and Modified New York City agar, and on Mueller Hinton agar without the addition of blood. It can survive and grow slowly at temperatures ranging from 25 to 42 °C. It is best transported on chocolate agar slopes and stored freeze-dried, frozen at −70 °C or in liquid nitrogen.

The organism is oxidase positive and catalase negative. It is capable of utilizing glucose with no gas formation and, unlike gonococci, it also utilizes maltose although occasional strains are maltose negative on primary isolation. It does not utilize lactose, sucrose or fructose. Meningococci produce γ-glutamyl aminopeptidase, but not prolyl aminopeptidase or β-galactosidase.

The Cell Envelope

The meningococcal cell is contained within a permeable polysaccharide capsule which overlays a multilayered envelope, very similar to that of *N.*

Principles and Practice of Clinical Bacteriology. Edited by A.M. Emmerson, P.M. Hawkey and S.H. Gillespie
© 1997 John Wiley & Sons Ltd

gonorrhoeae (see Chapter 7b) and other Gram-negative bacteria. This envelope consists of three layers: an outer membrane layer which contains proteins, lipooligosaccharides and phospholipids; a thin but rigid peptidoglycan layer; and an inner cytoplasmic membrane which contains, among other enzymes, enzymatic components of the electron transport chain and oxidative phosphorylation. Pili – long filamentous protein projections – also extend outwards from the cell envelope. The cell envelope has been extensively studied for pathogenesis, classification, immune response and vaccine development purposes. Many of the prominent components of the cell envelope, particularly the outer membrane components, show wide structural and antigenic diversity which have been exploited for epidemiological purposes in classifying clinical isolates.

Classification Systems of Clinical Isolates

For epidemiological purposes, several classification systems have been developed for *N. meningitidis*. The most widely used and well established is the one which divides strains immunologically into serogroups, serotypes, serosubtypes and immunotypes, based on antigenic differences in their capsules, class 2 or 3 outer membrane proteins, class 1 outer membrane protein and lipooligosaccharides, respectively. For example, a serogroup B serotype 4 serosubtype 15 and immunotype 10 is written as B : 4 : P1.15 : L10. These classification antigens deserve detailed analysis because they form the basis of the present meningococcal vaccines or are currently being considered as candidate antigens.

Other classification tools have also been used, such as those exploiting restriction fragment length polymorphism (RFLP) (Fox *et al.*, 1991) and multilocus enzyme electrophoresis (MLEE) based on isoenzymes. The latter typing (electrotyping, ET) scheme is based on the presence and electrophoretic mobility of isoforms of cytosolic enzymes whose molecular weights vary between different strains of meningococci. MLEE has enabled subdivision of genetically related strains of group A to

clones (or subgroups) and groups B and C to clusters (complexes) (Achtman, 1994). Using this method, it was possible to trace the movement of a certain clone (clone III-I) of group A meningococci from China to Nepal in 1983, to India and Pakistan in 1985, to Mecca in 1987 and to the meningitis belt of Africa and other parts of the world by 1989 (Caugant *et al.*, 1987; Moore, 1992).

Capsular Polysaccharides: The Serogroup Antigens

Meningococci possess a structurally and antigenically heterogeneous capsular polysaccharide which forms the basis of the classification into at least 13 serogroups. These are A, B, C, D, 29E, H, I, K, L, W135, X, Y and Z. While virtually all disease-associated isolates are capsulated, occasionally non-capsulated (or non-groupable) strains are isolated from carriers or patients. Group A capsule is composed of mannosamine phosphate; that of serogroups B, C, Y and W135 contains sialic acid, which is believed to be an important survival/virulence factor (Jarvis and Verdos, 1987). Serogroup C capsular polysaccharide is a homopolymer of $(2–9)$-α-N-acetylneuraminic acid and only differs from the $2–8$-α-N-acetyl-neuraminic acid oligomer of serogroup B capsular polysaccharide by one linkage. Whereas the former is immunogenic in humans and generates protective antibodies, the latter is poorly immunogenic. It is interesting that serogroup C strains seem to be more rapidly spreading than serogroup B and occur more frequently in clustered outbreaks in crowded institutions, whereas serogroup B is more widespread in the community. The structure and biosynthesis of serogroup B capsule have been the subject of extensive studies and the gene complex involved in its biosynthesis has been identified (Frosch *et al.*, 1989).

Group A meningococci are now rare in the more developed countries, but are the major pathogens in the 'meningitis belt' of Africa and a number of Asian countries, where they are responsible for the epidemics. In the UK group A was responsible for the epidemics in the first half of the century, whereas in the second half this serogroup became increasingly uncommon and was replaced by serogroup B (up to 70%) and serogroup C (20–30%), with occasional isolates of serogroups A, W135, X, Y, Z/29E and ungroupable strains. In Europe and the American continent, groups B and C are currently responsible for about 85% of cases, with serogroups Y and W135 accounting for most of the remainder. Serogroups H, I and K have been reported in China. In the USA, until the late 1980s serogroup B meningococci accounted for 50% of the cases and serogroup C for 35%. However, in 1989–1991, the two serogroups were almost equally distributed (46% and 45%, respectively) (Jackson and Wenger, 1993). In Norway in 1975, less than 50% of isolates were serogroup B strains but by 1981 these had reached 89.1%, only to drop again to 71.5% by 1990 (Lystad and Aasen, 1991). Serogroup A strains, however, were responsible for 24% of the cases in Norway in 1975 but by 1990 had almost disappeared. Serogroup B meningococci also dominate in the current epidemics in Central and Latin America and in South Australia.

The Class 1, 2 and 3 Outer Membrane Proteins: The Serotype and Serosubtype Antigens

The meningococcal outer membrane contains a number of major outer membrane proteins (OMPs) which are divided on the basis of their apparent molecular weights on sodium dodecyl sulphate-polyacrylamide gel electrophoresis (SDS-PAGE), and on their peptide analysis, into five structural classes (classes 1–5) (Tsai *et al.*, 1981). All meningococci possess a class 2 or class 3 protein in their outer membrane, the expression of the two classes being mutually exclusive. These proteins are therefore regarded as alleles of a single gene locus, *porB* (Hitchcock, 1989), and they function as porins (Blake and Gotschlich, 1987) allowing entry of nutrients and are essential to the viability of the bacterium. Despite their common functions, they exhibit a large degree of antigenic diversity between different strains, which is the basis of the serotype classification of meningococci. Strains of *N. meningitidis* are subdivided into over 20 different serotypes, designated by numbers. However, many isolates cannot be typed with the available monoclonal antibodies.

Strains are further subtyped to more than 10 serosubtypes by the immunological differences between the class 1 protein (designated P1.*n.*). The class 1 protein is a product of the *porA* gene (Barlow *et al.*, 1989) and is expressed by most but not all meningococcal isolates (Woods and Cannon, 1990; Achtman *et al.*, 1992). This is interesting not only because such strains cannot be subtyped, but also they will not be affected by bactericidal antibodies generated with class 1 protein-based vaccines (see below).

The above serotyping and serosubtyping systems are largely dependent on monoclonal antibodies, which require multiple assays. The main shortcoming of this typing and subtyping scheme is that not all isolates can be typed or subtyped with the currently available battery of monoclonal antibodies. However, recent advances in molecular technology are overcoming this problem. The genes encoding the classes 1, 2 and 3 proteins have all now been sequenced. Comparisons of the deduced amino acid sequences of a number of variants have established the differences in primary structure that account for the antigenic differences between the proteins from different strains, some of which have been confirmed by the analysis of overlapping peptides with monoclonal antibodies. The determination of these primary structures has also enabled the prediction of a possible secondary structure for these proteins in which the most variable amino acid sequences are restricted to specific regions, the so-called variable regions (VRs), and exposed on the cell surface (Van der Ley *et al.*, 1991). This molecular approach to the analysis of serotyping and subtyping antigens is superior to serological typing because it can identify types which are missed serologically, the so-called nontypables (Feavers *et al.*, 1992; Maiden *et al.*, 1992). The new methodology is based on amplification of part of the genes encoding the variable regions using the polymerase chain reaction (PCR) and may lead to the development of techniques for the rapid identification and typing of meningococcal isolates directly from clinical specimens.

Similar to the prevalent serogroup profile, there is a trend for each serotype and subtype to change with time within one geographical location. This is particularly obvious among serogroups B and C. For example, until recently, Group B : 15 : P1.7,16 strains were found to be responsible for the majority of infections in England and Wales. However, there are currently more serologically non-typable and non-subtypable strains isolated in these two countries than most types and subtypes identified. Among 923 group B isolates in 1992 there were 423 non-typables and 140 non-subtypables; and among 929 group B isolates in 1993 there were 570 non- typables and 162 non-subtypables (Jones and Kaczmarski, 1993, 1994), reflecting the emergence of new strains which may or may not represent major genetic and/or antigenic shifts. Most of these newly emerging non-typable strains seem to be genotypically related to serotype 4 (Jones and Kaczmarski, 1995).

In Norway, the dominating serotype and subtype of serogroup B strain causing disease has been for many years group B : 15 : P1.7,16 (Lystad and Aasen, 1991), although changes are occurring and an increase in strains expressing P1.4 subtype antigen has been noted. In Central and South America, the predominant strain is group B : 4 : P1.15, which is responsible for over 95% of cases (Sierra *et al.*, 1991). It has recently been proposed that the generation and spread of new antigenic variants probably result from the horizontal transfer of DNA between strains (Hobbs *et al.*, 1994). The functional significance of such recombination events is, however, not clear. They may result from selective pressure on surface components involved with host cells, and therefore serve as immune evasion mechanisms, or may just reflect random transformation events during periods of frequent colonization (Morelli *et al.*, 1994).

With increased international travel, global dissemination of outbreak-associated strains is common. A typical example is the international epidemic of group A meningococcal disease which occurred in association with the Haj, the annual Moslem pilgrimage to Mecca in Arabia. In 1987, a major explosive outbreak of group A meningococcal infection caused thousands of cases of invasive disease. The infected Hajis caused numerous secondary infections in their home countries in different parts of the world, such as the Persian Gulf states, Pakistan, the UK, the USA and Israel, although these did not develop into widespread outbreaks. These meningococcal strains were from the same clone (A III-I) expressing P1.9. The intercontinental spread of a particular clone of serogroup B : 15 : P1.16 (clone ET-5) which was responsible for outbreaks in Norway, Iceland, Denmark, the Netherlands and the UK has also been documented, with outbreaks occurring in South Africa and Latin America (Caugant *et al.*, 1987). This strain emerged in northwestern Europe and dominated the previously prevalent B : 2a : P1.2 and B : 2b : P1.2 of the 1970s.

Other Class Proteins

The class 4 OMP, which appears to be highly conserved between meningococcal strains, shows considerable homology with the equivalent protein (PIII) of *N. gonorrhoeae* (Klugman *et al.*, 1989). The class 5 proteins are another group of surface-exposed proteins, encoded by *opa* genes which are fairly constant in sequence except for two hyper-variable regions (Aho *et al.*, 1991); they also undergo phase variation. Another class 5 protein called class 5C (or Opc), the amino acid sequence of which shows only 22% homology with that of Opa proteins (Olyhoek *et al.*, 1991), is widely distributed in serogroups A, B, C, W135 and Y. Opc protein has been implicated in adhesion to epithelial and endothelial cells (Virji *et al.*, 1993). Interestingly, *N. meningitidis* isolated from the nasopharynx of patients and healthy carriers express large amounts of Opc whereas, generally, isolates from blood or cerebrospinal fluid (CSF) express less. It has been suggested that the expression of Opc may be an important virulence mechanism for meningococci whereby a small proportion of the organisms express large amounts of this highly immunogenic protein that enables them to invade from the nasopharynx.

Iron-regulated Proteins

When grown under iron restriction, e.g. in the presence of an iron chelator such as desferrioxamine, meningococci express several proteins which appear to be suppressed (partially or totally) under iron-sufficient growth conditions. Many of these proteins, which vary in terms of their molecular mass and cellular localization, are believed to be directly related to iron acquisition from the host's iron-binding proteins and other iron sources. These iron-regulated proteins include two transferrin-binding proteins (Tbp1 and Tbp2) (Ala'Aldeen, 1996), two lactoferrin-binding proteins (Schryvers and Morris, 1988), a 37 kDa periplasmic iron-binding protein (Fbp) (Chen *et al.*, 1993), an 85 kDa haemoglobin–haptoglobin utilization protein (Hpu) (Lewis and Dyer, 1995), two RTX cytotoxin-related proteins (a 120 kDa FrpA and a 200 kDa FrpC) (Thomson and Sparling, 1993; Thomson *et al.*,

1993) and a 70 kDa protein (FrpB) of uncertain function (Ala'Aldeen *et al.*, 1990a, 1994a).

Although pathogenic neisseria are not able to produce siderophores, they are capable of removing iron from both human transferrin and lactoferrin through a saturable receptor-mediated mechanism which is highly specific for human transferrin and lactoferrin, respectively (Schryvers and Gonzalez, 1989). These receptors do not bind or utilize the iron load of transferrin and lactoferrin molecules of other animal species. This may explain the inability of the organism to adapt to the nasopharynx of non-human hosts. It has been demonstrated that transferrin binds directly to the surface of *in vivo* and *in vitro* grown meningococci (Figure 7c.1) (Ala'Aldeen, 1996). During this process these glycoproteins are not internalized, which differs from the mammalian cell transferrin receptor. The binding of iron-loaded transferrin to the meningococcal surface is an energy-independent process,

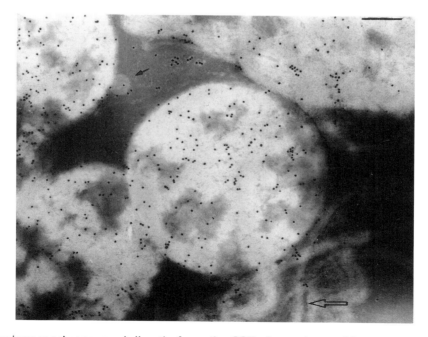

Figure 7c.1. Meningococci recovered directly from the CSF of a patient, without laboratory subculturing and labelled with gold-labelled human transferrin. Electron-dense particles represent the specific binding of transferrin molecules by the transferrin receptors. Also note the presence of pili (open arrow) and outer membrane blebs (closed arrow). Bar = 250 nm.

whereas iron uptake from transferrin is energy dependent.

Lipooligosaccharide (Endotoxin)

Meningococcal endotoxin (lipooligosaccharides, LOS) consist of an outer membrane-bound glycolipid which differs from the lipopolysaccharides (LPS) of the Enterobacteriaceae by lacking the O side chains, thus resembling the rough form of LPS (Griffiss *et al.*, 1988). It consists of three main components, namely an oligosaccharide core linked to a hydrophobic lipid A (the toxic component) and an oligosaccharide side chain (the immunogenic component). Structural and immunogenic heterogeneity within the oligosaccharide side chain has been used to classify strains to 12 immunotypes designated L*n*. Although individual strains of meningococci can produce more than one immunotype of LOS (e.g. L3,7,9), some immunotypes are more common among some serogroups than others, e.g. immunotypes L8–L11 are found within serogroup A, whereas groups B and C are associated with L1–L9 (Verheul *et al.*, 1993). Immunotype L3,7,9 is the most prevalent immunotype within groups B and C, followed by immunotypes L2 and L1,8.

Meningococcal LOS consists of a conserved (cross-reactive) and a variable (immunotype-specific) group of epitopes, as determined by monoclonal antibodies (Mandrell *et al.*, 1986). The quantitative and qualitative expression of these variable epitopes can vary not only between various strains, but also between different cells within the same culture and on the same cell, depending on the growth conditions. Although it is not entirely clear whether these immunotype differences between strains have any bearing on the invasive capability of the individual organism, some LOS immunotypes (such as L1,8,10) appear to be expressed on epidemiologically related carrier isolates, whereas others (such as L3,7,9) seem to be expressed mainly by disease isolates (Jones *et al.*, 1992; Mackinnon *et al.*, 1993).

Pili

Meningococci express two distinct classes of pili (class I and class II) which are extremely heterogeneous in terms of molecular and antigenic structure. Even a single strain can express more than one pilin in the course of infection (Stephens *et al.*, 1985). They are involved in the initial attachment of the organism to the nasopharyngeal cells and also enhance the organism's competence to accept foreign DNA. Pili, which consist of pilin glycopeptide polymers, are expressed *in vivo* (Figure 7c.1) and in *in vitro* primary isolates.

PATHOGENESIS AND PATHOPHYSIOLOGY OF DISEASE

Early in the twentieth century a close relationship was noted between the carrier rate in a population and the onset, rise and decline of an epidemic of meningitis (Glover, 1918). It is thought that transmission from one person to another is probably via the respiratory tract, but precise data supporting this hypothesis or on the mechanism involved are not available. It is known that, following exposure, the usual host–parasite relationship is one of commensalism but a small proportion of individuals will develop one of a variety of clinical syndromes. To become established in the nasopharynx, meningococci must be able to adhere to nasopharyngeal cells. Pili probably play an important part in this process, and they have been shown to be associated with attachment to human nasopharyngeal cells *in vitro* (Stephens and Farley, 1991). The outer membrane proteins Opa and Opc also appear to play a role in the colonization and invasion of human epithelial and endothelial cells (Virji *et al.*, 1993). However, it is unclear how the organism reaches the circulation. It is likely that meningococci adhere to non-ciliate columnar cells of the nasopharynx and pass through these cells by endocytosis to reach the subepithelial cells. The bacteria then reach the bloodstream, where they are confronted by a hostile environment. If they survive and multiply, they may cause bacteraemia, leading to different clinical syndromes depending on the host's defensive capabilities and other ill-understood factors.

During meningococcal septicaemia, there are signs and symptoms of circulatory failure, multiorgan dysfunction, coagulopathy and metabolic imbalances. There is increased vascular permeability and vasodilatation, which result in capillary leak syndrome with peripheral oedema. Loss of intravascular fluid and plasma proteins results in hypovolaemia and reduced venous return, and hence reduced cardiac output, hypotension and reduced perfusion of vital organs. Persistent hypovolaemia, and the associated vomiting and diarrhoea, will eventually lead to systemic hypoxia, acidosis and grossly impaired electrolyte and metabolic imbalance with multi-organ dysfunction.

The Role of Endotoxin

The lipid A moiety of the endotoxin is thought to be responsible for much of the acute symptoms, extensive tissue damage and multi-organ dysfunction through stimulating the release of inflammatory mediators, including tumour necrosis factor α (TNF-α) and a series of interleukins and other cytokines. In addition, meningococcal endotoxin seems to trigger a number of major intravascular cascade systems, including coagulation, fibrinolysis, complement and kallikrein–kinin (van Deventer *et al.*, 1990; Brandtzaeg, 1995). Although endotoxin is largely membrane associated, it is shed from live organisms in large quantities via the outer membrane vesicles (blebs), which also contain outer membrane proteins. This bleb shedding is known to occur *in vitro* (in broth cultures) and *in vivo* (Figure 7c.1). Increasing levels of circulating endotoxin are associated with increasing seriousness of disease and very high levels (>700 ng/l) are associated with fulminant septic shock, disseminated intravascular coagulation (DIC) and high fatality rate (Brandtzaeg, 1995). Endotoxin seems to trigger, directly or indirectly, the release of extremely high levels of monocyte tissue factor activity as detected in severely septicaemic patients, suggesting that

monocytes are responsible for the overwhelming DIC (Osterud and Flaegstad, 1983).

Coagulopathy

Coagulopathy is indicated by the presence of prolonged kaolin partial thromboplastin time, prothrombin time and thrombin time; reduced platelet count, plasma fibrinogen, plasminogen and α_2-antiplasmin; increased fibrin degradation products, fibrinopeptide A and plasminogen activator inhibitor I; and reduced functional levels of coagulation factor V, antithrombin III, protein C, protein S and extrinsic pathway inhibitor (Brandtzaeg, 1995). Severity of disease is also predicted from markedly increased levels of immunoreactive plasminogen activator inhibitor I, and figures exceeding 1850 μg/l almost always reflect a fatal outcome (Brandtzaeg, 1995). The fibrinolytic cascade seems to be activated early in the disease, which is then downregulated by increasing levels of plasminogen activator inhibitor I, resulting in the formation of microthrombi in various body organs, including the skin and the suprarenal glands. The uncontrolled and excessive consumption of coagulation factors then results in a haemorrhagic diathesis with disseminated tissue haemorrhages.

Activated Complement Cascades

The complement cascade, a major line of antimeningococcal acute host defence, is also triggered, probably by the effect of endotoxin alone. Both the classical and alternative pathways seem to be activated during meningococcal disease; however, during severe septic shock, the alternative pathway seems to dominate. Although complement-mediated bacteriolysis is an effective protective antibacterial mechanism, it is believed to have some indirect detrimental effect via the release of the C3a, C4a and C5a anaphylatoxins, and/or the release of membrane-bound endotoxin which may follow the attack of the membrane attack complex (Frank *et al.*, 1987). Increased levels of C3 activation products and terminal complement complexes are thought to reflect the severity of disease (Brandtzaeg, 1995).

Cytokines

It is interesting that during septic shock increased levels of endotoxin, TNF-α, interleukin 1β (IL-1β), IL-6 and IL-8 are detected in the peripheral blood and reflect disease severity. During meningococcal meningitis without septicaemia there may be a compartmentalized CSF rise of endotoxin levels, associated in about half of the cases with CSF rise of TNF-α and IL-1β, which all reflect severity of meningitis (Brandtzaeg *et al.*, 1992a, 1992b). The rise in IL-6 and IL-8 does not seem to be compartmentalized.

Consequences of the Bacterial Insults

General

The uncontrolled and complicated cascades of organism- or endotoxin-induced events, including inflammatory mediators and coagulopathies, eventually lead to capillary leakage syndrome, circulatory collapse, myocarditis, renal failure, adult respiratory distress syndrome, adrenal haemorrhage, haemorrhagic skin and serosal surface lesions, muscular infarction and other organ dysfunctions. Of these, circulatory failure is the most prominent cause of death in overwhelming meningococcal disease. Myocardial dysfunction is due probably to a combination of many effects, including direct effect of the bacterium and its endotoxin, inflammatory mediators, impaired coronary artery perfusion, hypoxia, acidosis, hypocalcaemia, hypokalaemia, hypomagnesaemia and hypophosphataemia.

Outcome of disease can be predicted from the initial renal function (e.g. serum creatinine level), and those who develop uraemia or anuria early in the disease will have much poorer prognosis than those who develop only a mild degree of renal impairment (Brandtzaeg *et al.*, 1989). Adrenal haemorrhages, the so-called 'Waterhouse–Fredrichsen syndrome' which is observed in a large percentage of fatal cases, is not unique to fulminant meningococcal septicaemia as it occurs in other overwhelming Gram-negative endotoxaemia with DIC. The resulting adrenal insufficiency is an additional contributing factor for the circulatory collapse.

Haemorrhagic skin lesions (petechiae and ecchymoses), which vary in size and severity, reflect the meningococcal predilection for the dermal blood vessels and the severity of DIC and state of septicaemia. There is vascular damage (with or without vasculitis) with endothelial cell injury or death, with meningococci identifiable and/or cultivable from lesion biopsies.

The central nervous system

Bacterial endotoxin and peptidoglycan are believed to be mainly responsible, directly or indirectly through inflammatory mediators, for the meningeal inflammation, blood–brain barrier dysfunction and the changes in CSF. These include cellular, biochemical and hydrodynamic changes of the CSF. Increased CSF secretion and impaired absorption and blood–brain barrier dysfunction can lead to the accumulation of CSF, raised intracranial pressure and reduced cerebral blood flow. Increased CSF lactate indicates brain tissue hypoxia. In patients with meningococcal septicaemia and meningitis, the brain tissue hypoxia, which is worsened by the shock-induced under-perfusion, vasculitis and DIC, may result in neuronal injury and varying degrees of brain tissue damage.

Immunity

Bactericidal antibodies

Protection has been correlated with the presence of bactericidal antibodies (Frasch, 1983) and various lines of evidence highlight the importance of humoral bactericidal activity in host defence against *N. meningitidis*. For example, the peak incidence of the disease occurs in children under one year of age, who as a group have few or no bactericidal antibodies. Meningococcal disease is up to 10 000 times more common in terminal complement component-deficient individuals than in normal healthy individuals, with a much higher frequency of second episodes of the illness

(Andreoni *et al.*, 1993). Passive immunization with antibodies (serum therapy) and active immunization with some capsular polysaccharides (which stimulates antibody response and not T-helper cell response) have been successful in the treatment and prevention of the disease. Further evidence emerged following a study reported by Goldschneider and colleagues (1969a, 1969b) where pre-immune sera were obtained from new recruits of the American armed forces and examined for susceptibility using serum bactericidal activity and immunofluorescence. Unlike the control group, the majority of those who lacked bactericidal activity against prevalent strains acquired meningococci. Thus, bactericidal assays have become established as the best available test to determine the protective ability of specific antisera raised against vaccine candidates. However, it is not certain to what extent the *in vitro* experimental conditions reflect events occurring *in vivo* nor whether the above data apply to infections with all serogroups. The data linking bactericidal antibodies with protection relate primarily to the group A and C polysaccharides but have been extended to include bactericidal antibodies against OMPs.

Natural immunity

The mechanisms responsible for the development of natural immunity against meningococci remain unclear. The majority of the adult population have bactericidal antibodies against most prevalent invasive meningococcal strains (Goldschneider *et al.*, 1969a, 1969b). About half of the newborn infants seem to inherit these antibodies from their mothers and remain relatively protected for the first few months of life. After the first six months, these bactericidal antibodies are no longer detectable. Toddlers older than two years gradually accumulate bactericidal antibodies over the following decade. It is not entirely clear how these specific bactericidal antibodies are generated, but they are likely to be produced by carriage of meningococci, including invasive or non-invasive strains, commensal neisseriae and other organisms which share cross-reactive antigens with prevalent

meningococcal strains. Carriage of strains of *N. meningitidis* or the commensal *N. lactamica* is considered an effective, but not absolute, immunization process during which bactericidal antibodies are generated which may protect against invasive meningococcal strains of different serogroups, serotypes and serosubtypes. Although the majority of the meningococcal strains isolated from carriers are groupable and indistinguishable from invasive ones, often non-groupable strains are isolated. Both forms of the organism are capable of generating bactericidal antibodies which can protect against homologous and heterologous strains from different serogroups (Reller *et al.*, 1973). These indicate that non-capsular antigens are capable of generating cross-protective antibodies. Also, *Escherichia coli* serotype K1, *Pasteurella haemolytica* serotype A-2 and *Moraxella nonliquefaciens* have immunochemically identical polysaccharide antigens to that of Group B meningococci (Adlam *et al.*, 1987) and the polysaccharide capsule of serogroup A cross-reacts with *Bacillus pumilis*.

IgA and IgA protease

During infection, IgA antibodies are generated against a variety of different cell wall components, including the capsular polysaccharide, LOS, class OMPs and some iron-regulated proteins (Ala'Aldeen and Griffiss, 1995). IgA has been shown to block the bactericidal activity of convalescent sera containing bactericidal IgG and IgM antibodies, and the removal of IgA from non-bactericidal acute sera will restore the killing effect of IgM antibodies present in these sera (Griffiss and Bertram, 1977). It is interesting to note that the ability of IgA to inhibit IgG binding is dependent on the relative ratios of the two antibodies, although inhibition of IgM binding is not competitive (Griffiss and Goroff, 1983). It is believed that epidemics of meningococcal disease occur in populations with elevated levels of blocking IgA which may be induced by cross-reactive enteric bacteria (Griffiss, 1995). Meningococci also produce proteases that cleave secretory and serum IgA1 (but not IgA2) from the hinge region, which may further enhance the blocking effect of the antibodies by generating functionally useless antigen-binding Fab fragments.

Complement

It has long been established that late complement components are vital for complete protection against invasive meningococcal disease (Andreoni et al., 1993). Both the classical and alternative pathways are important for protection. Those with complement deficiencies, including C2, C3, C4b, C5–9 and properdin, are at high risk of developing meningococcal disease and/or suffering more severe disease. Those with late complement component deficiency are particularly at much greater risk of acquiring meningococcal disease and developing second episodes of disease. It is interesting that these patients suffer from disease at an older age with lower mortality rate, and with group Y being the most frequently isolated serogroup, whereas men suffering from the X-linked properdin deficiency are at much greater risk of developing severe disseminated meningococcal disease with a very high mortality rate (Densen et al., 1987). This highlights the importance of the early complement components and the initiation of complement activation and, by inference, the role of the alternative pathway in meningococcal lysis.

Cellular immune response

While the great majority of the studies have focused on the role of serum bactericidal activity in the host defence against meningococcal disease, much less attention has been given to the killing of bacteria by phagocytosis, and therefore little is known about the relative importance of phagocyte-mediated killing of meningococci as compared with serum bactericidal activity. Halstensen and colleagues (1989) reported a close association between the opsonin activity, duration and severity of symptoms and the anti-OMP IgG levels.

Finally, for most antigens, an efficient humoral immune response resulting in the production of antibodies and the generation of memory response requires help from T lymphocytes. However, T cells respond to peptide antigens associated with molecules of the major histocompatibility complex (HLA in humans) and so will not be stimulated by polysaccharide vaccines. This may explain why the protective efficacy of these vaccines is short lived and ineffective in young children. A way to overcome this problem is to conjugate the polysaccharide-containing B cell epitopes to carrier proteins containing epitopes for recognition by T cells. This may be achieved by using proteins containing T cell epitopes as carriers in conjugate vaccines (see page 298).

EPIDEMIOLOGY

Compulsory notification of disease in the UK, imposed in 1912, helped to demonstrate the rise and fall of epidemics, which shows one large peak in reported cases (a few thousands) during the period of the First World War and an even higher one (exceeding 12 000 cases) which coincided with the second World War. Currently, we are experiencing a worldwide epidemic with a clear increase in the number of cases reported in the past decade. The occurrence of cases is generally unpredictable, but occasional clustering occurs in various geographical areas, particularly during the periods of increased disease activity. Baseline incidence rate between epidemics in the industrialized countries is between one and three cases per 100 000 population, compared with 10–25 per 100 000 in non-industrialized countries. Attack rates are highest in those aged under five years, and in winter and spring, possibly due to prevalence of viral respiratory infections which are thought to act as predisposing factors (Moore et al., 1990). In the UK notification of the disease has more than doubled since the early 1980s. Despite a downward trend in the number of isolated strains in the early 1990s, the Public Health Laboratory Services Meningococcal Reference Unit reported around 1300 confirmed cases from England and Wales for the last three to four years and the Office of Population Censuses and Surveys received slightly more disease notifications for the same years (Jones and Kaczmarski, 1993,

1994, 1995); 50–60% of cases occurred in children under five years of age, of which around 40% were in children aged less than one year. The highest incidence of cases occurred in the month of January and the lowest in August/September. In the USA, approximately 2600 cases of meningococcal disease have occurred annually over the past few years (1.1 cases per 100 000 population), with an overall case–fatality rate of 12% (Jackson and Wenger, 1993). The highest rate of attack occurs in the months of February and March and the lowest in September; 46% of cases affect those of two years of age or younger.

In Third World countries more than 310 000 people are thought to suffer from meningococcal diseases annually, of which it is estimated 35 000 cases are fatal. Over 300 million people live in countries within the 'meningitis belt' of Savannah Africa, which is a vast area extending from Ethiopia in the east to The Gambia in the west, and from the Sahara in the north to the tropical rain forest of central Africa in the south. This belt has expanded since it was first described in 1963 (Lapeyssonie, 1963), and it now includes 15 countries, namely Ethiopia, Sudan, Central African Republic, Chad, Cameroon, Nigeria, Niger, Benin, Togo, Ghana, Burkina Faso, Mali, Guinea, Senegal and The Gambia (Greenwood, 1987). In 1988 and 1989, 80% of meningococcal isolates in the African continent occurred in these 15 countries, and in 1989 more than half the reported cases were from Ethiopia (Riedo *et al.*, 1995). During epidemics, attack rates in some countries of the meningitis belt reach as high as 1000 cases per 100 000 population, which contrasts with 5–25 cases per 100 000 in the industrialized countries (Rey, 1991). In many regions of the meningitis belt, epidemics occur in cycles, with intervals between epidemics in the majority of cases less than 12 years (range 2–25 years) (Riedo *et al.*, 1995). Epidemics last for approximately two to four years (Lapeyssonie, 1963), and occur mainly in the hot dry months, possibly due to the influence of dry air on the integrity of the mucosal membranes of the nasopharynx. Some northern African countries (like Egypt) also experience fluctuating epidemics. Large-scale epidemics have also occurred in many countries of Asia (e.g. Pakistan, India and China), and Central and Latin America (e.g. Cuba, Chile and Brazil). In Cuba, the attack rate reached levels of more than 50 cases per 100 000 population (Sierra *et al.*, 1991).

Age and Sex

Age-specific rates for meningococcal infection in England and Wales between 1984 and 1991 show a sudden rise in the attack rate of invasive meningococcal infection among infants in the first few months of life which peaks at the age of six months (more than 50 cases per 100 000) and remains relatively high for the first 12–24 months of life (Jones, 1995). The attack rate falls dramatically to 10 cases per 100 000 at the age of two years and continues to decline until it reaches the overall adult rate of 0.4 cases per 100 000, only to produce a second but smaller peak (less than five cases per 100 000) amongst the 17–18-year-olds. Boys are probably at a slightly higher risk of invasive disease in the first few years of life whereas among the teenagers this is reversed. It is interesting that during epidemics the average age of patients is older than between epidemics.

Carriage

As an obligate human pathogen, the natural habitat of the meningococcus is the human nasopharynx. Although seasonal variation, temperature and humidity seem to have a clear impact on invasive meningococcal disease, they have very little, if any, effect on prevalence of carriage. It is interesting that the highest attack rate of invasive meningococcal disease in Europe and the USA is in the first year of life, whereas the highest carriage rate is found among teenagers and young adults (Cartwright, 1995). This implies that infected children are victims of the grown-ups who maintain the organism in the community. While it is difficult to estimate true carriage rate in different groups in any community at any one time, it is known that several factors could influence carriage in the population. These include factors related to the parasite, the host and the environment. Some serogroups of *N. meningitidis* (see above), e.g. serogroup 29E, are regarded to be of low pathogenicity and are isolated from carriers, whereas serogroups A, B and C are responsible for over 90% of the invasive meningococcal infections worldwide. Carriage is more common in the second and third decades of life, and more common among smokers than non-smokers. The body's immune status, changes in the oropharyngeal flora and concurrent viral upper respiratory tract infections are also believed to influence carriage. Mycoplasma and viral infections, particularly influenza A infection, are increasingly blamed for predisposition of carriage and invasive meningococcal disease. Carriage rates are known to be much higher among family members and close contacts of infected patients and in closed communities with overcrowding conditions, such as military recruits' training camps, prisons and schools. Baseline carriage rates of 5–15% are considered usual; however, epidemics are thought to occur when the rate exceeds 20%. During epidemics carriage rate could reach as high as 50% or more, and among homosexuals it could exceed 40%. Finally, it is difficult to obtain an estimate of the actual duration of meningococcal carriage, but it has been shown to be as short as several days to as long as several months or a few years (Cartwright, 1995). Patients with invasive disease may carry the organisms for days or weeks before becoming ill.

CLINICAL MANIFESTATIONS

Meningococci are capable of causing a wide range of different clinical syndromes which can vary in severity from a transient mild sore throat to meningitis, and to acute meningococcal septicaemia which can cause death within hours of the appearance of symptoms. Bacteraemia with or without sepsis, meningococcal septicaemia with or without meningitis, meningoencephalitis, chronic meningococcaemia, pneumonia, septic arthritis, pericarditis, myocarditis, endocarditis, conjunctivitis, panophthalmitis, genitourinary tract infection, pelvic infection, peritonitis, and proctitis are all among the diseases caused by meningococci. Meningitis and/or septicaemia are by far the most

common presentations of disease. In 1994, 42% of the total clinical isolates in England and Wales were from cases of septicaemia, and the remainder were from cases of meningitis (Jones and Kaczmarski, 1995). It is important to remember that the clinical picture can progress from one end of the spectrum to the other during the course of disease.

Acute Meningococcal Septicaemia With or Without Meningitis

Acute meningococcal diseases may present initially with a series of non-specific manifestations which, combined, may provide indicative diagnostic clues. This may include signs of septicaemia, meningitis or both. Presentation with severe meningococcal septicaemia is less common but deadlier than meningitis.

The majority of cases occur in young children and present with rapid onset of raised temperature which may be accompanied by vomiting, photophobia, convulsions, skin rash, lethargy, irritability, drowsiness, reluctance to feed, diarrhoea and other more localized signs and symptoms. In older children and adults, headache, restlessness, generalized muscular pain and arthralgia are also found. The onset may be preceded by prodromal symptoms mimicking viral upper respiratory tract infections. On examination, the patient is often distressed, with temperature ranging from normal to 41 °C.

Meningococcal septicaemia is most often associated with characteristic meningococcal rash (Figure 7c.2). These, when present, can be of macular, maculopapular, petechial, purpuric, ecchymotic or necrotic nature and can appear anywhere in the body, including the trunk, extremities, pressure sites, palm, sole, face, palate and conjunctiva. Adjacent lesions can coalesce and form confluent purpura, petechiae, haemorrhagic bullae or even gangrenous necrotic skin and subcutaneous lesions. In severe cases, DIC with intense peripheral vasoconstriction may cause peripheral gangrene which can involve fingers, toes or even entire limbs.

In severe cases, patients present in shock with tachycardia, progressively impaired peripheral perfusion, increased respiratory rate, hypoxia,

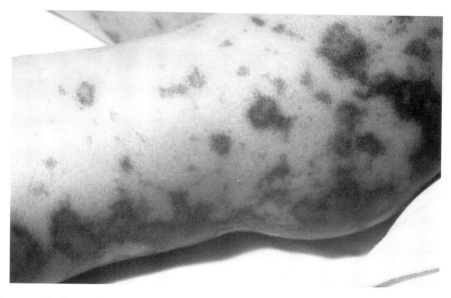

Figure 7c.2. Characteristic meningococcal rash in a child with meningococcal septicaemia. Note petechiae coalescing in places. (Courtesy of Dr H. Vyas, Nottingham.)

cyanosis, acidosis, electrolyte imbalance, elevated plasma lactate levels, hypotension, progressive circulatory failure with oliguria or anuria. Progressively impaired central perfusion leads to a decline in the level of consciousness and may lead to coma. Poor prognostic signs include extensive and rapidly progressing necrotic skin lesions, hypotension, shock, multi-organ failure, decreasing level of consciousness, and signs of DIC.

Varying degrees of respiratory failure and acute respiratory distress syndrome are found in most patients with meningococcal septicaemic shock. These are caused by various factors, including pulmonary oedema due to capillary leak syndrome, and pulmonary vascular occlusion due to DIC. Reversible oliguria or renal failure occurs in severe cases due to hypovolaemia and impaired organ perfusion. In cases of prolonged shock, tubular and cortical necrosis can cause irreversible renal failure.

Meningitis

Signs and symptoms of meningococcal meningitis include general (non-specific) and localized (specific) ones. Patients often remain alert, but signs of cerebral involvement such as convulsions, declining level of consciousness and coma may be present. In the young and previously healthy, localized signs of meningeal irritation may occur early in the disease. Most, but not all, patients present with clear signs of meningeal irritation. Of these, neck stiffness is by far the most important; however, it is present in less than half of the patients (Carpenter, 1962). In infants and young children neck stiffness is difficult to test for, but often the head is retracted when the child is left to take the most comfortable position. This is observed in association with a bulging fontanelle due to increased intracranial pressure, and the child is clearly irritable and lies on his side with his back to the light (photophobia). A positive Kernig's sign, the inability to extend the knee when the hip is flexed in supine position, is another important and pathognomonic sign of meningeal irritation. Attempts to flex the neck in a sudden movement with the patient in a sitting position with the legs outstretched will induce a reflex flexion of both hips and knees (Brudziniski's sign).

Other Manifestations

Acute or chronic meningococcal septic (or rarely immunoreactive) arthritis is relatively common and may complicate any of the acute meningococcal diseases. It usually affects one or more joints and manifests at any stage of disease (Schaad, 1980). Occasionally, arthritis is the only presenting complaint, which most often involves a single large joint such as the knee or the hip. Meningococci may be seen in Gram stains and isolated in cultures of joint aspirates.

Upper and lower respiratory tract infection, such as otitis media, pharyngitis, bronchitis and pneumonia, can occur as part of disseminated meningococcal disease or as primary infections. Primary pneumonia is typically caused by serogroup Y meningococci and has a good prognosis. Blood cultures, sputum, lung biopsy (not performed routinely) and trachea aspirate can yield the organism. Culture-positive nasopharyngeal swabs can be misleading and therefore are not recommended.

Similarly, other organs may be attacked by meningococci as part of meningococcal septicaemia and/or as a primary organ infection. These include pericarditis, myocarditis and endocarditis. Myocarditis is thought to be present in most cases of overwhelming septicaemia. Also, meningococcal urethritis and endocervicitis in sexually active women and proctitis in homosexuals can occur. Meningococci seem to be responsible for 2% of all bacterial conjunctivitis and this may proceed to systemic meningococcal disease in nearly one-third of cases (Barquet et al., 1990).

Chronic Meningococcal Disease

Finally, chronic meningococcal disease (chronic meningococcaemia) is a rare but long-recognized clinical entity which presents as chronic intermittent high temperature, joint pain, headache with or without skin lesions, affecting adults more than children (Benoit, 1963). The condition can last months and cause a variety of complications. The organism may be isolated from the blood in the first few weeks of the illness.

Transient Meningococcaemia

Relatively mild culture-positive flu-like illness can present with non-specific symptoms such as raised temperature, joint pain with or without rash and can persist for days or weeks. Such mild bacteraemia may resolve completely without treatment, or progress to acute severe disease or persist as chronic meningococcaemia.

Complications

A significant number of the patients who recover end up with permanent neurological sequelae, including mental retardation, cerebellar ataxia, cranial nerve deficits, deafness (due to auditory nerve damage), persistent headache, hydrocephalus, dementia, convulsions, peripheral nerve lesions, subdural empyema and psychoneurological complications.

Mortality

Mortality rate from meningococcal disease varies between 7% and 70% depending on a number of factors, including the severity of disease, the speed at which it develops, the organs involved, the age and immune status of the patient, socioeconomic status, the standard of health care and the speed by which the disease is diagnosed and antibiotics administered. In those patients who present with signs of severe septicaemia, particularly in underdeveloped countries, the mortality rate can reach up to 70% (deMorais et al., 1974). In developed countries, 15–30% of septicaemic patients die despite treatment in advanced intensive care units.

The overall mortality from meningococcal meningitis in Europe and North America is 5–15% despite the sensitivity of the organism to many antibiotics and despite the high standard of health care in these two continents. Children seem to have a better chance of recovery from meningococcal meningitis than adults. Mortality rate for children under the age of five is around 5%, compared with 10–15% in adults.

The average case–mortality rate in England

and Wales for the last few years has been 12%, which represents an average of the rate for meningitis (around 7%) and septicaemia (around 20%) (Jones, 1995). The mortality rate for patients with septicaemic shock remains very high (50–60%) despite state-of-the-art intensive care facilities. These figures have not changed for the last two or three decades. Most deaths occur in the first two or three days of admission to hospital. Very rapid development of septicaemia is a poor prognostic sign. Often patients, particularly those with septicaemia and septic shock, die within a few hours of the appearance of the first symptoms.

LABORATORY DIAGNOSIS

Specimens

Cerebrospinal fluid

In cases of meningitis, performing a lumbar puncture and taking blood cultures are essential. Any signs and symptoms suggestive of meningitis should prompt the clinician to perform a lumbar puncture without delay. However, this procedure is not an absolute must in all cases of meningococcal disease and its risks must be weighed against its benefits. In cases of raised intracranial pressure, lumbar puncture is associated with grave risks and therefore should not be performed (Mellor, 1992). Mild increase in intracranial pressure is present in virtually all patients with meningococcal meningitis, and is not a contraindication for lumbar puncture. However, when clinically evident, it is considered severe enough to prevent lumbar puncture attempts. Even after a markedly increased intracranial pressure, papilloedema may appear late in the process (24–48 hours); therefore, more acute signs of raised intracranial pressure should be looked for. These include severe deterioration in the level of consciousness, bradycardia, abnormal blood pressure and respiratory depression. Lumbar puncture should be avoided in the presence of septicaemic shock, as this may aggrevate the circulatory collapse, and it is important to remember that, in cases of meningococcal septicaemia

without signs of meningitis, the CSF examination may not reveal any cellular or biochemical abnormality.

Direct microscopy In meningitis, depending on white cell count and bacterial load, the CSF may remain clear or become very cloudy. Two hundred white cells per cubic millimetre (0.2×10^9 cells/l) can make the CSF look turbid. The leucocyte count (predominantly polymorphonuclear cells) can reach as high as thousands or even 10 000 mm^3, as can the bacterial cell count (not measured routinely). Protein content is raised and may even reach levels as high as 10 g/l, and glucose levels fall below 40% of plasma glucose levels or even be undetectable. Raised lactate dehydrogenase and neuraminidase levels can also be detected in the CSF of patients with meningococcal meningitis.

Direct microscopy of CSF deposit often provides the first positive diagnostic clue which can guide the choice of antibiotic. The Gram stain may reveal Gram-negative diplococci in more than two-thirds of the cases presenting with meningitis, provided the patient had not received antibiotics prior to lumbar puncture. Diplococci are seen both inside and outside the pus cells. The serogroup of the causative organism can be obtained without delay by probing the CSF deposit with capsular polysaccharide-specific antibodies conjugated to fluorescein isothiocyanate.

Recovery of organism from the CSF remains the ultimate diagnostic goal. The organism is often isolated in cases with septicaemia without signs of meningitis whose CSF could otherwise be normal. Following the recent awareness campaigns in the UK and the increased awareness of general practitioners of meningococcal disease, many patients will have received antibiotics before they arrive in hospital. This dramatically reduces the chances of recovering *N. meningitidis* from the CSF.

Blood

Blood cultures may yield the organism in up to 60% of cases if taken before antibiotics are administered. This rate is markedly reduced after the first dose of penicillin. *Neisseria meningitidis* may grow in conventional (simple) broth culture systems without producing visible turbidity, therefore, in all patients with suspected meningococcal disease, blind subculture (usually after 12–18 hours) of the broth onto solid media is strongly recommended. If negative, the procedure may be repeated after 48 hours of incubation.

Throat and nasopharynx

Throat and nasopharyngeal culture may also reveal the organism in more than half of cases, which can support but not necessarily confirm the diagnosis. With the increasing use of antibiotics prior to admission, these specimens may be the only source where isolates can be obtained. Therefore, it is very important that throat swabs are taken, by the general practitioner or the hospital doctor, as soon as the disease is suspected, irrespective of whether the first dose of penicillin is administered or not. Swabs must be transported to the laboratory as soon as possible in order to maximize the chances of recovery of the organism.

Skin lesions

Skin lesions may also yield the causative organism. Petechial lesions can be injected with a small volume of sterile saline and aspirated with a hypodermic needle and inoculated into a broth medium. Alternatively, skin biopsies can be Gram stained and processed for culture immediately. In patients with meningococcal septicaemia, the organisms can be recovered from skin biopsies even after the start of antibiotics (van Deuren et al., 1993).

Isolation of *N. meningitidis*

No effort should be spared to isolate the causative organism and, where possible, all the relevant culture specimens should be taken before antibiotics are administered. Recovery and identification of the organism are important for clinical and epidemiological reasons. Isolation of the organism will confirm the diagnosis, influence the choice of antibiotics, provide useful epidemio-logical information and boost the confidence of the clinicians in managing meningococcal disease. Meningococci can be isolated from a number of possible sources, including the CSF, blood, throat or nasopharyngeal swabs, skin lesions, joint aspirates, eye swabs, or any other body fluid or tissue specimens.

Identification

Isolates must be identified to species level in the local laboratory and further classified in a reference laboratory. Meningococci must be differentiated from other oxidase-positive, Gram-negative diplococci, using biochemical and immunological tests. The rapid carbohydrate utilization test (RCUT) provides fast and reliable identification. In this test, a heavy bacterial inoculum is suspended in broth containing individual sugars, and meningococci will ferment glucose and maltose (but not lactose and sucrose) within an hour or so. γ-Glutamyl aminopeptidase activity can be detected in rapid tests, such as Gonocheck (Du Pont de Nemours, Inc.), where adding meningococcal colonies to the rehydrated substrates will produce a yellow reaction. On isolates from the nasopharynx, throat, eyes, rectum or other sites where gonococci and respiratory neisseriae can also be carried, precise identification must be attempted. Coagglutination tests (e.g. Phadebact Monoclonal GC Test, Launch Diagnostics Ltd), using specific anti-gonococcal antibodies conjugated to protein A of non-viable staphylococci, will identify or exclude gonococci but not meningococci.

The serogroup of the organism is identified by detecting the capsular polysaccharide antigen using immunological tests, including latex agglutination, coagglutination and counter-immuno-electrophoresis.

It is important to remember that there is always a potential risk of acquiring meningococcal infection through handling live organisms while performing biochemical or antibiotic sensitivity tests. Therefore, any work with live cultures of *N. meningitidis* should be performed in class I safety cabinets.

Detection of Meningococcal Antigens, Antibodies and DNA

In culture-negative CSF, presumptive diagnosis can be obtained by detecting very low levels of meningococcal antigens using various immunological and biochemical techniques. Using specific antibodies, the capsular polysaccharide antigens of serogroups A, C, W135 and Y can be reliably identified in the CSF of more than three-quarters of cases. This test is not reliable for serogroup B due to the capsule's poor immunogenicity and its cross-reaction with the capsule of *E. coli* serotype K1, which is another common cause of meningitis in young infants.

High titres of specific anti-meningococcal antibodies in a single specimen of serum, or rising titres in paired sera, can also provide a retrospective diagnosis. These are measured by enzyme-linked immunosorbent assay with crude preparations of outer membrane vesicles as antigens (Jones and Kaczmarski, 1995).

Meningococcal DNA can be detected from the CSF, whole blood and plasma during the acute stage of the disease, and diagnostic PCR tests are under development in many centres. Reasonably good results have been obtained with CSF (Ni *et al.*, 1992) but it may be a few years before this technique becomes fully evaluated, and established for both CSF and blood. An obvious shortcoming of this technique is the fact that it requires expensive equipment and reagents; therefore, it is unlikely to become widely available in most hospitals in the developed world, let alone in the Third World.

Other Investigations

Peripheral white cell count varies from subnormal levels to over 45×10^9 cells/l. In patients presenting with skin rash and septicaemia, clotting parameters must be monitored. In these cases, prothrombin and activated partial thromboplastin times are usually prolonged. Diminished plasma fibrinogen and increased fibrinogen degradation product titre are detected.

Poor prognostic peripheral blood parameters include low blood white cell count ($<10 \times 10^9$ cells/l), thrombocytopenia, grossly abnormal coagulation indices (Algren *et al.*, 1993) and raised serum creatinine.

MANAGEMENT

In the pre-antibiotic era, particularly following the great success of the use of anti-diphtheria antiserum in treating cases of diphtheria, therapeutic administration of immune sera became fasionable for a number of infectious diseases, including meningococcal meningitis. Good results were obtained with anti-meningococcal antisera administered intrathecally, intracisternally or intravenously, with clear reduction in mortality rates (Flexner, 1913). The first use of antibiotics was in the latter part of 1935, following the discovery of the sulphonamides, which were then replaced by penicillin the following decade. For the past five decades, penicillin has become established as the mainstay of specific antimeningococcal treatment.

Chemotherapy

The choice of antibiotic treatment varies depending on a number of interrelated factors, including those relating to the patient, organism, pharmacokinetics of the antibiotics (CSF penetration), circumstances, epidemiological data, affordability and hospital facilities. The standard approach, particularly in meningitis, is blindly to cover for most of the possible causative organisms using relatively broad-spectrum antibiotics until the diagnosis is confirmed, and then switch to penicillin.

The start of chemotherapy

Treatment should commence as soon as the disease is suspected. Parenteral penicillin given by the general practitioner before referral to hospital, or by hospital doctors on arrival before laboratory confirmation (or even before performing lumbar puncture if this was delayed), has been shown to reduce mortality rate (Cartwright *et al.*, 1992; Strang and Pugh, 1992). One megaunit of penicillin given intramuscularly, or up to 100 mg/kg benzylpenicillin given intravenously, is recommended. It is wise, however, to place an intravenous cannula as soon as possible and obtain a throat or nasopharyngeal swab and two sets of blood cultures, one from each arm, before antibiotics are commenced.

Blind treatment

It is widely recommended now that until positive laboratory identification of the organism is made, the patient must be treated blindly with a broad-spectrum bactericidal antibiotic that is effective against all other possible causes of pyogenic meningitis. Recently, third-generation cephalosporins, such as cefotaxime (200 mg/kg per day) or ceftriaxone (100 mg/kg per day), have replaced the conventional penicillin and chloramphenicol combination in many developed countries. Although these cephalosporins do not necessarily improve morbidity or mortality, they offer the advantage of using a single, relatively non-toxic, therapeutic agent which penetrates the CSF extremely well. They are effective against *N. meningitidis*, *Streptococcus pneumoniae*, *Haemophilus influenzae*, *E. coli* and *Streptococcus agalactiae* (group B streptococci). Furthermore, penicillin- and chloramphenicol-resistant *H. influenzae* are now widespread and penicillin-insensitive and/or penicillin-resistant strains of meningococci (minimum inhibitory concentration, MIC, ≥ 0.12 mg/l) have now emerged in many countries, including Spain, South Africa, the UK, Canada and the USA (Sutcliffe *et al.*, 1988; Riley *et al.*, 1991; Jackson *et al.*, 1994; Woods *et al.*, 1994) and possibly other countries such as Greece, Switzerland, Romania and Belgium (Woods *et al.*, 1994). The mechanism of resistance does not seem to involve β-lactamase production, but it is believed to be due to reduced affinity of penicillin-binding proteins 2 as a result of some possible changes in the nucleotide sequence of its gene, *penA* (Zang *et al.*, 1990; Saez-Nieto *et al.*, 1992). Until the mid-1980s no such strains were known

and by the end of the decade nearly half of the strains in Spain showed some degree of insensitivity to penicillin. However, these strains remain sensitive to the third-generation cephalosporins.

Cefuroxime, a second-generation cephalosporin, and ceftazidime, another third-generation cephalosporin, are also effective in treating meningococcal meningitis. However, these two agents are not recommended for blind treatment, especially as ceftazidime is not very effective against *Streptococcus pneumoniae*. The major shortcoming of the cephalosporins is that they are not effective against *Listeria monocytogenes*, although a relatively uncommon cause of meningitis, and they are very expensive. In many underdeveloped countries, where cephalosporins are not affordable, the combination of penicillin and chloramphenicol is still used.

Specific antibiotic treatment

Penicillin remains the drug of first choice and is highly effective in penicillin-sensitive strains. The drug's penetration to the CSF is poor in the absence of inflamed blood–brain barrier; however, when high and frequent (meningitic) doses of penicillin are given, good therapeutic levels are achieved. Neonates under the age of two months are given up to 60 mg/kg 6-hourly, whereas children between two months and six years are given up to 75 mg/kg every 4 hours and children above the age of six years and adults should receive up to 2.4 g/kg every 4 hours. Temptation to reduce doses upon clinical improvement must be resisted because the CSF penetration of penicillin reduces as the inflamed blood–brain barrier recovers.

Meningococci are usually highly sensitive to benzylpenicillin (MIC 0.003–0.06 mg/l). Strains with MIC between 0.12 and 1.0 mg/l are considered of reduced sensitivity, although many of these still respond to therapeutic (high meningitic) doses of intravenous penicillin. Meningococci are also highly sensitive to many, but not all, other penicillin derivatives such as ampicillin, amoxycillin and anti-pseudomonal penicillins (MICs <0.06 mg/l). Penicillin V is not very effective

(MIC of 0.25 mg/l) and meningococci are highly resistant to the penicillinase-resistant penicillins, such as methicillin (MIC ⩾6.0 mg/l).

All meningococcal strains isolated in 1994 in England and Wales were susceptible to therapeutic doses of penicillin, with 93% of strains showing an MIC of less than 0.1 mg/l and with the remainder having an MIC of 0.16–0.64 mg/l (Jones and Kaczmarski, 1995). In countries where penicillin-resistant meningococcal strains are not yet isolated, the cephalosporins can be replaced with high-dose parenteral benzylpenicillin as soon as laboratory diagnosis is made. However, irrespective of the country and the prevalence of resistant strains, it is safe practice to test for sensitivity of the organism for penicillin before the antibiotics are switched.

In cases of penicillin allergy or an organism's penicillin insensitivity, the cephalosporins should be continued, unless history suggests anaphylaxis. Chloramphenicol, which is bactericidal to meningococci and achieves high concentration levels in the CSF, is a good alternative to penicillin in the poorer countries. It is given at doses of 100 mg/kg per day (maximum of 4 g per day), or as single long-acting chloramphenicol injections in oil. The latter is as effective as a five-day parenteral penicillin course for treating meningococcal meningitis. Single injection of chloramphenicol in oil is not as effective against pneumococcal meningitis and, therefore, should not be used for blind treatment of pyogenic meningitis.

Antibiotic treatment should be given for a total of seven days (Radetsky, 1990). Five-day courses have also been successful; however, in the presence of acute complications, treatment is usually extended to 10–14 days. It is interesting that, recently, it was clearly demonstrated that following antibiotic administration the increased levels of circulating free endotoxin and endotoxin-activated inflammatory mediator systems decline very rapidly (Brandtzaeg, 1995).

Management of Septic Shock

Management of meningococcal septicaemia is a medical emergency and requires intensive care facilities for the first 48 hours until the patient is clinically and physiologically stable. Clinical and laboratory signs of septic shock must be recognized immediately and those with rapidly progressing disease, rapidly spreading skin rash, increasing tachycardia and tachypnoea, oliguria, low peripheral blood white cell count and signs of DIC require urgent intervention. Hypotension, which may develop late, is not always present on admission, particularly in children and, therefore, could be a misleading parameter for septic shock (Nadel et al., 1995). An increasing gap between core and peripheral temperature is a poor sign, suggesting worsening underperfusion.

Hypovolaemia and electrolyte imbalance should be monitored and corrected with colloid, electrolyte supplement and inotropes as soon as possible. Hypokalaemia, despite acidosis, hypocalcaemia and hypoglycaemia, are seen in the early phase of disease and ought to be corrected with care and may require dialysis, especially if severe oliguria or renal failure was present. It is very important to ensure that high concentration of oxygen is given in all cases. A child's ventilation can deteriorate very rapidly, and pulmonary oedema and/or respiratory distress syndrome may develop soon after admission and therefore all children must be electively ventilated even if no signs of underventilation or respiratory failure were evident (Nadel et al., 1995). Further, children requiring colloid support of 40–80 ml/kg, or those who are obtunded, should also be electively ventilated. The use of fresh frozen plasma in systemic meningococcal disease is controversial (Busund et al., 1993); however, where evidence of severe DIC is present, it is administered and it may also serve to correct complement insufficiencies. Low doses of heparin are also often given.

Management of Raised Intracranial Pressure

Attempts to correct raised intracranial pressure, if present, is made only after systemic shock is brought under control. In severe meningitis, extensive measures may be needed to reduce intracranial pressure. Electrolyte imbalance, hypovolaemia and cardiac output must be corrected. While colloids are administered to correct the hypovolaemia, subsequent crystalloids are restricted. Other measures such as hyperventilation (maintaining pCO_2 between 3.5 and 4.5 kPa) and careful use of mannitol are also important. Patients must be managed in an intensive care unit, nursed in a quiet room with the head slightly raised above the rest of the body.

Other Measures

Monitoring cardiac output using echocardiography is useful. Supportive measures are required to correct any other organ dysfunction and/or other complications. Dexamethasone is thought to reduce the severity of neurological complications in pyogenic meningitis and therefore recommended by many authors. However, data on the use of steroids in meningococcal meningitis are extremely limited and those so far published are inconclusive. In patients who are already hypocortisolaemic, corticosteroids may be of benefit. Similarly, other anti-inflammatory agents have been investigated for their benefit in reducing neurological sequelae, with no breakthroughs so far.

There are a number of potentially therapeutic agents that may be useful in correcting the pathophysiology of the disease which are under investigation and not yet available. These include, among other things, agents that minimize or neutralize the inflammatory response to bacteria and its toxins or reverse the coagulopathies.

PREVENTION AND CONTROL

Control of meningococcal outbreaks consists of a number of interrelated measures which include management of individual cases, notification of known and suspected cases, administration of chemoprophylaxis to close contacts, good clinical surveillance, small- or large-scale vaccination and information dissemination. Concerted efforts are required among the hospital physician, the microbiologist, the public health specialist and the general practitioner to prevent secondary cases and control fear and anxiety among case contacts.

In all cases of suspected meningococcal disease, attempts should be made to obtain positive culture from CSF, blood, throat swab or any other appropriate specimens, while the patient is in the hospital, or retrospectively by sending paired sera or other clinical materials for the detection of antigen, antibody or DNA to a reference laboratory. All meningococcal isolates should be sent to such a reference laboratory for a full identification of individual strains. While in the hospital, patients should be isolated for the first 24 hours following antibiotic administration. The risk of acquiring disease from patients is minimal in the ward, but is greater in the laboratory, particularly for those who handle live cultures (see above).

Notification of all strongly suspected and proven cases of meningococcal diseases to the appropriate public health authorities at the earliest opportunity is essential, so that close contacts of the index case are identified. Detailed information is needed on full clinical and epidemiological aspects of these cases. In many countries the disease is notifiable by law, and as soon as an outbreak is recognized an active surveillance must follow. Outbreaks are identified when two or more meningococcal cases are associated in time, place and identity of the meningococcal isolates. Outbreaks can occur within individual families, communities or institutions.

Contacts of the index case are approximately one thousand times more at risk of developing disease than the rest of the community and are therefore given prophylactic antibiotics to eradicate possible carriage. Close contacts include household and kissing contacts who had been exposed to the index case over the previous 10 days (incubation period is 2–10 days), and also include infants and young children in play groups and nurseries. Nasopharyngeal culture of close contacts is unnecessary, delays antibiotic administration and may have undesirable social implications. It is important to inform adequately close contacts about the disease and the need for compliance with prophylaxis. They must receive clear instructions to seek medical advice immediately, should they develop any signs or symptoms of meningococcal disease. It is interesting that nearly one-third of immediate family contacts of patients carry an organism which in 90% of cases has the same identity as that of the index strain.

Chemoprophylaxis

In the 1940s and until the 1960s sulphonamides were the mainstay of treatment and eradication of carriage. However, sulphonamide-resistant strains are now prevalent worldwide. About one-third of all isolates in England and Wales in 1994 were resistant to sulphonamides, with MICs $\geqslant 10$ mg/l (Jones and Kaczmarski, 1995), whereas only three case isolates (out of 1129 isolates) in these two countries in the same year were resistant to rifampicin (MIC $\geqslant 5$ mg/l) and none were resistant to ciprofloxacin (MIC <0.02 mg/l). A two-day course of 12-hourly oral rifampicin (600 mg in adults, 10 mg/kg in children and 5 mg/kg in infants) is highly effective in up to 95% of cases. However, failure due to lack of compliance, drug resistance or recurrence is known. Rifampicin should not be used during pregnancy and in patients suffering from liver diseases. Also the drug is expensive, causes discoloration of body fluids and soft contact lenses and it interferes with the function of the oral contraceptive pill. Alternatives are single doses of ciprofloxacin (500 mg orally, not in young children) and ceftriaxone (250–500 mg intramuscularly, 125 mg in children under the age of 12 years) and they are highly effective. The latter, which has been shown to be more effective than rifampicin (Schwartz *et al.*, 1988), offers the greater advantage of being licensed for use in pregnancy and young children. Minocycline (100 mg orally twice daily for three days) is also effective; however, it should not be given to children and pregnant women because of its vestibular toxicity and its ability to discolour the growing teeth.

Prophylactic antibiotics are given to the identified close contacts all at the same time as soon as the index case is diagnosed. The throat of the index case is also cleared of organisms by giving these antibiotics before discharge from hospital. Random administration of antibiotics to school contacts, which should be coordinated by the department of public health medicine, is only advised in infants' nurseries and play groups but not for older children, unless they are close contacts. Except in exceptional circumstances, infants under the age of three months are not usually given prophylaxis. Finally, close contacts of cases caused by serogroups A or C may be offered the currently available capsular polysaccharide vaccines. Vaccines against serogroup B are not yet available (see below).

Vaccines

An ideal meningococcal vaccine should be safe, offer long-lasting immunity to all age groups, cross-protect against all meningococcal serogroups and serotypes, be given orally or nasally and be easily incorporated into the World Health Organization's Expanded Program on Immunization. So far no such vaccine has been developed. Nevertheless, there are vaccines available against four out of 13 serogroups of meningococci. These are based on the capsular polysaccharide of groups A, C, Y and W135. However, these vaccines are believed to offer only a relatively short-lived immunity against their homologous serogroups and they do not affect carriage rates or interrupt transmission of infection within a community (Hassan-King *et al.*, 1988; Masterton *et al.*, 1988; Moore *et al.*, 1988). Furthermore, they offer little protection to children under the age of two years, the most vulnerable age group, and hence they are not suitable for including in paediatric immunization programmes. No polysaccharide vaccine yet exists against serogroup B meningococcal disease and this is seen as a major obstacle to the wider use of meningococcal vaccines in Europe and American continents.

Group A and C Capsular Polysaccharide

The first successful vaccines produced were against group A and C *N. meningitidis* using high-molecular-weight (>100 kDa) capsular polysaccharide of these strains (Gotschlich *et al.*, 1969). A series of large-scale field trials were conducted in the 1970s among different age groups in different parts of the world, including Europe,

Africa and Latin America, which showed that the capsular polysaccharide vaccine is effective in controlling epidemics of group A disease in almost all age groups. It soon became clear that antibody responses among infants to the group A and C capsular polysaccharide vaccines depended on a number of factors, including the age of the infant, the molecular weight of the antigen, the number of doses of antigen, and the prior experience of the infant, with naturally occurring antigens cross-reactive with the meningococcal capsular polysaccharide. It became evident that children under the age of two years do respond, particularly to serogroup A capsular polysaccharide, with small increases in specific antibodies. The strength of the response and its duration increased with age and in adults 100% seroconversion was achieved which lasted longer than in children. For example, Reingold *et al.* (1985) showed that the group A capsular polysaccharide vaccine efficacy in children vaccinated at less than four years of age almost disappeared over the following three years, whereas those who were four years of age or older when vaccinated showed evidence of vaccine-induced clinical protection for three years after vaccination.

The group C capsular polysaccharide vaccine, when administered routinely among recruits of the US Army to prevent severe outbreaks, has virtually eradicated the group C meningococcal disease in this population. Subsequent trials and antibody response studies among children confirmed this success among age groups above two years but not among children under two years of age (Tauney *et al.*, 1974; Peltola *et al.*, Ceesay *et al.*, 1993). It is interesting that more recent data show that although anticapsular antibodies and bactericidal activity in adults decline substantially by two years following vaccination, both persist at a level significantly above prevaccination levels for up to 10 years (Zangwill *et al.*, 1994).

On the basis of these results, serogroup C capsular polysaccharide vaccines are now recommended for general use in epidemics except for children under the age of 18 months. In contrast, serogroup A capsular polysaccharide vaccines are recommended to be given during epidemics in all age groups, including infants, with a booster dose given to those under the age of 18 months. These vaccines are now given to those who are at increased risk of meningococcal disease, including those with late complement component deficiencies and those with functional or anatomical asplenia. These vaccines are also offered to military recruits in the UK and USA and to all Hajis before they arrive in Mecca. However, it is important that, due to significant shortcomings, these capsular polysaccharide vaccines are not useful for routine immunization of infants. Production of improved capsular polysaccharide vaccines, particularly against group A and C meningococcal infections, is still a research priority. A vaccine capable of inducing protective immunity among infants is needed so that it can be added to the routine childhood immunization as part of the Expanded Program on Immunization.

Vaccines in Development

Conjugated group A and C polysaccharide vaccines

The success of linking Hib capsular polysaccharide to a protein carrier, resulting in a vaccine which induces a thymus-dependent (T-cell dependent) IgG response in young children, and thus immunological memory, has encouraged the development of capsular polysaccharide–protein conjugate vaccines for serogroup A and C meningococci. Considerable work has therefore been done to couple A and C capsular polysaccharides to proteins so as to change the character of the antigen from thymus independent to thymus dependent (Cruse and Lewis, 1989). A series of Phase I and II immunogenicity clinical trials have recently been conducted on conjugated serogroup A and C capsular polysaccharide vaccines in countries like The Gambia and the UK. It will be some time before such vaccines are fully evaluated.

Group B capsular polysaccharide

Group B meningococcal capsular polysaccharide consists of repeated residues of α-(2−8)-linked oligomers of sialic acid, which serves as an important virulence factor and protective cell component for the organism. Candidate vaccines based on the native group B polysaccharide induce a transient antibody response of predominantly IgM isotype. This poor immunogenicity of the group B capsular polysaccharide could be due to sensitivity to neuraminidases or immunotolerance of the host due to its similarity to sialic acid moieties in human brain tissues (Finne *et al.*, 1983), which has caused considerable concern regarding the possible induction in humans of adverse autoimmune consequences by administration of serogroup B capsular polysaccharide-based vaccines. Nevertheless, attempts are ongoing to produce a capsular polysaccharide-based group B vaccine.

Outer membrane proteins

In view of the problems associated with the currently available capsular polysaccharide vaccines and the poor immunogenicity of group B capsular polysaccharide, much of the attention has focused on non-capsular antigens, including constitutively expressed and iron-regulated OMPs. It is important to know that recurrence of meningococcal disease is extremely rare in the absence of immunodeficiencies, irrespective of the serogroups of the infective organisms. This indicates that non-capsular antigens can generate long-lasting cross-protective immunity.

Constitutively expressed outer membrane proteins Among the constitutively expressed OMPs, the class proteins (especially class 1, 2 and 3 proteins) have attracted most of the attention. These proteins show considerable interstrain antigenic variation, hence are used as a basis for the serotyping and subtyping scheme for characterizing strains of *N. meningitidis*. However, they are still considered attractive candidate vaccine antigens because within a particular epidemiological setting the majority of strains causing disease belong to only a limited number of types and subtypes. Antibodies against the class 1 OMP as well as the mutually exclusive class 2 and 3 OMPs have been

detected in both immunized and infected individuals; however, the presence of antibodies does not necessarily correlate with protection (Mandrell and Zollinger, 1989; Wedege *et al.*, 1991; Orren *et al.*, 1992). An obvious drawback of vaccines based entirely on serotype and serosubtype antigens is the fact that the predominant types and subtypes associated with disease in any one area change from time to time.

In the past decade, a number of serogroup B meningococcal vaccines based on serotype/subtype antigen-enriched OMPs were developed and tested in clinical trials (Bjune *et al.*, 1991; Sierra *et al.*, 1991; Zollinger *et al.*, 1991). Following large-scale placebo-controlled, randomized double-blind trials, only the vaccines produced in Norway and Cuba showed significant protective efficacy. The Norwegian vaccine consisted of OMPs from the Norwegian epidemic strain of *N. meningitidis*, B:15:P1.7,16 and was given to children aged 14–16 years. It produced a point estimate of protective efficacy of 57% after a 30-month follow-up and, therefore, was considered insufficiently effective for general use (Bjune *et al.*, 1991). The Cuban vaccine consisted of group C capsular polysaccharide mixed with OMPs from a Cuban epidemic strain, B:4:P1.15. When given to children aged 10–16 years, it offered an estimated point efficacy of 83% after 16 months of follow-up (Sierra *et al.*, 1991) and, as a result, the vaccine is now incorporated into the routine childhood vaccination programme in Cuba. Although the Cuban trial did not directly address efficacy in children aged less than 10 years, follow-up studies of the mass vaccination have suggested that the overall protective efficacy based on vaccine coverage and incidence of disease in children under six years old is about 93% (Sierra *et al.*, 1991). However, when the Cuban vaccine was tested in a case–control study in Brazil, protective efficacy was reported to vary with age. The vaccine was effective in children aged four years and older, but not in younger children (De Moraes *et al.*, 1992).

Comparative clinical trials between the Norwegian and Cuban vaccine preparations have recently been conducted in Iceland and Chile in order to resolve the discrepancies. This subject has recently been reviewed more extensively (Ala'Aldeen and Griffiths, 1995).

Transferrin receptors and other iron-regulated outer membrane proteins

This field has expanded very rapidly over the past few years and iron-regulated proteins have attracted considerable attention as possible vaccine candidates. Among the iron-regulated proteins, the transferrin-binding proteins (Tbps), Tbp1 and Tbp2 have attracted most of the attention as vaccine candidates. It is now clear that the transferrin receptor is formed, partly or wholly, by Tbp1 and Tbp2 (Ala'Aldeen, 1996). Tbp1 is a ~98 kDa transmembrane protein and loses its biological and much of its immunological properties when exposed to denaturing conditions. Tbp2 (~65–90 kDa) is a lipoprotein anchored to the outermost layer of the cell membrane (Legrain et al., 1993) and shows considerable molecular and antigenic heterogeneity amongst different strains of N. meningitidis. Tbp2 retains its transferrin-binding activity and strong immunogenic properties following denaturation. It is interesting that humans recovering from natural infection responded with cross-reactive anti-Tbp2 antibodies (Ala'Aldeen et al., 1994). Tbp1 and Tbp2 have compatible characteristics with a safe and broadly cross-reactive vaccine candidate. It is clear that both Tbps are surface exposed and immunogenic in humans and animals. The Tbps seem to possess a combination of important epitopes which can generate protective antibodies capable of killing the organism by complement-mediated bactericidal activity and/or nutritional starvation. Antibodies to their native structure are bactericidal to homologous and many heterologous strains. These include strains from various serogroups, serotypes and serosubtypes with no obvious correlation between the bactericidal activity and the identity of the strains or the molecular mass of the heterogeneous Tbp2 molecule (Ala'Aldeen, 1996). It is possible that a mixture of more than one Tbp2 isotype (depending on the prevalent meningococcal strains in any one country) with stabilized native Tbp1 molecules will be required in order to enhance and broaden the protective efficacy of any Tbp-based vaccines (Ala'Aldeen, 1996).

REFERENCES

Achtman, M. (1994) Clonal spread of serogroup A meningococci: a paradigm for the analysis of micro-evaluation in bacteria. Molecular Microbiology, 11, 15–22.

Adlam, C., Knights, J.M., Mugridge, A. et al. (1987) Production of colominic acid by Pasteurella haemolytica serotype A2 organisms. FEMS Microbiological Letters, 42, 23–25.

Aho, E.L., Dempsey, J.A., Hobbs, M.M. et al. (1991) Characterization of the opa (class 5) gene family of Neisseria meningitidis. Molecular Microbiology, 5, 1429–1437.

Ala'Aldeen, D.A.A. (1996) Transferrin receptors of Neisseria meningitidis: promising candidates for a broadly cross-protective vaccine. Journal of Medical Microbiology, 44, 235–241.

Ala'Aldeen, D.A.A. and Griffiths, E. (1995) Vaccine development against meningococcal disease. In Molecular and Clinical Aspects of Bacterial Vaccine Development (eds D.A.A. Ala'Aldeen and C.E. Hormaeche), pp. 1–39. Wiley, Chichester.

Ala'Aldeen, D.A.A., Davies, H.A., Wall, R.A. et al. (1990) The 70 kilodalton iron regulated protein of Neisseria meningitidis is not the human transferrin receptor. FEMS Microbiological Letters, 69, 37–42.

Ala'Aldeen, D.A.A., Davies, H.A. and Borriello, S.P. (1994a) Vaccine potential of meningococcal FrpB: studies on surface exposure and functional attributes of common epitopes. Vaccine, 12, 535–541.

Ala'Aldeen, D.A.A., Stevenson, P., Griffiths, E. et al. (1994b) Immune responses in man and animals to meningococcal transferrin-binding proteins: implications for vaccine design. Infection and Immunity, 62, 2894–2900.

Algren, J.T., Lal, S., Cutliff, S.A. and Richman, B.J. (1993) Predictors of outcome in acute meningococcal infection in children. Critical Care Medicine, 21, 447–452.

Andreoni, J., Kayhty, H. and Densen, P. (1993) Vaccination and role of capsular polysaccharide antibody in prevention recurrent meningococcal disease in late complement component-deficient individuals. Journal of Infectious Diseases, 168, 227–231.

Barlow, A.K., Heckels, J.E. and Clarke, I.N. (1989) The class 1 outer membrane protein of Neisseria meningitidis: gene sequence and structural and immunological similarities to gonococcal porins. Molecular Microbiology, 3, 131–139.

Barquet, N., Gasser, I., Domingo, P. et al. (1990) Primary meningococcal conjunctivitis: report of 21 patients and review. Reviews of Infectious Diseases, 12, 838–847.

Benoit, F.L. (1963) Chronic meningococcaemia: case report and review of the literature. American Journal of Medicine, 35, 103–112.

Bjune, G., Hoiby, E.A., Gronnesby, J.K. et al. (1991) Effect of outer membrane vesicle vaccine against group B meningococcal disease in Norway. Lancet, 338, 1093–1096.

Blake, M.S. and Gotschlich, E.C. (1987) Functional and immunologic properties of pathogenic neisserial surface proteins. In Bacterial Outer Membranes as Model Systems (ed. M. Inouye), pp. 377–400. Wiley, Chichester.

Brandtzaeg, P. (1995) Pathogenesis of meningococcal infections. In Meningococcal Disease (ed. K. Cartwright), pp. 71–114. Wiley, Chichester.

Brandtzaeg, P., Halstensen, A., Kierulf, P. et al. (1992a) Molecular mechanisms in the compartmentalized inflammatory response presenting as meningococcal meningitis or septic shock. Microbial Pathogenesis, 13, 423–431.

Brandtzaeg, P., Ovstebo, R. and Kierulf, P. (1992b) Compartmentalization of lipopolysaccharide-production correlates with the clinical presentation in meningococcal disease. Journal of Infectious Diseases, 166, 650–652.

Busund, R., Straume, B. and Revhaug, A. (1993) Fatal course in severe meningococcemia: clinical predictors and effect of transfusion therapy. Critical Care Medicine, 21, 1699–1705.

Carpenter, R.R. (1962) The clinical spectrum of bacterial meningitis. American Journal of Medicine, 33, 262–275.

Cartwright, K. (1995) Meningococcal carriage and disease. In Meningococcal Disease (ed. K. Cartwright), pp. 114–146. Wiley, Chichester.

Cartwright, K., Reilly, S., White, D. and Stuart, J. (1992) Early treatment with parenteral penicillin in meningococcal disease. British Medical Journal, 305, 143–147.

Caugant, D.A., Frohom, L.O., Bovre, K. et al. (1987) Intercontinental spread of Neisseria meningitidis of the ET-5 complex. Antonie Van Leeuwenhoek, 53, 389–394.

Ceesay, S.J., Allen, S.J., Menon, A. et al. (1993) Decline in meningococcal antibody levels in African children 5 years after vaccination and the lack of an effect of booster immunisation. Journal of Infectious Diseases, 167, 1212–1216.

Chen, C.Y., Berish, S.A., Morse, S.A. et al. (1993) The ferric iron-binding protein of pathogenic Neisseria spp. functions as a periplasmic transport protein in iron acquisition from human transferrin. Molecular Microbiology, 10, 311–318.

Cruse, J.M. and Lewis, R.E. (1989) Conjugate vaccines. Contributions to Microbiology and Immunology, 10, 1–196.

De Moraes, J.C., Perkins, B.A., Camargo, M.C. et al. (1992) Protective efficacy of a serogroup B meningococcal vaccine in Sao Paulo, Brazil. Lancet, 340, 1074–1078.

deMorais, J.S., Munford, R.S., Risi, J.B. et al. (1974) Epidemic disease due to serogroup C Neisseria meningitidis in Sao Paulo, Brazil. Journal of Infectious Diseases, 129, 568–571.

Densen, P., Weiler, J.M., Griffiss, J.M. et al. (1987) Familial properdin deficiency and fatal meningococcemia. New England Journal of Medicine, 316, 922–926.

Feavers, I.M., Suker, J., McKenna, A.J. et al. (1992) Molecular analysis of the serotyping antigens of Neisseria meningitidis. Injection and Immunity, 60, 3620–3629.

Finne, J., Leinonen, M. and Makela, P.H. (1983) Antigenic similarities between brain components and bacteria causing meningitis. Lancet, ii, 355–357.

Flexner, S. (1913) The results of the serum treatment in thirteen hundred cases of epidemic meningitis. Journal of Experimental Medicine, 17, 553–576.

Fox, A.J., Jones, D.M., Gray, J.J. et al. (1991) An epidemiologically valuable typing method for Neisseria meningitidis by analysis of restriction fragment length polymorphisms. Journal of Medical Microbiology, 34, 265–270.

Frank, M.M., Joiner, K. and Hammer, C. (1987) The function of antibodies and complement in the lysis of bacteria. Reviews of Infectious Diseases, 9, S537–545.

Frasch, C.E. (1983) Immunisation against Neisseria meningitidis. In Medical Microbiology (eds C. Easmon and J. Jeljaszewics), pp. 115–144. Academic Press, London.

Frosch, M., Weisberger, C. and Meyer, T.F. (1989) Molecular characterisation and expression in Escherichia coli of the gene complex encoding the polysaccharide capsule of Neisseria meningitidis. Proceedings of the National Academy of Sciences of the USA, 86, 1669–1673.

Glover, J.A. (1918) The cerebrospinal fever epidemic of 1917 at 'X' depot. Journal of the Royal Army Medical Corps, 30, 23–36.

Goldschneider, I., Gotschlich, E.C. and Artenstein, M.S. (1969a) Human immunity to the meningococcus. II. Development of natural immunity. Journal of Experimental Medicine, 129, 1327–1348.

Goldschneider, I., Gotschlich, E.C. and Artenstein, M.S. (1969b) Human immunity to the meningococcus. I. The role of human antibody. Journal of Experimental Medicine, 129, 1307–1326.

Gotschlich, E., Liu, T.Y. and Artenstein, M.S. (1969) Human immunity to the meningococcus. III. Preparation and immunochemical properties of the group A, group B and group C meningococcal polysaccharides. *Journal of Experimental Medicine*, **129**, 1349–1365.

Greenwood, B.M. (1987) The epidemiology of acute bacterial meningitis in tropical Africa. In *Bacterial Meningitis* (eds J.D. Williams and J. Burnie), pp. 61–91. Academic Press, London.

Griffiss, J.M. (1995) Mechanisms of host immunity. In *Meningococcal Disease* (ed. K. Cartwright), pp. 35–70. Wiley, Chichester.

Griffiss, J.M. and Bertram, M.A. (1977) Immunoepidemiology of meningococcal disease in military recruits. II. Blocking of serum bactericidal activity by circulating IgA early in the course of invasive disease. *Journal of Infectious Diseases*, **136**, 733–739.

Griffiss, J.M. and Goroff, D.K. (1983) IgA blocks IgM and IgG initiated immune lysis by separate molecular mechanisms. *Journal of Immunology*, **130**, 2882–2885.

Griffiss, J.M., Schneider, H., Mandrell, R.E. *et al.* (1988) Lipooligosaccharides: the principal glycolipids of the *Neisseria* outer membrane. *Reviews of Infectious Diseases*, **10**, S287–295.

Halstensen, A., Sjursen, H., Vollest, S.E. *et al.* (1989) Serum opsonins to serogroup B meningococci in meningococcal disease. *Scandinavian Journal of Infectious Diseases*, **21**, 267–276.

Hassan-King, M.K.A., Wall, R.A. and Greenwood, B.M. (1988) Meningococcal carriage, meningococcal disease and vaccination. *Journal of Infection*, **16**, 55–59.

Hitchcock, P.J. (1989) Unified nomenclature for pathogenic *Neisseria* species. *Clinical Microbiology Reviews*, **2**, S64–S65.

Hobbs, M.M., Seiler, A., Achtman, M. *et al.* (1994) Microevaluation within a clonal population of pathogenic bacteria: recombination, gene duplication and horizontal gene exchange in the Opa gene family of *Neisseria meningitidis*. *Molecular Microbiology*, **12**, 171–180.

Jackson, L.A. and Wenger, J.D. (1993) Laboratory-bases surveillance for meningococcal diseases in selected areas, United States. *Morbidity and Mortality Weekly Report*, **42**, 21–30.

Jackson, L.A., Tenover, F.C., Baker, C. *et al.* (1994) Prevalence of *Neisseria meningitidis* relatively resistant to penicillin in the United States, 1991. *Journal of Infectious Diseases*, **169**, 438–441.

Jarvis, G.A. and Verdos, N.A. (1987) Sialic acid of group B *Neisseria meningitidis* regulates alternative complement pathway activation. *Infection and Immunity*, **55**, 174–180.

Jones, D. (1995) Epidemiology of meningococcal disease in Europe and the USA. In *Meningococcal Disease* (ed. K. Cartwright), pp. 146–157. Wiley, Chichester.

Jones, D.M. and Kaczmarski, E.B. (1993) Meningococcal infections in England and Wales: 1992. *Communicable Diseases Report*, **3**, R129–131.

Jones, D.M. and Kaczmarski, E.B. (1994) Meningococcal infections in England and Wales: 1993. *Communicable Diseases Report*, **4**, R97–R101.

Jones, D.M. and Kaczmarski, E.B. (1995) Meningococcal infections in England and Wales: 1994. *Communicable Diseases Report*, **5**, R125–R130.

Jones, D.M., Borrow, R., Fox, A.J. *et al.* (1992) The lipooligosaccharide immunotype as a virulence determinant of sulphonamide resistant B15:P1.7,16 meningococci. In *8th International Pathogenic Neisseria Conference* (*Abstract Book*) (eds C.J. Conde-Glex *et al.*), p. 186. Instituto Nacional De Salud Publica, Cuernavaca.

Klugman, K.P., Gotschlich, E.C. and Blake, M.S. (1989) Sequence of the structural gene (*rmp*M) for the class 4 outer membrane protein of *Neisseria meningitidis*, homology of the protein to gonococcal protein III and *Escherichia coli* Omp A and construction of meningococcal strains that lack class 4 protein. *Infection and Immunity*, **57**, 2066–2071.

Lapeyssonie, L. (1963) La meningite cerebro-spinale en Afrique. *Bulletin of the World Health Organization*, **28** (Suppl.), 3–114.

Legrain, M., Mazarin, V., Irwin, S.W. *et al.* (1993) Cloning and characterization of *Neisseria meningitidis* genes encoding the transferrin-binding proteins Tbp 1 and Tbp 2. *Gene*, **130**, 73–80.

Lewis, L.A. and Dyer, D.W. (1995) Identification of an iron-regulated outer membrane protein of *Neisseria meningitidis* involved in the utilization of hemoglobin complexed to haptoglobin. *Journal of Bacteriology*, **177**, 1299–1306.

Lystad, A. and Aasen, S. (1991) The epidemiology of meningococcal disease in Norway 1975–1991. *NIPH Annals*, **14**, 57–66.

Mackinnon, F.G., Borrow, R., Gorringe, A.R. *et al.* (1993) Demonstration of lipooligosaccharide immunotype and capsule as virulence factors for *Neisseria meningitidis* using an infant mouse intranasal infection model. *Microbial Pathogenesis*, **15**, 359–366.

Maiden, M.C.J., Bygraves, J.A., McCarvil, J. *et al.* (1992) Identification of meningococcal serosubtypes by polymerase chain reaction. *Journal of Clinical Microbiology*, **30**, 2835–2841.

Mandrell, R.E. and Zollinger, W.D. (1989) Human immune response to meningococcal outer membrane protein epitopes after natural infection or vaccination. *Infection and Immunity*, **57**, 1590–1598.

Mandrell, R., Schneider, H., Apicella, M. *et al.* (1986) Antigenic and physical diversity of *Neisseria gonorrhoeae* lipooligosaccharides. *Infection and Immunity*, **54**, 63–69.

Masterton, R.G., Youngs, E.R., Wardle, J.C.R. *et al.* (1988) Control of an outbreak of group C meningococcal meningitis with a polysaccharide vaccine. *Journal of Infection*, **17**, 177–182.

Mellor, D.A. (1992) The place of computed tomography and lumber puncture in suspected bacterial meningitis. *Archives of Disease in Childhood*, **67**, 1417–1419.

Moore, P.S. (1992) Meningococcal meningitis in sub-Saharan Africa: a model for the epidemic process. *Clinical Infectious Diseases*, **14**, 515–525.

Moore, P.S., Lee, L.H., Telzak, E.E. *et al.* (1988) Group A meningococcal carriage in travellers returning from Saudi Arabia. *Journal of the American Medical Association*, **260**, 2686–2689.

Moore, P.S., Hierhoizer, J., Dewitt, W. *et al.* (1990) Respiratory viruses and mycoplasma as co-factors for epidemic group A meningococcal meningitis. *Journal of the American Medical Association*, **264**, 1271–1275.

Morelli, G., Valle, J.D., Lammel, C.J. *et al.* (1994) Immunogenicity and evolutionary variability of epitopes within IgA1 protease from serogroup A. *Neisseria meningitidis*. *Molecular Microbiology*, **11**, 175–187.

Nadel, S., Levin, M. and Habibi, P. (1995) Treatment of meningococcal disease in childhood. In *Meningococcal Disease* (ed. K. Cartwright), pp. 207–243. Wiley, Chichester.

Ni, H., Knight, A.I., Cartwright, K. *et al.* (1992) Polymerase chain reaction for diagnosis of meningococcal meningitis. *Lancet*, **340**, 1432–1434.

Olyhoek, A.J.M., Sarkari, J., Bopp, M. *et al.* (1991) Cloning and expression in *Escherichia coli* of *opc*, the gene for an unusual class 5 outer membrane protein from *Neisseria meningitidis*. *Microbial Pathogenesis*, **11**, 249–257.

Orren, A., Warren, R.E., Potter, P.C. *et al.* (1992) Antibodies to meningococcal class 1 outer membrane proteins in South African complement-deficient and complement-sufficient subjects. *Infection and Immunity*, **60**, 4510–4516.

Osterud, B. and Flaegstad, T. (1983) Increased tissue thromboplastin activity in monocytes of patients with meningococcal infection: related to unfavourable prognosis. *Thrombosis and Haemostasis*, **49**, 5–7.

Peltola, H., Safary, A., Kayhty, H. *et al.* (1985) Evaluation of two tetravalent (ACYW135) meningococcal vaccines in infants and small children: a clinical study comparing immunogenicity of O-acetyl negative and O-acetyl positive group C polysaccharides. *Paediatrics*, **76**, 91–96.

Radetsky, M. (1990) Duration of treatment in bacterial meningitis: a historical inquiry. *Pediatric Infectious Disease Journal*, **9**, 2–9.

Reingold, A.C., Broom, C.V., Hightower, A.W. *et al.* (1985) Age-specific differences in duration of clinical protection after vaccination with meningococcal polysaccharide A vaccine. *Lancet*, **ii**, 114–117.

Reller, B.L., MacGregor, R.R. and Beaty, H.N. (1973) Bactericidal antibody after colonization with *Neisseria meningitidis*. *Journal of Infectious Diseases*, **127**, 56–62.

Rey, M. (1991) Improving the early control of outbreaks of meningococcal disease. In *Neisseria 1990* (eds M. Achtman, P. Kohl, C. Marchal *et al.*), pp. 117–122. Walter de Gruyter, Berlin.

Riedo, F.X., Plikaytis, B.D. and Broome, C.V. (1995) Epidemiology and prevention of meningococcal disease. *Pediatric Infectious Disease Journal*, **14**, 643–657.

Riley, G., Brown, S. and Krishnan, C. (1991) Penicillin resistance in *Neisseria meningitidis*. *New England Journal of Medicine*, **324**, 997.

Saez-Nieto, J.A., Lujan, R., Berron, S. *et al.* (1992) Epidemiology and molecular basis of penicillin-resistant *Neisseria meningitidis*: a 5-year history (1985–1989). *Clinical Infectious Diseases*, **14**, 394–402.

Schaad, U.B. (1980) Arthritis in disease due to *Neisseria meningitidis*. *Reviews of Infectious Diseases*, **2**, 880–887.

Schryvers, A.B. and Gonzalez, G.C. (1989) Comparison of the abilities of different protein sources of iron to enhance *Neisseria meningitidis* infection in mice. *Infection and Immunity*, **57**, 2425–2429.

Schryvers, A.B. and Morris, L.J. (1988) Identification and characterization of the human lactoferrin-binding protein from *Neisseria meningitidis*. *Infection and Immunity*, **56**, 1144–1149.

Schwartz, B., Al-Tobaiqi, A., Al-Ruwais, A. *et al.* (1988) Comparative efficacy of ceftriaxone and rifampicin in eradicating pharyngeal carriage of Group A *Neisseria meningitidis*. *Lancet*, **i**, 1239–1242.

Sierra, G.V.G., Campa, H.C., Varcacel, N.M. *et al.* (1991) Vaccine against group B *Neisseria meningitidis*: protection trial and mass vaccination results in Cuba. *NIPH Annals*, **14**, 195–210.

Stephens, D.S. and Farley, M.M. (1991) Pathogenic events during infection of human nasopharynx with *Neisseria meningitidis* and *Haemophilus influenzae*. *Reviews of Infectious Diseases*, **13**, 22–33.

Stephens, D.S., Whitney, A.M., Rothbard, J. *et al.* (1985) Pili of *Neisseria meningitidis*: analysis of structure and investigation of structural and antigenic relationships to gonococcal pili. *Journal of Experimental Medicine*, **161**, 1539–1553.

Strang, J.R. and Pugh, E.J. (1992) Meningococcal infections: reducing the case fatality rate by giving penicillin before admission to hospital. *British Medical Journal*, **305**, 141–143.

Sutcliffe, E.M., Jones, D.M., El-Sheikh, S. *et al.* (1988) Penicillin-insensitive meningococci in the UK. *Lancet*, **i**, 657–658.

Tauney, A.E., Galvai, P.A., deMorais, J.S. *et al.* (1974) Disease prevention by meningococcal serogroup C polysaccharide vaccine in preschool children. *Pediatric Research*, **8**, 429.

Thomson, S.A. and Sparling, P.F. (1993) Cytotoxin-related FrpA protein of *Neisseria meningitidis* is excreted extracellularly by meningococci and by Hly BD⁺ *Escherichia coli*. *Infection and Immunity*, **61**, 2908–2911.

Thomson, S.A., Wang, L.I., West, A. *et al.* (1993) *Neisseria meningitidis* produces iron-regulated proteins related to the RTX family of exoproteins. *Journal of Bacteriology*, **175**, 811–818.

Tsai, C., Frasch, C. and Mocca, L. (1981) Five structural classes of major outer membrane proteins in *Neisseria meningitidis*. *Journal of Bacteriology*, **146**, 69–78.

Van der Ley, P., Heckels, J.E., Virji, M. *et al.* (1991) Topology of outer membrane proteins in pathogenic *Neisseria* species. *Infection and Immunity*, **59**, 2963–2971.

van Deuren, M., van Dijke, B.J., Koopman, R.J.J. *et al.* (1993) Rapid diagnosis of acute meningococcal infections by needle aspiration or biopsy of skin lesions. *British Medical Journal*, **306**, 1229–1230.

van Deventer, S.J.H., Buller, H.R., ten Cate, J.W. *et al.* (1990) Experimental endotoxemia in humans: analysis of cytokine release and coagulation, fibrinolytic, and complement pathways. *Blood*, **76**, 2520–2526.

Verheul, A.F.M., Snippe, H. and Poolman, J.T. (1993)

Meningococcal lipooligosaccharides: virulence factor and potential vaccine components. *Microbiological Reviews*, **57**, 34–49.

Vieusseaux, M. (1806) Mémoire sure le maladie qui a regne a Geneve ou printemps de 1805. *Journal Médicine Chirugie et Pharmacologie*, **II**, 163–165.

Virji, M., Makepeace, K., Achtman, M. *et al.* (1993) Meningococcal Opa and Opc proteins: their role in colonisation and invasion of human epithelial and endothelial cells. *Molecular Microbiology*, **10**, 499–510.

Wedege, E., Bjune, G., Frøholm, L.O. *et al.* (1991) Immunoblotting studies of vaccinee and patient sera from a Norwegian serogroup B meningococcal vaccination trial. *NIPH Annals*, **14**, 183–186.

Weichselbaum, A. (1887) Ueber die aetiologie der akuten Meningitis Cerebrospinalis. *Fortschritte der Medizin*, **5**, 573–575.

Woods, C.R., Smith, A.L., Wasilauskas, B.L. *et al.* (1994) Invasive disease caused by *Neisseria meningitidis* relatively resistant to penicillin in North Carolina. *Journal of Infectious Diseases*, **170**, 453–456.

Woods, J.P. and Cannon, J.G. (1990) Variation in expression of class 1 and class 5 outer membrane proteins during nasopharyngeal carriage of *Neisseria meningitidis*. *Infection and Immunity*, **58**, 569–572.

Zang, Q.Y., Jones, D.M., Saez-Nieto, J.A. *et al.* (1990) Genetic diversity of penicillin-binding 2 genes of penicillin-resistant strains of *Neisseria meningitidis* revealed by fingerprinting of amplified DNA. *Antimicrobial Agents and Chemotherapy*, **34**, 1523–1528.

Zangwill, K.M., Stout, R.W., Carlone, G.M. *et al.* (1994) Duration of antibody response after meningococcal polysaccharide vaccination in US Air Force personnel. *Journal of Infectious Diseases*, **169**, 847–852.

Zollinger, W.D., Boslego, J., Moran, E. *et al.* (1991) Meningococcal serogroup B vaccine protection trial and follow-up studies in Chile. *NIPH Annals*, **14**, 211–212.

8

HAEMOPHILUS

Tony J. Howard

INTRODUCTION

This genus represents a group of Gram-negative bacilli that are typically unable to grow on culture media without the presence of whole blood or one of its constituents. They are obligatory parasites that usually inhabit the upper respiratory tract. The major pathogen is *Haemophilus influenzae*. This is associated with a wide spectrum of disease which includes invasive infections such as meningitis, bacteraemia, pneumonia, epiglottitis and septic arthritis, which are mainly seen in childhood and localized respiratory infections which occur at all ages. Other human pathogens include *H. influenzae* biogroup *aegyptius* which is responsible for acute epidemic conjunctivitis and Brazilian purpuric fever, *H. ducreyi* which causes the venereal disease, chancroid, and a number of other species of low pathogenicity, e.g. *H. parainfluenzae*, *H. haemolyticus*, *H. parahaemolyticus*, *H. aphrophilus* and *H. segnis* which are occasionally associated with abscesses or infective endocarditis.

HISTORICAL

The first recorded observation of haemophili was probably made by Robert Koch in 1883 when he described the occurrence of a profusion of minute rods in pus from patients with conjunctivitis whilst he was engaged on cholera research in Egypt. Haemophili were first cultured by Richard Pfeiffer in 1891. Pfeiffer had been working at the Koch Institute in Berlin from 1887. At the beginning of the 1889–1892 influenza pandemic he began a series of small-scale studies in relation to this disease and in 1890 published a photomicrograph of minute bacilli seen in the sputum of affected cases without ascribing much significance to the findings. He later extended his work on influenza and in January 1892 published a report identifying a small bacillus as the cause of this disease. At this stage primary culture of this organism had been achieved by spreading sputum onto 1.5% sugar agar; however, subculture could not be established until a few months later when Pfeiffer found that this could be achieved by adding a drop of human blood to the agar surface. There was initially strong support for Pfeiffer's contention that the influenza bacillus was the cause of influenza; however, observations at variance with this theory were recorded by other workers who described outbreaks of influenza without being able to cultivate Pfeiffer's bacillus and cases where the organism could be isolated in the absence of clinical influenza. By the 1918–1919 pandemic the view that the influenza bacillus was the causative

Principles and Practice of Clinical Bacteriology. Edited by A.M. Emmerson, P.M. Hawkey and S.H. Gillespie
© 1997 John Wiley & Sons Ltd

agent still had its protagonists; however, an increasing number of workers were promoting the filter-passer hypothesis, arguing that an agent smaller than a bacterium was responsible. The debate was finally resolved when Smith, Andrews and Laidlaw described the influenza virus in 1933; however, *H. influenzae* has retained the specific epithet which commemorates the initial confusion regarding its role. As well as being linked to influenza, soon after its discovery the influenza bacillus was observed to be associated with a range of other respiratory and invasive infections in patients with chronic bronchitis, and at the turn of the century this led to the suggestion that chronic bronchitis was one of the sequels of influenza. The role played by this organism in chronic obstructive airways disease (COAD) began to be unravelled by later workers (Mulder, 1938; May 1952). Invasive pyogenic infections such as meningitis, lobar pneumonia and septic arthritis were recognized to be essentially diseases of childhood. In 1931 Margaret Pittman demonstrated that these were caused by a specific capsular type which was epidemiologically distinct from infections caused by other types of this organism.

DESCRIPTION OF THE GENUS

The organisms are small non-motile, non-sporing Gram-negative rods that are facultative anaerobes but grow poorly in the absence of oxygen. Addition of 5–10% carbon dioxide to the incubation atmosphere enhances the growth of many strains and is a cultural requirement for some. Sugars are fermented, with gas production in some species. Nitrates are reduced to nitrites. The G + C content of DNA of the *Haemophilus* genus is 37–44 mol%.

The inability to culture *Haemophilus* spp. in the absence of blood or blood products relates to two nutritional requirements, originally referred to as X and V factors and later identified as haemin and nicotinamide adenine dinucleotide (NAD) or nicotinamide adenine dinucleotide phosphate (NADP) respectively. Different species may require either or both of those factors and the

pattern of X and V dependence forms an important criterion for speciation (Table 8.1). X factor can also comprise protoporphyrin IX and other iron-containing protoporphyrins. This group of compounds is required because of the inability of X-dependent strains to convert δ-aminolaevulinic acid to protoporphyrin, a process involving several enzyme-mediated steps, some or all of which may be defective (White and Granick, 1963; Biberstein *et al.*, 1963).

Demonstration of X and V requirements is usually undertaken using a disk test wherein the presence or absence of growth is observed around paper disks impregnated with X or V, or X and V, factors placed on a nutrient agar. Unfortunately, no nutrient medium is probably entirely free of X factor and the disk test may be erroneous in up to 20% of cases, usually wrongly ascribing *H. influenzae* to *H. parainfluenzae*. More accurate results are obtained using the porphyrin test (Kilian, 1974). This test demonstrates the ability of an organism to synthesize porphobilinogen and other porphyrins from δ-aminolaevulinic acid. A loopful of bacteria from colonies on a plate culture is transferred to a solution of δ-aminolaevulinic acid and incubated for 4 hours at 37 °C. Production of porphyrins is indicated by red fluorescence following exposure to ultraviolet radiation at 360 nm (using a Wood's lamp) or development of a red colour in the lower water phase on addition of Kovac's reagent. A negative result confirms X dependence. A summary of cultural and biochemical characters which distinguish various *Haemophilus* spp. is provided in Table 8.1.

Haemophilus influenzae

This is a small Gram-negative rod or coccobacillus $0.3–0.5 \times 1–2$ μm in size. On occasions it may exhibit marked pleomorphism. Long filamentous forms are sometimes seen in clinical samples and ageing cultures and spherical and irregularly shaped cells in specimens from patients treated with antibiotics (Figure 8.1). It is non-motile, non-sporing and non-acid fast. A small proportion of strains are capsulate.

Table 8.1 DISTINGUISHING CHARACTERS OF *HAEMOPHILUS* SPP. ASSOCIATED WITH INFECTIONS IN MAN

Character	*H. influenzae*	*H. influenzae* biogroup *aegyptius*	*H. haemolyticus*	*H. para-influenzae*	*H. para-haemolyticus*	*H. aphrophilus*	*H. para-phrophilus*	*H. segnis*	*H. ducreyi*
X[a] requirement	+	+	+	–	–	–[b]	–	–	+
V requirement	+	+	+	+	+	–	+	+	–
CO_2 (5%) requirement	–	–	–	–	–	+	+	–	–
Haemolysis	–	–	+	–	+	–	–	–	–/w
Haemagglutination	–/w	+	–	–	–	–	–	–	–
Fermentation reactions:									
glucose, acid	+	+L	+	+	+	+	+	w	–/w
glucose, gas	–	–	±L	–/+	±L	+	+	–	–
sucrose, acid	+	–	+	+	+	+	+	w	–
xylose, acid	–	–	–	–	–	–	+	–[c]	–
lactose, acid	–	–	–	–	–	+	+	–	–
mannose, acid	–	–	+	+	–	+	+	–	–

w, weak positive; L, positive only after incubation for one day; –/w, some strains negative some weakly positive; ±, some strains positive, some negative.

[a] Based on the porphyrin test.

[b] A requirement for haemin on primary isolation but porphyrin test positive (usually weakly).

[c] Most strains negative, occasional strains positive.

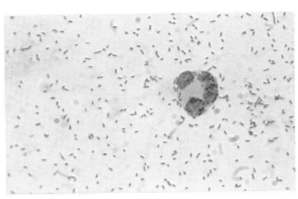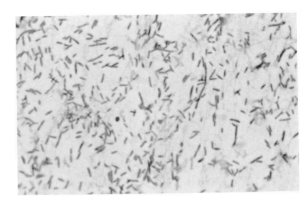

Figure 8.1. Gram-stains of *H. influenzae* in CSF: (a) typical coccobacillary morphology; (b) filamentous and spherical forms.

Cultural characteristics

Haemophilus influenzae grows aerobically and only poorly anaerobically. Growth is enhanced by a moist atmosphere supplemented with 5–10% carbon dioxide Temperature range for growth is 20–42 °C with an optimum between 35 and 37 °C. The growth on blood agar is restricted by the limited availability of V factor and colonies are small in size. Growth also varies according to the source of the blood and is very poor on sheep blood.

Growth on blood agar is improved by heating for a few minutes at 75–100 °C to prepare 'chocolate agar'. This inactivates NADase and releases extra V factor into the medium Similar results are also obtained with transparent media where red cells are disrupted and NADase enzymes inactivated either by peptic digestion (Fildes agar) (Fildes, 1920) or heat (Levinthal's agar) (Alexander, 1965). Blood agar can also be supplemented by applying a streak of *Staphylococcus aureus* across the surface of an inoculated plate or by supplementing the medium directly with 10 mg/1 of crystalline β-NAD. Nutrient agar supplemented with 10 mg/1 of haemin and 10 mg/1 β-NAD will also support good growth. Defined media for *H. influenzae* have also been described (Butler, 1962; Wolin, 1963; Herriott *et al.*, 1970); how-

ever, none supports the growth of all strains (Tebbutt, 1984). After 24 hours at 37 °C on 'chocolate agar' the colonies of non-capsulate strains of *H. influenzae* are usually 0.5–1 mm in diameter, circular, low convex, smooth, pale, grey and transparent. On Fildes agar they are transparent and have a slightly blue iridescence. They have a fishy, seminal smell. The colonies of capsulate strains are larger, 1–3 mm in diameter, high convex and mucoid. On transparent media they exhibit strong iridescence consisting of red, orange, green and blue shades which alter with the angle of observation. This is best seen in young cultures (12–18 hours) by looking obliquely at colonies on a transparent medium illuminated with a bright, concentrated light source from beneath (Figure 8.2, see Plate 1).

Biochemical reactions

Haemophilus influenzae ferments glucose and xylose but not sucrose, lactose or mannose. It produces acid but not gas. It is catalase positive, oxidase positive and reduces nitrates to nitrites. Differential results for the indole, urease and ornithine decarboxylase reactions allows strains within the species to be grouped into eight distinct biotypes (Table 8.2) (Kilian, 1976; Oberhofer and Back, 1979; Gratten, 1983; Sottnek and Albritton, 1984). G + C content of DNA is 39 mol%.

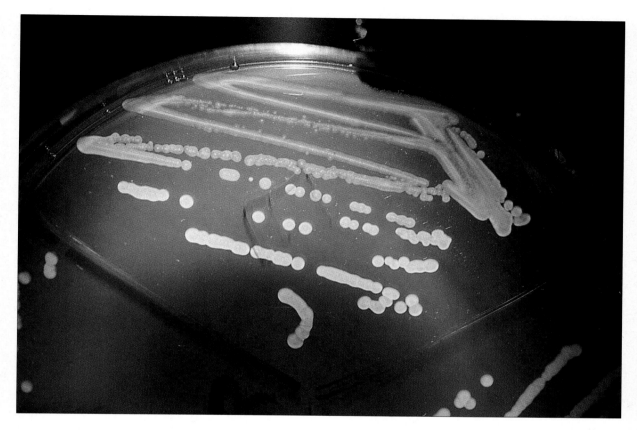

Plate 1 *H. influenzae* type b exhibiting iridescence on a transparent agar medium. (Publication of this figure is sponsored by Eli Lilly & Co. Ltd, Basingstoke, Hampshire, UK.)

Encapsulation

A minority of strains of *H. influenzae* possess a polysaccharide capsule. Based on the antigenicity of this structure these strains can be divided into six types, labelled a–f. The type b capsule is a ribosylphosphate polymer (PRP) and strains possessing it are responsible for most of the invasive infections which occur in childhood.

Capsulation is an unstable property and repeated subculture may lead to the emergence of slower-growing, pleomorphic, capsule-deficient mutants which have a rough colonial appearance They produce capsular material but do not export it to the bacterial surface (Catlin and Tartagni, 1969). The genes for type b capsulation are chromosomal and are clustered in a region of around 36 kb designated *cap*b. This consists of a duplication of two 18 kb segments of DNA linked by a 1 kb bridge region containing the gene *bexA*, which is essential for the export of capsular polysaccharide (Kroll *et al.*, 1988). Loss of capsulation is associated with reduction to only a single copy of the 18 kb segment and disruption of the *bexA* gene.

Infections Caused by *H. influenzae*

Pathogenesis

Haemophilus influenzae is exclusively a human parasite which resides principally in the upper respiratory tract. The species is responsible for two quite distinct spectra of clinical disease. It produces invasive infections in children which mainly comprise meningitis, epiglottitis, pneumonia and septic arthritis and a range of local infections which affect all ages. The latter usually arise in the presence of some physiological or anatomical abnormality and mainly affect the respiratory tract. They include purulent exacerbations of COAD, acute otitis media and acute sinusitis.

Invasive disease For *H. influenzae* to establish systemic infections it must gain attachment to the mucosal surface of the respiratory tract, pass across epithelial and endothelial barriers, invade the bloodstream and then localize in the tissues, producing cell damage in the target organ. Initial attachment is facilitated by the possession of fimbriae by many strains; however, these structures may not be the only adhesins since non-fimbriated bacteria also adhere to epithelial cells of human airways (Read *et al.*, 1991) and do not seem to compete with the same receptor (Loeb *et al.*, 1988). Following colonization, switching from the fimbriated to non-fimbriated phenotype may be an important event in the subsequent development of disease as non-fimbriated variants can better invade the epithelium (Farley *et al.*, 1990). Encapsulation offers no significant advantage to the organism in attachment and may actually decrease the efficiency of this process. A similar consideration may apply to the next phase of invasion: passage through epithelial and endothelial cells and translocation across cellular barriers. Both endothelial and epithelial cells endocytose capsulated strains less efficiently than capsule-deficient variants (St Geme and Falkow, 1991). Presence of type b capsule becomes a critical factor as organisms gain access to the bloodstream. Type b strains are able to resist the intracellular clearing mechanisms, particularly those that are complement mediated, more effectively than other serotypes or non-capsulate strains. Subsequent multiplication and development of a high-grade bacteraemia allows establishment of infection in the target organ. In the case of meningitis, the site of bacterial entry is probably the choroid plexus. What the molecular basis is for the increased virulence conferred by PRP is still ill understood. Lipopolysaccharide is also likely to contribute to the invasive potential of *H. influenzae*. Experimental evidence suggests that it facilitates survival of the organism in the nasopharynx, dissemination from the nasopharynx to the bloodstream, and end organ damage.

Respiratory disease This is mainly caused by non-typable strains. These are highly adept at colonizing the respiratory mucosa and carriage of these organisms probably occurs at some time in all individuals. The organism occupies areas of the upper respiratory tract rich in non-ciliated

TABLE 8.2   CHARACTERS OF EIGHT BIOTYPES OF *HAEMOPHILUS INFLUENZAE*

Character	Biotype							
	1	2	3	4	5	6	7	8
Indole production	+	+	−	−	+	−	+	−
Urease activity	+	+	+	+	−	−	−	−
Ornithine decarboxylase	+	−	−	+	+	+	−	−

epithelium, a process facilitated by fimbriae and other adhesins. In health, the normal local defence mechanisms usually prevent dissemination from the nasopharynx, particularly via the mucociliary clearance. Impairment of these defences, e.g. by the epithelial damage, impaired ciliary function and outflow obstruction associated with viral infection, may result in local bacterial proliferation. Bacterial products such as lipopolysaccharide and a low molecular weight heat-stable compound (Wilson *et al.*, 1985) will then result in increased mucus production, further disruption of ciliary activity and additional damage to the epithelial surface. This will lead to enhanced spread of the organism within the respiratory tract and will increase further the associated tissue damage.

Epidemiology

Normal carriage

Haemophilus influenzae is part of the normal commensal flora of the human oro- and nasopharynx. The frequency with which it has been demonstrated in the upper respiratory tract has varied markedly in different studies and rates between 25% and 82% have been recorded (Sell *et al.*, 1973; Dawson and Zimmerman, 1952). The majority of colonizing strains are non-capsulate and several different strains may be carried at any one time. The duration of carriage of one strain is a few months at most and frequent recolonization with different strains takes place. *Haemophilus influenzae* type b has generally been shown to be present in only 1–5% of populations studied and other capsular types (usually d, e and f) in 1–10%. Introduction of large-scale immunization

with conjugate *H. influenzae* type b vaccines may result in a major reduction in the carriage of type b strains in a population (Takala *et al.*, 1991).

Systemic disease due to H. influenzae type b

The relative proportions of different invasive diseases due to *H. influenzae* type b seen in a UK population are shown in Table 8.3. The clinical presentation varies according to age. In children meningitis predominates, whereas in adults pneumonia is commonest. The age distribution of cases seen in the UK prior to vaccination is shown in Table 8.4. The highest attack rate occurred in infants aged 5–11 months. A small increase in susceptibility is also seen in ageing adults.

Substantial variations are seen in relation to geographical location (Table 8.5) and very high levels of disease have been recorded in certain native populations. In some areas of Alaska 7% of Eskimo children developed *H. influenzae* type b disease during the first two years of life. The age distribution, particularly for meningitis, also shows geographical variation with disease occurring at earlier ages in non-industrialized settings where incidence of the disease is high. In Africa, and amongst the native populations of Alaska, the USA and Australia, most disease is seen in the first year of life, 30–40% of infections occurring in the first six months. Epiglottitis occurs in slightly older age groups than meningitis, most cases presenting between two and four years of age. It is rarely seen in societies where *H. influenzae* type b infections predominate present in young infants.

Factors associated with increased risk of invasive *H. influenzae* type b disease are summarized

TABLE 8.3 CLINICAL PRESENTATION OF INVASIVE DISEASE DUE TO *H. INFLUENZAE* TYPE b[a]

	Children (n = 300) (%)	Adults (n = 37) (%)
Meningitis	59	5
Epiglottitis	17	14
Bacteraemia	8	16
Septic arthritis	5	8
Pneumonia	4	46
Cellulitis	3	–
Other	4	11

[a] Unpublished data from Wales 1980–1992.

TABLE 8.4 INCIDENCE OF INVASIVE INFECTIONS DUE TO *H. INFLUENZAE* TYPE b PER 100 000 POPULATION IN A UK POPULATION PRIOR TO THE INTRODUCTION OF LARGE-SCALE IMMUNIZATION

Age (years)	Cases/100 000 population/year
<1	57
1–4	29
5–15	0.5
16–64	0.1
65–74	0.4
≥75	0.9

in Table 8.6. Increasing family size, overcrowding crèche/nursery attendance and household contact with a case presumably all act by increasing the probability that a susceptible subject will come in contact with the organism.

A national survey conducted in the USA demonstrated that attack rates varied with the age of the household contacts; the estimated risk within 30 days was 40% for children under two years of age,

2% for children aged two and three years, 0.1% for children aged four and five years and 0% for those aged six years and over. For children aged under six years this represents a relative risk of *H. influenzae* type b disease up to 800 times greater than the background level (Ward *et al.*, 1979). Most information regarding the risk in nurseries comes from studies in US day care centres. The risk in these settings appears to be much lower than for household contacts. For children aged less than two years the risk over 60 days has been calculated to be 1% – about 25 times the background level of disease (Broome *et al.*, 1987); however, there is uncertainty regarding the accuracy of this estimate.

The contribution that immunosuppressive conditions such as asplenia or immunoglobulin deficiencies has played in the overall occurrence of *H. influenzae* type b disease has been small in the past; however, the reduction of *H. influenzae* type b disease by immunization programmes may increase their relative importance in the future. The striking association of *H. influenzae* type b disease with certain racial groups has prompted studies in relation to a possible genetic predisposition. Alleles of the immunoglobulin genes km(1) and G2m(n) and the enzyme uridine monophosphokinase have received much attention but it is unlikely that they play a significant role in the epidemiology of these infections (Mäkelä *et al.*, 1992).

Season of the year also affects the incidence of invasive *H. influenzae* type b disease, infections being more common in the winter months This suggests that cofactors, particularly intercurrent

TABLE 8.5 THE INCIDENCE OF *H. INFLUENZAE* TYPE b DISEASE IN CHILDREN UNDER FIVE YEARS IN POPULATIONS NOT EXPOSED TO LARGE-SCALE VACCINATION

Location	Year(s) of study	Cases per year per 100 000 population	Reference
England (five regions)	1990–91	26	Nazareth *et al.* (1992)
Wales	1990–91	33	Nazareth *et al.* (1992)
Finland	1985–86	52	Takala *et al.* (1989)
USA (California)	1976–78	60	Granoff and Basden (1980)
Apache Indians (USA)	1973–81	254	Losonsky *et al.* (1984)
Alaskan Eskimos	1971–77	491	Ward *et al.* (1981)
Australian aborigines	1985–86	1100	Hansman *et al.* (1986)

TABLE 8.6   RISK FACTORS ASSOCIATED WITH INVASIVE *H. INFLUENZAE* TYPE b DISEASE

Age
Season
Family size
Low economic status
Crèche/nursery attendance
Household/nursery contact with a case
Race
Genetic factors
Immunosuppression including haematological malignancies, Hodgkin's disease and HIV infection
Asplenia: functional (e.g. sickle cell disease) or anatomical
Immunoglobulin and complement deficiencies

viral infections, may play an important role in the pathogenesis of these infections.

Invasive diseases due to serotypes other than type b

These infections are rare. The spectrum of disease is similar to that seen with type b infections, with meningitis being the commonest presentation.

Invasive diseases due to non-typable strains

The epidemiology of these infections differs in a number of ways from those associated with type b strains. In the absence of *H. influenzae* type b vaccination, invasive infections due to non-typable *H. influenzae* occur about 10 times less frequently than those due to type b. The highest attack rate is seen in neonates, particularly those born prematurely, with a mortality of nearly 50% in this population. Most infants have evidence of symptomatic infection at birth or within the first few hours of life with pneumonia and respiratory distress dominating the clinical presentation. Some studies have demonstrated a predominance of strains of biotype IV in this situation.

Infections in adults are uncommon, however, they occur with a similar frequency to those caused by type b strains. Pneumonia and bacteraemia are the commonest presentations and those are usually associated with some form of underlying disease, particularly malignancy or chronic lung disease. Increased susceptibility is seen in older age groups.

Localized respiratory infections

These comprise the majority of infections caused by non-typable strains. They include otitis media, sinusitis and acute exacerbations of COAD. They occur with much greater frequency than invasive disease. They are often initiated by viral infections and thus have a seasonal occurrence which correlates with the circulation of respiratory viruses in a population. Acute otitis media occurs in childhood with a peak incidence between 6 and 24 months. *Haemophilus influenzae* and *Streptococcus pneumoniae* are the two commonest bacterial pathogens associated with each of these conditions. Non-typable *H. influenzae* are also important causes of purulent conjunctivitis.

CLINICAL CONDITIONS

Meningitis

There are no specific features that allow *Haemophilus* meningitis to be distinguished from other bacterial causes on clinical grounds. In children, antecedent upper respiratory infection and otitis media are common, but both may be seen in association with meningitis caused by other organisms. Characteristically, *Haemophilus* meningitis arises after a few days' mild illness though the onset may be abrupt and fulminating. Occasionally, the presentation may resemble acute meningococcal septicaemia with widespread petechiae, collapse and bilateral adrenal haemorrhage.

The mortality associated with *Haemophilus* meningitis is usually around 3–5%. The incidence of long-term sequelae has varied from study to study. Neurological deficits have been noted in 10–30% of subjects when long-term follow-ups have been assessed.

Although uncommon, *Haemophilus* meningitis may also present in the adult. In contrast to the disease in children, predisposing factors are commonly present. These may consist of local disorders such as cranial trauma or surgery, or general conditions such as diabetes or alcoholism. The more frequent association with underlying disease may be the explanation for a much higher mortality (10–30%) than that seen in children.

Epiglottitis

The second most common form of invasive disease, epiglottitis, is characterized by a fulminant course and is a paediatric emergency. Following several days of a mild and non-specific upper respiratory tract illness there is sudden onset of intense sore throat, fever and rapidly progressive dyspnoea, dysphagia, inspiratory stridor and hoarseness. On presentation, the child will be restless, anxious and drooling from the mouth and is often seen adopting a sitting position, leaning forward in an attempt to reduce the airway obstruction. Abrupt deterioration may occur within a few hours of onset, leading to death as a result of respiratory obstruction, toxaemia or a combination of the two. A concomitant pneumonia may also be present.

Most fatalities occur before resuscitation can be instituted and mortality following effective medication is low.

Septic Arthritis

Prior to immunization in the UK *H. influenzae* was the commonest cause of septic arthritis in children under five years of age. It occurs most commonly in children under two years of age and usually affects the large joints, particularly knees, ankles and elbows.

The condition is rare in adults but when it does arise exhibits certain features that differ from those seen when the disease occurs in childhood. Type b strains are those most commonly involved although non-typable strains may also be implicated. Predisposing conditions are often present, commonly comprising: pre-existing joint disease, particularly rheumatoid arthritis; diabetes; alcoholism; or immunoglobulin deficiencies. In general, involvement of a wider range of joints tends to occur in adults in comparison with children and multiple involvement is more common.

Osteomyelitis

In contrast to septic arthritis, *Haemophilus* osteomyelitis is rare. It is mainly seen in children less than two years of age and the long bones, particularly the humerus, are most commonly affected.

Pneumonia

Haemophilus pneumonia is again a disease that, prior to vaccination, was most commonly seen in infancy, particularly in association with diseases in other sites such as otitis media, epiglottitis or meningitis.

In general, unilateral disease is more common than bilateral disease and pleural effusions are found in a high percentage of cases. Extension of the disease to produce a suppurative pericarditis has been described in approximately 5% of cases.

Pneumonia in adults represents a wider spectrum of disease than in children. Pneumonia secondary to type b strains with similar characteristics to those observed in children may be encountered but is rare. In patients with diabetes, alcoholism or immunoglobulin defects *Haemophilus* pneumonia often presents with more than one lobe affected, commonly with a pleural effusion, and in a small percentage of cases may proceed to cavitation. Type b organisms may be responsible for these infections but in the compromised host non-typable strains predominate. The outcome of these infections is related to the nature of the underlying disease. The overall mortality of bacteraemic disease is high.

Cellulitis

This is a rare but characteristic presentation of disease due to *H. influenzae* type b and is usually seen in children under two years of age. The cellulitis presents as a well-defined lesion that often has a bluish or purplish hue. The sites involved include cheek, periorbital area, head and neck and upper and lower extremities. Abscess formation may occasionally occur. *H. influenzae* cellulitis in adults is very rare. It is associated with type b infection and usually occurs in association with disease in other sites. It is said to present less frequently with the characteristic colour seen in children.

LABORATORY DIAGNOSIS

Collection of Specimens

Invasive infections associated with *H. influenzae* are often accompanied by bacteraemia and blood cultures should always be taken prior to starting antibiotic therapy. Other specimens that may indicate *Haemophilus* infection include: cerebrospinal fluid (CSF); pus; joint, pleural, bronchial or pericardial aspirates; and sputum. Rarely *H. influenzae* may cause urinary tract infection and can be isolated from urine. This is usually seen in children with renal tract abnormalities.

Dry swabs should be moistened with saline before sampling and transported to the laboratory in bacteriological transport medium. All specimens should be kept at room temperature and processed without undue delay.

Direct Examination

Haemophilus influenzae stains poorly with neutral red as a counterstain and better results are obtained using safranin or dilute carbol fuchsin. A Gram stain of CSF provides a rapid method of diagnosing *Haemophilus* meningitis. When present in CSF *H. influenzae* usually appears as typical coccobacilli; however, occasionally they appear as pleomorphic, long, filamentous forms.

Capsule Detection

Large numbers of haemophili in CSF can be confirmed as type b strains by the capsular swelling reaction. A drop of the CSF is mixed with a drop of a *H. influenzae* type b antiserum on a glass slide and examined microscopically. A positive result is indicated by the presence of swollen and sharply delineated organisms compared with controls.

Antigen Detection

The demonstration of type b capsular antigen in CSF, serum or urine may provide an early indication of *Haemophilus* infection. Methods include countercurrent immunoelectrophoresis (CIE), latex agglutination (Wellcogen *H. influenzae* b test, Wellcome) and staphylococcal coagglutination (Phadebact CSF tests, Pharmacia). The latter two tests are more sensitive than CIE. Urine must be concentrated 25- to 50-fold by membrane filtration to increase sensitivity. The latter can be undertaken using a Minicon B15 concentrator (Amicon Corp).

Some caution is necessary in the interpretation of these tests. False positive reactions may be obtained due to a cross-reacting antigen from other organisms (particularly *Streptococcus pneumoniae*) or as a result of recent immunization with a type b polysaccharide vaccine.

Culture

The best general-purpose medium for the isolation of *H. influenzae* is 'chocolate agar'. This can be used unsupplemented for specimens that are likely to contain this organism in pure culture, e.g. CSF, pus or normally sterile body fluids. Specimens from the respiratory tract will usually contain oropharyngeal bacteria that may hinder isolation. Addition of bacitracin (300 mg/1) to the medium will improve selectivity. No attempt should be made to obtain a throat swab from a child with acute epiglottitis as the interference may precipitate respiratory obstruction. Laboratory diagnosis should be made by blood culture or the demonstration of type b antigen in serum or urine.

Blood cultures are satisfactory using conventional media, or radiometric or infrared BACTEC (Becton Dickinson) systems (Shanson, 1990). Examining broths for turbidity may be unreliable for the detection of *H. influenzae* and conventional media should be routinely subcultured if *Haemophilus* infection is a possibility. Routine subculture should also be undertaken if the Oxoid Signal System is used as *H. influenzae* may not produce sufficient pressure to give a positive indication of growth (Fox *et al.*, 1988).

Antimicrobial Sensitivity

The species is naturally sensitive to a wide range of antibiotics, including ampicillin or amoxycillin, many of the newer cephalosporins, tetracyclines, sulphonamides, trimethoprim, rifampicin, fluoroquinolones and chloramphenicol. It has lesser intrinsic sensitivity to penicillin, erythromycin and 'first-generation' cephalosporins. Over the last 20 years antibiotic resistance to most of these agents has emerged. The most important of these has been resistance to ampicillin. This is usually due to the production of a TEM-1 like β-lactamase enzyme, encoded by the transposon TnA. The TnA sequence may be found within either large or small plasmids (30 and 3 MDa respectively) or in chromosomal DNA. Rare isolates producing a different β-lactamase, ROB-1, have also been described. The prevalence of β-lactamase-producing strains of *H. influenzae* varies in different parts of the world and is commoner in type b organisms compared with other serotypes and non-typable strains. In the UK around 5–10% of non-typable and 15–20% of type b strains are β-lactamase producers. Less commonly, ampicillin resistance may also be encountered in strains which do not produce β-lactamase. This is due to alteration of one or more penicillin-binding proteins (PBPs), particularly PBP5. This form of resistance results in decreased susceptibility to a number of β-lactam antibiotics in addition to ampicillin. Conjugative plasmids are also responsible for resistance to chloramphenicol and tetracycline. Chloramphenicol resistance is usually mediated by the production of a chloramphenicol acetyltransferase enzyme. Most chloramphenicol-resistant strains

are resistant to tetracycline and some may be β-lactamase producers. Such multiply resistant strains are generally uncommon; however, a high incidence has been reported in patients with meningitis in Spain (Campos *et al.*, 1986).

Antibiotic Sensitivity Tests

Sensitivity test media require appropriate supplementation to support the growth of haemophili. A number of suitable formulations have been described for undertaking disk diffusion, broth and agar dilution techniques (Needham, 1988).

The accuracy of routine sensitivity tests with *H. influenzae* can be enhanced by incorporating a test for β-lactamase production. The acidometric paper strip method (Slack *et al.*, 1977) and the nitrocefin test (Kammer *et al.*, 1975) both give results within a few minutes. In the former test material from several colonies is transferred to a paper strip impregnated with penicillin and bromocresol purple (intralactam strip, Mast) and moistened with distilled water; if the organism produces β-lactamase the penicillin will be hydrolysed to penicilloic acid and the colour of the strip will change from purple to yellow. In the second test, several colonies are applied to blotting paper impregnated with a nitrocefin solution. This is a chromogenic cephalosporin which is readily hydrolysed by a variety of β-lactamases when it changes from a yellow to a red colour.

MANAGEMENT OF DISEASES CAUSED BY *H. INFLUENZAE* TYPE B

Treatment

Early treatment of meningitis with an appropriate antibiotic given intravenously in high dosage is crucial. Chloramphenicol is effective and has long been the favoured choice in many units. It is given in a dosage of 75–100 mg/kg in four divided doses. Oral therapy should not be given in the acute stages of the illness as vomiting or impaired absorption may result in low serum levels; however, oral treatment with the same dosage can be used satisfactorily once this phase has passed and the patient's condition has stabilized (Tuomanen, 1981). Since oral absorption can vary, serum levels of the drug should be monitored. The patient should also be kept hospitalized to ensure compliance and to observe for any complications of meningitis.

Chloramphenicol-resistant type b strains remain rare in most parts of the world; however, their occurrence and the avoidance of potential chloramphenicol toxicity has prompted the increasing use of third-generation cephalosporins, particularly cefotaxime 200 mg/kg day in four divided doses or ceftriaxone 75–100 mg/kg once daily or divided into 12 hourly doses (total daily dose not to exceed 4 g). The clinical efficacy of these agents is equivalent to that of chloramphenicol. Intravenous ampicillin at a dose of 200–300 mg/kg in four divided doses is also effective; however, the common occurrence of ampicillin-resistant strains of *H. influenzae* type b means that this agent must not be used alone for the treatment until it is clearly established that the strain responsible is unequivocally sensitive to this drug.

Antibiotic therapy is only one component of the clinical management of patients with *Haemophilus* meningitis and full supportive care is required to achieve the most favourable outcome. Unconscious patients may require respiratory ventilation and appropriate fluid and electrolyte balance must be maintained. Use of steroids has been controversial; however, dexamethasone 0.15 mg/kg 6-hourly given over the first four days of therapy has been shown to have a significant effect on reducing deafness (Lebel *et al.*, 1988). A subdural effusion will require surgical drainage either via needle aspiration or craniotomy.

Chloramphenicol or a third-generation cephalosporin are also the antibiotics of choice for other invasive infections due to *H. influenzae* type b. Maintenance of a patient's airway is essential in the management of patients with acute epiglottitis. This can be achieved by endotracheal or naso-tracheal incubation, which should be undertaken by experienced anaesthetic staff. Facilities must be on hand to undertake emergency tracheotomy if required. High-dose steroids may help to reduce soft tissue oedema.

Immunization

It has long been recognized that antibodies directed towards *H. influenzae* type b capsular polysaccharide (PRP) play a major role in promoting immunity to this organism and this is reflected in the inverse relationship between naturally occurring antibodies and the age incidence of disease (Figure 8.3). With the exception of

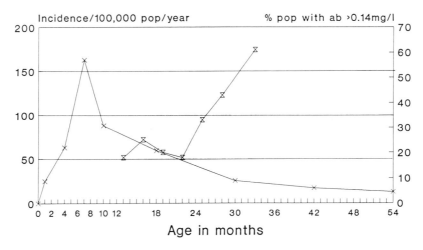

Figure 8.3. The incidence of invasive Hib disease in North Wales, 1980–1990 (*x*) and the occurrence of PRP antibodies in children less than three years of age, *n* = 109 (⊠). (Unpublished data.)

young infants (who are protected by maternal antibodies) antibody levels are at their lowest in children under two years of age, when the risk of invasive *H. influenzae* type b infections is at its highest.

The earliest vaccine directed towards the prevention of *H. influenzae* type b disease consisted of purified PRP prepared from the supernatant of *H. influenzae* type b broth cultures. This was found to be safe and immunogenic in children over two years of age. However, the immune response to it in younger children was unsatisfactory. These results correlated with clinical efficacy in field trials. In a study involving 100 000 children in Finland, although 90% efficacy was recorded in children over 18 months of age, little protection was seen in younger subjects (Peltola *et al.*, 1984).

The inability of the PRP antigen to produce an effective immune response in infants was overcome by the development of conjugate vaccines which link the capsular polysaccharide hapten to a protein 'carrier'. In contrast to purified PRP preparations which predominantly invoke T cell-independent responses, these elicit an immune response characterized by T helper cell activation. They thus produce higher concentrations of PRP antibodies than the purified PRP vaccines, are immunogenic in young infants, and induce anamnestic (booster) responses. Four conjugate vaccines are currently available. Each varies

according to the protein carrier, the length of the linkage between the two and the coupling procedure used (Table 8.7). Of these four vaccines, PRP-D is the least immunogenic. Although it proved highly effective in a trial involving Finnish children (Eskola *et al.*, 1990), poor results were achieved when it was administered to an Eskimo population (Ward *et al.*, 1994). The protective efficacy of the other three vaccines has been uniformly excellent in all populations studied.

Mass immunization of children with a PRP conjugate vaccine was introduced in the UK in October 1992, in conjunction with the diphtheria–pertussis–tetanus and polio primary immunizations. Initially a catch-up exercise for older children up to 48 months of age was also conducted. This programme has resulted in the virtual disappearance of invasive *H. influenzae* type b infections in children in the UK (Figure 8.4) and reflects the dramatic impact of large-scale PRP–conjugate vaccine usage on these diseases already observed in other parts of the world. As well as combining PRP–conjugate vaccination with the childhood immunization programme, the vaccine should also be administered to the following:

(1) Unimmunized household contacts of a case of invasive *H. influenzae* type b disease who are less than four years of age.
(2) The index case, irrespective of age. This is to

TABLE 8.7   *HAEMOPHILUS INFLUENZAE* TYPE b VACCINES

Vaccine	Manufacturer (tradename)	Polysaccharide	Linker	Protein carrier
PRP-D	Connaught (ProHIBiT)	Heat sized to 200–2000 kDa	6-carbon	Diphtheria toxoid
HbOC	Lederle–Praxis (HibTITER)	20-unit oligosaccharide	None	CRM$_{197}$[a]
PRP-OMP	Merck, Sharp & Dohme (Pedvax HIB)	Native	Complex thioether	Outer member protein complex of *N. meningitidis*
PRP-T	Institute Merieux (Act-HIB)	Native	6-carbon	Tetanus toxoid

[a] CRM$_{197}$ is a non-toxic, naturally occurring diphtheria toxin.

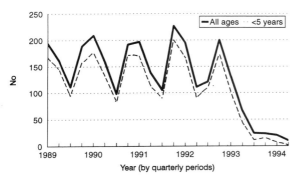

Figure 8.4. Invasive disease due to *H. influenzae* type b. (Laboratory reports to the Communicable Disease Surveillance Centre, Colindale, 1989–1994.)

prevent a second episode of invasive disease. Such an occurrence is uncommon but well recognized. It may result from relapse or reinfection following the failure of primary antibiotic therapy to eliminate the organisms from the nasopharynx and an inadequate immune response to the infecting organism.

Others groups at higher risk of *H. influenzae* type b infection than the normal population such as those with HIV infection or with asplenia should also be considered for vaccination.

When a case occurs in a playgroup, nursery or crèche, the opportunity should be taken to identify and vaccinate any unimmunized children under four years of age.

Chemoprophylaxis

Rifampicin in a dosage of 20 mg/kg (up to a maximum of 600 mg) given orally once daily for four days is effective in eradicating carriage of *H. influenzae*. It has been used to prevent secondary infection in household and nursery contacts, to limit hospital outbreaks and to prevent second episodes in an index case, although its efficacy in these situations is not proven and anecdotal reports of failures of rifampicin prophylaxis in household and day care centre contacts have been published. Its use should be considered when a case arises in a household containing an unimmunized child less than four years of age. All members of the household (including the index case) should receive the drug under these circumstances. The children at risk should also be immunized.

HAEMOPHILUS INFLUENZAE BIOGROUP AEGYPTIUS

Organisms within this group conform to biotype III of *H. influenzae* but exhibit a number of phenotypic differences from other strains of the species. These were previously thought to be sufficient to warrant separate species status but genetic analysis has confirmed that they are best considered as a subgroup of *H. influenzae* (Musser et al., 1990).

Biogroup *aegyptius* is more nutritionally exacting and grows more slowly than *H. influenzae*. Its colonies on heated blood agar reach only about 0.5 mm diameter in 48 hours. Better growth and higher rates of isolation are obtained on heated blood agar enriched with 1% Iso Vitalex. In contrast to other strains of *H. influenzae* biogroup *aegyptius* fails to ferment D-xylose, is sensitive to troleandomycin and shows stronger haemagglutinating activity with human or guinea-pig red blood cells. This organism has an affinity for the conjunctiva and is responsible for an acute contagious conjunctivitis.

A specific clone which is genetically related to serotype c strains (Musser et al., 1990) has been shown to be responsible for a fulminant invasive infection in children: Brazilian purpuric fever. This is characterized by fever with rapid progression to purpura, hypotensive shock and death. The condition is often preceded by a purulent conjunctivitis which has resolved before the onset of fever. Blood cultures are positive for *H. influenzae* biogroup *aegyptius*.

HAEMOPHILUS APHROPHILUS

This organism is carbon dioxide dependent and on primary isolation has an apparent requirement for X factor. The latter characteristic is often lost on subculture. It is a common commensal in the mouth and dental plaque and an occasional cause of jaw infections, endocarditis and brain abscess.

HAEMOPHILUS DUCREYI

This is the causative agent of the venereal disease, chancroid. It was first described by Ducreyi in 1889.

Description of the Organism

In Gram stains of purulent material, *H. ducreyi* may present a variety of morphological features, appearing as short, plump, bipolar staining Gram-negative bacilli, evenly staining coccobacilli or slender rods. Preparations prepared from solid media may appear as single bacilli, groups or small chains.

Cultural Requirements

Haemophilus ducreyi is a fastidious organism which grows only slowly on chocolate agar. Media which improve the yield include 30% rabbit blood agar and coagulated human or rabbit blood (Deacon *et al.*, 1956). Other media available for the isolation of this organism have been reviewed by Morse (1989). GC agar (Gibco) containing 1–2% haemoglobin, 5% fetal bovine serum, 10% CVA enrichment (Gibco) and 3 mg/l vancomycin has the highest sensitivity. The use of two different media may increase the chance of isolation. Cultures must be incubated in a moist atmosphere with additional carbon dioxide at 35–37 °C for up to five days.

Colonies are pinpoint in size at 24 hours and 1–2 mm in diameter at 48–72 hours. They have a tan, yellowish or greyish-yellow colour and can be pushed across the surface of a solid medium with an inoculating loop. Colonies are difficult to emulsify and suspensions difficult to prepare. Colonies may be variable in size and opacity, giving the appearance of a mixed culture.

Biochemical Reaction

Haemophilus ducreyi reduces nitrate to nitrite, gives a positive oxidase test with tetramethyl-*p*-phenylenediamine but not dimethyl-*p*-phenylenediamine, and is alkaline phosphatase positive.

It is catalase and indole negative. Reports of the action of *H. ducreyi* on carbohydrates have been conflicting.

Clinical Features

Infection is established in the mucosa or skin of the genital area via a break in the epithelium. Initially, small inflammatory papules develop surrounded by a narrow erythematous zone. Within two or three days a pustule forms that soon ruptures, resulting in a sharply circumscribed ulcer with ragged undermined edges and without induration. Chancroid ulcers are very vascular and have a friable base which bleeds easily on scraping. A painful, tender, usually unilateral inguinal lymphadenopathy ensues. Involved lymph nodes may become fluctuant and spontaneously rupture. The organism is found in the ulcer, its exudate and in the associated lymph nodes. The infection is encountered most commonly in developing countries.

Laboratory Diagnosis

A saline moistened swab can be used to take specimens from the base and margins of an ulcer. The organism may be identified on Gram stain although interpretation can be complicated by the polymicrobial flora often encountered in genital ulcers. Definitive diagnosis requires culture of the organism. Confirmation that suspicious colonies are *H. ducreyi* can be achieved using one of the several rapid test systems currently available. These include Minitek, API Zym and the Rapid IDNH system.

Antimicrobial Susceptibility and Treatment

Many strains exhibit resistance to one or more antimicrobial agents, and resistance to tetracyclines, sulphonamides and ampicillin is common. The latter is mediated by a TEM-1 type β-lactamase and can be demonstrated using chromogenic cephalosporin or an iodometric method. Erythromycin, ceftriaxone and co-amoxiclav are all effective in treatment.

HAEMOPHILUS HAEMOLYTICUS

This *Haemophilus* has been regarded by some as a variety of *H. influenzae*, from which it differs in forming zones of β-haemolysis around its colonies on blood agar. The haemolysis is strongest on sheep or ox blood, but is also seen on horse or human blood. The organism is found as a commensal in the oropharynx of healthy individuals. It is of very low pathogenicity.

HAEMOPHILUS PARAHAEMOLYTICUS

This organism resembles *H. parainfluenzae* in most characters but differs in forming β-haemolytic colonies. It is commonly present as a commensal in the mouth and throat and is occasionally found in cases of oral sepsis and endocarditis.

HAEMOPHILUS PARAINFLUENZAE

This organism differs from *H. influenzae* by being V but not X dependent, by its ability to ferment sucrose but not D-xylose and by its low pathogenicity. Morphologically it resembles *H. influenzae* but it forms larger, more opaque yellowish-white colonies on heated blood agar. It is normally present as a commensal in the mouth and throat. It occasionally causes endocarditis, is sometimes a component of a mixed flora encountered in lung or cerebral abscesses and may possibly play a pathogenic role in bronchopulmonary infections in patients with chronic obstructive airways disease and cystic fibrosis.

HAEMOPHILUS PARAPHROPHILUS

This is very similar in characteristics to *H. aphrophilus*, although requiring V and not X factor for growth. It is an oropharyngeal commensal that is occasionally associated with endocarditis and oral, lung or cerebral abscesses.

HAEMOPHILUS SEGNIS

This requires V but not X factor and grows very slowly, forming opaque whitish colonies up to 0.5 mm in diameter after 48 hours. It is commonly present as a commensal in the mouth, dental plaque and throat. It appears to be almost entirely non-pathogenic.

REFERENCES

Alexander, H.E. (1965) The haemophilus group. In *Bacterial and Mycotic Infections of Man*, 4th edn (ed. R.J. Dubos and J.G. Hirsch), pp. 724–741. Pitman Medical, London.

Biberstein, E.L., Mini, P.D. and Gills, M.G. (1963) Action of *Haemophilus* cultures on δ-aminolevulinic acid. *Journal of Bacteriology*, **86**, 814–819.

Broome, C.V., Mortimer, E.A. Katz, S.L. *et al.* (1987) Use of chemoprophylaxis to prevent the spread of *Haemophilus influenzae* type b disease in day care facilities. *New England Journal of Medicine*, **316**, 1226–1228.

Butler, L.O. (1962) A defined medium for *Haemophilus influenzae* and *Haemophilus parainfluenzae*. *Journal of General Microbiology*, **27**, 51–60.

Campos, J., Garcia-Tornel, S., Gairi, J.M. *et al.* (1986) Multiply resistant *Haemophilus influenzae* type b causing meningitis: comparative clinical and laboratory study. *Journal of Pediatrics*, **108**, 897–902.

Catlin, B.W. and Tartagni, V.R. (1969) Delayed multiplication of newly capsulated transformants of *Haemophilus influenzae* detected by immunofluorescence. *Journal of General Microbiology*, **56**, 387–401.

Dawson, B. and Zimmerman, K. (1952) Incidence and type distribution of capsulated *H. influenzae* strains. *British Medical Journal*, **i**, 740–742.

Deacon, W.E. Albritton, D.C., Olansky, S. *et al.* (1956) VDRL chancroid studies: a simple procedure for the isolation and identification of *Haemophilus ducreyi*. *Journal of Investigative Dermatology*, **26**, 399–406.

Eskola, J., Käyhty, H., Takala, A.K. *et al.* (1990). A randomised, prospective field trial of a conjugate vaccine in the protection of infants and young children against invasive *Haemophilus influenzae* type b disease. *New England Journal of Medicine*, **323**, 1381–1387.

Farley, M.M., Stephens, D.S., Kaplan, S.L. *et al.* (1990) Pilus and non-pilus-mediated interactions of *Haemophilus influenzae* type b with human erythrocytes and human nasopharyngeal mucosa. *Journal of Infectious Diseases*, **161**, 274–280.

Fildes, P. (1920) Peptic blood agar for culture of *B.*

influenzae and general purposes. *British Journal of Experimental Pathology*, **1**, 129.

Fox, H., Healing, D.E. and George, R.H. (1988) Evaluation of use of Signal system of blood culture in paediatrics. *Journal of Clinical Pathology*, **41**, 683–686.

Granoff, D.M. and Basden, M. (1980) *Haemophilus influenzae* infections in Fresno County California: a prospective study of the effects of age, race and contact with a case on incidence of disease. *Journal of Infectious Diseases*, **141**, 40–46.

Gratten, M. (1983) *Haemophilus influenzae* biotype VII. *Journal of Clinical Microbiology*, 1015–1016.

Hansman, D., Hanna, J. and Morey, F. (1986). High prevalence of invasive *Haemophilus influenzae* disease in Central Australia, 1986. *Lancet*, **i**, 927.

Herriott, H.M., Meyer, E.Y., Vogt, M. *et al.* (1970) Defined medium for growth of *Haemophilus influenzae*. *Journal of Bacteriology*, **101**, 513–516.

Howard, A.J., Dunkin, K.T., Musser, J.M. *et al.* (1991) Epidemiology of *Haemophilus influenzae* type b invasive diseases in Wales. *British Medical Journal*, **303**, 444–445.

Kammer, R.B., Preston, D.A., Turner, J.R. *et al.* (1975) Rapid detection of ampicillin-resistant *Haemophilus influenzae* and their susceptibility to sixteen antibiotics. *Antimicrobial Agents and Chemotherapy*, **8**, 91–94.

Kilian, M. (1974) A rapid method for the differentiation of *Haemophilus* strains: the porphyrin test. *Acta Pathologica et Microbiologica Scandinavica*, Sect. B, **82**, 835–842.

Kilian, M. (1976) A taxonomic study of the genus *Haemophilus* with the proposal of a new species. *Journal of General Microbiology*, **93**, 9–62.

Kroll, J.S. Hopkins, I. and Moxon, E.R. (1988) Capsule loss in *H. influenzae* type b occurs by recombination-mediated disruption of a gene essential for polysaccharide export. *Cell*, **53**, 347–356.

Lebel, M.H., Freij, B.J., Syrogiannopoulos, G.A. *et al.* (1988) Dexamethasone therapy for bacterial meningitis: results of two double blind placebo-controlled trials. *New England Journal of Medicine*, **319** 964–971.

Loeb, M.R. Connor, E. and Penney, D. (1988) A comparison of the adherence of fimbriated and non fimbriated *Haemophilus influenzae* type b to human adenoids in organ culture. *Infection and Immunity*, **56**, 484–489.

Losonsky, G.A., Santosham, M. Sehgal, V.M. *et al.* (1984) *Haemophilus influenzae* disease in the White Mountain Apaches: molecular epidemiology of a high risk population. *Pediatric Infectious Diseases*, **3**, 539–547.

Mäkelä, P.H., Takala, A.K., Peltola, H. *et al.* (1992) Epidemiology of invasive *Haemophilus influenzae*

type b disease. *Journal of Infectious Diseases*, **165**, (Suppl. 1), S2–6.

May, J.R. (1952) The bacteriology of chronic bronchitis. *Lancet*, **ii**, 1206–1207.

Morse, S.A. (1989) Chancroid and *Haemophilus ducreyi*. *Clinical Microbiology Reviews*, **2**, 137–157.

Mulder, J. (1938) *H. influenzae* (Pfeiffer) as a ubiquitous cause of common acute and chronical purulent bronchitis. *Acta Medica Scandinavica*, **94**, 98–140.

Musser, J.M., Kroll, J.S., Granoff, D.M. *et al.* (1990) Global genetic structure and molecular epidemiology of uncapsulated *Haemophiulus influenzae*. *Reviews of Infectious Diseases*, **12**, 75–111.

Nazareth, B., Slack, M.P.E., Howard, A.J. *et al.* (1992) A survey of invasive *Haemophilus influenzae* infections. *CDR Review*, **2**, 13–16.

Needham, C.A. (1988) *Haemophilus influenzae*: antibiotic susceptibility. *Clinical Microbiology Reviews*, **1**, 218–227.

Oberhofer, T.R. and Back, A.E. (1979) Biotypes of *Haemophilus* encountered in clinical laboratories. *Journal of Clinical Microbiology*, **10**, 168–174.

Peltola, H., Käyhty, H., Virtanen, M. *et al.* (1984) Prevention of *Haemophilus influenzae* type b bacteremic infections with the capsular polysaccharide vaccine. *New England Journal of Medicine*, **310**, 1561–1566.

Pittman, M. (1931) Variation and type specificity in the bacterial species *H. influenzae*. *Journal of Experimental Medicine*, **53**, 471–492.

Read, R.C., Wilson, R., Rutman, A. *et al.* (1991) Interaction of non typable *Haemophilus influenzae* with human respiratory mucosa in vitro. *Journal of Infectious Diseases*, **163**, 549–558.

Sell, S.H., Turner, D.J. and Federspiel, C.F. (1973) Natural infections with *Haemophilus influenzae* in children: types identified. In *Haemophilus influenzae* (ed. S.H.W. Sell and D.T. Karzon), pp. 3–12. Vanderbillt University Press.

Shanson, D.C. (1990) Blood culture technique: current controversies. *Journal of Antimicrobial Chemotherapy*, 25 (Suppl. C), 17–29.

Slack, M.P.E., Wheldon, D.B. and Turk, D.C. (1977) A rapid test for beta-lactamase production by *H. influenzae*. *Lancet*, **ii**, 906.

Sottnek, F.O. and Albritton, A.L. (1994) *Haemophilus influenzae* biotype VIII. *Journal of Clinical Microbiology*, **20**, 815–816.

St Geme, J.W., III and Falkow S. (1991) Loss of capsule expression by *Haemophilus influenzae* type b results in enhanced adherence to and invasion of human cells. *Infection and Immunity*, **59**, 1325–1333.

Takala, A.K., Eskola, J., Peltola, H. *et al.* (1984) Epidemiology of invasive *Haemophilus influenzae* type b disease among children in Finland before vaccination with *Haemophilus influenzae* type b conjugate vaccine. *Pediatric Infectious Diseases*, **8**, 297–302.

Takala, A.K., Eskola, J., Leinonen, M. *et al.* (1991) Reduction of oropharyngeal carriage of *Haemophilus influenzae* type b (Hib) in children immunised with an Hib conjugate vaccine. *Journal of Infectious Diseases*, **164**, 982–986.

Tebbutt, G.M. A chemotyping scheme for clinical isolates of *Haemophilus influenzae*. *Journal of Medical Microbiology*, **17**, 335–345.

Tuomanen, E.I. (1981) Oral chloramphenicol in the treatment of *Haemophilus influenzae* meningitis. *Journal of Pediatrics*, **99**, 968–974.

Ward, J.I. Fraser, D.W. Baraff, L.J. *et al.* (1979) *Haemophilus influenzae* meningitis: a national study of secondary spread in household contacts. *New England Journal of Medicine*, **301**, 122–126.

Ward, J.I., Margolis, H.S., Lum, M.K.W. *et al.* (1981) *Haemophilus influenzae* disease in Alaskan Eskimos: characteristics of a population with an unusual incidence of invasive disease. *Lancet*, **i**, 1281–1285.

Ward, J., Brenneman, G., Letson, G.W. *et al.* (1990) Limited efficacy of a *Haemophilus influenzae* type b conjugate vaccine in Alaska native infants. *New England Journal of Medicine*, **323**, 1393–1401.

White, D.C. and Granick, S. (1963) Haemin biosynthesis in *Haemophilus*. *Journal of Bacteriology*, **85**, 842–850.

Wilson, R., Roberts, D.E. and Cole, P.J. (1985) Effect of bacterial products on human ciliary function in vitro. *Thorax*, **40**, 125–131.

Wolin, H.L. (1963) Defined medium for *Haemophilus influenzae* type b. *Journal of Bacteriology*, **85**, 253–254.

9

BORDETELLA

R.C. Matthews and Noel W. Preston

INTRODUCTION

Small Gram-negative bacilli, associated with respiratory tract infections in man and animals, were classified for many years as *Haemophilus* because of their liking for blood in laboratory media. Indeed, many species of these organisms fail to grow on media devoid of blood components.

However, although the causative organism of pertussis (whooping cough) grows well on special media containing blood, and was designated *Haemophilus pertussis*, it does not need the growth factors X (haematin) and V (co-dehydrogenase) which are characteristic requirements in the genus *Haemophilus* (Hornibrook, 1940). From the 1960s, therefore, a new genus name (*Bordetella*, in honour of Bordet (Bordet and Gengou, 1906) who reported the first isolation in 1906) has been adopted for the whooping cough bacillus (*B. pertussis*) and related species (*B. parapertussis* and *B. bronchiseptica*).

CLASSIFICATION

Three species are placed by many taxonomists in the genus *Bordetella*. However, apart from being small Gram-negative rods which cause respiratory tract infections, and sharing a number of antigens, they are significantly different from each other phenotypically and genotypically.

Bordetella pertussis

By far the most important human pathogen in the genus is the usual causative organism of pertussis infection, from which the species name *B. pertussis* is derived. It is shorter and thinner than coliform organisms, but biochemical activity is very limited and is unhelpful in identification.

Normal habitat

There is no known animal or environmental reservoir of *B. pertussis*; natural infection occurs only in the human host, so it is potentially possible for the disease to be eradicated (see below). The main source of infection is the typical clinical case of pertussis (Thomas and Lambert, 1987). There is little evidence of symptom-free carriers (Anonymous, 1992); and, if the microbe cannot be isolated by efficient attempts at swabbing and culture, there must be little risk of transmission.

Bordetella parapertussis

A much less frequent cause of whooping cough is an antigenically related species designated *B.*

Principles and Practice of Clinical Bacteriology. Edited by A.M. Emmerson, P.M. Hawkey and S.H. Gillespie
© 1997 John Wiley & Sons Ltd

TABLE 9.1   COMPARISON OF *B. PERTUSSIS* and *B. PARAPERTUSSIS*

Property of species	B. pertussis	B. parapertussis
Incubation time for visible colonies	3 days	2 days
Growth on nutrient agar	None	Good
Pigment diffusing in medium	None	Brown
Slide agglutination with:		
pertussis antiserum	Strong	Weak
parapertussis antiserum	Weak	Strong
130 kb DNA fragment[a]	Present	Absent
Cause of whooping cough	Usual	Rare

[a] Conserved band after PFGE of *Xba* I-generated macrorestriction digests (see text).

parapertussis. This organism is readily distinguished from *B. pertussis* by its growth on nutrient agar in two days, with the production of a characteristic brown diffusible pigment (Table 9.1). A bacterial suspension from charcoal–blood–agar is agglutinated more strongly by parapertussis than by pertussis antiserum.

The epidemiology, diagnosis and treatment of infection with this species are the same as for *B. pertussis*, and will not be described separately. The incidence is so low, however, and the illness usually mild, that most countries have not felt the need to produce a prophylactic vaccine against it (Preston and Matthews, 1995).

Bordetella bronchiseptica

Colonies of this species are visible on nutrient agar after overnight incubation. It also differs from the other species by being motile and by producing an obvious alkaline reaction in the Hugh and Leifson medium which is used to differentiate oxidative from fermentative action on sugars. Hence, it is placed by some taxonomists in the genus *Alkaligenes*; however, it is distinguished readily from the intestinal commensal *Alkaligenes faecalis* by its rapid hydrolysis of urea.

Although it is rarely encountered in human infection, *B. bronchiseptica* is a common respiratory

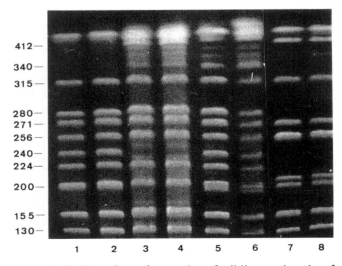

Figure 9.1. PFGE of *B. pertussis* isolates from four pairs of siblings, showing four different DNA types (lanes 1 and 2, 3 and 4, 5 and 6, 7 and 8 respectively); sizes of fragments (kb) on left (Khattak *et al.*, 1992). (Reproduced by permission of the *British Medical Journal*.)

pathogen of animals, especially laboratory stocks of rodents. Because it shares antigens with other species of *Bordetella*, animals must be checked for freedom from *Bordetella* antibody before they are used in the preparation of specific antisera. Sheep or donkeys, therefore, have sometimes been used in preference to rodents.

Genetic diversity of Bordetella *spp.*

The ready differentiation of the three species of *Bordetella* by their phenotypic properties is found also in their genetic diversity. Digestion of DNA with the rare-cutting enzyme *Xba* I followed by pulsed-field gel electrophoresis (PFGE) showed that

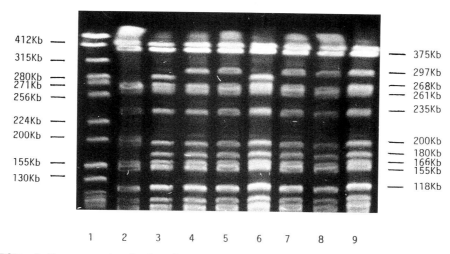

Figure 9.2. PFGE of *B. parapertussis* showing three DNA types (lanes 4, 5, 7–9; lanes 3 and 6; lane 2) compared with *B. pertussis* type 1 (lane 1) (Khattak and Matthews, 1993a). (Reproduced by permission of the American Society of Microbiology.)

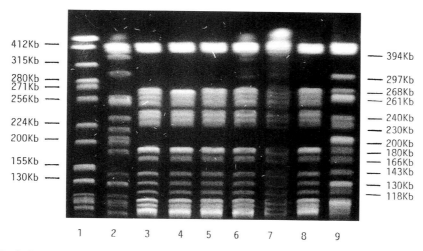

Figure 9.3. PFGE of *B. bronchiseptica* showing three DNA types (lanes 3–8; lane 2; lane 9) compared with *B. pertussis* type 1 (lane 1) (Khattak and Matthews, 1993a). (Reproduced by permission of the American Society of Microbiology.)

each produced species-specific macrorestriction profiles, with some variation between different isolates of the same species (Khattak and Matthews, 1993a) (Figures 9.1–9.3). Examination of 130 isolates of *B. pertussis* generated 21 types, with variable bands between 200 and 412 kb and a conserved band at 130 kb. *Bordetella parapertussis* (10 isolates) and *B. bronchiseptica* (eight isolates) each yielded three types but also had seven and five conserved bands respectively.

PATHOGENICITY

As with many other diseases, pertussis involves two stages: microbial colonization of the respiratory epithelium, and subsequent proliferation with tissue damage.

Colonization (Adhesion)

Ciliated epithelium of the respiratory tract is the main site of attachment of *B. pertussis*. Colonization is facilitated by the agglutinogens.

Agglutinogens

Strains of *B. pertussis* produce different combinations of three surface antigens (1, 2 and 3) which are detectable by bacterial agglutination with absorbed antisera and are therefore designated agglutinogens. Three serotypes cause human disease (types 1,2; 1,2,3; 1,3) and a degraded organism (type 1) can infect and kill mice.

Strains possessing agglutinogen 2 (types 1,2 and 1,2,3) are highly fimbriate, giving them a colonizing advantage in the respiratory tract. These serotypes predominate in non-vaccinated communities. The surface of type 1,3 organisms, however, is mainly agglutinogen 3; they are agglutinated only feebly by antibody to agglutinogen 1 (agglutinin 1). Hence, a child vaccinated with type 1,2 organisms can still be infected with type 1,3. Conversely, a child with only agglutinin 3 is still susceptible to type 1,2 infection. Thus, the prevalent serotype in vaccinated communities varies with the antigenic composition of the vaccine in use (Preston, 1988).

Figure 9.4 illustrates these features on bacteria which have been treated with antibody labelled with 10 nm gold particles (Preston *et al.*, 1990): Figure 9.4(a) shows gold particles along the bundles of agglutinated fimbriae on cells of serotype 1,2,3 treated with gold-labelled agglutinin 2; Figure 9.4(b) shows a non-fimbriate bacterium of serotype 1,3 labelled only on the cell surface after treatment with gold-labelled agglutinin 3.

However, non-fimbriate type 1,3 organisms can colonize in the presence of agglutinins 1 and 2,

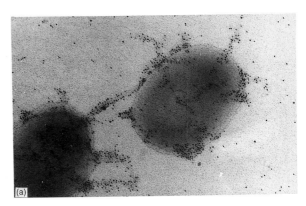

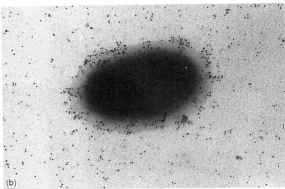

Figure 9.4. Immunoelectron microscopy of *B. pertussis* cells after application of antibody labelled with 10 nm gold particles. (a) Cells of serotype 1,2,3 with gold particles along the bundles of agglutinated fimbriae after treatment with gold-labelled agglutinin 2. (b) A non-fimbriate bacterium of serotype 1,3 labelled only on the cell surface after treatment with gold-labelled agglutinin 3. (Preston *et al.*, 1990). (Reproduced by permission of the Pathological Society of Great Britain and Ireland.)

suggesting that agglutinogen 3 is an alternative adhesin. Indeed, there is no known difference in virulence between these serotypes; but their different agglutinogen content leads to serotype-specific immunity, so that all three agglutinogens should be present in vaccine (Manclark, 1991).

Other putative adhesins are filamentous haemagglutinin (FHA) in association with pertussis toxin (PT) (Tuomanen, 1988) and a 69 kDa outer membrane protein (OMP) (Robinson and Ashworth, 1988). But these are found on all strains of *B. pertussis*, so a major protective role for them would be difficult to reconcile with past inadequacies of vaccine deficient in one or more of the type-specific agglutinogens (Preston, 1993). Moreover, a Swedish trial found no correlation between anti-FHA or anti-PT titres in vaccinated children and subsequent protection against pertussis (Ad hoc group, 1988). Also, although vaccination of mice with the 69 kDa OMP protects them against intracerebral challenge, there is no evidence that antibody to it has a protective role in the child (Robinson and Ashworth, 1988).

Toxins in Human Disease

Several toxins of *B. pertussis* have likely roles in pathogenesis (Goldman, 1988). A tracheal cytotoxin may paralyse the cilia of the respiratory epithelium, so that the airway has to be cleared by paroxysms of coughing. Adenylate cyclase may impair cell function by enhancing intracellular cyclic AMP. But pertussis is not an invasive disease: the target cells are those which the bacteria have colonized (Goldman, 1988), and there is little opportunity for neutralization of toxin between release from the bacteria and action on the respiratory epithelium. Antitoxic immunity alone cannot be expected to protect against pertussis. Protection has been shown to depend on the prevention of colonization by the type-specific agglutinins. Evidence of such serotype-specific immunity in children was first reported 30 years ago (Preston, 1963), and has persisted over three decades (Miller *et al.*, 1992; Preston and Carter, 1992).

The most widely discussed toxic product of this organism is one that is now called pertussis toxin (PT) (Preston, 1988). It has various effects in mice – producing lymphocytosis, hyperinsulinaemia, hypoglycaemia and sensitization to histamine. But in the human host, apart from a varied degree of lymphocytosis, there is little evidence of these metabolic disturbances (Furman *et al.*, 1988; Cherry *et al.*, 1988). Moreover, although vaccination with PT protects mice against experimental infection, anti-PT levels in vaccinated children do not correlate with immunity (Ad hoc group, 1988).

Animal Models of Disease

Marmosets and rabbits can be infected intranasally with fresh isolates of *B. pertussis* from human cases (Preston, 1988; Stanbridge and Preston, 1974; Preston *et al.*, 1980). Like the child, they exhibit catarrh, persistence of colonization in the nasopharynx for many weeks, change of serotype during colonization, and inability of the degraded type 1 organism to establish itself as the predominant serotype. Also, all three hosts produce a similar range of agglutinin response to vaccination, and active immunization shows evidence of serotype specificity.

The mouse brain model, which has been used internationally for over 40 years in the evaluation of pertussis vaccine potency, does not show these features and there is increasing recognition of its inadequacy (Manclark, 1991). Fresh clinical isolates of *B. pertussis* are avirulent in the mouse brain. Only a few atypical laboratory strains are virulent. Strain W.18–323 is the standard intracerebral challenge strain for mice and this is atypical both phenotypically and genotypically (Preston, 1988; Khattak and Matthews, 1993b). As the challenge strain can be of any serotype, including the degraded serotype 1, this potency test gives no assurance that the vaccine contains agglutinogens 2 and 3 which are necessary for human prophylaxis (Preston, 1993). Moreover, the mouse shows a more limited range of agglutinin response so that the serotype specificity of active immunity is not seen in this model (Preston, 1988), the common agglutinogen 1 apparently having a dominant role. However, by passive protection with individual agglutinins, type-specific immunity has been demonstrated even in mouse brain (Preston and Evans, 1963).

Because of the many differences between mouse and man, in bacterial pathogenicity and immune response, the mouse brain model is unreliable for determining which components of *B. pertussis* are necessary for active immunization of the child.

EPIDEMIOLOGY

In non-vaccinated communities, pertussis is a major cause of morbidity and mortality world-wide, being most severe in young children. The likelihood of becoming infected depends on the degree of contact: 80–90% for non-immune siblings exposed in the household, but less than 50% for non-immune child contacts at school. Although adults are susceptible to pertussis, the incidence is low, the illness is usually mild and atypical, and transmission of infection to others is infrequent (Anonymous, 1992). Most patients are children below the age of 15 years, and epidemics occur at intervals of about four years (Figure 9.5), reflecting the time necessary to build up a new susceptible population after the 'herd' immunity produced by an outbreak.

CLINICAL FEATURES

Whooping Cough

Pertussis (severe cough) is the dominant feature of a clinical condition that has been recognized for centuries, in which a child has many bouts of paroxysmal coughing each day, the bouts being characteristically more frequent during the night and followed by a long high-pitched inspiratory whoop (whooping cough) and vomiting. During a paroxysm, the tongue is protruded, fluid flows from the eyes, nose and mouth, and the face becomes increasingly cyanotic with an anoxia that may affect the brain. Such attacks are exhausting for both the patient and the parents but, in between, the child does not usually appear ill.

If a typical attack is witnessed, there may be little hesitation in reaching a clinical diagnosis of pertussis. It is in the first two years of life that the disease is most severe and sometimes lethal. However, the illness is often mild and atypical, especially in older children and adults, in younger children who have been incompletely immunized, and in very young infants partially protected by maternal antibody. In particular the whoop is often absent in young infants.

Even in typical cases, the characteristic paroxysmal stage is preceded by an incubation period of one to two weeks and a catarrhal stage of another one to two weeks of vague respiratory symptoms and occasional coughing. During this time the clinical diagnosis is uncertain, though the child is infectious.

Although a fatal outcome is usually avoided in countries where modern intensive care facilities are available, the severe coughing can cause long-term respiratory damage, and anoxia can lead to neurological sequelae.

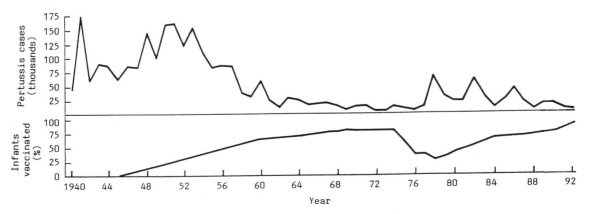

Figure 9.5. Pertussis in Britain since 1940 (Preston, 1993). (Reproduced by permission of Birkhauser Verlag.)

Pseudo-whooping Cough

In atypical cases, the laboratory has a vital role in diagnosis, because similar coughing may be caused by several other microbes including a variety of viruses, but that illness is usually mild and of shorter duration. The term 'pseudo-whooping cough' has been applied to such disease (Stott and Davis, 1981), because of the danger that false diagnosis may create a popular impression of pertussis as a trivial disease: 'in the absence of positive bacterial culture, whooping cough should not be diagnosed for an illness of less than three weeks' duration'. With genuine pertussis, the coughing is likely to persist for months rather than weeks.

DIAGNOSTIC METHODS

Bacterial Culture

There is broad agreement that the 'gold standard' for the diagnosis of pertussis is bacterial culture from nasopharyngeal specimens. Contrary to popular belief, such cultures yield positive results in as many as 80% of cases (Cherry et al., 1988), provided specimen collection and laboratory techniques are optimal (Anonymous, 1992).

Although the organisms are thriving on the ciliated epithelium of the lower respiratory tract, coughing brings them up to the nasopharynx, from which they can be recovered by a pernasal swab (Abbott et al., 1982). Postnasal throat swabs, or 'cough plates' held in front of the patient's mouth, give a poor yield because the slow-growing bordetellae are overgrown by the numerous commensal organisms. Approach through the nose, with a delicate and flexible pernasal swab, is a painless procedure which encounters only diphtheroid and staphylococcal commensals. These are usually readily suppressed by penicillin (0.25 u/ml) in the charcoal–blood–agar medium. If the patient has been exposed to penicillin, however, better inhibition of commensals may be achieved with cephalexin, 30 μg/ml. Higher concentrations of either antibiotic agent will suppress many strains of bordetellae. With the tip directed downwards and towards the mid-line, the pernasal swab is passed gently along the floor of the nose until it meets the resistance of the posterior wall of the nasopharynx (Figure 9.6). Practice with a co-operative adult may be helpful and, because the swab tickles the nose, a child's head must be held firmly to avoid jerking. Some staff may object to the technique because it often precipitates a paroxysm of coughing and subsequent vomiting but this actually helps to confirm the diagnosis and, at least, it is a bout which can be anticipated.

After withdrawal from the patient, the swab should be rubbed immediately onto a segment of charcoal–blood–agar and the Petri dish should then be returned to the laboratory for completion of 'plating' and incubation (see below). A minimum of seven days should be allowed before these cultures are discarded as negative. Various transport media have been recommended for transit of the swab to the laboratory, but these result in a decrease in the isolation rate attainable by inoculation of the plate at the bedside (Abbott et al., 1982).

A single swab may yield a negative culture, but

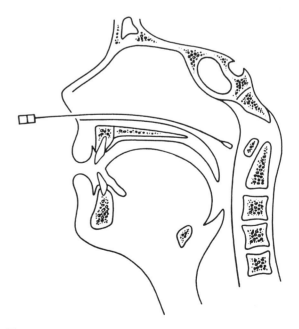

Figure 9.6. Pernasal swab obtaining sample of nasopharyngeal flora (Abbott *et al.*, 1982). (Reproduced by permission of the Association of Clinical Pathologists.)

the sensitivity of the technique is increased by taking specimens on several successive days. So rarely has a positive culture been obtained from a healthy person, other than one incubating the disease, that a false positive result by this method can be discounted (Preston, 1988). Although the densest bacterial growth is obtained during the catarrhal and early paroxysmal stages of the disease, colonies can still be grown from swabs taken up to three months from the onset, if coughing persists. So, contrary to popular belief, the infection can still be transmitted to non-immune contacts throughout this period.

Culture conditions

Bordetella pertussis does not grow on nutrient agar, and it fails to produce discrete colonies on ordinary blood agar. Bordet–Gengou medium contains starch and a high concentration of blood, to absorb toxic metabolites. It yields discrete colonies after incubation for three days (or longer on primary isolation). However, charcoal–blood–agar (in which the inclusion of absorbent charcoal allows the concentration of blood to be reduced to only 10%) gives smoother growth which is less prone to erroneous serological results (Abbott *et al.*, 1982; Preston, 1988).

The optimum growth temperature is 35–36 °C. The organism is a fairly strict aerobe requiring free access to air, and adequate humidity must be provided throughout the lengthy incubation (Abbott *et al.*, 1982). Colonies are convex, greyish white, with a shiny surface and butyrous consistency. Together with the microscopic morphology, the colonial appearance provides firm evidence of identity to an experienced worker, but confirmation should be sought with serology. A saline suspension of colonies is rapidly agglutinable with a polyvalent pertussis antiserum containing agglutinins 1, 2 and 3 (see above), but it agglutinates weakly or not at all with a parapertussis antiserum (depending on how thoroughly the latter has been cross-absorbed).

Typing

Because the serotypes of *B. pertussis* undergo spontaneous variation, even during the course of infection in a single host (Preston, 1988), this typing system cannot be used as an epidemiological tool.

Nevertheless, it is important that isolates from pertussis patients be sent to a national reference laboratory for serotyping by slide agglutination with antisera to the three agglutinogens (Preston, 1970). The prevalent serotype in a community is a useful guide to any deficiency in vaccine composition or immunization schedule (Preston, 1993).

In contrast, genetic fingerprinting by PFGE appears to be relatively stable (Khattak *et al.*, 1992). Isolates from pairs of siblings with whooping cough were indistinguishable from each other (Figure 9.1). Of the 21 types identified among 130 isolates, the three commonest types were DNA type 1 (31%), DNA type 2 (9%) and DNA type 3 (15%). The predominant type varied in different countries (Khattak *et al.*, 1992; Knowles *et al.*, 1993). In an outbreak in Montreal, type 5 predominated (30% of isolates) and an unusual new type emerged (20%) (Knowles *et al.*, 1993).

There is no apparent correlation between serotype and PFGE type. The latter is a much more costly and time-consuming technique and, unlike serotyping, is not used routinely. Unfortunately DNA fingerprints produced by frequent-cutting enzymes, which can be resolved by conventional agarose gel electrophoresis, have so far proved incapable of discriminating between strains of *B. pertussis*.

Antimicrobial Sensitivities

Although *B. pertussis* is sensitive to various antimicrobial agents *in vitro*, most of them have been found to be without therapeutic effect *in vivo*, possibly because of the superficial nature of the infection and the abundant mucous secretion. Sensitivity tests are therefore unhelpful. Erythromycin is usually considered to be the drug of choice.

Detection of Bacterial Antigens

Direct fluorescence

Direct fluorescent antibody testing of nasopharyngeal secretions has the theoretical advantage of detecting bacteria killed by previous antibiotic therapy but false negative results are likely if the organisms are scanty. More serious are false positive results with antigenically related organisms such as staphylococci, yeasts, haemophili, moraxellae and legionellae (Preston, 1988; Adamson *et al.*, 1989), some of which resemble bordetellae microscopically. The test antiserum against bordetellae should therefore be absorbed with these organisms; but appropriate reagents are not readily available, and this diagnostic method is therefore unreliable (Centers for Disease Control, 1990).

Counterimmunoelectrophoresis (CIE)

Antigens can also be detected in the serum and the urine by methods such as CIE (Boreland and Gillespie, 1984), but the specificity of these tests was not determined and reports on the sensitivity showed levels well below the 80% achievable by correct cultural procedures. A more recent CIE-based assay with a monoclonal antibody showed higher sensitivity but its specificity was uncertain as nearly half of the CIE-positive cases were culture negative (Boreland *et al.*, 1988).

Polymerase chain reaction (PCR)

A more promising approach may be the application of PCR to nasopharyngeal secretions from suspected cases. Using primers directed against a *Bordetella*-specific tandemly repeated sequence, 98 samples from 332 suspected cases were PCR positive and 66 culture positive (Glare *et al.*, 1990). As methods for avoiding false positives become more sophisticated, this approach may have some real clinical value though the cost implications are such that it is unlikely to replace culture.

Detection of *Bordetella* Antibody

Tests for antibody in sera and nasopharyngeal secretions have been widely used in the diagnosis of pertussis, especially in the USA. It is generally recognized, however, that the serological response to pertussis infection is often slow and weak, especially in very young children, so that false

negative results with serology can be expected in the early stages of illness when bacterial culture is most likely to be positive. Conversely, positive serological results are ambiguous, at any stage, because antigens are shared with other organisms (see above). Even with insensitive tests such as bacterial agglutination, pertussis antibodies are readily detected in the sera of healthy persons. The most helpful serological result, diagnostically, is a more than four-fold rise in antibody titre between samples taken two to three weeks apart, but this is not usually demonstrable unless the first sample is taken before the onset of the paroxysmal stage. More sensitive techniques such as enzyme-linked immunosorbent assay (against antigens such as FHA or PT, of uncertain purity – see below) are liable to increase the number of false positive results, and thus give unjustified respectability to a diagnosis which should actually be 'pseudo-whooping cough'.

There is a need for the specificity of any serological technique to be assessed by comparison with the 'gold standard' of bacterial culture.

Diagnostic Accuracy and Vaccine Efficacy

A false diagnosis of pertussis may be of little consequence to the individual patient because, sadly, there is no reliable therapy or antibiotic prophylaxis for contacts; and transmission is mainly from cases that are typical clinically (Thomas and Lambert, 1987). Much more serious is false diagnosis in trials to assess the efficacy of vaccines (which cannot be expected to protect against non-pertussis infection): as diagnostic accuracy increases, from clinical to serological to culture, so the reported efficacy of whole-cell pertussis vaccine rises from about 65% to 80% to 95% (Preston, 1988; Cherry *et al.*, 1988).

MANAGEMENT

Antimicrobial Therapy

When pertussis infection is well established, antibiotic agents have little or no clinical effect.

However, if erythromycin is given *before* the paroxysmal stage, the severity of the illness may be reduced. A minimum of 14 days' therapy is required (Bass, 1985), and this may eliminate the organisms and thus reduce the exposure of contacts. Shorter periods of treatment merely suppress the organism, and positive cultures can still be obtained.

Erythromycin is sometimes recommended for the prophylaxis of non-vaccinated infants, but it seems unrealistic to expect such treatment to be maintained for the several months that the older sibling or adult may remain infectious.

Fever may indicate secondary lung infection with other bacteria such as pyogenic cocci or *Haemophilus*, for which appropriate antibiotic therapy should be provided (see Chapters 1, 2 and 8).

Medical Support

Cyanosis and anoxia may be reduced by avoiding sudden noises, excitement or excessive medical examination, which tend to precipitate paroxysms; but mucus and vomit should be removed to avoid their inhalation. Cough suppressants, bronchodilators and corticosteroids have been used for prevention of paroxysms, but they may cause harm through retention of secretions. Pertussis immunoglobulin has been given, but with little evidence of benefit. This may be because these preparations have not been assessed for the presence of all three agglutinins. Lack of effective therapy for whooping cough emphasizes the great importance of the highest possible uptake of pertussis vaccine.

CONTROL

Isolation of the Patient and Prevention of Cross-infection

Large inocula of bacteria are disseminated during paroxysms of coughing so that transmission is thought to be mainly from typical cases of whooping cough amongst young children, rather than from the milder cases amongst older children and adults (Preston and Matthews, 1996a). However, because a patient is infectious before the most characteristic symptoms develop, and because the coughing may persist for many weeks or months when a child is no longer seriously ill, control of the disease by isolation is unrealistic.

Vaccines

Whole-cell vaccines

During the last half-century, suspensions of whole bacterial cells, killed by heat or chemicals, have been used worldwide. They should be adsorbed on to adjuvant, such as aluminium hydroxide, to enhance the immune response (especially important for agglutinogen 3) (Preston, 1988) and to minimize adverse reactions (Pollock *et al.*, 1984) (Table 9.2). As mentioned already, the vaccine should contain all three agglutinogens (Manclark, 1991); but, because the agglutinin 3 response is usually the weakest, type 1,3 organisms are the last to be eliminated from a community with an effective vaccination programme.

After three or more doses, the *efficacy* of the vaccine against accurately diagnosed pertussis infection (see above) is very high – about 95%. This emphasizes the importance, in vaccine trials, of optimal techniques for swabbing and bacterial culture, and the need for national and international reference facilities to confirm the identity of isolates and to type them.

The *safety* of pertussis vaccine was questioned repeatedly by the mass media in Britain, and some other countries, during the 1970s; and this led to a sharp decline in vaccine uptake (Figure 9.5). Despite continued improvement in the general health of the population, three large epidemics then followed before the slow restoration of confidence in the vaccine during the 1980s began to take effect. Minor reactions can be expected as

TABLE 9.2 ADSORBED PERTUSSIS VACCINE BETTER THAN PLAIN

Type of vaccine	Immune response	Adverse reactions
Plain (without adjuvant)	Weaker	More
Adsorbed (on to adjuvant)	Stronger	Less

part of the immune response (Preston, 1993) (they are reduced by the use of adsorbed vaccine) but the real concern was a possible association of pertussis vaccination with brain disorder. The National Childhood Encephalopathy Study (1981) showed a clustering of neurological disorders within seven days of vaccination. However, there was a corresponding decrease in the risk of disorder during the next 21 days: the vaccine merely 'brings out something that is to occur anyway but is just moved forward in time because of the immunization' (Cherry *et al.*, 1988). Moreover, subsequent analysis of the study's data revealed faulty categorization of some infants so that, even for the first seven days, there was no significant difference in recent vaccination between cases and controls (Bowie, 1990). It is time for pertussis vaccine encephalopathy to be recognized as 'the myth that it is' (Cherry, 1990; Wentz and Marcuse, 1991).

The only firm *contraindication* is a severe local or general reaction to a previous dose. A feverish illness (but not minor infections) is cause for postponement until the person is well. Previous neurological illness is reason to seek the advice of a paediatrician: for example, because pyrexia may follow vaccination, and so trigger convulsions, it may be wise to accompany the vaccine with a prophylactic antipyretic agent (Anonymous, 1990) in children with a history of febrile fits. Allergy is not a contraindication. There is no age limit: children who missed vaccination in infancy may receive the normal three-dose course; and it may sometimes be advisable to vaccinate adults such as obstetric and paediatric doctors and nurses (Anonymous, 1992).

Acellular vaccines

Although whole-cell pertussis vaccine is now seen as highly effective and very safe, the scares of the 1970s provoked intensive research on a component (acellular) vaccine from which potentially harmful toxins had been excluded. In Japan, extracts containing FHA and PT have constituted a vaccine which has been used for over 10 years, but without reliable evidence of efficacy there (Preston, 1993).

A trial of this vaccine in Sweden (Ad hoc group, 1988) showed only modest efficacy, unrelated to the anti-FHA or anti-PT titre in the vaccinees. Traces of agglutinins may have provided some immunity, but these were not assayed.

Other countries are developing vaccines containing agglutinogens (Miller *et al.*, 1992). However, acellular vaccine is likely to be more costly than whole-cell vaccine, and it would have to be tested in millions of children to show that it was no less safe and no less effective (Baxter and Gibbs, 1987). Such trials should really be made in at least two countries (Preston and Matthews, 1996b): one with a prevalence of serotype 1,2 infection, and one with serotype 1,3.

Vaccination schedules and herd immunity

Two doses of vaccine are not sufficient to provide a reliable degree of immunity, especially against type 1,3 infection: many such partially immunized children have developed culture-positive pertussis infection. Three doses, at monthly intervals during the first six months of life, give lasting immunity; but most countries recommend one or two further doses at 18 months and/or five years of age. An infant vaccination uptake of 85–90% over a period of 10–15 years provides a high level of population (or herd) immunity amongst the children who are the main source of pertussis infection. If the microbe dies before it finds a new susceptible host, infants too young for immunization are protected indirectly by this herd immunity, and the disease is virtually eliminated. By compulsory vaccination, with the first dose at three months of age, many countries of the Middle East and the former communist block of Eastern Europe achieved this goal (Preston, 1993).

However, the optimal age for the first dose is controversial. In spite of the effective development of herd immunity against diphtheria and poliomyelitis worldwide, and against pertussis in the above-mentioned areas, when the first dose has been given at three months, some countries have felt the urge to vaccinate children even earlier to reduce the incidence of infant deaths. However, a neonatal dose may not only give a poorer response, but be detrimental to the subsequent response at the usual age (Baraff *et al.*, 1984). Compared with starting at three months, a start at two months has given a weaker immune response (Booy *et al.*, 1992) either from the inhibitory effect of maternal antibody or from immunological immaturity. Evidence from the USA is unhelpful because most children are vaccinated much later than the recommended ages of two, four and six months (Alford *et al.*, 1992). In Canada, there is concern over serotype 1,3 pertussis infections occurring in some children who had actually received three doses starting at two months (Knowles *et al.*, 1993). In Britain, it is too soon to assess the long-term efficacy, against type 1,3 infection in particular, of a recently introduced schedule with doses at two, three and four months. However, preliminary evidence that the first dose is tending to be received at nearly three months (Ramsay *et al.*, 1993), rather than two months, may be good for herd immunity.

The problems of achieving effective herd immunity do not differ between developing and developed countries. Advocates of the vaccination of pregnant women, to provide young infants with passive immunity, merely complicate the situation by postponing to an unknown older age the time when the infant will be sufficiently free from maternal antibody to mount an effective immune response.

Vaccination incentives

Compulsory vaccination has been highly effective in many countries. A subtle form of compulsion, practised in the USA, requires up-to-date vaccination for school entry; but this has the disadvantage of leaving the majority unprotected until about five years of age (Alford *et al.*, 1992). Several countries have benefited from favourable publicity for vaccination by cooperation of the mass media (Preston, 1993). A shrewd incentive was adopted throughout Britain in 1990, whereby family doctors received payment for achieving target rates of vaccine uptake. After the previous influence of the mass media (Figure 9.5), recovery of vaccination

rates was peaking at little more than 80% nationally but the rate was over 90% by 12 months of age in 1993 (district range 79–98%) (Ritchie *et al.*, 1992; White *et al.*, 1993).

If high rates of effective vaccination of children can be achieved and maintained, this will gradually produce herd immunity among older siblings so that transmission to infants too young to have been vaccinated will be avoided, with virtual elimination of disease.

REFERENCES

Abbott, J.D., Macaulay, M.E. and Preston, N.W. (1982) Bacteriological diagnosis of whooping cough. ACP broadsheet 105. British Medical Association, London.

Adamson, P.C., Wu, T.C., Meade, B.D. *et al.* (1989) Pertussis in a previously immunized child with human immunodeficiency virus infection. *Journal of Pediatrics*, **115**, 589–592.

Ad hoc group for the study of pertussis vaccines (1988) Placebo-controlled trial of two acellular pertussis vaccines in Sweden. *Lancet*, **i**, 955–960.

Alford, D., Kelly, J., Halpin, T.J. *et al.* (1992) Retrospective assessment of vaccination coverage among school-aged children. *Morbidity and Mortality Weekly Report*, **41**, 103–107.

Anonymous (1990) Prophylactic paracetamol with childhood immunisation? *Drug and Therapeutics Bulletin*, **28**, 73–74.

Anonymous (1992) Pertussis: adults, infants, and herds. *Lancet*, **339**, 526–527.

Baraff, L.J., Leake, R.D. Burstyn, D.G. *et al.* (1984) Immunologic response to early and routine DTP immunization in infants. *Pediatrics*, **73**, 37–42.

Bass, J.W. (1985) Erythromycin for pertussis: probable reasons for past failures. *Lancet*, **ii**, 147.

Baxter, D.N. and Gibbs, A.C.C. (1987) How are the sub-unit pertussis vaccines to be evaluated? *Epidemiology and Infection*, **99**, 477–484.

Booy, R., Aitken, S.J.M., Taylor, S. *et al.* (1992) Immunogenicity of combined diphtheria, tetanus, and pertussis vaccine given at 2, 3 and 4 months versus 3, 5 and 9 months of age. *Lancet*, **339**, 507–510.

Bordet, J. and Gengou, O. (1906) Le microbe de la coqueluche. *Annals de L'Institut Pasteur, Paris*, **20**, 731–741.

Boreland, P.C. and Gillespie, S.H. (1984) Counter-immunoelectrophoresis in the diagnosis of whooping cough. *Journal of Clinical Pathology*, **37**, 950–951.

Boreland, P.C., Gillespie, S.H. and Ashworth, L.A.E. (1988) Rapid diagnosis of whooping cough using monoclonal antibody. *Journal of Clinical Pathology*, **41**, 573–575.

Bowie, C. (1990) Lessons from the pertussis vaccine court trial. *Lancet*, **335**, 397–399.

Centers for Disease Control (1990) Pertussis surveillance: United States, 1986–1988. *Morbidity and Mortality Weekly Report*, **39**, 57–66.

Cherry, J.D. (1990) Pertussis vaccine encephalopathy: it is time to recognize it as the myth that it is. *Journal of the American Medical Association*, **263**, 1679–1680.

Cherry, J.D., Brunell, P.A., Golden, G.S. *et al.* (1988) Report of the Task Force on pertussis and pertussis immunization 1988. *Pediatrics*, **81**, 939–984.

Furman, B.L., Sidey, F.M. and Smith, M. (1988) Metabolic disturbances produced by pertussis toxin. In *Pathogenesis and Immunity in Pertussis*. (ed. A.C. Wardlaw and R. Parton), pp. 147–172. Wiley, Chichester.

Glare, E.M., Paton, J.C., Premier, R.R. *et al.* (1990) Analysis of a repetitive DNA sequence from *Bordetella pertussis* and its application to the diagnosis of pertussis using the polymerase chain reaction. *Journal of Clinical Pathology*, **28**, 1982–1987.

Goldman, W.E. (1988) Tracheal cytotoxin of *Bordetella pertussis*. In *Pathogenesis and Immunity in Pertussis* (ed. A.C. Wardlaw and R. Parton), pp. 231–246. Wiley, Chichester.

Hornibrook, J.W. (1940) Nicotinic acid as a growth factor for *H. pertussis*. *Proceedings of the Society for Experimental Biology and Medicine*, **45**, 598–599.

Khattak, M.N. and Matthews, R.C. (1993a) Genetic relatedness of *Bordetella* species as determined by macrorestriction digests resolved by pulsed-field gel electrophoresis. *International Journal of Systematic Bacteriology*, **43**, 659–664.

Khattak, M.N. and Matthews, R.C. (1993b). A comparison of the DNA fragment patterns of the mouse-virulent challenge strains and clinical isolates of *Bordetella pertussis*. *Journal of Infection*, **27**, 119–124.

Khattak, M.N., Matthews, R.C. and Burnie, J.P. (1992) Is *Bordetella pertussis* clonal? *British Medical Journal*, **304**, 813–815.

Knowles, K., Lorange M., Matthews, R. *et al.* (1993) Serotyping of outbreak and vaccine strains of *Bordetella pertussis*. *Abstr. 33rd ICAAC*, New Orleans.

Manclark, C.R. (ed.) (1991) Proceedings of an informal consultation on the World Health Organization requirements for diphtheria, tetanus, pertussis and combined vaccines. DHHS publication no. (FDA) 91-1174. United States Public Health Service, Bethesda, MD.

Miller, E., Vurdien, J.E. and White, J.M. (1992) The epidemiology of pertussis in England and Wales. *Communicable Disease Report*, **2**, R152–154.

National Childhood Encephalopathy Study (1981) *Whooping cough: Reports from the Committee on Safety of Medicines and the Joint Committee on Vaccination and Immunisation*, pp. 79–169. HMSO, London.

Pollock, T.M., Miller, E., Mortimer, J.Y. *et al.* (1984) Symptoms after primary immunisation with DTP and with DT vaccine. *Lancet*, **ii**, 146–149.

Preston, N.W. (1963) Type-specific immunity against whooping-cough. *British Medical Journal*, **ii**, 724–726.

Preston, N.W. (1970) Technical problems in the laboratory diagnosis and prevention of whooping-cough. *Laboratory Practice*, **19**, 482–486.

Preston, N.W. (1988) Pertussis today. In *Pathogenesis and Immunity in Pertussis* (ed. A.C. Wardlaw and R. Parton), pp. 1–18. Wiley, Chichester.

Preston, N.W. (1993) Eradication by vaccination: the memorial to smallpox could be surrounded by others. *Progress in Drug Research*, **41**, 151–189.

Preston, N.W. and Carter, E.J. (1992) Serotype specificity of vaccine-induced immunity to pertussis. *Communicable Disease Report*, **2**, R155–156.

Preston, N.W. and Evans, P. (1963) Type-specific immunity against intracerebral pertussis infection in mice. *Nature*, **197**, 508–509.

Preston, N.W. and Matthews, R.C. (1995) Immunological and bacteriological distinction between parapertussis and pertussis. *Lancet*, **345**, 463–464.

Preston, N.W. and Matthews, R.C. (1996a) Transmission of pertussis: do adults have an important role? *Lancet*, **347**, 129.

Preston, N.W. and Matthews, R.C. (1996b) Components of acellular pertussis vaccines. *Lancet*, **347**, 764.

Preston, N.W., Timewell, R.M. and Carter, E.J. (1980) Experimental pertussis infection in the rabbit: similarities with infection in primates. *Journal of Infection*, **2**, 227–235.

Preston, N.W., Zorgani, A.A. and Carter, E.J. (1990) Location of the three major agglutinogens of *Bordetella pertussis* by immuno-electronmicroscopy. *Journal of Medical Microbiology*, **32**, 63–68.

Ramsay, M.E.B., Rao, M., Begg, N.T. *et al.* (1993) Antibody response to accelerated immunisation with diphtheria, tetanus, pertussis vaccine. *Lancet*, **342**, 203–205.

Ritchie, L.D., Bisset, A.F,, Russell, D. *et al.* (1992) Primary and preschool immunisation in Grampian: progress and the 1990 contract. *British Medical Journal*, **304**, 816–819.

Robinson, A. and Ashworth, L.A.E. (1988) Acellular and defined-component vaccines against pertussis. In *Pathogenesis and Immunity in Pertussis* (ed. A.C.

Wardlaw and R. Parton), pp. 399–417. Wiley, Chichester.

Stanbridge, T.N. and Preston, N.W. (1974) Experimental pertussis infection in the marmoset: type specificity of active immunity. *Journal of Hygiene (Cambridge)*, **72**, 213–228.

Stott, N.C.H. and Davis, R.H. (1981) Pertussis vaccination and pseudo whooping cough. *British Medical Journal*, **282**, 1871.

Thomas, M.G. and Lambert, H.P. (1987) From whom do children catch pertussis? *British Medical Journal*, **295**, 751–752.

Tuomanen, E. (1988) *Bordetella pertussis* adhesins. In *Pathogenesis and Immunity in Pertussis* (ed. A.C. Wardlaw and R. Parton), pp. 75–94. Wiley, Chichester.

Wentz, K.R. and Marcuse, E.K. (1991) Diphtheria–tetanus–pertussis vaccine and serious neurologic illness. *Pediatrics*, **87**, 287–297.

White, J.M., Leon, S. and Begg, N.T. (1993) 'COVER' (Cover of vaccination evaluated rapidly); 26 *Communicable Disease Report*, **3**, R117–118.

10

BRUCELLOSIS

E.J. Young

INTRODUCTION

Brucellosis is primarily a disease of animals (zoonosis), but it was first recognized for the illness it causes in humans. In 1859 Jeffery Allen Marston, an Assistant Surgeon in the Royal Artillery, reported the first reliable description of human brucellosis based on his personal experience with the disease. In 1886, Sir David Bruce, another British Army physician, isolated the organism later called *Brucella melitensis*, the causative agent of Malta fever as the disease was known, from postmortem spleen tissue. Between 1904 and 1907, the Mediterranean Fever Commission, established to investigate epidemic brucellosis in Malta, published landmark studies on the nature of the disease. In the Third Report (1905), Sir Themistocles Zammit, a Maltese physician, described that a large proportion of native goats were chronically infected with *B. melitensis* and shed organisms in their milk. Evidence that ingestion of fresh goat's milk was the mode of transmission of the disease from animals to man was detailed in the Seventh Report (1907).

In 1895, the Danish physician Bernhard Bang isolated *B. abortus* from cyetic tissues of cattle suffering contagious abortions. Human infection with the agent of Bang's disease was reported in the USA in 1922 by Keefer and in 1924 by Orpan in Great Britain; however, the relatedness of these organisms was not immediately recognized.

In 1914, Jacob Traum, a bacteriologist with the US Department of Agriculture, isolated *B. suis* from aborted swine, and four years later Alice Evans, an American bacteriologist, discovered a close taxonomic relationship between the agents of Malta fever and Bang's disease. Evans suggested that these bacteria formed a distinct genus, and she proposed the name *Brucella* to honour Bruce. The development of an agglutination test in 1897 by Sir Almroth Wright provided the means to diagnose brucellosis by measuring specific antibodies in the serum. The fourth species of *Brucella* capable of causing human infection was discovered in 1966 by the American virologist Leland Carmichael. He and his colleagues isolated *Brucella canis* from kennel-bred dogs suffering contagious abortions.

DESCRIPTION OF THE ORGANISM

Morphology

Brucella are small, Gram-negative coccobacilli which lack flagella, endospores or capsules. *Brucella melitensis*, *B. abortus*, *B. suis* and *B.*

Principles and Practice of Clinical Bacteriology. Edited by A.M. Emmerson, P.M. Hawkey and S.H. Gillespie
© 1997 John Wiley & Sons Ltd

neotomae are naturally smooth organisms, whereas *B. canis* and *B. ovis* are naturally rough. When cultured *in vitro*, especially in liquid media, smooth to rough variation can occur spontaneously.

The cell wall consists of an outer layer of lipopolysaccharide–protein approximately 9 mm thick. Thin-section electron micrographs reveal an electron-dense layer 3–5 nm thick consisting of a highly cross-linked muramyl-mucopeptide complex associated with lipoproteins. Matrix and porin proteins penetrate the peptidoglycan layer at irregular intervals. A low-density periplasmic space separates the peptidoglycan layer from the cell membrane.

Classification

The genus *Brucella* contains six nomen species which are classified according to their principal animal hosts. Strains within the species *B. melitensis*, *B. abortus* and *B. suis* which vary in their biochemical reactions, and in some cases in preferred host species, are further subdivided into biotypes or biovars (Table 10.1). However, taxonomic studies using DNA–DNA and DNA–rRNA hybridization indicate that the genus should be reclassified to comprise a single species, *B. melitensis*, with other nomen species classified as biovars (Verger *et al.*, 1985). Nevertheless, by current convention the original nomen species scheme is generally retained for epidemiological

considerations. In fact, genomic fingerprints and restriction fragment length polymorphisms of conserved gene loci indicate that the present taxonomy is relevant. The omp2 locus is conserved in all the *Brucella* spp. and complete sequence analysis of this locus has revealed nucleotide differences among the species (Ficht *et al.*, 1990; Marquis and Ficht, 1993). Phylogenetically *Brucella* spp. appear to have a common origin with free-living, soil-dwelling bacteria. Based on 5S and 16S rRNA sequences, *Brucella* is now included in the α_2 group of the family Proteobacteriaceae together with *Agrobacterium tumefacium* and *Rochalimeae quintana* (Moreno *et al.*, 1990; Minnick and Stiegler, 1993).

Genetics

Studies using restriction endonuclease techniques suggest that *B. melitensis* contains two independent chromosomes (Michaux *et al.*, 1993). Although much remains to be learned, the genes for structural proteins (Ficht *et al.*, 1989) and functional enzymes (Bricker *et al.*, 1990; Essenberg *et al.*, 1993) have been cloned. Naturally occurring plasmids or temperate bacteriophages have not been found among *Brucella* spp. The reason for this is unclear; however, recent studies have shown that under laboratory conditions the brucellae can accept plasmids from strains of bacteria of other genera, and that they are stable

TABLE 10.1 PATHOGENICITY OF *BRUCELLA* SPECIES AND BIOVARS

Nomen Species	Biovars	Preferred hosts	Pathogenicity for man
B. melitensis	1, 2, 3	Goats, sheep	High
B. abortus	1–6, 9	Cattle	Moderate
B. suis	1	Swine	High
	2	Swine	Low
	3	Swine	High
	4	Reindeer, caribou	Moderate
	5	Rodents	High
B. canis	None	Dogs	Moderate/Low
B. ovis	None	Sheep	None
B. neotomae	None	Desertwood rats	None

over many generations even after passage in animals (Verger *et al.*, 1993).

PATHOGENESIS

Antigens

O-Polysaccharide

A variety of surface and cytoplasmic antigens of *Brucella* have been identified. The major surface component is endotoxin, which in smooth strains consists of a somatic *O*-polysaccharide linked via a core oligosaccharide to lipid A, which anchors the molecule in the outer cell membrane. The immunodominant epitopes of the smooth lipopolysaccharide (sLPS) reside within the *O*-side chain and include the A and M antigens described by Wilson and Miles (1932). The structure of the *B. abortus* *O*-polysaccharide (A epitope) consists of an unbranched, linear homopolymer of α-(1,2)-linked *N*-formylperosamine residues (Caroff *et al.*, 1984a). This polysaccharide is essentially identical to the *O*-side chain of *Yersinia enterocolitica* $O:9$, which accounts for the cross-reactions between these organisms (Caroff *et al.*, 1984b). The structure of the *B. melitensis* *O*-polysaccharide (M epitope) is closely related to that of *B. abortus*; however, the linear polymer is made up of repeating units composed of five *N*-formyl pentosaminyl residues, four of them being α-(1,2) and one α-(1,3)-linked (Bundle *et al.*, 1987).

Lipid A

Unlike the endotoxins from Enterobacteriaceae which separate into the aqueous phase of phenol/water extracts, *Brucella* endotoxin is recovered from the phenol phase. The lipid A of *Brucella* LPS is characterized by a large proportion of long-chain saturated fatty acids ($>C_{16}$), very small amounts of hydroxylated fatty acids, no —OH myristic acid, and a proportion of amide- and ester-linked fatty acids that is different from that in enterobacteria such as *Escherichia coli* (Moreno *et al.*, 1979). *Brucella* endotoxin also differs from enterobacterial endotoxins in some of its biological

activities. For example, it is only weakly pyrogenic for rabbits, does not induce the dermal Shwartzman reaction, and is many times less potent in eliciting interleukin 1 (IL-1) and TNF-α from human monocytes (Goldstein *et al.*, 1992). Paradoxically, *Brucella* endotoxin is less toxic than enterobacterial endotoxins for LPS-responsive (C_3H/HeN) mice, but is more toxic for LPS-hyporesponsive (C_3H/HeJ) mice (Moreno *et al.*, 1981).

Host Defences

Route of infection

Intact skin is an effective barrier to the entry of *Brucella*, but even minute abrasions can permit the ingress of viable bacteria. The low pH of gastric juice provides some protection against oral infection, and antacids or histamine-blocking drugs appear to increase susceptibility to brucellosis (Steffen, 1977). Normal human serum has moderate anti-*Brucella* activity, and complement opsonizes organisms for phagocytosis. Human neutrophils destroy some *Brucella* strains, but they lack activity against *B. melitensis* (Young *et al.*, 1985). Bacteria that escape killing by neutrophils enter the lymphatics, where they localize within organs rich in elements of the reticuloendothelial system (RES). Initially, *Brucella* survive and even replicate within macrophages of the RES.

Immune response

Recovery from intracellular infection depends upon the interaction between macrophages and specifically sensitized thymic lymphocytes by a process that is only partially understood (Smith, 1990). Processed bacterial antigen is expressed on the macrophage membrane in association with major histocompatibility complex (MHC) class II determinants resulting in the release of cytokines and enhanced intracellular bacteriolysis (Splitter and Everlith, 1986; Jiang and Baldwin, 1993). Interferon γ (INF-γ) is believed to be an important mediator of acquired cellular resistance against facultative intracellular pathogens, and treatment of mice with anti-INF-γ monoclonal antibodies results in increased growth of *Brucella* in the tissues of mice (Zhan and Cheers, 1993). Although humoral antibodies appear to play some role in resistance to *Brucella*, cell-mediated immunity appears to be the principal mechanism of recovery. In studies in cattle with natural resistance to bovine brucellosis, mammary macrophages and blood monocyte-derived macrophages were shown to control intracellular replication of *B. abortus* significantly better than mononuclear phagocytes from susceptible cattle (Price *et al.*, 1990).

Intracellular survival

Brucella spp. are facultative intracellular pathogens which have evolved mechanisms to evade destruction by phagocytic cells of the host. Although these mechanisms are poorly understood, several virulence factors have been proposed. *O*-Polysaccharide is considered important, since smooth strains of brucellae resist phagocytosis and killing more effectively than rough strains. Furthermore, *B. abortus* LPS and lipid A are less active than enterobacterial endotoxins in activating nitroblue tetrazolium reduction and lysozyme release in human neutrophils (Rasool *et al.*, 1992). In addition, virulent strains of *B. abortus* contain a copper–zinc superoxide dismutase which converts oxygen radicals to hydrogen peroxide and oxygen (Tatum *et al.*, 1992). Two nucleotide-like substances (5'-guanosine monophosphate and adenine) have been recovered from culture filtrates of *B. abortus* which suppress iodinization of the myeloperoxidase–H_2O_2–halide killing mechanism of neutrophils (Canning *et al.*, 1986). Whether similar adaptations to the intracellular milieu operate among other *Brucella* spp. is unknown.

EPIDEMIOLOGY

Brucellosis exists worldwide in domestic and wild animals, and is especially prevalent in countries bordering the Mediterranean, throughout the Arabian Gulf, the Indian subcontinent, and in parts of Mexico, Central and South America. *Brucella abortus* occurs primarily in cattle and other bovidae, such as buffalo and yaks. Goats and sheep are the preferred hosts of *B. melitensis*, although in some countries camels may be a reservoir. *Brucella suis* biovars 1–3 are found in swine, whereas, biovar 4 is confined to reindeer and caribou. *Brucella canis* occurs in dogs, especially under conditions of intense, confined breeding. Pathogenicity of *B. canis* for man is low and infections have occurred primarily among laboratory workers. *Brucella ovis*, an ovine pathogen, and *Brucella neotomae*, which has been isolated infrequently from desert wood rats, are not known to cause disease in man.

Animals remain chronically infected, with organisms localized in reproductive organs, resulting in abortions and sterility. *Brucella* are shed in large quantities in the animal's milk, urine, faeces, and in cyetic products. Persons in contact with diseased animals, such as farmers, veterinarians and abattoir workers, can contract brucellosis from direct inoculation through abrasions in the skin, via the conjunctivae of the eyes, and from inhalation of infected aerosols. Laboratory-acquired infections have been reported among personnel handling cultures of *Brucella*. Ingestion of dairy products, such as fresh cheese prepared from the milk of infected animals, is probably the most common source of human infection with *B. melitensis*, and may occur in persons who have had no direct contact with animals (Young, 1983). Human-to-human transmission of brucellosis is extremely rare, although *Brucella* has been recovered from banked human spermatozoa, so the potential for venereal transmission exists (Vandercam *et al.*, 1990).

CLINICAL FEATURES

Presentation

The onset of symptoms of human brucellosis can be acute or insidious, and the manifestations are protean. Patients present with non-specific complaints, such as malaise, anorexia, fatigue, weight loss, joint pains and depression. Objective physical abnormalities are few; notably fever, lymphadenopathy and occasionally hepatosplenomegaly. Fever is present in the majority of patients with active infection. Patients infected with *B. melitensis* may demonstrate an undulant fever pattern if followed for a sufficient time without intervention with antibiotics or antipyretics. When dealing with patients suspected of brucellosis, clinicians should attempt to elicit a history of animal exposure, travel to endemic countries, or ingestion of 'exotic' foods, such as dairy products prepared from raw milk. Brucellosis can involve any organ system, especially those rich in elements of the RES, such as lymph nodes, spleen, liver and bone marrow.

Nervous System

Depression and mental inattention are common findings in brucellosis, but direct invasion of the central nervous system occurs in less than 5% of cases. *Brucella* meningitis can be acute or chronic, and there is little to distinguish it from other forms of lymphocytic meningitis. Peripheral nervous system complications include neuropathy, neuritis and radiculitis.

In spite of adequate treatment and no objective evidence for relapse or localized complications, a small percentage of patients will experience a delayed recovery from brucellosis. Such patients generally continue to complain of the same symptoms that afflicted them during the acute stages of the disease. Chronic fatigue is the hallmark of this condition, which is generally attributed to a premorbid neurosis (Spink, 1951). Often the presence of low titres of brucella antibodies suggests that these patients suffer from chronic brucellosis; however, rarely do they improve with additional antibiotic therapy. The management of such patients is particularly difficult when there are potential financial or other gains to be derived from pending industrial or occupational injury claims.

Skeletal System

Osteoarticular complications of brucellosis are common, occurring in 20–60% of cases (Mousa *et al.*, 1987). Sacroiliitis is the most frequent joint manifestation, affecting patients of all ages, and usually occurring in association with systemic signs of brucellosis (Gotuzzo *et al.*, 1982; Ariza *et al.*, 1993). In the absence of a positive culture, the diagnosis can be delayed because X-rays and radionuclide bone scans may be negative during the early stages of infection. Eventually, blurring of the joint space is evident, and brucella serological tests are uniformly positive.

Arthritis of peripheral joints is the next most frequent complication, principally involving large joints, such as the hips, knees and ankles. Spondylitis is reported in less than 4% of cases (Ariza *et al.*, 1985), and is principally a disease of older men. Radiographic changes appear months after the onset of infection, whereas radionuclide bone scans typically show areas of increased uptake. The earliest lesions on radiographs is sclerosis and epiphysitis of the anterosuperior angle of the vertebra. This progresses to narrowing of the disk space and eventually vertebral osteomyelitis. Computed tomography is particularly useful for documenting bone destruction and for determining the condition of the spinal canal and paravertebral soft tissue (Tekkok *et al.*, 1993). The osteoarticular manifestations of brucellosis respond to antimicrobial therapy without sequelae and surgery is reserved for drainage of rare paraspinal abscesses.

Gastrointestinal System

Brucellosis resembles typhoid fever, with systemic symptoms predominating over gastrointestinal complaints. Nevertheless, more than two-thirds of patients complain of nausea, anorexia, vomiting, weight loss and abdominal discomfort. Inflammation of Peyer's patches, the ileal and colonic mucosa have been described. The liver is probably always involved; however, liver function tests are usually only mildly elevated. The spectrum of histological lesions of the liver are varied depending in part on the infecting *Brucella* species. Non-specific mononuclear cell infiltrates, granulomas and abscesses have each been reported. Cholecystitis, pancreatitis and peritonitis are rare complications.

Cardiovascular System

Endocarditis occurs in less than 2% of cases, but accounts for the majority of brucellosis-related deaths. The aortic valve is infected most often and aneurysms of the sinus of Valsalva are common. Myocarditis, pericarditis and infected aortic aneurysms have been reported.

Respiratory System

A variety of pulmonary complications have been reported, including bronchitis, pneumonia, lung nodules, abscesses and empyema.

Genitourinary System

With appropriate methods *Brucella* can be isolated from urine; however, urinary tract lesions are rare. Interstitial nephritis, glomerulonephritis, pyelonephritis and IgA nephropathy have been described. Unilateral orchitis is common in men. Abortion can occur in pregnant women; however, the incidence is no greater in brucellosis than in other bacteraemic infections. Pregnant women can be treated successfully if the disease is diagnosed early.

LABORATORY DIAGNOSIS

Bacteriological Diagnosis

The diagnosis of brucellosis is made with certainty when brucellae are grown from blood or other tissues.

Isolation

Brucella can be cultured in any high-quality peptone-based media, but growth is enhanced by the addition of blood or serum. They grow aerobically, but *B. ovis* and some biovars of *B. abortus* require an atmosphere of 10% carbon dioxide for primary isolation. Primary isolation of *Brucella* from clinical samples may require prolonged incubation.

Cultures of bone marrow are reported to have a higher yield than peripheral blood (Gotuzzo *et al.*,

1986). A biphasic medium (Casteneda's method) is also said to increase the yield without the need for subcultures. *Brucella* spp. grow relatively slowly *in vitro*, especially on primary isolation; however, rapid isolation methods have shortened the recovery times from weeks to days with a yield near 80% (Arnow *et al.*, 1984). Many clinical laboratories now employ the BACTEC system, which relies on the detection of $^{14}CO_2$ produced by ^{14}C-labelled substrate. Using seeded samples of *B. melitensis* an inverse linear relationship was found between the log of the initial concentration of bacteria and the time to detection in the BACT/ALERT system (Solomon and Jackson, 1992). Moreover, seeded cultures of *B. abortus* required several days longer to detect when small inocula were used in the BACTEC NR730 system (Zimmerman *et al.*, 1990). Studies comparing BACTEC systems with lysis concentration techniques indicate comparable rates of recovery, but shorter isolation times with the latter method (Etemadi *et al.*, 1984; Kolman *et al.*, 1991; Navas *et al.*, 1993). A rapid diagnostic test using synthetic oligonucleotides as primers in the polymerase chain reaction (PCR) has been devised (Fekete *et al.*, 1992; Herman and de Ridder, 1992).

Regardless of the method used, clinicians are urged to notify the laboratory that brucellosis is suspected so that cultures are not discarded prematurely and that appropriate precautions are taken to protect personnel (for example, ACDP Category 3 containment).

Identification

Brucella is always catalase positive, but oxidase and urease activities and H_2S production are variable. Differentiation of *Brucella* spp. is accomplished by selective inhibition of growth on media containing dyes, such as thionin and basic fuchsin, agglutination by monospecific antisera, oxidation of various substrates, and lysis by brucellaphages (Tables 10.2 and 10.3).

The identification of *Brucella* spp. and biovars is best left to reference laboratories equipped with biological safety cabinets for the protection of personnel. Many clinical laboratories now employ

TABLE 10.2   CHARACTERISTICS OF *BRUCELLA* SPECIES AND BIOVARS

Nomen species	Biovars	Requirement for CO_2	Production of H_2S	Urease activity	Growth on media containing dyes[a]		Agglutination by monospecific antiserum[b]		
					Thionin	Basic fuchsin	A	M	R
B. melitensis	1	−	−	Variable	+	+	−	+	−
	2	−	−	Variable	+	+	+	−	−
	3	−	−	Variable	+	+	+	+	−
B. abortus	1	(+)	+	Slow	−	+	+	−	−
	2	(+)	+	Slow	−	−	+	−	−
	3	(+)	+	Slow	+	+	+	−	−
	4	(+)	+	Slow	−	(+)	−	+	−
	5	−	−	Slow	+	+	−	+	−
	6	−	(+)	Slow	−	+	+	−	−
	9	−	+	Slow	+	+	−	+	−
B. suis	1	−	+	Rapid	+	(−)	+	−	−
	2	−	−	Rapid	+	−	+	−	−
	3	−	−	Rapid	+	+	+	−	−
	4	−	−	Rapid	+	(−)	+	+	−
	5	−	−	Rapid	+	−	−	+	−
B. canis		−	−	Rapid	+	−	−	−	+
B. ovis		+	−	−	+	(−)	−	−	+
B. neotomae		−	+	Rapid	−	−	+	−	−

+, positive; −, negative; (+), most strains positive; (−), most strains negative.
[a] Dye concentration, 20 μg/ml.
[b] A, monospecific for *B. abortus* A antigen; *M*, monospecific for *B. melitensis* M antigen; R, monospecific for rough *Brucella* antigen.

TABLE 10.3   OXIDATIVE METABOLISM AND BACTERIOPHAGE LYSIS OF *BRUCELLA* SPECIES AND BIOVARS

Nomen species		L-Alanine	L-Aspargine	L-Glutamic acid	L-Arginine	L-Citruline	DL-Ornithine	L-Lysine	D-Ribose	D-Xylose	D-Galactose	D-Glucose	i-Erythnitol	Lysis at RTD by bacteriophage[a]		
														Tb	Wb	Bk
B. melitensis	1, 2, 3	+	+	+	−	−	−	−	−	−	−	+	+	NL	NL	L
B. abortus	1–6, 9	+	+	+	−	−	−	−	+	−	+	+	+	L	L	L
B. suis	Biovar 1	±	−	−	+	+	+	+	+	+	+	+	+	NL	L	L
	Biovar 2	−	±	±	+	+	+	−	+	+	+	+	+	NL	L	L
	Biovar 3	±	−	+	+	+	+	+	+	+	−	+	+	NL	L	L
	Biovar 4	−	−	+	+	+	+	+	+	+	−	+	+	NL	L	L
	Biovar 5	−	+	+	+	+	+	+	+	+	−	+	+	NL	L	L
B. canis		±	−	+	+	+	+	+	+	−	±	+	±	NL	NL	NL
B. ovis		±	+	+	−	−	−	−	−	−	−	−	−	NL	NL	NL
B. neotomae		±	+	+	−	−	−	−	±	−	+	+	+	NL	L	L

+, oxidized by all strains; −, not oxidized by any strain; ±, oxidized by some strains.
[a] L, lysis; NL, no lysis at routine test dilution (RTD) by *Brucella* phages; Tb, Tblisi; Wb, Weybridge; Bk, Berkeley.

rapid identification systems based on patterns of biochemical profiles. Such automated identification systems should be used with caution, because characteristics of *Brucella* spp. have not been incorporated into the databases of some commercial rapid identification systems, and isolates of brucellae have been misidentified as *Morxella* spp. or *Haemophilus* spp. (Peiris *et al.*, 1992; Barham *et al.*, 1993).

Serological Diagnosis

In the absence of a positive culture, a presumptive diagnosis of brucellosis can be made by demonstrating the presence of high or rising titres of antibodies to *Brucella* in the serum. The immune response in brucellosis is characterized by an initial rise in IgM isotype antibodies commencing approximately one week after infection. By the second week a switch to IgG synthesis occurs, after which both classes of immunoglobulins continue to rise. Following antimicrobial therapy, the titre falls slowly, with IgG declining faster than IgM. Low levels of IgM antibodies can persist for months to years after infection and do not necessarily indicate persistent disease (Gazapo *et al.*, 1989). If the level of IgG antibodies does not fall, or is found to increase, chronic localized infection or relapse should be considered (Ariza *et al.*, 1992a).

Standard agglutination test

A variety of serological tests have been used to measure antibodies to *Brucella*; however, the serum agglutination test (SAT) remains the standard against which other tests are compared (Young, 1991). The SAT measures the total quantity of agglutinating antibodies (IgM plus IgG), and does not differentiate between immunoglobulin classes. To determine the titre of IgG antibodies, serum is treated with a disulphide-reducing agent (e.g. 2-mercaptoethanol or dithiothreitol), which destroys the agglutinability of IgM but does not alter IgG (Buchanan and Faber, 1980).

The standard SAT antigen is prepared from *B. abortus* strain 19, and it detects antibodies against all the major species (*B. abortus*, *B. melitensis*

and *B. suis*). This antigen will not detect antibodies against *B. canis*, which is a naturally rough species lacking sLPS. Owing to shared epitopes, cross-reactions can occur with antibodies to *Vibrio cholerae*, *F. tularensis*, and *Yersinia enterocolitica* serotype O:9; however, the titres are generally low and do not confound the diagnosis.

The majority of patients with active brucellosis will have SAT titres $\geq 1:160$, with a portion of the antibody being IgG. However, no single titre is *always* diagnostic, depending in part on the stage of illness or prior exposure to *Brucella*. Therefore, regardless of the serological test used, the results must be analysed in light of epidemiological, clinical and other laboratory information (Young, 1991).

Alternative techniques

Other serological tests have been devised to measure antibodies to *Brucella*, including a very sensitive enzyme-linked immunosorbent assay (ELISA). Unfortunately, no standardized *Brucella* antigen preparation exists for the ELISA, making comparisons of results between laboratories difficult.

MANAGEMENT

Antimicrobial Sensitivity

Numerous antimicrobial agents are active *in vitro* against *Brucella*, but a relative few are effective in treating human brucellosis (Hall, 1990). The tetracyclines, especially long-acting analogues such as doxycycline and minocycline, remain the drugs of choice; however, clinical relapse unrelated to antibiotic resistance has led to a preference for combination drug therapy (Montejo *et al.*, 1993).

The diagnosis of brucellosis should be confirmed by recovering the causative agent or by demonstrating high titres of specific antibodies in the serum. Not all patients will require hospitalization; however, those with severe symptoms and those with life-threatening complications are best treated in hospital. Antimicrobial chemotherapy must be continued for a minimum of six weeks (Joint FAO/WHO Report, 1986). Patients should be encouraged to continue therapy even after symptoms have resolved, as failure to complete a full course of treatment is the most common cause of relapse.

Traditionally, tetracycline (500 mg orally four times a day for six weeks) plus streptomycin (1 g intramuscularly once daily for two to three weeks) was the preferred combination. Recently, generic tetracycline has been replaced by doxycycline (100 mg orally twice daily for six weeks) because of the reduced dosage and lower incidence of adverse reactions. Although the addition of rifampicin (600–1200 mg orally per day) appears to be equally effective (Ariza et al., 1992b), many authorities still prefer the combination of doxycycline and an aminoglycoside. Gentamicin has largely replaced streptomycin, and is usually given in a dose of 5 mg/kg intramuscularly in divided doses for the first 10–14 days of therapy. Laboratory studies have shown that the addition of an aminoglycoside to other agents produces a more rapid killing of Brucella in vitro (Rubinstein et al., 1991).

The fixed combination of trimethoprim/sulphamethoxazole (TMP/SMZ) has also been used to treat brucellosis, but high rates of relapse have been reported unless the drug is continued for three to six months. Nevertheless, TMP/SMZ has certain advantages, such as the treatment of pregnant women or young children, for whom the tetracyclines are contraindicated because of the risk of staining deciduous teeth.

Fluoroquinolone compounds also have anti-Brucella activity in vitro, but are complicated by a high rate of relapse and possibly the selection of resistant strains. For this reason, quinolones, as in the case of rifampicin, are best reserved as adjunctive therapy to be used in combination with a tetracycline.

Treatment of complications

Patients with evidence of meningitis should have computed tomography of the brain followed by lumbar puncture. Although Brucella is rarely recovered from cerebrospinal fluid (CSF), the presence of specific antibodies in CSF is sufficient evidence of neurobrucellosis. Treatment of neurobrucellosis should continue for three to six months. Patients with Brucella endocarditis may not be cured with antimicrobial chemotherapy alone, and valve replacement surgery may be required.

Prognosis

Before the advent of effective antimicrobial therapy, brucellosis was a chronic, relapsing disease with a mortality of about 2%. Although serious illness can be caused by any Brucella spp., B. melitensis is generally the most virulent and accounts for the majority of fatalities. Life-threatening complications include infection of the central nervous system and the heart (Mousa et al., 1988; Lulu et al., 1988).

With appropriate treatment, the majority of patients with brucellosis recover uneventfully, although some will experience a prolonged remission of symptoms. Chronic brucellosis, defined as symptoms persisting for more than 12 months after diagnosis (Spink 1951), is now uncommon. Relapses generally occur before 12 months and are associated with persistently high titres of IgG antibodies and/or positive blood cultures. Chronic localized infections, such as osteomyelitis or deep tissue abscesses, are also characterized by elevated titres of antibody and positive cultures from the infection site. However, the majority of patients with persistent non-specific complaints lack objective evidence of infection and are thought to suffer from psychoneuroses.

PREVENTION

The prevention of human brucellosis depends on the elimination of the disease from domestic animals. In the USA the Cooperative State/Federal Brucellosis Eradication Program is credited with the control of bovine brucellosis (Brown, 1977; Nicoletti, 1980). This programme mandates the identification of infected herds through serological testing, quarantine of reactors, slaughter of infected animals, and protection of non-reactors by immunization. Following the Second World War mandatory pasteurization of milk for human consumption further ensured protection of the milk supply. An effective vaccine exists for cattle (*B. abortus* strain 19); however, it can induce a transient rise in antibodies in uninfected animals and is capable of causing disease if accidentally injected into humans.

In countries where *B. melitensis* is enzootic the control of caprine and ovine brucellosis is complicated by the nomadic grazing habits of goats (Escalante and Held, 1969). Uncontrolled importation of animals from brucella enzootic areas has been shown to impact on the incidence of brucellosis in animals and man (Hafez, 1986). Since fresh unpasteurized goat's milk cheese is the principal vehicle for transmitting *B. melitensis*, physicians in countries where the brucellosis is controlled or eradicated must be alert to the possibility of contaminated foods imported from brucella enzootic areas (Young and Suvannoparrat, 1975; Thapar and Young, 1986). In recent years ingestion of imported unpasteurized goat milk products has accounted for the majority of cases of human brucellosis in the state of Texas (Taylor and Perdue, 1989). An effective vaccine exists for goats and sheep (*B. melitensis* strain Rev-1), but it has the same shortcomings as the vaccine for *B. abortus*.

Infection with *B. suis* is primarily an abattoir-associated disease (Buchanan *et al.*, 1974) and no effective vaccine exists for the immunization of swine.

REFERENCES

Ariza, J., Gudiol, F., Valverde, J. *et al.* (1985) Brucellar spondylitis: a detailed analysis based on current findings. *Reviews of Infectious Diseases*, **7**, 656–664.

Ariza, J., Pellicer, T., Pallares, R. *et al.* (1992a) Specific antibody profile in human brucellosis. *Clinical Infectious Diseases*, **14**, 131–140.

Ariza, J., Gudiol, F., Pallares, R. *et al.* (1992b) Treatment of human brucellosis with doxycycline plus rifampin or doxycycline plus streptomycin. *Annals of Internal Medicine*, **117**, 25–30.

Ariza, J., Pujol, M., Valverde, J. *et al.* (1993) Brucellar sacroiliitis: findings in 63 episodes and current relevance. *Clinical Infectious Diseases*, **16**, 761–765.

Arnow, P.M., Smaron, M. and Ormiste, V. (1984) Brucellosis in a group of travelers to Spain. *Journal of the American Medical Association*, **251**, 505–507.

Barham, W.B., Church, P., Brown, J.E. *et al.* (1993) Misidentification of *Brucella* species with use of rapid bacterial identification systems. *Clinical Infectious Diseases*, **17**, 1068–1069.

Bricker, B.J., Tabatabi, L.B., Judge, B.A. *et al.* (1990) Cloning, expression, and occurrence of the *Brucella* Cu–Zn superoxide dismutase. *Infection and Immunity*, **58**, 2935–2939.

Brown, G.M. (1977) The history of the brucellosis eradication program in the United States. *Annali Sclavo*, **19**, 21–34.

Buchanan, T.M. and Faber, L.C. (1980) 2-Mercaptoethanol brucella agglutination test: usefulness for predicting recovery from brucellosis. *Journal of Clinical Microbiology*, **11**, 691–693.

Buchanan, T.M., Hendricks, S.L., Patton, C.M. *et al.* (1974) Brucellosis in the United States, 1960–1972: an abattoir-associated disease. Part III. Epidemiology and evidence for acquired immunity. *Medicine*, **53**, 427–439.

Bundle, D.R., Cherwonogrodzky, J.W., Caroff, M. *et al.* (1987) The lipopolysaccharides of *Brucella abortus* and *Brucella melitensis*. *Annals of the Pasteur Institute/Microbiology*, **138**, 92–97.

Canning, P.C., Roth, A. and Deyoe, B.L. (1986) Release of 5′-guanosine-monophosphate and adenine by *Brucella abortus* and their role in the intracellular survival of the bacteria. *Journal of Infectious Diseases*, **154**, 464–470.

Caroff, M., Bundle, D.R., Perry, M.B. *et al.* (1984a) Antigenic S-type lipopolysaccharide of *Brucella abortus* 1119–3. *Infection and Immunity*, **46**, 384–388.

Caroff, M., Bundle, D.R. and Perry, M.B. (1984b) Structure of the O-chain of the phenol-phase soluble cellular lipopolysaccharide of *Yersinia enterocolitica* O:9. *European Journal of Biochemistry*, **139**, 195–199.

Escalante, J.A. and Held, J.R. (1969) Brucellosis in Peru. *Journal of the American Veterinary Medical Association*, **155**, 2146–2152.

Essenberg, R.C. and Sharma, Y.K. (1993) Cloning of genes for proline and leucine biosynthesis from *Brucella abortus* by functional complementation in *Escherichia coli*. *Journal of General Microbiology*, **139**, 87–93.

Etemadi, H., Raissadat, A., Pickett, M.J. *et al.* (1984) Isolation of *Brucella* species from clinical specimens. *Journal of Clinical Microbiology*, **20**, 586.

Fekete, A., Bantle, J.A., Halling, S.M. *et al.* (1992) Amplification fragment length polymorphism in *Brucella* strains by use of polymerase chain reaction with arbitrary primers. *Journal of Bacteriology*, **174**, 7778–7783.

Ficht, T.A., Bearden, S.W., Sowa, B.A. *et al.* (1989) DNA sequence and expression of the 36-kilodalton outer membrane protein gene of *Brucella abortus*. *Infection and Immunity*, **57**, 3281–3291.

Ficht, T.A., Bearden, S.W., Sowa, B.A. *et al.* (1990) Genetic variation at the omp 2 porin locus of the brucellae: species-specific markers. *Molecular Microbiology*, **4**, 1135–1142.

Gazapo, E., Lahos, J.G., Subiza, J.L. *et al.* (1989) Changes in IgM and IgG antibody concentrations in brucellosis over time: importance for diagnosis and follow-up. *Journal of Infectious Diseases*, **159**, 219–225.

Goldstein, J., Hoffman, T., Frasch, C. *et al.* (1992) Lipopolysaccharide (LPS) from *Brucella abortus* is less toxic than that from *Escherichia coli*, suggesting the possible use of *B. abortus* or LPS from *B. abortus* as a carrier in vaccines. *Infection and Immunity*, **60**, 1385–1389.

Gotuzzo, E., Alarcon, G.S., Bocanegra, T.S. *et al.* (1982) Articular involvement in human brucellosis: a retrospective analysis of 304 cases. *Seminars in Arthritis and Rheumatism*, **12**, 245–255.

Gotuzzo, E., Carrillo, C., Guerra, J. *et al.* (1986) An evaluation of diagnostic methods for brucellosis: the value of bone marrow cultures. *Journal of Infectious Diseases*, **153**, 122–125.

Hafez, S.M. (1986) The impact of uncontrolled animal importation and marketing on the prevalence of brucellosis in Saudi Arabia. *Annals of Saudi Medicine*, **6**, 15–18.

Hall, W.H. (1990) Modern chemotherapy for brucellosis in humans. *Reviews of Infectious Diseases*, **12**, 1060–1099.

Herman, L. and de Ridder, H. (1992) Identification of *Brucella* spp. by using the polymerase chain reaction. *Applied and Environmental Microbiology*, **58**, 2099–2101.

Jacobs, F., Abramowicz, D., Vereerstraeten, P. *et al.* (1990) Brucella endocarditis: the role of combined medical and surgical treatment. *Reviews of Infectious Diseases*, **12**, 740–744.

Jiang, X. and Baldwin, C.L. (1993) Effect of cytokines on intracellular growth of *Brucella abortus*. *Infection and Immunity*, **61**, 124–129.

Joint FAO/WHO Expert Committee on Brucellosis, Sixth Report (1986) World Health Organization Technical Report Series 740, Geneva.

Kolman, S., Maayan, M.C., Gotesman, G. *et al.*(1991) Comparison of the Bactec and lysis concentration methods for recovery of *Brucella* species from clinical specimens. *European Journal of Clinical Microbiology and Infectious Diseases*, **10**, 647–648.

Lulu, A.R., Araj, G.F., Khateeb, M.I. *et al.* (1988) Human brucellosis in Kuwait: a prospective study of 400 cases. *Quarterly Journal of Medicine*, **66**, 39–54.

Marquis, H. and Ficht, T.A. (1993) The omp 2 gene locus of *Brucella abortus* encodes two homologous outer membrane proteins with properties characteristic of bacterial porins. *Infection and Immunity*, **61**, 3785–3790.

McLean, D.R., Russell, N. and Khan, M.Y. (1992) Neurobrucellosis: clinical and therapeutic features. *Clinical Infectious Diseases*, **15**, 582–590.

Mediterranean Fever Commission Reports (1905–1907) Royal Society of London, Harrison & Sons, London (7 parts).

Michaux, S., Paillisson, J., Carles-Nurit, M.J. *et al.* (1993) Presence of two independent chromosomes in the *Brucella melitensis* 16M genome. *Journal of Bacteriology*, **175**, 701–705.

Minnick, M.F. and Stiegler, G.L. (1993) Nucleotide sequence and comparison of the 5S ribosomal RNA genes of *Rochalimaea henselae*, *R. quintana*, and *Brucella abortus*. *Nucleic Acid Research*, **21**, 2518.

Montejo, J.M., Alberola, I., Glez-Zarate, P. *et al.* (1993) Open, randomized therapeutic trial of six antimicrobial regimens in the treatment of human brucellosis. *Clinical Infectious Diseases*, **16**, 671–676.

Moreno, E., Pitt, M., Jones, L. *et al.* (1979) Purification and characterization of smooth and rough lipopolysaccharide from *Brucella abortus*. *Journal of Bacteriology*, **138**, 361–369.

Moreno, E., Berman, D.T. and Boettcher, L.A. (1981) Biologic activities of *Brucella abortus* lipopolysaccharides. *Infection and Immunity*, **31**, 362–370.

Moreno, E., Stackbrandt, E., Dorsch, M. *et al.* (1990) *Brucella abortus* 16S rRNA and lipid A reveal a phylogenetic relationship with members of the alpha-2 subdivision of the class *Proteobacter*. *Journal of Bacteriology*, **172**, 3569–3576.

Mousa, A.R.M., Muhtaseb, S.A., Almudallal, D.S. *et al.* (1987) Osteoarticular complications of brucellosis: a study of 169 cases. *Reviews of Infectious Diseases*, **9**, 531–543.

Mousa, A.R.M., Elhag, K.M., Khogali, M. *et al.* (1988) The nature of human brucellosis in Kuwait: study of 379 cases. *Reviews of Infectious Diseases*, **10**, 211–217.

Navas, E., Guerrero, A., Cobo, J. *et al.* (1993) Faster isolation of *Brucella* spp. from blood by isolator compared with BacteC NR. *Diagnostic Microbiology and Infectious Diseases*, **16**, 78–81.

Nicoletti, P. (1980) The epidemiology of bovine brucellosis. *Advances in Veterinary Science and Comparative Medicine*, **24**, 70–98.

Peiris, V., Faser, S., Fairhurst, M. *et al.* (1992) Laboratory diagnosis of brucella infection: some pitfalls. *Lancet*, **339**, 1415–1416.

Price, R.E., Templeton, J.W., Smith, R. *et al.* (1990) Ability of mononuclear phagocytes from cattle naturally resistant or susceptible to brucellosis to control in vitro intracellular survival of *Brucella abortus*. *Infection and Immunity*, **58**, 879–886.

Rasool, O., Frear, E., Moreno, E. *et al.* (1992) Effect of *Brucella abortus* lipopolysaccharide on oxidative metabolism and lysozyme release by human neutrophils. *Infection and Immunity*, **60**, 1699–1702.

Rubinstein, E., Lang, R., Shasha, B. *et al.* (1991) In vitro susceptibility of *Brucella melitensis* to antibiotics. *Antimicrobial Agents and Chemotherapy*, **35**, 1925–1927.

Smith, R. (1990) T-lymphocyte-mediated mechanisms of acquired protective immunity against brucellosis in cattle. In *Advances in Brucellosis Research* (ed. L.G. Adams), pp. 164–190. Texas A&M University Press, College Station.

Solomon, H.M. and Jackson, D. (1992) Rapid diagnosis of *Brucella melitensis* in blood: some operational characteristics of the BACT/ALERT. *Journal of Clinical Microbiology*, **30**, 222–224.

Spink, W.W. (1951) What is chronic brucellosis? *Annals of Internal Medicine*, **35**, 358–374.

Splitter, G.A. and Everlith, K.M. (1986) Collaboration of bovine T lymphocytes and macrophages in T-lymphocyte response to *Brucella abortus*. *Infection and Immunity*, **51**, 776–783.

Steffen, R. (1977) Antacids: a risk factor in traveller's brucellosis? *Scandinavian Journal of Infectious Diseases*, **9**, 311–312.

Tatum, F.M., Detilleux, P.G., Sacks, J.M. *et al.* (1992) Construction of Cu–Zn superoxide dismutase deletion mutants of *Brucella abortus*: analysis of survival in vitro in epithelial and phagocytic cells and in vivo in mice. *Infection and Immunity*, **60**, 2863–2869.

Taylor, J.P. and Perdue, J.N. (1989) The changing epidemiology of human brucellosis in Texas, 1977–1986. *American Journal of Epidemiology*, **130**, 160–165.

Tekkok, I.H., Berker, M., Ozzan, O.E. *et al.* (1993) Brucellosis of the spine. *Neurosurgery*, **33**, 838–844.

Thapar, M.K. and Young, E.J. (1986) Urban outbreak of goat cheese brucellosis. *Journal of Pediatric Infectious Diseases*, **5**, 640–643.

Vandercam, B., Zech, F., de Cooman, S. *et al.* (1990) Isolation of *Brucella melitensis* from human sperm. *European Journal of Clinical Microbiology and Infectious Diseases*, **9**, 303–304.

Verger, J.M., Grimont, F., Grimont, P.A.D. *et al.* (1985) *Brucella* a monospecific genus as shown by desoxyribonucleic acid hybridization. *International Journal of Systematic Bacteriology*, **35**, 292–295.

Verger, J.M., Grayon, M., Chaslus-Dancla, E. *et al.* (1993) Conjugative transfer and in vitro/in vivo stability of the broad-host-range Inc P R751 plasmid in *Brucella* spp. *Plasmid*, **29**, 142–146.

Wilson, G.S. and Miles, A.A. (1932) The serological differentiation of smooth strains of the *Brucella* group. *British Journal of Experimental Pathology*, **13**, 1–13.

Young, E.J. (1983) Human brucellosis. *Reviews of Infectious Diseases*, **5**, 821–842.

Young, E.J. (1991) Serologic diagnosis of human brucellosis: analysis of 214 cases by agglutination tests and review of the literature. *Reviews of Infectious Diseases*, **13**, 359–372.

Young, E.J. and Suvannoparrat, U. (1975) Brucellosis outbreak attributed to ingestion of unpasteurized goat cheese. *Journal of the American Medical Association*, **135**, 240–243.

Young, E.J., Borchert, M., Kretzer, F. *et al.* (1985) Phagocytosis and killing of *Brucella* by human polymorphonuclear leukocytes. *Journal of Infectious Diseases*, **151**, 682–690.

Zhan, Y. and Cheers, C. (1993) Endogenous gamma interferon mediates resistance to *Brucella abortus* infection. *Infection and Immunity*, **61**, 4899–4901.

Zimmerman, S.J., Gillikin, S., Sofat, N. *et al.* (1990) Case report and seeded blood culture study of *Brucella* bacteremia. *Journal of Clinical Microbiology*, **28**, 2139–2141.

11

LEGIONELLA

T.G. Harrison

INTRODUCTION

In July 1976 a dramatic outbreak of an acute, febrile respiratory illness occurred in the city of Philadelphia among approximately 4400 Legionnaires (veterans of the US army) who had gathered to attend the 58th convention of the Pennsylvania Branch of the American Legion. There was a total of 182 convention-associated cases of whom 29 died, and as most of the victims were military veterans the outbreak aroused considerable media interest. The newspapers used colourful names to describe the illness: 'Philly Killer', 'Legion Fever', 'Legion Malady' and 'Legionnaires' disease'. Surprisingly the latter of these was adopted by the scientific community and this name has, in part, helped to perpetuate media interest in this uncommon form of pneumonia ever since.

The search for the cause of the Philadelphia outbreak was exhaustive and only after more than six months of investigations was the isolation of the causative organism reported (McDade *et al.*, 1977). In order to isolate the organism investigators had inoculated guinea-pigs with autopsy material from a Legionnaires' disease patient. Tissue from the guinea-pigs that developed fever were used to inoculate embryonated hens' eggs. Using these rickettsial isolation techniques

McDade and colleagues (1977) were able to demonstrate the presence of Gram-negative bacilli in preparations of the infected eggs. Convalescent sera from patients (91%) identified in the outbreak reacted with antigens prepared from these bacteria in an indirect immunofluorescent antibody test. These results were consistent with the view that the bacterium was the aetiological agent of Legionnaires' disease (LD).

Investigators at the Centers for Disease Control, Atlanta, recognized epidemiological similarities between the Philadelphia outbreak, where an air-conditioning system was implicated as the source of infection, and several earlier outbreaks of illness including one in Washington, DC, during 1965, one in Pontiac, Michigan, during 1968 and one in the same Philadelphia hotel in 1974 which occurred amongst delegates to a convention of the Independent Order of Odd Fellows. Retrospective examination of stored sera collected from patients during these outbreaks revealed that these outbreaks had also been caused by this organism (McDade *et al.*, 1977). Thus although newly recognized, LD was clearly not a new illness. Outbreaks of LD have now been recognized to have occurred since the 1940s.

The realization that a hitherto unrecognized bacterium was responsible for an illness with

Principles and Practice of Clinical Bacteriology. Edited by A.M. Emmerson, P.M. Hawkey and S.H. Gillespie
© 1997 John Wiley & Sons Ltd

significant morbidity and mortality led to a period
of intense interest in all aspects of the organism. It
was quickly appreciated that in addition to air-
conditioning systems water distribution systems
were also important sources of infection. It was
also established that legionellae occur widely in
both natural and man-made aquatic environments.
As knowledge of the habitat expanded so did the
number of *Legionella*-like organisms identified.

DESCRIPTION OF THE ORGANISM

Taxonomy

The causative agent of LD was initially designated
the Legionnaires' disease bacterium (McDade
et al., 1977). DNA/DNA homology studies on the
few clinical and environmental isolates then available revealed that they were members of a distinct

TABLE 11.1   MEMBERS OF THE FAMILY LEGIONELLACEAE

Legionella species	Multiple serogroups	Causes human illness[a]
1. *L. adelaidensis*		−
2. *L. anisa*		+ (sporadic cases and an outbreak of Pontiac fever)
3. *L. birminghamensis*		−
4. *L. bozemanii*	2	+ (sporadic cases and nosocomial outbreaks)
5. *L. brunensi*		−
6. *L. cherrii*		−
7. *L. cincinnatiensis*		+
8. *L. dumoffii*		+ (sporadic cases and a single documented outbreak)
9. *L. erythra*	2[b]	−
10. *L. fairfieldensis*		−
11. *L. feeleii*	2	+ (sporadic cases and an outbreak of Pontiac fever)
12. *L. geestiana*		−
13. *L. gormanii*		+
14. *L. gratiana*		−
15. *L. hackeliae*	2	+
16. *L. israelensis*		−
17. *L. jamestowniensis*		−
18. *L. jordanis*		+
19. *L. lansingensis*		+
20. *L. londiniensis*		−
21. *L. longbeachae*	2	+ (many cases in South Australia − sporadic elsewhere)
22. *L. maceachernii*		+
23. *L. micdadei*		+ (sporadic cases and local outbreaks in USA)
24. *L. moravica*		−
25. *L. nautarum*		−
26. *L. oakridgensis*		+ (serological evidence only)
27. *L. parisiensis*		−
28. *L. pneumophila*[c]	16	+ (the majority of sporadic and epidemic cases)
29. *L. quarteirensis*		−
30. *L. quinlivanii*	2	−
31. *L. rubrilucens*		−
32. *L. sainthelensi*	2[d]	+
33. *L. santicrucis*		−
34. *L. shakespearei*		−
35. *L. spiritensis*	2	−
36. *L. steigerwaltii*		−
37. *L. tucsonensis*		+
38. *L. wadsworthii*		+
39. *L. worsleiensis*		−

[a] Evidenced by isolation of the organism unless otherwise indicated.
[b] *L. erythra* Sgp 2 is serologically indistinguishable from *L. rubrilucens*.
[c] *L. pneumophila* comprises three subspecies; subsp. *pneumophila*; subsp *fraseri* and subsp *pascullei*.
[d] *L. sainthelensi* Sgp 2 is serologically indistinguishable from *L. santicrucis*.

species, and the family Legionellaceae and the genus *Legionella* were subsequently defined in 1979 for a single species *Legionella pneumophila* (Brenner *et al.*, 1979).

The decision, taken at that time, to create a new family was based on phenotypic evidence: *Legionella pneumophila* was distinct from other Gram-negative bacteria in nutritional requirements and cell wall composition. Since this time 38 other species of *Legionella* have been identified (Dennis *et al.*, 1993) (Table 11.1) and the validity of the family Legionellaceae has been substantiated both phenotypically and phylogenetically (Harrison and Saunders, 1994). However, classification at the genus level has been controversial. The generally held view is that all the species are phenotypically very similar and so should all be placed into the genus *Legionella*. On the basis of limited phenotypic evidence (e.g. colony autofluorescence) and a different interpretation of DNA homology data, some workers maintain that the family should be divided into three genera: *Legionella*, *Fluoribacter* and *Tatlockia*. Alternative names have been formally proposed and consequently *L. bozemanii*, *L. dumoffii*, *L. gormanii*, *L. micdadei* and *L. maceachernii* may be found cited in the literature as *F. bozemanae*, *F. dumoffi*, *F. gormanii*, *T. micdadei* and *T. maceachernii* respectively.

Recent phylogenetic studies (Harrison and Saunders, 1994) have again demonstrated that the species of the family Legionellaceae are monophyletic, showing no discrete divisions. Furthermore if the family were to be divided in this way many genera with only one or two species would be created. The phenotypic data do not support this view, as although identification of members of the genus is relatively simple, distinguishing between many of the species is very difficult and often requires the application of molecular techniques.

Definition

Legionellae are nutritionally fastidious, pleomorphic Gram-negative, non-spore-forming organisms. *In vivo* they are short rods or coccobacilli measuring 0.3–0.9 μm in width and 2.0–6.0 μm in length; on artificial media they may be seen as rods or occasionally as filamentous, 6.0–20.0 μm or more in length. They are usually poorly motile with one or two polar flagella, although non-motile strains do occur. Branched-chain fatty acids predominate in the cell wall, which also contains large amounts of ubiquinones with more than 10 isoprene units in the side chain. L-Cysteine and iron salts are required for growth *in vitro*, carbohydrates are not fermented or oxidized and nitrate is not reduced to nitrite. Legionellae are urease negative, catalase positive and give variable results in the oxidase test. The legionellae have a genome size of approximately 2.5×10^9 Da and a G + C content of 39–42%, the exception being *L. geestiana* which has a G + C content of 52%.

PATHOGENICITY

As discussed below legionellae appear to be primary pathogens of protozoans which can from time to time give rise to infection in humans and possibly other animals. However, despite more than 10 years of research the mechanisms underlying this pathogenicity are still only poorly understood and what data there are relate mainly to *L. pneumophila*.

Infection by legionellae occurs following inhalation of a fine-particle aerosol (<5 μm) containing organisms which are both viable and virulent. Once within the lungs legionellae are taken up by alveolar macrophages and multiply intracellularly. The uptake by, and survival within, monocytes and macrophages of the Philadelphia-1 strain of *L. pneumophila* has been extensively studied by Horwitz and colleagues (Horwitz, 1983; Horwitz and Maxfield, 1984; Horwitz and Silverstein, 1980, 1981; Bellinger-Kawahara and Horwitz, 1990). They have demonstrated that the major outer membrane protein (MOMP) of the organism fixes complement component C3 and then attaches to the host cell via the complement receptors CR1 and CR3. Phagocytosis continues by an unusual mechanism termed 'coiling phagocytosis' in which long phagocytic pseudopods coil round the organism. Within the macrophage the bacterium remains in the phagosome and neither phagosome/

lysosome fusion nor phagosome acidification takes place. Although initially thought to be highly significant the importance of this sequence of events is not now clear as other workers have reported that some virulent strains of *L. pneumophila* are taken up by conventional phagocytosis and that a typical phagolysosome is formed (Rechnitzer, 1989). Multiplication of the legionellae continues until the host cell is packed with organisms and finally disrupts, releasing legionellae to infect further host cells. Although cytotoxic activity has been observed for *L. pneumophila* (Quinn *et al.*, 1989) it is not clear whether it is the action of a toxin or physical disruption that causes the host cell to lyse.

The host limits infection primarily by cell-mediated immune mechanisms. Once activated by cytokines macrophages are poor hosts for legionellae; phagocytic activity is reduced by about 50%, possibly through decreased expression of CR1 and CR3, and intracellular iron is decreased by down-regulation of the transferrin receptor expression (Bellinger-Kawahara and Horwitz, 1990). Studies using polymorphonuclear leucocyte (PMN)-depleted guinea-pigs suggest that PMNs also play an important role in host defence. Although this observation is consistent with the large numbers of PMNs seen in histology specimens from LD patients, *in vitro* studies have not been able to elucidate the mechanism by which this occurs.

Although a strong humoral response accompanies infection this appears to provide little protection and possibly may be detrimental, promoting uptake of *L. pneumophila* by macrophages (Horwitz and Silverstein, 1981).

Virulence Factors

A wide range of putative virulence factors have been studied but despite considerable research little progress has been made. Molecules studied to date include cell surface components, peptide toxins and enzymes (Dowling *et al.*, 1992). Only those where significant results have been obtained are discussed here.

The MOMP is a cation-selective porin, and distinct but closely related molecules are found in all species of *Legionella*. As described above,

MOMP is central to the phagocytic process. Horwitz (1988) has speculated that, at least in the case of the Philadelphia-1 strain of *L, pneumophila*, acidification of the monocyte phagosome might be inhibited by insertion of the MOMP porin into the phagosome membrane. This theory, however, awaits experimental confirmation.

A second surface protein to receive considerable attention is the 24 kDa protein designated the macrophage infectivity potentiator (Mip). Cianciotto and colleagues (1990a) using a pair of isogenic strains (one of which was deficient in Mip) demonstrated that Mip was required for the full expression of virulence by *L. pneumophila*. It appears that Mip is required either for optimal internalization of the legionellae by macrophages or for resistance to the bactericidal mechanisms active shortly after phagocytosis. It is, however, noteworthy that the Mip-deficient mutant did multiply in macrophages and did produce illness in guinea-pigs. Clearly, Mip can only contribute in part to the virulence of a strain. The Mip protein is conserved in, and specific to, *L. pneumophila* but 24–31 kDa Mip-like proteins have been found in the other *Legionella* spp. (1990b). Whether or not these other Mip-like proteins contribute to virulence of these other species has not yet been determined.

Cellular Constituents

The cell wall of legionellae is typical of a Gram-negative organism, being trilaminar with an outer membrane, peptidoglycan layer and cytoplasmic membrane; however, the composition of the cell wall is unusual. The subunits of peptidoglycan are extensively cross-linked producing a highly stable layer which confers some resistance to degradation by lysozyme (Amano and Williams, 1983). The lipopolysaccharide (LPS) composition of *Legionella* has also been shown to be unusual, the monosaccharide and the fatty acid composition being particularly complex in structure (Sonesson *et al.*, 1989). Furthermore, *L. pneumophila* LPS has been shown to have very little endotoxin-like activity compared with *Salmonella* LPS (Wong *et al.*, 1979).

Legionella contains large amounts (>80%) of branched-chain fatty acids and only small amounts of hydroxy acids. Although qualitatively similar, the fatty acid profiles of some *Legionella* spp. show marked and consistent quantitative differences. In addition, all species contain unusual members of the ubiquinone group of respiratory isoprenoid-quinones, which contain 9–15 isoprenyl unit side chains. The combination of fatty acid profiling and ubiquinone analysis has proved a valuable, although not routine, tool for the identification of legionellae (Wait, 1988).

As noted above, the *L. pneumophila* LPS is unusual in composition and has little endotoxin-like activity in comparison with typical LPS. However, it has been suggested that differences in LPS structure between strains might account for differences in virulence. Monoclonal antibodies (mAbs) have been used extensively to differentiate between strains of *L. pneumophila* serogroup 1. Dournon and colleagues (1988) were the first to notice that strains (designated MAB2$^+$) which reacted with one such mAb, directed against an LPS epitope (Petitjean *et al.*, 1990), were more likely to be isolated from patients than were strains which did not react (MAB2$^-$ strains). This has led to the widely held view that MAB2$^+$ strains are more virulent than MAB2$^-$ strains. There is some evidence that MAB2$^-$ strains infect human monocytes less well than do MAB2$^+$ strains; however, some recent studies have not confirmed this (Edelstein and Edelstein, 1993). An alternative explanation, indicated by Dennis and Lee's (1988) studies, is that MAB2$^+$ strains survive better in aerosols than MAB2$^-$ strains and hence are more likely to be inhaled in a viable state by a susceptible individual than are MAB2$^-$ strains.

The legionellae produce a number of proteolytic enzymes and aminopeptidases. One such protease, a 38–42 kDa zinc metalloprotease has been studied in detail and variously called tissue destructive protease (Conlan *et al.*, 1988), zinc metalloprotease (Quinn *et al.*, 1989) and major secretory protein (Szeto and Shuman, 1990). This molecule has been shown to be cytotoxic and haemolytic; it is elaborated intracellularly by growing *L. pneumophila* and experimentally causes pulmonary lesions which closely resemble those seen in infection (Quinn *et al.*, 1989; Conlan *et al.*, 1988; Szeto and Shuman, 1990; Williams *et al.*, 1993). Studies using guinea-pig models of LD to determine if this protease is a virulence factor have yielded conflicting results. Blander and colleagues (1990) concluded that while the enzyme is immunoprotective it is not a virulence factor. In contrast, Moffat and colleagues (1994) found that although deletion of the protease did not completely abolish virulence it did attenuate the infection and delay death in the guinea-pigs.

EPIDEMIOLOGY

Normal Habitat

Extensive environmental studies indicate that legionellae are ubiquitous organisms occurring over a wide geographical area in river mud, streams, lakes, rivers, warm spa water, water in hydrothermal areas, numerous other natural bodies of water and, most recently, subterrestial groundwater sediments (Fliermans *et al.*, 1981; Fliermans and Tyndall, 1993). Legionellae have also been isolated from diverse man-made habitats including air-conditioning systems, potable water supplies, ornamental fountains and plumbing fixtures and fittings in hospital, shops and homes (Tobin *et al.*, 1981; Colbourne *et al.*, 1988; Stout *et al.*, 1992).

Early studies indicated that legionellae could be detected by immunofluorescence (IF) in most natural bodies of water examined but could only be isolated and cultured from a few of these (Fliermans *et al.*, 1981). Initially, because of the questionable specificity of the reagents used in the IF, only the isolation rate was considered to be an accurate indication of the likely incidence of legionellae. The isolation rate is, in part, dependent on the temperature of the body of water examined. Legionellae can readily be isolated and cultured from water between about 20 and 40 °C; below this temperature they can remain viable but cannot easily be cultured (Colbourne *et al.*, 1988). Hence isolation rates probably give a poor estimate of the true incidence of legionellae. It is now clear that legionellae are very widely distributed, being found in almost all natural bodies of fresh water, although they may be present at only low numbers and possibly in a 'dormant' state (Colbourne *et al.*, 1988).

The ubiquitous nature of legionellae, even in low nutrient environments, appears to contrast with exacting requirements for culture and isolation of the organism in the laboratory. The explanation seems to be that legionellae naturally grow in association with other microorganisms. Tison and colleagues (1980) first demonstrated that *L. pneumophila* could grow in mineral salts medium at 45 °C in association with cyanobacteria (*Fischerella* sp.). In the same year Rowbotham (1980) observed that when legionellae were phagocytosed by *Acanthamoeba* trophozoites *in vitro*, they could survive and multiply within the amoebal vacuole. It has subsequently been shown that other protozoa such as species of *Hartmanella*, *Naegleria* and *Valkampfia* can also be parasitized. It is now widely acknowledged that these host−parasite relationships are central to the propagation and distribution of legionellae within the environment. Indeed increasing evidence, such as the isolation of legionellae from amoebae taken directly from the environment (Harf and Monteil, 1988), have led to the suggestion that legionellae may not be free-living bacteria *per se* (Fields, 1991). This close association has several potential benefits for legionellae, such as the provision of adequate concentrations of nutrients in otherwise nutrient-poor conditions; the protection from adverse external conditions within, for example, amoebal cysts (Kilvington and Price, 1990); and possibly a mode of distribution with the amoebal cyst acting as a carrier.

In common with most other aquatic bacteria legionellae colonize surfaces at the aqueous/solid interface. Here, together with their protozoal hosts, other bacteria and algae they form a complex consortium of organisms loosely termed 'biofilm'. It is believed that biofilm formation provides nutritional advantages and protection from adverse environmental influences to its constituent organisms compared with their planktonic counterparts.

In man *Legionella* infection can vary in severity from a mild flu-like illness to acute life-threatening pneumonia. There is no evidence of person-to-person spread, the only documented way to acquire infection being by inhalation of aerosol containing virulent organisms. The pneumonic form of the disease, LD, is well characterized but the mild non-pneumonic form is ill defined and encompasses any condition which is not LD but where there is some evidence of *Legionella* infection. The term 'Pontiac fever' is sometimes used interchangeably with non-pneumonic legionellosis; however, it is more appropriately applied specifically for those cases characterized by a self-limiting, flu-like illness with a high attack rate and short incubation period (see section on Pontiac fever, below). The data presented below relate only to LD; that is, where there is clear evidence of pneumonia and the criteria for laboratory diagnosis have been met (Memorandum, 1990).

Incidence and Risk Factors

Although cases of LD have been reported from many countries throughout the world the incidence of the disease is largely unknown, as active surveillance systems are in place in only a few countries. Certainly LD is not a common cause of pneumonia and in most areas probably accounts for less than 5% of all pneumonia cases requiring admission to hospital (Woodhead *et al.*, 1986). Much higher figures have been reported but in these series diagnosis often relied only on serology using antigens whose specificity has not been established or is known to be poor (MacFarlane *et al.*, 1982).

In England and Wales surveillance is organized through a voluntary reporting scheme where about 300 laboratories report cases to the PHLS Communicable Disease Surveillance Centre (CDSC). Further information is then sought from the reporting physician. In the 14 years from 1980 to 1993 a total of 2480 cases of LD were reported to the CDSC, suggesting an incidence in England and Wales of approximately 3.5 cases per million per year (D. Dedman; personal communication). Although the annual number of cases reported to the CDSC over this period has changed little (Figure 11.1) there is some suggestion of a decline over the last few years. Whether this is due to a real decrease or reduced reporting is not clear. A recent history of travel is reported in 44% of cases, most of these (40%) being travel abroad. Of the 60% UK cases, the infection was acquired while in hospital in 15% and in the local community in the remainder.

LD is seen in patients of all ages (1–92 years) but is most frequent in adults over 40 years old and very rare in children (Figure 11.2). There are many more cases among males than among females (ratio of 2.7 : 1). Significant risk factors include a compromised immune system, recent surgery, congestive heart failure, chronic bronchitis, liver cirrhosis, renal insufficiency and heavy smoking. Not surprisingly, therefore, in certain patient groups, such as organ transplant patients, the incidence is much higher than 5% and LD may even be the main cause of lung infections. The overall mortality is approximately 13% but this can be much higher in immunocompromised patients.

A seasonal variation in the incidence of LD has been recognized in many parts of the world (Breiman, 1993). In England and Wales most cases are seen in late summer and early autumn, although there have been several major outbreaks during the winter and early spring following periods of unseasonably warm weather.

Although highly publicized, outbreaks of LD are uncommon and only account for 25% of cases. There is, however, some evidence to suggest that many of the remaining 75% of cases are associated with a common source of infection, although this is not recognized at the time. Cooling towers have been identified as the source in most of the major outbreaks of LD but overall water distribution systems are the most frequently implicated sources.

Travel-associated LD

Almost half the annual cases of LD, both sporadic and epidemic, are travel associated. The majority of these are linked to Mediterranean holiday resorts. Where investigations have been undertaken, hotel water systems have been most frequently identified as the likely source. The incidence of cases appears to be highest in those countries and areas where the tourist industry is still developing. Although countries such as Spain, with long-established tourist industries, account for the highest numbers of cases, the rate of infection has declined from about six per million

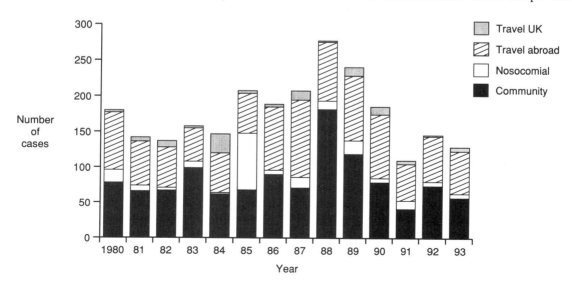

Figure 11.1. Legionnaires' disease: England and Wales 1980–1993. (Data provided by CDSC, PHLS.)

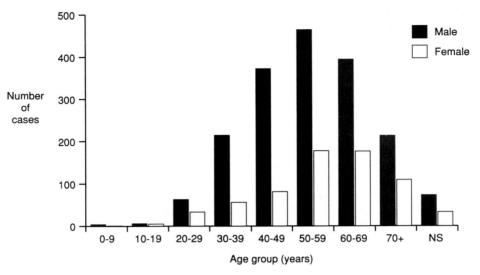

Figure 11.2. Age and sex distribution of cases of Legionnaire's disease: England and Wales 1980–1993. (Data provided by CDSC, PHLS.)

visitors in 1989–1991 to about four per million visitors in 1992. This contrasts with Turkey, which has a less-developed tourist industry, where the rate of infection at 18 per million visitors has remained static over the same period (Joseph et al., 1993).

Nosocomially Acquired LD

Hospitals often have large and complex water distribution systems and a population of susceptible patients. It is not surprising therefore that nosocomially acquired LD is a significant problem. About 9% of reported cases per annum in England and Wales are hospital acquired. Although this is only a small number of cases annually the fatality rate of approximately 30% is high. A second striking feature is that a very much larger proportion of infections are caused by non-L. pneumophila Sgp 1 MAB2$^+$ strains (see below) than is reported overall (Joseph et al., 1994). Both observations are probably a reflection of the immunocompromised status of most patients in the nosocomial group.

The majority of these cases are recognized as part of an outbreak many of which are considered to be caused by contaminated water systems. It is likely that many of the sporadic cases are caused in this way but most are not investigated in detail.

Legionella spp. able to Cause Human Infection

To date 18 species have been reported as pathogenic for humans (Table 11.1). However, infections caused by species other than L. pneumophila are rare and are almost always seen in patients who are immunocompromised (Dournon, 1988). One exception to this is L. longbeachae Sgp 1 in South Australia which is now recognized to be a significant cause of community acquired pneumonia there. The reservoir for the organisms appears to be potting composts prepared from composted wood where it is found growing in association with amoebae (Steele, 1993).

The majority of sporadic and almost all outbreak associated cases of LD are caused by the so-called 'virulent' strains (i.e. MAB2$^+$) of L. pneumophila Sgp 1. Strains of L. pneumophila Sgp 1 which are MAB2$^-$ together with strains of other L. pneumophila serogroups account for most of the other cases. With a few exceptions (Table 11.1) other *Legionella* spp. are only seen as the cause of rare sporadic cases of LD. It does, however, seem likely that under appropriate circumstances any *Legionella* species could cause infection.

CLINICAL FEATURES

Legionnaires' Disease

Although overall an uncommon form of pneumonia, in the context of severe community-acquired pneumonias LD is much more significant, probably being the second commonest form, accounting for 14–37% of cases (Hubbard *et al.*, 1993). LD has no special features that clearly distinguish it from other pneumonias but the clinical picture is usually suggestive of the diagnosis (Mayaud and Dournon, 1988).

The onset of LD is generally more insidious than in typical pneumococcal pneumonia, with fever, headaches and malaise being the first manifestations. In about half of the cases gastrointestinal abnormalities are present. Respiratory signs often only appear later in the course of the disease. A cough is rare and if present it is generally non-productive early in the illness, although later small amounts of purulent, and sometimes bloody sputum, may be expectorated. Lung examination usually reveals abnormalities at this stage of the disease with at least rales and very often consolidation being evident. A small pleural effusion, sometimes suspected from the presence of thoracic pain, is present in about one-third of patients but is difficult to recognize on clinical examination. Progression of the lung infection may be rapid and be responsible for increasing dyspnoea and acute respiratory failure (Mayaud and Dournon, 1988).

A frequently reported but non-specific feature of LD is the presence in many cases of gastrointestinal symptoms or neurological signs. In the series studied by Mayaud *et al.* (1984) diarrhoea was present in about 50% of cases and appeared early in the course of the disease. Nausea, vomiting or right lower abdominal pain with tenderness were each seen in 20–30% patients. Nervous system manifestations, which were dominated by alterations of the mental status such as disorienta-

tion and confusion, were found in about 25% of cases (Mayaud and Dournon, 1988).

Routine laboratory findings are not particularly helpful. Abnormalities of liver function are frequently found, with elevated serum levels of transaminases, alkaline phosphatase and bilirubin. Proteinuria, haematuria and renal insufficiency are infrequent in patients receiving early treatment. Elevation of creatinine phosphokinase and aldolase blood levels, suggestive of muscle damage, is seen in some patients.

The prognosis for patients treated with appropriate antibiotics within seven days of onset is good and they usually recover even if they are immunocompromised (Mayaud *et al.*, 1984). In contrast, the prognosis is poor in patients not treated before acute respiratory failure and shock develop. This is usually late in the course of the illness. In such cases rhabdomyolysis, acute renal failure, pancytopenia, disseminated intravascular coagulation, icterus or coma are not infrequent (Mayaud and Dournon, 1988). However, in most instances patients die from the respiratory distress syndrome and not from the extrapulmonary manifestations of the disease.

Pontiac Fever

Pontiac fever is an acute, non-pneumonic, flu-like illness which is usually self-limiting (Glick *et al.*, 1978). The attack rate is usually very high (>90%) and the disease affects previously healthy, and often young, individuals. The incubation period is short, varying from a few hours to two to three days and the illness resolves spontaneously, usually within two to six days. Outbreaks of Pontiac fever have been reported to be caused by *L. pneumophila*, *L. feeleii*, *L. micdadei* and *L. anisa* (Glick *et al.*, 1978; Goldberg *et al.*, 1989). Although the subject of considerable speculation, the explanation for the differences between LD and Pontiac fever remain unclear.

DIAGNOSTIC METHODS

Although in most instances the clinical picture of LD allows sufficient suspicion of the diagnosis for appropriate treatment to be initiated, evidence from laboratory tests is essential for a definitive diagnosis. There are three approaches to the laboratory diagnosis of *Legionella* infections: culture of the causative organism; identification of the organism, its components or products in clinical specimens; and demonstration of significant levels of antibody directed against the organism in patients' sera.

Specimens for Culture

Culture of legionellae from clinical specimens is relatively easy and, in situations where clinical awareness is high, has a sensitivity of 50–80% (Dournon, 1988; Winn, 1993). Furthermore diagnosis by culture and isolation has several advantages over any other approach. Firstly, isolation of a *Legionella* species provides definitive proof of the diagnosis as colonization without infection has not been demonstrated (Bridge and Edelstein, 1983). Secondly, isolation may be the only way to establish a diagnosis, for example if the patient does not produce antibodies or if there are no reagents available to detect the infecting species/serogroup. Thirdly, isolation of the infecting strain allows subtyping to be undertaken, providing valuable epidemiological data for the control and prevention of further cases of infection.

Given these clear advantages it is perhaps surprising that overall only 13% of cases reported to the CDSC between 1980 and 1993 were confirmed by isolation of the organism. The explanation for this disappointing observation is not entirely clear but may in part be due to the fact that the diagnosis of legionellosis is often only considered after both the initiation of antibiotic therapy and the failure to identify more common pathogens.

Specimens for culture should be taken as early as possible and ideally before antibiotic treatment is initiated. Lower respiratory tract specimens are most likely to yield positive results but sputa are quite satisfactory provided the specimens are pretreated (Dournon, 1988). The pretreatments used to reduce contaminants exploit the property

that legionellae are generally more tolerant to heating and resistant to low pH exposure than are other organisms found in the respiratory tract. Isolation is usually attempted using BCYE agar with and without selective antibiotics; dilution of the specimen may also help. Many combinations of antibiotics have been tried but for the culture of strains from clinical specimens a mixture of polymixin, vancomycin, cefamandole and anisomycin have proved very effective (Dournon, 1988).

Microscopic and Colonial Appearance

A bacterium which is Gram negative, catalase positive and grows on complete BCYE but not on the same medium lacking supplemental L-cysteine can be presumptively identified as a *Legionella* spp. Colonies usually first appear after three to six days of incubation but may be visible in about 36 hours from specimens where large numbers of legionellae are present with few contaminating organisms. Growth tends to be delayed by about 12–24 hours where selective agars are used.

Colonies of *Legionella* are convex, have an entire edge, glisten and have a characteristic granular or 'ground-glass' appearance which is most pronounced in young colonies. Colony colour varies considerably and in large part depends upon the thickness and formulation of growth medium used. In general, however, coloration varies from a blue/green when the colonies are first visible becoming pink/purple as they grow larger. As the colonies age they become less characteristic, being white/grey and smoother; however, the pink/purple coloration can still be seen at their edges. As the name suggests, the colonies of *L. erythra* have a slight red coloration.

All species of *Legionella*, with the exception of *L. oakridgensis*, are weakly motile, having one or two polar flagella. The flagella can be easily demonstrated by one of the many described 'silver-plating stains', based on Fontana's stain for spirochaetes. Furthermore the flagella from all species share common antigens and can be visualized using a suitable antiflagellar serum. Expression of flagellae appears to depend on the growth phase (most abundant in late log phase), the temperature of incubation and the 'passage' history of the isolate.

Plasmids of various sizes (12 to >120 kb) have been found in most species of *Legionella*. Plasmid-bearing isolates are frequently obtained from environmental sources but less commonly from clinical specimens. It has been suggested that the plasmids may enhance survival in the natural habitat and in support of this view one 36 MDa plasmid has been shown to mediate resistance to ultraviolet radiation (Tully, 1991).

Growth Requirements

Legionellae will grow in the temperature range of 29–40 °C with an optimum of 35 °C. However, they will withstand considerably higher temperatures, of 50 °C and above, for a considerable time (>30 minutes) – a characteristic which is exploited in their culture and isolation from clinical and environmental specimens (Dennis, 1988). They grow well aerobically on BCYE agar, particularly when supplemented with α-ketoglutarate. The function of the charcoal in the medium seems to be to prevent superoxide formation. Amino acids such as arginine, threonine, methionine, serine, isoleucine, valine and cystine form the major sources of energy for the organism. Legionellae show an absolute requirement for L-cysteine although *L. oakridgensis* appears not to require L-cysteine as a culture medium supplement after primary isolation. Trace metals such as calcium, cobalt, copper, magnesium, manganese, nickel, vanadium and zinc enhance growth. Although legionellae do not appear to require iron in greater amounts than do other organisms, the presence of soluble iron stimulates growth.

Studies by Rowbotham (1990, 1993) have shown that some legionellae (described as *Legionella*-like amoebal pathogens (LLAPs)) can be obtained from environmental and clinical samples by co-cultivation with amoebae but cannot be grown *in vitro*. Other LLAPs have been identified which can be cultured *in vitro* but require BCYE supplemented with 10 mg/l sodium selenite for growth.

Differentiation of Species

There are a number of simply demonstrated phenotypic characteristics which allow the Legionellaceae to be subdivided into groups of species, or in some cases into individual species (Table 11.2). As in most cases these characteristics have been determined using small numbers of strains of each species, or even a single isolate; the stability of these phenotypic markers is uncertain. Identification of an isolate should, therefore, always be confirmed by an alternative method such as chemical analysis of cellular components, serological identification or molecular analysis.

Antigenic Properties

Legionellae can be subdivided into serogroups (Sgp) by their reaction with hyperimmune antisera containing antibodies directed against the somatic LPS, or 'O', antigens. To date 60 serogroups have been recognized among the 39 species, although in the cases of *L. erythra* Sgp 2 and *L. sainthelensi* Sgp 2 these are indistinguishable from *L. rubrilucens* and *L. santicrucis* respectively (Table 11.1). There is considerable antigenic overlap between some of the serogroups, particularly within the blue-white autofluorescent species complex, and therefore hyperimmune antisera require extensive absorption to render them serogroup specific. There is also significant antigenic heterogeneity within many serogroups. Thus strains of one serogroup may react to different degrees with a serogroup-specific antiserum. Thomason and Bibb (1984) examined this phenomenon in detail using five cross-absorbed polyclonal antisera and 176 *L. pneumophila* Sgp 1 strains. They identified 17 subsets that fell broadly into three subgroups. Serogroup heterogeneity is most clearly revealed using monoclonally derived antibodies (mAbs) which identify type specific epitopes. Panels of such mAbs have been used extensively to subgroup strains of *L. pneumophila* Sgp 1 for epidemiological purposes (Joly *et al.*, 1986).

In addition to O antigens legionellae have flagellar antigens. As noted above, flagella from

TABLE 11.2 SUMMARY OF PHENOTYPIC CHARACTERISTICS AND BIOCHEMICAL REACTIONS HELPFUL IN DIFFERENTIATING BETWEEN *LEGIONELLA* SPP. (MODIFIED FROM HARRISON AND SAUNDERS, 1994).

Test	Result	Relevant species	Comment
Subculture onto BCYE Subculture onto BCYE-Cys	Supports growth Does not support growth	All species[a]	Blood agar is not a suitable substitute for BCYE-Cys, particularly for environmental specimens, as non-legionellae may grow on BCYE but not on blood agar
Gram's stain	Gram negative	All species	Legionellae will readily counterstain with 0.1% basic fuchsin
Catalase test	Positive	All species (*L. pneumophila* only weakly)	Some species possess a peroxidase rather than a catalase but they still give a positive result in the test if 3% H_2O_2 is used
Oxidase test	Negative	All species	Positive results are sometimes recorded but this is probably due to contamination with BCYE medium
Hippurate hydrolysis	Positive Negative	*L. pneumophila* positive All other species negative	Some strains, particularly of subsp. *fraseri*, are said to be negative in this test
Colony autofluorescence under long-wavelength UV (~365 nm)	Red fluorescence	*L. erythra* and *L. rubrilucens*	Red fluorescence may only be seen after prolonged or reduced temperature (~30 °C) incubation
	Blue-white fluorescence	*L. anisa, L. bozemanii, L. cherrii, L. dumoffii, L. gormanii, L. gratiana, L. parisiensis, L. steigerwaltii, L. tucsonensis*	Many of these species are phenotypically and antigenically very similar to others in the group
	No fluorescence	All other species	
Bromocresol-purple spot test	Positive Negative	*L. micdadei, L. maceachernii* positive. All other species negative	These species are serologically distinct

[a] Except some LLAPs (see section on growth requirements for details).

all species share common antigens – a property which can be useful in the identification of new or unknown strains of *Legionella*. It has also been shown that *Legionella* flagella can be subtyped using panels of mAbs (Saunders and Harrison, 1988). The existence of phase variation has not yet been investigated.

Alternatives to Culture

Despite the many advantages of culture, the time taken to obtain results by this method is measured in days. In contrast, the direct demonstration of *Legionella* antigen or nucleic acids in clinical specimens can be achieved within a few hours of specimen collection. Furthermore a diagnosis may be established by visualization or detection of the organism in tissue even when they are no longer viable, after antibiotic therapy or retrospectively in fixed tissues.

Microscopy

Bacteriological stains such as Gimenez and modified Warthin–Starry have been used successfully to detect legionellae in clinical material. However, such stains may reveal any bacterial species and so a specific diagnosis cannot be established. Immunofluorescence using rabbit hyperimmune antisera has been used to diagnose LD since legionellae were first recognized but the poor sensitivity and, particularly, the poor specificity of this method have severely limited its use. More recently the problem of specificity has been overcome by using reagents made from monoclonal antibodies, the most widely used of these being directed against the *L. pneumophila* MOMP (Gostings *et al.*, 1984). This reagent reacts with all the serogroups of *L. pneumophila* and so obviates the need for repeated testing of a specimen with several different antisera. The clinical utility of this reagent has been evaluated (Edelstein *et al.*, 1985) and the specificity has been found to be excellent, allowing a diagnosis to be confidentially established very rapidly. The sensitivity is, however, still considerably lower than that of culture.

Antigen detection

The presence of a soluble antigen in the urine of patients with legionellosis has formed the basis for a range of radioimmunoassays, latex agglutination tests and, particularly, enzyme linked immuno-assay (ELISAs). Studies have shown that antigen may be detectable in the urine very early in the course of the illness, often allowing a diagnosis to be established shortly after admission to hospital (Birtles *et al.*, 1990). Although test kits are available commercially some are cumbersome to use (e.g. they use radioisotopes) and others have performed badly in the laboratory. Until such a time as a simple and reliable test is available this excellent diagnostic method is limited to reference centres.

Molecular methods

A commercial nucleic acid hybridization test for the detection of *L. pneumophila* has been introduced and was shown to be reasonably sensitive for the detection of legionellae in clinical specimens (Finkelstein *et al.*, 1993); however, questions concerning the kit's specificity (Laussucq *et al.*, 1988) and the use of radioisotopes have limited its utility. The recent development of PCR-based techniques for the detection of bacterial nucleic acids in clinical specimens offers the possibility of both highly sensitive and highly specific *Legionella* genus-specific assays (Kessler *et al.*, 1993)

although tests suitable for routine use appear some way off yet.

Diagnosis by Estimation of Antibody Levels

The estimation of antibody levels is still the most commonly employed method for the diagnosis of LD: in 84% of cases of LD reported to the CDSC between 1980 and 1992 a diagnosis of LD was established only by serology.

Historically the indirect immunofluorescent antibody test (IFAT) was the method used to establish that *L. pneumophila* was the causative agent of LD (McDade *et al.*, 1977). Since this time several variants of this test have been thoroughly evaluated for the diagnosis of infection caused by *L. pneumophila* Sgp 1, and the IFAT has become the reference test for LD diagnosis (Harrison and Taylor 1988). The test predominantly used in the UK employs a formolized yolk-sac antigen (FYSA) and fluoroscienisothiocyanate (FITC)-labelled anti-human conjugate capable of detecting IgG, IgM and IgA. This test has been shown to have excellent sensitivity (approximately 80%) and specificity (>99%) (Harrison and Taylor, 1988), the later being particularly important in a disease of low prevalence such as LD, if a positive result is to have any real significance.

It is important that a conjugate capable of detecting all three major classes of immunoglobulin is used if sensitivity is to be maximized. There is no value in determining specific IgM levels as a marker of recent infection as IgM can, and usually does, persist for months or even years after infection. Conversely if only IgG is present it may be reasonable to conclude that infection is not recent.

One possible area of concern is false positive results, the mechanism of which is not known, which have recently been reported to occur with sera from patients with *Campylobacter* infections. This cross-reaction appears real and significant (Marshall *et al.*, 1994) although in practice it does not often cause any diagnostic confusion.

Although reagents for IFATs to detect infection caused by species and serogroups of *Legionella* other than *L. pneumophila* Sgp 1 are commercially available there are very few evaluation data for these tests and results obtained using them should be treated with considerable caution.

In addition to the IFAT many other assays have been developed for the serological diagnosis of LD, including ELISAs (Wreghitt *et al.*, 1982), direct agglutination tests (Harrison and Taylor, 1982) and haemagglutination tests (Lennette *et al.*, 1979). With one exception few of these tests have been widely used. The exception is a rapid microagglutination test (Harrison and Taylor, 1982) which, largely because of its speed, simplicity and, most importantly availability, has been used widely in the UK. Again, because of the paucity of culture-proven cases caused by *Legionella* other than *L. pneumophila* Sgpl, the rapid micro-agglutination test (RMAT) has been only thoroughly evaluated for the diagnosis of infections caused by this serogroup, although some data are available for *L. pneumophila* Sgp5 (Constantine and Wreghitt, 1991).

Antibiotic Treatment

Legionellae are susceptible to a wide range of antibiotics *in vitro* but these findings are not necessarily predictive of their *in vivo* efficacy. As legionellae are facultative intracellular organisms some antibiotics that are active *in vitro* are not active *in vivo* because their intracellular penetration is poor. Furthermore the media used to culture legionellae inhibit the activity of some antibiotics, making a valid determination of minimum inhibitory concentrations (MICs) and minimum bactericidal concentration (MBCs) difficult (Edelstein and Meyer, 1980; Dowling *et al.*, 1984).

A limited number of antibiotics including erythromycin, rifampicin and several fluoroquinolones have been shown to be effective in animal and cell culture models of infection (Vildé *et al.*, 1986). Furthermore these studies have shown that any combination of these drugs has a synergistic effect. Despite good evidence that the fluoroquinolones are more active than erythromycin, in the absence of any prospective studies, the drug of choice remains erythromycin. Rifampicin

is usually added to this if the patient does not respond (Plouffe, 1993).

PREVENTION AND CONTROL OF INFECTION

Five essential elements must be in place if legionellae are to give rise to infection. A virulent strain must be present in an environmental reservoir; conditions must be such that it can multiply to significant numbers; a mechanism must exist for creating an aerosol containing the organisms from the reservoir; the aerosol must be disseminated; and finally a susceptible human must inhale the aerosol. Prevention of infection depends upon breaking this 'chain of causation' (Breiman, 1993).

As discussed above, legionellae can be found in low numbers in almost all aquatic environments. It is probably not possible to eradicate legionellae from such a system because of regrowth from residual biofilm or reseeding from other environmental sources. However, it is feasible to ensure that the numbers of organisms remain at a low level, and it is the aim of most preventative procedures to break this link of the chain. Legionellae grow best in water at temperatures between 20 and 40 °C, particularly where there is an accumulation of organic and inorganic material. Thus the strategy is to keep the systems clean by regular maintenance; to keep cold water at below 20 °C and hot water above 50 °C; to avoid the use of certain materials in the construction of water systems; and, where appropriate, to use a programme of treatment with biocides and other chemicals.

Aerosols can be generated from many sources such as cooling towers, showers, taps, nebulizers, and other domestic and industrial equipment. The use of effective drift eliminators in cooling towers can considerably reduce the release of aerosol. However, in some instances, for example showers, there is little that can be done but to avoid their use. Where the population at risk is particularly susceptible, e.g. transplant patients, this approach is sometimes taken. Approved codes of practice and guidelines detailing all aspects of design, maintenance and running of water systems and cooling towers have been provided from a number of governmental and professional bodies and much excellent advice is now available (Health and Safety Commission, 1991, 1992; Department of Health, 1991).

REFERENCES

Amano, K.I. and Williams, J.C. (1983) Peptidoglycan of *Legionella pneumophila*: apparent resistance to lysozyme hydrolysis correlates with a high degree of peptide cross-linking. *Journal of Bacteriology*, **153**, 520–526.

Bellinger-Kawahara, C. and Horwitz, M.A. (1990) Complement component C3 fixes selectively to the major outer membrane protein (MOMP) of *Legionella pneumophila* and mediates phagocytosis of liposome–MOMP complexes by human monocytes. *Journal of Experimental Medicine*, **172**, 1201–1210.

Birtles, R.J., Harrison, T.G., Samuel, D. *et al.* (1990) Evaluation of urinary antigen ELISA for diagnosing *Legionella pneumophila* serogroup 1 infection. *Journal of Clinical Pathology*, **43**, 685–690.

Blander, S.J., Szeto, L., Shuman, H.A. *et al.* (1990) An immunoprotective molecule, the major secretory protein of *Legionella pneumophila*, is not a virulence factor in a guinea pig model of Legionnaires' disease. *Journal of Clinical Investigation*, **86**, 817–824.

Breiman, R.F. (1993) Modes of transmission in epidemic and nonepidemic *Legionella* infection: directions for further study. In *Legionella: Current Status and Future Perspectives* (ed. J.M. Barbaree, F. Breiman and A.P. Dufour), pp. 30–35. American Society of Microbiology, Washington, DC.

Brenner, D.J., Steigerwalt, A.G. and McDade, J.E. (1979) Classification of the Legionnaires' disease bacterium: *Legionella pneumophila*, genus novum, species nova, of the Family Legionellaceae, familia nova. *Annals of Internal Medicine*, **90**, 656–658.

Bridge, J.A. and Edelstein, P.H. (1983) Oropharyngeal colonization with *Legionella pneumophila*. *Journal of Clinical Microbiology*, **18**, 1108–1112.

Cianciotto, N.P., Eisenstein, I., Mody, C.H. *et al.* (1990a) A mutation in the *mip* gene results in an attenuation of *Legionella pneumophila* virulence. *Journal of Infectious Diseases*, **162**, 121–126.

Cianciotto, N.P., Bangsborg, J.M., Eisenstein, B.I. *et al.* (1990b) Identification of *mip*-like genes in the genus *Legionella*. *Infection and Immunity*, **58**, 2912–2918.

Colbourne, J.S., Dennis, P.J., Trew, R.M. *et al.* (1988) *Legionella* and public water supplies. *Water Science and Technology*, **20**, 5–10.

Conlan, J.W., Williams, A. and Ashworth, L.A.E. (1988) *In vivo* production of a tissue-destructive

protease by *Legionella pneumophila*. *Journal of General Microbiology*, **134**, 143–149.

Constantine, C.E. and Wreghitt, T.G. (1991) A rapid micro-agglutination technique for the detection of antibody to *Legionella pneumophila* serogroup 5. *Journal of Medical Microbiology*, **34**, 29–31.

Dennis, P.J. (1988) Isolation of legionellae from environmental specimens. In *A Laboratory Manual for Legionella* (ed. T.G. Harrison and A.G. Taylor), pp. 31–44. Wiley, Chichester.

Dennis, P.J. and Lee, J.V. (1988) Differences in aerosol survival between pathogenic and non-pathogenic strains of *Legionella pneumophila* serogroup 1. *Journal of Applied Bacteriology*, **65**, 135–141.

Dennis, P.J., Brenner, D.J., Thacker, W.L. *et al.* (1993) Five new *Legionella* species isolated from water. *International Journal of Systematic Bacteriology*, **43**, 329–337.

Department of Health and Social Security and the Welsh Office (1991) *The Control of Legionellae in Health Care Premises: A Code of Practice*. HMSO, London.

Dournon, E. (1988) Isolation of legionellae from clinical specimens. In *A Laboratory Manual for Legionella* (ed. T.G. Harrison and A.G. Taylor), pp. 13–30. Wiley, Chichester.

Dournon, E., Bibb, W.F., Rajagopalan, P. *et al.* (1988) Monoclonal antibody reactivity as a virulence marker for *Legionella pheumophila* serogroup 1 strains. *Journal of Infectious Disease*, **157**, 496–501.

Dowling, J.N., McDevitt, D.A. and Pasculle, A.W. (1984) Disk diffusion antimicrobial susceptibility testing of members of the family Legionellaceae including erythromycin-resistant variants of *Legionella micdadei*. *Journal of Clinical Microbiology*, **19**, 723–729.

Dowling, J.N., Saha A.K. and Glew, R.H. (1992) Virulence factors of the family Legionellaceae. *Microbiological Reviews*, **56**, 32–60.

Edelstein, P.H. and Edelstein, M.A.C. (1993) Intracellular growth of *Legionella pneumophila* serogroup 1 monoclonal antibody type 2 positive and negative bacteria. *Epidemiology and Infection*, **111**, 499–502.

Edelstein, P.H. and Meyer, R.D. (1980) Susceptibility of *Legionella pneumophila* to twenty antimicrobial agents. *Antimicrobial Agents and Chemotherapy*, **18**, 403–408.

Edelstein, P.H., Beer, K.B., Sturge, J.C. *et al.* (1985) Clinical utility of a monoclonal direct fluorescent reagent specific for *Legionella pneumophila*: comparative study with other reagents. *Journal of Clinical Microbiology*, **22**, 419–421.

Fields, B.S. (1991) The role of amoebae in legionellosis. *Clinical Microbiology Newsletter*, **13**, 92–93.

Finkelstein, R., Brown, P., Palutke, W.A. *et al.* (1993) Diagnostic efficacy of a DNA probe in pneumonia caused by *Legionella* species. *Journal of Medical Microbiology*, **38**, 183–186.

Fliermans, C.B. and Tyndall, R.L. (1993) Association of *Legionella pneumophila* with natural ecosystems. In *Legionella: Current Status and Emerging Perspectives* (ed. J.M. Barbaree, F. Breiman and A.P. Dufour), pp. 284–285. American Society for Microbiology, Washington, DC.

Fliermans, C.B., Cherry, W.B., Orrison, L.H. *et al.* (1981) Ecological distribution of *Legionella pneumophila*. *Applied and Environmental Microbiology*, **41**, 9–16.

Glick, T.H., Gregg, M.B., Berman, B. *et al.* (1978) Pontiac fever: an epidemic of unknown etiology in a health department: 1. Clinical and epidemiological aspects. *American Journal of Epidemiology*, **107**, 149–160.

Goldberg, D.J., Wrench, J.G., Collier, P.W. *et al.* (1989) Lochgoilhead fever: an outbreak of non-pneumonic legionellosis due to *Legionella micdadei*. *Lancet*, **i**, 316–318.

Gostings, L.H., Cabrian, K., Sturge, J.C. *et al.* (1984) Identification of a species-specific antigen in *Legionella pneumophila* by a monoclonal antibody. *Journal of Clinical Microbiology*, **20**, 1031–1035.

Harf, C. and Monteil, H. (1988) Interactions between free-living amoebae and *Legionella* in the environment. *Water Science Technology*, **20**, 235–239.

Harrison, T.G. and Saunders, N.A. (1994) Taxonomy and typing of legionellae. *Reviews in Medical Microbiology*, **5**, 79–90.

Harrison, T.G. and Taylor, A.G. (1982) A rapid microagglutination test for the diagnosis of *Legionella pneumophila* (serogroup 1) infection. *Journal of Clinical Pathology*, **35**, 1028–1031.

Harrison, T.G. and Taylor, A.G. (1988) The diagnosis of Legionnaires' disease by antibody levels. In *A Laboratory Manual for Legionella* (ed. T.G. Harrison and A.G. Taylor), pp. 124–135. Wiley, Chichester.

Health and Safety Commission (1991) *The Prevention or Control of Legionellosis (Including Legionnaires' Disease): Approved Code of Practice.* HMSO, London.

Health and Safety Commission (1992) *The Notification of Cooling Tower and Evaporative Condensers Regulations 1992. Statutory Instrument, 1992 No. 225. Health and Safety.* HMSO, London.

Horwitz, M.A. (1983) The Legionnaires' disease bacterium (*Legionella pneumophila*) inhibits phagosome–lysosome fusion in human monocytes. *Journal of Experimental Medicine*, **158**, 2108–2126.

Horwitz, M.A. (1988) Phagocytosis and intracellular biology of *Legionella pneumophila*. In *Bacteria–Host Cell Interaction* (ed. M.A. Horwitz), pp. 283–302. Liss, New York.

Horwitz, M.A. and Maxfield, F.R. (1984) *Legionella pneumophila* inhibits acidification of its phagosome in human monocytes. *Journal of Cell Biology*, **99**, 1936–1943.

Horwitz, M.A. and Silverstein, S.C. (1980) Legionnaires' disease bacterium (*Legionella pneumophila*) multiplies intracellularly in human monocytes. *Journal of Clinical Investigation*, **66**, 441–450.

Horwitz, M.A. and Silverstein, S.C. (1981) Activated human monocytes inhibit the intracellular multiplication of legionnaires' disease bacteria. *Journal of Experimental Medicine*, **154**, 1618–1633.

Hubbard, R.B., Mathur, R.M. and MacFarlane, J.T. (1993) Severe community-acquired legionella pneumonia: treatment, complications and outcome. *Quarterly Journal of Medicine*, **86**, 327–332.

Joly, J.R., McKinney, R.M., Tobin, J.O'H. *et al.* (1986) Development of a standardized subgrouping scheme for *Legionella pneumophila* serogroup 1 using monoclonal antibodies. *Journal of Clinical Microbiology*, **23**, 768–771.

Joseph, C.A., Harrison, T.G. and Watson, J.M. (1993) Legionnaires' disease surveillance: England and Wales, 1992. *Communicable Diseases Report*, **3**, R124–126.

Joseph, C.A., Watson, J.M., Harrison, T.G. *et al.* (1994) Nosocomial Legionnaires' disease in England and Wales, 1980–92. *Epidemiology and Infection*, **112**, 329–345.

Kessler, H.H., Reinthaler, F.F., Pschaid, A. *et al.* (1993) Rapid detection of *Legionella* species in bronchoalveolar lavage fluids with the Enviro Amp Legionella PCR amplification and detection kit. *Journal of Clinical Microbiology*, **31**, 3325–3328.

Kilvington, S. and Price, J. (1990) Survival of *Legionella pneumophila* within *Acanthamoeba polyphagia* cysts following chlorine exposure. *Journal of Applied Bacteriology*, **68**, 519–525.

Laussucq, S., Schuster, D., Alexander, W.J. *et al.* (1988) False-positive DNA probe test for *Legionella* species associated with a cluster of respiratory illnesses. *Journal of Clinical Microbiology*, **26**, 1442–1444.

Lennette, D.A., Lennette, E.T., Wentworth, B.B. *et al.* (1979) Serology of Legionnaires' disease: comparison of indirect fluorescent antibody, immune adherence hemagglutination, and indirect hemagglutination tests. *Journal of Clinical Microbiology*, **10**, 876–879.

MacFarlane, J.T., Finch, R.G., Ward, M.J. *et al.* (1982) Hospital study of adult community-acquired pneumonia. *Lancet*, **ii**, 255–258.

Marshall, L.E., Boswell, T.C. and Kudesia, G. (1994) False positive legionella serology in campylobacter infection: campylobacter serotypes, duration of antibody response and elimination of cross-reactions in the indirect fluorescent antibody test. *Epidemiology and Infection*, **112**, 347–357.

Mayaud, C. and Dournon, E. (1988) Clinical features of Legionnaires' disease. In *A Laboratory Manual for Legionella* (ed. T.G. Harrison and A.G. Taylor), pp. 5–11. Wiley, Chichester.

Mayaud, C., Carett, M.F., Dournon, E. *et al.* (1984) Clinical features and prognosis of severe pneumonia caused by *Legionella pneumophila*. In *Legionella: Proceedings of the 2nd International Symposium* (ed. C. Thornsberry, A. Balows, J.C. Feeley *et al.*), pp. 11–20. American Society for Microbiology, Washington, DC.

McDade, J.E., Shepard, C.C., Fraser, D.W. *et al.* (1977) Legionnaires' disease: isolation of a bacterium and demonstration of its role in other respiratory disease. *New England Journal of Medicine*, **297**, 1197–1203.

Memorandum from a WHO meeting (1990) Epidemiology, prevention and control of legionellosis: memorandum from a WHO meeting. *Bulletin of the World Health Organization*, **68**, 155–164.

Moffat, J.F., Edelstein, P.H., Regular, D.P. *et al.* (1994) Effects of an isogenic Zn-metalloprotease-deficient mutant of *Legionella pneumophila* in a guinea-pig pneumonia model. *Molecular Microbiology*, **12**, 693–705.

Petitjean, F., Dournon, E., Strosberg, A.D. *et al.* (1990) Isolation, purification and partial analysis of the lipopolysaccharide antigenic determinant recognised by a monoclonal antibody to *Legionella pneumophila* serogroup 1. *Research in Microbiology*, **141**, 1077–1094.

Plouffe, J.F. (1993) Evolution of chemotherapy and diagnostic tests. In *Legionella: Current Status and Future Perspectives* (ed. J.M. Barbaree, F. Breiman and A.P. Dufour), pp. 294–295. American Society for Microbiology, Washington, D.C.

Quinn, F.D., Keen, M.G. and Tompkins, L.S. (1989) Genetic immunological, and cytotoxic comparison of *Legionella* proteolytic activities. *Infection and Immunity*, **57**, 2719–2725.

Rechnitzer, C. and Blom, J. (1989) Engulfment of the Philadelphia strain of *Legionella pneumophila* within pseudopod coils in human phagocytes. *APMIS*, **97**, 105–114.

Rowbotham, T.J. (1980) Preliminary report on the pathogenicity of *Legionella pneumophila* for freshwater and soil amoebae. *Journal of Clinical Pathology*, **33**, 1179–1183.

Rowbotham, T.J. (1983) Isolation of *Legionella pneumophila* from clinical specimens via amoeba, and the interaction of those and other isolates with amoeba. *Journal of Clinical Pathology*, **36**, 978–986.

Rowbotham, T.J. (1993) *Legionella*-like amoebal pathogens. In *Legionella: Current Status and Emerging Perspectives* (ed. J.M. Barbaree, F. Breiman and A.P. Dufour), pp. 137–140. American Society for Microbiology, Washington, DC.

Saunders, N.A. and Harrison, T.G. (1988) The application of nucleic acid probes and monoclonal antibodies to the investigation of *Legionella* infections. In *A Laboratory Manual for Legionella* (ed. T.G. Harrison and A.G. Taylor), pp. 137–153. Wiley, Chichester.

Sonesson, A., Jantzen, E., Bryn, K. *et al.* (1989) Chemical composition of a lipopolysaccharide from *Legionella pneumophila*. *Archives of Microbiology*, **153**, 72–78.

Steele, T.W. (1993) Interactions between soil amoebae and soil legionellae. In *Legionella: Current Status and Future Perspectives* (ed. J.M. Barbaree, F. Breiman and A.P. Dufour), pp. 140–142. American Society for Microbiology, Washington, DC.

Stout, J.E., Yu, V.L., Yee, Y.C. *et al.* (1992) *Legionella pneumophila* in residential water supplies: environmental surveillance with clinical assessment for Legionnaires' disease. *Epidemiology and Infection*, **109**, 49–57.

Szeto, L. and Shuman, H.A. (1990) The *Legionella pneumophila* major secretory protein, a protease, is not required for intracellular growth or cell killing. *Infection and Immunity*, **58**, 2585–2592.

Thomason, B.M. and Bibb, W.F. (1984) Use of absorbed antisera for demonstration of antigenic variation among strains of *Legionella pneumophila* serogroup 1. *Journal of Clinical Microbiology*, **19**, 794–797.

Tison, D.L., Pope, D.H., Cherry, W.B. *et al.* (1980) Growth of *Legionella pneumophila* in association with blue-green algae (Cyanobacteria). *Applied and Environmental Microbiology*, **39**, 456–459.

Tobin, J.O'H., Swann, R.A. and Bartlett, C.L.R. (1981) Isolation of *Legionella pneumophila* from water systems: methods and preliminary results. *British Medical Journal*, **282**, 515–517.

Tully, M. (1991) A plasmid from a virulent strain of *Legionella pneumophila* is conjugative and confers resistance to ultraviolet light. *FEMS Microbiology Letters*, **90**, 43–48.

Vildé, J.L., Dournon, E. and Rajagopalan, P. (1986). Inhibition of *Legionella pneumophila* multiplication within human macrophages by antimicrobial agents. *Antimicrobial Agents and Chemotherapy*, **30**, 743–748.

Wait, R. (1988) Confirmation of the identity of legionellae by whole cell fatty-acid and isoprenoid quinone profiles. In *A Laboratory Manual for Legionella* (ed. T.G. Harrison and A.G. Taylor), pp. 69–101. Wiley, Chichester.

Williams, A., Rechnitzer, C., Lever, M.S. *et al.* (1993) Intracellular production of *Legionella pneumophila* tissue-destructive protease in alveolar macrophages. In *Legionella: Current Status and Emerging Perspectives* (ed. J.M. Barbaree, R.F. Breiman and A.P.

Dufour), pp. 88–90. American Society for Microbiology, Washington, DC.

Winn, W.C. (1993) *Legionnella* and the clinical microbiologist. In *Infectious Disease Clinics of North America*, pp. 377–392. Saunders, Philadelphia.

Wong, K.H., Moss, C.W., Hochstein, D.H. *et al.* (1979) 'Endotoxicity' of the legionnaires' disease bacterium. *Annals of Internal Medicine*, **90**, 624–627

Woodhead, M.A., MacFarlane, J.T., Macrae, A.D. *et al.* (1986) The rise and fall of Legionnaires' disease in Nottingham. *Journal of Infection*, **13**, 293–296.

Wreghitt, T.G., Nagington, J. and Gray, J. (1982) An ELISA test for the detection of antibodies to *Legionella pneumophila*. *Journal of Clinical Pathology*, **35**, 657–660.

12

IDENTIFICATION OF ENTEROBACTERIACEAE

Peter M. Hawkey

The family Enterobacteriacae is the most widely studied family of organisms in the world. They have a worldwide distribution and, whilst largely found in animals, medical microbiologists are inclined to gain a distorted view of the family as they only encounter species associated with human disease, such as *Escherichia coli*, *Proteus mirabilis*, *Salmonella* spp. and *Klebsiella* spp. The genera *Erwinia* and *Pectobacteria* are major plant pathogens causing blights, wilts and rots in many different crops. *Yersinia ruckeri* is a major pathogen of farmed salmon, and the salmonellae are pathogens of cattle, sheep and poultry. Various species of Enterobacteriaceae have been isolated from the gut contents of animals ranging from fleas to elephants, some being adapted to very specific hosts, e.g. *Proteus myxofaciens* in the gut of gypsy moth larvae.

The family is numerically important to the medical microbiologist, as they may account for 80% of clinically significant Gram-negative bacilli and about 50% of isolates from cases of septicaemia. The family now has over 20 genera and more than 100 species, of which about 50 are definitely or probably associated with human disease (Farmer *et al.*, 1985). Taxonomy now makes use of information on the relationship of isolates from examining a wide range of semantides (large information-bearing molecules). These are DNA, both in terms of sequences of genes and DNA/DNA hybridization studies, RNA, particularly 16S rRNA phylogenetic trees, and proteins both as functional enzymes and as electrophoretic cellular protein patterns. The synthesis of this information has led to the development of a clear and scientifically robust taxonomy of the Enterobacteriaceae. These developments are comprehensively and authoritatively reviewed by Farmer and colleagues in a review which although now some 15 years old is still the most useful (Farmer *et al.*, 1985). Changes in taxonomy are often reluctantly accepted by medical microbiologists, but this is an evolving area and much of that which is familiar remains. I urge the reader to embrace the newer names and use them – they will become familiar in time. Although there appear to be a number of unfamiliar genera, such as *Ewingella*, *Obesum bacterium* and *Xenorhabdus*, these organisms are very rarely encountered. In clinical material 99% of isolates are represented by 23 species, whereas the remaining 1% belong to 74 species (Farmer *et al.*, 1985). The adage from the authors, 'when you hear hoof beats, think horses, not zebras', is indeed true.

Principles and Practice of Clinical Bacteriology. Edited by A.M. Emmerson, P.M. Hawkey and S.H. Gillespie
© 1997 John Wiley & Sons Ltd

There are four reasons why clinical microbiologists may wish to identify microorganisms:

(1) to help predict the likely outcome of the infection;
(2) to identify potential cross-infection risks and cross-infection retrospectively;
(3) to attempt to predict likely sensitivity to antimicrobials;
(4) to obtain research information on new disease associations with microorganisms.

The level to which an identification is made is very much a question of the clinical significance of the cultured bacteria. In the case of a moist, non-inflamed surgical wound from which a mixture of faecal bacteria, such as enterococci, *Escherichia coli*, *Klebsiella* spp., *Proteus mirabilis* and *Pseudomonas aeruginosa* are cultured, identification of the individual isolates of Enterobacteriaceae is inappropriate and a report of mixed faecal flora should be made. Isolates of Enterobacteriaceae from blood cultures, normally sterile sites (e.g. cerebrospinal fluid, peritoneum, deep tissues), infections at different sites requiring linking (e.g. isolate from a blood culture and urine), enteric pathogens (e.g. *Salmonella enteritidis*, *Shigella sonnei*) and if epidemiologically important (e.g. multi-resistant *Klebsiella pneumoniae*) should be identified to species level.

With the development of newer technologies the utilization of identification as a predictor of pathogenicity, e.g. identification of *Shigella dysenteriae*, will be replaced by identification of the genes responsible for pathogenicity, regardless of the host background. In the example cited, this will identify isolates of *E. coli* of similar pathogenic potential to *Shigella* which might easily be missed if biochemical identification methods are used. Species identification of some Enterobacteriaceae combined with antimicrobial sensitivity data may predict responses to certain agents. This is true of the use of cefotaxime/ceftazidine to treat bacteraemia and pneumonia caused by *Enterobacter* spp. because of the selection of derepressed mutants expressing the chromosomal gene *amp*C encoded by the β-lactamase found in that species.

There are other species-specific β-lactamase associations which have been extensively reviewed recently (Livermore, 1995). These predictions are not confined to β-lactams: *Serratia marcescens* was found to be the only species of Enterobacteriaceae that carries the *aac*(6')-Ic gene that encodes the aminoglycoside-inactivating enzyme AAC(6')-Ic, when 186 strains of 10 species of *Serratia* were probed with a specific DNA probe (Snelling *et al.*, 1993). The enzyme confers resistance to aminoglycosides, such as tobramycin, netilmicin and amikacin, and aminoglycoside-sensitive strains of *S. marcescens* can express the gene fully after exposure to these substrates, leading to treatment failure. Some species of the Enterobacteriaceae are 'intrinsically' resistant to certain antimicrobials and this can be used to help in the presumptive identification of isolates in the clinical laboratory. Table 12.1 lists this information.

Suspicion that an isolate cultured from a clinical specimen belongs to the Enterobacteriaceae arises from the following characteristics:

- Gram-negative bacillus $0.5-2$ μm $\times$ $2-4$ μm
- cytochrome oxidase negative
- ferments glucose
- nitrates reduced to nitrites
- facultative anaerobe

Some species have characteristic appearances on solid media which may give a clue as to identity: swarming – *Proteus* spp.; pronounced mucoid capsule – *Klebsiella*/*Enterobacter* spp. However, definitive identification relies on the use of the fermentation of carbohydrate tests and a number of other tests to identify the presence or absence of specific enzymes, e.g. amino acid decarboxylases, urease, phenylalanine deaminase. Microbiologists at the end of the nineteenth century, such as Escherich and Gärtner (who discovered *Salmonella enteritidis* in 1888) relied heavily on the use of agglutination tests to differentiate Enterobacteriaceae. It was workers such as the American bacteriologist Theobald Smith and Herbert Durham, at the University of Cambridge, who appreciated the value of carbohydrate fermentation tests in identification. Durham reviewed the state of knowledge in 1900 (Durham, 1900) and,

TABLE 12.1 INTRINSIC ANTIMICROBIAL RESISTANCE ENCOUNTERED IN CLINICALLY SIGNIFICANT ENTERO-BACTERIACEAE. RESISTANCE TO AGENTS SHOWN IN PARENTHESES IS ONLY SEEN IN HYPER-PRODUCERS OF β-LACTAMASE

Species	Agents to which most strains are resistant	Common chromosomal β-lactamase[a]
Citrobacter diversus	Ampicillin,[b] cefuroxime, cephalothin,[c] cefoxitin (piperacillin,[d] ticarcillin[e])	'K1 type'[f]
Citrobacter freundii	Ampicillin, cephalothin, cefoxitin (piperacillin, cefotaxime, ceftazidine, aztreonam)	AmpC
Enterobacter spp.	Ampicillin, cephalothin, cefoxitin (piperacillin, cefotaxime, ceftazidine, aztreonam)	AmpC
Klebsiella pneumoniae	Ampicillin, ticarcillin	SHV-1
Klebsiella oxytoca	Ampicillin, ticarcillin (piperacillin, cefuroxime, cefotaxime, aztreonam)[g]	K1
Morganella morganii	Polymyxins, nitrofurantoin, ampicillin, cephalothin, cefuroxime (ticarcillin, piperacillin, cefotaxime, ceftazidine)	AmpC
Proteus mirabilis	Polymyxins, tetracycline, nitrofurantoin	
Proteus vulgaris/ penneri	Polymyxins, nitrofurantoin, ampicillin, cefuroxime, cephalothin, cefoxitin (piperacillin, ticarcillin)	'K1 type'[h]
Providencia stuartii/ rettgeri	As *M. morganii*, plus tetracycline except *Prov. stuartii* resistant to gentamicin/tobramycin	AmpC
Serratia marcescens	Polymyxins,[j] ampicillin, cephalothin, cefuroxime (ticarcillin, piperacillin, cefotaxime)	AmpC

[a] Expression of these genes varies, so resistance in individual strains may vary according to induction or mutation to hyperproduction. Representative of: [b] amoxycillin; [c] cephalexin, cefazolin, cephradine; [d] azlocillin/mezlocillin; [e] carbenicillin. [f] Some strains have AmpC-like enzymes (Jones *et al.*, 1994). [g] Hyperproduction of K1 only occurs in 10–20% of isolates, rarer than *Enterobacter* spp. AmpC. [h] 'Cefuroximases' classified by Bush *et al.* (1995) as 2e. [j] Frequently forms 'target zones' around disc.

using a range of fermentable vegetable extracts, as well as other tests, recognized 10 distinct 'types' which accord broadly with many of the genera now recognized in the Enterobacteriaceae.

Initially, laboratories prepared their own identification media and the choice and quality control were highly individualistic. In the late 1960s, miniaturized, disposable, commercially prepared systems such as the API and Enterotube systems became available. These offered rapid, reliable identification and in the case of the API20E system used freeze-dried reagents that were rehydrated by inoculation with a suspension of the bacterium to be identified. Traditionally, laboratories relied on either flow charts or tables for translating test results into a species identification. Various systems were devised to save time, one of the best known being the 'Identicards' (notched record cards probed with a knitting needle) described in *Cowan and Steele's*

Manual for the Identification of Medical Bacteria (Barrow and Feltham, 1993). The widely used API20E system for the identification of Enterobacteriaceae translates the results from 21 individual tests into an octal number. The tests are arranged in groups of three and the positive and negative results for each converted into a single octal, representing the results for that group of three tests, as shown in Table 12.2. A seven-digit

TABLE 12.2 OCTAL CONVERSION OF BINARY CODE

Binary	Conversion formula	Octal
– – –	0 + 0 + 0 =	0
+ – –	0 + 0 + 1 =	1
– + –	0 + 2 + 0 =	2
+ + –	0 + 2 + 1 =	3
– – +	4 + 0 + 0 =	4
+ – +	4 + 0 + 1 =	5
– + +	4 + 2 + 0 =	6
+ + +	4 + 2 + 1 =	7

TABLE 12.3 BIOCHEMICAL REACTIONS OF THE COMMONLY ENCOUNTERED CLINICALLY SIGNIFICANT ENTEROBACTERIACEAE (AFTER FARMER ET AL., 1985)

Species	Indole production	Methyl red	Voges–Proskauer	Citrate (Simmons')	Hydrogen sulphide (TSI)	Urea hydrolysis	Phenylalanine deaminase	Lysine decarboxylase	Arginine dihydrolase	Ornithine decarboxylase	Motility (36°C)	Gelatine hydrolysis (22°C)	D-Glucose, gas	Lactose fermentation	Sucrose fermentation	D-Mannitol fermentation	Dulcitol fermentation	Adonitol fermentation	D-Sorbitol fermentation	L-Arabinose fermentation	Raffinose fermentation	L-Rhamnose fermentation	D-Xylose fermentation	Melibiose fermentation	DNAse, 25°C	ONPGᵃ
Escherichia coli	+	+	–	–	–	–	–	+	>	>	+	–	+	+	>	+	>	–	+	+	>	>	+	>	–	+
Shigella serogroups A, B and C	>	+	–	–	–	–	–	–	–	–	–	–	–	–	–	+	–	–	>	>	>	–	–	>	–	–
Shigella sonnei	–	+	–	–	–	–	–	–	–	+	–	–	–	–	–	+	–	–	–	+	–	>	–	–	–	+
Salmonella, most serotypes	–	+	–	+	+	–	–	+	>	+	+	–	+	–	–	+	+	–	+	+	–	+	+	+	–	–
Salmonella typhi	–	+	–	–	+	–	–	+	–	–	+	–	–	–	–	+	–	–	+	+	–	–	>	+	–	–
Salmonella paratyphi A	–	+	–	–	>	–	–	–	>	+	+	–	+	–	–	+	+	–	–	+	–	+	–	+	–	–
Citrobacter freudii	+	+	–	+	>	>	–	–	>	>	+	–	+	>	>	+	>	–	+	+	>	+	+	>	–	+
Citrobacter diversus	+	+	–	+	–	>	–	–	>	+	+	–	+	>	>	+	>	+	+	+	–	+	+	–	–	+
Klebsiella pneumoniae	–	>	+	+	–	+	–	+	–	–	–	–	+	+	+	+	>	+	+	+	+	+	+	+	–	+
Klebsiella oxytoca	+	>	+	+	–	+	–	+	–	–	–	–	+	+	+	+	>	+	+	+	+	+	+	+	–	+
Enterobacter aerogenes	–	–	+	+	–	–	–	+	–	+	+	–	+	+	+	+	–	+	+	+	+	+	+	+	–	+
Enterobacter cloacae	–	–	+	+	–	>	–	–	+	+	+	–	+	+	+	+	>	>	+	+	+	+	+	+	–	+
Hafnia alvei	–	>	>	>	–	–	–	+	–	+	>	–	+	–	>	+	–	–	–	+	–	+	+	–	–	+
Serratia liquefaciens	–	+	+	+	–	–	–	+	–	+	+	+	>	>	+	+	–	>	+	+	+	>	+	>	>	+
Serratia marcescens	–	>	+	+	–	>	–	+	–	+	+	+	>	–	+	+	–	–	+	–	>	–	–	–	+	+
Proteus mirabilis	–	+	>	>	+	+	+	–	–	+	+	+	+	–	>	–	–	–	–	–	–	–	+	–	>	–
Proteus vulgaris	+	+	–	>	+	+	+	–	–	–	+	+	>	–	+	–	–	–	–	–	–	–	+	–	>	–
Providencia rettgeri	+	+	–	+	–	+	+	–	–	–	+	–	>	–	>	+	–	+	–	–	–	>	>	–	–	>
Providencia stuartii	+	+	–	+	–	>	+	–	–	–	>	–	–	–	>	>	–	–	–	–	–	–	+	–	>	–
Providencia alcalifaciens	+	+	–	+	–	–	+	–	–	–	+	–	+	–	–	–	–	+	–	–	–	–	–	–	–	–
Morganella morganii	+	+	–	–	–	+	+	–	–	+	+	–	+	–	–	–	–	–	–	–	–	–	>	–	>	–
Yersinia enterocolitica	>	>	–	–	–	>	–	–	–	+	–	–	–	+	+	+	–	–	+	+	–	–	+	<	–	+
Yersinia pestis	–	>	–	–	–	–	–	–	–	–	–	–	–	–	–	+	–	–	>	+	>	>	+	>	–	>
Yersinia pseudotuberculosis	–	+	–	–	–	+	–	–	–	–	–	–	–	–	–	+	–	–	–	+	>	+	+	>	–	>

ᵃONPG, *o*-nitrophenyl-*β*-D-galactopyranoside; >90% positive = +; 10–90% positive = V; <10% positive = –; after 48 hours incubation at 37°C.

number is generated, which can either be looked up in a code book or searched for on a computer database. The database can be derived from a large number of isolates and a probability of correct identification can be given, taking into account unusual biochemical properties of biotypes of species. The API20E system (bioMerieux SA, Marcy l'Etoile, France) has been in use for nearly 25 years and in a recent evaluation was still found to provide a good level of accuracy of identification (78.7% at 24 hours) which, although slightly lower than earlier evaluations, is acceptable (O'Hara et al., 1992).

Because of the special requirements for the identification of enteric pathogens, such as Salmonella spp. and Shigella spp., shortened sets of biochemical tests are used to screen isolates. These are described in the relevant chapter and range from single tubes of media, like triple sugar iron agar, to disposable cupule systems to detect pre-formed enzymes, such as API Z (bioMerieux Sa, Marcy l'Etoile, France). The practical details of using these various systems for identification are described in detail elsewhere (Pedler, 1989).

More recently, the principles enshrined in packaged disposable kits has been further developed into automated systems. Generally, these use pre-prepared cartridges of freeze-dried reagents which, after rehydration and inoculation, are incubated and continuously monitored by an automated spectrophometer. Most systems use 'conventional' biochemical tests with colour changes or release of fluorophores, but growth inhibition by antibiotics and dyes are also included. The Biolog system determines carbon source utilization profiles and the Midi microbial identification system utilizes an automated high-resolution gas chromatography system coupled to a computer. These systems are described and reviewed in detail elsewhere (Stager and Davis, 1992). It is easy for microbiologists to lose sight of the basic biochemical characteristics of the species of the Enterobacteriaceae when using automated systems. Should problems arise, back-up systems should be available and the microbiologist should be aware of the key biochemical

properties of the commonly encountered and clinically significant Enterobacteriaceae, which are shown in Table 12.3.

Individual laboratories should make choices as to the level of identification performed on isolates, and which system to use. When making comparisons of identification systems, there are many factors to be considered and the final choice will be different for different types of laboratories (D'Amato et al., 1981).

REFERENCES

Barrow, G.I. and Feltham, R.K.A. (eds) (1993) *Cowan and Steel's Manual for the Identification of Medical Bacteria*, 3rd edn. Cambridge University Press, Cambridge, UK.

Bush, K., Jacoby, G.A. and Medeiros, A.A. (1995) A functional classification scheme for β-lactamases and its correlation with molecular structures. *Antimicrobial Agents and Chemotherapy*, **39**, 1211–1233.

D'Amato, R.F., Holmes, B. and Bottone, E.J. (1981) The systems approach to diagnostic microbiology. *Critical Reviews in Microbiology*, **9**, 1–44.

Durham, H.E. (1900) Some theoretical considerations upon the nature of agglutinins, together with further observations upon *Bacillus typhi abdominalis*, *Bacillus enteritidis*, *Bacillus coli communis*, *Bacillus lactis aeruginosa* and some other bacilli of allied character. *Journal of Experimental Medicine*, **5**, 354–388.

Farmer, J.J., Davis, B.R., Hickman-Brenner, F.W. *et al.* (1985) Biochemical identification of new species and biogroups of Enterobacteriaceae isolated from clinical specimens. *Journal of Clinical Microbiology*, **21**, 46–76.

Jones, M.E., Avison, M.B., Damidinsuren, E., McGovan, A.P. and Bennett, P.M. (1994) Heterogeneity at the β-lactamase structural gene *ampC* amongst *Citrobacter* spp. assessed by polymerase chain reaction analysis: potential for typing at a molecular level. *Journal of Medical Microbiology*, **41**, 209–214.

Livermore, D. (1995) β-Lactamases in laboratory and clinical resistance. *Clinical Microbiology Reviews*, **8**, 557–584.

O'Hara, C.M., Rhoden, D.L. and Miller, J.M. (1992) Reevaluation of the API 20E identification system versus conventional biochemicals for identification of members of the family Enterobacteriaceae: a new look at an old product. *Journal of Clinical Microbiology*, **30**, 123–125.

Pedler, S.J. (1989) Bacteriology of intestinal disease. In

Medical Bacteriology: A Practical Approach (eds P.M. Hawkey and D.A. Lewis). IRL Press at Oxford University Press, Oxford, pp. 139–166.

Snelling, A.M., Hawkey, P.M., Heritage, J., Downey, P., Bennett, P.M. and Holmes, B. (1993) The use of a DNA probe and PCR to examine the distribution of the *aac*(6')-Ic gene in *Serratia marcescens* and other Gram-negative bacteria. *Journal of Antimicrobial Chemotherapy*, **31**, 841–854.

Stager, C.E. and Davis, J.R. (1992) Automated systems for identification of microorganisms. *Clinical Microbiology Reviews*, **5**, 302–327.

12a

ESCHERICHIA COLI

Nathan M. Thielman and Richard L. Guerrant

INTRODUCTION

First described as *Bacterium coli commune* by Dr Theodor Escherich in 1885, the ubiquitous *Escherichia coli* is now recognized as one of the most versatile pathogens in both animals and humans. Escherich recognized its role as a human pathogen nine years later when he suggested that the organism caused ascending bladder infections in young women. *Escherichia* is the type genus for the family Enterobacteriacae and *E. coli* is the type species (Farmer *et al.*, 1985). In addition to *E. coli*, the genus comprises four other species: *E. blattae*, *E. hermannii*, *E. vulneris* and *E. fergusonii*, *E. adecarboxylata* having been reassigned to a new genus, *Leclercia*. *Escherichia blattae*, as the name suggests, has been recovered from the cockroach gut and does not cause human infection. *Escherichia vulneris* is particularly associated with wounds of the limbs, whereas *E. fergusonii* and *E. hermannii* are occasionally isolated from clinical specimens. *Escherichia coli* has emerged as an important diarrhoeal pathogen with remarkably diverse phenotypes and pathogenic mechanisms, as well as a significant cause of septicaemia in adults and neonates. *Escherichia coli* is the most widely studied living organism and much that is known about it is summarized in a recent monograph (Neidhardt, 1996).

DESCRIPTION OF THE ORGANISM

Escherichia coli is a short, non-spore-forming and often fimbriate Gram-negative bacillus which grows readily on simple culture media or synthetic media with glycerol or glucose as the sole carbon source. With the exception of many enteroinvasive strains, on routine culture *E. coli* is often first identified as a lactose-fermenting Gram-negative rod. With further biochemical analysis, these oxidase-negative organisms are distinguished from other lactose fermenters by indole production (except *E. vulneris*), lack of citrate utilization, positive methyl red test, negative Voges–Proskauer reaction and usually positive lysine and ornithine decarboxylase reactions. The characteristics of *Escherichia* spp. are shown in Table 12a.1.

Normal Habitat

The primary habitat of *E. coli* and the other species (with the exception of *E. blattae*) is the large bowel and tissues of warm-blooded animals. The organism can be found in soils and water, but this is invariably a result of faecal contamination. *Escherichia coli* has been used as an indicator of faecal pollution of water for nearly 100 years. Human and animal food should be regarded as a secondary habitat, although proliferation of bacteria

Principles and Practice of Clinical Bacteriology. Edited by A.M. Emmerson, P.M. Hawkey and S.H. Gillespie
© 1997 John Wiley & Sons Ltd

TABLE 12a.1   BIOCHEMICAL CHARACTERISTICS OF MEMBERS OF THE GENUS *ESCHERICHIA*

Test	*E. coli*	(Inactive)	*E. vulneris*	*E. hermannii*	*E. fergusonii*	*E. blattae*
Indole	+	V	–	+	+	–
Methyl red	+	+	+	+	+	+
Lysine decarboxylase	+	V	V	–	+	+
Arginine dihydrolase	V	–	V	–	+	–
Ornithine decarboxylase	V	–	–	+	+	+
Yellow pigment	–	–	V	+	–	–
Fermentation of:						
Adonitol	–	–	–	–	+	–
Cellobiose	–	–	+	+	+	–
Mannitol	+	+	+	+	+	–
Sorbitol	+	V	–	–	–	–
Arabitol	–	–	–	–	+	–

+, >90% strains positive; V, 10–90% strains positive; – <10% strains positive.

can occur if the food is mishandled, leading to food poisoning.

PATHOGENIC MECHANISMS AND CLINICAL FEATURES OF INFECTION

Diarrhoeal Disease

Nearly all of the mechanisms whereby diarrhoeal disease is caused are found in *E. coli*. Table 12a.2 summarizes these mechanisms, as well as the major clinical syndromes, genetic determinants, experimental models, and the predominant serotypes of enterovirulent *E. coli*.

Enterotoxigenic E. coli *(ETEC)*

By some estimates, ETEC, which produces heat-labile and/or heat-stable enterotoxins, causes over 600 million cases of diarrhoea worldwide annually, with 700 000 deaths in children younger than five years (Elsinghorst and Kopecko, 1992). The majority of ETEC disease affects impoverished populations living in developing countries and it remains the major cause of diarrhoea in travellers to these regions (Guerrant and Bobak, 1991).

After ingestion of contaminated food or water, ETEC colonizes the proximal small intestine and attaches via fimbrial colonization factor antigens (CFAs). This virulence determinant allows for *in*

situ multiplication and infection, whereas enterotoxin secretion largely accounts for the watery diarrhoea characteristic of ETEC. Both appear to be necessary to cause disease. CFAs in human ETEC strains are primarily protein fimbriae with subunits of 14–22 kDa. They are capable of agglutinating erythrocytes in the presence of D-mannose, expressed at 37 °C, but not at 18 °C, and correlate closely with certain O serogroups (Schlager and Guerrant, 1988). While CFA/I represents a single fimbrial antigen, CFA/II and CFA/IV are comprised of different fimbrial coli surface (CS) antigens. These CS antigens haemagglutination patterns, enterotoxin associations and genetic determinants of the major CFAs are detailed in Table 12a.3.

Of the four different enterotoxins (LT/I, LT/II, STa and STb) produced by ETEC, LT/I and STa are well-established secretagogues in humans. The cholera-like LTs (molecular weight 84–86 kDa) are proteins comprised of one A polypeptide and five identical B polypeptides. After binding to GM1 ganglioside receptors on intestinal brush border, the enzymatically active A1 subunit catalyses adenosine diphosphate (ADP) ribosylation of a regulatory subunit of adenylate cyclase, resulting in cAMP accumulation and ultimately fluid secretion. LTs from strains of *E. coli* isolated from humans and piglets which are neutralized by antitoxin against cholera toxin belong to the LT/I groups. LT/II toxins are biologically similar to

LT/I toxins in that they activate adenylate cyclase, but differ in that they are not neutralized by antibodies to cholera toxin (Chang *et al.*, 1987) and bind best to GD1 receptors rather than GM1. The prototypical LT/II toxin, produced by strain SA53 (isolated from a water buffalo in Thailand), is now designated as LT/IIa. LT/IIb, antigenically distinguishable from LT/IIa, has been isolated from humans and animals (Seriwatana *et al.*, 1988). Though the structural genes for LT/I reside on a plasmid, chromosomal genes appear to affect its level of expression (Ghosh *et al.*, 1992) and those that encode LT/II toxins are chromosomal (Pickett *et al.*, 1989).

In contrast, heat-stable (ST) toxins are much smaller (16–18 amino acids for STa), less antigenic than LT toxins, and they produce intestinal secretion by a distinctly different mechanism. STa activates guanylate cyclase in the brush border of intestinal epithelial cells in jejunum and ileum, leading to increased levels of cyclic GMP (Hughes *et al.*, 1978). The exact mechanism by which cyclic GMP leads to fluid secretion remains unclear, but it may involve phosphorylation of membrane-bound proteins important for ion transport. The methanol-insoluble STb toxin, recognized predominantly from animal isolates, is larger and causes cyclic nucleotide-independent bicarbonate secretion in piglet loops, but its role in human diarrhoeal disease is uncertain.

Enterohaemorrhagic E. coli *(EHEC)*

EHEC that produce one or more of the Shiga-like toxins (SLTs) are emerging as an increasingly important cause of diarrhoea in both developed and developing regions. In the northwestern United States, a region particularly prone to epidemics of EHEC, over 500 people were stricken within several months in outbreaks related to the ingestion of hamburgers at fast-food restaurants. In addition, outbreaks have been associated with a wide range of foods, such as contaminated pickles, rehydrated onions, unpasteurized dairy products and even apple cider (Su and Brandt, 1995). Cattle appear to be the primary reservoir of EHEC strains which produce

diarrhoea in humans (Su and Brandt, 1995). While person-to-person transmission has been documented in smaller outbreaks in child day-care facilities (Belongia *et al.*, 1993), major outbreaks affecting thousands in South Africa and Swaziland have been caused by the EHEC strain *E. coli* O157 associated with contaminated water supplies (Isaacson *et al.*, 1993).

The hallmark of EHEC illness is bloody diarrhoea, often associated with haemorrhagic colitis and the absence of fever. Its most important sequela, the haemolytic uraemic syndrome or HUS (a constellation of microangiopathic haemolytic anaemia, thrombocytopenia and acute renal failure), occurs most frequently in children between one and four years of age and the elderly (Cohen and Giannella, 1992). Whereas HUS occurs in approximately 10% of patients in sporadic cases of haemorrhagic colitis (Griffin *et al.*, 1988) following outbreaks this syndrome may occur in as many as 24–40% of patients with *E. coli* O157 : H7 infection (Pavia *et al.*, 1990).

Several studies point to pre-existing EHEC infection in 75–95% of children presenting with HUS (Karmali *et al.*, 1985; Lopez *et al.*, 1989). However, because HUS commonly occurs seven days after the onset of haemorrhagic colitis, the likelihood of recovering EHEC strains in stool cultures at the onset of the syndrome is diminished. Reported risk factors for the development of HUS in patients with EHEC diarrhoea include the extremes of age (Griffin *et al.*, 1988), leucocytosis (Pavia *et al.*, 1990), reduced P1 antigen expression on red blood cells (Taylor *et al.*, 1990), and the use of antimotility agents (Cimolai *et al.*, 1990).

The type of toxin secreted by infecting *E. coli* may also affect the incidence of HUS; it has been observed that strains that produced SLT/II alone more commonly produced disease associated with HUS than those which produced SLT/I alone or with SLT/II (Ostroff *et al.*, 1989; Kleanthous *et al.*, 1990).

The toxins of EHEC, first shown to be cytotoxic in Vero cells (and thus named verotoxins, VT), bear both structural and functional resemblance to Shiga toxin, and as such are alternatively termed Shiga-like toxins (SLTs). The terms VT and

TABLE 12a.2 TEN POSSIBLE ENTERIC VIRULENCE TYPES OF *E. COLI*

Types of *E. coli* enteropathogens

	Genetic code	Mechanism	Model	Predominant O serogroups	Type of diarrhoea
Enterotoxigenic (ETEC)					
LT (I/II)	Plasmid Plasmid (LT-I) Chromosomal (LT-II)	CFA/I–V → colonize Adenylate cyclase → secretion	MRHA 18 h rabbit ileal loop CHO/Y1 cells	1, 6, 7, 8, 9, 11, 15, 20, 25, 27, 60, 63, 75, 80, 85, 88, 89, 99, 101, 109, 114, 128, 139, 153	Acute watery
STa	Plasmid	Guanylate cyclase → secretion	4–6 h rabbit ileal loop Suckling mice	11, 12, 15, 20, 25, 27, 60, 63, 75, 78, 80, 85, 88, 89, 99, 101, 109, 114, 115, 139, 148, 149, 153, 159, 166, 167	Acute watery
STb	Plasmid	Cyclic nucleotide-independent HCO_3^- secretion	Piglet loop		
Enterohemorrhagic (EHEC)					
SLT I/II/IIvh/IIvp	Phage/?plasmid (some also have *eae*, see below)	Glycosidase cleaves adenosine-4324 in 28S rRNA of 60S ribosomal subunits to halt protein synthesis	HeLa cell cytotoxicity	157, 26, 103, 111, 113 *et al.*	Bloody (±HUS)
Enteroinvasive (EIEC)	Plasmid (140 MDa) + chromosomal	Cell invasion and spread 68–80 kDa EIET (chromosomal)	Sereny test	11, 28, 29, 112, 115, 121, 124, 136, 143, 144, 147, 152, 164, 173	Acute dysenteric
Enteropathogenic (EPEC)	1. Plasmid (60 MDa; EAF, bfpA)	BFP → efficient Localized adherence (LA)	LA to HEp-2 cells	18, 26, 44, 55, 86, 111, 114, 119, 125, 126, 127, 128, 142, 157, 158	Acute + persistent
	2. Chromosomal (cfm)	Tyrosine kinase and intracellular Ca^{2+}-dependent actin condensation	Fluorescence actin staining (FAS)		
	3. Chromosomal (*eaeA*)	94 kDa intimin → intimate, effacing adherence			

Enteroaggregative (EAggEC)	Plasmid (60 MDa; AA)	BFP → aggregative adherence (AA)	AA to HEp-2 cells	3(17–2), 15, 44(042), 51, 77, 78, 86, 91, 92(221)	Persistent (?Acute)
	Plasmid (60 MDa; AA)	2–5 kDa EAST-1, guanylate cyclase EALT pore forming Ca^{2+} ionophore	Using chambers	111, 113, 126, 141, 146, ?(346)	
Diffusely adherent (DAEC)	Chromosomal (daaC probe)	Fimbrial adhesin (F1845)	Diffuse adherence to HEp-2 cells	75(F1845), ?(189), 11, 15(57–1), 126(AIDA–I)	?Acute ?Persistent
	Plasmid	Afimbrial adhesin (homologous to *Shigella* IcsA)			
Enteric colonizing	Plasmid	CFA/I–V ?Hydrophobic → colonize	MRHA $(NH_4)_2SO_4$ hydrophobicity	–	?Persistent
GU/NS/normal flora	Chromosomal/plasmid	Type 1 pili P-fimbriae S-fimbriae AFA-I	MSHA bind P blood group Ag	1, 2, 4, 6, 7, 25, 45, 75, 81	None

Underline, pathogenicity in humans established in outbreaks or volunteer studies; HUS, haemolytic uraemic syndrome.

TABLE 12a.3   THE MAJOR FIMBRIAL ADHESINS OF ETEC

Fimbrial adhesin determinant	Coli surface (CS) antigens	Mannose-resistant haemagglutination reactions	Enterotoxin association	Genetic
CFA/I Plasmid	–	h+/b+	ST	60 MDa
CFA/II	CS1 or CS2 + CS3 rCS3 alone	h+/b+	ST or LT	Plasmid
CFA/IV	CS4 or CS5 + CS6 CS6 alone	CS4 and CS5: hA+/b+; CS6: none	ST or LT	Plasmid

With type A human red blood cells (h); with bovine red blood cells (b).

SLT are both used widely; SLT/I is identical to VT1 and SLT/II corresponds to VT2. At least two immunologically distinct SLTs have been described. Whereas the 70 kDa SLT/I is virtually identical to Shiga toxin with one A and five B subunits and is neutralizable by antiserum against Shiga toxin, the somewhat smaller (60 kDa) SLT/II is neither neutralized by anti-Shiga toxin antibodies nor monoclonal antibodies to SLT/II.

In addition to its potent cytotoxic activity, the bacteriophage-mediated SLT causes diarrhoea and intestinal morphological changes in rabbits (Pai et al., 1986). It has been suggested that the enterotoxic activity of SLT is related to impaired absorptive activity of villus cells as a result of impaired protein synthesis. Studying the morphological effects of SLT on rabbit intestine, Keenan et al. found that villus cells, which bear more SLT binding sites than crypt cells, are expelled into the intestinal lumen prematurely, perhaps because of SLT-induced apoptosis (Keenan et al., 1986). The preferential effects of SLT on villus cells over crypt cells in the intestine were demonstrated by electrolyte studies in isolated rabbit jejunal epithelium in which SLT caused significant impairment of sodium chloride absorption (a function of the villus cell) while anion secretion (crypt cell function) remained intact (Kandel et al., 1989). In addition, SLTs are cytotoxic for vascular endothelium, and it may be that the features of HUS arise through its interactions with the endothelium (Gyles, 1992).

In addition to toxin production, intimate attachment of EHEC appears to play a role in pathogenesis. A gene functionally homologous to that found in EPEC (see below), the eae gene, demonstrated in EHEC 0157:H7, appears to be important for inducing F-actin accumulation in HEp-2 cells and for mediating intimate attachment to colonic epithelial cells in the newborn piglet EHEC model (Donnenberg et al., 1993a).

Enteroinvasive E. coli (EIEC)

EIEC, recognized primarily as an important cause of diarrhoea in developing regions, occasionally causes diarrhoea in travellers to these regions and has been implicated in several outbreaks in developed countries (Gordillo et al., 1992). Like Shigella spp., EIEC causes dysentery, with scanty stools of blood and mucus. The syndrome may be accompanied by fever, abdominal cramping, malaise and toxaemia, and is occasionally preceded by watery diarrhoea.

EIEC, like Shigella, penetrate and proliferate within epithelial cells, leading to eventual colonic epithelial cell destruction. This trait is primarily mediated by a large (120–140 MDa) plasmid which has extensive sequence homology with the invasion plasmid of Shigella spp. (Calderwood et al., 1987), but requires the chromosomal determinants of certain O group antigens for full expression of its invasive virulence (Schlager and Guerrant, 1988; see Ch. 12b). In addition, some strains of EIEC secrete a chromosomally mediated 68–80 kDa enterotoxin.

Adherent E. coli

Adherent E. coli are recognized by their ability to adhere to HEp-2 (human laryngeal epidermoid

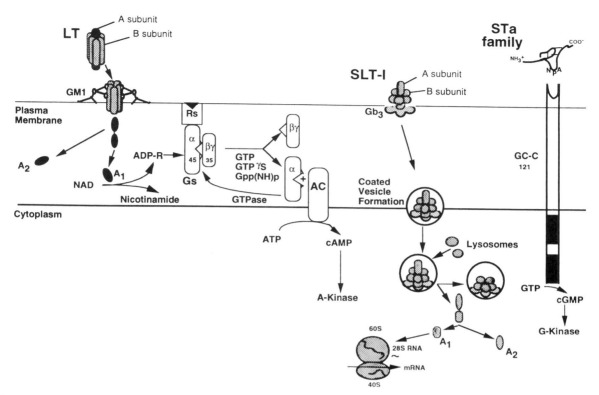

Figure 12a.1. Molecular pathogenesis of the major toxins associated with *E. coli*. Mechanisms of action of the major toxins of *E. coli*. *Heat-labile toxin (LT)*, an analogue of cholera toxin, binds to a monosialoganglioside receptor via its B subunits, after which the A1 subunit is released from Bs and A2 by cleavage of a disulphide bond. This enzymatically active peptide catalyses the dissolution of NAD to nicotinamide and ADP-ribose, allowing for the ADP ribosylation of Gsa which then dissociates from the $\beta\gamma$ subunit and activates adenylate cyclase. Cyclic AMP formation, catalysed by adenylate cyclase, stimulates water and electrolyte secretion by intestinal epithelial cells via protein kinase A, prostaglandin synthesis, and possibly platelet activating factor. *Shiga-like toxins (SLTs) I and II* produced by EHEC bind to globotriosyl ceramide (Gb3) via B subunits and undergo receptor mediated endocytosis. The A subunit is released into the cytoplasm where it is proteolytically degraded to A1 and A2 fragments. The former binds to the 60S ribosome and cleaves an adenine residue at position 4324 in 28S ribosomal RNA, thereby halting protein synthesis and causing cell death. *Heat-stable enterotoxin (ST)*, an 18–19 amino acid peptide, appears to bind to an extracellular domain of guanylate cyclase to increase cyclic GMP which activates G kinase, ultimately leading to altered sodium and chloride transport via phosphorylation of membrane proteins.

carcinoma) cells. At present there are at least three well-characterized HEp-2 adherent phenotypes:

(1) Enteropathogenic *E. coli* (EPEC) produce local attaching and effacing lesions on epithelial cells.

(2) Enteroaggregative *E. coli* (EAggEC) adhere in a 'stacked brick' pattern to both HEp-2 cells and glass slides.

(3) Diffusely adherent *E. coli* (DAEC) adhere in a diffuse pattern to HEp-2 cells only.

There are also reports of a potential new category of enterovirulent *E. coli*, cell-detaching *E. coli*, which caused detachment of HEp-2 (and multiple other cell lines) from glass coverslips, found in Aboriginal children in tropical Western Australia (Gunzburg *et al.*, 1993).

Enteropathogenic E. coli *(EPEC)* EPEC causes acute and persistent diarrhoea among children in developing countries, and has been reported as the leading cause of infant diarrhoea in some regions (Clausen and Christie, 1982; Gomes *et al.*, 1989; Echeverria *et al.*, 1991b). In addition, it has been implicated in nosocomial neonatal diarrhoea with high mortality in Africa (Senerwa *et al.*, 1989).

Recognized as focally adherent microcolonies in tissue culture or identified by characteristic fluorescent actin staining of epithelial cells (Shariff *et al.*, 1993), EPEC ultimately causes degeneration of the microvillus brush border and cupping and pedestal formation of the plasma membrane at sites of bacterial attachment in humans (Rothbaum *et al.*, 1982) and in animal models (Moon *et al.*, 1983). The organism first attaches non-intimately to intestinal epithelium via an inducible bundle-forming pilus (Giron *et al.*, 1991a). The major structural subunit of this organelle is encoded by the *bfp*A gene carried on a large plasmid common to EPEC and bears homology to genes encoding type IV fimbriae of other pathogenic bacteria (Donnenberg *et al.*, 1992). Following initial adherence, EPEC attach intimately to epithelial cells and, in a step chromosomally encoded by a cfm region, activate host cell tyrosine kinases and cause the release of calcium from intracellular stores, effecting a profound rearrangement of the cytoskeleton. Epithelial cells lose their microvillus architecture as filamentous actin, myosin, α-actin, talin and ezrin condense directly beneath the adherent *E. coli* (Donnenberg *et al.*, 1993b). The intimate attaching step, coincident with but separable from these cytoskeletal changes, is mediated by a 94 kDa outer membrane protein 'intimin', which bears significant homology to the predicted amino acid, sequences of intimin and invasin proteins of *Yersinia pseudotuberculosis* and *Y. enterocolitica* (Yu and Kaper, 1992). The chromosomal gene cluster, *eae*A, which encodes this protein has clearly been identified as a virulence trait in EPEC strains infecting human volunteers (Donnenberg *et al.*, 1993a). In addition to *eae*A, the *eae*B gene and one other locus appear to be required for intimate attachment (Donnenberg *et al.*, 1993c).

Enteroaggregative E. coli *(EAggEC)* EAggEC coalesce in a characteristic 'stacked brick' pattern on HEp-2 cells. This phenotype has been convincingly implicated as a cause of persistent diarrhoea in children from the developing world (Vial *et al.*, 1988; Bhan *et al.*, 1989). Some EAggEC strains have variably caused diarrhoea in adult human volunteer studies (Mathewson *et al.*, 1986). In gnotobiotic piglets, EAggEC strains have caused diarrhoea with histopathological correlates of aggregative colonization of intact epithelium, hyperaemia of the distal small bowel and caecum, and swelling of small intestinal villi (Tzipori *et al.*, 1992).

While the exact mechanism by which EAggEC causes diarrhoea remains to be elucidated, putative pathogenic determinants include toxin production and fimbrial adherence. The precise role of the novel EAggEC heat-stable toxin (EAST) has yet to be defined as has the recently identified 120 kDa heat-labile protein that is antigenically related to the C-terminal region of *E. coli* haemolysin (Savarino *et al.*, 1991). The latter induces host cell calcium-dependent protein phosphorylation which, via cytoskeletal derangements, may lead to secretion (Baldwin *et al.*, 1992).

Diffusely adherent E. coli *(DAEC)* The role of DAEC in acute or persistent diarrhoea remains controversial. While epidemiological investigations have suggested a role for DAEC in diarrhoeal illnesses of Mayan children in Mexico (Giron *et al.*, 1991b) and of nosocomial diarrhoea in both children and adults in France (Jallat *et al.*, 1993), others have not found a statistically significant correlation of DAEC with diarrhoea (Gomes *et al.*, 1989; Echeverria *et al.*, 1992). In a recent study of Aboriginal children in Western Australia, DAEC were associated with diarrhoea only in children 18 months of age or older (Gunzburg *et al.*, 1993). Similarly, in a study of Chilean children, an association with DAEC and diarrhoea was seen only in older children, with the strongest correlation in those 48 to 60 months of age (Levine *et al.*, 1993). When the probe-positive DAEC strains 57-1 (O15:HM) and C18845 (O75:NM) were given to adult volunteers neither demonstrated significant pathogenicity (Tacket *et al.*, 1990).

At least two different genetic determinants are responsible for the manner in which diffusely adherent *E. coli* attach to epithelial cells. Originally isolated from strain 2787 (O126:H27), a 6.0 kb plasmid-derived fragment encodes the 100 kDa afimbrial adhesin (AIDA-I) that confers diffuse adherence in many DAEC. The AIDA-I precursor displays significant homology to the virG (icsA) protein of *Shigella flexneri* which participates in its intercellular spread (Benz and Schmidt, 1993). In other strains, a pilus adhesin whose genetic determinant (F1845) may be encoded by either chromosomal or plasmid DNA confers the diffusely adherent phenotype.

Colonizing E. coli

Colonization of the relevant intestinal tissue is key in the pathogenesis of any infectious diarrhoeal disease, and there is some evidence to suggest that colonization alone may cause secretory diarrhoea. For example, strain 1392, originally enterotoxigenic, but since shown to express only the colonization factor antigen (CFA/II), has caused diarrhoea in human volunteer studies (Levine *et al.*, 1986) and in the reversible ileal tie adult rabbit diarrhoea model (RITARD) (Wanke and Guerrant, 1987). In the latter, colonization by this organism was associated with reduced disaccharidase activity as well as an impairment of normal water and electrolyte absorption (Schlager *et al.*, 1990). The potential role for colonization alone in causing persistent diarrhoea in children in tropical regions remains to be defined.

Urinary Tract Infections

The vast majority of acute and many chronic urinary tract infections are caused by *E. coli*, with only a few serogroups (O1, O2, O4, O6, O7 and O75) predominating (Roberts and Phillips, 1979). Important virulence properties, including increased adherence to uroepithelial cells, resistance to serum bactericidal activity, presence of aerobac-

tin, higher quantity of K antigen and production of haemolysin, are seen more frequently in strains which cause urinary tract infections than in those found in normal faecal flora (Svanborg-Eden *et al.*, 1981). It is widely held that uropathogenic *E. coli* are selected from the faecal flora by the presence of such virulence traits. One of the most important host factors in the pathogenesis of uncomplicated urinary tract infections is the presence of a short urethra in women with resultant frequent colonization with coliforms. When normal urinary flow is altered by obstruction or the presence of a foreign body, urinary tract infections may be more complicated.

The adherence factor most consistently associated with uropathogenic *E. coli*, the P pilus, is expressed on 80% of mannose-resistant haemagglutinating *E. coli* strains isolated from patients with pyelonephritis, compared with 19% from those with acute cystitis, 14% with asymptomatic bacteriuria, and 7% from faecal isolates of healthy children (Vaisanen *et al.*, 1981). This adhesin recognizes the disaccharide α-D-galactosyl-(1–4) β-D-galactose on the P blood group antigen (enabling it to bind to red blood cells) and on uroepithelial cells from the majority of the population (Kallenius *et al.*, 1981). Less well established are the role of other chromosomally mediated non-P receptor fimbrial adhesins (also termed X-specific adhesins) such as S fimbriae which bind to the Tamm–Horsfall protein present in urine, 075X, capable of binding to fibronectin and collagen, and type 1 fimbriae which appear to be involved in non-specific binding of bacteria to mannose-rich mucoid slime of the bladder in urinary tract infections (Hacker, 1992). In addition, the presence of K antigen has been associated with upper urinary tract infections, and antibody to the K antigens protected against infection in experimental animals (Kaijser and Ahistedt, 1977).

Neonatal Meningitis

Newborn infants are particularly predisposed to meningitis, and *E. coli*, along with Group B streptococci, account for the majority of these infections. Eighty per cent of these infections are caused by organisms carrying the K1 capsular antigen (McCracken *et al.*, 1974). Epidemiological studies have shown that pregnancy is associated with an increased rate of carriage of K1 *E. coli*, that subsequent colonization of the newborn intestinal flora occurs in about 30% of newborns, and that these strains are implicated in cases of neonatal meningitis. Two-thirds of strains responsible for meningitis belong to serogroups O1, O7, O16 and O18ac (Schiffer *et al.*, 1976).

While the means by which K1 *E. coli* causes meningitis remains to be explained, observations of immunological cross-reactivity and polysaccharide structure homology to *Neisseria meningitidis* Group B may indicate similarity of pathogenic mechanisms or tissue tropism. K1 antibodies are infrequently found in adults, and K1 antigen appears to be poorly immunogenic; however, anti-K1 sIgA is present in human colostrum, and therefore may afford some protection for the newborn (Schiffer *et al.*, 1976).

Bacteraemia

Despite the overall frequency with which *E. coli* colonizes mucosal surfaces and causes diarrhoeal disease and urinary tract infections, bloodstream infection remains a relatively rare complication of *E. coli* infections. Nevertheless, *E. coli* is the most commonly isolated Gram-negative bacterium causing bacteraemia and a leading cause of nosocomial bacteraemia (Weinstein *et al.*, 1983). Case fatality rates from nosomial *E. coli* bacteraemia may be as high as 25% (Stamm *et al.*, 1977). The most common source for bacteraemia is a urinary tract infection, especially when obstructed.

K1 *E. coli* is the most frequently isolated capsulated type from bacteraemic patients (Cross *et al.*, 1984). In a rat model the 50% lethal dose was more than 10^5-fold higher for the K1-encapsulated parent compared with non-encapsulated strains for certain O serotypes (Cross *et al.*, 1986).

As with other Gram-negative bacteria, the lipopolysaccharide of *E. coli* is an important pathogenicity factor and may cause fatal septic shock and disseminated intravascular coagulation. The pathogenesis of these phenomena involves the complex interactions of tumour necrosis factor α, platelet-activating factor, interleukins, leukotrienes, thromboxanes and activators of the complement cascade with the endothelium (Bone, 1991). With recent concern over the efficacy and expenses of specific anti-endotoxin therapy for the treatment of Gram-negative sepsis, future therapeutic strategies may target some of these mediators.

Miscellaneous Infections

Given the ubiquity of this organism, it is not surprising that *E. coli* has been found in a variety of other infections. Not infrequently alimentary-related surgical wound infections, pneumonia (often related to colonization of endotracheal tubes) and peritonitis due to *E. coli* occur. Patients with vascular disease, particularly those with diabetes mellitus, are prone to polymicrobial infections in distal extremities, often involving *E. coli* and anaerobes. *E. coli* has been implicated in endocarditis (Carruthers, 1977), suppurative thrombophlebitis (Garrison *et al.*, 1982), septic arthritis, endophthalmitis (Faraawi and Fong, 1988), intra-abdominal abscess (Altemeier *et al.*, 1973), spontaneous bacterial peritonitis (Wilcox and Dismukes, 1987), liver abscess, brain abscess, osteomyelitis and prostatitis. *Escherichia hermannii* and *E. fergusonii* are rarely encountered in clinical material. *Escherichia vulneris* typically infects and colonizes wounds on the arms and legs. *Escherichia hermannii* has been recovered from a range of clinical specimens but is not thought to be a primary pathogen; the pathogenic role of *E. fergusonii* is not yet clear (Farmer *et al.*, 1985).

EPIDEMIOLOGY

Escherichia coli usually occurs as a harmless commensal of the mammalian (and to an undetermined extent avian) intestinal flora. Some strains adhere to intestinal mucosa, whereas others are transients in the gut lumen. It is typically found in densities of 10^6 cfu/g colon contents. *Escherichia coli* is one of the first bacteria to colonize the neonatal gut, usually from the mother in both humans and animals. Man is subject to continual immigrations of strains into the gut, usually from raw meat and poultry handling (Cooke, 1974). As described above, *E. coli*, and to a lesser extent related bacteria like *E. vulneris*, are opportunistic pathogens of humans at a wide range of sites. Much of the epidemiology of *E. coli* in both man, animals and the environment has been accomplished using serotyping, usually of O and H antigens.

From a relatively small number of human strains causing extraintestinal disease and from *E. coli* isolated from normal faeces, Kauffmann first identified 20 O (somatic lipopolysaccharide), 55 K (capsular) and 19 H (flagellar) antigens in his typing scheme. Since then this typing system has grown to include 173 O, 80 K and 56 H antigens (Orskov and Orskov, 1984). While all three were once defined on the basis of bacterial agglutination testing and immunogenicity, the current serotyping scheme establishes O and H antigens based on bacterial agglutination; the K antigen is determined by gel immunoprecipitation or phage typing (Orskov and Orskov, 1984).

Some *E. coli* strains causing diarrhoea lack capsular K antigenicity and can be differentiated from non-pathogenic *E. coli* by analysis of their O and H serogroups. However, because the capacity to cause disease is often encoded by transmissible genetic virulence traits (or plasmids or phages), demonstration of these traits is becoming more important than serotyping in defining strains of *E. coli* as enteropathogens. The majority of *E. coli* strains that cause extraintestinal disease have neutral O antigens (Orskov and Orskov, 1992).

Biotyping has been used, but the discrimination is low. Bacteriophage typing has also been applied from time to time, and has been used to attempt to subtype O157 strains. A variety of molecular typing methods have been applied to *E. coli*. Subtypes of O157:H7 *E. coli* have been successfully defined by digesting genomic DNA with *Eco*RI and *Pvu*II and probing the restriction fragment length polymorphism (RFLP) pattern with DNA probes for the SLTI and II genes (Samadpour, 1995). Ribotyping has been used in a number of studies of nosocomial *E. coli* in neonatal units, and when compared in such a setting with arbitrarily primed polymerase chain typing both methods performed well (Alos *et al.*, 1993).

DIAGNOSTIC METHODS

Members of the genus grow well on most microbiological media. *E. coli* form characteristic deep red colonies on MacConkey's agar, whilst haemolysis/discoloration around the colony is seen on blood agar. The culture of *E. coli* from urine requires the use of quantitative culture methods, described in detail elsewhere (Lewis, 1989). In addition, the use of CLED (cysteine, electrolyte-deficient agar) is recommended as 1–2% of *E. coli* organisms isolated from urine are cysteine requiring; broths used for identification will also require additional cysteine (McIver and Tapsall, 1990).

Because *E. coli* O157, the most common serogroup of EHEC isolated from humans, and other SLT-producing strains, generally do not ferment sorbitol, sorbitol MacConkey (SMAC) medium is widely used to screen for EHEC in faecal specimens. Inclusion of rhamnose and cefixime in this medium improves selectivity by inhibiting the growth of other sorbitol non-fermenters such as occasional non-O157 *E. coli* and certain *Proteus* spp. (Chapman *et al.*, 1991). Enrichment culture followed by immunogenetic separation using magnetic beads coated with O157 antibody has been shown to be a highly sensitive isolation method (Chapman and Siddons, 1996). A recently described indirect haemagglutination assay consisting of sheep erythrocytes coated with lipopolysaccharide from *E. coli* O157 appears to be a practical and specific test for the serological diagnosis of *E. coli* O157 infections in children with HUS one week after onset of diarrhoea. While *E. coli* O157 strains have been most frequently associated with EHEC infections, at least 33 additional clinically relevant EHEC serotypes can be identified by toxin production or gene probe in stool specimens or cultures (Brook and Bannister, 1991).

EIEC may be difficult to identify by standard bacteriological methods because of variability in biochemical reactions, including late or non-lactose fermentation and indole production (Echeverria *et al.*, 1991a). They are, however, lysine decarboxylase negative and usually non-motile. The classical invasion assay, the Sereney test (in which invasion is demonstrated with the provocation of keratoconjunctivitis in the guinea-pig eye), has been largely replaced by specific radio-labelled and biotinylated DNA probes (Gicquelais *et al.*, 1990).

In addition to the HEp-2 and HeLa cell adherence assays for identifying EAggEC strains, a DNA probe derived from a 1 kb fragment from a plasmid of strain 17-2 appears to be useful as a specific tool for identifying some, but not all, EAggEC (Baudry *et al.*, 1990).

Antimicrobial Sensitivities

Most isolates of *E. coli* are generally sensitive to antimicrobials active against Gram-negative bacteria. However, the species readily acquires plasmids carrying antibiotic resistance determinants. In the UK about 40% of isolates are resistant to ampicillin usually by virtue of plasmid-mediated TEM-1 β-lactamase and about 20% are resistant to trimethoprim due to plasmid-mediated trimethoprim-resistant dihydrofolate reductase (Grüneberg, 1990). Resistance to older, infrequently used agents, such as sulphonamides and tetracycline, remains high. Antimicrobial-resistant strains can be isolated from animals and this represents a potential reservoir of resistance genes. Quinolones (e.g. ciprofloxacin) and extended spectrum β-lactams (ESBLs), e.g. ceftazidime, are generally highly active but 'mutant' TEM and SHV β-lactamases which destroy ESBLs and *gyr*A mutations conferring resistance to all current quinolones are increasingly recognized and will present therapeutic problems in the future.

MANAGEMENT OF INFECTION

Infections caused by *E. coli* respond to treatment with appropriate antibiotics, although the mortality in septicaemia can be high, especially in the immunocompromised and elderly.

Prevention of infection, particularly enteric, relies on the provision of good sanitation and provision of clean water, together with good food-handling practices. In the hospital *E. coli* can readily spread via the faecal–oral route and hand-washing with good environmental cleaning is important in controlling outbreaks.

Though the issue remains unsettled, some consider antibiotic use in EHEC disease as a potentially significant risk factor for HUS. In addition to controversial epidemiological data suggesting that use of trimethoprim–sulphamethoxazole may predispose patients to HUS (Pavia *et al.*, 1990), there are reports of this drug and others increasing *in vitro* toxin production in clinical isolates of EHEC (Walterspiel *et al.*, 1992). In contrast to the above, a retrospective case–control survey of patients with *E. coli* O157:H7-associated diarrhoea suggested that prolonged appropriate antibiotic therapy was associated with lack of progression to HUS (Cimolai *et al.*, 1990). In addition, in a randomized controlled study, trimethoprim–sulphamethoxazole given to children with *E. coli* O157:H7 enteritis yielded no difference in the incidence of HUS, but the small sample size precludes generalizing these findings and underscores the need for further investigation of the role of antimicrobial therapy in EHEC infections (Prouix *et al.*, 1992).

REFERENCES

Alos, J.I., Lambert, T. and Courvalin, P. (1993) Comparison of two molecular methods for tracing nosocomial transmission of *Escherichia coli* K1 in a neonatal unit. *Journal of Clinical Microbiology*, **31**, 1704–1709.

Altemeier, W.A., Culbertson, W.R., Fullen, W.D. and Shook, C.D. (1973) Intraabdominal abscesses. *American Journal of Surgery*, **125**, 70–79.

Baldwin, T.J., Knutton, S., Sellers, L. *et al.*, (1992) Enteroaggregative *Escherichia coli* strains secrete a heat-labile toxin antigenically related to *E. coli* hemolysin. *Infection and Immunity*, **60**, 2092–2095.

Baudry, B., Savarino, S.J., Vial, P., Kaper, J.B. and Levine, M.M. (1990) A sensitive and specific DNA probe to identify enteroaggregative *Escherichia coli*, a recently discovered diarrheal pathogen. *Journal of Infectious Diseases*, **161**, 1249–1251.

Belongia, E.A., Osterholm, M.T., Soler, J.T. *et al.* (1993) Transmission of *Escherichia coli* O157:H7 infection in Minnesota child day-care facilities. *Journal of the American Medical Association*, **269**, 883–888.

Benz, I. and Schmidt, M.A. (1993) Diffuse adherence of enteropathogenic *Escherichia coli* strains: processing of AIDA-I. *International Journal of Medical Microbiology, Virology, Parasitology and Infectious Diseases*, **278**, 197–208.

Bhan, M.K., Raj, P., Levine, M.M. *et al.* (1989) Entero-aggregative *Escherichia coli* associated with persistent diarrhea in a cohort of rural children in India. *Journal of Infectious Diseases*, **159**, 1061–1064.

Bone, R.C. (1991) The pathogenesis of sepsis. *Annals of Internal Medicine*, **115**, 457–469.

Brook, M.G. and Bannister, B.A. (1991) Verocytotoxin producing *Escherichia coli*. *British Medical Journal*, **303**, 800–801.

Calderwood, S.B., Auclair, F., Donohue-Rolfe, A., Keusch, G.T. and Mekalanos, J.J. (1987) Nucleotide sequence of the Shiga-like toxin genes of *Escherichia coli*. *Proceedings of the National Academy of Sciences USA*, **84**, 4364–4368.

Carruthers, M.M. (1977) Endocarditis due to enteric bacilli other than salmonellae: case reports and literature review. *American Journal of the Medical Sciences*, **273**, 203–211.

Chang, P.P., Moss, J., Twiddy, E.M. and Holmes, R.K. (1987) Type II heat-labile enterotoxin of *Escherichia coli* activates adenylate cyclase in human fibroblasts by ADP ribosylation. *Infection and Immunity*, **55**, 1854–1858.

Chapman, P.A. and Siddons, C.A. (1996) A comparison of immunomagnetic separation and direct culture for the isolation of venocytotoxin-producing *Escherichia coli* O157 from cases of bloody diarrhoea, non-bloody diarrhoea and asymptomatic contacts. *Journal of Medical Microbiology*, **44**, 267–271.

Chapman, P.A., Siddons, C.A., Zadik, P.M. and Jewes, L. (1991) An improved selective medium for the isolation of *Escherichia coli* O157. *Journal of Medical Microbiology*, **35**, 107–110.

Cimolai, N., Carter, J.E., Morrison, B.J. and Anderson, J.D. (1990) Risk factors for the progression of *Escherichia coli* O157:H7 enteritis to hemolytic–uremic syndrome. *Journal of Pediatrics*, **116**, 589–592.

Clausen, C.R. and Christie, D.L. (1982) Chronic diarrhea in infants caused by adherent *Escherichia coli*. *Journal of Pediatrics*, **100**, 358–361.

Cohen, M.B. and Giannella, R.A. (1992) Hemorrhagic colitis associated with *Escherichia coli* O157:H7. *Advances in Internal Medicine*, **37**, 173–195.

Cooke, E.M. (1974) *Escherichia coli and Man.* Churchill Livingstone, Edinburgh.

Cross, A.S., Gemski, P., Sadoff, J.C., Orskov, F. and Orskov, I. (1984) The importance of the K1 capsule in invasive infections caused by *Escherichia coli*. *Journal of Infectious Diseases*, **149**, 184–193.

Cross, A.S., Kim, K.S., Wright, D.C., Sadoff, J.C. and Gemski, P. (1986) Role of lipopolysaccharide and capsule in the serum resistance of bacteremic strains of *Escherichia coli*. *Journal of Infectious Diseases*, **154**, 497–503.

Donnenberg, M.S., Giron, J.A., Nataro, J.P. and Kaper, J.B. (1992) A plasmid encoded type IV fimbrial gene of enteropathogenic *Escherichia coli* associated with localized adherence. *Molecular Microbiology*, **6**, 3427–3437.

Donnenberg, M.S., Tacket, C.O., James, S.P. *et al.* (1993a) Role of the *eae*A gene in experimental enteropathogenic *Escherichia coli* infection *Journal of Clinical Investigation*, **92**, 1412–1417.

Donnenberg, M.S., Tzipori, S., McKee, M.L. *et al.* (1993b) The role of the eae gene of enterohemorrhagic *Escherichia coli* in intimate attachment in vitro and in a porcine model. *Journal of Clinical Investigation*, **92**, 1418–1424.

Donnenberg, M.S., Yu, J. and Kaper, J.B. (1993c) A second chromosomal gene necessary for intimate attachment of enteropathogenic *Escherichia coli* to epithelial cells. *Journal of Bacteriology*, **175**, 4670–4680.

Echeverria, P., Sethabutr, O. and Pitarangsi, C. (1991a) Microbiology and diagnosis of infections with *Shigella* and enteroinvasive *Escherichia coli*. *Reviews of Infectious Diseases*, **13**, S220–S225.

Echeverria, P., Orskov, F., Orskov, I. *et al.* (1991b) Attaching and effacing enteropathogenic *Escherichia coli* as a cause of infantile diarrhea in Bangkok. *Journal of Infectious Diseases*, **164**, 550–554.

Echeverria, P., Serichantalerg, O., Changchawalit, S. *et al.* (1992) Tissue culture-adherent *Escherichia coli* in infantile diarrhea. *Journal of Infectious Diseases*, **165**, 141–143.

Elsinghorst, E.A. and Kopecko, D.J. (1992) Molecular cloning of epithelial cell invasion determinants from enterotoxigenic *Escherichia coli*. *Infection and Immunity*, **60**, 2409–2417.

Faraawi, R. and Fong, I.W. (1988) *Escherichia coli* emphysematous endophthalmitis and pyelonephritis; case report and review of the literature. *American Journal of Medicine*, **84**, 636–639.

Farmer, J.J., Davis, B.R., Hickman-Brenner, F.W. *et al.* (1985) Biochemical identification of new species and biogroups of Enterobactenaceae isolated from clinical specimens. *Journal of Clinical Microbiology*, **21**, 46–76.

Garrison, R.N., Richardson, J.P. and Fry, D.E. (1982) Catheter associated septic thronbophlebitis. *Southern Medical Journal*, **75**, 917–919.

Ghosh, A.R., Nair, G.B., Naik, T.N. *et al.* (1992) Entero-adherent *Escherichia coli* is an important diarrhoeagenic agent in infants aged below 6 months in Calcutta, India. *Journal of Medical Microbiology*, **36**, 264–268.

Gicquelais, K.G., Baldini, M.M., Martinez, J. *et al.* (1990) Practical and economical method for using biotinylated DNA probes with bacterial colony blots to identify diarrhea-causing *Escherichia coli*. *Journal of Clinical Microbiology*, **28**, 2485–2490.

Giron, J.A., Ho, A.S. and Schoolnik, G.K. (1991a) An inducible bundle-forming pilus of enteropathogenic *Escherichia coli*. *Science*, **254**, 710–713.

Giron, J.A., Jones, T., Millan-Velasco, F. *et al.* (1991b) Diffuse-adhering *Escherichia coli* (DAEC) as a putative cause of diarrhea in Mayan children in Mexico. *Journal of Infectious Diseases*, **163**, 507–513.

Gomes, T.A., Blake, P.A. and Trabulsi, L.R. (1989) Prevalence of *Escherichia coli* strains with localized, diffuse, and aggregative adherence to HeLa cells in infants with diarrhea and matched controls. *Journal of Clinical Microbiology*, **27**, 266–269.

Gordillo, M.E., Reeve, G.R., Pappas, J. *et al.* (1992) Molecular characterization of strains of enteroinvasive *Escherichia coli* O143, including isolates from a large outbreak in Houston, Texas. *Journal of Clinical Microbiology*, **30**, 889–893.

Griffin, P.M., Ostroff, S.M., Tauxe, R.V. *et al.* (1988) Illnesses associated with *Escherichia coli* O157:H7 infections: a broad clinical spectrum. *Annals of Internal Medicine*, **109**, 705–712.

Gruneberg, R.N. (1990) Changes in the antibiotic sensitivities of urinary pathogens, 1971–1989. *Journal of Antimicrobial Chemotherapy*, **26** (Suppl. F), 3–11.

Guerrant, R.L. and Bobak, D.A. (1991) Bacterial and protozoal gastroenteritis. *New England Journal of Medicine*, **325**, 327–340.

Gunzburg, S.T., Chang, B.J., Elliott, S.J., Burke, V. and Gracey, M. (1993) Diffuse and enteroaggregative patterns of adherence of enteric *Escherichia coli* isolated from aboriginal children from the Kimberley region of Western Australia. *Journal of Infectious Diseases*, **167**, 755–758.

Gyles, C.L. (1992) *Escherichia coli* cytotoxins and enterotoxins. *Canadian Journal of Microbiology*, **38**, 734–746.

Hacker, J. (1992) Role of fimbrial adhesins in the pathogenesis of *Escherichia coli* infections. *Canadian Journal of Microbiology*, **38**, 720–727.

Hughes, J.M., Murad, F., Chang, B. and Guerrant, R.L. (1978) Role of cyclic GMP in the action of heat-stable enterotoxins of *Escherichia coli*. *Nature*, **271**, 755–756.

Isaacson, M., Canter, P.H., Effler, P. *et al.* (1993) Haemorrhagic colitis epidemic in Africa. *Lancet*, **341**, 961.

Jallat, C., Livrelli, V., Darfeuille-Michaud, A., Rich, C. and Joly, B. (1993) *Escherichia coli* strains involved in diarrhea in France: high prevalence and heterogeneity of diffusely adhering strains. *Journal of Clinical Microbiology*, **31**, 2031–2037.

Kaijser, B. and Ahlstedt, S. (1977) Protective capacity of antibodies against *Escherichia coli* and K antigens. *Infection and Immunity*, **17**, 286–289.

Kallenius, G., Svenson, S., Mollby, R. *et al.* (1981) Structure of carbohydrate part of receptor on human uroepithelial cells for pyelonephritogenic *Escherichia coli*. *Lancet*, **ii**, 604–606.

Kandel, G., Donohue-Rolfe, A., Donowitz, M. and Keusch, G.T. (1989) Pathogenesis of *Shigella* diarrhea. XVI. Selective targetting of Shiga toxin to villus cells of rabbit jejunum explains the effect of the toxin on intestinal electrolyte transport. *Journal of Clinical Investigation*, **84**, 1509–1517.

Karmali, M.A., Petric, M., Lim, C. *et al.* (1985) The association between idiopathic hemolytic uremic syndrome and infection by verotoxin-producing *Escherichia coli*. *Journal of Infectious Diseases*, **151**, 775–782.

Keenan, K.P., Sharpnack, D.D., Collins, H., Formal, S.B. and O'Brien, A.D. (1986) Morphologic evaluation of the effects of Shiga toxin and *E. coli* Shiga-like toxin on the rabbit intestine. *American Journal of Pathology*, **125**, 69–80.

Kleanthous, H., Smith, H.R., Scotland, S.M. *et al.* (1990) Haemolytic uraemic syndromes in the British Isles, 1985–8: association with verocytotoxin producing *Escherichia coli*. Part 2: Microbiological aspects. *Archives of Disease in Childhood*, **65**, 722–727.

Levine, M.M., Morris, J.G., Losonsky, G., Boedeker, E. and Rowe, B. (1986) Fimbriae (pili) adhesins as vaccines. In *Protein–Carbohydrate interactions in Biological Systems*. *Molecular Biology of Microbial Pathogenicity*. Academic Press, London.

Levine, M.M., Ferreccio, C., Prado, V. *et al.* (1993) Epidemiologic studies of *Escherichia coli* diarrheal infections in a low socioeconomic level peri-urban community in Santiago, Chile. *American Journal of Epidemiology*, **138**, 849–869.

Lewis, D.A. (1989) Bacteriology of urine. In *Medical Bacteriology: A Practical Approach* (eds P.M. Hawkey and D.A. Lewis), pp. 1–19. IRL Press, at Oxford University Press, Oxford.

Lopez, E.L., Diaz, M., Grinstein, S. *et al.* (1989) Hemolytic uremic syndrome and diarrhea in Argentine children: the role of Shiga-like toxins. *Journal of Infectious Diseases*, **160**, 469–475.

Mathewson, J.J., Johnson, P.C., DuPont, H.L., Satterwhite, T.K. and Winsor, D.K. (1986) Pathogenicity of enteroadherent *Escherichia coli* in adult volunteers. *Journal of Infectious Diseases*, **154**, 524–527.

McCracken, G., Jr, Sarff, L.D., Glode, M.P. *et al.*

(1974) Relation between *Escherichia coli* K1 capsular polysaccharide antigen and clinical outcome in neonatal meninnitis. *Lancet*, **ii**, 246–250.

McIver, C.J. and Tapsall, J.W. (1990) Assessment of conventional and commercial methods for identification of clinical isolates of cysteine-requiring strains of *Escherichia coli* and *Klebsiella* species. *Journal of Clinical Microbiology*, **28**, 1947–1951.

Moon, H.W., Whipp, S.C., Argenzio, R.A., Levine, M.M. and Giannella, R.A. (1983) Attaching and effacing activities of rabbit and human enteropathogenic *Escherichia coli* in pig and rabbit intestines. *Infection and Immunity*, **41**, 1340–1351.

Neidhardt, F.C. (ed.) (1996) *Escherichia coli and Salmonella: Cellular and Molecular Biology*, 2nd edn. American Society for Microbiology, Washington.

Orskov, F. and Orskov, I. (1984) Serotyping of *Escherichia coli*. In *Methods in Microbiology*, pp. 43–112. Academic Press, London.

Orskov, F. and Orskov, I. (1992) *Escherichia coli* serotyping and disease in man and animals. *Canadian Journal of Microbiology*, **38**, 699–674.

Ostroff, S.M., Tarr, P.I., Neill, M.A. *et al.* (1989) Toxin genotypes and plasmid profiles as determinants of systemic sequelae in *Escherichia coli* O157:H7 infections. *Journal of Infectious Diseases*, **160**, 994–998.

Pai, C.H., Kelly, J.K. and Meyers, G.L. (1986) Experimental infection of infant rabbits with verotoxin-producing *Escherichia coli*. *Infection and Immunity*, **51**, 16–23.

Pavia, A.T., Nichols, C.R., Green, D.P. *et al.* (1990) Hemolytic–uremic syndrome during an outbreak of *Escherichia coli* O157:H7 infections in institutions for mentally retarded persons: clinical and epidemiologic observations. *Journal of Pediatrics*, **116**, 544–551.

Pickett, C.L., Twiddy, E.M., Coker, C. and Holmes, R.K. (1989) Cloning, nucleotide sequence, and hybridization studies of the type IIb heat-labile enterotoxin gene of *Escherichia coli*. *Journal of Bacteriology*, **171**, 4945–4952.

Prouix, F., Turgeon, J.P., Delage, D., Lafleur, L. and Chicoine, L. (1992) Randomized, controlled trial of antibiotic therapy for *Escherichia coli* O157:H7 enteritis. *Journal of Pediatrics*, **121**, 299–303.

Roberts, A.P. and Phillips, R. (1979) Bacteria causing symptomatic urinary tract infection or asymptomatic bacteriuria. *Journal of Clinical Pathology*, **32**, 492–496.

Rothbaum, R., McAdams, A.J., Giannella, R. and Partin, J.C. (1982) A clinicopathologic study of enterocyte-adherent *Escherichia coli*: a cause of protracted diarrhea in infants. *Gastroenterology*, **83**, 441–454.

Samadpour, M. (1995) Molecular epidemiology of *Escherichia coli* O:157:H7 by restriction fragment length polymorphism using Shiga-like toxin genes. *Journal of Clinical Microbiology*, **33**, 2150–2154.

Savarino, S.J., Fasano, A., Robertson, D.C. and Levine, M.M. (1991) Enteroaggregative *Escherichia coli* elaborate a heat-stable enterotoxin demonstrable in an in vitro rabbit intestinal model. *Journal of Clinical Investigation*, **87**, 1450–1455.

Schiffer, M.S., Oliveira, E., Glode, M.P. *et al.* (1976) A review: relation between invasiveness and the K1 capsular polysaccharide of *Escherichia coli*. *Pediatric Research*, **10**, 82–87.

Schlager, T.A. and Guerrant, R.L. (1988) Seven possible mechanisms for *Escherichia coli* diarrhea. *Infectious Disease Clinics of North America*, **2**, 607–624.

Schlager, T.A., Wanke, C.A. and Guerrant, R.L. (1990) Net fluid secretion and impaired villous function induced by colonization of the small intestine by nontoxigenic colonizing *Escherichia coli*. *Infection and Immunity*, **58**, 1337–1343.

Senerwa, D., Olsvik, O., Mutanda, L.N. *et al.* (1989) Enteropathogenic *Escherichia coli* serotype O111:HNT isolated from preterm neonates in Nairobi, Kenya. *Journal of Clinical Microbiology*, **27**, 1307–1311.

Seriwatana, J., Echeverria, P., Taylor, D.N. *et al.* (1988) Type II heat-labile enterotoxin-producing *Escherichia coli* isolated from animals and humans. *Infection and Immunity*, **56**, 1158–1161.

Shariff, M., Bhan, M.K., Knutton, S. *et al.* (1993) Evaluation of the fluorescence actin staining test for detection of enteropathogenic *Escherichia coli*. *Journal of Clinical Microbiology*, **31**, 386–389.

Stamm, W.E., Martin, S.M. and Bennet, J.V. (1977) Epidemiology of nosocomial infecting due to gram-negative bacili: aspects relevant to development and use of vaccines. *Journal of Infectious Diseases*, **136** (Suppl.), S151–S160.

Su, C. and Brandt, L.J. (1995) *Escherichia coli* O157:H7 infections in humans. *Annals of Internal Medicine*, **123**, 698–714.

Svanborg-Eden, C., Hagberg, L. and Hanson, L.A. (1981) Adhesion of *Escherichia coli* in urinary tract infection. *CIBA Foundation Symposium*, **80**, 161–187.

Tacket, C.O., Moseley, S.L., Kay, B., Losonsky, G. and Levine, M.M. (1990) Challenge studies in volunteers using *Escherichia coli* strains with diffuse adherence to HEp-2 cells. *Journal of Infectious Diseases*, **162**, 550–552.

Taylor, C.M., Milford, D.V., Rose, P.E., Roy, T.C. and Rowe, B. (1990) The expression of blood group P1 in post-enteropathic haemolytic uraemic syndrome. *Pediatric Nephrology*, **4**, 59–61.

Tzipori, S., Montanaro, J., Robins-Browne, R.M. *et al.* (1992) Studies with enteroaggregative *Escherichia coli* in the gnotobiotic piglet gastroenteritis model. *Infection and Immunity*, **60**, 5302–5306.

Vaisanen, V., Elo, J., Taligren, L.G. *et al.* (1981) Mannose-resistant haemagglutination and P antigen recognition are characteristic of *Escherichia coli* causing primary pyelonephritis. *Lancet*, **ii**, 1366–1369.

Vial, P.A., Robins-Browne, R., Lior, H. *et al.* (1988) Characterization of enteroadherent-aggregative *Escherichia coli*, a putative agent of diarrheal disease. *Journal of Infectious Diseases*, **158**, 70–79.

Walterspiel, J.N., Ashkenazi, S., Morrow, A.L. and Cleary, T.G. (1992) Effect of subinhibitory concentrations of antibiotics on extracellular Shiga-like toxin 1. *Infection*, **20**, 25–29.

Wanke, C.A. and Guerrant, R.L. (1987) Small-bowel colonization alone is a cause of diarrhea. *Infection and Immunity*, **55**, 1924–1926.

Weinstein, M.P., Reller, L.B., Murphy, J.R. and Lichtenstein, K.A. (1983) The clinical significance of positive blood cultures: a comprehensive analysis of 500 episodes of bacteremia and fungemia in adults. I. Laboratory and epidemiologic observations. *Reviews of Infectious Diseases*, **5**, 35–53.

Wilcox, C.M. and Dismukes, W.E. (1987) Spontaneous bacterial peritonitis: a review of pathogenesis, diagnosis, and treatment. *Medicine*, **66**, 447–456.

Yu, J. and Kaper, J.B. (1992) Cloning and characterization of the *eae* gene of enterohaemorrhagic *Escherichia coli* O157:H7. *Molecular Microbiology*, **6**, 411–417.

12b

SHIGELLA

A.M. Emmerson and Stephen H. Gillespie

INTRODUCTION

The disease caused by *Shigella* spp. was recognized by Hippocrates as a condition characterized by the frequent passage of stools containing blood and mucus. He also recognized some aspects of the epidemiology, noting that after a dry winter and a wet spring the number of cases became more frequent in the summer. It was not until 1875 when the cause of amoebic dysentery was discovered and later when Shiga isolated the organism which was later to be known as *Shigella dysenteriae* that the two dysenteric diseases could be clearly differentiated (Shiga, 1898).

Dysentery has always played an important part in human history, influencing the course of military campaigns. Although the mortality rate among soldiers with bacillary dysentery was approximately 2.5%, the high attack rate meant that almost as many men died of this cause as the effects of battle. At crucial times large numbers of soldiers were infected and incapable of performing military duties. When people are herded together in gaols or on ships, epidemic dysentery may sweep through the population with devastating effect. Dysenteric disease remains an ever-present danger in the refugee camps of modern times.

The first of the genus to be identified was *S. dysenteriae*, which for many years was known as Shiga's bacillus (Shiga, 1899). *Shigella flexneri* was originally described by Flexner in 1900. *Shigella sonnei* was first isolated in 1904 but it was not until 1915 that its pathogenic potential was recognized by Sonne.

DESCRIPTION OF THE ORGANISM

Shigellae are small Gram-negative rods, non- or late lactose fermenting; they are facultative anaerobes which ferment sugars without gas production. Although non-motile under conventional tests recent studies have shown the presence of flagellar genes and expression of a motile phenotype under certain conditions (Girón, 1995). For details of the biochemical features of *Shigella* spp. see Table 12b.1.

Shigellae do not survive as well as salmonellas in clinical specimens and so should be plated onto isolation medium as quickly as possible. Some selective media, deoxycholate citrate agar (DCA) or Wilson and Blair designed for the isolation of *Salmonella*, can be too inhibitory for *Shigella*; thus it is useful to use a non-inhibitory medium such as MacConkey, salmonella–shigella (SS) or xylose–lactose–decarboxylate (XLD) in parallel (see below).

Principles and Practice of Clinical Bacteriology. Edited by A.M. Emmerson, P.M. Hawkey and S.H. Gillespie
© 1997 John Wiley & Sons Ltd

TABLE 12b.1 TYPICAL BIOCHEMICAL REACTIONS OF *SHIGELLA* SPP. AND *E. COLI*

	Indole	LDC	ODC	Motility	Glucose with gas	ONPG	D-Mannitol
S. sonnei	−	−	+	−	−	+	+
S. dysenteriae	−[a]	−	−	−	−	−	−
S. boydii	−	−	−	−	−	−	+
S. flexneri	−	−	−	−	−	−	+
E. coli	+	+	±	+	+	+	+

[a] *Shigella dysenteriae* type 2 is positive.

CLASSIFICATION

The genus *Shigella* is part of the Enterobacteriaceae family, which have been classified together on the basis of the disease that they cause. The shigellae have been shown to be closely related to *Escherichia coli* by DNA hybridization, isoenzyme analysis, and the presence of Shiga-like toxin (Brenner *et al.*, 1969; Crosa *et al.*, 1973; Goullet, 1980). They are most closely related to the enteroinvasive *E. coli*, which are also capable of producing a dysenteric illness.

The genus *Shigella* contains four species: *S. dysenteriae*, *S. flexneri*, *S. boydii* and *S. sonnei*. The species are differentiated on the basis of simple biochemical tests and serology of their lipopolysaccharides (LPS): *S. dysenteriae* are non-mannitol fermenters and their O-polysaccharide LPS is unrelated antigenically to the other shigellas. *Shigella flexneri* and *S. boydii* ferment mannitol but the latter are antigenically distinct from *S. flexneri*. All *S. flexneri* O-specific polysaccharides of the LPS antigens have a common rhamnose-containing tetrasaccharide (Robbins *et al.*, 1992). Included among the *S. boydii* are variants some of which are capable of producing gas from glucose. *Shigella sonnei* differs from the other members of the genus in that it ferments lactose in late cultures through possession of ONPG (see Table 12b.1). The O side chain is composed of a repeating disaccharide containing an unusual monosaccharide altruronic acid (Robbins *et al.*, 1992). This antigen is identical to that of *Pleisiomonas shigelloides* 017 which make up the majority of human isolates (See Chapter 16) and is the source of the cross-reactions between these two species.

The O-polysaccharide of the LPS is used to divide the species into serotypes as follows: *S. dysenteriae* into 12 serotypes, *S. flexneri* into 13, *S. boydii* into 18 and a single serotype of *S. sonnei*.

PATHOGENESIS

Shigella spp. are largely limited to mucosal infection of the distal ileum and colon; intestinal perforation, although rare, has been reported (Azad *et al.*, 1986); toxic megacolon may occur in up to 3% of patients in developing countries (Bennish, 1991). Bacteraemia is the most important lethal complication (Streulens *et al.*, 1990); meningitis and pneumonia due to general spread are rare (Bennish, 1991). Seizures are common especially with *S. dysenteriae* infection and these resemble febrile seizures although they occur in children over five years old (Rawashdeh *et al.*, 1994; Thapa *et al.*, 1995).

To establish an infection *Shigella* must invade the enteric epithelium via the basolateral epithelial surface. The organisms are unable to establish infection through intact tight junctions (Mounier *et al.*, 1992), they gain access to the basolateral side via M cells, the specialized antigen-presenting cells of the lymphoid follicles (Perdomo *et al.*, 1994a; Wassef *et al.*, 1989). Subsequent killing of macrophages in the submucosa leads to release of cytokines (Zychlinsky *et al.*, 1992, 1994) which attracts large numbers of polymorphonuclear leucocytes (PMNs). A path for *Shigella* invasion is opened via the tight junctions which are broken down by the PMNs (Perdomo *et al.*, 1994b) (Figure 12b.1).

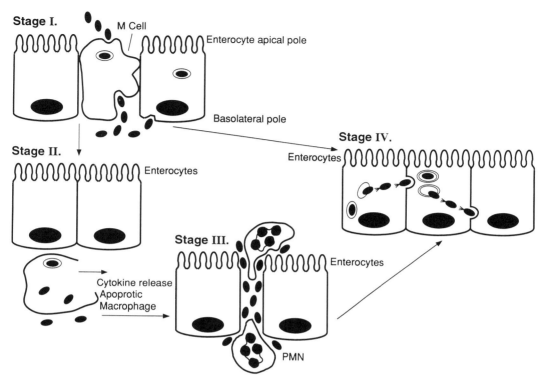

Figure 12b.1. Proposed invasion pathway for *Shigella* spp.

Once inside the enterocyte *Shigella* lyse the phagolysosomal membrane, escaping into the cytoplasm where they multiply (Sansonetti *et al.*, 1986). The bacteria spread in the cytoplasm and infect adjacent cells. This capacity is mediated by a 120 kDa protein which polymerizes intracellular actin. Expression of this protein is under the control of the *virG* (*icsA*) gene (Bernardini *et al.*, 1989). The recent description of flagella and motility under physiological conditions may also play a part in intercellular infection (Girón, 1995). Bacterial multiplication results in the death of the mucosal cell.

The presence of a 220 kb plasmid is essential for expression of an invasive phenotype (Sasakawa *et al.*, 1992). It possesses a series of genes forming one or more regulons which come under complex regulatory control of genes on the plasmid and the chromosome. Loss of the virulence plasmid is associated with loss of the invasive phenotype. Most of the structural genes needed for adherence, invasion and intercellular spread are located on this plasmid. Invasion is coded by the *ipa* genes and intercellular spread by the *ics* genes. Regulatory genes include *vacC*, *vacB*, and *kcpA*, which are located on the chromosome and are post-transcriptional regulators of *ipa* and *ipc*. *virF* activates *virB* and both genes are found on the plasmid (Sasakawa *et al.*, 1992). The *virR* gene found on the chromosome mediates temperature control of *virF*, *virB* gene expression.

Shigella dysenteriae type 1 produces a potent (Shiga toxin) exotoxin which enhances local vascular damage. It is structurally closely related to the Shiga-like toxins of *E. coli*. It produces fluid accumulation in the rabbit ileal loop model but does not appear to be necessary for intracellular killing of mucosal epithelial cells. Systemic distribution of the toxin results in microangiopathic renal damage with subsequent development of the haemolytic uraemic syndrome (Obrig *et al.*, 1988). The Shiga toxin is a bipartite molecule with an enzymatic A subunit activated by proteolytic cleavage, and a multimeric receptor-binding B subunit (O'Brien *et al.*, 1992). The binding subunits, like-cholera toxin, bind to a host cell surface glycolipid, in this case Gb3, which possesses a Gal α-1,4-Gal as the carbohydrate moiety. Shiga toxin exerts its lethal effect by inhibiting the host cell 60S ribosomal subunit by cleaving a specific adenosine residue of the 28S rRNA.

EPIDEMIOLOGY

There are more than 200 million cases of bacillary dysentery annually, of which 5 million require admission to hospital and over half a million die (Bennish and Wojtynial, 1991). Infection is spread by the faecal–oral route with great ease as the infective dose is low (10^2–10^3 cfu). *Shigella* spp. are obligate human pathogens and do not infect other hosts, although experimental infections can be achieved in other primates. Most cases of bacillary dysentery spread from person to person and this may occur rapidly, especially in closed communities and when individuals are brought together in large numbers and sanitary arrange-

ments are inadequate. Dysentery is a disease of poverty and the incidence of infection can be correlated with poor housing quality and sanitary facilities. When large populations are suddenly displaced through war, civil strife or natural disaster there is a rapid increase in the numbers of cases as an inevitable consequence of inadequate sanitation and water supply. Epidemics of disease may be both water- and food-borne, and can be associated with faecally contaminated wells.

Shigellosis is a disease of children under five years old in developing countries, reaching a peak at between 18 and 23 months (Henry, 1991). Disease is more severe in children who are malnourished (Bennish, 1991). In one study all of the fatal cases were severely malnourished (Thapa *et al.*, 1995). Patients suffered convulsions, bacteraemia, renal failure, intestinal perforation and toxic mega-colon (Thapa *et al.*, 1995; Rawashdeh *et al.*, 1994). *Shigella* dysentery has a significant effect on childhood mortality and on growth in excess of dysenteric illnesses of other aetiologies (Henry, 1991; Bennish, 1991).

In developing countries *S. flexneri* and *S. dysenteriae* are most frequently isolated, whereas *S. sonnei* and *S. flexneri* predominate in developed countries. The change in pattern of infection

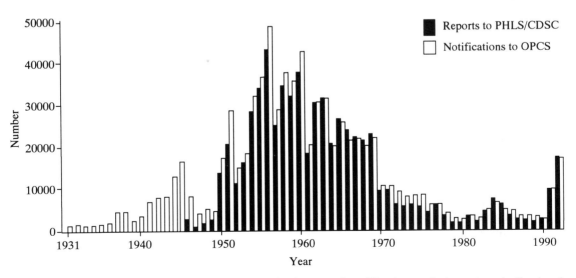

Figure 12b.2.   Laboratory reports of *S. sonnei* infections and notifications of dysentery in England and Wales. (Reproduced from the *Communicable Disease Report*, 23 April 1993.)

occurred in industrialized countries more than 50 years ago and resulted in a fall in mortality from dysentery as the more virulent forms became less common (Figure 12b.2). Haemolytic uraemic syndrome is associated with infection with *S. dysenteriae*.

In industrialized countries the scale of bacillary dysentery is not clearly established as many cases do not come to medical attention or are neither investigated bacteriologically nor notified to public health authorities. Infection is more common in children than in adults. *Shigella* is an important cause of traveller's diarrhoea making up to 10% of cases, especially in individuals returned from developing countries (Vila *et al.*, 1994).

CLINICAL FEATURES

Dysentery is an infection, not a toxaemia, and symptoms result from changes in the bowel wall caused by multiplication of the organisms after ingestion. The incubation period appears to be two to three days on average.

Clinical features vary markedly among the different types of shigellae, sonne dysentery being the mildest. Diarrhoea is frequently the only symptom in sonne dysentery and consists of several loose stools in the first 24 hours. This acute stage passes off rapidly and in most cases by the second day the condition has largely subsided. From then on the frequent bowel movement is more of a social inconvenience. In some, the infection can be a mild and trivial affair; for others the symptoms are more severe and vomiting can lead to dehydration, especially among the young. Fever is usually absent but sometimes, at the onset, there is a sharp rise in temperature and general signs and symptoms may suggest meningeal involvement. Cerebrospinal fluid (CSF) findings have always been normal, although *S. sonnei* septicaemia has been recorded.

Abdominal pain is not usually a prominent symptom although the illness may mimic appendicitis or even intussusception in babies. In some severe cases, the onset may be sudden, with vomiting, headache, rigors, severe colic and exhausting diarrhoea. This may lead to dehydration, tetany and meningeal signs.

While the illness caused by *S. flexneri* and *S. dysenteriae* may be no worse than sonne dysentery, in most cases the patient is more acutely ill with constitutional upset. Diarrhoea is severe and persistent. Faecal material soon gives way to mucus and blood and it is some days before faecal material returns. Abdominal pain and tenderness are frequent features and the patient is toxic and febrile. The pulse is rapid and weak and the patient becomes feeble, the skin punched, the tongue coated and urine scanty. The patient suffers from great thirst and cramps in the limbs; confusion or delirium may ensue. Generally, symptoms gradually subside over a period of 10–14 days but relapses do occur, with a flare-up of the dysenteric diarrhoea and rapid death. Fulminant choleraic or gangrenous forms are usually due to *S. dysenteriae*. Bacteraemia, pneumonia, meningitis, seizures and the haemolytic uraemic syndrome are recognized complications.

During the acute stage of the disease *Shigella* organisms are excreted in large numbers in the faeces but during recovery the numbers fall, although the organism may remain in the faeces for several weeks after the symptoms have subsided.

LABORATORY DIAGNOSIS

The organisms are usually present in large numbers in the intestinal mucus or the faeces in the early stages. Freshly passed stools should be examined, although rectal swabs showing marked faecal staining may be used. If the specimen includes blood and mucus these should be plated directly. When faeces are kept alkaline, shigellae may survive for days but in acid stools they die in a few hours. If there is likely to be much delay it may be useful to collect faeces into a buffered 30% glycerol saline solution. Nothing is to be gained by culturing urine or blood, since these are invariably negative. Numerous water-borne epidemics are on record and in several instances shigellas have been isolated from water itself.

Microscopic examination of the mucus in the early stages of acute bacillary dysentery shows a marked predominance of polymorphonuclear cells and red cells.

Faecal material is plated out directly onto DCA, SS agar or XLD medium. Shigellae appear as small colourless or slightly pink colonies on DCA and as pink or red colonies on XLD. Some strains have a pink or yellow periphery on XLD. A few strains grow poorly on inhibitory medium and it is advisable to use MacConkey agar and to examine any non-lactose-fermenting colonies after overnight incubation. A preliminary identification can often be made by slide agglutination with specific antisera from the growth on the primary plate. In any event full biochemical and serological tests must be performed on subcultures that have been checked for purity.

The biochemical identification of *Shigella* is complicated by the similarity of some strains of other genera, in particular strains of *Hafnia*, *Providencia*, *Aeromonas* and atypical *E. coli*; non-lactose-fermenting or anaerogenic strains of *E. coli* are a common problem.

Isolates are always non-motile, oxidase and lysine decarboxylase negative. *Shigella* of Group A (*S. dysenteriae*), Group B (*S. flexneri*) and Group C (*S. boydii*) are non-lactose fermenters. *S. sonnei* (Group D) is a late lactose fermenter. Group A organisms do not ferment mannitol while Groups B, C and D do. Acid is produced from a number of carbohydrates. Gas production is restricted to some subtypes of *S. flexneri*.

For more detailed biochemical tests see *Identification of Shigella*, ACP Broadsheet 60 (1968) and Barrow and Feltham (1993).

If slide agglutination is negative with appropriate antisera, a full biochemical identification is required.

Serological methods are little used in the diagnosis of dysentery but they may be of value in the retrospective investigation of outbreaks. Bacterial agglutination tests are unreliable and are no longer used. Typing methods for the subdivision of serotypes (e.g. bacteriophage or colicine methods) are sometimes carried out to help trace the source of the infection. Colicine typing of *S. sonnei* is more convenient for epidemiological purposes.

Safety

Most potential isolates belong to Advisory Committee on Dangerous Pathogens (ACDP) Group 2 and good laboratory practice is all that is required. Should *S. dysenteriae* be suspected, then all manipulations should be carried out in a Class I microbiological safety cabinet in the containment level 3 laboratory. Since the infecting dose is between 10 and 100 colonies great care must be taken to avoid environmental contamination. Gloves should be worn and the bench surfaces should be disinfected (e.g. with clear phenol) before removing the used gloves, followed by careful handwashing. Aerosolization is also a problem – avoid splashes.

Antimicrobial Sensitivities

The earliest reports described *Shigella* spp. as susceptible to sulphonamides but within a few years resistant strains began to appear. Between 1947 and 1950 antibiotic-resistant strains become predominant in many countries. It is likely that, given time, resistance to all useful antibiotics will be selected. For the years 1979–1983 the frequency of resistance in Groups A, B and C was 48% for ampicillin, 52% for chloramphenicol, 73% for sulphonamides, 72% for streptomycin, 69% for tetracyclines and 17% for trimethoprim (Gross *et al.*, 1984). In more recent years a high frequency of plasmid-mediated resistance has been observed in enterobacteria, including shigellae. Many of these resistances are now found on single plasmids which are readily transferable either via conjugation or transposition. Since 1980, outbreaks of dysentery due to multi-resistant *S. dysenteriae* type 1 have occurred in several countries in South East Asia.

Most cases of shigellosis, especially those caused by *S. sonnei*, are mild and do not require antibiotic therapy. Symptomatic treatment with the maintenance of hydration is all that is required. However, treatment with a suitable antibiotic is necessary in the very young, the aged or the debilitated and in severe infections. Because of the high incidence of antibiotic resistance among shigellae it is necessary to determine the resistance pattern of the strain before starting treatment where possible.

Drug Resistance Tests

Shigella isolates can be tested using Stokes' comparative disc diffusion method (Stokes, 1958) or the agar plate dilution method. Disc concentrations are as follows: ampicillin (10 μg), nalidixic acid (30 μg), furazolidone (30 μg), streptomycin (30 μg), sulphonamides (250 μg), tetracycline (10 μg) and trimethoprim (1.25 μg).

During the last decade, quinolones such as norfloxacin, ciprofloxacin, ofloxacin and fleroxacin have emerged as drugs of choice for the treatment of various bacterial enteric infections, including shigellosis. Controlled trials have shown that the quinolones in varying regimens, from a single dose (Salam *et al.*, 1994) to five days' treatment, significantly reduce the intensity and severity of traveller's diarrhoea as well as shigellosis (Wiström and Norrby, 1995). Quinolone resistance is presently uncommon among shigellae but it is inevitable that resistance will develop and increase with increased usage of these agents.

Antimotility drugs such as diphenoxylate (Lomotil) are not recommended in the treatment of diarrhoea, although loperamide, a synthetic antidiarrhoeal agent, has been shown to decrease the number of unformed stools and shortens the duration of diarrhoea caused by *Shigella* in adults treated with ciprofloxacin (Murphy *et al.*, 1993).

MANAGEMENT OF INFECTION

Oral Rehydration Therapy

Oral rehydration therapy (ORT) is the cornerstone of worldwide efforts to reduce mortality from acute diarrhoea, and while toxaemia plays a major role in the severity of illness in shigellosis, dehydration has to be corrected. The World Health Organization (WHO)/UNICEF oral rehydration formula (ORS) contains glucose and sodium in a molar ratio of 1.2 : 1. Potassium chloride is added to replace potassium lost in the stool. Trisodium citrate dihydrate (or sodium bicarbonate) corrects metabolic acidosis caused by faecal loss of bicarbonate. Oral rehydration therapy has proved to be a simple, safe and cost-effective means of preventing and managing dehydration in the community (Richard *et al.*, 1993).

When patients, especially babies and elderly persons, are acutely ill, there is much loss of fluids and salts in vomit and in stools, and replacement of fluids may need to be controlled by electrolyte estimations. Intravenous administration need seldom be continued for more than 24 hours but children suffering from the haemolytic–uraemic syndrome may require dialysis. Patients with tetany may respond to intravenous normal saline alone or with the addition of 20% calcium gluconate.

On clinical grounds, antibiotics are not required for mild or moderate cases; this applies to virtually every case of dysentery seen in Britain, where 98% of cases are due to *S. sonnei*. In severe forms of dysentery due to *S. dysenteriae* and *S. flexneri* where shigellae have penetrated intestinal epithelial cells in large numbers, the use of antibiotics such as ciprofloxacin, pivmecillinam or ceftriaxone (Bennish and Salam, 1992) to kill these intracellular organisms may prevent severe destruction of the intestinal wall. Persistent hiccough or the passage of sloughs in the stools are ominous signs. The choleraic and gangrenous types of bacillary dysentery are almost invariably fatal.

Biotherapy is the use of live organisms or their metabolic products for treatment. The most commonly available sources are fermented milk products such as yoghurt, kefir and buttermilk. Unless pasteurized these products contain live bacteria and they have been used for the prevention and treatment of gastrointestinal complaints. Kefir is traditionally made from goats' milk by the addition of kefir granules consisting of *Lactobacillus* spp. and a yeast (*Torula kefir*). *Saccharomyces boulardii* is a non-pathogenic yeast which is sometimes used to treat diarrhoea. It does not multiply in the gut and there is no permanent colonization of the bowel (Roffe, 1996).

INFECTION CONTROL

The mild and often fleeting nature of the clinical illness associated with sonne dysentery means that patients, often children, remain ambulant and are free to continue their daily activities and act as dispersers of the organism. When the arrangements for the disposal of human faeces are crude or non-existent heavy contamination of the environment is inevitable, but even with modern sanitation the disease can spread easily and rapidly if there is a break in hygiene standards. The dose of *Shigella* needed to cause infection is very small (less than 200 organisms) and, given moist alkaline, cool and shady conditions, large numbers will survive for many days. Even on dried linen, organisms will survive in the dark for long periods. Environmental contamination, particularly in and around toilet facilities, remain an important focus for continuing outbreaks of dysentery.

Shigellae are sensitive to heat and are killed in 1 hour at 55 °C. At laboratory temperatures below this level, they survive for varying periods of time and, unless strict care is exercised, a laboratory bench will remain a rich source of contamination. Shigellae are readily killed by disinfectants: in 6 hours by 0.5% clear phenolics or in 15–30 minutes by 1% phenol. A handwash of 1% benzalkonium chloride will kill *S. sonnei* in 1 minute in a dilution of 1 in 64. A solution of 3% (1 in 30) is a useful hand decontamination fluid which is safe to use on children's hands and has been used to control outbreaks of sonne dysentery in pre-school institutions.

Drinking water should be protected and kept well away from toilet facilities as shigellae can survive in tap or sterilized water for as long as four to six weeks. Water-borne outbreaks tend to be explosive, especially in developing countries. Handwashing, although very important, cannot be guaranteed to remove all dysentery bacilli from hands, which readily become recolonized from inanimate objects. Symptomatic staff should, where possible, remain off work until they no longer have to go to the toilet during working hours.

Spread by Personal Contact

Without doubt, sonne dysentery spreads by direct contact in Britain and is largely a disease of young children. This reflects the intimate nature of contact between young children and decreases with age as the standard of hygiene increases. Symptomless excreters play a much less important role in the spread of disease than the acute case. Although splashing occurs with contamination of the toilet area, door handles etc., it is likely that hand-to-hand contact facilitates spread among young children. Supervised handwashing with benzalkonium hand disinfection is important. Likewise staff-to-patient and patient-to-staff transmission can occur.

Control must therefore depend on the exclusion of acute cases from communal water closets and the institution of supervised hand hygiene for the young. Children without symptoms can be allowed to stay at school provided their hygiene is supervised. The use of antibiotics prophylactically in an attempt to limit the spread should be avoided.

Vaccines

Serum antibodies do not seem to be protective against intestinal shigella infection. Killed shigellae induced humoral immunity only and research and clinical trials are under way with live attenuated strains. There are conflicting reports about the efficacy of live vaccines. Non-invasive strains or recombinants can be produced which proliferate, do not invade, are safe and do not revert. The development of appropriate vaccines is a complex task (Black, 1993).

REFERENCES

Azad, M.A.K., Islam, M. and Butler, T. (1986) Colonic perforation in *Shigella dysenteriae* 1 infection. *Pediatric Infectious Diseases Journal*, **5**, 103–104.

Barrow, G.I. and Feltham, R.K.A. (eds) (1993) *Cowan and Steel's Manual for the Identification of Medical Bacteria*, 3rd edn. Cambridge University Press, Cambridge, UK.

Bennish, M.L. (1991) Mortality due to shigellosis: community and hospital data. *Reviews of Infectious Diseases*, **13** (Suppl. 4), S219–S224.

Bennish, M.L. and Salam, M.A. (1992) Rethinking options for the treatment of shigellosis. *Journal of Antimicrobial Chemotherapy*, **30**, 243–247.

Bennish, M.J. and Woityniak, B.J. (1991) Mortality due to shigellosis: community and hospital data. *Reviews of Infectious Diseases*, **13** (Suppl. 4), S245–S251.

Bernardini, M.L., Mounier, J., d'Hautville, H., Coquis-Rondon, M. and Sansonetti, P.J. (1989) Identification of *icsA*, a plasmid locus which governs bacterial intra- and intercellular spread through interaction with F-actin. *Proceedings of the National Academy of Sciences USA*, **86**, 3867–3871.

Black, R.E. (1993) Epidemiology of diarrhoeal disease: implication for control by vaccines. *Vaccine*, **11**, 100–106.

Brenner, D.J., Fanning, G.F., Johnston, K.E., Citarella, R.V. and Falkow, S. (1969) Polynucleotide sequence relationships among members of the Enterobacteriaciae. *Journal of Bacteriology*, **98**, 637–650.

Broadsheet 60 (1968) Identification of *Shigella*. Association of Clinical Pathologists. *Journal of Clinical Pathology*, 1–10.

Christie, A.B. (1987) Bacillary dysentery. In *Infectious Diseases*, vol. 1, 4th edn, Ch. 6. Churchill Livingstone, Edinburgh.

Crosa, J.H., Brenner, D.J., Ewing, W.H. and Falkow, S. (1973) Molecular relationships among the Salmonellae. *Journal of Bacteriology*, **115**, 307–315.

Flexner S. (1900) On the etiology of tropical dysentery. *Bulletin of Johns Hopkins Hospital*, **11**, 231–242.

Girón, J.A. (1995) Expression of flagella and motility by *Shigella*. *Molecular Microbiology*, **18**, 63–75.

Goullet, P. (1980) Esterase electrophoretic pattern relatedness between *Shigella* and *Escherichia coli*. *Journal of General Microbiology*, **117**, 493–500.

Gross, R.J., Threlfall, E.J., Ward, L.R. and Rowe, B. (1984) Drug resistance in *Shigella dysenteriae*, *S. flexneri* and *S. boydii* in England and Wales: increasing incidence of resistance to trimethoprim. *British Medical Journal*, **288**, 784–786.

Henry, F.J. (1991) The epidemiological importance of dysentery in communities. *Reviews of Infectious Diseases*, **13** (Suppl.), S238–S244.

Mounier, J., Vasselon, T., Hellio, R., Lesourd, M. and Sansonetti, P.J. (1992) *Shigella flexneri* enters human colonic Caco-2 epithelial cells through the basolateral pole. *Infection and Immunity*, **60**, 237–248.

Murphy, G.S., Bodfudatta, L., Echeverria, P., Tyansuphaswadikul, S., Hoge, C.W., Imlarp, S. and Tamura, K. (1993) Ciprofloxacin and loperamide in the treatment of bacillary dysentery. *Annals of Internal Medicine*, **118**, 582–586.

O'Brien, A.D., Tesh, V.L., Donohue-Rolfe, A., Jackson, M.P., Olnsess, S., Sandvig, K., Lindberg, A.A. and Keusch, G.T. (1992) Shiga toxin: biochemistry, genetics, mode of action and role in pathogenesis. *Current Topics in Microbiology*, **180**, 65–94.

Obrig, T.G., del Vecchi, P.J., Brown, J.E., Morgan, T.P., Rowland, B.M., Judge, T.K. and Rothamn, S.W. (1988) Direct cytotoxic action of Shiga toxin on human vascular endothelial cells. *Infection and Immunity*, **56**, 2373–2378.

Perdomo, O.J.J., Cavaillon, J.-M., Heurre, M., Ohayon, H., Gounon, P. and Sansonetti, P.J. (1994a) Acute inflammation causes epithelial invasion and mucosal destruction in experimental shigellosis. *Journal of Experimental Medicine*, **180**, 1307–1319.

Perdomo, O.J.J., Gounon, P. and Sansonetti, P.J. (1994b) Polymorphonuclear leukocyte transmigration promotes invasion of colonic epithelial monolayer by *Shigella flexneri*. *Journal of Clinical Investigation*, **93**, 633–643.

Rawashdeh, M.O., Adabneh, A.M. and Shurman, A.A. (1994) Shigellosis in Jordanian children: a clinico-epidemiological prospective study. *Journal of Tropical Pediatrics*, **40**, 355–359.

Richards, L., Claeson, M. and Pierce, N.F. (1993) Management of acute diarrhea in children: lessons learned. *Pediatric Infectious Diseases Journal*, **12**, 5–9.

Robbins, J.B., Chu, C. and Schneerson, R. (1992) Hypothesis for vaccine development: protective immunity to enteric diseases caused by non-typhoidal salmonellae and shigella may be conferred by serum IgG antibodies to the O-specific polysaccharide of their lipopolysaccharide. *Clinical Infectious Diseases*, **15**, 346–361.

Roffe, C. (1996) Biotherapy for antibiotic-associated and other diarrhoeas. *Journal of Infection*, **32**, 1–10.

Salam, I., Katelaris, P., Leigh-Smith, S. and Farthing, M.J.G. (1994) Randomised trial of single-dose ciprofloxacin for travellers' diarrhoea. *Lancet*, **344**, 1537–1539.

Sansonetti, P.J., Ryter, A., Clerc, P., Maurelli, A.T. and Mounier, J. (1986) Multiplication of *Shigella flexneri* within HeLa cell: lysis of phagocytic vacuole and plasmid mediated contact hemolysis. *Infection and Immunity*, **51**, 461–469.

Sasakawa, C., Buysse, J.M. and Watanabe, H. (1992) The large virulence plasmid of *Shigella*. *Current Topics in Microbiology*, **180**, 21–44.

Shiga, K. (1898) Ueber den dysenteriebacillus (*Bacillus dysenteriae*). *Zentralblatt der Bacteriologie*, **24**, 817–828.

Sonne, C. (1915) Ueber die Bacteriologie der giftarmen Dysenteribacillen (Paradysenteribacillen). *Zentralblatt für Bacteriologie l, Originale Abteilung*, **75**, 408–456.

Stokes, E.J., Ridgway, G.L. and Wren, M.W.D. (1993) *Clinical Microbiology*, 7th edn, Edward Arnold, London.

Streulens, M.J., Mondonl, G., Roberts, M. and Williams, P.H. (1990) Role of bacterial and host factors in the pathogenesis of *Shigella* septicaemia. *European Journal of Clinical Microbiology and Infectious Diseases*, **9**, 337–344.

Thapa, B.R., Venkateswarlu, K., Malik, A.K. and Panagrahi, D. (1995) Shigellosis in children from North India: a clinicopathological study. *Journal of Tropical Pediatrics*, **41**, 303–307.

Vila, J., Gascon, J., Abdalla, S., Marco, F., Moreno, A., Corachan, M. and Jimenez de Anta, T. (1994) Antimicrobial resistance of *Shigella* isolates causing traveller's diarrhoea. *Antimicrobial Agents and Chemotherapy*, **38**, 2668–2670.

Wassef, J.S., Keren, D.F. and Mailloux, J.L. (1989) Role of M cells in initial antigen uptake and in ulcer formation in the rabbit intestinal loop model of shigellosis. *Infection and Immunity*, **57**, 858–863.

Wiström, J. and Norrby, S.R. (1995) Fluroquinolones and bacterial enteritis, when and for whom? *Journal of Antimicrobial Chemotherapy*, **36**, 23–39.

Zychlinsky, A., Prevost, M.C. and Sansonetti, P.J. (1992) *Shigella flexneri* induces apoptosis in infected macrophages. *Nature*, **358**, 167–170.

Zychlinsky, A., Fitting, C., Cavaillon, J.-M. and Sansonetti, P.J. (1994) Interleukin-1 is released by murine macrophages during apoptosis induced by *Shigella flexneri*. *Journal of Clinical Investigation*, **94**, 1328–1332.

12c

SALMONELLA

Stephen H. Gillespie

INTRODUCTION

Infection with organisms of the *Salmonella* spp. is an important public health problem throughout the world. The number of cases of salmonellosis is rising and typhoid continues to exact a considerable death toll in developing countries.

DESCRIPTION OF THE ORGANISM

Classification

Taxonomists, it appears, cut their teeth on the Enterobacteriaceae. They were simple to cultivate and submitted themselves readily to biochemical testing (Barrow and Fletham, 1992). The consequence of this earlier enthusiasm is a proliferation of genera and species which, in the modern age, dominated as it is by the results of molecular studies, would never be dignified with genus or species designation. DNA–DNA homology studies indicate that *Salmonella* and *Escherichia coli* are 90% homologous – sufficiently similar to cause them to be classified in the same species. Although this has been proposed it is unlikely to happen as the genus *Salmonella* has an important clinical identity making it useful in day-to-day microbiological practice. *Salmonella* are fermenta-tive facultatively anaerobic, oxidase-negative Gram-negative rods. They are generally motile, aerogenic, non-lactose fermenting, urease negative, citrate utilizing and acetyl methyl carbinol negative (see Table 12c.1).

The species has previously been divided into a large number of serotypes which have conventionally been written in a way which appears to give the status of a species, e.g. *Salmonella dublin*, or *Salmonella montevideo*. This represents the other extreme of classification. Two approaches are commonly used: to designate all salmonellae in the species *Salmonella enterica* or to divide the genus into three species: *Salmonella typhi*, *Salmonella cholera-suis*, and *Salmonella enteritidis*. The latter species is then subdivided into the serotypes of the Kaufmann–White scheme of which there are more than 2200 (Ewing, 1986). Although this is a logical approach one may expect that microbiological reports will still contain '*Salmonella typhimurium*' for some time to come.

Population Structure of *Salmonella* spp.

The population structure of *Salmonella* spp. has been studied by a number of techniques including multilocus enzyme electophoresis (MLEE) (Selander *et al.*, 1986; Selander and Smith, 1991).

Principles and Practice of Clinical Bacteriology. Edited by A.M. Emmerson, P.M. Hawkey and S.H. Gillespie
© 1997 John Wiley & Sons Ltd

TABLE 12c.1   CHARACTERISTICS OF *SALMONELLA* SPP.

Test	*Salmonella* spp.	*Shigella* spp.
Urease	−	−
Motility	+[a]	−
Indole	−	−
Gas from glucose	+[b]	−
Mannitol	+	+[c]
ONPG	−[d]	−[e]
H$_2$S	+[d]	−
Citrate	+[f]	−
Lysine decarboxylase	+	−
Ornithine decarboxylase	+	−[e]

[a] Rare strains which are non-motile are reported.
[b] *Salmonella typhi* negative.
[c] *Shigella dysenteriae* does not ferment mannitol.
[d] Some exceptions.
[e] *Shigella sonnei* positive.
[f] Up to 25% citrate negative.

These studies show that many of the common serotypes are genotypically diverse and polyphyletic. However the population structure of *Salmonella* is essentially clonal. For each common serotype most disease is caused by a few clones which have an intercontinental or global distribution (Beltran *et al.*, 1988). Among strains of *S. typhi* the majority of clinical isolates belong to two clones distinguished by MLEE (Reeves *et al.*, 1989). The phylogenetic lineage of *S. typhi* is old but the distinctive characteristics of clones of this serovar including adaption to infection in man may be recent developments. These data invalidate the concept that the serological classification of the Kaufmann–White scheme has any biological significance.

PATHOGENICITY

Salmonella typhi

Natural history of infection

After ingestion *S. typhi* must pass through the stomach, which provides a considerable barrier to infection. Organisms cannot be cultured from the stomach 30 minutes after ingestion, and antacids and H$_2$ antagonists reduce the number of organisms required to initiate infection. Bacteria will multiply in the intestine but stools are only intermittently positive to culture during the first week and even after experimental infection with 10^5 to 10^7 cfu the presence of organisms in the stools during the first five days did not necessarily indicate that illness would develop (Hornick *et al.*, 1970). The organisms penetrate the intestinal epithelial barrier without causing apparent inflammation, probably via the M cells, a process which happens quickly (<1 minute) (Gerichter, 1960). They are then transported to the mesenteric lymph nodes, later disseminating via the lymphatics and bloodstream to grow intracellularly within the cells of the reticulo-endothelial system. This time corresponds roughly to the incubation period. After approximately one week there is a secondary bacteraemia and typhoid bacilli reinvade the gut via the liver and gall-bladder, settling in Peyer's patches. Multiplication continues with thinning and ulceration of the gut wall. This may lead to the complications of perforation or haemorrhage (see p. 405).

The virulence antigens of S. typhi

Almost all virulent *S. typhi* organisms possess a Vi antigen – a polysaccharide composed of *N*-acetylglucosamine uronic acid. Organisms lacking the antigen require a much higher dose to infect; antibodies to Vi are detected in patients recovering from typhoid and when Vi antigen is used as a vaccine protective immunity is conferred (Acharya *et al.*, 1987). In most instances capsular antigens prevent phagocytosis but *S. typhi* is readily phagocytosed and lives successfully in the intracellular environment. It is possible that Vi antigen acts as a scavenger of free radicals inside the phagocyte.

The macrophage has an important role to play in the pathogenesis of typhoid fever. This was recognized as long ago as 1898 by Mallory, who stated: 'the typhoid bacillus produces a mild diffusible toxine, partly within the intestinal tract, and partly within the blood and organs of the body. The toxine produced proliferation of the endothelial cells which acquire for a time malignant properties. The new formed cells are epithelioid in character, have irregular, lightly stained, eccentrically situated nuclei, abundant sharply defined acidophilic protoplasm and are characterized by marked phagocytic properties' (Mallory, 1898). In volunteer experiments patients were made tolerant of endotoxin by repeated injection of small doses to the extent that they could tolerate 2.5 μg with no ill-effect. In spite of this the volunteers became ill when challenged with *S. typhi*, exhibiting the characteristic clinical features of the disease (Greisman *et al.*, 1964). Like other members of the Enterobacteriaceae *S. typhi* and other salmonellas possess a lipopolysaccharide with a lipid A core. Stimulation of cells of the monocyte lineage results in the release of tumour necrosis factor α (TNF-α) and other cytokines. This gives rise to the fever, chills and rigors common in the clinical presentation and explains the phenomena so carefully recorded by previous workers.

Lipopolysaccharides also assist salmonellae by defending the organism against the effects of complement pathway. The long 'O' side chain on the molecule means that activated complement (membrane attack complex) is unable to damage the outer membrane. The *rck* gene, encoded on the *S. typhimurium* virulence plasmid, codes for a protein which acts to prevent the formation and insertion of fully polymerized tubular C9 complexes into the outer membrane.

Other *Salmonella* spp.

Invasion

Our understanding of the molecular mechanisms whereby salmonellae invade intestinal epithelial cells has been expanded radically in recent years. Many intestinal pathogens invade by triggering actin rearrangement, which results in the formation of pseudopodia and phagocytosis of the bacterium. *Salmonella typhimurium* and *S. cholera-suis* cause a change in appearance of the host cell surface, giving it a ruffle. Actin rearrangement accompanies internalization of the bacterium, all of which returns to normal immediately afterwards. The ruffling/internalization process appears to be mediated by genes found in the *inv* locus (*invA–H*). Disruption in *invA* and *invE* prevented the organism triggering the ruffling process reducing its ability to invade (Altmeyer *et al.*, 1993). The genes of this cluster have considerable sequence homology with the *Yops* locus of *Yersinia*. The G + C percentage of the *inv* locus is much closer to the overall G + C percentage of *Yersinia* spp. (46%) than to that of *Salmonella* (G + C = 52%), opening the intriguing possibility that these genes were originally acquired form *Yersinia*.

The *inv* locus is not alone in being responsible for invasion. Another locus located near to *inv* is *hil* (the hyperinvasion locus) and, when deleted, invasion decreases by 1000-fold.

Intracellular survival

Intracellular survival is an important pathogenicity determinant of *Salmonella* spp. A repertoire of antigens is expressed by organisms growing in an intracellular environment. It is estimated that as many as 200 genes may be involved. The processes of intracellular survival are now beginning to be understood. These genes enable the organisms to survive in conditions of low pH, in the presence of free radicals and to overcome the deleterious effects of host defensins and lysosomal enzymes.

One of the systems which has been studied in detail is the *PhoP/PhoQ* operon. This codes for a two-component regulatory system. Genes activated by *PhoP/PhoQ* are known as *pag* genes, of which *pag A–C* have begun to be characterized. Those repressed by *PhoP/PhoQ* are known as *prg* genes, of which there are at least six *prg A–H*. Mutants which constitutively produce PhoP and a mutant in which *PhoP/PhoQ* is disrupted are both avirulent, demonstrating the importance of regulating the complex process of adaptation to the intracellular environment (Behlau and Miller, 1993). PhoQ is a sensor and PhoP is a transcriptional activator. The system responds to metabolic signals such as carbon starvation, low pH, oxygen tension (Groisman *et al.*, 1989). *PagC* appears only to be induced while inside macrophages and not inside epithelial cells, leading to the idea that the PhoP–PhoQ system is specific for intra-macrophage survival (Guiney *et al.*, 1995).

The acid tolerance response (ATR) is thought to be controlled by the iron regulator Fur. It is activated at pH <5.0, enabling the organisms to survive if they have had time to adapt and turn on this system.

Virulence plasmids

Jones *et al.* 1982 originally identified a cryptic plasmid capable of conferring a virulent phenotype on *S typhimurium*. It is now recognized that non-typhoid salmonellae associated with extraintestinal invasion – *S. typhimurium*, *S. enteritidis*, *S. dublin*, *S. cholera-suis* and *S. gallinarum-pullorum* – possess plasmids of differing sizes which contain genes important for invasive infection. All of these plasmids possess *spv* genes contained on an 8 kb regulon. The regulon consists of the positive regulator *spvR* and four structural genes: *spvA*, *spvB*, *spvC* and *spvD*. Efficient transcription of SpvR depends on an alternative σ factor RpoS which is encoded on the chromosome. The activity of RpoS increases as the organisms enter the post-exponential phase of growth (Abe

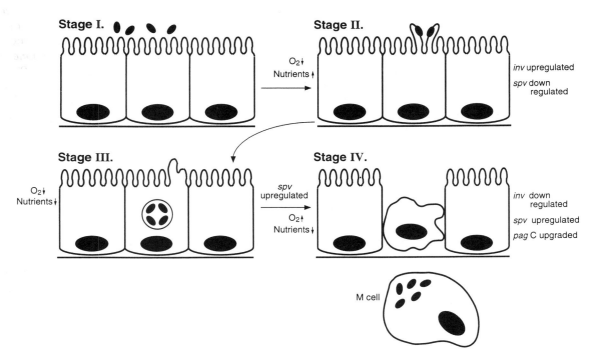

Figure 12c.1. Proposed pathway for *Salmonella* invasion showing changes in the regulation of genes involved in the process.

et al., 1994). The expression of *spv* genes is regulated by the growth phase of the bacteria: during early exponential growth in rich media these genes are not expressed, but the synthesis of SpvA begins in the transition period between late logarithmic and early post-exponential phase growth. The other proteins are expressed later. It appears that nutrient starvation, iron limitation and pH, rather than cell density, is the stimulus for *spv* expression (Valone *et al.*, 1993).

The *spv* genes enhance the growth of *Salmonella* strains within macrophages and non-professional phagocytic cells, including epithelial cells (Hefferman *et al.*, 1985). The nature of the initial signal for its induction is unknown.

The way in which all of these factors may interact is illustrated in Figure 12c.1.

EPIDEMIOLOGY

Typhoid

The incidence of typhoid is falling world-wide but it still remains a major threat to human health. The World Health Organization estimate there are 16 000 000 cases of typhoid each year and more than 600 000 deaths (Ivanoff *et al.*, 1994). Typhoid is predominantly a disease of the developing world: the incidence in the Far East is approximately 1000/100 000. In some developing countries the majority of cases are reported to be in the 5–14-year age group whereas other reports show a more even distribution but confirm that typhoid is an uncommon but serious infection in patients over 30 (Butler *et al.*, 1991). In industrialized countries the majority of *S. typhi* infections are acquired abroad. Infection is acquired by ingestion of contaminated food, water or contact with a patient or carrier of the disease. In addition *S. typhi* can be a laboratory-acquired infection.

Non-typhoid *Salmonellosis*

Infective dose

The stomach acts as a barrier to *Salmonella* infection; consequently patients with achlorhydria, or who are taking antacids or H_2 antagonists, the young and the very old are more susceptible to infection. Similarly ingestion of organisms in food, especially fatty food, is more likely to result in infection as the organisms are protected from the deleterious effects of gastric acid. This has been seen most recently in the outbreak of *Salmonella* infection associated with contaminated chocolate. Endoscopy with a contaminated instrument can also circumvent this natural defence (Beecharn *et al.*, 1979). A large number of experimental studies have been performed to determine the infective dose, and the lowest dose causing infection varied from 10^5 to 10^{10} (Blaser and Newman, 1982). An exception to these relatively high doses was a single study where patients were infected with *S. sofia* and *S. bovis-morbificans* by the nasal route. The minimum infective dose in this instance was only 25 organisms (McKenzie and Livingstone, 1968).

There are many factors which have contributed to the changing epidemiology of non-typhoid *Salmonella* infection. There has been increased consumption of processed food and use of commercial food services, especially fast food, increasing the risk of exposure to *Salmonella* transmitted by food handlers (Hederg *et al.*, 1994). The importance of hygienic practices in the food and catering industries is emphasized when controls fail and an epidemic results. Non-typhoid salmonellae are found in the intestines of food animals. Infection can spread among animals while they are being transported for slaughter and contamination can be spread from infected to uninfected carcasses in the abattoir if inappropriate practices are adopted. Raw meat should be adequately cooked before ingestion and this can be a particular problem in frozen chickens if they are not adequately defrosted before cooking is commenced. Cooked food and raw meat should be stored separately in refrigerators and food items which have been cooked and chilled should be adequately reheated before eating.

Changes in farming practices, and a move to more industrial-scale farm size and feeding make infection more likely to occur and difficult to eradicate when it does. Chickens and eggs are now the biggest source of food-borne *Salmonella* infection (Duguid and North, 1991).

Patients of all ages are affected by salmonellosis but the main burden of disease falls on the elderly and those that are immunocompromised.

Outbreaks in hospitals and institutions

Outbreaks of salmonellosis may occur in many situations but individuals in institutional care, for example hospitals and old people's homes, are particularly vulnerable and outbreaks characteristically take two forms. The point source outbreak is caused by ingestion of a contaminated food item by a large number of patients. In this instance cases are closely related in time and a common source is usually identified, e.g. a turkey at a Christmas party.

If a case of salmonellosis is admitted to the ward, *Salmonella* spreads readily if good control of infection practices are not in place. In this instance cases continue to arise sporadically over a number of days. Nursing and medical staff play a role in perpetuating such an outbreak through inadequate infection control practices or because they become infected and become asymptomatic carriers.

CLINICAL FEATURES

Infection with organisms of the genus *Salmonella* results in three main syndromes: infection localized to the intestine, often known as salmonellosis, invasive or bacteraemic disease and enteric fever.

Salmonellosis

Symptoms of salmonellosis can develop in as little as 6 hours and usually appear within 24 hours after ingestion of the organisms. Patients complain of nausea, vomiting and diarrhoea. Fever and abdominal pain are also common but the degree of each of these symptoms varies considerably between patients. In salmonellosis patients complain of symptoms related to enteritis and to dysentery; blood in the stool is not uncommon. Abdominal pain is usually mild or moderate but can be sufficiently severe to mimic an acute abdomen in some cases. After symptoms subside patients

continue to excrete organisms in their stools for up to three months. Approximately 1–3% may excrete organisms for more than a year.

In some patients, especially the elderly or immunocompromised, invasive disease may develop. This is more likely to occur with the *S. cholera-suis* serotype. In community outbreaks the majority of patients will suffer no serious effects but a small proportion, usually the elderly, will suffer invasive disease with a significant mortality. Bacteraemia may result in the seeding of other organs. The bones, including the vertebral column, may become infected, producing an acute osteomyelitis. In patients with sickle cell disease osteomyelitis is common and may be very difficult to treat.

Invasive salmonellosis has become an important problem among those infected with HIV, who are estimated to be between 20 and 100 times more at risk of infection than the general population (Angulo and Swerdlow, 1995; Gruenewald *et al.*, 1994). Salmonella septicaemia usually occurs late in the course of HIV disease in industrialized countries. Salmonella septicaemia was the leading cause of treatable and preventable death in HIV-infected individuals in a study from Kenya (Gilks *et al.*, 1990). Bacteraemia in HIV-positive patients in the Côte d'Ivoire was associated with a mortality rate of 62% (Vugia *et al.*, 1993). Recurrent *Salmonella* septicaemia is rare in immuno-competent subjects but is a common problem in HIV-infected individuals, especially in those who do not complete an adequate course of antimicrobials. It is now considered an AIDS-defining illness.

Typhoid

The incubation period for typhoid is longer than that of salmonellosis: usually one week. Historical accounts of typhoid written before the development of antimicrobial chemotherapy emphasized four main stages, lasting roughly one week each. The first week was characterized by rising fever, the second by rose spots, abdominal pain and splenomegaly, and the third by the abdominal complications of haemorrhage or perforation followed by recovery in the fourth week (Stuart and Pullen, 1946).

The disease classically begins with an intermittent fever pattern which becomes more sustained over the first few days of infection. Most patients report fever or rigors, and headache; a smaller proportion report nausea, vomiting, abdominal cramps and cough. Patients can present paradoxically with either diarrhoea or constipation. Given the diversity of these clinical symptoms and the lack of a strong clinical pattern, patients should be suspected of having typhoid with an appropriate history or ingestion of suspect food.

On examination a fever is usually present and careful recording may demonstrate the stepwise progression characteristic of this syndrome. The abdomen may be tender and approximately half of patients will have a palpable liver and/or spleen. There is a relative bradycardia. Careful inspection of the skin may reveal the presence of rose spots which characteristically begin around the umbilicus, but this sign is difficult to elucidate in a patient with dark skin. Signs in the chest or meningismus may suggest an alternative diagnosis, emphasizing the fact that clinical diagnosis of typhoid may be difficult. Paratyphoid fever shares many of these clinical features.

In countries where schistosomiasis is endemic, retained eggs may be a source for recurrent typhoid infection as it is thought that *S. typhi* binds to the egg surface and later multiplies to cause a relapse.

Differential diagnosis

Many infections may mimic typhoid and it is important to exclude malaria in those with an appropriate travel history. A detailed travel history should be taken to generate a full differential diagnosis, which might include the conditions listed in Table 12c.2.

Complications

The case fatality rate with antimicrobial chemotherapy is less than 5% but is higher in children under the age of one year and older adults (Butler *et al.*, 1991). In young children seizures may occur as a result of fever, hypoglycaemia or electrolyte

TABLE 12c.2   DIFFERENTIAL DIAGNOSIS OF TYPHOID

Malaria
Yersinia enterocolitica, Y. pseudotuberculosis infection
Campylobacter infections
Amoebiasis
Brucellosis
Tuberculosis
Plague
Intestinal anthrax
Melioidosis
Oroya fever
Rat-bite fever
Leptospirosis
Relapsing fever
Rickettsial infections

imbalance. The most important complications are intestinal perforation or haemorrhage. The pathophysiological background to these complications has already been described. Intestinal perforation results in release of colonic bacteria into the peritoneum with consequent peritonitis. Haemorrhage results from severe ulceration of Peyer's patches. In the period before antimicrobial therapy the mortality of intestinal perforation was approximately 90%. The appearance of chloramphenicol reduced this to around 60%. With modern intensive care facilities and surgery the mortality rate is much lower (Bitar and Tarpley, 1985). Even in developing countries when optimal facilities are not available the mortality associated with intestinal perforation treated medically and surgically is approximately 25% (Butler *et al.*, 1985, 1991).

Typhoid may be complicated by acute pneumonia causing diagnostic confusion. Meningitis, cholecystitis and hepatitis are rare complications but should be considered when the appropriate clinical features are present. Like other salmonella infections osteomyelitis or other localized infection may develop.

LABORATORY DIAGNOSIS

Specimens

A multiplicity of specimens are submitted for the isolation of *Salmonella*, including specimens of food and sewage, in addition to specimens from patients. Salmonellosis is most conveniently diagnosed by culture of diarrhoeal stool. Three stools should be submitted for culture to maximize the clinical yield. When patients are febrile or enteric fever is suspected, blood culture should be performed (see below).

In enteric fever culture of the stool may be negative in up to half of patients during the first week of infection, but is more likely to be positive from the second week of illness. A positive isolate of *S. typhi* from stool alone is not diagnostic in the absence of characteristic clinical features, as up to 10% of patients become chronic carriers after acute infection. A definitive diagnosis is made by culture of enteric fever organisms from a sterile site. Blood culture is positive in up to 75% in patients but a higher yield is obtained by culturing bone marrow, with the added advantage that a positive culture can usually be obtained even when the patient has commenced antimicrobial therapy. *Salmonella typhi* can be isolated from the urine, especially after the second week of illness. Chronic excretion of this organism in the urine can cause diagnostic confusion in a patient being investigated for urinary tract infection. The organism can also be isolated from jejunal juice obtained from a duodenal string test (Hoffman *et al.*, 1984). Positive cultures can also be obtained from rose spots, although in practice it is rarely necessary to perform this technique. Clot culture has a venerable place in the mythology of microbiology, enabling a bacterial culture and serological test to be performed on a single sample. It should not now be performed, as it has clearly been shown that routine clot culture is not cost effective if a sensitive blood culture method is used (Duthie and French, 1990).

The diagnosis of *Salmonella* spp. can be conveniently divided into four phases: initial isolation, screening identification, definitive identification, and typing.

Initial Isolation

The problem with isolating *Salmonella* spp. from stools is in ensuring adequate sensitivity and selection. Salmonellae will grow on strongly inhibitory media but *Shigella* spp., which are often sought at the same time, are more readily inhibited. Thus a compromise must be made. In order to maximize diagnostic yield a fluid enrichment medium such as selenite F is usually inoculated in parallel with the plates, allowing these to be subcultured if the plates show no suspicious colonies. Selenite F is inhibitory to enterococci and *Escherichia coli* due to the presence of sodium selenite. Salmonellae are able to grow continuously in this medium, and although the other species will slowly begin to multiply useful selective enrichment does occur. Care must be taken with the quality control of this medium as the degree of inhibition can vary widely and may reduce the diagnostic yield. The inhibition is also most pronounced at low oxygen tension so the medium should be poured into universal bottles to a depth greater than 5 cm (Gillespie, 1994).

Deoxycholate citrate agar (DCA) is highly selective but may inhibit some shigellae. The growth of coliforms and Gram-positive organisms is strongly inhibited due to sodium citrate and sodium deoxycholate in the medium. Lactose and an indicator system are included and H_2S-producing organisms will reduce the ferric ammonium citrate in the medium to produce a black centre to the colonies. Typically salmonellae produce pale colonies with a black centre, but this appearance can be mimicked by *Proteus* spp. and some *Citrobacter* organisms. Xylose lysine deoxycholate agar (XLD) is a popular medium and as it is less inhibitory than DCA and is often used in parallel to optimize the yield of shigellae. The medium contains three sugars – xylose, lactose and sucrose – together with lysine. The colour changes which occur in the colonies depend on the biochemical reactions of the organisms. Organisms which ferment two or more of the sugars will produce bright yellow colonies. Those which do not ferment the sugars or decarboxylate the lysine will appear as colourless colonies. Organisms which ferment none or one of the sugars and decarboxylate lysine will appear as red colonies. Since, like DCA, this medium also contains ferric ammonium citrate a black centre will be found on those colonies which produce H_2S.

Wilson and Blair medium is a more reliable modification of the original bismuth sulphite agar. It is highly inhibitory to other species and is particularly useful for the isolation of *S. typhi* from heavily contaminated specimens. Selection depends on the presence of brilliant green, sodium sulphite and bismuth ammonium citrate. *Salmonella typhi* has a characteristic silvery sheen with an adjacent brown-black zone in the agar.

Screening Identification

A large number of suspect colonies must be examined to maximize the diagnostic yield. To limit the number of full biochemical tests which must be performed, a screening test is used to exclude organisms such as *Citrobacter* and *Proteus*. Several techniques are used, including short sugar series, the Kligler iron medium and Kohn's tubes. Commercial screening tests such as the API Z are also available. Kligler's is the most popular of the composite media; it contains sucrose and an excess of lactose, ferric ammonium citrate and a suitable indicator. Organisms which ferment glucose but not lactose are inoculated: there is an initial acid production which turns the medium yellow, but under the aerobic conditions of the slope this reverts to alkaline. When lactose is also fermented there is sufficient acid, so that the medium does not revert. The medium is blackened by H_2S-producing organisms and gas produced by sugar fermentation disrupts the medium. This can be used along with indole and urease tests, and together the results are used to select those organisms which should be definitively identified. The growth on the slope may be used for serological testing. Alternatively commercial tests use the substrate for several biochemical reactions which when inoculated with a heavy suspension of organism change colour rapidly, due to the action of pre-formed enzymes.

Definitive Identification

The definitive identification of *Salmonella* spp. depends on obtaining biochemical and serological confirmation of the diagnosis. The techniques employed for biochemical identifications are similar to those already described (see page 367). Serological identification depends on determining which lipopolysaccharide 'O' (sOmatic) and flagellar 'H' antigens are present. These are usually identified using a bank of polyclonal and specific antisera by simple bacterial agglutination. 'Species' identification is then made by reference to the Kauffmann–White scheme (Ewing, 1986). Negative 'O' agglutination may be found and this may be due to the presence of an unusual or new serotype. Negative agglutination may also occur due to the presence of a capsular antigen (e.g. Vi) and this can be overcome by heating the culture for 1 hour at 100 °C. The flagellar antigens are diphasic in many serotypes. Phase 1 antigens are specific whereas phase 2 antigens may share antigens with other serotypes. When salmonellae are found to have organisms in the non-specific phase, variation can be induced by Craigie tube or Jameson filter methods (see Gillespie, 1994).

Typing

For many diagnostic purposes and control of infection serotyping is sufficient. For adequate surveillance of food-borne infections and outbreaks in hospitals and institutions more sophisticated typing methods must be employed. Phage typing systems have been developed for the organisms most commonly implicated in food-borne outbreaks. Molecular methods such as ribotyping, pulse field gel electrophoresis, restriction fragment length polymorphism (RFLP) and IS200 typing have been used to subdivide serotypes of *Salmonella* such as *S. enteritidis* (Olsen *et al.*, 1994). RAPD has recently been applied successfully to this last serotype (Fadl *et al.*, 1995).

Laboratory Diagnosis of Typhoid

Widal test

The Widal test uses O and H antigens from *S. typhi* and *S. paratyphi* in a simple bacterial agglutination test to aid the diagnosis of enteric fever. Although simple to perform the test is difficult to interpret, requiring a detailed knowledge of the patient's medical, travel and vaccination history. Acute and convalescent serum should be obtained and a positive diagnosis made on the basis of a four-fold rise or fall in *S. typhi* 'O' and 'H' antibodies. In patients with previous exposure to typhoid or vaccination 'H' antibodies may be high due to previous infection or vaccination. The 'O' antibody concentrations fall about six months after previous infection or vaccination. Cross-reacting antibodies produced by exposure to other serotypes may be a problem but this is usually identified by including a non-specific salmonella antigen preparation in the test battery. If paired sera are not available a single serum may be valuable if it yields an antibody concentration significantly in excess of the community norm for the patient test. Thus, a patient from an industrialized country with a titre of 180 was likely to have acute infection whereas this figure would be equivocal for a patient likely to have previous exposure. Methods which detect IgM antibodies to *S. typhi* lipopolysaccharide (LPS) have been evaluated and are superior to the Widal test; however, these are not widely available as a routine.

Antigen detection

The 'O', 'H' and Vi antigens may be detected in blood and urine of patients with typhoid. Co-agglutination, counterimmunoelectroimmunophoresis and ELISA techniques for their detection have been described (Shetty *et al.*, 1985; Barrett *et al.*, 1982). Sensitivity of over 90% have been reported and, although valuable, these techniques cannot replace culture with the increasingly unpredictable susceptibility pattern of enteric fever organisms.

TREATMENT

Salmonella spp. are susceptible to a range of antimicrobial agents, including chloramphenicol, 4-fluoroquinolones ampicillin, trimethoprim, aminoglycosides and third-generation cephalosporins. Salmonellosis rarely requires systemic antimicrobials unless infection is complicated by bacteraemia or localized infection such as

osteomyelitis. Traditionally chloramphenicol is the first-line agent for the treatment of typhoid but clinical trials indicate ampicillin, co-trimoxazole, third-generation cephalosporins and trimethoprim are effective (Girgiz *et al.*, 1995). More recently 4-fluoroquinolones, including ciprofloxacin and ofloxacin, have been introduced for the treatment of typhoid and have proved to be very effective and are now probably the first choice agent for the treatment of typhoid and bacteraemic salmonellosis. Short courses of 15 mg/kg ofloxacin for three days are effective in the treatment of multiple drug-resistant infection (Nguyen *et al.*, 1995).

Multiple drug-resistant *S. typhi* was first described in Mexico in the 1960s, probably arising from uncontrolled antibiotic use. It is now commonplace in *S. typhi*, and non-typhoid *Salmonella* in the Indian subcontinent, Latin America, Africa and the countries of the Far East (Rasaily *et al.*, 1994; Coovadia *et al.*, 1992; Bhutta *et al.*, 1991).

Treatment of Chronic Carriers

Chronic carriage is common in patients recovering from typhoid who have not been treated with antibiotics. Chloramphenicol therapy reduces chronic carriage rates to less than 10%. Chronic carriage rates after 4-fluorquinolone therapy are thought to be less than 5%. In some circumstances eradication of chronic carriage might be necessary. Before embarking on this course the real benefits to the patient in the context of the risk posed to pubic health should be carefully considered. Thus, treatment of a single asymptomatic person living alone might not be necessary but a food handler with no other means of employment would require it. Chronic carriage may be eradicated by further courses of specific antimicrobial therapy and clinicians vary widely in the regimens which are recommended.

PREVENTION AND CONTROL

Vaccination

In 1896 Almoth Wright described the first use of a typhoid vaccine given to two officers in the Indian

Medical Service. Initial attempts at large-scale vaccination of soldiers in India and in the Boer War led to controversy about its efficacy, which continued over the next 50 years. It was not until the 1960s that controlled field trials were performed (Woodward, 1980). These studies were with heat- or phenol-killed organisms and the most successful demonstrated protection of 65–88% for up to seven years.

The first effective oral typhoid vaccine was made by attenuating a virulent strain of *S. typhi* Ty2, yielding the strain Ty21A after radiation. It has been shown to be effective in a number of field trials and produces approximately 70% protection, lasting for up to seven years (Levine *et al.*, 1987). The genome has multiple mutations and the organism was originally thought to have been attenuated because of a specific mutation in the galE enzyme essential for production of the 'O' polysaccharide. Volunteer studies with another *S. typhi* strain with a single galE mutation was not attenuated and caused disease, suggesting that the mechanism of attenuation is elsewhere.

An alternative vaccine approach is to use purified Vi antigen. This idea had been proposed many years ago but unpromising results from early field trials discouraged its use (Woodward, 1980). A more modern preparation does show effective protection and has entered clinical use as a single-dose vaccination. Like Ty21A approximately 70% protection is afforded for up to seven years (Acharya *et al.*, 1987). It has the advantage that it is inexpensive to produce by a semisynthetic procedure using pectin from citrus fruit.

The most modern approach is to use strains of *Salmonella* with defined mutations in metabolic pathways. These strains arose out of a need to produce attenuated organisms for teaching purposes. It was only later that their potential as vaccine candidates was recognized (Hoiseth and Stocker, 1981). Work has continued in developing auxotrophic mutants, harbouring defined mutations in genes coding for enzymes in the prechorismate biosynthetic pathway (*aro* mutants). These strains are unable to scavenge essential aromatic metabolites such as *para*-aminobenzoic acid. As these substances are not available in mammalian tissues the organism is attenuated. As attenuation comes though metabolic handicap these mutants should also be attenuated in immunocompromised populations. These are now promising vaccine candidates for typhoid but can also be manipulated to carry foreign genes, opening the prospect for oral vaccination against a wide range of diseases (Chatfield *et al.*, 1992, 1995). The best-characterized strains are CVD906 and CVD908, which are mutants of Ty2 and ISP 1820 respectively in which *aroC* and *aroD* mutations have been induced. In a study CVD906 induced symptoms in some volunteers but CVD908 did not, nor was it isolated from the blood. At a dose of 5×10^7 it induced seroconversion to the LPS of *S. typhi* in 83% of volunteers. In addition IgA to flagellin was detected in 100% of the subjects (Tacket *et al.*, 1992). Further studies are now under way with this candidate.

Many other attenuation strategies are under investigation. These include mutations in adenylate cyclase *cya* and cAMP receptor *crp*; these affect the expression of genes involved in carbohydrate and amino acid metabolism. Two component regulatory systems, the *ompB* operon and *phoP/phoQ* system, have been investigated.

Prevention of Salmonellosis in the Food Industry

Central to the prevention of transmission of salmonellosis via food is the cooperation of farmers, veterinarians, abattoir workers and agriculture ministries. Similarly good practice in food preparation facilities is necessary to minimize the risks of transmission. Coupled with these measures all outbreaks should be investigated using epidemiological techniques both as a local and national surveillance programme. The final defence against salmonellosis must be the consumer both in preparation of food at home and in the exercise of choice in purchase of commercially prepared food.

Prevention of Salmonellosis in the Hospital Environment

Salmonellosis can be a particular problem in hospitals and similar institution because of the presence of elderly or immunocompromised patients. Common source outbreaks require urgent investigation of the patients to determine the presence of a pathogen and to provide specimens for typing and also the food which should be investigated to indicate the source and breakdown in the hygienic arrangements.

As salmonellosis is transmitted by the faecal−oral route it can be readily contained using source isolation in a single room with enteric precautions.

REFERENCES

Abe, A., Matsui, H., Danbara, H., Tanaka, K., Takahashi, H. and Kawahara, K. (1994) Regulation of *spvR* gene expression of *Salmonella* virulence plasmid pKDSC50 in *Salmonella choleraesuis*. *Molecular Microbiology*, **12**, 779−787.

Acharya, I.L., Lowe, C.U., Thapa, R. *et al.* (1987) Prevention of typhoid fever in Nepal with the Vi capsular polysaccharide of *Salmonella typhi*. *New England Journal of Medicine*, **317**, 1101−1104.

Altmeyer, R.M., McKern, J.K., Bossio, J.C., Rosenshine, I., Finlay, B.B. and Galan, J.A. (1993) Cloning and molecular characterization of a gene involved in *Salmonella* adherence and invasion of cultured epithelial cells. *Molecular Microbiology*, **7**, 89−98.

Angulo, F.J. and Swerdlow, D.L. (1995) Bacterial enteric infections in persons infected with human immunodeficiency virus. *Clinical Infectious Diseases*, **21** (Suppl. 1), S84−93.

Barrett, T.J., Snyder, J.D., Blake, P.A. and Feeley, J.C. (1982) Enzyme-linked immunosorbent assay for detection of *Salmonella typhi* Vi antigen in urine from typhoid patients. *Journal of Clinical Microbiology*, **15**, 235−237.

Barrow, G.I. and Feltham, R.K.A. (1992) *Cowan and Steel's Manual for the Identification of Medical Bacteria*, 3rd edn. Cambridge University Press, Cambridge, UK.

Beecham, H.J., III, Cohen, M.L. and Parkin, W.E. (1979) *Salmonella typhimurium* transmission by fibre-optic upper gastointestinal endoscopy. *Journal of the American Medical Association*, **241**, 1013−1015.

Behlau, I. and Miller, S.I. (1993) A *PhoP*-repressed gene promotes *Salmonella typhimurium* invasion of epithelial cells. *Journal of Bacteriology*, **175**, 4474−4484.

Beltran, P., Musser, J.M., Helmuth, R. *et al.* (1988) Toward a population genetic analysis of *Salmonella*: genetic diversity and relationships among strains of serotypes of *S. cholera-suis*, *S. derby*, *S. dublin*, *S. enteritidis*, *S. heidelberg*, *S. infantis*, *S. newport* and *S. typhimurium*. *Proceedings of the National Academy of Sciences of the USA*, **85**, 7752−7757.

Bhutta, Z.A., Naqvi, S.H., Razzaq, R.A. and Farooqui, B.J. (1991) Multidrug resistant typhoid in children: presentation and clinical features. *Reviews of Infectious Diseases*, **13**, 832−836.

Bitar, R. and Tarpley, J. (1985) Intestinal perforation in typhoid fever: a historical and state of the art review. *Reviews of Infectious Diseases*, **7**, 257−271.

Blaser, M.J. and Newman, L.S. (1982) A review of human salmonellosis: I. Infective dose. *Reviews of Infectious Diseases*, **4**, 1096−1106.

Butler, T., Knight, J., Nath, S.K, Speelman, P., Roy, S.K. and Azad, M.A.K. (1985) Typhoid fever complicated by intestinal perforation: a persisting fatal disease requiring surgical management. *Reviews of Infectious Diseases*, **7**, 244−256.

Butler, T., Islam, A., Kabir, I. and Jones, P.K. (1991) Patterns of morbidity and mortality in typhoid fever dependent on age and gender: review of 552 hospitalized patients with diarrhoea. *Reviews of Infectious Diseases*, **13**, 85−90.

Chatfield, S., Li, J.L., Sydenham, M., Douce, G. and Dougan, G. (1992) *Salmonella* genetics and vaccine development. In *Molecular Biology of Bacterial Infection: Current Status and Future Perspectives* (eds Hormaeche, Penn and Smythe), pp. 299−312. Society for General Microbiology Symposium, Cambridge University Press, Cambridge, UK.

Chatfield, S.N., Roberts, M., Dougan, G., Hormaeche, C. and Khan, C.M.A. (1995) The development of oral vaccine against parasitic diseases using live attenuated *Salmonella*. *Parasitology*, **110**, S17−S24.

Coovadia, Y.M., Gathiram, V., Bhamjee, A. *et al.* (1992) An outbreak of multi-drug resistant *Salmonella typhi* in South Africa. *Quarterly Journal of Medicine*, **82**, 91−100.

Duguid, J.P. and North, R.A.E. (1991) Eggs and salmonella food poisoning: an evaluation. *Journal of Medical Microbiology*, **34**, 65−72.

Duthie, R. and French, G.L. (1990) Comparison of methods for the diagnosis of typhoid fever. *Journal of Clinical Pathology*, **43**, 863−865.

Ewing, W.H. (1986) *Edward's and Ewing Identification of Enterobacteriaceae*, 4th edn. Elsevier Science, New York.

Fadl, A.A., Nguyen, V.A. and Khan, M.I. (1995) Analysis of *Salmonella enteritidis* isolates by arbitrarily primed PCR. *Journal of Clinical Microbiology*, **33**, 987−989.

Gerichter, C.B. (1960) The dissemination of *Salmonella typhi*, *S. paratyphi A* and *S. paratyphi B* through the organs of the white mouse by oral infection. *Journal of Hygiene (Camb.)*, **58**, 307−319.

Gilks, C.F., Brindle, R.J., Otieno, L.S. *et al.* (1990) Life threatening bacteraemia in HIV-1 seropositive adults admitted to hospital in Nairobi, Kenya. *Lancet*, **336**, 545–549.

Gillespie, S.H. (1994) Examination of faeces for bacterial pathogens. In *Medical Microbiology Illustrated*, Ch. 17, pp. 192–210. Butterworth–Heinemann, Oxford.

Girgis, N.L., Sultan, Y., Hammad, O. and Farid, Z. (1995) Comparison of the efficacy, safety and cost of cefixime, ceftriaxone, and aztreonam in the treatment of multi-drug resistant *Salmonella typhi* septicemia in children. *Pediatric Infectious Disease Journal*, **14**, 603–605.

Greismann, S.E., Hornick, R.B. and Woodward, T.E. (1964) The role of endotoxin during typhoid fever and tularaemia in man III. Hyper-reactivity to endotoxin during infection. *Journal of Clinical Investigation*, **48**, 613–629.

Gruenewald, R., Blum, S. and Chan, J. (1994) Relationship between human immunodeficiency virus infection and salmonellosis in 20 to 59-year old residents of New York City. *Clinical Infectious Diseases*, **18**, 358–363.

Guiney, D.G., Libby, S., Fang, F.C., Krause, M. and Fiere, J. (1995) Growth phase regulation of plasmid virulence genes in *Salmonella*. *Trends in Microbiology*, **3**, 275–279.

Hedberg, C.W., MacDonald, K.L. and Osterholm, M.T. (1994) Changing epidemiology of food-borne disease: a Minnesota perspective. *Clinical Infectious Diseases*, **18**, 671–682.

Heffernan, E.J., Fierer, J., Chikami, G. and Guiney, D. (1985) Natural history of oral *Salmonella dublin* infection in BALB/c mice: effect of an 80 kilobase plasmid on virulence. *Journal of Infectious Diseases*, **155**, 1254–1259.

Hoffman, S.L., Punjabi, N.H., Rockill, R.C., Sutomo, A., Rivai, A.R. and Pulunsih, S.P. (1984) Duodenal string-capsule culture compared with bone marrow, blood and rectal swab culture for the diagnosis of typhoid and paratyphoid fever. *Journal of Infectious Diseases*, **149**, 157–161.

Hoiseth, S.K. and Stocker, B.A.D. (1981) Aromatic-dependent *Salmonella typhimurium* are non-virulent and effective as live vaccines. *Nature*, **291**, 238–240.

Hornick, R.B., Griesman, S.E., Woodward, T.E., Du Pont, H.L., Dawkins, A.T. and Snyder, M.J. (1970) Typhoid fever: pathogenesis and immune control. *New England Journal of Medicine*, **283**, 686–691.

Ivanoff, B., Levine, M.M. and Lambert, P.H. (1994) Vaccination against typhoid fever: present status. *Bulletin of the World Health Organization*, **71**, 957–971.

Jones, G.W., Rabert, D.K., Svinarich, D.M. and Whitfield, H.J. (1982) Association of adhesive, invasive and virulent phenotypes of *Salmonella typhimurium* with autonomous 60-megadalton plasmid. *Infection and Immunity*, **38**, 476–486.

Levine, M.M., Ferreccio, C., Black, R.E., Chilean Typhoid Committee and Germanier, R. (1987) Large-scale field trail of Ty21A live oral typhoid vaccine in enteric coated capsule formulation. *Lancet*, **i**, 1049–1052.

MacKenzie, C.R. and Livingstone, D.J. (1968) Salmonellae in fish and food. *South African Medical Journal*, **42**, 99–1003.

Mallory, F.B. (1898) A histological study of typhoid fever. *Journal of Experimental Medicine*, **3**, 611–638.

Nguyen, M.D., Pham, T.T., Walsh, A.I. *et al.* (1995) Short course of ofloxacin for treatment of multidrug resistant typhoid *Clinical Infectious Diseases*, **20**, 917–923.

Olsen, J.E., Stor, M.N., Threlfall, E.J. and Brown, D.J. (1994) Clonal lines of *Salmonella enterica* serotype *enteritidis* by IS200, ribo-, pulsed-field gel electrophoresis and RFLP typing. *Journal of Medical Microbiology*, **40**, 15–22.

Raily, R., Dutta, P., Saha, M.R., Lahiri, M. and Pal, S.C. (1994) Multi-drug resistant typhoid fever in hospitalized children: clinical bacteriological and epidemiological profiles. *European Journal of Epidemiology*, **10**, 41–46.

Reeve, M.W., Evins, G.M., Heiba, A.A., Plikaytis, B.D. and Farmer, J.J. III (1989) Clonal nature of *Salmonella typhi* and its genetic relatedness to other salmonellae as shown by multi-locus enzyme electrophoresis and proposal of *Salmonella bongori* comb nov. *Journal of Clinical Microbiology*, **27**, 313–320.

Selander, R.K. and Smith, N.H. (1990) Molecular population genetics of *Salmonella*. *Reviews in Medical Microbiology*, **1**, 219–228.

Selander, R.K., Caugant, D.A., Ochman, H., Musser, J.M., Gilmore, M.N. and Whittam, T.S. (1986) Methods of multi-locus electrophoresis for bacterial population genetics and systematics. *Applied Environmental Microbiology*, **51**, 873–884.

Shetty, N.P., Srinivasa, H. and Bhat, P. (1985) Coagglutination and counter immunoelectrophoresis in the rapid diagnosis of typhoid fever. *American Journal of Clinical Pathology*, **84**, 80–84.

Stuart, B.M. and Pullen, R.L. (1946) Typhoid: clinical analysis of three hundred and sixty cases. *Archives of Internal Medicine*, **78**, 629–661.

Tacket, C.O., Hone, D.M., Losonsky, G.A., Guers, L., Edelman, R. and Levine, M.M. (1992) Clinical acceptibility and immunogenicity of CVD908 *Salmonella typhi* vaccine stain. *Vaccine*, **10**, 443–446.

Valone, S.E., Chikami, G.K. and Miller, V.L. (1993) Stress induction of the virulence proteins (SpvS, -B, -C) from native plasmid pSDL2 of *Salmonella dublin*. *Infection and Immunity*, **61**, 705–713.

Vugia, D.J., Kiehlbauch, J.A., Yeboue, K. *et al.* (1993) Pathogens and predictors of fatal septicaemia in septicaemia associated with human immuno-deficiency virus. *Journal of Infectious Diseases*, **168**, 564–570.

Woodward, W.E. (1980) Volunteer studies of typhoid fever and vaccines. *Transactions of the Royal Society of Tropical Medicine and Hygiene*, **74**, 553–556.

12d

KLEBSIELLA, CITROBACTER, ENTEROBACTER AND SERRATIA

C.A. Hart

INTRODUCTION

These four genera are all members of the family Enterobacteriaceae but exhibit different degrees of relatedness to each other and to other members of the family. For example, *Serratia* spp. are 25% related to the other three genera, and *Enterobacter* spp. (except *E. aerogenes*) are 45% related to *Klebsiella*. Interestingly *Citrobacter freundii* and *C. diversus* are only 50% related (Brenner, 1984). The phenotypic characteristics of the genera are shown in Table 12d.1. They are all oxidase-negative (catalase-positive) Gram-negative rods which are facultative anaerobes.

All four genera are associated with nosocomial infections and infection in the immunocompromised host. However, *Klebsiella* spp. are much more frequently associated with infection, being responsible for 3% of community-acquired and 9% of hospital-acquired cases of septicaemia in one hospital (Eykyn *et al.*, 1990). The other three genera were together responsible for 0.9% of community-acquired and 4% of nosocomial episodes of septicaemia.

KLEBSIELLA SPECIES

The genus *Klebsiella* is named after the German bacteriologist Edwin Klebs (1834–1913). In the UK literature several other species have been differentiated on biochemical properties (Table 12d.2), including *K. pneumoniae* (Friedlander's bacillus), *K. aerogenes*, *K. ozaenae* and *K. rhinoscleromatis*. Based on DNA homology studies these should all be included in the species *K. pneumoniae*. However, to maintain continuity with previous literature the old names are used to designate subspecies. For example, *K. aerogenes* is *K. pneumoniae* subsp. *aerogenes* and Friedlander's bacillus is *K. pneumoniae* subsp. *pneumoniae*. Other species in the genus are *K. oxytoca*, *K. terrigena* and *K. planticola* (Orskov, 1984). The latter two are soil and plant bacteria not associated with human disease and will not be discussed further.

DESCRIPTION OF THE ORGANISM

Klebsiella spp. are straight bacilli, $0.3–1 \ \mu m \times 0.6–6 \ \mu m$, non-motile, and most isolates possess a thick polysaccharide capsule and fimbriae. Their DNA mol. % G + C is 53–58.

They are facultative anaerobes that have no particular growth factor requirement. They hydrolyse sugars fermentatively, mostly with release of carbon dioxide rather than hydrogen. *Klebsiella* spp. usually hydrolyse urea and most can utilize

Principles and Practice of Clinical Bacteriology. Edited by A.M. Emmerson, P.M. Hawkey and S.H. Gillespie
© 1997 John Wiley & Sons Ltd

TABLE 12d.1   BIOCHEMICAL CHARACTERISTICS OF THE GENERA OF *KLEBSIELLA, CITROBACTER, ENTEROBACTER* AND *SERRATIA*

	Klebsiella spp.	*Citrobacter* spp.	*Enterobacter* spp.	*Serratia* spp.
Motile	−	+	+	+
Indole	V (*K. oxytoca*)	+	−	−
Methyl red	V	+	−	V
Voges–Proskauer	V	−	+	+
H₂S production	−	+	−	−
Arginine decarboxylase	−	+	V	−
Lysine decarboxylase	+	−	V	+
Ornithine decarboxylase	−	V	+	V
Gelatinase	−	−	+	+
Urease	+	V	V	+
Acid from:				
Adonitol	+	V	V	V
Inositol	+	−	V	+

+ ≥90% strains positive
V 10–90% strains positive
− ≤ 10% strains positive

TABLE 12d.2   BIOCHEMICAL CHARACTERISTICS OF *KLEBSIELLA* SPP.

	Klebsiella pneumoniae			*Klebsiella oxytoca*	*Klebsiella terrigena*	*Klebsiella planticola*
	subsp. pneumoniae	subsp. aerogenes	subsp. rhinoscleromatis			
Indole production	−	−	−	+	−	+ (60%)
Pectate degradation	−	−	−	+	−	−
β-Galactosidase	+	+	−	+	+	+
Growth at 10 °C	−	−	−	+	+	+
Gentisate utilization	−	−	−	+	+	−
Methyl red	+	−	+	−	+	V
Voges–Proskauer	+	−	−	+	+	+
Urease	+	+	−	+	+	+
Gas from glucose	+	+	−	+	+	+
Growth in KCN	−	+	+	+	+	+
Grow on Simmon's citrate	+	+	−	+	+	+
Acid from dulcitol	+	V	−	V	−	−
Acid from lactose	+	+	−	+	+	+
Lysine decarboxylase	+	+	−	+	+	+
Histamine assimilation	−	−	−	−	+	+
Melezitose assimilation	−	−	−	+ (75%)	+	−

+ ≥90% strains positive
V 10–50% strains positive
− ≤ 10% strains positive

citrate and glucose as sole carbon sources *Klebsiella oxytoca* differs from *K. pneumoniae* in being indole positive and able to liquefy gelatin, degrade pectate and utilize gentisate and *m*-hydroxybenzoate. All are lactose fermenters and those that are the most efficient carry *lac* genes on both chromosome and plasmid.

Capsule

A key characteristic of *Klebsiella* spp. is the production of mucoid colonies when grown on solid media. This is enhanced when the media contain an excess of carbohydrate. The mucoid character is due to the thick polysaccharide capsule

(Figure 12d.1) which absorbs a large amount of water. The capsular material may also diffuse freely into the surrounding medium as extracapsular polysaccharide. There are at least 77 different capsular (K) serotypes and subtypes with similar antigenicity, but different polysaccharide backbones have been described (Allen *et al.*, 1987b). Despite this antigenic diversity the range of monosaccharide units is limited to L-fucose, L-rhamnose, D-mannose, D-glucose, D-galactose, D-glucuronic acid or D-galacturonic acid, some with *O*-acetyl and pyruvate ketal groups (Sutherland, 1985). *Klebsiella pneumoniae* subsp. *pneumoniae* is predominantly serotype 3, as is *K. pneumoniae* subsp. *rhinoscleromatis*. *Klebsiella pneumoniae* subsp. *ozaenae* encompasses serogroups 3, 4, 5 and 6, but each of the serogroups has been associated with *K. pneumoniae* subsp. *aerogenes*.

The genetic control of *Klebsiella* capsular synthesis is complex. A 29 kb chromosomal fragment from *K. pneumoniae* K2 Chedid was able to induce K2 capsular biosynthesis in capsuleless mutants of *K. pneumoniae*, but an extra plasmid encoded *rmp*A gene was required for its expression in *Escherichia coli* (Aravawa *et al.*, 1991). Two genes *rcs*A (regulation of capsule synthesis) and *rcs*B have been cloned from the chromosome of *K. pneumoniae* subsp. *aerogenes* K21 that cause expression of a mucoid character in *E. coli*. This, however, is due to activation of synthesis of colanic acid which is antigenically similar to the K21 capsular polysaccharide (Allen *et al.*, 1987a). Capsular polysaccharide biosynthesis is greater under nitrogen than carbon limitation and increased at lower (c. 30 °C) temperatures (Mengistu *et al.*, 1994). The initial biosynthesis takes place in the cytoplasm and utilizes UTP and ATP. The assembled polysaccharide is transported across the inner membrane using an undecaprenyl phosphate (P-C55) carrier (Troy, 1979). How it traverses the periplasmic space and outer membrane and forms the capsule is unclear. Group II capsules of *E. coli* are homopolymers of a single monosaccharide (Jann and Jann, 1990). These are transported across the periplasmic space utilizing so-called traffic

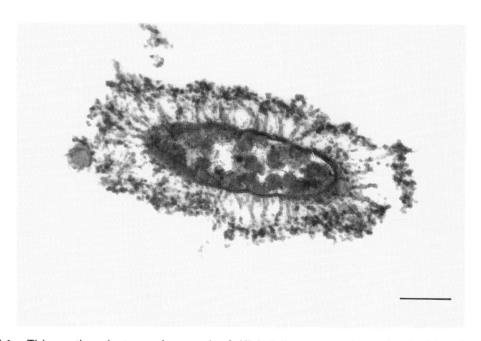

Figure 12d.1. Thin-section electron micrograph of *Klebsiella pneumoniae* stained with ruthenium red to demonstrate the capsule. (bar = 1 μm.)

ATPases or ABC (ATP-binding cassette) transporters (Pavelka *et al.*, 1991; Ames and Joshi, 1990). A further set of polypeptides are required for translocation of these group II *E. coli* capsular polysaccharides across the outer membrane and to tether them in place (Boulnois and Roberts, 1990). Unfortunately the capsules of *Klebsiella* spp. are more closely related to those of group I *E. coli*; for example, the klebsiellar K5 and K54 antigens are structurally identical to *E. coli* K55 and K28 respectively (Altman and Dutton, 1985). The capsular polysaccharides appear to form fibres protruding radially from the bacterial surface (Figure 12d.1). The presence of the capsule imparts a net negative charge to the bacterium and render it highly hydrophilic.

Adhesins

Klebsiella spp. possess both fimbrial and non-fimbrial adhesins (Tarkkanen *et al.*, 1992; Pruzzo *et al.*, 1989). The fimbriae can be of type 1 or type 3 (mannose-resistant haemagglutination), and occasionally P fimbriae.

A mannose-inhibitable non-fimbrial adhesin has been found on unencapsulated *Klebsiella* spp. (Pruzzo *et al.*, 1989), as has a plasmid-encoded non-fimbrial adhesin (29 kDa) which facilitates adhesion of *Klebsiella* to epithelial cells (Darfeuille-Michaud *et al.*, 1992). The situation is reversed for certain *K. pneumoniae* capsular serotypes that have mannose disaccharide units in their polysaccharide (Athamna *et al.*, 1991). Here the disaccharide acts as the receptor (rather than adhesin) for a mannose/*N*-acetylglucosamine-specific lectin on the surface of macrophages.

Lipopolysaccharide

The repertoire of O antigens on *K. pneumoniae* LPS is limited to 8 (O types 1, 3–5, 7–9 and 12), 0:1 being the most common.

Other Toxins

Klebsiella pneumoniae strains carrying genes for, or expressing heat-labile and heat-stable entero-toxins have been described (Betley *et al.*, 1986); their clinical importance is unclear.

Iron Scavenging

Klebsiella pneumoniae is able to scavenge iron from its surrounding medium using either enterochelin (phenolate siderophore), which is more important in pathogenic isolates, or aerobactin (hydroxamate siderophore).

NATURAL HABITAT

Although *Klebsiella* spp. are listed as part of the enteric flora in healthy individuals; if they are present it is only in small numbers ($<10^2$ cfu/g faeces). Premature babies and especially those in neonatal intensive care units (Tullus *et al.*, 1988; Hart, 1993), hospitalized patients even when moderately (Le Frock *et al.*, 1979) or severely ill (Kerver *et al.*, 1987), those with chronic disease and elderly individuals are relatively easily colonized by *Klebsiella* spp. This colonization may also extend to the oropharynx (Mackowiak *et al.*, 1979). Administration of antimicrobials that affect the colonization resistance (Van der Waaij, 1982) of the intestinal tract also predisposes to colonization by *Klebsiella* and other Enterobacteriaceae. In one study it was found that the half-life for carriage of aminoglycoside-resistant *K. pneumoniae*, but not of *K. oxytoca* in elderly patients, was 100 days and some subjects excreted bacteria for over 200 days (Hart and Gibson, 1982). *Klebsiella* spp. can be part of the normal flora of a variety of other animals and are widely distributed in the inanimate environment, usually *K. oxytoca*, *K. planticola* and *K. terrigena* or *K. pneumoniae* from human or animal excreta.

PATHOGENICITY

Apart from rhinoscleroma and ozaena, infections with *K. pneumoniae* are nosocomial and opportunist. Rhinoscleroma is a chronic granulomatous infection of the upper airways although contiguous skin and the trachea may also be affected. Lesions are characterized by a submucosal infiltrate of plasma cells and histiocytes called Mickulicz cells. These are foamy macrophages with vacuoles containing *K. pneumoniae* subsp. *rhinoscleromatis*. The infective dose, portal of entry and incubation period remain unknown. It is not clear how a bacterium with a hydrophilic capsule resistant to phagocytosis enters macrophages and survives.

The pathogenesis and pathogenic determinants of nosocomial and opportunistic *K. pneumoniae* infections are shown in Figure 12d.2. Most of our information on transmission of *K. pneumoniae* comes from studies of outbreaks of nosocomial infection. Reservoirs of *K. pneumoniae* tend to be the intestinal tract of other hospitalized patients (Le Frock *et al.*, 1979; Kerver *et al.*, 1987; Hart and Gibson, 1982), although other sites such as the oropharynx, skin (the nearer the perineum the heavier the colonization) and vagina may be carriage sites (Hart and Gibson, 1982). Although *K. pneumoniae* can be transmitted via surgical instruments, urinary catheters, food (Donowitz *et*

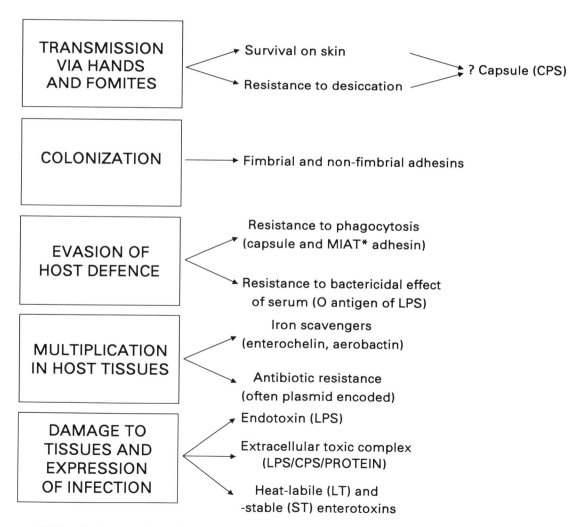

Figure 12d.2. Pathogenesis of nosocomial and opportunistic *K. pneumoniae* infection. MIAT*, mannose-inhibitable adhesin/phage T7 receptor.

al., 1981) and even expressed breast milk (Cooke *et al.*, 1980), hands are by far the most important route (Knittle *et al.*, 1975; Casewell and Phillips, 1977). *Klebsiella* spp. appear to be able to survive on skin better than, for example, *E. coli* or *Citrobacter* spp. (Hart *et al.*, 1981; Casewell and Desai, 1983), perhaps because of the hydrophilic capsule. This has been disputed by others (Fryklund *et al.*, 1995).

In most cases infection is preceded by intestinal colonization which, it is presumed, is mediated by fimbriae. Although there is considerable heterogeneity among the mannose-inhibitable type 1 fimbriae, the receptor binding moiety (29 kDa subunit) is highly conserved (Abraham *et al.*, 1988). These fimbriae appear to be important in attachment to respiratory and urinary tract mucosal cells (Williams and Tomas, 1990). Some *K. pneumoniae* possess plasmid-encoded proteins that mediate autoagglutination and attachment to plastic surfaces (Denoya *et al.*, 1986).

Klebsiella pneumoniae becomes established in other mucosal sites by migration and can enter the blood by translocation. Once in the bloodstream or in tissues it must evade the host's non-specific immune system. There is no doubt that the hydrophilic capsule inhibits phagocytic uptake of bacteria (Denoya *et al.*, 1986). Heavily encapsulated *K. pneumoniae* are more virulent than less encapsulated strains in experimentally infected mice (Williams *et al.*, 1983). Specific antibody can opsonize the bacteria and facilitate phagocytosis but the ability of virulent *K. pneumoniae* to shed capsular material may render this process less efficient. The capsule may also render bacteria resistant to opsonization and killing by the alternative complement cascade (Domenico *et al.*, 1982). The presence of long polysaccharide chains on LPS contributes greatly to resistance to serum killing (Merino *et al.*, 1992), perhaps by sterically hindering binding of the complement membrane attack complex to the outer membrane. Once in tissues the iron scavengers, in particular enterochelin, allow the bacteria to grow even when iron is scarce (Tarkkanen *et al.*, 1992). The presence of antibiotic resistance plasmids is also of assistance in allowing *Klebsiella* to grow in the tissues

of patients receiving antibiotics. The tissue damage by *Klebsiella* is probably due to both release of toxic molecules by the bacteria and the host's response, in particular frustrated activated phagocytes releasing toxic oxygen radicals. The major bacterial determinant is endotoxin released either as LPS alone or in complexes with capsular polysaccharide (Straus, 1987; Williams and Tomas, 1990).

EPIDEMIOLOGY

Klebsiella spp. are important nosocomial pathogens worldwide. In a UK prevalence survey, *Klebsiella* spp. were responsible for 8.3% of urinary tract infection, 4% of wound infections and 3.5% of pneumonias (Meers *et al.*, 1980). In the USA the importance of *K. pneumoniae* as a cause of nosocomial bacteraemia has declined from 9.1% of cases in 1975 to 4.5% in 1985–1989 (Pittet, 1993). In neonatal intensive care units *Klebsiella* spp. appear in the top three or four pathogens in developed (Gladstone *et al.*, 1990) and developing countries (Rajab and De Louvois, 1990). Explosive life-threatening outbreaks of septicaemia due to multidrug-resistant *Klebsiella* spp. occur with monotonous regularity (Morgan *et al.*, 1984; Donowitz *et al.*, 1981; Fryklund *et al.*, 1995). In this setting septicaemia usually follows intestinal colonization with *Klebsiella* spp. which, it is suggested, can result from use of ampicillin rather than cephalosporins in the unit (Tullus and Burman, 1989). Outbreaks of infection are a feature in compromised patients often with multidrug-resistant organisms (Casewell *et al.*, 1977; Curie *et al.*, 1978). *Klebsiella* spp. have been reported to be responsible for 14% of cases of bacteraemia associated with intravascular devices (Eykyn *et al.*, 1990).

Rhinoscleroma is found in Eastern Europe, and occasionally in Italy, Switzerland, Spain and southern France. It is also endemic in Africa, Latin America and parts of the Middle and Far East. It is commoner in women than men and usually presents in early adulthood. It is associated with poor and crowded living conditions with poor sanitation.

Pneumonia due to *K. pneumoniae* subsp. *pneumoniae* is an uncommon occurrence and generally occurs as a community-acquired infection in elderly debilitated males.

Epidemiological Typing Methods

The major typing method for *Klebsiella* spp. is capsular serotyping. Although this was originally done by the Quellung reaction, other techniques such as immunofluorescence (Murcia and Rubin, 1979) or counter-current immunoelectrophoresis (Palfreyman, 1978) are more readily applicable. An analysis of *K. pneumoniae* isolated from blood showed that K2 (8.9% of isolates), K21 (7.8%) and K55 (4.8%) were the commonest serotypes and that 25 serotypes accounted for 70% of the isolates (Cryz *et al.*, 1986). In a UK survey K21 (42% of isolates) and K2 (16.5 %) were the commonest isolates from nosocomial infections (Casewell and Talsania, 1979). Other methods available for typing *Klebsiella* spp. are biotyping (Simoons-Smit *et al.*, 1987), antimicrobial susceptibility patterns, Klebecin typing (Edmondson and Cooke, 1979) and a variety of molecular methods including pulsed-field gel electrophoresis of digested chromosomal DNA (Gouby *et al.*, 1994).

CLINICAL FEATURES

Nosocomial *Klebsiella* infections can occur at almost any site and the clinical features do not differ from those caused by any of the Enterobacteriaceae. *Klebsiella* spp. have also been associated with some para-infective conditions such as ankylosing spondylitis, anterior uveitis and rheumatoid arthritis (Sahly *et al.*, 1994) but their role is unclear.

Rhinoscleroma begins as a painless chronic inflammatory swelling which causes nasal or respiratory tract obstruction. The nasal lesions enlarge locally to produce the so-called Hebra nose, which is grossly distorted and splayed. Local spread and local metastatic foci, often with lymph node involvement, are frequently described. Ozaena is seldom seen nowadays and there are doubts over its status as a disease entity.

DIAGNOSIS

The nosocomial *Klebsiella* spp. are simple to detect by standard cultural techniques and their isolation from normally sterile sites or in significant numbers from sites with a normal flora provides evidence of infection.

The diagnosis of rhinoscleroma depends upon the typical histopathological appearance (Mickulicz cells) which can be made more specific by using anti-capsular antibody (Meyer *et al.*, 1983). The differential diagnosis of rhinoscleroma includes espundia, rhinosporidiosis, leprosy, yaws and malignancy.

ANTIMICROBIAL SUSCEPTIBILITY

Klebsiella spp. seem to have a particular propensity to acquire, build up and maintain antibiotic resistance plasmids (Hart *et al.*, 1981). Most *Klebsiella* are intrinsically resistant to ampicillin but acquisition of plasmid-encoded resistance has resulted in outbreaks of nosocomial infection. In the 1970s and 1980s outbreaks of infection due to gentamicin- and tobramycin- (but not amikacin-) resistant *K. pneumoniae* were reported in increasing numbers (Casewell *et al.*, 1977; Curie *et al.*, 1978; Morgan *et al.*, 1984). With the introduction of second- and third-generation cephalosporins, isolates of *K. pneumoniae* resistant to cefuroxime, ceftazidime and cefotaxime soon emerged. Initially this was chromosomally encoded (Hart and Percival, 1982) but subsequently plasmid-encoded extended-spectrum β-lactamases caused large outbreaks of infection especially in adult intensive care units (Jacoby and Medeiros, 1991; Hibbert-Rogers *et al.*, 1994). In general, these extended-spectrum β-lactamases have arisen by evolution of TEM and SHV genes (Hibbert-Rogers *et al.*, 1994). Resistance to fluoroquinolones can be high; for example, in one French hospital 97% of β-lactamase-resistant *K. pneumoniae* were resistant to ciprofloxacin (Bergogne-Bérézin *et al.*, 1993). It appears that *Klebsiella* spp. do not remain predictably susceptible to a new antibiotic beyond a relatively short 'honeymoon period'.

TREATMENT AND PREVENTION

Because *K. pneumoniae* can be resistant to so many different antimicrobial agents, empirical therapy must be based on knowledge of local susceptibility patterns. Prevention of nosocomial infection requires adherence to infection control policies, and handwashing is an important part of this. Passive immunization with anticapsular antibody or active immunization with capsular polysaccharides has had some effect in treating and preventing *Klebsiella* infection in burns patients (see references in Cryz, 1986).

K. pneumoniae subsp. *rhinoscleromatis* is sensitive *in vitro* to many antibiotics, including streptomycin, cotrimoxazole, gentamicin and tobramycin. However, ciprofloxacin or ofloxacin appear to be the drugs of choice but they must be given for long periods (months). Surgical removal of lesions will also be necessary.

CITROBACTER SPECIES

The genus *Citrobacter* was first named in 1932, but until recently the name did not gain full acceptance (Sakazaki, 1984). Species in the present genus have been previously named *Levinia amalonatica*, *Escherichia freundii*, *Salmonella hormaechii*, *S. ballerup* and the Ballerup/Bethesda group. Currently 11 species are recognized: *C. koseri* (formerly *C. diversus*), *C. freundii*, *C. amalonaticus*, *C. formeri*, *C. youngae*, *C. braakii*, *C. werkmanii*, *C. sedlakii* and unnamed species 9, 10 and 11 (O'Hara *et al.*, 1995).

DESCRIPTION OF THE ORGANISM

Citrobacter are rods (1 μm $\times$ 2–6 μm), usually non-encapsulated, but some *C. freundii* strains produce Vi capsular antigen (Houng *et al.*, 1992). They are motile by means of peritrichous flagella and some possess class 1 fimbriae (Abraham *et al.*, 1988). All are lactose fermenters but some isolates of *C. freundii* are late lactose fermenters. This together with their ability to produce H_2S in the butt of triple sugar or Kligler's iron-agar has led to their being confused with *Salmonella* but *C.*

freundii is indole positive. At least 42 O antigens, one of which cross-reacts with *E. coli* 0157 (Bettelheim *et al.*, 1993) and 90 H-antigens are expressed by the genus. The mol. % G + C of their DNA is 51–52.

NORMAL HABITAT

Citrobacter spp. are found in the intestinal tract of man and other animals and are widely distributed in the environment. *Citrobacter koseri* appears to become established with some ease in the neonatal intestine and even in the mother's or nurse's intestinal flora (Williams *et al.*, 1984; Goering *et al.*, 1992). In contrast, spontaneous loss of intestinal carriage of other *Citrobacter* spp. that were multidrug resistant occurred more readily than that of *Klebsiella* or *E. coli* (Hart and Gibson, 1982).

PATHOGENICITY

The virulence determinants of *Citrobacter* spp. are little understood. It is presumed that they colonize the intestine and other sites using fimbriae. Production of capsule (Vi) and *E. coli* 0157 lipopolysaccharide is more related to confusing microbiologists than causing disease. Some strains of *C. freundii* carry the *eae* (enteropathogenic *E. coli* attaching and effacing) gene and are associated with murine colonic hyperplasia (Frankel *et al.*, 1994). Recently an outbreak of gastroenteritis and haemolytic uraemic syndrome was associated with *C. freundii* producing verotoxin 2 (Tschäpe *et al.*, 1995). Expression of a 32 kDa outer membrane protein was found among isolates of *C. koseri* causing neonatal meningitis (Li *et al.*, 1990).

EPIDEMIOLOGY AND INFECTIONS

Citrobacter spp. are an infrequent cause of bacteraemia; in a UK survey 0.7% of episodes were caused by *C. freundii* and *C. koseri* equally (Eykyn *et al.*, 1990), and it does not appear in the 'top 10' bacteraemic isolates from 1975 to 1989 in the USA (Pittet, 1993). *Citrobacter koseri* does, however, appear to be an important neonatal pathogen

(Williams *et al.*, 1984; Goering *et al.*, 1992). In common with other Enterobacteriaceae, *Citrobacter* spp. can cause meningitis, bacteraemia pneumonia, urinary tract infection and wound infections.

Most infections are sporadic and the reservoir for *Citrobacter* spp. is the intestinal tract. Spread is most likely to be by hands, although *Citrobacter* spp. survive less well on skin than *Klebsiella* or *Enterobacter* spp. (Hart *et al.*, 1981). For epidemiological purposes *Citrobacter* spp. have been differentiated by biotype, O-serotyping, plasmid profiles (Williams *et al.*, 1984; Goering *et al.*, 1992), outer membrane protein profiles (Tschäpe *et al.*, 1995) and analysis of chromosomal DNA (Morris *et al.*, 1986).

DIAGNOSIS

Citrobacter spp. can be easily grown from most infected sites. One of the major pitfalls in the laboratory is distinguishing them from *Salmonella* spp. and *E. coli*.

ANTIMICROBIAL SUSCEPTIBILITY

Antibiotic susceptibilities are not entirely predictable but in one survey all isolates of *C. freundii* and *C. koseri* were sensitive to ciprofloxacin and imipenem and over 50% were sensitive to gentamicin and trimethoprim (Reeves *et al.*, 1993). A particular feature of *Citrobacter* spp. is the carriage of inducible cephalosporinases and the frequency of emergence of de-repressed mutants overproducing such enzymes (Stapleton *et al.*, 1995). These enzymes are chromosomally encoded, not inhibited by clavulanate, able to hydrolyse third-generation cephalosporins and are induced by their substrates. Approximately 10% of hospitalized children were found to be excreting *Citrobacter* spp. expressing these enzymes (Berkowitz and Metchock, 1995).

TREATMENT AND PREVENTION

Antimicrobial chemotherapy will depend upon the local susceptibility pattern. However, treatment with fluorinated quinolones, imipenem or amikacin is likely to be successful depending on the site of infection. Prevention is by appropriate infection control measures (Williams *et al.*, 1984).

ENTEROBACTER SPECIES

Enterobacter cloacae was first described as *Bacterium cloacae* and as *Cloaca cloacae* but renamed *E. cloacae* when the genus was established (Richard, 1984).

Enterobacter spp. are biochemically active and *E. aerogenes* is similar to *K. pneumoniae*. *Enterobacter* spp. differ from *Klebsiella* spp. in being motile and from *Serratia* spp. by being negative for lipase, Tween 80 esterase and DNAase. Currently there are 11 species in the genus: *E. cloacae*, *E. aerogenes*, *E. agglomerans*, *E. gergoviae*, *E. sakazakii*, *E. taylorae*, *E. asburiae*, *E. intermedium*, *E. amnigenus*, *E. dissolvens* and *E. nimipressuralis*. The role of the latter five species in human infection is unclear. *Enterobacter amnigenus* and *E. intermedium* are environmental bacteria that do not grow at 41 °C.

DESCRIPTION OF THE ORGANISM

Enterobacter spp. are 0.6–1.0 μm × 1.2–3.0 μm long, motile by means of peritrichous flagella and possess class 1 fimbriae (Abraham *et al.*, 1988). They ferment glucose with production of acid and gas, and are methyl red negative and Voges–Proskauer positive. Although the optimal growth temperature is 30 °C most clinical isolates grow well at 37 °C. *Enterobacter cloacae* has 53 O antigens and 56 H antigens. Approximately 80% of *E. aerogenes* isolates are encapsulated. The capsule is usually thinner than that of *Klebsiella* but shares some antigens (e.g. K68, K26, K59). *Enterobacter agglomerans* and *E. sakazakii* produce a yellow diffusible pigment at 20 °C on agar; the mol. % DNA G + C content is 52–60.

NORMAL HABITAT

Enterobacter spp. are found in soil and water but *E. cloacae* and *E. aerogenes* can be a minority component of the intestinal flora of man and other animals, and in sewage (up to 10^7 cfu/g).

PATHOGENICITY

Enterobacter spp. are important nosocomial and opportunistic pathogens. There is little information on their virulence determinants. It is presumed that they adhere to mucosal surfaces using fimbriae.

EPIDEMIOLOGY

Enterobacter spp. and in particular E. cloacae (the most common) and E. aerogenes are associated with sporadic and occasionally epidemic nosocomial infection (Gaston, 1988). Enterobacter sakazakii has been particularly associated with neonatal sepsis (Arseni et al., 1987) and E. taylorae is a rare cause of nosocomial infection. Enterobacter spp. are responsible for 1.5% (Eykyn et al., 1990) to 6% (Pittet, 1993) of bacteraemic episodes in adults. Common source outbreaks have been linked to enteral feeds and dextrose infusions (Maki et al., 1976), probably due to an ability to grow in concentrated glucose solutions. Hospital cross-infection can produce outbreaks, for example, by contamination of urinals (Mummery et al., 1974) or by transfer on hands in neonatal units (Haertl and Bandlow, 1993; Ahmet et al., 1995). Enterobacter spp. survive as well as Klebsiella spp. on hands (Hart et al., 1982).

For epidemiological purposes, Enterobacter spp. have been subdivided by biotype, antibiogram, cloacin typing, phage typing (Gaston, 1988), plasmid profile, pyrolysis mass spectrometry (Ahmet et al., 1995) and a variety of molecular biological techniques including pulsed-field gel electrophoresis (Haertl and Bandlow, 1993) and repetitive element polymerase chain reaction (Georghiou et al., 1995).

ANTIMICROBIAL SUSCEPTIBILITY

All isolates of E. cloacae and E. aerogenes are resistant to cephradine, cefuroxime and amoxycillin, but most UK isolates remain sensitive to cefotaxime, ceftazidime, cefpirome, imipenem, gentamicin and ciprofloxacin (Reeves et al., 1993). The presence of plasmid-encoded resistance is not uncommon. Like Citrobacter spp., Enterobacter spp. have the capacity to produce both inducible and derepressed chromosomally encoded cephalosporinases. Recently strains of E. aerogenes resistant to imipenem have emerged (de Champs et al., 1993). These were found to hyper-express a chromosomally encoded cephalosporinase, a variety of plasmid-encoded β-lactamases (TEM types) and to have lost an outer membrane (porin) protein.

TREATMENT AND PREVENTION

Treatment depends upon the local antimicrobial susceptibility patterns and prevention is by adherence to appropriate control of infection procedures.

SERRATIA SPECIES

The type species, Serratia marcescens, was first described by Bizio in 1823 as a cause of red discoloration of cornmeal porridge: 'bleeding polenta'. The red pigment produced by S. marcescens is water insoluble, not light fast and is called prodigiosin (Yu, 1979). It has been responsible for the appearance of 'blood' on foodstuffs throughout history. Its presence in sputum has also led to a misdiagnosis of bronchiectasis or even bronchial carcinoma. Serratia marcescens has also been used extensively as a biological tracer. The earliest experiment was in the House of Commons in 1906 and involved gargling with a solution of S. marcescens and then declaiming to an audience of agar plates (doubtless more attentive and receptive than the usual audience!).

Serratia spp. are indole negative, produce lecithinase and lipase and are more likely to be gelatinase and DNAase positive than the other Enterobacteriaceae (Grimont and Grimont, 1984). The genus contains nine species, namely: S. marcescens, S. liquefaciens, S. rubidaea (previously S. marinorubra), S. ficaria, S. fonticola, S. odorifera, S. plymuthica, S. grimesii and S. proteomaculans subsp. quinovora. Of these, S. marcescens, S. liquefaciens and S. rubidaea are most often associated with human infection. Serratia fonticola is found in water, S. ficaria shuttles between fig tree and fig wasp but can cause human infection, and S. plymuthica and S.

proteomaculans subsp. *quinovora* are rare causes of human disease.

DESCRIPTION OF THE ORGANISM

Serratia spp. are straight rods 0.5–0.8 μm × 0.9–2.0 μm. Most are motile by means of peritrichous flagella. In a survey of respiratory tract isolates, over 17% of *Serratia* spp. possessed type 3 fimbriae (Hornick *et al.*, 1991). Mucoid colonies of *S. plymuthica* occur regularly but most other *Serratia* spp. are non-capsulate. *Serratia odorifera* does possess a microcapsule which cross-reacts with *Klebsiella* K4 or K68 antisera. There are 21 somatic antigens (O1–O21), 25 flagellar (H1–H25) antigens, and 16–50% of strains have the serotype O14 : H12. Prodigiosin is produced by two biogroups of *S. marcescens* and most *S. rubidaea* and *S. plymuthica* between 20 °C and 35 °C. Colonies of these bacteria are completely red or have a red centre or margin. Most species produce a fishy–urinary odour; *S. odorifera* and *S. ficaria* smell musty. All *Serratia* spp. are Voges–Proskauer positive (except for 40% of *S. plymuthica*) and hydrolyse tributyrin; mol. % DNA G + C content is 52–60.

NORMAL HABITAT

Serratia spp. are widely distributed in the environment (water, soil, plants) and can be found in the rodent gut (Grimont and Grimont, 1984) and occasionally in the human intestinal tract. *Serratia* spp. appear to colonize the premature neonate's intestinal tract when in intensive care but are rarely found in staff or mothers (Christensen *et al.*, 1982; Newport *et al.*, 1985).

ANTIMICROBIAL SUSCEPTIBILITY

As for *Enterobacter* spp., *Serratia* spp. are generally resistant to cefuroxime, cephradine and amoxycillin but sensitive to ceftazidime, imipenem, cefpirome and ciprofloxacin (Reeves *et al.*, 1993). Susceptibility to cefotaxime and gentamicin is less predictable. *Serratia* spp. are also relatively resistant to disinfectants, *S. marcescens*

being the most resistant and *S. plymuthica* the least. *Serratia* spp. can also express chromosomally encoded cephalosporinases.

Serratia spp. are able to acquire and maintain resistance plasmids; incompatibility groups B, C, F_I, F_{II}, H_2, M, N, P and W have been detected (Grimont and Grimont, 1984). Plasmids appear to be able to move from genus to genus and one American hospital outbreak of infection due to gentamicin-resistant *S. marcescens* was followed by another due to similarly resistant *K. pneumoniae* carrying the same plasmid (Thomas *et al.*, 1977). Recently plasmid-encoded resistance to imipenem has been described in clinical isolates of *S. marcescens* (Ito *et al.*, 1995).

PATHOGENICITY

Other than class 3 fimbriae no other virulence determinants have been ascribed to *Serratia* spp. However, their ability to survive in disinfectant solution, to grow at relatively low temperatures and to adhere to plastics can provide a reservoir for infection. They are not part of the adult normal flora but can colonize premature neonates (Christensen *et al.*, 1982; Newport *et al.*, 1985).

Prodigiosin production seems unrelated to pathogenicity since up to 80% of clinical isolates are non-producers. *Serratia marcescens* produces a pore-forming haemolysin which allows the bacterium to acquire haemoglobin and haem using an extracellular scavenger protein (Letoffe *et al.*, 1994).

EPIDEMIOLOGY AND INFECTIONS

Serratia spp. are nosocomial and opportunist pathogens, *S. marcescens* being the most important. The inanimate environment, especially when moist, is the major reservoir of *S. marcescens* as is the premature neonate's intestinal tract (Christensen *et al.*, 1982; Newport *et al.*, 1985). Transmission has been by fomites such as disinfectant and cleansing solutions, contact lenses, hand lotions, urinary catheters, catheter hubs, parenteral fluids, mechanical respirators and fibre-optic bronchoscopes (Yu, 1979). Spread appears to be via hands although *Serratia* spp. tend to be infrequently detected on hands (Christensen *et al.*, 1982; Newport *et al.*, 1985). Community-acquired *S. plymuthica*, *S. ficaria* and *S. proteamaculans* subsp. *quinovora* infections have resulted from contamination from soil and plant material.

Infections can be sporadic or epidemic. *Serratia* spp. is a relatively rare cause of bacteraemia, causing 0.4% of cases in one large UK hospital (Eykyn *et al.*, 1990). In the USA in 1975, *Serratia* spp. were responsible for 3.8% of cases of nosocomial bacteraemia but since then have not appeared in the top 10 isolates (Pittet, 1993).

Epidemiological typing methods for *Serratia* spp. include serotyping (Newport *et al.*, 1985), bacteriocin susceptibility, phage typing and bio-typing (Grimont and Grimont, 1984), antibio-grams (Christensen *et al.*, 1982) and a variety of molecular techniques including polymerase chain reaction of repetitive intergenic consensus sequences (Lin *et al.*, 1994).

CLINICAL FEATURES

Serratia spp. can cause urinary tract infection, pneumonia, meningitis (rarely), endophthalmitis, bacteraemia and wound infections. One particularly striking 'non-illness' is the red diaper syndrome due to excretion of *S. marcescens* in the infant stool (Yu, 1979).

DIAGNOSIS

Serratia spp. are easily cultured on most media from infected sites. Some strains of *S. plymuthica* do not grow well at 37 °C.

TREATMENT AND PREVENTION

Specific treatment depends upon the susceptibility of the isolate but most are still susceptible to ciprofloxacin, imipenem and ceftazidime. Prevention is by appropriate infection control measures. Especial care must be taken with storage of disinfects, plastic blood containers and contact lenses.

REFERENCES

Abraham, S.N., Sun, D., Dale, J.B. and Beachey, E.H. (1988) Conservation of the D-mannose-adhesion protein among type 1 fimbriated members of the family Enterobacteriaceae. *Nature*, **336**, 682–684.

Ahmet, Z., Houang, E. and Hurley, R. (1995) Pyrolysis mass spectrometry of cephalosporin-resistant *Enterobacter cloacae*. *Journal of Hospital Infection*, **31**, 99–104.

Allen, P., Hart, C.A. and Saunders, J.R. (1987a) Isolation from *Klebsiella* and characterization of two *rcs* genes that activate colanic acid capsular biosynthesis in *Escherichia coli*. *Journal of General Microbiology*, **133**, 331–340.

Allen, P.M., Williams, J.M., Hart, C.A. and Saunders, J.R. (1987b) Identification of two chemical types of K21 capsular polysaccharide from Klebsiellae. *Journal of General Microbiology*, **133**, 1365–1370.

Altman, E. and Dutton, G.G.S. (1985) Chemical and structural analysis of the capsular polysaccharide from *Escherichia coli* O9 : K28(A) : H-(K28 Antigen). *Carbohydrate Research*, **178**, 293–303.

Ames, G.F.L. and Joshi, A.K. (1990) Energy coupling in bacteria and periplasmic permeases. *Journal of Bacteriology*, **171**, 4133–4137.

Arakawa, Y., Ohta, M., Wacharotayankun, R. *et al.*, (1991) Biosynthesis of *Klebsiella* K2 capsular polysaccharide in *Escherichia coli* HB101 requires the functions of *rmp*A and chromosomal *cps* gene cluster of the virulent strain *Klebsiella pneumoniae* Chedid (O1 : K2). *Infection and Immunity*, **59**, 2043–2050.

Arseni, A., Malamon-Ladas, E., Koutsia, C., Xanthou, M. and Trikka, E. (1987) Outbreak of colonization of neonates with *Enterobacter sakazakii*. *Journal of Hospital Infection*, **9**, 143–150.

Athamna, A., Ofek, I., Keisari, Y., Markowitz, S., Dutton, G.G.S. and Sharon, N. (1991) Lectinophagocytosis of encapsulated *Klebsiella pneumoniae* mediated by surface lectins of guinea-pig alveolar macrophages and human monocyte derived macrophages. *Infection and Immunity*, **59**, 1673–1682.

Bergogne-Bérézin, E., Decré, D. and Joly-Guillon, M.-L. (1993) Opportunistic nosocomial multiply resistant bacterial infections: their treatment and prevention. *Journal of Antimicrobial Chemotherapy*, **32** (Suppl. A), 39–48.

Berkowitz, F.E. and Metchock, B. (1995) Third generation cephalosporin-resistant gram negative bacilli in the feces of hospitalized children. *Pediatric Infectious Disease Journal*, **14**, 97–100.

Betley, M.J., Miller, V.L. and Mekalanos, J.J. (1986) Genetics of bacterial enterotoxins. *Annual Review of Microbiology*, **40**, 577–605.

Bettelheim, K.A., Evangelidis, H., Pearce, J.C., Sowers, E. and Strockbine, N.A. (1993) Isolation of a *Citrobacter freundii* strain which carries the *Escherichia coli* 0157 antigen. *Journal of Clinical Microbiology*, **31**, 760–761.

Borgstein, J., Sada, E. and Cortes, R. (1993) Ciprofloxacin for rhinoscleroma and ozaena. *Lancet*, **342**, 122.

Boulnois, G.J. and Roberts, I.S. (1990) Genetics of capsular polysaccharide production in bacteria. *Current Topics in Microbiology*, **150**, 1–18.

Brenner, D.J. (1984) Family 1: Enterobacteriaceae. In *Bergey's Manual of Systematic Bacteriology*, Vol. 1 (eds N.R. Krieg and J.G. Holt), pp. 408–420. Williams & Wilkins, Baltimore.

Casewell, M.W. and Desai, N. (1983) Survival of multi-resistant and other Gram negative bacilli on finger-tips. *Journal of Hospital Infection*, **4**, 350–360.

Casewell, M.W. and Phillips, I. (1977) Hands as a route of transmission for *Klebsiella* species. *British Medical Journal*, **ii**, 1315–1317.

Casewell, M. and Talsania, H.G. (1979) Predominance of certain *Klebsiella* capsular types in hospitals in the United Kingdom. *Journal of Infection*, **1**, 77–79.

Casewell, M.W., Dalton, M.T., Webster, M. and Phillips, I. (1977) Gentamicin-resistant *Klebsiella aerogenes* is a urological ward. *Lancet*, **ii**, 444–446.

Christensen, G.D., Korones, S.B., Reed, L., Bulley, R., McLaughlin, B. and Bisno, A.L. (1982) Epidemic *Serratia marcescens* in a neonatal intensive care unit: importance of the gastrointestinal tract as reservoir. *Infection Control*, **3**, 127–133.

Cooke, E.M., Sazegar, T., Edmondson, A.S., Brayson, J.C. and Hall, D. (1980) *Klebsiella* species in hospital food and kitchens: a source of organisms in the bowel of patients. *Journal of Hygiene*, **84**, 97–101.

Cryz, S.J., Mortimer, P.M., Mansfield, V. and Germainer, R. (1986) Seroepidemiology of *Klebsiella* bacteremic isolates and implications for vaccine development. *Journal of Clinical Microbiology*, **23**, 687–690.

Curie, K., Speller, D.C.E., Simpson, R.A., Stephens, M. and Cooke, D.I. (1978) A hospital epidemic caused by a gentamicin-resistant *Klebsiella aerogenes*. *Journal of Hygiene*, **80**, 115–123.

Darfeuille-Michaud, A., Jallat, C., Aubel, D. *et al.* (1992) R-plasmid encoded adhesive factor in *Klebsiella pneumoniae* strains responsible for human nosocomial infections. *Infection and Immunity*, **60**, 44–55.

de Champs, C., Henquell, C., Guelon, D., Sirot, D., Gazuy, N. and Sirot, J. (1993) Clinical and bacteriological study of nosocomial infections due to *Enterobacter aerogenes* resistant to imipenem. *Journal of Clinical Microbiology*, **31**, 123–127.

Denoya, C.D., Trevisan, A.R. and Zorzopoulos, J. (1986) Adherence of multi-resistant strains of *Klebsiella pneumoniae* to cerebrospinal fluid shunts: correlation with plasmid content. *Journal of Medical Microbiology*, **21**, 225–231.

Domenico, P., Johanson, W.G. and Straus, D.C. (1982) Lobar pneumonia in rats produced by *Klebsiella pneumoniae*. *Infection and Immunity*, **37**, 327–355.

Donowitz, L.G., Marsik, F.J., Fisher, K.A. and Wenzel, R.P. (1981) Contaminated breast milk: a source of *Klebsiella* bacteremia in a newborn intensive care unit. *Journal of Infectious Diseases*, **3**, 716–720.

Edmondson, A.S. and Cooke, E.M. (1979) The development and assessment of a bacteriocin typing method for *Klebsiella*. *Journal of Hygiene*, **82**, 207–223.

Eykyn, S.J., Gransden, W.R. and Phillips, I. (1990) The causative organisms of septicaemia and their epidemiology. *Journal of Antimicrobial Chemotherapy*, **25** (Suppl. c), 41–58.

Frankel, G., Candy, D., Everest, P. and Dougan, G. (1994) Characterization of the C-terminal domains of intimin-like proteins of enteropathogenic and enterohemorrhagic *Escherichia coli*, *Citrobacter freundii* and *Hafnia alvei*. *Infection and Immunity*, **62**, 1835–1842.

Fryklund, B., Tullus, K. and Burman, L.G. (1995) Survival on skin and surfaces of epidemic and non-epidemic strains of enterobacteria from neonatal special care units. *Journal of Hospital Infection*, **29**, 201–208.

Gaston, M.A. (1988) *Enterobacter*: an emerging nosocomial pathogen. *Journal of Hospital Infection*, **11**, 197–208.

Georghiou, P.R., Hanill, R.J., Wright, C.E. *et al.* (1995) Molecular epidemiology of infections due to *Enterobacter aerogenes*: identification of hospital outbreak-associated strains by molecular techniques. *Clinical Infectious Diseases*, **20**, 84–94.

Gladstone, I.M., Ehrenkranz, A.R.A., Edberg, S.C. and Baltimore, R.S. (1990) A ten year review of neonatal sepsis and comparisons with previous 50-year experience. *Pediatric Infectious Disease Journal*, **9**, 819–825.

Goering, R.V., Ehrenkranz, N.J., Sanders, C.C. and Sander, W.E. (1992) Long term epidemiological analysis of *Citrobacter diversus* in a neonatal intensive care unit. *Pediatric Infectious Disease Journal*, **11**, 99–104.

Gouby, A., Neuwirth, C., Bourg, G. *et al.* (1994) Epidemiological study by pulsed-field gel electrophoresis of an outbreak of extended-spectrum β-lactamase producing *Klebsiella pneumoniae* in a geriatric hospital. *Journal of Clinical Microbiology*, **32**, 301–305.

Grimont, P.A.D. and Grimont, F. (1984) Genus VIII: *Serratia*. In *Bergey's Manual of Systematic Bacteriology*, Vol. 1 (eds N.R. Krieg and J.G. Holt), pp. 477–494. Williams & Wilkins, Baltimore.

Haertl, R. and Bandlow, G. (1993) Epidemiological fingerprinting of *Enterobacter cloacae* by small-fragment restriction endonuclease analysis and pulsed-field gel electrophoresis of genomic restriction fragments. *Journal of Clinical Microbiology*, **31**, 128–133.

Hart, C.A. (1993) *Klebsiellae* and neonates. *Journal of Hospital Infection*, **23**, 83–86.

Hart, C.A. and Gibson, M.F. (1982) Comparative epidemiology of gentamicin-resistant enterobacteria: persistence of carriage and infection. *Journal of Clinical Pathology*, **35**, 452–457.

Hart, C.A. and Percival, A. (1982) Resistance to cephalosporins among gentamicin-resistant Klebsiellae. *Journal of Antimicrobial Chemotherapy*, **9**, 275–286.

Hart, C.A., Gibson, M.R. and Buckles, A. (1981) Variation in skin and environmental survival of hospital gentamicin-resistant enterobacteria. *Journal of Hygiene*, **87**, 277–285.

Hibbert-Rogers, L.C.F., Heritage, J., Todd, N. and Hawkey, P. (1994) Convergent evolution of TEM-26: a β-lactamase with extended spectrum activity. *Journal of Antimicrobial Chemotherapy*, **33**, 707–720.

Hornick, D.B., Allen, B.C., Horn, M.A. and Clegg, S. (1991) Fimbrial types among respiratory isolates belonging to the family Enterobacteriaceae. *Journal of Clinical Microbiology*, **21**, 1795–1800.

Houng, H.S., Noon, K.F., Ou, J.T. and Barron, L.S. (1992) Expression of Vi antigen in *Escherichia coli* K12: characterization of ViaB from *Citrobacter freundii* and identity of ViaA with KesB. *Journal of Bacteriology*, **174**, 5910–5915.

Ito, H., Arakawa, Y., Ohsuka, S., Wacharotayankum, R., Kato, N. and Ohta, M. (1995) Plasmid mediated dissemination of the metallo-β-lactamase gene *bla*IMP among clinically isolated strains of *Serratia marcescens*. *Antimicrobial Agents and Chemotherapy*, **39**, 824–829.

Jacoby, G.A. and Medeiros, A.A. (1991) More extended spectrum β-lactamases. *Antimicrobial Agents and Chemotherapy*, **35**, 1697–1704.

Jann, B. and Jann, K. (1990) Structure and biosynthesis of capsular antigen of *Escherichia coli*. *Current Topics in Microbiology and Immunology*, **150**, 19–42.

Kerver, A.J., Rommes, J.H., Mevissen-Verhage, E.A.E. *et al.* (1987) Colonization and infection in surgical intensive care patients: a prospective study. *Intensive Care Medicine*, **13**, 347–351.

Knittle, M.A., Eitzman, D.V. and Baer, H. (1975) Role of hand contamination in the epidemiology of gram-negative nosocomial infections. *Journal of Pediatrics*, **86**, 433–437.

Le Frock, J.L., Ellis, C.A. and Weinstein, L. (1979) Impact of hospitalization on the aerobic microflora. *American Journal of Medical Science*, **277**, 269–274.

Letoffe, S., Ghigo, J.M. and Wandersman, C. (1994) Iron acquisition from heme and hemoglobin by *Serratia marcescens* extracellular protein. *Proceedings of the National Academy of Sciences USA*, **91**, 9876–9880.

Li, J., Musser, J.M., Beltran, P., Kline, M.W. and Selander, R.K. (1990) Genotypic heterogeneity of strains of *Citrobacter diversus* expressing a 32-kilodalton outer membrane protein associated with neonatal meningitis. *Journal of Clinical Microbiology*, **28**, 1760–1765.

Lin, P.Y., Lau, Y.J., Hu, B.S. *et al.* (1994) Use of PCR to study the epidemiology of *Serratia marcescens* isolates in nosocomial infection. *Journal of Clinical Microbiology*, **32**, 1935–1938.

Mackowiak, P.A., Martin, R.M. and Smith, J.W. (1979) The role of bacterial interference in the increased prevalence of Gram-negative bacilli among alcoholics and diabetics. *American Review of Respiratory Disease*, **120**, 589–593.

Maki, D.G., Rhame, F.S., Mackel, D.C. and Bennet, J.V. (1976) Nationwide epidemic of septicaemia caused by contaminated intravenous products. 1. Epidemiological and clinical features. *American Journal of Medicine*, **60**, 471–485.

Meers, P.D., Ayliffe, G.A.J., Emmerson, A.M. *et al.* (1980) Report on the National Survey of Infection in Hospitals 1980. *Journal of Hospital Infection*, **2** (Suppl.), 1–48.

Mengistu, Y., Edwards, C. and Saunders, J.R. (1994) Continuous culture studies on the synthesis of capsular polysaccharide by *Klebsiella pneumoniae* K1. *Journal of Applied Bacteriology*, **76**, 424–430.

Merino, S., Camprubi, S., Alberts, S., Benedi, V. and Tomas, J. (1992) Mechanism of *Klebsiella pneumoniae* resistance to complement-mediated killing. *Infection and Immunity*, **60**, 2529–2535.

Meyer, P.R., Shum, T.K., Becker, T.S. and Taylor, C.R. (1983) Scleroma (rhinoscleroma). A histologic immunohistochemical study with bacteriologic correlates. *Archives of Pathology and Laboratory Medicine*, **107**, 377–383.

Morgan, M.E.I., Hart, C.A. and Cooke, R.W.I. (1984) Klebsiella infection in a neonatal intensive care unit: role of bacteriological surveillance. *Journal of Hospital Infection*, **5**, 377–385.

Morris, J.G., Lin, F.Y.C., Morrison, C.B. *et al.* (1986) Molecular epidemiology of neonatal meningitis due to *Citrobacter diversus*: a study of isolates from hospitals in Maryland. *Journal of Infectious Diseases*, **154**, 409–414.

Mummery, R.V., Rowe, B. and Gross, R.J. (1974) Urinary tract infections due to atypical *Enterobacter cloacae*. *Lancet*, **ii**, 1333.

Murcia, A. and Rubin, S.J. (1979) Reproducibility of an indirect immunofluorescent-antibody technique for capsular serotyping of *Klebsiella pneumoniae*. *Journal of Clinical Microbiology*, **9**, 208–213.

Newport, M.T., John, J.F., Michel, Y.M. and Levkoff, A.H. (1985) Endemic *Serratia marcescens* infection in a neonatal intensive care nursery associated with gastrointestinal colonization. *Pediatric Infectious Diseases*, **4**, 160–167.

O'Hara, C.M., Roman, S.B. and Miller, J.M. (1995) Ability of commercial identification systems to identify newly recognized species of *Citrobacter*. *Journal of Clinical Microbiology*, **33**, 242–245.

Orskov, I. (1984) Genus V: *Klebsiella*. In *Bergey's Manual of Systematic Bacteriology*, Vol. 1 (eds N.R. Krieg and J.G. Holt), pp. 461–465. Williams & Wilkins, Baltimore.

Palfreyman, J.M. (1978) *Klebsiella* serotyping by counter-current immunoelectrophoresis. *Journal of Hygiene*, **81**, 219–225.

Pavelka, M.S., Wright, L.F. and Silver, R.P. (1991) Identification of two genes *kps*M and *kps*T in region 3 of the polysialic acid gene cluster of *Escherichia coli* K1. *Journal of Bacteriology*, **173**, 4603–4610.

Pittet, D. (1993) Nosocomial bloodstream infections. In *Prevention and Control of Nosocomial Infections*, 2nd edn (ed. R.P. Wenzel), pp. 512–555. Williams & Wilkins, Baltimore.

Pruzzo, C., Guzman, C.A., Caegari, L. and Satta, G. (1989) Impairment of phagocytosis by the *Klebsiella pneumoniae* mannose-inhibitable adhesin-T7 receptor. *Infection and Immunity*, **57**, 975–982.

Rajab, A. and De Louvois, J. (1990) Survey of infection in babies at Khoula hospital Oman. *Annals of Tropical Paediatrics*, **10**, 39–43.

Reeves, D.S., Bywater, M.J. and Holt, H.A. (1993) The activity of cefpirome and ten other antimicrobial agents against 2858 clinical isolates collected from 20 centres. *Journal of Antimicrobial Chemotherapy*, **31**, 345–362.

Richard, C. (1984) Genus VI: *Enterobacter*. In *Bergey's Manual of Systematic Bacteriology*, Vol. 1 (eds N.R. Krieg and J.G. Holt), pp. 465–469. Williams & Watkins, Baltimore.

Sahly, H., Kekow, J., Podshun, R., Schaff, M., Gross, W.L. and Ullman, U. (1994) Comparison of the antibody responses to the 77 klebsiellar types in ankylosing spondylitis and various rheumatic diseases. *Infection and Immunity*, **62**, 4838–4843.

Sakazaki, R. (1984) Genus IV: *Citrobacter*. In *Bergey's Manual of Systematic Bacteriology*, Vol. 1 (eds N.R. Krieg and J.G. Holt), pp. 458–461. Williams & Wilkins, Baltimore.

Simoons-Smit, A.M., Verweij-van Vught, A.M.J.J., De Vries, P.M.J.M. and Maclaren, D.M. (1987) Comparison of biochemical and serological typing results and antimicrobial susceptibility patterns in the epidemiological investigation of *Klebsiella* spp. *Epidemiology and Infection*, **99**, 625–634.

Stapleton, P., Shannon, K. and Phillips, I. (1995) The ability of β-lactam antibiotics to select mutants with derepressed β-lactamase synthesis from *Citrobacter freundii*. *Journal of Antimicrobial Chemotherapy*, **36**, 483–496.

Straus, D.C. (1987) Production of an extracellular toxic complex by various strains of *Klebsiella pneumoniae*. *Infection and Immunity*, **55**, 44–48.

Sutherland, I.W. (1985) Biosynthesis and composition of gram-negative bacterial extracellular and wall polysaccharides. *Annual Review of Microbiology*, **39**, 243–270.

Tarkkanen, A.M., Allen, B.C., Williams, P.H. *et al.* (1992) Fimbriation, capsulation and iron scavenging systems of *Klebsiella* strains associated with human urinary tract infection. *Infection and Immunity*, **60**, 1187–1192.

Thomas, F.E., Jackson, R.T., Melly, A. and Alford, R.H. (1977) Sequential hospital-wide outbreaks of resistant serratia and klebsiella species. *Archives of Internal Medicine*, **137**, 581–584.

Troy, F.A. (1979) The chemistry and biosynthesis of selected bacterial capsular polymers. *Annual Review of Microbiology*, **33**, 519–560.

Tschäpe, H., Prager, R., Streckel, W., Fruth, A., Tietze, E. and Böhme, G. (1995) Verotoxinogenic *Citrobacter freundii* associated with severe gastroenteritis and cases of haemolytic uraemic syndrome in a nursery school: green butter as the infection source. *Epidemiology and Infection*, **114**, 441–450.

Tullus, K. and Burman, L.G. (1989) Ecological effect of ampicillin and cefuroxime in neonatal units. *Lancet*, **i**, 1405–1407.

Tullus, K., Berglund, B., Fryklund, B., Kuhn, I. and Burman, L.G. (1988) Epidemiology of faecal strains of the family Enterobacteriaceae in 22 neonatal units and influence of antibiotic policy. *Journal of Clinical Microbiology*, **26**, 1166–1170.

Van der Waaij, D. (1982) Colonization resistance of the digestive tract: clinical consequences and implications. *Journal of Antimicrobial Chemotherapy*, **10**, 263–270.

Williams, P. and Tomas, J.M. (1990) The pathogenicity of *Klebsiella pneumoniae*. *Reviews of Infectious Diseases*, **1**, 196–204.

Williams, P., Lambert, P.A., Brown, M.R.W. and Jones, R.J. (1983) The role of the O and K antigens in determining the resistance of *Klebsiella aerogenes* to serum killing and phagocytosis. *Journal of General Microbiology*, **129**, 2181–2191.

Williams, W.W., Mariano, J., Spurrier, M. *et al.* (1984) Nosocomial meningitis due to *Citrobacter diversus* in neonates: new aspects of the epidemiology. *Journal of Infectious Diseases*, **150**, 229–236.

Yu, V.L. (1979) *Serratia marcescens*: historical perspective and clinical review. *New England Journal of Medicine*, **300**, 887–893.

12e

PROTEUS, *PROVIDENCIA* AND *MORGANELLA*

Peter M. Hawkey

TAXONOMY AND GENERAL DESCRIPTION OF THE GENERA

For many years these three genera have been grouped as the tribe Proteeae on the basis that all members are capable of oxidative deamination of aromatic amino acids such as phenylalanine and tryptophan. Other characteristics which suggest an oxidase-negative non-lactose-fermenting bacterium may belong to this tribe are: swarming (*Proteus*), motility, methyl red (MR)+/ Voges–Proskauer (VP)–, H₂S positive, urease positive (except *Providencia*), protease/lipase production (*Proteus*) and resistance to polymxyins.

DNA homology studies have shown that *Proteus morganii*, as it was previously known, has but 20% homology with the other members of the Proteeae (Brenner *et al.*, 1978), and in consequence the separate genus *Morganella* was created and existing and new species redistributed amongst *Proteus* and *Providencia*. Because of the similarities in pathogenicity and natural habitat clinical microbiologists do still tend to group these bacteria together. *Proteus mirabilis* and *Proteus vulgaris* were originally described in 1885 and although the taxonomic status of *P. mirabilis* has been stable, *P. vulgaris* has undergone some

changes. DNA hybridization studies by Hickman *et al.* (1982) suggested that *P. vulgaris* can be divided into three groups, biogroup (BG) 1 strains being named as *Proteus penneri*; and BG 2 and 3. BG2 strains can generally be distinguished from *P. penneri* by analysis of electrophoretic protein patterns, however BG3 strains are heterogeneous, which is confirmed by hybridization studies. As the type strain of *P. vulgaris* (NCTC 4175) belongs to a very rare genomospecies its replacement has been requested (Brenner *et al.*, 1995). *Proteus myxofaciens* is not a human pathogen and is only reported to have been isolated from gypsy moth larvae (Farmer *et al.*, 1985). The bacterium, previously known as *Proteus morganii*, described by Morgan in 1906 from the faeces of children with diarrhoea, was reassigned to its own genus *Morganella* (Brenner *et al.*, 1978). Subsequently three DNA relatedness groups have been identified and two subspecies *morganii* and *sibonii* have been suggested (Jensen *et al.*, 1992).

There are currently five recognized species, based on DNA hybridization studies and phenotypic and protein characteristics, in the genus *Providencia*. The genus was named after Providence, Rhode Island, where C.A. Stuart worked on this group of bacteria. The new species *Providencia rustigianii* and *Providencia heimbachae* were

---

Principles and Practice of Clinical Bacteriology. Edited by A.M. Emmerson, P.M. Hawkey and S.H. Gillespie

430

TABLE 12e.1 KEY BIOCHEMICAL CHARACTERISTICS OF THE SPECIES BELONGING TO THE GENERA *PROTEUS*, *PROVIDENCIA* AND *MORGANELLA*

Test or property[a]	P. mirabilis	P. myxofaciens[b]	P. penneri	P. vulgaris[c] BG2	BG3	M. morganii[d]	Prov. alcalifaciens	Prov. rustigianii	Prov. heimbachae	Prov. stuartii	Prov. rettgeri
Indole	−[e]	−	−	+	+	+	+	+	−	+	+
Citrate	V[e]	V	−	−	−	−	+	V	V	+	+
H₂S	+[e]	−	V	+	+	−	−	−	−	−	−
Urease	+	+	+	+	+	+	−	−	−	V[g]	+
Ornithine decarboxylase	+	−	−	−	−	+	−	−	−	−	−
Gelatinase	+	+	>	+	>	−	−	+	−	−	−
Lipase	+	+	>	>	>	−	−	−	−	−	−
Swarming[h]	+	+	+	+	+	−	−	−	−	−	−
Fermentation of:											
Mannose	−	−	−	−	−	+	+	+	+	+	+
Maltose	−	+	+	+	+	−	−	−	−	−	−
Xylose	+	−	+	+	+	−	−	−	−	−	>
Salicin	−	−	−	+	−	−	−	−	−	−	+
Inositol	−	−	−	−	−	−	+	−	>	+[f]	+
Adonitol	−	−	−	−	−	−	+	−	+	−[f]	+
Arabitol	−	−	−	−	−	−	−	−	−	−	+
Trehalose	+	+	>	>	>	−	−	+	−	+	−
Galactose								−	+	+	+
Rhamnose							−	−	+	−	>
Aesculin hydrolysis	−	−	−	+	−	−	−	−	−	−	>

[a] Tests in bold type are useful in differentiating the three genera.
[b] Only occurs as pathogen of gypsy moth larvae.
[c] BG, biogroup.
[d] Biogroup 1 strains are lysine decarboxylase positive (plasmid mediated) non-motile and glycerol positive.
[e] +, 90–100% positive; V, 10–90% positive; −, 0–10% positive.
[f] BG4 inositol negative and BG6 adonitol positive, both rare;
[g] Plasmid encoded property.
[h] 37 °C on nutrient or blood agar.

grouped within *Providencia alcalifaciens* but neither are found in human clinical specimens (Müller *et al.*, 1986).

The remaining species are easily distinguished (see Table 12e.1); however, the occurrence of plasmid-encoded urease activity in some strains of *Providencia stuartii*, which were previously confused with *Proteus* (now *Providencia*) *rettgeri* should be noted (Farmer *et al.*, 1985). These changes have been summarized by Farmer *et al.* (1985), where full biochemical descriptions of the species will be found.

The biochemical characteristics useful in differentiating the genera of the tribe Proteeae are shown in Table 12e.1 in bold type. One of the most striking features of the genus *Proteus* in culture is their ability to swarm on solid media (i.e. a form of active, surface motility); this is associated with considerable cellular polymorphism (Falkinham and Hoffman, 1984). The size of typical vegetative cells in broth culture is $1-3 \times 0.4-0.6$ μm, whereas in young swarming cultures long, curved multinucleate, multiflagellated cells $10-80$ μm are seen, which then migrate rapidly ($2-10$ μm/s) in close cell-to-cell

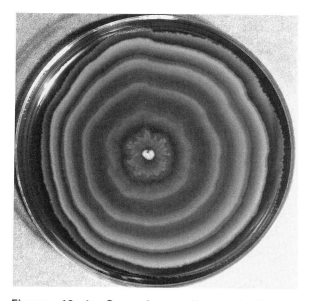

Figure 12e.1. Swarming culture of *Proteus mirabilis* (blood agar, 22°C incubated for 40 h) demonstrating 'bulls-eye' appearance

contact. After a defined period swarm cells stop moving and coordinately revert to the short vegetative form; this leads to the 'bulls-eye' appearance of swarming *P. mirabilis* cultures (Figure 12e.1).

All members of the genus possess flagella and are mobile, usually by virtue of the possession of peritrichous flagella, with the exception of some strains of *M. morganii*. The flagella of *P. mirabilis* are variable in morphology.

The major antigenic determinates of the Proteeae are somatic (O) and flagellar (H) antigens. Typing schemes for detecting O antigens have been described in detail for the various species: *P. mirabilis/P. vulgaris* (Penner and Hennessy, 1980), *M. morganii* (Penner and Hennessy, 1979), *Prov. rettgeri* (Penner *et al.*, 1974), *Prov. stuartii/ Prov. alcalifaciens* (Penner *et al.*, 1976).

PATHOGENICITY OF PROTEEAE

It has long been recognized that the possession of urease (a nickel metallo-enzyme) by a number of the members of the Proteeae represents a likely pathogenicity factor (Mobley and Hausinger, 1989). A wide range of biochemically and genetically distinct ureases are found amongst all of the urease-positive members of the Proteeae (Jones and Mobley, 1987), many of which have now been cloned and sequenced. The gene in *P. mirabilis* is chromosomal and consists of the structural genes *ureABC*; *ureD* is upstream and *ureEFG* downstream. These four genes are thought to be involved in nickel acquisition and enzyme assembly. The *ureR* gene lies upstream of *ureD* and is a positive regulator in the presence of urea (Island and Mobley, 1995). This gene cluster interestingly shows considerable homology, and organizational similarities to urease gene clusters on plasmids in *Escherichia coli*, *Prov. stuartii* and *Salmonella cubana* suggesting common routes of evolution (D'Orazio and Collins, 1993). A mouse model of pyelonephritis was developed and mice infected with urease-defective *P. mirabilis* required a 1000-fold higher ID_{50}, and much less renal tissue damage and urolithiasis occurred, suggesting that urease has a major pathogenic role in urinary tract infections (Johnson *et al.*, 1993).

The formation of urinary stones results from the pH rise that occurs in urine due to the release of ammonium ions from urea as a result of the activity of bacterial ureases. The stones are a mixture of struvite $(MgNH_4PO_4.6H_2O)$ and carbonate apatite $(Ca_{10}(PO_4)_6CI_3)$, which precipitate at $pH > 6.5$ (Mobley and Hausinger, 1989). It has been observed that *P. mirabilis* is particularly associated with blocked urinary catheters rather than other urease-producing bacteria (Mobley and Warren, 1987). The capsular polysaccharide from *P. mirabills* particularly enhances struvite formation, possibly by weakly concentrating Mg^{2+} because of its structure and anionic nature (Dumanski *et al.*, 1994). The most frequently encountered member of the Proteeae in infected/colonized urinary catheters is *Prov. stuartii* (Mobley *et al.*, 1988). It appears this is not due to increased entry of *Prov. stuartii* into the catheter system but to the ability of *Prov. stuartii* to adhere to catheter material via mannose-resistant *Klebsiella*-like haemagglutinins (MR/K), whereas strains only found in patients for a short duration expressed mannose-sensitive haemagglutinins (Mobley *et al.*, 1988). *Proteus mirabilis* also expresses MR/K type fimbriae which probably contribute to catheter adherence, but also produce *P. mirabilis* fimbriae (PMF), uroepithelial cell adhesin (UCA), ambient temperature fimbriae (ATF) and mannose-resistant/*Proteus*-like fimbriae (MR/P) (Bahrani *et al.*, 1994). The association of MR/P fimbriae and the development of pyelonephritis was made by Silverblatt and Ofek in 1978 (cited in Bahrani *et al.*, 1994), and the relevant gene has been cloned; the use of *mrp*A-negative mutants in a mouse model of ascending urinary tract infection confirms the important role of MR/P fimbriae in the pathogenesis of acute pyelonephritis (Bahrani *et al.*, 1994). Recently the gene encoding UCA has been cloned and amino acid sequence homology was found between a range of different pilins in other bacteria, such as *Haemophilus*, *Bordetella* and *E. coli* pilins F17, G and 1C (Cook *et al.*, 1995). UCA seems to be distinct from MR/P and may be responsible for uroepithelial cell adhesion. The use of a Tn5-based transposon mutagenesis system in

P. mirabilis to produce swarm cell-negative mutants in the mouse model has shown the importance of hyperflagellated swarm cells in establishing ascending infections of the urinary tract (Allison *et al.*, 1994). During swarm cell differentiation a number of virulence factors are produced, including an extracellular metalloprotease with activity against IgA (Senior *et al.*, 1991). Molecular analysis of the *zap*A gene, which encodes a metalloprotease thought to be similar to that enzyme, shows it to be a member of the serralysin family of proteases; *zap*A$^-$ mutants will be useful in investigating its role in the virulence of *P. mirabilis* (Wassif *et al.*, 1995).

Siderophores are essential for bacteria to acquire iron, particularly when multiplying in an animal host. The Proteeae are unique amongst the Enterobacteriaceae in possessing amino acid deaminases which result in the production of α-keto and α-hydroxycarboxylic acids, such as phenylpyruvic and indolylpyruvic acids; these in turn, bind actively to iron and have been demonstrated to have siderophore activity (Drechsel *et al.*, 1993).

Whilst definitive evidence for the enteropathogenic role of Proteeae is generally lacking, some studies have suggested possible roles for *M. morganii* and *P. mirabilis*. A study of traveller's diarrhoea demonstrated an association with *Prov. alcalifaciens* (Haynes and Hawkey, 1989). It has further been shown that strains of *Prov. alcalifaciens* isolated from the faeces of patients suffering from diarrhoea in Bangladesh are capable of invading HEp-2 cell monolayers, with actin condensation (Albert *et al.*, 1995).

EPIDEMIOLOGY

Habitat

Most of the Proteeae are widely distributed in nature, being frequently found in the faeces of animals and man as well as associated materials such as decomposing meat and sewage. All of the clinically significant species were found in a study of faecally contaminated calf bedding, bovine meat being suggested as a possible route of colonization of the human gut (Hawkey *et al.*, 1986b). Faeces have been reported as a source for nosocomial infections caused by *P. mirabilis* (Burke *et al.*, 1971), *M. morganii* (Senior and Leslie, 1986) and *Prov. stuartii* (Hawkey *et al.*, 1982). Maternal vaginal carriage of *P. mirabilis* (probably secondary to faecal carriage) has been described as a significant source of neonatal infections (Bingen *et al.*, 1993). Groin skin colonization has been reported as a probable source of urinary tract infection in the elderly (Ehrenkranz *et al.*, 1989). The carriage of *P. mirabilis* in the prepuce of 22% of uncircumcised and 1.7% of circumcised male infants is thought to explain the occurrence of *P. mirabilis* infections in male babies (Glennon *et al.*, 1988).

Proteus mirabilis and less frequently *P. vulgaris*, possibly due to its low carriage rate in faeces (Senior and Leslie, 1986), are associated with urinary tract infections and the infected urine, particularly when patients have an indwelling catheter, can be a source for cross-infection; infected urine can therefore be regarded as a habitat for Proteeae, (Kippax, 1957; Hickman and Farmer, 1976; Warren, 1986). Similarly *Prov. stuartii* (Hawkey *et al.*, 1982) and *M. morganii* (McDermott and Mylotte, 1984) nosocomial infection can be acquired from infected urine, although in the case of the last organism infected wounds may be a significant source (Williams *et al.*, 1983).

Providencia alcalifaciens which can be isolated from both human and animal faeces, over the years has often been regarded as not being a human pathogen. However, early workers such as C.A. Stuart and Patricia Carpenter (Central Public Health Laboratory, London) thought it could cause diarrhoeal illness (Penner *et al.*, 1979). Recently it has been shown that the species is found much more frequently in travellers with diarrhoea returning to the UK (Haynes and Hawkey, 1989) and some evidence for enteropathogenicity has emerged.

Human Infections

The most common infection caused by Proteeae is

infection of the urinary tract, and *P. mirabilis* is by far the most common species of Proteeae isolated from the urinary tract, and is the third most frequently isolated species of Enterobacteriaceae in the clinical laboratory (Hickman and Farmer, 1976). Whilst the association of Proteeae with urinary tract infection, particularly the anatomically abnormal or catheterized urinary tract (*P. mirabilis* and *Prov. stuartii* in particular), is very well documented (Warren *et al.*, 1982; Hawkey, 1984; Ehrenkranz *et al.*, 1989), detailed prospective epidemiological studies using strain typing are rare. It seems likely that faecal carriage can be a source for subsequent infection of the abnormal tract (Hawkey *et al.*, 1982). The colonized groin area of geriatric patients has also been proposed as a source for all Proteeae (Ehrenkranz *et al.*, 1989) although this needs to be proven by typing studies. Cross-infection of both multiple and an endemic strain amongst catheterized patients in the hospital setting via hands and fomites (e.g. jugs, specific gravity cylinders) has been documented particularly for *Prov. stuartii* (Hawkey *et al.*, 1982; Rahav *et al.*, 1994). In neonatal units, the vaginal carriage of *P. mirabilis* (Bingen *et al.*, 1993) and rectal/vaginal carriage in a nurse (Burke *et al.*, 1971) and probable subsequent spread via hands have led to serious outbreaks of septicaemia, meningitis and omphalitis. Cross-infection by *M. morganii* is rare, but episodes in which infected wounds co-infected with *P. mirabilis* have acted as a source with subsequent transfer to other patients have been described and documented with strain typing (Williams *et al.*, 1983). In a review of 19 cases of *M. morganii* bacteraemia the most common source was found to be an infected wound and extensive use of cephalosporins (to which *M. morganii* is often resistant) was thought to be an important factor leading to the development of infection and (McDermott and Mylotte, 1984). The source and route of transmission of *Prov. alcalifaciens* in human diarrhoeal illness have not been investigated, but are likely to be via food or asymptomatic faecal carriage leading to transient hand carriage. Ribotyping has also been applied to an outbreak of *Prov. stuartii* catheter infection, suggesting multiple sources of infecting bacteria (Rahav *et al.*, 1994).

Epidemiological Typing Methods

A wide range of epidemiological typing methods have been applied to Proteeae, the oldest and most widely used being O serotyping. A number of schemes have been described; these were consolidated and refined by using passive haemagglutination by Professor J. Penner at the University of Toronto and are referenced in the first section. Although discrimination and typability are good by this method a large set of antisera is required. In the case of the swarming *Proteus* spp. use has been made for many years of the Dienes test. Originally described by Dienes in 1946, a line of demarcation appears between two swarming strains if they are different, whereas identical strains swarm into one another (Figure 12e.2). The phenomenon appears to be largely due to both sensitivity to and production of bacteriocins (Senior, 1977). It is an easily applied method, but discrimination is not always good and reliability can be a problem (Hickman and Farmer, 1976).

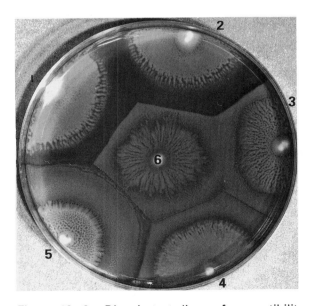

Figure 12e.2. Diene's test, lines of compatibility are seen between isolates 1 and 2; 3 and 6 indicating that they are indistinguishable but different from each other. Isolates 4 and 5 are incompatible and different from the other two groups of isolates (1 and 2; 3 and 6). Blood agar, incubated for 48 h at 22 °C.

Bacteriocin typing schemes have been described for Proteeae, one of the most extensive being produced for *Proteus* (Senior, 1976). Bacteriophage typing has also been described (Hickman and Farmer, 1976). The almost universal applicability of molecular typing methods to different bacterial species has resulted in their being applied to a wide range of nosocomial outbreaks of cross-infection. A recent comparison of ribotyping and arbitrarily primed polymerase chain reaction typing (AP-PCR) in investigating *P. mirabilis* cross-infection in a maternity hospital concluded that AP-PCR was equivalent to ribotyping and easier to perform (Bingen *et al.*, 1993).

CLINICAL MANIFESTATIONS

The urinary tract is the most commonly infected site, although infection of the anatomically normal and uncatheterized tract is rare. Pyelonephritis and urinary stone formation are common features of infection with *P. mirabilis* for the reasons described above. *Providencia stuartii*, *Proteus mirabilis* and *M. morganii* are the most frequently found species in the catheterized urinary tract; often more than one species of Proteeae is present and usually mixed with other bacterial species. *Providencia stuartii* is the species which persists best; in a prospective study of bacteriuria in 20 catheterized patients, the mean duration of new episodes was 10.4 weeks for *Prov. stuartii*, 5.5 weeks for *P. mirabilis* and 2.9 weeks for enterococci (Warren *et al.*, 1982).

The frequent presence of *Prov. stuartii* in catheter bags has been shown to explain the condition in which the bag turns deep purple in colour, termed the purple urine bag syndrome (PUBS). Some strains of *Prov. stuartii* possess an indoxyl suphatase which degrades high levels of urinary indoxyl sulphate (usually in patients with bacterial overgrowth of the small bowel) to indoxyl, which condenses to form the insoluble dyes indirubin (red) and indigo (blue). These dyes are soluble in the plasticizers of the bag wall and stain it purple (Dealler *et al.*, 1988).

Proteus mirabilis has been reported as causing a number of other infections, such as bacteraemia arising from the infected/colonized urinary tract (Muder *et al.*, 1992), nosocomial wound infections (Chow *et al.*, 1979; Williams *et al.*, 1983) and meningitis in neonates arising from infected umbilical stumps (Burke *et al.*, 1971); it is also found with other bacteria in brain abscess derived from middle ear infections. Chronic colonization of the ear may cause local infections and local spread results in its isolation from brain abscesses. Other members of the Proteeae, notably *M. morganii*, are associated with soft tissue infections, such as wound infections (Tucci and Isenberg, 1981; Williams *et al.*, 1983; McDermott and Mylotte, 1984). In studies of bacteruria *P. mirabilis* is the most frequently reported of the Proteeae, because it is the most frequently encountered member of the tribe in clinical specimens (McDermott and Mylotte, 1984). *Proteus vulgaris* and *P. penneri* cause a similar spectrum of infections to *P. mirabilis* but are somewhat rarer. In long-term care and geriatric facilities, where patients with urinary catheters are common, *Prov. stuartii* is the most frequent cause of bacteremia (Hawkey, 1984; Muder *et al.*, 1992). *Providencia stuartii* has been noted to cause nosocomial pneumonia and wound and burn infections, but these are quite rare (Hawkey, 1984). The role of Proteeae in diarrhoeal disease has long been debated (Penner *et al.*, 1979) and most species at some time have been suggested as putative causative agents. In a recent study of travellers with diarrhoea returning to the UK from Mediterranean countries, 10% had *Prov. alcalifaciens* in faecal samples, whereas only 1.3% of controls with diarrhoea who had not travelled were positive (Haynes and Hawkey, 1989). Evidence for enteropathogenicity of *Prov. alcalifaciens* has now emerged (see above).

LABORATORY DIAGNOSIS

Isolation

All members of the Proteeae likely to be encountered in clinical material are capable of growth on commonly used laboratory media (nutrient, blood and MacConkey's agar) incubated at 37 °C in room air. A number of selective media have been developed for the isolation of Proteeae (Penner, 1981). PIM agar, which has been used in a number

of studies, utilizes clindamycin and colistin as the selective agents and tryptophan/tyrosine as differential agents (Hawkey *et al.*, 1986a).

Identification of Proteeae is generally reliably achieved using one of the recognized commercial identification systems, either automated or manual. It is worth noting that *Prov. stuartii* may pose problems and be misidentified by most systems if supplementary tests are not included (Cornaglia *et al.*, 1988). A modified MacConkey's agar which detects phosphatase activity has been shown to alleviate this problem (Thaller *et al.*, 1992). The biochemical characteristics of the Proteeae species are shown in Table 12e.1. Changes in taxonomy and identification methods appear to have resulted in a decrease in reports of nosocomial *Prov. rettgeri* infections, at the same time as an increase in *Prov. stuartii*. This is most likely due to the recognition of urease-positive *Prov. stuartii* rather than selection of *Prov. stuartii* which are resistant to many widely used antimicrobials (Hawkey, 1984). Much effort can be expended by the laboratory in identifying and carrying out antimicrobial sensitivity tests on isolates of Proteeae from specimens where the isolates have little or no clinical relevance. In the case of blood culture isolates, the pathogenic status of those isolates is clear; however, from colonized wounds and catheter urines the clinical condition of the patient is paramount in deciding the laboratory tests used and the level of reporting. One study has shown that the Proteeae may be selectively under-reported by some microbiology laboratories from catheter urine specimens, with the potential for missed treatment of bacteraemic patients (Damron *et al.*, 1986).

Resistance to Antimicrobials and Chemotherapy of Proteeae

β-Lactam antibiotics are widely used to treat infections caused by bacteria belonging to the family Enterobacteriacae. In the case of the Proteeae, *P. mirabilis*, unlike the other species (except *Prov. alcalifaciens*, which is generally very susceptible to antibiotics [Penner, 1981]), does not appear to produce a chromosomal cephalosporinase or AmpC type penicillinase

(Livermore, 1995). In consequence, many cases of infection caused by *P. mirabilis* can often be treated with ampicillin or older cephalosporins such as cephradine or cephalexin. *Prov. stuartii* carries a number of intrinsic plasmid-mediated antibiotic resistance determinants and may be difficult to treat (Hawkey, 1984; Warren, 1986). The extended-spectrum cephalosporins are suitable for treating infections caused by the *Providencia* spp., *M. morganii* and *P. vulgaris*, although plasmid-mediated extended-spectrum β-lactamases have rarely been reported from the Proteeae. The TEM family of β-lactamases is found in most of the species of Proteeae at varying frequencies, often dictated by local usage of ampicillins (Hawkey, 1984). Imipenem resistance is very rare in the Proteeae with the exception of occasional isolates of *P. mirabilis*, when altered penicillin-binding proteins appear to be responsible (Neuwirth *et al.*, 1995).

Most isolates of Proteeae are susceptible to aminoglycosides, provided none of the plasmid-mediated aminoglycoside-inactivating enzymes are present (e.g. APH(3')). *Providencia stuartii* and probably some strains of *Prov. rettgeri* carry a chromosomally encoded gentamicin 2'-*N*-acetyltransferase (AAC(2')) which is not always expressed. The enzyme probably plays a role in the maintenance of peptidoglycan structure (Payie *et al.*, 1995). Commonly used antibiotics for the treatment of urinary tract infections caused by Proteeae are trimethoprim and fluoroquinolones, such as ciprofloxacin, which are effective subject to sensitivity testing of individual isolates. Caution should be observed in using chloramphenicol to treat brain abscesses caused by *P. mirabilis* as most strains carry an inducible chloramphenicol acetylase gene (Charles *et al.*, 1985) which will result in treatment failure. *Providencia stuartii* has been regarded by some workers to be resistant to the disinfectant chlorhexidine. It has been suggested that chlorhexidine inhibits membrane-bound ATPase and this may provide an understanding for resistance, although a study of *Prov. stuartii* mutants resistant to high levels of chlorhexidine failed to confirm this (Chopra *et al.*, 1987). Proteeae are usually intrinsically resistant to

the polymyxins and nitrofurantoins, possibly due to particular properties of their bacterial membranes.

REFERENCES

Albert, M.J., Ansaruzzaman, M., Bhuiyan, N.A., Neogi, P.K.B. and Faruque, A.S.G. (1995) Characteristics of invasion of HEp-2 cells by *Providencia alcalifaciens*. *Journal of Medical Microbiology*, **42**, 186–190.

Allison, C., Emödy, L., Coleman, N. and Hughes, C. (1994) The role of swarm cell differentiation and multicellular migration in the uropathogenicity of *Proteus mirabilis*. *Journal of Infectious Diseases*, **169**, 1155–1158.

Bahrani, F.K, Massad, G., Lockatell, C.V. *et al.* (1994) Construction of an MR/P fimbrial mutant of *Proteus mirabilis*: role in virulence in a mouse model of ascending urinary tract infection. *Infection and Immunity*, **62**, 3363–3371.

Bingen, E., Boissinot, C., Desjardins, P. *et al.* (1993) Arbitrarily primed polymerase chain reaction provides rapid differentiation of *Proteus mirabilis* isolates from a paediatric hospital. *Journal of Clinical Microbiology*, **31**, 1055–1059.

Brenner, D.J., Farmer, J.J., III, Fanning, G.R. *et al.* (1978) Deoxyribonucleic acid relatedness of *Proteus* and *Providencia* species. *International Journal of Systematic Bacteriology*, **28**, 269–282.

Brenner, D.J., Hickman-Brenner, F.W., Holmes, B. *et al.* (1995) Replacement of NCTC 4175, the current type strain of *Proteus vulgaris*, with ATCC 29905. *International Journal of Systematic Bacteriology*, **45**, 870–871.

Burke, J.P., Ingall, D., Klein, J.O., Gezon, H.M. and Finland, M. (1971) *Proteus mirabilis* infections in a hospital nursery traced to a human carrier. *New England Journal of Medicine*, **284**, 115–121.

Charles, I.G., Harford, S., Brookfield, J.F.Y. and Shaw, W.V. (1985) Resistance to chloramphenicol in *Proteus mirabilis* by expression of a chromosomal gene for chloramphenicol acetyltransferase. *Journal of Bacteriology*, **164**, 114–122.

Chopra, I., Johnson, S.C. and Bennett, P.M. (1987) Inhibition of *Providencia stuartii* cell envelope enzymes by chlorhexidine. *Journal of Antimicrobial Chemotherapy*, **19**, 743–751.

Chow, A.W., Taylor, P.R., Yoshikawa, T.T. and Guze, L.B. (1979) A nosocomial outbreak of infections due to multiply resistant *Proteus mirabilis*: role of intestinal colonisation as a major reservoir. *Journal of Infectious Diseases*, **139**, 621–627.

Cook, S.W., Mody, N., Valle, J. and Hull, R. (1995) Molecular cloning of *Proteus mirabilis* uroepithelial cell adherence (*uca*) genes. *Infection and Immunity*, **63**, 2082–2086.

Cornaglia, G., Dainelli, B., Berlutti, F. and Thaller, M.C. (1988) Commercial identification systems often fail to identify *Providencia stuartii*. *Journal of Clinical Microbiology*, **26**, 323–327.

Damron, D.J., Warren, J.W., Chippendale, G.R. and Tenney, J.H. (1986) Do clinical microbiology laboratories report complete bacteriology in urine from patients with long-term urinary catheters? *Journal of Clinical Microbiology*, **24**, 400–404.

Dealler, S.F., Hawkey, P.M. and Millar, M.R. (1988) Enzymatic degradation of urinary indoxyl sulphate by *Providencia stuartii* and *Klebsiella pneumoniae* causes the purple urine bag syndrome. *Journal of Clinical Microbiology*, **26**, 2152–2156.

D'Orazio, S.E.F. and Collins, C.M. (1993) Characterisation of a plasmid-encoded urease gene cluster found in members of the family Enterobacteriaceae. *Journal of Bacteriology*, **175**, 1860–1864.

Drechsel, H. Thieken, A., Reissbrodt, R., Jung, G. and Winkelmann, G. (1993) α-Keto acids are novel siderophores in the genera *Proteus*, *Providencia*, and *Morganella* and are produced by amino acid deaminases. *Journal of Bacteriology*, **175**, 2727–2733.

Dumanski, A.J., Hedelin, H., Edin-Liljegren, A., Beauchemin, D. and McLean, R.J.C. (1994) Unique ability of the *Proteus mirabilis* capsule to enhance mineral growth in infectious urinary calculi. *Infection and Immunity*, **62**, 2998–3003.

Ehrenkranz, N.J., Alfonso, B.C., Eckert, D.G. and Moskowitz, L.B. (1989) Proteeae species bacteriuria accompanying Proteeae species groin skin carriage in geriatric outpatients. *Journal of Clinical Microbiology*, **27**, 1988–1991.

Falkinham, J.O., III and Hoffman, P.S. (1984) Unique developmental characteristics of the swarm and short cells of *Proteus vulgaris* and *Proteus mirabilis*. *Journal of Bacteriology*, **158**, 1037–1040.

Farmer, J.J., III, Davis, B.R., Hickman-Brenner, F.W. *et al.* (1985) Biochemical identification of new species and biogroups of Enterobacteriaceae isolated from clinical specimens. *Journal of Clinical Microbiology*, **21**, 46–76.

Glennon, J., Ryan, P.J., Keane, C.T. and Rees, J.P. (1988) Circumcision and periurethral carriage of *Proteus mirabilis* in boys. *Archives of Disease in Childhood*, **63**, 556–557.

Hawkey, P.M. (1984) *Providencia stuartii*: a review of a multiply antibiotic-resistant bacterium. *Journal of Antimicrobial Chemotherapy*, **13**, 209–226.

Hawkey, P.M., Penner, J.L., Potten, M.R. *et al.* (1982) Prospective survey of fecal, urinary tract, and environmental colonization by *Providencia stuartii* in two geriatric wards. *Journal of Clinical Microbiology*, **16**, 422–426.

Hawkey, P.M., McCormick A. and Simpson, R.A. (1986a) Selective and differential medium for the primary isolation of members of the Proteeae. *Journal of Clinical Microbiology*, **23**, 600–603.

Hawkey, P.M., Penner, J.L., Linton, A.H., Hawkey, C.A., Crisp, L.J. and Hinton, M. (1986b) Speciation, serotyping, antimicrobial sensitivity and plasmid content of Proteeae from the environment of calf-rearing units in South West England. *Journal of Hygiene*, **97**, 405–417.

Haynes, J. and Hawkey, P.M. (1989) *Providencia alcalifaciens* and travellers diarrhoea. *British Medical Journal*, **299**, 94–95.

Hickman, F.W. and Farmer, J.J., III (1976). Differentiation of *Proteus mirabilis* by bacteriophage typing and the Dienes reaction. *Journal of Clinical Microbiology*, **3**, 350–358.

Hickman, W.W., Steigerwalt, A.G., Farmer, J.J., III and Brenner, D.J. (1982) Identification of *Proteus penneri* sp. nov., formerly known as *Proteus vulgaris* indole negative or as *Proteus vulgaris* biogroup I. *Journal of Clinical Microbiology*, **15**, 1097–1102.

Island, M.D. and Mobley, H.L.T. (1995) *Proteus mirabilis* urease operon fusion and linker insertion analysis of *ure* gene organisation, regulation and function. *Journal of Bacteriology*, **177**, 5653–5660.

Jensen, K.T., Frederiksen, W., Hickman-Brenner, R.W., Steigerwalt, A.G., Riddle, C.F. and Brenner, D.J. (1992) Recognition of *Morganella* subspecies with proposal of *Morganella morganii* supsp. *morganii* subsp. nov. and *Morganella morganii* subsp. *sibonii* subsp. nov. *International Journal of Systematic Bacteriology*, **42**, 613–620.

Johnson, D.E., Russell, R.G., Lockatell, C.V., Zulty, J.C., Warren, J.W. and Mobley, H.L. (1993) Contribution of *Proteus mirabilis* urease to persistence, urolithiasis, and acute pyelonephritis in a mouse model of ascending urinary tract infection. *Infection and Immunity*, **61**, 2748–2754.

Jones, B.D. and Mobley, H.L.T. (1987) Genetic and biochemical diversity of ureases of *Proteus*, *Providencia* and *Morganella* species isolated from urinary tract infection. *Infection and Immunity*, **55**, 2198–2203.

Kippax, P.W. (1957). A study of *Proteus* infections in a male urological ward. *Journal of Clinical Pathology*, **10**, 211–214.

Livermore, D.M. (1995) β-lactamases in laboratory and clinical resistance. *Clinical Microbiology Reviews*, **8**, 557–584.

McDermott, C. and Mylotte, J.M. (1984) *Morganella morganii*: epidemiology of bacteremic disease. *Infection Control*, **5**, 131–137.

Mobley, H.L.T. and Hausinger, R.P. (1989) Microbial ureases: significance, regulation and molecular characterization. *Microbiological Reviews*, **53**, 85–108.

Mobley, H.L.T. and Warren, J.W. (1987) Urease-positive bacteriuria and obstruction of long-term urinary catheters. *Journal of Clinical Microbiology*, **25**, 2216–2217.

Mobley, H.L.T., Chippendale, G.R., Tenney, J.H. *et al.* (1988) MR/K hemagglutination of *Providencia stuartii* correlates with adherence to catheters and with persistence in catheter-associated bacteriuria. *Journal of Infectious Diseases*, **157**, 264–271.

Müller, H.E., O'Hara, C.M., Fanning, G.R., Hickmann-Brenner, F.W., Swenson, J.M. and Brenner, D.J. (1986) *Providencia heimbachae*, a new species of Enterobacteriaceae isolated from animals. *International Journal of Systematic Bacteriology*, **36**, 252–256.

Muder, R.R., Brennen, C., Wagener, M.M. and Goetz, A.M. (1992) Bacteremia in a long-term-care facility: a five-year prospective study of 163 consecutive episodes. *Clinical Infectious Diseases*, **14**, 647–654.

Neuwirth, C. Siebor, E., Duez, J.M., Pechinot, A. and Kazmierczak, A. (1995) Imipenem resistance in clinical isolates of *Proteus mirabilis* associated with alterations in penicillin-binding proteins. *Journal of Antimicrobial Chemotherapy*, **36**, 335–342.

Payie, K.G., Rather, P.N. and Clarke, A.J. (1995) Contribution of gentamicin 2'-N-acetyltransferase to the O acetylation of peptidoglycan in *Providencia stuartii*. *Journal of Bacteriology*, **177**, 4303–4310.

Penner, J.L. (1981) The tribe Proteeae. In *The Prokaryotes: A Handbook on Habitats, Isolation and Identification of Bacteria* (eds M.P. Starr, H. Stolp, H.G. Truper, A. Balows and H.G. Schlegel). Springer-Verlag, Heidelberg, pp. 1204–1224.

Penner, J.L. and Hennessy, J.N. (1979) O Antigen grouping of *Morganella morganii* (*Proteus morganii*) by slide agglutination. *Journal of Clinical Microbiology*, **10**, 8–13.

Penner, J.L. and Hennessy, J.N. (1980) Separate O-grouping schemes for serotyping clinical isolates of *Proteus vulgaris* and *Proteus mirabilis*. *Journal of Clinical Microbiology*, **12**, 304–309.

Penner, J.L., Hinton, N.A. and Hennessy, J. (1974) Serotyping of *Proteus rettgeri* on the basis of O antigens. *Canadian Journal of Microbiology*, **20**, 777–789.

Penner, J.L., Hinton, N.A., Hennessy, J.N. and Whitely, G.R. (1976) Reconstruction of the somatic (O-) antigenic scheme for *Providencia* and preparation of O-typing antisera. *Journal of Infectious Diseases*, **133**, 283–291.

Penner, J.L., Fleming, P.C., Whiteley, G.R. and Hennessy, J.N. (1979). O-serotyping *Providencia alcalifaciens*. *Journal of Clinical Microbiology*, **10**, 761–765.

Rahav, G., Pinco, E., Silbaq, F. and Bercovier, H. (1994) Molecular epidemiology of catheter-associated bacteriuria in nursing home patients. *Journal of Clinical Microbiology*, **32**, 1031–1034.

Senior, B.W. (1976) Typing of *Proteus* strains by proticine production and sensitivity. *Journal of Medical Microbiology*, **10**, 7–17.

Senior, B.W. (1977) The Dienes phenomenon: identification of the determinants of compatibility. *Journal of General Microbiology*, **102**, 235–244.

Senior, B.W. and Leslie, D.L. (1986) Rare occurrence of *Proteus vulgaris* in faeces: a reason for its rare association with urinary tract infections. *Journal of Medical Microbiology*, **21**, 139–144.

Senior, B., Loomes, L. and Kerr, M. (1991) The production and activity *in vivo* of *Proteus mirabilis* Iga protease in infections of the urinary tract. *Journal of Medical Microbiology*, **35**, 203–207.

Thaller, M.C., Berlutti, F., Pantanella, F., Pompei, R. and Satta, G. (1992) Modified MacConkey medium which allows simple and reliable identification of *Providencia stuartii*. *Journal of Clinical Microbiology*, **30**, 2054–2057.

Tucci, V. and Isenberg, H.D. (1981) Hospital cluster epidemic with *Morganella morganii*. *Journal of Clinical Microbiology*, **14**, 563–566.

Warren, J.W. (1986) *Providencia stuartii*: a common cause of antibiotic-resistant bacteriuria in patients with long-term indwelling catheters. *Reviews of Infectious Diseases*, **8**, 61–67.

Warren, J.W., Tenney, J.H., Hoopes, J.M., Muncie, H.L. and Anthony, W.C. (1982) A prospective microbiological study of bacteriuria in patients with chronic indwelling urethral catheters. *Journal of Infectious Diseases*, **146**, 719–723.

Wassif, C., Cheek, D. and Belas, R. (1995). Molecular analysis of a metalloprotease from *Proteus mirabilis*. *Journal of Bacteriology*, **177**, 5790–5798.

Williams, E.W., Hawkey, P.M. Penner, J.L., Senior, B.W. and Barton, L.J. (1983) Serious nosocomial infection caused by *Morganella morganii* and *Proteus mirabilis* in cardiac surgery unit. *Journal of Clinical Microbiology*, **18**, 5–9.

12f

YERSINIA

M. Prentice

INTRODUCTION

The genus *Yersinia* contains three species which are well-established human pathogens. *Yersinia pestis* is responsible for plague, an often fulminant systemic zoonosis. *Y. pseudotuberculosis* and *Y. enterocolitica* cause yersiniosis, a self-limiting gastrointestinal illness that may have serious complications in special circumstances.

The characteristic signs of bubonic plague leave reliable historical records of epidemics (Christie and Corbel, 1990). The first pandemic (worldwide spread of the infection) began in the reign of the Roman Emperor Justinian in AD 541. The second pandemic, subsequently called the Black Death, began in Central Asia in the 1340s, before spreading across the whole of Europe, Asia and North Africa, killing a third of the population (Ziegler, 1982). The third pandemic began in the Yunan province of China in the 1870s and later spread to Hong Kong where in 1894 Alexandre Yersin and Shibasaburo Kitasato isolated the causative agent. During the third pandemic infection spread to ports in India, Africa, South America and the western coast of North America.

DESCRIPTION OF THE ORGANISM

Taxonomy

Yersinia pseudotuberculosis was first reported in 1889 from caseating lesions in rodents and was for many years classified with *Yersinia pestis* in the genus *Pasteurella* (Bercovier and Mollaret, 1984). *Yersinia enterocolitica* was first reported as a *Y. pseudotuberculosis*-like organism isolated from enteric specimens and skin lesions of patients in the USA (Schleifstein and Coleman, 1939) and later named *Bacterium enterocoliticum*. In the 1960s European microbiologists identified another heterogeneous group of bacteria resembling but distinct from *Yersinia* (then *Pasteurella*) *pseudotuberculosis* and termed them *Pasteurella* X. In 1964 Frederiksen pointed out similarities between *Pasteurella* X and *Bacterium enterocoliticum* and proposed the new species name *Yersinia enterocolitica* to cover this biochemically disparate group. *Yersinia intermedia*, *Y. frederiksenii*, *Y. kristensenii*, *Y. aldovae* *Y. mollaretti* and *Y. bercovieri* have subsequently been split off from *Y. enterocolitica sensu stricto* within the group of *Y.*

Principles and Practice of Clinical Bacteriology. Edited by A.M. Emmerson, P.M. Hawkey and S.H. Gillespie

enterocolitica-like organisms on biochemical and genetic grounds. They are of doubtful pathogenicity and little clinical significance. Apart from *Y. ruckeri*, a fish pathogen, DNA relatedness among *Yersinia* spp. is at least 40% and *Y. pestis* and *Y. pseudotuberculosis* have DNA relatedness of over 90%. The molar G + C ratio of *Yersinia* is 46–50%, consistent with that for Enterobacteriaceae (Bercovier and Mollaret, 1984).

Physiological Characteristics

The organisms are Gram-negative coccobacilli or short rods with rounded ends 1–3 μm long and 0.5–0.8 μm in diameter (Bercovier and Mollaret, 1984; Mair and Fox, 1986). They are non-sporing and only *Y. pestis* strains (grown *in vivo* or at 37 °C) form a capsule (Brubaker, 1991). *Yersinia pestis* in particular demonstrates bipolar staining and pleomorphism. *Yersinia pestis* is non-motile but all other species are motile at 25 °C and non-motile at 37 °C. All species are facultative anaerobes and produce catalase but not oxidase.

All yersiniae grow on nutrient agar forming smaller colonies than other Enterobacteriaceae. All have a growth optimum of less than 37 °C (25–29 °C) and grow over a range of 4–42 °C. *Yersinia pestis* requires 48 hours incubation to produce 1 mm colonies at 25–37 °C whereas the enteropathogenic yersiniae produce visible colonies after 24 hours. *Yersinia pestis* colonies are opaque, smooth and round with irregular edges whereas other *Yersinia* spp. rapidly produce smooth-edged colonies with an elevated centre. Yersiniae are non-haemolytic on blood agar. Although *Y. enterocolitica* grows well on MacConkey agar and other enteric media, *Y. pestis* and *Y. pseudotuberculosis* grow poorly on MacConkey agar on primary isolation (however, laboratory-adapted *Y. pseudotuberculosis* strains may flourish) (Mair and Fox, 1986). Iron is required for the growth of all yersiniae and is important in pathogenicity.

PATHOGENICITY

Yersinia pestis must cause disseminated infection in the mammalian host for transmission by a flea vector or the respiratory route. *Yersinia pseudotuberculosis* and *Y. enterocolitica* are more likely to be transmitted if the host remains alive to spread the infection by chronic faecal excretion. The main virulence factors are listed in Table 12e.1. All the pathogenic yersiniae share a tropism for lymphoid tissue and an ability to avoid the non-specific immune response of the host. Although they grow well in macrophage cell lines, in animal models of disease they are predominantly extracellular (Cornelis, 1992).

Pathogenicity Factors Unique to *Y. pestis*

Isolates of *Y. pestis* possess two plasmids not found in other *Yersinia* spp. (Brubaker, 1991) that encode virulence factors; the 100 kb Tox plasmid and the 9.5 kb Pst plasmid (see Table 12f.1). In addition to promoting disseminated infection by fibrinolysis, the plasminogen activator produced by the Pst plasmid also affects expression of other virulence factors encoded by the Lcr plasmid found in all pathogenic yersiniae (see below). Virulent *Y. pestis* strains possess the property of pigmentation. This describes the brown coloration colonies acquire on haemin-containing media by storing haemin in the outer membrane. White (non-pigmented) *Y. pestis* mutants arise spontaneously on plating a fully virulent strain on media containing haemin and are of greatly reduced virulence in mice, but virulence is restored in mice that are overloaded with iron or haemin (Jackson and Burrows, 1957). The mammalian host restricts the availability of iron required for the growth of invading microbial pathogens by sequestration and successful pathogens have evolved systems for evading this restriction. The pigmented phenotype is genetically linked with other iron metabolism-related virulence factors. It is thought to be important for survival in the flea gut and may also serve as an initial iron source in the early stages of infection and promote uptake into eukaryotic cells and subsequent intracellular survival (Perry, 1993).

TABLE 12f.1   VIRULENCE FACTORS OF *YERSINIA*

Yersinia species	Virulence factor	Gene (if cloned)	Gene Location	Action
Y. pestis only	Fraction 1 antigen (Galyov *et al.*, 1990) Murine exotoxin (Brubaker, 1991)	*caf 1*	100 kb Tox plasmid	Inhibits phagocytosis Lethal for mice and rats only
	Plasminogen activator (Brubaker, 1991)	*pla*	9.5 kb Pst plasmid	Dissemination from subcutaneous injection
Y. pestis and *Y. pseudo-tuberculosis*	pH 6 antigen (Lindler and Tall, 1993)	*psaA*	Chromosomal	Forms fimbriae facilitating cell entry
All pathogenic yersiniae	Low calcium response (Cornelis, 1992; Straley *et al.*, 1993)	*yadA*, *yopH*, *lcrV*, etc.	70 kb Lcr/pYV plasmid	Complex operon: see text
	Lipopolysaccharide (Brubaker, 1991; Skurnik and Toivanen, 1993)	*rfb*	Chromosomal	Endotoxin activity Serum resistance
Mouse-lethal strains of all three species	HMWP (high molecular weight proteins) Carniel *et al.*, 1992; de Almeida *et al.*, 1993)	*irp2*	Chromosomal	Iron metabolism related. Possibly synthesis of yersiniabactin
Mouse-lethal *Y. enterocolitica* and *Y. pseudo-tuberculosis*	Yersiniabactin (Heesemann *et al.*, 1993)		Chromosomal	Siderophore (not yet demonstrated in *Y. pestis*)
Entero-pathogenic yersiniae only	Inv protein Ail protein (Cornelis, 1992)	*inv* *ail*	Chromosomal	Invasion of mammalian epithelial cells
Y. enterocolitica only	Myf antigen (Iriarte *et al.*, 1993)	*myfA*	Chromosomal	Homologous to pH6 antigen, i.e. fimbrial structure
	ST toxin (Cornelis, 1992)	*yst*	Chromosomal	Resembles *E. coli* ST toxin

Pathogenicity Factors Shared by *Y. pestis* and *Y. pseudotuberculosis*

The pH 6 antigen is a fibrillar protein first described in *Y. pestis* grown at pH ≤ 6.7 and > 37 °C. Its expression is associated with a more rapidly progressive illness after *Y. pestis* infection in mice (Lindler and Tall, 1993).

Pathogenicity Factors Common to All Pathogenic Yersiniae

The YV (associated with *Yersinia* virulence) or Lcr (Low calcium response) plasmid is a 70 kb plasmid essential for virulence in all three pathogenic species. It controls a complex reaction in which *in vitro* vegetative growth is restricted when yersiniae are grown at 37 °C in low calcium concentrations (<2.5 mM Ca^{2+}). At the same time a series of proteins encoded by the virulence plasmid is produced and in some cases secreted in quantity. The growth restriction is reversed either by reduction of temperature to 26 °C or by the addition of Ca^{2+}. The proteins produced include Yops (Cornelis, 1992; Straley *et al.*, 1993) (originally an acronym for Yersinia outer membrane proteins: they are now known not to be membrane anchored) and the adhesin YadA. Eleven Yops have been identified in *Y. enterocolitica*, most of which have homologues in the other species. In *Y. pestis* all Yops apart from Lcr V (the cytoplasmic V antigen) are hydrolysed after excretion by the outer membrane plasminogen activator encoded by the Pst plasmid. The functions of some Yops are now known. YopE is cytotoxic for HeLa cells, YopH is a tyrosine phosphatase with potential disruptive effects on macrophage regulation, and YopM inhibits platelet aggregation. YadA forms a fibrillar matrix on the surface of the enteropathogenic yersiniae, making them adherent to eukaryotic cells and promoting intestinal colonization. It is produced at 37 °C irrespective of the Ca^{2+} concentration. In *Y. pestis* the *yadA* gene is inactive, suggesting that YadA and most of the Yops (hydrolysed in *Y. pestis*) are adaptations to the more chronic form of parasitism seen in gastrointestinal yersiniosis. Regulation by Ca^{2+} was originally thought to mean that Yops would be induced by the calcium-restricted intracellular environment of the host after invasion had occurred, but as mentioned above there is increasing evidence that yersiniae spread and multiply extracellularly where Ca^{2+} concentrations are greater than 2.5 mM, and current research is directed to resolving how Yops are induced *in vivo* in this environment (Cornelis, 1992).

Lipopolysaccharide from *Y. pestis* has endotoxin-like properties and is partially responsible for serum resistance, although the organism is rough (lacks extended O-group chains, only one serotype) (Brubaker, 1991). The enteropathogenic yersiniae can produce longer O-group side chains corresponding to the different serotypes, and *rfb* genes partially responsible for this in *Y. enterocolitica* and *Y. pseudotuberculosis* have been cloned (Skurnik and Toivanen, 1993).

Pathogenicity Factors in Mouse-lethal Yersiniae Belonging to All Three Species

Two high molecular weight proteins (HMWP1 and HMWP2) are synthesized only in conditions of iron starvation (such as those encountered after host invasion). The gene for HMWP2, *irp2*, is linked to the gene for pigmentation in *Y. pestis*,

but unlike pigmentation is expressed in all three pathogenic species. It has a narrower distribution than the pYV plasmid, only being found in the highly virulent 'American' *Y. enterocolitica* O:8 strains and more virulent strains of *Y. pseudotuberculosis* (Carniel *et al.*, 1992; de Almeida *et al.*, 1993). It may be involved in synthesis of the siderophore yersiniabactin (Heesemann *et al.*, 1993).

Siderophores (small non-protein molecules secreted by the bacterial cell to chelate iron and be reabsorbed via a receptor) are well known in Enterobacteriaceae. Yersiniabactin is produced by *Y. pseudotuberculosis* and mouse-lethal *Y. enterocolitica* (it has not yet been demonstrated in *Y. pestis*). Enteropathogenic low-virulence *Y. enterocolitica* strains unable to produce yersiniabactin can, however, utilize siderophores produced by other bacteria (e.g. desferrioxamine B) (Perry, 1993) and these substances potentiate their virulence.

Pathogenicity Factors in Enteropathogenic Yersiniae

The chromosomal genes found in *Y. enterocolitica* *inv* (*inv*asion) and *ail* (*a*ttachment-*inv*asion *l*ocus) when introduced into non-invasive *Escherichia coli*. confer the ability to penetrate cultured human epithelial cells. Only pathogenic serotypes of *Y. enterocolitica* produce these two proteins (Cornelis, 1992). *Yersinia pseudotuberculosis* produces Inv but not Ail and neither protein is produced by *Y. pestis*. Synthesis of Inv is maximal at 28 °C and that of Ail at 37 °C. *Yersinia enterocolitica* produces a heat-stable enterotoxin which has the same mode of action as the heat-stable toxin STa of *E. coli* (see page 376) (Cornelis, 1992) and a fibrillar adhesin Myf (Iriarte *et al.*, 1993).

EPIDEMIOLOGY

Normal Habitat

Yersinia pestis is primarily a rodent pathogen usually transmitted by the bite of an infected flea and therefore has two main habitats: in the stomach or proventriculus of various flea species at ambient temperature, or in the bloodstream or tissues of a rodent host at body temperature. There is an inanimate reservoir in the soil of rodent burrows after their inhabitants have died (Bercovier and Mollaret, 1984) but *Y. pestis* has exacting nutritional requirements that make it less well equipped to survive in the environment than the other *Yersinia* spp. *Yersinia pseudotuberculosis* and *Y. enterocolitica* are spread by the enteric route and their habitat is either in the host's gut or its associated lymphatic tissue, or in the food and water by which the host is infected. *Y. enterocolitica* strains lacking virulence determinants and other avirulent *Yersinia* spp. are frequently found in the environment (including human foods) and can be isolated in equal frequency from the stools of asymptomatic and symptomatic humans (Van Noyen *et al.*, 1981). Outbreaks of disease related to food or water supplies contaminated with fully virulent *Y. enterocolitica* are well described (Cover and Aber, 1989; Lee *et al.*, 1990).

Yersinia pestis has been isolated from all continents and plague is enzootic in Africa, North and South America and Asia (Middle East, Far East, and countries of the former USSR), following the third pandemic (Christie and Corbel, 1990; Butler, 1983, 1989). Many different combinations of rodent and flea vector species have been described. Classically, efficient flea vectors feeding on an infected host permit the establishment of *Y. pestis* in the proventriculus. Subsequent 'blocking' of the gastrointestinal tract with an overgrowth of *Y. pestis* and regurgitation of infected blood introduces the pathogen into the bloodstream of a new host (Christie and Corbel, 1990; Butler, 1983). Sylvatic plague with a cycle of infection in rodents outside urban areas is the rule. Between 1977 and 1991, 14 752 cases of plague with 1391 deaths were reported to the World Health Organization. Most of the cases were from Africa and Asia. The USA, which contains a relatively large enzootic focus, contributed only 255 human cases over this period because the areas involved are rural and largely uninhabited. In 1994 the first outbreaks of plague in India for almost 30 years

occurred in two neighbouring districts in the north west of the country. Many facts about these outbreaks were unclear at the time but doubts about the diagnosis have subsequently been settled (Ramalingaswami, 1995). There may have been 58 deaths (Mavalankar, 1995). Generally, urban plague requires contact with infected fleas from urban rodents. Worldwide the urban black rat *Rattus rattus* is the most important reservoir and *Xenopsylla cheopis* (the oriental rat flea) is the most efficient vector for human disease (Christie and Corbel, 1990; Butler, 1983). Transmission can also occur from human to human by the human flea *Pulex irritans* or by the respiratory route from human to human or domestic animal to human (Benenson, 1990).

Yersinia pseudotuberculosis also causes a zoonosis of wild and domestic animals with man as an incidental host (Bercovier and Mollaret, 1984; Butler, 1983). Disease incidence is highest in the winter months and results from contact with sick or asymptomatic animals, or ingestion of food or water contaminated with their excreta. *Yersinia enterocolitica* exists worldwide in the environment as commensal biotype 1A strains but the disease-causing serotypes are more frequently identified with a specific host. Serotype O:9 and O:3 strains are the predominant types associated with diarrhoea in northern Europe and disease is more common in autumn/winter (Cover and Aber, 1989; Butler, 1983; Tauxe *et al.*, 1987; Prentice *et al.* 1991). Human disease is linked to asymptomatic infection in pigs and consumption of pork products (Tauxe *et al.*, 1987) and in Belgium, Scandinavia and other northern European countries (Cover and Aber, 1989; Tauxe *et al.*, 1987; Working Group, 1981) *Y. enterocolitica* ranks with *Campylobacter* as a cause of diarrhoea. In the UK infection is less common but there was evidence of increasing incidence during the late 1980s (Prentice *et al.*, 1991). In the USA sporadic infection is uncommonly reported but outbreaks are well recognized, and serotype O:3 strains are now more commonly isolated than the highly pathogenic O:8 biotype 1B strains which used to predominate (Lee *et al.*, 1990).

CLINICAL FEATURES

Plague

Lymphadenitis in the regional lymph nodes draining the area of the flea bite produces a tense tender swelling or bubo after two to six days incubation in cases of bubonic plague. Fever and prostration are usual and progression to septicaemic plague with meningitis or secondary pneumonia can occur. Pneumonic plague may result in transmission of infection by aerosol. Primary septicaemia can occur in the absence of a bubo. Untreated bubonic plague has a mortality of 50–90% and untreated meningitis or septicaemia is usually fatal (Christie and Corbel, 1990; Butler, 1983).

Yersiniosis

Yersinia pseudotuberculosis (Christie and Corbel, 1990; Bercovier and Mollaret, 1984; Butler, 1983, Benenson, 1990) causes mesenteric adenitis and chronic diarrhoea in animals that resolves spontaneously or progresses to a fatal septicaemia with widespread caseating lesions developing in lymphatic tissue. Humans develop a mesenteric adenitis that may simulate appendicitis (pseudoappendicitis). With improvements in water quality infection has become rare. Far Eastern scarlatiniform fever is an epidemic form of *Y. pseudotuberculosis* characterized by a rash, arthralgia and polyarthritis reported from the eastern territories of the former USSR and Japan.

Yersinia enterocolitica causes an enteritis and occasionally pseudoappendicitis (as a result of terminal ileitis rather than mesenteric adenitis) with an incubation period of 1–11 days (Cover and Aber, 1989). Infection can occasionally be chronic and relapsing (Hoogkamp-Korstanje *et al.*, 1988). Most infections are in children under five years of age. Pseudoappendicitis is more common in young adults. Spontaneous resolution is the norm but certain groups such as iron-overloaded patients (e.g. thalassaemia, haemochromatosis, iron supplement overdose), those with liver disease or diabetes and the elderly are at increased risk of a septicaemic illness with a fatal outcome

(Cover and Aber, 1989; Prentice *et al.*, 1991). *Yersinia enterocolitica* may be a more common cause of mycotic aneurysm than *Salmonella* spp. in some populations (Prentice *et al.* 1993). Medical interventions associated with systemic disease include the use of desferrioxamine (iron chelation therapy in thalassaemia) and blood transfusion. The latter occurs when a blood donor has asymptomatic bacteraemia at the time of donation and depends on the ability of *Y. enterocolitica* to grow at 4 °C in stored blood (Prentice, 1992). Immunological complications are important especially in northern Europe, where HLA-B27 is frequent (Hermann *et al.*, 1993). Reactive arthritis follows several weeks after diarrhoea, with other complications such as erythema nodosum and glomerulonephritis. *Yersinia enterocolitica* antibodies are found in autoimmune thyroid disease patients in these countries (Cover and Aber, 1989).

LABORATORY DIAGNOSIS

Plague

In known endemic areas the clinical features described above are well recognized and a presumptive diagnosis may be made on the appearance of bipolar staining Gram-negative rods from a bubo aspirate, cerebrospinal fluid (CSF) or sputum. Recent events in India have shown that diagnosis may not be easy in countries where plague is rarely seen. For example *Burkholderia pseudomallei* (causing melioidosis, prevalent in South East Asia) may have a similar bipolar staining appearance and may cause both respiratory symptoms and lymphadenopathy. In the USA pneumonic plague has been misdiagnosed as hantanvirus pulmonary syndrome (Centers for Disease Control, 1994). Diagnostic techniques include direct immunofluorescence using antibody to the F1 antigen, detection of rising titres in a passive haemagglutination test for F1 antibody (WHO Expert Committee, 1970) and antigen detection by gene probes (McDonough *et al.*, 1988). Culture of non-contaminated samples (blood, lymph nodes) can be performed as for other yersiniae (below) and animal inoculation is employed for contaminated specimens. Microscopy and culture are the most widely available diagnostic techniques for plague and culture is essential for epidemiological investigation of new outbreaks. However, *Y. pestis* is a Hazard Group 3 (P3) pathogen and clinical material and cultures should be handled in a Class 1 protective cabinet within a Hazard Group 3 facility by workers wearing protective clothing, gloves, face mask and goggles or a visor. The reference laboratory in the USA is the plague Section, Division of Vector-Borne Infectious Diseases, Centers for Disease Control, PO Box 2087, Fort Collins, CO 80522 USA. Facilities for the diagnosis of imported cases in the United Kingdom are available at the Laboratory of Enteric Pathogens, Central Public Health Laboratory, 61 Colindale Avenue, London NW9 5HT (Cheasty and Rowe, 1994).

Yersiniosis

Isolation from clinical material free from contamination (blood culture, lymph nodes) is by culture on conventional media (blood agar, nutrient agar) incubated at 25 °C and 37 °C (Mair and Fox, 1986). Growth occurs in conventional and proprietary blood culture broths but prolonged incubation may be required for primary isolation. For isolation from faeces, routine enteric media such as MacConkey, desoxycholate or SS agar incubated at 25–30 °C for 48 hours can be used. A selective medium specifically for yersiniae, cefsulodin–irgasan–novobiocin (CIN) agar, incubated at 30 °C, is commercially available. Cold enrichment by incubation in phosphate-buffered saline at 4 °C for three weeks is extremely effective at encouraging the overgrowth of yersiniae in mixed culture with other Enterobacteriaceae. This is impractical in a routine diagnostic service and may promote the isolation of commensal yersiniae (Van Noyen *et al.*, 1981). *Yersinia pseudotuberculosis* is rarely isolated from faeces culture even in proven cases of human infection, and diagnosis is usually serological (Mair and Fox, 1986). Gene probes and polymerase chain reaction (PCR) techniques for detection of pYV plasmid (Wren, 1990) or chromosomal target genes (Nakajima *et al.*, 1992) have been described.

Identification of *Yersinia*

Table 12f.2 gives the main reactions distinguishing the species- and other genus-specific characteristics have been mentioned under the general description above. The API-20E kit (bioMerieux) incubated at 28 °C reliably identifies *Y. enterocolitica* and *Y. pseudotuberculosis* (Sharma *et al.*, 1990). Further

TABLE 12f.2   CHARACTERISTICS OF *YERSINIA* SPECIES

Test	Y. pestis	Y. pseudotuberculosis	Y. enterocolitica	Y. intermedia	Y. frederiksenii	Y. kristensenii
Motility (37 °C)	–	–	–	–	–	–
Motility (25 °C)	–	+	+	+	+	–
Ornithine decarboxylase	–	–	+	+	+	+
Lysine decarboxylase	–	–	–	–	–	–
Urease	–	+	+	+	+	+
Gelatinase	–	–	–	–	–	–
Voges–Proskauer (25 °C)	–	–	+	+	+	–
Indole	–	–	d	+	+	d
Simmon's Citrate	–	–	–	+	d	–
Acid production						
Glucose	+	+	+	+	+	+
Rhamnose	–	+	–	+	+	–
Sucrose	–	–	+	+	+	–
Melibiose	d	+	–	+	–	–
Sorbitol	–	–	+	+	+	+

All species are catalase positive, oxidase negative; none forms H_2S in TSI medium.
+, 90% or more of strains positive; –, 90% or more strains negative; d, 11–89% strains positive.
Adapted from Bercovier and Mollaret (1984). Biochemical tests incubated at 28 °C for three days unless indicated.

biochemical characterization of *Y. enterocolitica*-like strains into five biovars and different species is possible (Bercovier and Mollaret, 1984; Corbel, 1990). In the clinical laboratory dealing with fresh isolates the possession of the pYV-related property of pigmentation and small colony growth on Congo red–magnesium oxalate agar (CR-MOX) at 37 °C gives useful information about clinical significance. As a plasmid-related property this may be lost on repeated subculture but simultaneous testing for non-plasmid-derived factors associated with virulent serotypes (such as the absence of pyrazinamidase and the inability to ferment salicin or aesculin) overcomes this (Farmer *et al.*, 1992). Phage typing schemes for *Y. enterocolitica* and *Y. pseudotuberculosis* are available. The main serotypes associated with disease in Europe are O : 9, O : 3 and O : 5,27. These are of low virulence with little capacity to cause systemic disease outside the risk groups outlined above. Biotype 1B, serotype O : 8 strains mainly found in North America have the capacity to cause severe disease in non-iron-overloaded hosts, presumably because they possess the iron-related virulence factors of yersiniabactin and high-molecular weight proteins.

Serology

A passive haemagglutination test using *Y. pestis* Fraction 1 antigen (unique to *Y. pestis*) is available in countries where plague is endemic (Butler, 1983; WHO Expert Committee, 1970). Whole cell agglutination antibody is diagnostic for infection with serogroups I, III and V of *Y. pseudotuberculosis* but groups II and IV share O antigen sugars with group B and D salmonellae (Mair and Fox, 1986). High titres may be obtained soon after onset of symptoms. *Yersinia enterocolitica* agglutinating antibodies are more likely to be found in convalescence (Mair and Fox, 1986). *Y. enterocolitica* O : 9 strains share polysaccharide antigens with *Brucella abortus* and cross-reactions between O : 5,27 strains and *E. coli* also occur. ELISA assays have demonstrated elevated classes or subclasses of immunoglobin in patients with autoimmune complications (Hoogkamp-Korstanje *et al.*, 1992).

Antimicrobial Sensitivities

Yersinia pestis in vitro is sensitive to most agents active against Gram-negative bacteria. Resistance in human isolates is unusual and resistance has not emerged during therapy (Butler, 1983). Antibiotics active *in vitro* include streptomycin, chloramphenicol, tetracycline, ampicillin, cotrimoxazole and cephalothin. A similar spectrum is seen for *Y. pseudotuberculosis* (Soriano and Vega, 1982) but *Y. enterocolitica* strains have a constitutive penicillinase and may also possess a chromosomally mediated inducible cephalosporinase (Pham *et al.*, 1991). The newer third-generation cephalosporin, quinolone and penem antimicrobials are active *in vitro* against all *Yersinia* spp. (Soriano and Vega, 1982; Lyons *et al.*, 1991), including *Y. pestis* (Bonacorsi *et al.*, 1994).

TREATMENT

Streptomycin is the most effective treatment for plague, at a dose of 1 g twice daily (30 mg/kg per day) for 10 days (Butler, 1983, 1989; Benenson, 1990; Tauxe *et al.*, 1987). Oral tetracycline is recommended for plague meningitis at a dose of 4 g per day (60 mg/kg per day) in four divided doses for 10 days after a loading dose of 25 mg/kg.

Yersiniosis is usually a self-limiting condition but for chronic or relapsing illness with *Y. enterocolitica*, focal disease outside the gastrointestinal tract or septicaemia, cotrimoxazole or ciprofloxacin has been recommended (Hoogkamp-Korstanje, 1988). Opinions are divided on the efficacy of third-generation cephalosporins *in vivo* (Soriano *et al.*, 1988). *Yersinia pseudotuberculosis* is treated with similar agents and, as β-lactamases are absent, ampicillin is also used (Mair and Fox, 1986).

PREVENTION AND CONTROL

The control of plague is based on reducing the likelihood of people being bitten by infected fleas or exposed to aerosols from humans or animals with plague pneumonia. A detailed summary of the international and patient-centred measures in force to prevent the spread of plague from and within enzootic areas is available (Benenson, 1990). It is an internationally quarantinable disease. Current vaccines are restricted in application by local and systemic reactions and short duration of protective immunity, and indicated only for those working with live *Y. pestis* in laboratories or likely to be in contact with rats and fleas in endemic areas (Butler, 1983; Benenson, 1990).

Person-to-person spread of yersiniosis has been described but is rarely demonstrated. Most documented outbreaks have been food or water borne (Cover and Aber, 1989; Tauxe *et al.*, 1987; Prentice *et al.*, 1991). Control is based on the avoidance of consumption of contaminated food and water. The food industry has to be particularly alert to avoid contamination of products whose safety is assured by refrigeration with psychrotrophic yersiniae able to grow at 4 °C. The rare syndrome of *Y. enterocolitica* donor blood contamination follows a similar pattern and control measures have proved difficult to devise. The need for bacteriological investigation of transfusion reactions must be emphasised (Prentice, 1992; McDonald *et al.*, 1996).

REFERENCES

Benenson, A.S. (ed.) (1990) *Control of Communicable Diseases in Man*, 15th edn. American Public Health Association, Washington, DC.

Bercovier, H. and Mollaret, H.H. (1984) Genus XIV. Yersinia. In *Bergey's Manual of Systematic Bacteriology* (eds N.R. Krieg and J.G. Holt), pp. 498–506. Williams & Wilkins, Baltimore.

Bonacorsi, S.P., Scavizzi, M.R., Guiyoule, A. *et al.* (1994) Assessment of a fluoroquinolone, 3 beta-lactams, 2 aminoglycosides, and a cycline in treatment of murine *Yersinia pestis* infection. *Antimicrobial Agents and Chemotherapy*, **38**, 481–486.

Brubaker, R.R. (1991) Factors promoting acute and chronic diseases caused by yersiniae. *Clinical Microbiology Reviews*, **4**, 309–324.

Butler, T. (1983) *Plague and Other Yersinia Infections*. Plenum Press, New York.

Butler, T. (1989) The black death past and present. 1. Plague in the 1980s. *Transactions of the Royal Society of Tropical Medicine and Hygiene*, **83**, 458–460.

Carniel, E., Guiyoule, A., Guilvout, I. *et al* (1992)

Molecular cloning, iron-regulation and mutagenesis of the *irp2* gene encoding HMWP2, a protein specific for the highly pathogenic *Yersinia*. *Molecular Microbiology*, **6**, 379–388.

Centers for Disease Control (1994) Human plague – United States 1993–4. *MMWR*, **43**, 242–246.

Cheasty, T. and Rowe, B. (1994) Plague: bacteriology and laboratory aspects. *PHLS Microbiology Digest*, **11**, 220–223.

Christie, A.B. and Corbel, M.J. (1990) Plague and other yersinial diseases. In *Bacterial Diseases*, 8th edn (ed. G.R. Smith and C.S.F. Easmon), pp. 399–421. Edward Arnold, London.

Corbel, M.J. (1990) *Yersinia*. In *Systematic Bacteriology*, 8th edn (ed. M.T. Parker and B.L. Duerden), pp. 495–512. Edward Arnold, London.

Cornelis, G.R. (1992) Yersiniae, finely tuned pathogens. In *Molecular Biology of Bacterial Infection: Current Status and Future Perspectives* (ed. C.E. Hormaeche, C.W. Penn and C.J. Smith), pp. 231–264. Cambridge University Press, Dublin.

Cover, T.L. and Aber, R.C. (1989) *Yersinia enterocolitica*. *New England Journal of Medicine*, **321**, 16–24.

de Almeida, A.M.P., Guiyoule, A., Guilvout, I. *et al.* (1993) Chromosomal *irp2* gene in *Yersinia*: distribution, expression, deletion and impact on virulence. *Microbial Pathogenesis*, **14**, 9–21.

Farmer, J.J., Carter, G.P., Miller, V.L. *et al.* (1992) Pyrazinamidase, CR-MOX agar, salicin fermentation-esculin hydrolysis, and *d*-xylose fermentation for identifying pathogenic serotypes of *Yersinia enterocolitica*. *Journal of Clinical Microbiology*, **30**, 2589–2594.

Frederiksen, W. (1964). A study of some *Yersinia pseudotuberculosis*-like bacteria (*Bacterium enterocoliticum'* and 'Pasteurella X'). *Proceedings of the 14th Scandinavian Congress of Pathology and Microbiology*, pp. 103–104. Norwegian Universities Press, Oslo.

Galyov, E.E., Smirnov, O.Y., Karlishev, A.V. *et al.* (1990) Nucleotide-sequence of the *Yersinia pestis* gene encoding F1 antigen and the primary structure of the protein – putative T-cell and B-cell epitopes. *Febs Letters*, **277**, 230–232.

Heesemann, J., Hantke, K., Vocke, T. *et al.* (1993) Virulence of *Yersinia enterocolitica* is closely associated with siderophore production, expression of an iron-repressible outer membrane polypeptide of 65,000 Da and pesticin sensitivity. *Molecular Microbiology*, **8**, 397–408.

Hermann, E., Yu, D.T.Y., Meyer zum Buschenfelde, K.-H. *et al.* (1993) HLA-B27-restricted CD8 T cells derived from synovial fluids of patients with reactive arthritis and ankylosing spondylitis. *Lancet*, **342**, 646–650.

Hoogkamp-Korstanje, J.A.A. (1988) Antibiotics in *Yersinia enterocolitica* infections. *Journal of Antimicrobial Chemotherapy*, **20**, 123–131.

Hoogkamp-Korstanje, J.A.A., de Koning, J. and Heeseman, J. (1988) Persistence of *Yersinia enterocolitica* in man. *Infection*, **16**, 81–85.

Hoogkamp-Korstanje, J.A.A., de Koning, J., Heesemann, J. *et al.* (1992) Influence of antibiotics on IgA and IgG response and persistence of *Yersinia enterocolitica* in patients with *Yersinia*-associated spondylarthropathy. *Infection*, **20**, 53–57.

Iriarte M., Vanooteghem, J.C., Delor, I. *et al.* (1993) The Myf fibrillae of *Yersinia enterocolitica*. *Molecular Microbiology*, **9**, 507–520.

Jackson, S. and Burrows, T.W. (1957) The virulence enhancing effect of iron on non-pigmented mutants of virulent strains of *Pasteurella pestis*. *British Journal of Experimental Pathology*, **37**, 577–583.

Lee, L.A., Gerber, A.R., Lonsway, D.R. *et al.* (1990) *Yersinia enterocolitica* O:3 infections in infants and children associated with the preparation of chitterlings. *New England Journal of Medicine*, **322**, 984–987.

Lindler, L.E. and Tall, B.E. (1993) *Yersinia pestis* pH 6 antigen forms fimbriae and is induced by intracellular association with macrophages. *Molecular Microbiology*, **8**, 311–324.

Lyons, M.M., Prentice, M.B., Cope, D. *et al.* (1991) Antimicrobial susceptibility of pathogenic *Yersinia enterocolitica* strains in the British Isles. In *Current Investigations of the Microbiology of Yersiniae* (ed. T. Une, T. Maruyama and M. Tsubokura), pp. 251–254. Karger, Basel.

Mair, N.S. and Fox, E. (1986) *Yersiniosis*. Public Health Laboratory Service, London.

Mavalankar, D.V. (1995) Indian plague epidemic – unanswered questions and key lessons. *Journal Of the Royal Society of Medicine*, **88**, 547–551.

McDonald, C.P., Barbara, J.A.J., Hewitt, P.E. *et al.* (1996) *Yersinia enterocolitica* transmission from a red-cell unit 34 days old. *Transfusion Medicine*, **6**, 61–63.

McDonough, K.A., Schwan, T.G., Thomas, R.E. *et al.* (1988) Identification of a *Yersinia pestis*-specific DNA probe with potential for use in plague surveillance. *Journal of Clinical Microbiology*, **26**, 2515–2519.

Nakajima, H., Inoue, M., Mori, T. *et al.* (1992) Detection and identification of *Yersinia pseudotuberculosis* and pathogenic *Yersinia enterocolitica* by an improved polymerase chain reaction. *Journal of Clinical Microbiology*, **30**, 2484–2486.

Perry, R.D. (1993) Acquisition and storage of inorganic iron and hemin by the yersiniae. *Trends in Microbiology*, **1**, 142–147.

Pham, J., Bell, S.M. and Lanzarone, J.Y.M. (1991) A study of the β-lactamases of 100 clinical isolates of *Yersinia enterocolitica*. *Journal of Antimicrobial Chemotherapy*, **28**, 19–24.

Prentice, M.B. (1992) *Yersinia enterocolitica* and blood transfusion. *British Medical Journal*, **305**, 663–664.

Prentice, M.B., Cope, D. and Swann, R.A. (1991) Epidemiology of *Yersinia enterocolitica* in the British Isles 1986–1989. In *Current Investigations of the Microbiology of Yersiniae* (ed. T. Une, T. Maruyama and M. Tsubokura). Karger, Basel.

Prentice, M.B., Fortineau, N., Lambert, T. *et al.* (1993) *Yersinia enterocolitica* and mycotic aneurysm. *Lancet*, **341**, 1535–1536.

Ramalingaswami, V. (1995) Plague in India. *Nature Medicine*, **1**, 1237–1239.

Schleifstein, J.I. and Coleman, M.B. (1939) An unidentified microorganism resembling *B. lignieri* and *Past. pseudotuberculosis*, and pathogenic for man. *New York State Journal of Medicine*, **39**, 1749–1753.

Sharma, N.K., Doyle, P.W., Gerbasi, S.A. *et al.* (1990) Identification of *Yersinia* species by the API 20E. *Journal of Clinical Microbiology*, **28**, 1443–1444.

Skurnik, M. and Toivanen, P. (1993) *Yersinia enterocolitica* lipopolysaccharide: genetics and virulence. *Trends in Microbiology*, **1**, 148–152.

Soriano, F. and Vega, J. (1982) The susceptibility of *Yersinia* to eleven antimicrobials. *Journal of Antimicrobial Chemotherapy*, **10**, 543–547

Soriano, F., Ponte, C. and Fernandez-Roblas, R. (1988) Antibiotics in yersiniosis. *Journal of Antimicrobial Chemotherapy*, **21**, 261–262.

Straley, S.C., Skrzypek, E., Plano, G.V. *et al.* (193) Yops of *Yersinia* spp. pathogenic for humans. *Infection and Immunity*, **61**, 3105–3110.

Tauxe, R.V., Vandepitte, J., Wauters, G. *et al.* (1987) *Yersinia enterocolitica* infections and pork: the missing link. *Lancet*, **i**, 1129–1132.

Van Noyen, R., Vandepitte, J., Wauters, G. *et al.* (1981) *Yersinia enterocolitica*: its isolation by cold enrichment from patients and healthy subjects. *Journal of Clinical Pathology*, **34**, 1052–1056.

Williams, J.E., Gentry, M.K., Braden, C.A. *et al.* (1988) A monoclonal antibody for the specific diagnosis of plague. *Bulletin of the World Health Organization*, **66**, 77.

Working Group on Yersiniosis (1981) Yersiniosis. In Euro Report 60 (ed. J. Alonzo). World Health Organization, Copenhagen.

WHO Expert Committee on Plague (1970) *Fourth Report*, p. 447. World Health Organization, Geneva.

World Health Organization (1993) Human plague in 1991. *Weekly Epidemiological Record*, **68**, 21–23.

Wren, B.W. and Tabaqchali, S.T. (1990) Detection of pathogenic *Yersinia enterocolitica* by the polymerase chain reaction. *Lancet*, **336**, 693.

Ziegler, P. (1982) *The Black Death*. Penguin, London.

12g

VIBRIOS

B. Drasar

INTRODUCTION

A number of major texts have been written about cholera and cholera vibrios. The chapter provides an outline for the clinical microbiologist (Pollitzer, 1959; Barua and Burrows, 1974; Colwell, 1984; Barua and Greenough, 1992; Wachsmuth *et al.* (1994). The genus *Vibrio* (Pacini, 1854) is among the oldest still recognized by bacteriology. Taxonomy was reviewed by Baumann *et al.* (1984) and they listed 20 species, of which 12 had been isolated from clinical material. More recently, Farmer and Hickman-Brenner (1992) listed 34 species. However, of these 12 had been isolated from clinical material. These studies illustrate the way in which our knowledge of the genus *Vibrio* has advanced. Until recently, *Vibrio* consisted of a heterogeneous and poorly described group of organisms. However, a stricter definition of the genus, coupled with the transfer of some members to other well-understood groups, has allowed the taxonomy to be clarified. Some, such as *Campylobacter*, have been transferred to their own genera.

Vibrios are fermentative, Gram-negative bacteria that are oxidase positive. They are part of a widespread group of organisms, many of which are common in the environment. In clinical bacteriology we focus our attention mainly upon *Vibrio cholerae*, the cause of cholera, and *Vibrio parahaemolyticus*, a major cause of food poisoning. However, it is important to remember that these are not the only vibrios that can cause disease and indeed there are very many other vibrios that are not associated with human disease.

The genus as currently understood is comparatively well characterized, and consists of oxidase-positive fermentative organisms. All members are facultative anaerobes and grow well on culture media. It is usual to speak of these organisms as belonging to two groups: those isolated from clinical specimens, and the marine vibrios. However, this distinction is by no means clear.

All vibrios benefit by addition of sodium chloride to their media used for identification. An absolute requirement for sodium is not restricted to vibrios of marine origin. Indeed, many of those isolated from clinical material are thought to originate from marine sources. Of the 12 vibrios isolated from clinical specimens, most have also been associated with marine environments. They have been isolated from food poisoning associated with consumption of seafoods, and from wound infections resulting from contamination with a variety of marine materials (Table 12g.1).

Principles and Practice of Clinical Bacteriology. Edited by A.M. Emmerson, P.M. Hawkey and S.H. Gillespie

TABLE 12g.1   EXAMPLES OF DISEASE SYNDROMES ASSOCIATED WITH VIBRIOS

Species	Enteritis	Wound infection	Ear infection	Septicaemia
V. cholerae	+			
V. cholerae non-O1	+	+	+	+
V. mimicus	+		+	
V. fluvialis	+			
V. parahaemolyticus	+			+
V. vulnificus		+		+
V. damsela		+		+
V. metschnikovii		+		
V. alginolyticus		+	+	+

DESCRIPTION OF THE ORGANISM

The Family Vibrionaceae

The genus *Vibrio* is part of the family Vibrionaceae. The family also includes the genera *Photobacterium*, *Aeromonas* and *Plesiomonas*. Members of the family are usually oxidase positive and have polar flagella for motility. Peritrichous flagella may occasionally be produced.

Family definition

The organisms are rigid Gram-negative rods, motile by polar flagella in liquid media, but peritrichous flagella may be produced on solid media in some species. The are chemo-organotrophs; metabolism is both oxidative and fermentative. They utilize glucose fermentatively and are catalase positive; most species are oxidase positive and reduce nitrate to nitrite. They are facultative anaerobes without exacting nutritional requirements.

It is not certain that this family is a natural grouping in any evolutionary sense. It arose out of the wish to separate these organisms from the Enterobacteriaceae DNA homology studies suggest *Vibrio* and *Photobacterium* may be closely related. However, *Aeromonas* is more distantly related and may in fact be closer to *Pasteurella multocida* and the Enterobacteriaceae than to vibrios. Only in recent years has the extent and definition of the genus *Vibrio* become more delineated. In the past anaerobic vibrios, *V. fetus*,

V. faecalis and so forth were included; these organisms are now in the genus *Campylobacter* and are dealt with elsewhere (see Chapter 17b).

The Genus *Vibrio*

Historically, taxonomically and medically the genus *Vibrio* focuses on the organisms that cause cholera. These are largely members of the species *V. cholerae*; further species may occasionally cause clinically identical illness. Advances in molecular biology, immunology and bacterial taxonomy mean that *V. cholerae* is now among the best understood of bacterial species. The taxonomy of the organisms, the virulence mechanisms by means of which it causes disease, and the means of treating apparent cholera have all been thoroughly investigated.

Genus definition

The organisms are short asporogenous rods, with axis curved or straight, 0.5×3 μm. They are single or occasionally united in S shapes or spirals. They are motile by a single polar flagellum which is sheathed in certain if not all species. Some species produce lateral (peritrichous) flagella on solid media. Carbohydrates are fermented with the production of acid and no gas. A wide range of extracellular enzymes is produced, including amylase, chitinase, DNAase, gelatinase, lecithinase and lipase. They grow on simple mineral media. NaCl stimulates growth with an optimum of 1–3%. Some strains require NaCl for growth.

Temperature optima range from 18 to 37 °C and pH range is 6.0–9.0. They are sensitive to 0/129 (2,4-diamino–6,7-diisopropylpteridine). G + C content of DNA is 40–50 mol%.

PATHOGENESIS OF CHOLERA

Explanations of the pathogenesis of infection usually focus on interaction of the organism with its host. In this context, cholera is a comparatively simple disease. *Vibrio cholerae* enters the intestine and attaches to the mucosal surface. When attached, it produces cholera toxin, which attaches to the intestinal mucosal cells. An important function of mucosal cells is the control of ion transport; under normal conditions the net flow of ions is from the lumen to the tissue, which results in a net uptake of water. Cholera toxin disrupts ion fluxes without causing apparent damage to the mucosa (Gangarosa *et al.*, 1960). Cholera toxin decreases the net flow of sodium into the tissue. This produces a net flow of chloride and water out of the tissue into the lumen, causing the massive diarrhoea and electrolyte imbalance associated with infection.

What a bacterium can do to its host is only part of its life as a pathogen. An organism must be transmitted between hosts and establish itself in new hosts. The ability of an organism to survive in the external environment and to adapt to the internal environment provided by the host is an important aspect of its pathogenic armament-arium. When considered in this way, the pathogenesis of cholera and the ecology of *V. cholerae* are much more complex.

Transmission

Until the 1970s it was believed that the ecology of *V. cholerae* was restricted to its role as a human pathogen. That is to say, if infection of the human host could be eliminated the major ecological niche of *V. cholerae* would have been eliminated and the organism would no longer be able to survive. It is now clear that the human host represents only a small compartment of the ecology of the vibrio. Thus, even if the human infection were

eliminated, this would not materially influence the survival of the species. It is now clear the *V. cholerae* is a member of the autochthonous flora of brackish waters. It is able to persist and grow in a variety of aquatic environments in association with a variety of aquatic plants, zooplankton and blue-green algae. In some circumstances, it may be a member of the biofilm flora found on submerged surfaces. This ability to colonize many different bodies of water and to associate with different members of microbiota undoubtedly contributes to the patterns of endemic cholera. This environmental survival was originally investigated in the search for an explanation for seasonal patterns of cholera in endemic areas. However, it has much wider implications than this (Colwell, 1984; West, 1989; Drasar, 1992).

Infective Dose

When the interaction of a pathogen with a host is considered, this is often described as though it were a unitary process, i.e. that a bacterium and a person come into contact and this results in disease. The situation is much more complicated than this. For *V. cholerae* we are fortunate in having the results of volunteer studies in which the numbers of bacteria required to initiate infection in healthy adults were examined. The numbers of bacteria involved in the initiation of infection under these conditions were much larger than might have been expected for a major epidemic disease (Table 12g.2) (Cash *et al.*, 1974; Levine *et al.*, 1982, 1984; Suntharasamai *et al.*, 1992). These results can be interpreted in several ways. It may be that they indicate the scale of the importance of host factors in initiating infection. Thus, for example, neutralization of gastric acid bicarbonate decreases the numbers of bacteria required to initiate infection very considerably. Bacterial factors may also be important. The numbers of organisms required may reflect the size of bacterial population needed to ensure that the cells responsive to environmental signals are available. Thus, it may be that only a small fraction of laboratory-grown cells are immediately responsive to the environmental signals transmitted in the intestinal environment.

TABLE 12g.2 HUMAN CHALLENGE STUDIES WITH VIRULENT *V. CHOLERAE*. INOCULUM 10^6 BACTERIA. STOMACH ACID NEUTRALIZED

		Classical biotype		El Tor biotype	
		Inaba 569B	Ogawa 395	Inaba N16961	Ogawa E7946
0.	No response	4	3	0	1
1.	Positive stool culture	6	0	3	2
2.	Positive stool culture diarrhoea	28	12	25	6
3.	Positive stool culture severe diarrhoea (cholera)	14	10	10	1
	Total number of subjects	52	25	38	10

This would mean that not all cells were equally able to initiate the transcriptional regulation of those genes required for expression of virulence. It is also important to realize that these volunteer studies do not reflect the situation during an epidemic. Studies of epidemics caused by Classical and El Tor biotypes of *V. cholerae* suggest that in an epidemic most people are exposed to the organism. However, although many become temporary carriers, few develop clinical disease. The case–carrier ratio is 1 : 50 for Classical biotype and 1 : 90 for the El Tor biotype. It is not certain that these differences are significant: they may simply represent the different methodologies used in the studies.

Virulence Factors

Since the description of cholera toxin and the demonstration that the small intestinal mucosa remains intact in cholera, there has been a major resurgence of interest in the virulence factors of cholera vibrios. Prior to these discoveries, it was believed that the destruction of mucus by mucinase was the main virulence factor and that this caused destruction of the intestinal mucosa. A number of virulence factors have been described. Not all are firmly established as factors important in the disease. Some have been demonstrated in experimental systems. Others have been invoked to explain the side effects caused by genetically manipulated candidate cholera vaccine strains in some early studies. A general schema for the initiation of clinical infection is set out in Figure 12g.1.

Cholera toxin

Cholera toxin is the most important of the virulence factors produced by *V. cholerae*. Strains of *V. cholerae* 01 that do not produce cholera toxin

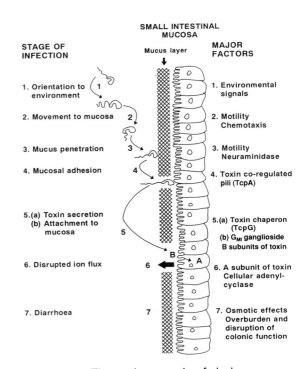

Figure 12g.1. The pathogenesis of cholera.

do not produce disease in human volunteers (Levine *et al.*, 1982). Such strains may cause a milder form of diarrhoea because of the presence of other toxins (Cash *et al.*, 1974; Levine *et al.*, 1988). This has proved a particular problem with candidate generally engineered vaccine strains. Cholera toxin consists of a number of subunits: one A or enzymatic subunit, and five identical B or binding subunits. The molecular weight of A subunit is 27 kDa and that of each of the B subunits is 11.7 kDa. The genes that code for the toxin subunits are part of the same operon. These genes are part of a coordinated regulated system that also controls the expression of toxin-coregulated type A pili and other virulence factors (DiRita *et al.*, 1991). The expression of these virulence factors is modulated by environmental influences. Environmental regulation of this system seems to be mediated by the toxR protein which spans the cytoplasmic membrane (DiRita, 1992). The system is further complicated by the fact that toxR is itself environmentally regulated and its expression at 37 °C may be downregulated in favour of the heat shock response (Figure 12g.2) (Parsot and Mekalanos, 1990).

Although the details of the regulatory system are not fully understood, it is certain that when *V. cholerae* colonize the intestine, the toxin is pro-

duced. It seems that A and B subunits are produced separately and then assembled in the bacterial cytoplasm. TcpG is a chaperon, which is involved in the assembly of toxin coregulated pili and may be involved in this process. Following assembly, the cholera toxin is transported to the periplasmic space and excreted by the bacterium. This is in contrast to the situation with heat-labile toxin of *Escherichia coli*, cells of which seem to have to lyse to release the toxin. When released into the intestine, cholera toxin binds to mucosal cells via the host G_{M1} ganglioside. The B subunits bind to the ganglioside and form a pseudoporin in the cell membrane, thus enabling the A subunit to enter the cell. Prior to insertion into the cell, the A subunit is nicked probably in the small intestinal environment after release by the bacterium. This nicking converts the A subunit into two smaller proteins, A1 and A2. It is the A1 subunit that enters the cells via the pore formed by the B subunits. The A subunit ADP ribosolates a membrane protein called G. This G protein regulates the activity of the host cell adenyl cyclase, and thus determines the level of cyclic AMP in the host cells. This brings about an uncontrollable rise in cyclic AMP levels. This has a variety of effects but in this context the most important is to alter the activities of sodium and chloride membrane transport systems (DiRita, 1992). These changes result in a disruption of the biodirectional ion fluxes in the mucosal membrane. The overall effect of this is to increase the relative concentrations of sodium and chloride ions in the lumen. Diarrhoea then results as a direct effect of the osmotic imbalance.

It is the osmotic imbalance which prevents, or at least much reduces, the active absorption of fluid that causes the diarrhoea. Further, cholera toxin may not be produced in large enough amounts to produce the diarrhoea in all individuals. The efflux of fluids must be sufficient to overcome the absorptive capacities of the colon. It is important to remember that the result of cholera toxin is a physiological lesion. Cells remain normal and are capable of carrying out normal functions, including absorption of salts and water. It is merely that the membrane fluxes from the cell to lumen are much exaggerated. It is for this reason that rehy-

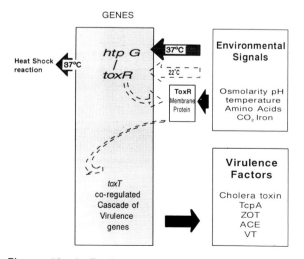

Figure 12g.2. Environmental control of virulence in *V. cholerae*.

dration together with a source of energy can correct the physiological disturbance by amplifying and reinforcing the ability of the membrane to absorb and reabsorb fluid.

Toxin coregulated pili

Attachment or adhesion to the intestinal mucosa is an essential part of the virulence mechanism of intestinal pathogens. Although this was demonstrated in *E. coli* many years ago, it is only recently that the mechanisms of attachment of *V. cholerae* have been elucidated. *Vibrio cholerae* produces a variety of haemagglutinins and pili which had been postulated to be important in virulence (Jones and Freter, 1976; Freter and Jones, 1976). But these do not occur uniformly in all virulent strains. Toxin-coregulated pili were not demonstrated in spite of many investigations, because of the conditions under which test organisms were grown. Only when strains grown on solid media were investigated were pili obvious. Since their discovery, it has been demonstrated that their production is regulated by the same cascade mechanism as is important for the production of toxin (Pearson *et al.*, 1993; Kaufman *et al.*, 1993). Thus, virulent *V. cholerae* produce their pili, which are important for their attachment, and a toxin that is important for the regulation of ion fluxes at the same time, when the correct environmental conditions trigger the transcription of the virulence genes. (DiRita, 1992; Parsot and Mekalanos, 1990). How toxin-coregulated pili bring about attachment of *V. cholerae* to the mucosal cells is not well understood. Most research has concentrated on the study of the regulation of the genes responsible for their production. Nevertheless, their importance in virulence has been established in volunteer studies. The strains that do not produce toxin-coregulated pili are avirulent in human volunteers (Herrington *et al.*, 1988).

Other virulence factors

Vibrio cholerae produces a number of other toxins in addition to cholera toxin. The existence of these toxins was first recognized when human volunteer studies were undertaken using mutagenized and biochemically engineered strains of *V. cholerae* that did not produce cholera toxin. Initial studies with live or vaccine strains showed that these strains that did not produce entire cholera toxin still produced symptoms. A number of toxins have been described, most recently zona occludens toxin (ZOT) (Fasano *et al.*, 1991; Baudry *et al.*, 1992). This toxin disrupts the tight junctions between mucosal cells. In effect, this increases the surface area of the mucosa available for ion and water loss. Such losses normally occur through the brush border but the action of this toxin exposes the sides of the cells and this may increase the efficiency of the virulence.

Vibrio cholerae has also been reported to produce verocell toxin (VT), which is analogous to the toxins produced by *Shigella dysenteriae*. Another enterotoxin, or accessory cholera enterotoxin (ACE), has also been described. *Vibrio cholerae* also produces haemolysin. The role of these additional toxins in the pathogenesis of cholera is not well understood. However, it is likely that they play a supporting role to cholera toxin. The variety of toxins produced by *V. cholerae* probably reflects its undoubted ability to produce a number of extracellular enzymes. These may well be important for the bacteria in non-intestinal environments such as aquatic systems, as part of the biofilm communities and in association with aquatic microflora and fauna. The production of extracellular enzymes and toxins may help the organism to digest a variety of substances and to increase the range of nutrients available to it.

Non-cholera Vibrios (non-01 *V. cholerae*)

Some of these strains also appear to produce cholera toxin together with ZOT (Karasawa *et al.*, 1993). Many others appear to produce cytolysins that are not cholera like (McCardell *et al.*, 1985). A few produce a toxin similar to heat-stable toxin of *E. coli* and some produce a shigella-like toxin (O'Brien *et al.*, 1984). Others produce no detectable enterotoxin at all and are probably non-pathogenic. Much research is still needed.

V. mimicus

These organisms were originally considered to be sucrose-negative *V. cholerae*. Some strains produce cholera toxin. Others produce an enterotoxin similar to the heat-stable toxin produced by non-01 *V. cholerae* and haemolysins similar to that produced by *V. parahaemolyticus* (Ramamurthy *et al.*, 1994).

V. parahaemolyticus

The factors necessary for pathogenesis have not yet been established. However, shigella-like toxin is produced (O'Brien *et al.*, 1984). An enterotoxin has been purified but it is not certain that this is responsible for the symptoms of *V. parahaemolyticus* food poisoning. The haemolysin is also thought to act as a virulence factor. Studies of this have revealed a regulatory system analogous to the toxR system in *V. cholerae* (Lin *et al.*, 1993).

EPIDEMIOLOGY OF CHOLERA

Cholera is a pandemic disease *par excellence*. Although it has undoubtedly been common in India since records began, and has spread to neighbouring countries on frequent occasions, the great days of cholera came after the resumption of world trade following the Napoleonic wars. Whether widespread cholera had occurred previously is not known. Writings of Europeans in India had from the earliest days of this intercourse made reference to this disease. Epidemics undoubtedly occurred among Europeans and European troops stationed in India (Orton, 1831; MacPherson, 1872; MacNamara, 1876). Until 1817, spread was probably limited but in that year the first pandemic started and reached Europe. This was rapidly followed by the second pandemic, which reached England through the port of Sunderland in 1831. It is notable that Snow, who later became famous for the elucidation of the water-borne transmission of cholera (Snow, 1849, 1855) was working as a doctor's apprentice in Newcastle at about this time. Early nineteenth-century Europe was ravaged by a series of epidemics of cholera. We do not know for certain what caused these epidemics although it is assumed to be *V. cholerae*. It was not until the fifth pandemic that Robert Koch (1884) succeeded in isolating and identifying the organism. Even when the organism had been isolated, there were many who did not believe that it was the cause of the disease, though few went so far as Pettenkoffer (1892) in their wish to demonstrate that *V. cholerae* was non-pathogenic. He drank a culture and did not get cholera. As we now know, this probably reflects the relative resistance of some people to cholera vibrios. Comparable studies in healthy volunteers have not always been successful in inducing disease. Pandemics of cholera occur worldwide; we are now probably about to embark on the eighth pandemic (Table 12g.3).

However, for most practical purposes it is the local epidemics in endemic areas that are of the greatest practical importance. Historically it is likely that endemic cholera has been restricted to the Ganges delta. However, in the recent pandemic – the seventh pandemic – many other endemic areas have been detected. How an area becomes an endemic focus is unclear; the answers probably relate to aspects of the ecology of *V. cholerae* that we do not fully understand. In endemic areas successive, usually seasonally related, epidemics of cholera occur.

Historically, cholera has been considered to be a water-borne disease (Feachem, 1981, 1982; Feachem *et al.*, 1981). Indeed, there is considerable evidence that water-borne transmission of cholera has been and is very important. However, in an epidemic situation, food-borne transmission is also very significant. *Vibrio cholerae* has often been isolated from seafood and shellfish and the vibrios are able to grow well in cooked rice and on other foods. However, external contamination of foods may be equally important. In the recent outbreak in Chile, cholera was transmitted by vegetables irrigated with untreated sewage. Similar transmission related to melons was seen in Peru (Crowcroft, 1994). Thus, both food and water can act as vehicles for transmission (Glass *et al.*, 1991; *Risks of Transmission of Cholera by Food*, 1991). Poor sanitation is undoubtedly important

TABLE 12g.3   THE CHRONOLOGY OF CHOLERA

At home	To 1817	Endemic on the Indian Subcontinent	
The historic pandemics	1817–1823 1829–1850 1852–1860 1863–1879	First pandemic Second pandemic Third pandemic Fourth pandemic	John Snow and the Broad Street Pump (1854)
The classical pandemics	1881–1896 1899–1923	Fifth pandemic Sixth pandemic	Robert Koch and the comma bacillus (1884)
The El Tor pandemic	1961 to date	Seventh pandemic	De and Chatterje cholera toxin (1953)
0139 Bengal	1992 to date	Eighth pandemic	

for maintaining transmission during epidemics. This probably explains why secondary transmission is rare when cases are imported into countries with good sanitation. Investigations of other outbreaks in an epidemic situation may demonstrate what vehicle is important.

Major questions remain about the epidemiology of cholera. Two questions are of particular importance:

(1) How does cholera survive in the interepidemic periods in endemic areas? That is, why are there cholera seasons?

There is linked to this a subsidiary question:

(1a) How do new endemic areas develop?
(2) How do pandemics arise?

Recent studies on the survival of *V. cholerae* have provided some clues to both of these questions. However, neither can be regarded as settled.

It seems likely that *V. cholerae* is a normal member of the autochthonous flora of natural aqueous habitats. A variety of members of the aquatic flora and fauna have been suggested as likely to produce the right habitat. These include the plants, crustaceans, amoebae and various forms of phytoplankton (Islam *et al.*, 1993, 1994; Thom *et al.*, 1992). These studies assume that the vibrios persist as active members of a biofilm microbiota. It is likely that the occurrence of starved and viable, but not culturable, forms is also important. These studies are particularly pertinent when considering the maintenance of endemic foci and the development of new endemic foci. If

we postulate that in endemic areas vibrios persist as part of the normal flora of a number of bodies of water it can be readily seen how local epidemics will arise. Seasonal variation can be explained in terms of variations in the aquatic microbiota, e.g. algal blooms linked to an increase in the numbers of *V. cholerae* in water. Further, colonization of lakes and watercourses in non-endemic areas may result in the development of new endemic areas and the range of areas in which cholera is endemic. Endemic foci associated with colonized water sources probably occur in Bangladesh (Tamplin *et al.*, 1990), Louisiana in the USA (Blake *et al.*, 1980) in parts of Africa (Glass *et al.*, 1991) and perhaps in Australia (Desmarchelier and Reichelt, 1981). It is possible that during the current South American outbreak, new endemic foci have been developed.

It has long been assumed that pandemics result from the spread of strains of *V. cholerae* from a source. The Ganges delta has been considered to be the ancestral home of vibrios. It has long been believed that pandemics spread from this area. Under this theory, a new, highly virulent strain of *V. cholerae* would develop in an endemic focus and then spread widely. However, application of ribotyping systems to cholera vibrios isolated during the seventh pandemic casts doubts on this. A variety of ribotypes have been demonstrated, each in part restricted to a particular area (Koblavi *et al.*, 1990). Thus, different types of *V. cholerae* El Tor occur on the Indian subcontinent, Africa and in South America. It has been suggested that this diversity of types represents the acquisition of virulence factors by *V. cholerae* normally resident in aquatic environments in the different areas. Studies on the possible eighth pandemic caused by *V. cholerae* 0139 suggest a single type is responsible for all the cases so far studied.

The reasons for the mechanisms of pandemic spread remain obscure. In the most recent pandemics rapid travel of persons by air and the movement of ballast water by ships can be seen as a means of moving local microbiotas around the world and possibly enhancing the range for colonization of *V. cholerae*. However, in past pandemics this did not occur. Carriers in cholera, in the long-term sense that they occur in typhoid, are very rare and, thus, spread by humans until the advent of rapid air transport does not seem to be an adequate explanation. Although the epidemiology of cholera has been studied since before the advent of microbiology and the pioneering studies of John Snow established many of the principles of epidemiology, our increased knowledge of the survival of the vibrio, its pathogenicity and the advent of molecular typing methods have not made our understanding that much clearer. For example, cholera had not been seen in South America for nearly 100 years and it was assumed that for some reason it would not occur there and that perhaps the population was not susceptible. The recent extension of the seventh pandemic to South America has made us realize that there is no area of the world in which cholera cannot become established. The advent of the new strain of *V. cholerae* 0139 has added a further question: how is it, and by what mechanism, do new pandemic strains occur during the history of cholera? Of the four pandemics for which a cause is known, three were caused by different organisms.

CLINICAL FEATURES OF CHOLERA

The presentation of cholera is diverse, with many asymptomatic cases and others with severe symptoms. The infection can be rapidly progressive. Patients may lose as much as 100% of their body weight in diarrhoea over three to four days, bringing about death in a few hours if not adequately treated, but a less fulminant course is usual. All of the symptoms arise as a result of the dehydration and electrolyte disturbance consequent on the loss of water and salts into the gut lumen. Diarrhoea is severe but abdominal pain is usually absent. Vomiting is often present in the early stages of cholera. Rarely ileus may occur on presentation and is associated with shock and this may mimic acute intestinal obstruction. The state of consciousness is altered but the patient can be roused to lucidity. There is generalized weakness and cardiac arrhythmias may arise.

Other species are associated with enteritis and wound or ear infection after contamination arising in marine environments. In some cases septicaemia may result. Examples of species associated with these syndromes is given in Table 12g.1.

LABORATORY DIAGNOSIS

Collection and Transport of Specimens

Many vibrios have been isolated from samples routinely submitted to clinical laboratories. When a suspected outbreak of cholera is being investigated, such samples may not be sufficient. The drying and acidification of specimens during their transport to the laboratory may prove to be a problem. Wherever possible samples should be dealt with with the minimum of delay. Alkaline peptone water used for the selective enrichment of vibrios can also be used for transport. This can act as an enrichment transport system. An alternative enrichment transport system using Tellurite–taurocholate peptone broth has been used successfully in Bangladesh. Of the routinely available transport media, Cary and Blair is the most satisfactory and may maintain the viability of vibrios for up to four weeks. In the absence of a suitable transport system blotting paper can be impregnated with liquid stool and packed in plastic bags. If these do not dry out, the vibrios will remain viable for about four weeks.

A rapid presumptive diagnosis can be achieved by mixing a drop of liquid faeces with a drop of specific antiserum. In patients with cholera the characteristic darting movement of the vibrios is inhibited.

Isolation

Vibrios can be isolated on normal laboratory media. Specialist media have been devised for the isolation of *V. cholerae* and these may be applicable to the isolation of other organisms. There are doubts about the cost-effectiveness of employing specialized media for the isolation of vibrios unless cholera is suspected. When a specialized medium, such as thiosulphate citrate bile salts sucrose agar (TCBS), has been employed in parallel with other media in routine clinical practice vibrios have been isolated, when present, on a variety of media. TCBS is extremely useful for isolating *V. cholerae*. But it should be remembered that some vibrio species do not grow well on TCBS. These include *V. metschnikovii*, *V. hollisae* and *V. cincinnatiensis*. Growth of *V. damsela* may also be reduced. The results obtained with TCBS produced by different manufacturers may be different and each batch should be quality controlled to ensure the isolation characteristics are understood. Vibrios can be identified using commercial identification systems such as API 20E or standard laboratory tests when standard peptone water sugars are used. Results are more reliable if these are supplemented by 1% NaCl. Indeed, 1% NaCl is essential as a growth factor for most of the clinically important vibrios. Exceptions to this are *V. cholerae* and *V. mimicus*.

Isolation Methods

A simple schema for the isolation of *V. cholerae* is set out in Table 12g.4. Although a number of vibrios have been isolated from clinical material, not all are of equal importance. In the routine laboratory, it is important that the system in place will ensure that *V. cholerae* is recognized if it occurs.

Different isolation techniques are necessary for halophilic and for non-halophilic vibrios. Enrichment methods designed principally for the isolation of *V. parahaemolyticus*, for example, are not ideal for the non-halophilic vibrios. If cholera vibrios are being looked for, the alkaline peptone water should not contain salt. This reduces overgrowth by other halophilic vibrios. It is also important to keep the pH alkaline: at a lower pH *Aeromonas* may so overgrow the vibrios that they cannot be isolated. This is particularly so with freshwater samples. Only one species of *Vibrio* is likely to be significant in any one clinical specimen. A method that permits isolation of both non-halophilic (*V. cholerae*) and halophilic (*V. parahaemolyticus*) vibrios is thus needed.

If the presence of a vibrio is suspected in patients with loose motions, about 5–10 ml of faecal material should be collected in a disposable container. The specimen should reach the laboratory as soon as possible. In the laboratory, inoculate about 2 g of faeces into 20 ml alkaline peptone water (peptone 10 g, NaCl 10 g, distilled water 1 litre, pH 8.6) and incubate for 5–8 h at 37 °C. This will enrich for halophilic vibrios. For *V. cholerae* alkaline peptone water without NaCl is used. At the same time, TCBS is streak inoculated with a heavy load of faecal material.

TABLE 12g.4   DETECTION OF *V. CHOLERAE* IN THE LABORATORY

Day 0	1. Streak inoculate selective (TCBS) and non-selective media
	2. Inoculate alkaline peptone water
	Incubate
Day 1	1. Suspicious colonies → agglutination with *V. cholerae* O1 antiserum
	↓
	Subculture for purity
	2. Alkaline peptone water
	↓
	Streak inoculate to selective and non-selective media
	Incubate
Day 2	1. Confirm agglutination results with pure culture; set up identification tests
	2. Test suspicious colonies isolated from alkaline peptone water

After 5–8 h incubation from the first alkaline peptone water inoculate, a new alkaline peptone water preparation with 1 ml of fluid from the top of the alkaline peptone water and a second TCBS plate with a loopful from the top and incubate overnight. Look for typical colonies on both TCBS plates (yellow or green colonies about 2 mm in diameter). Inoculate a third TCBS plate from the alkaline peptone water. If no colonies occur on this plate after overnight incubation the sample is probably negative. This schema can be adapted for other specimens.

Identification

Suspicious colonies are streak inoculated onto nutrient agar as a purity check. Vibrios may be identified by the tests shown in Table 12g.5. A small number of basic tests are needed to identify at the genus level.

Oxidase Colonies grown on nutrient agar should be tested using filter paper impregnated with 1% tetramethyl para-phenylene-diamine dihydrochloride. The oxidase test on growth from a plate containing a carbohydrate that is fermented by the organism can give a false negative.

0/129 sensitivity This is available as the phosphate (2,4-diamino-6,7-diisopropylpteridine phosphate) from BDH, product number 44169. Disks are prepared containing 10 and 150 μg and the test performed as for a disk diffusion sensitivity method on nutrient agar – *not* specialized sensitivity testing agars.

CLED Cystine–lactose–electrolyte-deficient medium was designed to prevent swarming of proteus. Being electrolyte deficient it is useful for distinguishing the non-halophilic vibrios (e.g. *V. cholerae*), which can grow on it, from the halophilic ones (e.g. *V. parahaemolyticus*), which cannot.

O/F Oxidation/Fermentation (tests) Media for these tests should have the sodium chloride concentration raised to 1%, which will support good growth of all the pathogenic *Vibrio* spp.

V. Cholerae 0:1, Non-0:1 NAG Vibrio

The definition of the species *V. cholerae* and the relationship of the species to the cholera vibrios that cause cholera has long been a source of confusion. Rather like *E. coli*, *V. cholerae* is a large and diverse species, not all members of which are pathogens. In the past it was customary to speak of cholera vibrios, non-cholera vibrios (NCVs) and non-agglutinable vibrios (NAGs). It is now clear that these organisms are all members of the same species. Taxonomic studies including DNA–DNA homology have shown that *V. cholerae* is a single, relatively homogeneous, closely related species (Citarella and Colwell, 1970). Like other Gram-negative bacteria, *V. cholerae* has a complex cell wall which includes lipopolysaccharides (LPS), the carbohydrate components of which are designated as O antigens. Most of the strains of *V. cholerae* isolated from cases of cholera belong to the O:1 serogroup. Within this serogroup are further subdivisions, three serogroups Inaba, Ogawa and Hijokima, and two biotypes, Classical and El Tor. Each biotype may include members of all serotypes. It should be remembered that not all O:1 strains cause cholera. Members of groups O:2 to O:138 may cause diarrhoea but are not thought to cause epidemic or endemic cholera. Although groups O:2 to O:138 are generally recognized to be less pathogenic than the Classical or El Tor biovars, they can cause symptoms very similar or identical to those of cholera and may cause epidemics of enteritis. Indeed, they are more commonly isolated in Britain from cases of enteritis than the El Tor or Classical biovars. Only *V. cholerae* O:1 is reportable to the World Health Organization as cholera. The Classical biovar has now almost died out and the current, seventh, cholera pandemic is caused by the El Tor biovar. Members of the recently isolated O:139 group cause a disease clinically indistinguishable from cholera and have been responsible for epidemics (Ramamurthy *et al.*, 1993; Albert *et al.*, 1993; Bhattacharya *et al.*, 1993; Cheasty and Rowe (1994). It is likely that these O:139 strains will be responsible for the eighth pandemic of cholera.

TABLE 12g.5 THE 12 *VIBRIO* SPECIES THAT ARE FOUND IN HUMAN CLINICAL SPECIMENS

Test	Percentage positive[a] for:											
	V. cholerae	*V. mimicus*	*V. metschnikovii*	*V. cincinnatiensis*	*V. hollisae*	*V. damsela*	*V. fluvialis*	*V. furnissii*	*V. alginolyticus*	*V. parahaemolyticus*	*V. vulnificus*	*V. carchariae*
D-Glucose, acid production	100	100	100	100	100	100	100	100	100	100	100	50
D-Glucose, gas production	0	0	0	0	0	10	0	100	0	0	0	0
Arginine, Moeller (1% NaCl)	0	0	60	0	0	95	95	100	0	0	0	0
Lysine, Moeller (1% NaCl)	99	100	35	60	0	50	0	0	99	100	99	100
Ornithine, Moeller (1% NaCl)	99	99	0	0	0	0	0	0	50	95	55	0
myo-Inositol	0	0	40	100	0	0	0	0	0	0	0	0
Sucrose	100	0	100	100	0	5	100	100	99	1	15	50
Nitrate → nitrite	99	100	0	100	100	100	100	100	100	100	100	100
Oxidase	100	100	0	100	100	95	100	100	100	100	100	100
Growth in nutrient broth with:												
0% NaCl	100	100	0	0	0	0	0	0	0	0	0	0
1% NaCl	100	100	100	100	99	100	99	99	99	100	99	100
Isolated from:												
1. Faeces	+++	++	-	-	+	-	+	+	±	++	±	-
2. Other samples	±	+	+	+	-	+	-	-	+	±	+	+

[a] After 48 hours incubation at 36 °C. Most of the positive reactions occur during the first 24 hours. NaCl 1% is added to the standard medium to enhance growth. Percentages approximate for guidance only. Boxes indicate useful tests.

TABLE 12g.6   THE BIOTYPES OF CHOLERA VIBRIOS (*V. CHOLERAE* O1)

	Biovar	
	Classical	El Tor
O1 antiserum	+	+
Voges–Proskauer reaction	–	+
Acetoin production[a]		
Haemolysis of sheep erythrocytes	–	+
Chick red cell agglutination	–	+
Polymyxin 50 i.u.	S	R
Classical phage IV	S	R
El Tor phage 5	R	S

[a]This difference is quantitative. Many classical strains produce trace amounts of acetoin not detected by the standard test.

Strains of *V. cholerae* can be divided into the two biotypes on the basis of the tests set out in Table 12g.6.

Serotyping   All strains of *V. cholerae* share a common H antigen. There are at least 139 O groups. Apart from O:1 and O:139 there is no link between the O group and pathogenicity. The O1 antiserum is available commercially as *V. cholerae* 'polyvalent' antiserum. Subtyping of O:1 strains may be done by testing for agglutination with absorbed Inaba and Ogawa antisera (Table 12g.7).

Vibrio mimicus

Until recently *V. mimicus* has been identified as *V. cholerae*. Organisms that are unable to ferment sucrose produce green colonies on TCBS but which are otherwise phenotypically similar to *V. cholerae* have been isolated from shellfish, brackish water and stools of human beings with diarrhoea in many parts of the world. Recent studies on more than 50 such organisms show that they have DNA relatedness to each other at species level but are related only distantly to *V. cholerae* (DNA–DNA homology 20–50%). Thus these bacteria would appear to be distinct species (Davis *et al.*, 1981). *Vibrio mimicus* shares O group serotypes with *V. cholerae*. Only some strains produce enterotoxin.

Vibrio parahaemolyticus

Some vibrios are halophilic, i.e. they have an obligate requirement for sodium chloride. This kind of vibrio is widely distributed in warm coastal and estuarine waters, requires sodium for growth and has been found in gastroenteritis outbreaks associated with the eating of seafoods throughout the world. The vibrio was first identified in Japan as a cause of food poisoning associated with shrimps. Further outbreaks have been associated with the eating of crabs, prawns and other seafoods.

TREATMENT

The nature of the life-threatening symptoms of cholera result from massive loss of water and salts. All other effects are probably consequent on the dehydration. Effective therapy concentrates on the replacement of fluids and prevention of further loss. Both oral and intravenous rehydration have their place in the management of cholera. Many cases of cholera, especially if diagnosed early, can be managed by oral rehydration. However, the volumes of fluid lost in severe cases may

TABLE 12g.7   SEROTYPING OF *V. CHOLERAE*

	O antigen	Type antigen	
V. cholerae	O:1		
Subtype			
Inaba	+	+	–
Ogawa	+	–	+
Hikojima	+	+	+
Non-cholera vibrios (NCVs)	O:1		
Non-agglutinable vibrios (NAGs)	to	Not applicable	
Non-01 *V. cholerae*	O:138		
0139: Bengal cholera	O:139		

be very large. Especially if diagnosis has been delayed, replacement of adequate volumes of fluid by mouth may prove difficult. Fluid losses of up to 20 litres per day have been reported. For these reasons, the use of intravenous rehydration methods may prove very valuable and should not be entirely excluded.

Rehydration therapy alone will lead to recovery from cholera (*Guidelines for Cholera Control*, 1986). However, it may be necessary to rehydrate for quite a long time. It must be remembered that cholera toxin becomes permanently bound to mucosal cells and thus ion fluxes are probably unbalanced throughout the life of that cell. For this reason, antibiotics are usually added to the treatment regime. The empirical evidence is that they reduce the time needed during which rehydration therapy has to be continued. The effect of antibiotics is to reduce the load of *V. cholerae* in the intestine. Elimination of the organism by antibiotics prevents the release and binding of more cholera toxin and thus only the limited amount of cholera toxin already released before antibiotic therapy is commenced continues to act on the intestine.

Though there is a role for antibiotics in the treatment of cholera, there is no role for antimotility agents. Such agents increase the retention of both vibrios and their attendant cholera toxin in the gut, and probably exacerbate the physiological effects. When using antibiotics it is important to remember that *V. cholerae*, like other bacteria, is able to develop antibiotic resistance. *Vibrio cholerae* is also able to acquire antibiotic resistance plasmids and, although they are not as stable hosts of plasmids as are some other organisms, this can be of considerable practical importance (Glass *et al.*, 1983). A number of antimicrobial agents have been used in endemic situations. These include tetracycline, doxycycline, furazolidone, trimethoprim–sulphamethoxazole and norfloxacin. Indeed, extensive use of tetracycline has resulted in many of the endemic strains becoming tetracycline resistant. Thus, although empirical therapy may be necessary, the performance of antibiotic resistance tests should also be a priority. *Vibrio cholerae* strains isolated from individuals under-

going antibiotic therapy should be maintained on media containing the antibiotics. It may be helpful to use a medium containing antibiotics in general use in isolation procedures. This would be in addition to standard media. Such procedures may be helpful in obtaining a more accurate picture of the effective antibiotic resistances in the population of *V. cholerae* in that many plasmids are unstable in *V. cholerae* in the absence of the selective pressure from antibiotics for their maintenance.

Cholera Vaccines

The first candidate cholera vaccine was produced within a year of the first isolation of *V. cholerae* by Koch. Since then, a variety of vaccines have been developed and used. The discovery of cholera toxin (De, 1959) provided a further stimulus to vaccine development. All types of vaccine have been tried. These include live parenteral vaccines, killed parenteral vaccines, oral killed vaccines, oral subunit vaccines and live oral vaccines. Oral vaccines include those developed by chemical mutagenesis such as Texas Star; those produced by using the techniques of molecular biology to disarm fully virulent strains; and those that use the ability of other organisms such as *Salmonella typhi* type 21A, which has an expression vector for genes encoding relevant *V. cholerae* antigens.

Conventional parenteral vaccines have been of little use in cholera. The level of protection afforded is low, perhaps 40–80% protection during the first two to three months after administration but no significant protection six months after. There is some evidence suggesting that the vaccine may be more effective when administered to the inhabitants of highly endemic areas. However, the vaccine is not at all satisfactory, and the World Health Organization has recommended that its use be discontinued. The advances in our understanding of the pathogenesis of cholera reawaken interest in oral vaccines. The isolation of the infection from systemic immune systems, and the lack of success from parenteral vaccines, made cholera a prime target for the development of oral vaccines. Studies have focused on the development of a live oral vaccine, although killed vaccines have also been investigated. Considerable advances have been made and several oral candidate vaccines have been developed and shown to protect in volunteer studies.

The first new vaccine to reach the field test stage was a killed oral vaccine (Clemens *et al.*, 1987). Killed vaccines were tested in an extensive field trial in Bangladesh (Clemens *et al.*, 1986). The basic vaccine consisted of a mixture of heat-killed and formalin-killed cells of *V. cholerae* O1 of both the Ogawa and Inaba subtypes. In this trial, the basic vaccine was administered alone or in combination with the B subunit of cholera toxin, and *E. coli* K12 preparation was administered as a control. These vaccines provided good, although short-term, protection against *V. cholerae*, both in the field trial and in adult volunteers.

These vaccines needed to be administered and boosted on two occasions by further vaccine. This would have disadvantages for large-scale use. However, their success demonstrated the possibility of a successful vaccination campaign using an oral vaccine.

The use of a live oral vaccine should overcome the problem of the need for multiple vaccine administration. Several such candidate vaccine strains have been developed and tested. The prototype strain of this approach was the vaccine strain Texas Star SR (Levine *et al.*, 1984). This strain,

isolated after nitrosoguanidine mutagenesis, produces B subunits only. Texas Star may be considered as establishing the principles by which the development and testing of candidate vaccines were governed. More recent strains have shown greater promise. A number of genetically engineered strains have been developed and tested (Table 12g.8) (Levine *et al.*, 1988). Those engineered with attenuated *V. cholerae* strain CVD103 HgR have shown the greatest promise. This strain is a derivative of CVD103 which was itself derived from wild-type O1 classical Inaba strain 569B. Strain 569B is pathogenic for volunteers. A gene coding for mercury resistance was introduced into CVD103 to produce CVD103 HgR. This marker enables us to differentiate vaccine strain from wild-type *V. cholerae* O1. In volunteer studies the efficacy was about 60%. This is better than currently available vaccines. In some groups, effective efficacy was much higher than this: up to 100% in some instances. The vaccine has undergone volunteer studies or clinical trials in the USA (Kokloff *et al.*, 1992), Switzerland, Thailand, Indonesia (Suharyono *et al.*, 1992), Peru (Gotuzzo *et al.*, 1993), Chile and Costa Rica. Apart from initial volunteer studies, most of these have been randomized placebo-controlled double-blind trials. As mentioned above, the vaccine shows good protective efficacy but, perhaps equally important in

TABLE 12g.8   CANDIDATE VACCINE STRAINS OF *V. CHOLERAE*

Strain number	Toxigenic status	Parent strain		
		Number	Biotype	Serotype
Texas Star SR	A^-B^+	3083	El Tor	Ogawa
JBK 70	A^-B^-	N16961	El Tor	Inaba
CVD 101	A^-B^+	395	Classical	Ogawa
CVD 102[a]	A^-B^+	CVD 101	Classical	Ogawa
CVD 103	A^-B^+	569 B	Classical	Inaba
CVD 103 Hg[b]	A^-B^+	CVD 103	Classical	Inaba
CVD 104	A^-B^{-d}	JBK 70	El Tor	Inaba
CVD 105	A^-B^{+d}	CVD 101	Classical	Ogawa
CVD 109	A^-B^{-e}	E7946	El Tor	Ogawa
CVD 110^{-c}	A^-B^+	CVD 109	El Tor	Ogawa

[a] Thymine-dependent mutant.
[b] Hg resistance inserted into *hylA* locus.
[c] Hg resistance and *CtxB* inserted into parent *HlgA* locus.
[c] Genes encoding El Tor haemolysin deleted.
[e] ACE ZOT and Ctx genes deleted.

terms of its large-scale application, there are no side effects. Occasional subjects reported diarrhoea but this was of no greater incidence than in the control groups. Studies have been undertaken in both adults and children. We now have a vaccine produced by the methods of molecular biology that is a significant improvement on vaccines produced by other methods and has considerable potential for use in control of cholera. It is likely that future generations of engineered vaccines will be even more useful but, at the present, the claims that molecular biology are able to produce a single-dose, live oral vaccine providing significant immunity after oral administration seem to have been amply fulfilled (Levine and Kaper, 1993).

It is worthwhile noting briefly a few considerations about immunity to cholera. It has long been assumed that the production of local intestinal immunity is what protects against infection. However, the best laboratory correlate with immunity is circulating vibriocidal antibody. The reasons for this are not clear. Nonetheless, field studies have shown that vibriocidal antibody in populations is the best indicator of the susceptibility of individuals to cholera, and further, such vibriocidal antibody is produced as a result of stimulation by effective vaccines (Wasserman et al., 1994). Antibody production is not the only important factor in determining susceptibility to cholera. There is undoubtedly a genetic element. Studies in Bangladesh have indicated that among those developing clinical cholera there is an excess of persons with O blood group (Levine et al., 1979). The reason for this has not been fully clarified, although it has been suggested that H substance might act as a receptor for the fucose-resistant adhesin of *V. cholerae*.

REFERENCES

Albert, M.J., Siddique, A.K., Islam, M.S. *et al.* (1993) Large outbreak of clinical cholera due to *Vibrio cholerae* non-O1 in Bangladesh (Letter.) *Lancet*, **341**, 704.

Barua, D. and Burrows, W. (eds) (1974) *Cholera*. Saunders, Philadelphia.

Barua, D. and Greenough, W.B. (eds) (1992) *Cholera* (Current Topics in Infectious Diseases). Plenum, New York.

Baudry, B., Fasano, A., Ketley, J.M. *et al.* (1992) Cloning of a gene (*ZOT*) encoding a new toxin produced by *Vibrio cholerae*. *Infection and Immunity*, **60**, 428–434.

Baumann, P., Furniss, A.L. and Lee, J.V. (1984) Section 5. Facultatively anaerobic gram-negative rods. In *Bergey's Manual of Systematic Bacteriology*, vol. 1 (ed. J.G. Holt and N.R. Krieg), pp. 518–538. Williams & Wilkins, Baltimore.

Bhattacharya, S.K., Bhattacharya, M.F., Balakrish Nair, G. *et al.* (1993) Clinical profile of acute diarrhoea cases infected with the new epidemic strain of *Vibrio cholerae* O139: designation of the disease as cholera. *Journal of Infection*, **27**, 11–15.

Blake, P.A., Allegra, D.T., Snyder, J.D. *et al.* (1980) Cholera: a possible endemic focus in the United States. *New England Journal of Medicine*, **302**, 305–309.

Cash, R.A., Music, S.I., Libonati, P. *et al.* (1974) Response of man to infection with *Vibrio cholerae*. I. Clinical, serologic, and bacteriologic responses to a known inoculum. *Journal of Infectious Diseases*, **129**, 45–52.

Cheasty, T. and Rowe, B. (1994) New cholera strains. *PHLS Microbiology Digest*, **11**, 73–76.

Citarella, R.V. and Colwell, R.R. (1970) Polyphasic taxonomy of the genus *Vibrio*. *Journal of Bacteriology*, **104**, 434–442.

Clemens, J.D., Harris, J.R., Khan, M.R. *et al.* (1986) Field trial of oral cholera vaccines in Bangladesh. *Lancet*, **ii**, 124–127.

Clemens, J.D., Stanton, B.F., Chakraborty, J. *et al.* (1987) B subunit-whole cell and whole cell-only oral vaccines against cholera: studies on reactogenicity and immunogenicity. *Journal of Infectious Diseases*, **155**, 79–85.

Colwell, R.R. (ed.) (1984) *Vibrios in the Environment*. Wiley, New York.

Crowcroft, N.S. (1994) Cholera: current epidemiology. In *Communicable Disease Report Review*, **4**, Review Number 13:R157–164. Public Health Laboratory Service, London.

Davis, B.R,, Fanney, G.R., Maddon, J.M. *et al.* (1981) Characterisation of biochemically atypical *Vibrio cholerae* strain and designation of a new pathogenic species *Vibrio mimicus*. *Journal of Clinical Microbiology*, **14**, 631–639.

De, S.N. (1959) Enterotoxicity of bacteria-free culture filtrate of *Vibrio cholerae*. *Nature*, **183**, 1533.

Desmarchelier, P.M. and Reichelt, J.L. (1981) Phenotypic characterization of clinical and environmental isolates of *Vibrio cholerae* from Australia. *Current Microbiology*, **5**, 123–127.

DiRita, V.J. (1992) Co-ordinate expression of virulence genes by ToxR in *Vibrio cholerae*. *Molecular Microbiology*, **6**, 451–458.

DiRita, V.J., Parsot, C., Jander, G. *et al.* (1991) Regulatory cascade controls virulence in *Vibrio cholerae*. *Proceedings of the National Academy of Sciences of the USA*, **88**, 5403–5407.

Drasar, B.S. (1992) Pathogenesis and ecology: the case of cholera. *Journal of Tropical Medicine and Hygiene*, **95**, 365–372.

Farmer, J.J. and Hickman-Brenner, F.W. (1992) The Genera *Vibrio* and *Photobacterium*. In *The Prokaryotes*, 2nd edn, Vol. 3 (ed. A. Balows, H.G. Trüper, M. Dworkin *et al.*), pp. 2952–3011. Springer-Verlag, New York.

Fasano, A., Baudry, B., Pumplin, D.W. *et al.* (1991) *Vibrio cholerae* produces a second enterotoxin which affects intestinal tight junctions. *Proceedings of the National Academy of Science of the USA*, **88**, 5242–5246.

Feachem, R.G. (1981) Environmental aspects of cholera epidemiology. I. A review of selected reports of endemic and epidemic situations during 1961–1980. *Tropical Diseases Bulletin of the Bureau of Hygiene and Tropical Diseases*, **78**, 675–698.

Feachem, R.G. (1982) Environmental aspects of cholera epidemiology. III. Transmission and control. *Tropical Diseases Bulletin of the Bureau of Hygiene and Tropical Diseases*, **79**, 1–47.

Feachem, R., Miller, C. and Drasar, B. (1981) Environmental aspects of cholera epidemiology. II. Occurrence and survival of *Vibrio cholerae* in the environment. *Tropical Diseases Bulletin of the Bureau of Hygiene and Tropical Diseases*, **78**, 865–880.

Freter, R. and Jones, G.W. (1976) Adhesive properties of *Vibrio cholerae*: nature of the interaction with intact mucosal surfaces. *Infection and Immunity*, **14**, 246–256.

Gangarosa, E.J., Beisel, W.R., Benyajati, C. *et al.* (1960) The nature of the gastrointestinal lesion in Asiatic cholera and its relation to pathogenesis: a biopsy study. *American Journal of Tropical Medicine and Hygiene*, **9**, 125–135.

Glass, R.I., Huq, M.I., Lee, J.V. *et al.* (1983) Plasmid-borne multiple drug resistance in *Vibrio cholerae* serogroup O1, biotype El Tor: evidence for a point-source outbreak in Bangladesh. *Journal of Infectious Diseases*, **147**, 204–209.

Glass, R.I., Claeson, M., Blake, P.A. *et al.* (1991) Cholera in Africa: lessons on transmission and control for Latin America. *Lancet*, **338**, 791–795.

Gotuzzo, E., Butron, B., Seas, C. *et al.* (1993) Safety, immunogenicity, and excretion pattern of single-dose live oral cholera vaccine CVD 103-HgR in Peruvian adults of high and low socioeconomic levels. *Infection and Immunity*, **61**, 3994–3997.

Guidelines for Cholera Control (1986) World Health Organization: Programme for Control of Diarrhoeal Diseases, 80.4 Rev 1.

Herrington, D.A., Hall, R.H., Losonsky, G. *et al.* (1988) Toxin, toxin-coregulated pili, and the *toxR* regulon are essential for *Vibrio cholerae* pathogenesis in humans. *Journal of Experimental Medicine*, **168**, 1487–1492.

Islam, M.S., Drasar, B.S. and Sack, R.B. (1993) The aquatic environment as a reservoir of *Vibrio cholerae*: a review. *Journal of Diarrhoeal Diseases Research*, **11**, 197–206.

Islam, M.S., Drasar, B.S. and Sack, R.B. (1994) The aquatic flora and fauna as reservoirs of *Vibrio cholerae*: a review *Journal of Diarrhoeal Diseases Research*, **12**, 87–96.

Jones, G.W. and Freter, R. (1976) Adhesive properties of *Vibrio cholerae*: nature of the interaction with isolated rabbit brush border membranes and human erythrocytes. *Infection and Immunity*, **14**, 240–245.

Karasawa, T., Mihara, T., Kurazono, H. *et al.* (1993) Distribution of the *zot* (zonula occludens toxin) gene among strains of *Vibrio cholerae* O1 an non-O1. *FEMS Microbiology Letters*, **106**, 143–145.

Kaufman, M.R. Shaw, C.E., Jones, I.D. *et al.* (1993) Biogenesis and regulation of the *Vibrio cholerae* toxin-coregulated pilus: analogies to other virulence factor secretory systems. *Gene*, **126**, 43–49.

Koblavi, S., Grimont, F. and Grimont, P.A. (1990) Clonal diversity of *Vibrio cholerae* O1 evidenced by rRNA gene restriction patterns. *Research in Microbiology*, **141**, 645–657.

Koch, R. (1884) Ueber die Cholerabacterian. *Deutsche Medizinische Wochenschrift*, **10**, 725–728.

Kotloff, K.L., Wasserman, S.S., O'Donnell, S. *et al.* (1992) Safety and immunogenicity in North Americans of a single dose of live oral cholera vaccine CVD 103-HgR: results of a randomized, placebo-controlled, double-blind crossover trial. *Infection and Immunity*, **60**, 4430–4432.

Levine, M.M. and Kaper, J.B. (1993) Live oral vaccines against cholera: an update. *Vaccine*, **11**, 207–212.

Levine, M.M., Nalin, D.R., Rennels, M.B. *et al.* (1979) Genetic susceptibility to cholera. *Annals of Human Biology*, **6**, 369–374.

Levine, M.M., Black, R.E., Clements, M.L. *et al.* (1982) The pathogenicity of nonenterotoxigenic *Vibrio cholerae* serogroup O1 biotype El Tor isolated from sewage water in Brazil. *Journal of Infectious Disease*, **145**, 296–299.

Levine, M.M., Black, R.E., Clements, M.L. *et al.* (1984) Evaluation in humans of attenuated *Vibrio cholerae* El Tor Ogawa strain Texas Star-SR as a live oral vaccine. *Infection and Immunity*, **43**, 515–522.

Levine, M.M., Kaper, J.B., Herrington, D. *et al.* (1988) Volunteer studies of deletion mutants of *Vibrio cholerae* O1 prepared by recombinant techniques. *Infection and Immunity*, **56**, 161–167.

Lin, Z., Kumagai, K., Baba, K. *et al.* (1993) *Vibrio parahaemolyticus* has a homolog of the *Vibrio cholerae toxRS* operon that mediates environmentally induced regulation of the thermostable direct hemolysin gene. *Journal of Bacteriology*, **175**, 3844–3855.

MacNamara, C. (1876) *A History of Asiatic Cholera*. Macmillan, London.

MacPherson, J. (1872) *Annals of Cholera from the Earliest Periods to the Year 1817*. Ranken, London.

McCardell, B.A., Madden, J.M. and Shah, D.B. (1985) Isolation and characterization of a cytolysin produced by *Vibrio cholerae* serogroup non-O1. *Canadian Journal of Microbiology*, **31**, 711–720.

O'Brien, A.D., Chen, M.E., Holmes, R.K. *et al.* (1984) Environmental and human isolates of *Vibrio cholerae* and *Vibrio parahaemolyticus* produce a *Shigella dysenteriae* 1 (Shiga)-like cytotoxin. *Lancet*, i, 77–78.

Orton, R. (1831) *The Epidemic Cholera of India: Madras*. Burgess & Hill, London.

Parsot, C. and Mekalanos, J.J. (1990) Expression of ToxR, the transcriptional activator of the virulence factors in *Vibrio cholerae*, is modulated by the heat shock response. *Proceedings of the National Academy of Sciences of the USA*, **87**, 9898–9902.

Pearson, G.D.N., Woods, A., Chiang, S.L. *et al.* (1993) CTX genetic element encodes a site-specific recombination system and an intestinal colonization factor. *Proceedings of the National Academy of Sciences of the USA*, **90**, 3750–3754.

Pettenkofer, von M. (1892) Ueber Cholera unt Berücksichtigung der jüngsten Cholera-Epidemic in Hamburg. *Münchener Medizische Wochenschrift*, **46**, 345–348.

Pollitzer, R. (1959) *Cholera*. WHO, Geneva.

Ramamurthy, T., Garg, S., Sharma, R. *et al.* (1993) Emergence of novel strain of *Vibrio cholerae* with epidemic potential in southern and eastern India. (Letter.) *Lancet*, **341**, 703–704.

Ramamurthy, T., Albert, M.J., Huq, A. *et al.* (1994) *Vibrio mimicus* with multiple toxin types isolated from human and environmental sources. *Journal of Medical Microbiology*, **40**, 194–196.

Risks of Transmission of Cholera by Food (1991) Health Programs Development, Veterinary Public Health Program. World Health Organization, Washington, DC.

Salyers, A.A. and Whitt, D.D. (1994) *Bacterial Pathogenesis: Molecular Approach*, Ch.12, pp. 141–156. American Society for Microbiology, Washington, DC.

Snow, J. (1849) *On Mode of Communication of Cholera*. John Churchill, London.

Snow, J. (1855) *On the Mode of Communication of Cholera*, 2nd edn. John Churchill, London.

Suharyono, Simanjuntak, C., Witham, N. *et al.* (1992) Safety and immunogenicity of single-dose live oral cholera vaccine CVD103-HgR in 5–9-year-old Indonesian children. *Lancet*, **340**, 689–694.

Suntharasamai, P., Migasena, S., Vongsthongsri, U. *et al.* (1992) Clinical and bacteriological studies of El Tor cholera after ingestion of known inocula in Thai volunteers. *Vaccine*, **10**, 502–505.

Tamplin, M.L., Gauzens, A.L., Huq, A. *et al.* (1990) Attachment of *Vibrio cholerae* serogroup O1 to zooplankton and phytoplankton of Bangladesh waters. *Applied and Environmental Microbiology*, **56**, 1977–1980.

Thom, S., Warhurst, D. and Drasar, B.S. (1992) Association of *Vibrio cholerae* with fresh water amoebae. *Journal of Medical Microbiology*, **36**, 303–306.

Wachsmuth, I.K., Blake, P.A. and Olsvik, O. (eds) (1994) Vibrio cholerae *and Cholera: Molecular to Global Perspectives*. American Society for Microbiology, Washington, DC.

Wasserman, S.S., Losonsky, G.A., Noriega, F. *et al.* (1994) Kinetics of the vibriocidal antibody response to live oral cholera vaccines. *Vaccine*, **12**, 1000–1003.

West, P.A. (1989), The human pathogenic vibrios: a public health update with environmental perspectives. *Epidemiology and Infection*, **103**, 1–34.

13

ACINETOBACTER AND OTHER GRAM-NEGATIVE NON-FERMENTATIVE BACILLI

E. Bergogne-Bérézin

INTRODUCTION

Among Gram-negative aerobic non-fermentative bacilli, besides *Pseudomonas* spp., several groups have gained prominence in the past decade because of the increased frequency of their recovery in clinical specimens and their increasing role in nosocomial infections. In a descending order of importance are *Acinetobacter* spp., *Stenotrophomonas* (*Xanthomonas*) *maltophilia*, *Flavobacterium* spp. and *Alcaligenes faecalis*. These bacteria possess several characteristics in common:

(1) *Epidemiology*. They are saprophytic bacilli, present in the environment (soil, water). As ubiquitous organisms, they may be recovered as well from the hospital environment and from colonized or infected patients or from staff (hand carriage).

(2) *Pathogenic role*. As opportunistic pathogens, these bacilli are responsible for nosocomial infections, mainly septicaemia, urinary tract infections and secondary meningitis. Their predominant role is in nosocomial pneumonia

and particularly in ventilator-associated pneumonia.

(3) *Antibiotic therapy*. They are responsible for infections which are difficult to treat due to their frequent multiple resistance to the major antibiotics. Various mechanisms of resistance have been recognized in these bacteria. Combination therapy is usually recommended for treatment based on careful antibiotic susceptibility testing.

(4) *Bacteriology and typing*. Gram-negative non-fermentative bacilli belonging to these genera are non-fastidious organisms, easily grown and identified thanks to reliable modern methods used. Their nomenclature has been clarified and speciation/subspeciation of these bacteria by genotypic analysis has resulted in reliable taxonomy with distinct strain types. In epidemiology, new molecular markers have emerged, allowing recognition of genotypically related strains involved in hospital outbreaks of infection. A schematic key to identification of non-fermentative aerobic Gram-negative bacilli is shown in Figure 13.1.

Principles and Practice of Clinical Bacteriology. Edited by A.M. Emmerson, P.M. Hawkey and S.H. Gillespie
© 1997 John Wiley & Sons Ltd

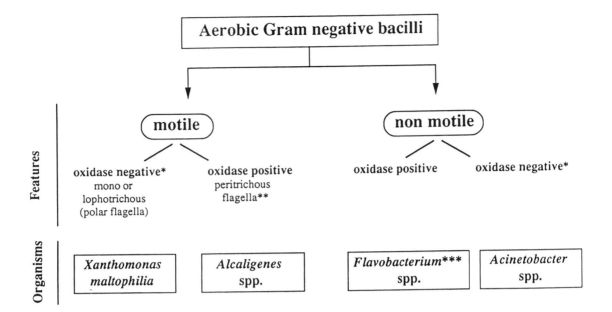

*oxidative metabolism of glucose.
**Alcaligenes : degenerated peritrichous flagella in the genus Alcaligenes, however functional.
***variably pigmented colonies (yellowish-orange pigment).

Figure 13.1. Key to identification of non-fermentative aerobic Gram-negative bacilli (genus Pseudomonas excluded).

ACINETOBACTER

INTRODUCTION

Acinetobacter spp. are Gram-negative bacteria commonly present in soil and water as free-living saprophytes, and are also isolated as commensals from skin, throat and various secretions of healthy people. There have been frequent changes in their taxonomy. Their pathogenic role in humans has been understood recently; Acinetobacter has emerged as an important nosocomial pathogen involved in outbreaks of hospital infections. The increasing number of these infections and the natural resistance of the strains have led to studies of epidemiology and resistance mechanisms in Acinetobacter.

DESCRIPTION OF THE GENUS

Definition

Acinetobacter strains are non-fermentative non-fastidious aerobic Gram-negative coccobacilli, usually found in diploid formation, and also in chains of variable length. They are not motile, as suggested by the Greek root of the word ακινετος (akinetos), i.e. 'unable to move'; but the cells display a 'twitching motility' presumably due to the presence of polar fimbriae. They are strictly aerobic and grow well on all common media, at temperatures between 20 and 30 °C, but for most strains the optimum is 33–35 °C. Growth at 41 and 44 °C can occur for a few species and is a discriminating character between species. Identification of Acinetobacter spp. is based upon oxidase-negative,

TABLE 13.1 EVOLUTION OF TAXONOMY AND DESIGNATION OF *ACINETOBACTER* SPP.

Genus *Moraxella*

	Group 2 — Oxidase negative										Group 1 — Oxidase positive	
Previous designations	*M. glucidolytica* var. var. nonliquefaciens var. liquefaciens[a] — *Bacterium anitratum, B5W, Diplococcus mucosus*							*M. lwoffi* var. nonliquefaciens var. liquefaciens[a] — *Mima polymorpha, Herellea vaginicola*			*M. lacunata* var. typica, var. atypica	*M. duplex* var. non-liquefaciens, var. liquefaciens
Previous nomenclatures	*Moraxella glucidolytica* — Genus *Acinetobacter*: one species, *Acinetobacter calcoaceticus* (Brisou and Prévôt, 1954)[b]							*Moraxella lwoffi*				
Biovars	*A. anitratus* (glucose acidified)							*A. lwoffi*[c] (glucose negative)				
(Bouvet and Grimont, 1986)	*A. calcoaceticus*	*A. baumannii*	UN[d]	*A. haemolyticus*	*A. junii*	UN[d]	*A. johnsonii*	*A. lwoffi*	UN[d]	*A. radioresistens*		
Genospecies[e]	1	2	3	4	5	6	7	8/9	10 11	12		

[a] All strains designated *liquefaciens* were proteolytic (gelatin hydrolysis which is recognized in *A. haemolyticus* and genospecies 6 in the current nomenclature).
[b] *Bergey's Manual* (1984).
[c] *A. alcaligenes* is haemolytic.
[d] UN, unnamed genospecies.
[e] The numbered genospecies are based on DNA–DNA hybridizations.

catalase-positive, indole-negative, nitrate-negative tests; production or not of acid from D-glucose, D-ribose, D-xylose, and L-arabinose (utilized oxidatively as carbon sources) has been cited above for strains formerly designated var. *anitratus* or var. *lwoffi* (Table 13.1).

Taxonomy

The history of the genus *Acinetobacter* has been confusing for many years and extensive taxonomic changes have occurred. Oxidase-negative non-motile Gram-negative diplobacilli have been classified into various genera, the most common being designated *Bacterium anitratum* (Schaub and Hauber, 1948), *Herellea vaginicola* and *Mima polymorpha* (Debord, 1939), *Achromobacter*, *Alcaligenes*, *Neisseria*, *Micrococcus calcoaceticus*, *Diplococcus*, B5W and *Cytophaga* (Juni, 1984). The genus *Acinetobacter*, as originally conceived by Brisou and Prévôt (1954), included oxidase-positive (*Moraxella*) and oxidase-negative strains, but in 1971 the Subcommittee of the Taxonomy of *Moraxella* and Allied Bacteria proposed that the genus *Acinetobacter* include only the oxidase-negative strains (Bøvre and Henriksen, 1976). In the 9th edition of *Bergey's Manual* (1984), classified in the family Neisseriaceae, the genus *Acinetobacter* comprised one species, *A. calcoaceticus*, and two varieties: var. *anitratus* (formerly *Herellea vaginicola*) and var. *lwoffi* (formerly *Mima polymorpha*). Recently, a taxonomic study of a large number of *Acinetobacter* strains by using modern methods of taxonomy (genetic transformations, DNA hybridizations and rRNA sequence comparisons), has resulted in a new classification of *Acinetobacter* spp. (Bouvet and Grimont, 1986): more than 15 species or genomic species (groups of strains at least 70% related by DNA hybridization with divergence values (ΔT_m) below 5 °C; Grimont and Bouvet, 1991) have been defined and new species have been created: *A. baumannii* (formerly *A. calcoaceticus* var. *anitratus* and *A. glucidolytica non liquefaciens*), *A. haemolyticus*, *A. junii*, *A. johnsonii* and *A. radioresistens* (Bouvet and Grimont, 1986). The new definition of *Acinetobacter* is based on phenotypic characters (biotyping) and

identification of genotypic species. A schematic presentation of the evolution of taxonomy and the main characteristics of these 'new' *Acinetobacter* spp. are shown in Tables 13.1 and 13.2 respectively. Species designation may also include previously used species designations: *A. anitratus* for glucose-positive strains, *A. lwoffi* for glucose-negative strains, and the designation '*Acinetobacter calcoaceticus*' is still widely used in the recent literature, remaining the reference name according to *Bergey's Manual* (Alexander *et al.*, 1988; Bleschemidt *et al.*, 1992; Gerner-Smidt *et al.*, 1992; Leonov *et al.*, 1990; Sato and Nakae, 1991; Urban *et al.*, 1993). The ability to produce acid from glucose (oxidation of glucose to produce gluconic acid) seems not to be regarded any more as a character of taxonomic significance.

Genetic Organization and Regulation

Acinetobacter has a circular chromosomal linkage map (Towner, 1991) and 29 genetic loci have now been mapped (Vivian, 1991). The three major modes of genetic transfer (transformation, conjugation, transduction) have been demonstrated in *Acinetobacter* and studies of the topological structure of the chromosome are in progress. *Acinetobacter* genes in appropriate vectors are already available.

Studies of organization and regulation of genes concerned with tryptophan biosynthesis and the β-ketoadipate degradative pathway have been carried out and similarities or homologies have been shown between *Acinetobacter* and *Pseudomonas* spp. with regard to genes regulating these metabolic pathways. Moreover, due to the clinical importance of antibiotic resistance in *Acinetobacter*, plasmids and transposons conferring antibiotic resistance have been transferred conjugally to recipient strains but the regulation of resistance genes is still under investigation (Lambert *et al.*, 1990; Towner, 1991).

PATHOGENESIS OF INFECTIONS

Virulence of *Acinetobacter* spp.

Among factors influencing the virulence of *Acinetobacter*, several characteristics seem to play a

TABLE 13.2 MAIN FEATURES FOR IDENTIFICATION OF THE MOST FREQUENTLY ISOLATED *ACINETOBACTER* SPP.

Bivoars	Genus *Acinetobacter*: *Acinetobacter calcoaceticus* (Brisou and Prévôt, 1954)[a]										
	A. anitratus (Glucose acidified)						*A. lwoffi*[b] (glucose negative)				
Genospecies	*A. calcoaceticus*	*A. baumannii*	UN[c]	*A. haemolyticus*	*A. junii*	UN[c]	*A. johnsonii*	*A. lwoffi*		UN[c]	*A. radioresistens*
(Bouvet and Grimont, 1986)	1[d]	2	3	4	5	6	7	8/9	10	11	12
Main characteristics	No growth at 41 °C	Growth at 44 °C	Growth at 41 °C but not at 44 °C	37 °C	37 °C	37 °C	–	37 °C	37 °C	37 °C	37 °C
Glucose (acidified)	Positive	Positive	Positive	Positive (52%)	Negative	Positive (66%)	Negative	Negative	Positive	Negative	Negative
Haemolysis	–	–	–	+(100%)	–	+(100%)	–	–	–	–	–
Gelatin hydrolysis	–	–	–	+(96%)	–	+(100%)	–	–	–	–	–
Utilization tests[e]											
DL-Lactate assimilation	+[f]	+	+	–[g]	+	–	+	+	+	+	–
Citrate	+	+	+	+(91%)	+(82%)	+	+	–	+	+	+
Malonate	+	+	+	–	–	–	–	–	–	–	+

[a] *Bergey's Manual* (1984).
[b] *A. alcaligenes* is haemolytic.
[c] UN, unnamed genospecies.
[d] The numbered genospecies are based on DNA–DNA hybridizations.
[e] Eleven other assimilation tests of carbon and energy sources can be used (Bouvet and Grimont, 1986; Gerner-Smidt, 1989).
[f] 100% positive strains.
[g] 0% positive strains.

role in enhancing the virulence of strains involved in infections. The presence of a polysaccharide capsule formed of L-rhamnose and D-glucose (Juni, 1984) renders the surface of strains more hydrophilic, but hydrophobicity is higher in *A. baumannii* isolated from catheters, or tracheal devices. The adhesiveness of *Acinetobacter* to human epithelial cells in relation to the presence of fimbriae correlates with twitching motility and/or is mediated by the capsular polysaccharide. A few enzymes (butyrate esterase, caprylate esterase and leucine arylamidase) seem to be involved in damaging tissue lipids. No DNAase, elastase, haemolysin, trypsin or chymotrypsin production has been detected in *Acinetobacter* strains. The lipopolysaccharide (LPS) component of the cell wall and the presence of lipid A are likely to participate in the pathogenicity of *Acinetobacter* in intensive care unit (ICU) patients (Avril and Mesnard, 1991).

Host predisposing factors

Various risk factors predisposing to severe infection common to *Acinetobacter* infections and other nosocomial agents have been identified over the last 10 years. Susceptible patients include those with severe underlying diseases: malignancy, burns, immunosuppression and major surgery. Age can play a role in the occurrence of *Acinetobacter* nosocomial infections, which are seen frequently in elderly patients (Ng *et al.*, 1989) and neonates as well (Stone and Des, 1986). The setting for infection is usually the medical or surgical ICU, renal or burns unit. Tubes, catheters and all kinds of artificial devices act as portals of entry at the site of infection. The role of antibiotics in predisposing to infection is probably in altering the normal flora and selecting resistant microorganisms. In French hospitals, *Acinetobacter* is found in 9.7% of nosocomial infections today (Joly-Guillou *et al.*, 1992b).

EPIDEMIOLOGY OF *ACINETOBACTER* SPP.

Strains of *Acinetobacter* are ubiquitous organisms: they are widely distributed in nature and can

be found in virtually 100% of soil and fresh-water samples when appropriate culture techniques are used (Von Gravenitz, 1985). As non-fastidious organisms, they utilize a wide variety of substrates as sole carbon source. In fresh-water samples, less than 1 to 7.9×10^4 cfu per 100 ml have been recorded, whereas in raw sewage effluents up to 10^6 cfu per 100 ml have been found. *Acinetobacter* can also be isolated from food and animals and forms part of the normal flora of fresh meats as well as contributing to the spoilage process of refrigerated meats. Human carriage has been demonstrated as well (Noble *et al.*, 1986).

Hospital Environment

The organism has been found in the inanimate environment, especially in moist situations such as room cold-air humidifiers, tap water, wash hand basins, water-baths, in moist Wright respirometers and all types of ventilatory equipment (Vieu *et al.*, 1979) which are capable of aerosolizing the organism: in angiography catheters, blood collection tubes and plastic urinals. The presence of *Acinetobacter* in mattresses in burns units made wet by fluids penetrating into the foam interior has been reported. *Acinetobacter* strains are likely to arise from the external environment rather than from an endogenous source.

Human Carriage

Acinetobacter can be a part of the bacterial flora of the skin in healthy adults and have been found in the axillae, groin and toe webs of normal individuals (Taplin *et al.*, 1963). Up to 25% of normal adults may harbour *Acinetobacter*, which is occasionally found in the oral cavity and respiratory tract (Glew *et al.*, 1977). Less frequently the organism can colonize the normal intestine, but this does not seem to constitute an important reservoir (Von Gravenitz, 1985). Both the skin of patients and staff have been implicated as the source of outbreaks of hospital infections; it has been shown that hand carriage of epidemic strains may occur on up to

29% of nurses, and transmission of *Acineto-bacter* strains from patients to the hands of staff has been demonstrated (French *et al.*, 1980). Movement of patients from ward to ward contributes to spread within the hospital and *Acinetobacter* spp. become established as part of the resident skin flora (Musa *et al.*, 1990), providing a source for hospital outbreaks.

CLINICAL MANIFESTATIONS

Acinetobacter has been isolated in various types of opportunistic infection including septicaemia, pneumonia, endocarditis, meningitis, skin and wound sepsis, and urinary tract infection (French *et al.*, 1980; Bergogne-Bérézin *et al.*, 1987; Ng *et al.*, 1989; Joly-Guillou *et al.*, 1992b). Although the organism has been frequently associated with nosocomial infection, some cases of community-acquired infections have also been reported, indicative of the primary pathogenicity of this organism (Rudin *et al.*, 1979). The distribution by site of *Acinetobacter* infections does not differ from other nosocomial Gram-negative bacteria. The main sites of infection in several surveys (Glew *et al.*, 1977, Joly-Guillou *et al.*, 1992a, 1992b) were the lower respiratory tract and the urinary tract, with rates of infection ranging from 15% to 30% of total infections caused by *Acinetobacter* (Table 13.3).

Respiratory Infection: Nosocomial Pneumonia

Nosocomial respiratory tract infection with *Acinetobacter* spp. occurs frequently in hospitals, especially in ICUs. Large outbreaks of *Acinetobacter* pneumonia have been described. All patients had severe underlying disease requiring assisted ventilation and most had a tracheostomy or were intubated, with either pneumonia of a lobar distribution, or tracheobronchitis, fever and purulent sputum yielding *Acinetobacter* as the sole or predominant organism. *Acinetobacter* represents 15.6% of the total Gram-negative bacilli involved in nosocomial pneumonia in France (Joly-Guillou *et al.*, 1992a). Microbiological diagnosis of nosocomial *Acinetobacter* pneumonia is mainly based on quantitative culture of samples taken by using a protected specimen brush (cut-off point $\geq 10^3$ cfu/ml) or by means of broncho-alveolar lavage (cut-off point $\geq 10^5$ cfu/ml). Community-acquired cases of pneumonia caused by *Acinetobacter* have been reported (Anstey *et al.*, 1992; Rudin *et al.*, 1979) and they may be more common than was previously recognized. As in other Gram-negative pneumonias, *Acinetobacter* pneumonia has been described in middle-aged or elderly patients with chronic underlying disease, alcoholics, but only rarely in previously healthy patients who develop a fulminant pneumonia with

TABLE 13.3   DISTRIBUTION OF *ACINETOBACTER* STRAINS BY SITES OF INFECTION

Clinical origin	USA[a]	France[b]		Belgium[c]
		University-Hospital Bichat–Claude Bernard	%(±SD) (n.s.)	
Year	NNIS (%) [1372] 1974–1977	1981	1991	89 ICU[d] 1991	% [237] 1990–1991
Urine	27	32	21	30.5(±15)	27
Tracheobronchial specimens	28.9	17.5	27	25.6(±13)	24.8
Pus, wounds	21.5	34	27.5	19.1(±16)	22.3
Blood cultures	9.3	6	7.5	7.5(±5)	7.6
Catheters	–	7	15.5	5(5)	–
Other (CNS, intra-abdominal area, burns, cardiovascular system etc.)	13.3	3	2	12(±7)	18.1

In brackets, number of strains; NS, not stated. After [a] Glew *et al.* (1977); [b] Joly-Guillou *et al.* (1992a); [c] Struelens *et al.* (1993); [d] Paediatric ICU: 15%; burn units: 8%; medical-surgical ICUs: 77%.

shock and severe hypoxaemia. The onset of the disease is rapid but non-specific with rapid prostration and respiratory distress.

Urinary Tract Infection (UTI)

Several reviews (Bergogne-Bérézin et al., 1987; Glew et al., 1977; Larson, 1984) have described Acinetobacter in 2–61% of nosocomially acquired UTI. A recent investigation in France has indicated an overall incidence of 30.5% of UTI (Joly-Guillou et al., 1992a). Factors predisposing patients to this infection do not differ from those of other nosocomial bacteria. Occasionally Acinetobacter spp. may cause community-acquired UTI in the absence of known predisposing factors.

Meningitis

Nosocomial meningitis is an infrequent manifestation of Acinetobacter infection. The first case report was in 1908 by Von Lingelsheim and the organism, then designated Diplococcus mucosus, was later renamed Mima by Debord (1939) because of its resemblance to the meningococcus on Gram stain. Cases of meningitis due to this organism have been reported after neurosurgical procedures, but rare cases of primary meningitis, especially in children, have also occurred. Acinetobacter meningitis may result from the introduction of the organism directly into the CNS following intracranial surgery, as well as after transnasal aspiration of craniopharyngioma, or lumbar puncture. The course of the disease has been described as a relatively indolent bacterial meningitis with meningeal signs, high fever, lethargy or headache. However, an acute clinical course may also occur. Problems may arise in diagnosis since the organism may mimic meningococci or Haemophilus influenzae due to its plemorphism.

Miscellaneous

Skin and wound infections, abscesses (Glew et al., 1977; Muller-Serieys et al., 1989), septicaemia (Ng et al., 1986), endocarditis (Gradon et al., 1992), peritonitis and burn wound infections

(Bergogne-Bérézin et al., 1987), have been described in the literature. Their rates vary depending on the hospital, the ward and the kind of patients involved.

LABORATORY DIAGNOSIS

Morphology

Acinetobacter is a non-motile Gram-negative rod which has an unusual morphology that can be of help in diagnosis: in smears, prepared from clinical specimens or from one-day blood agar plate, as well as in the stationary phase of growth, Acinetobacter appears quite spherical and in pairs (coccobacillary diplobacillus). Its usual size is 1–1.5 μm in diameter and 1.5–2.5 μm in length and, when grown in the presence of penicillin or in repeated subcultures, Acinetobacter strains are longer, club-shaped bacilli. They do not form spores and are not motile, but a 'twitching motility' has been cited as related presumably to the presence of polar fimbriae (Bergey's Manual, 1984). Another morphological characteristic of Acinetobacter is Gram stain, officially Gram negative but frequently difficult to destain, resulting in dark Gram-positive areas of the bacteria. This character together with the coccobacillary shape may help a trained microbiologist to suspect Acinetobacter although microscopic examination may sometimes lead to initial confusion with Moraxella or Neisseria strains. Electron microscopy of thin sections of cells have shown a cell wall structure typical of a Gram-negative bacteria and its chemical structure does not differ from that of other Gram negatives.

Cultural and Metabolic Characteristics

All strains grow well on common media at temperatures ranging from 26 to 30 °C, with an optimal temperature of 30 °–35 °C for most strains. They are strictly aerobic organisms; all are catalase positive and oxidase negative, the latter character being characteristic of the genus Acinetobacter, all other non-fermentative Gram-negative bacilli being oxidase positive. Most strains grow on

MacConkey agar or on Drigalski medium and lactose-negative colonies of *Acinetobacter* are 1–3 mm in diameter. On Mueller–Hinton agar medium, the colonies are smooth, non-pigmented, and generally iridescent; they are mucoid when the cells are encapsulated and the colonies are not inhibited by penicillin, unlike the genus *Moraxella* (previously confused with the genus *Acinetobacter*). Most strains can grow on a simple mineral medium such as the mineral base medium (MBM acetate) (Gilardi, 1985). In nutrient broth *Acinetobacter* growth is abundant and homogeneous.

Identification

Growth temperatures of 37, 41 and 44 °C in broth is a discriminating character between species (Table 13.2). Precise identification of species is based on the following characteristics:

- oxidization of glucose;
- gelatin hydrolysis;
- search for α-type haemolysis on horse or sheep blood agar (which is the result of phospholipase excretion);
- utilization tests (carbon/energy sources).

The nutritional abilities of *Acinetobacter* strains (mainly growth in a defined medium with ammonia as nitrogen source and a given carbon source) are considered today as essential properties for identification and biotyping of *Acinetobacter* spp. These utilization tests include: *trans*-aconitate, β-alanine, DL-aminobutyrate, arginine, azelate, citrate, glutarate, histidine, DL-lactate, D-malate and malonate. Responses for the most discriminant tests for identification of *Acinetobacter* spp. are shown in Table 13.4. Strains of species *A. calcoaceticus* and *A. baumannii* can utilize glucose by the oxidative pathway. All species use lactate except for *A. haemolyticus*, and all utilize citrate except for *A. lwoffi*. *Acinetobacter haemolyticus* and genospecies 6 are proteolytic but both acidify glucose only for about half of the strains. In fact many strains are unable to grow on glucose, but if they possess an aldose dehydrogenase they can acidify glucose media and media containing other sugars such as D-xylose, L-arabinose and D-galactose to their respective lactones. Nitrite and nitrate can serve as nitrogen sources since *Acinetobacter* possesses an assimilatory nitrate reductase (Juni, 1984).

TABLE 13.4 IDENTIFICATION TESTS FOR *ACINETOBACTER* BIOTYPING

Genomic species		Utilization tests				
Species designation	DNA Group	β-Alanine	Citrate	Glutamate	DL-Lactate	Malonate
A. calcoaceticus	1	+[a]	+	+	+	+
A. baumannii	2	+	+	+	+	+ (98)
Unnamed	3	+	+	+	+	+ (87)
A. haemolyticus	4	(−)	+ (91)[b]	(−)	(−)	(−)
A. junii	5	(−)	+ (82)	(−)	+	(−)
Unnamed	6	(−)	+	(−)	(−)	(−)
A. johnsonii	7	(−)	+	(−)	+	(−)
A. lwoffi	8	(−)	(−)	(−)	+	(−)
Unnamed	10	+	+	+	+	(−)
Unnamed	11	+	+	+	+	(−)
A. radioresistens	12	(−)	(−)	+	+	100

[a] 100% of positive strains; (−), 0% of positive strains.
[b] Figures in parentheses indicate percentage of positive strains of a given genospecies.
After Bouvet and Grimont (1986).

Typing Systems

In the last 30 years, outbreaks of *Acinetobacter* infection have been an increasing concern in hospitals. For epidemiological investigation of hospital outbreaks various typing methods have been devised for *Acinetobacter*. Due to the ubiquitous distribution of these bacteria, reliable typing methods would be valuable in epidemiological studies.

Phenotypic systems

The early typing systems were based on phenotypic characters, such as biotyping (Bouvet and Grimont, 1986), phage typing, serology or bacteriocin typing (Bergogne-Bérézin *et al.*, 1987). Determination of susceptibility patterns (Joly-Guillou *et al.*, 1988) has proved useful in differentiating outbreak strains when there are marked similarities in resistance patterns or when a new resistance emerges (French *et al.*, 1980; Devaud *et al.*, 1982). However, the main limitation of this epidemiological tool is its lack of specificity, as several distinct strains may share the same antibiogram pattern. Resistances may change rapidly within the same outbreak due to the acquisition of plasmids coding for antibiotic resistance, or the appearance of chromosomal mutants. Many strains possess a capsule which has been used for typing by an immunofluorescent antibody technique. In this scheme, 28 serotypes were recognizable, but there is little experience of its application in a clinical setting. Another method using agglutination reactions with rabbit antisera has been used and identified 20 serovars (Traub, 1989). A bacteriocin typing method has also been described (Andrews, 1986) and has been shown useful in epidemiological investigations. A phage-typing system has been developed at the Phage-typing Centre of the Pasteur Institute, Paris (Vieu *et al.*, 1979). The system was based on the use of two complementary series of bacteriophages, highly specific for *A. calcoaceticus*. The initial set of 21 phages used since 1976 for routine investigation of hospital outbreaks of *Acinetobacter* infections was enlarged by the addition of a further 14 phages. Approximately 2500 clinical strains from France and other European countries have been analysed and predominant phage types (17 and 124) were recognized in outbreaks.

Protein profiles

Whole cell and cell envelope protein electrophoresis (Dijkshoorn *et al.*, 1993) (sodium dodecyl sulphate–polyacrylamide gel electrophoresis (SDS–PAGE)) has been used to study the dissemination of *Acinetobacter* strains within hospitals: electrophoretic patterns of cell envelope proteins included 30–50 protein bands of clearly distinguishable staining intensities; all isolates within each outbreak were very similar in cell envelope protein profile.

Genotypic systems

With the recent development of molecular biology techniques, new typing systems based on genotypic characters have proved discriminative, stable and reproducible. Ribotyping (Dijkshoorn *et al.*, 1993; Gerner-Smidt, 1991) has been applied to *Acinetobacter*, based on DNA extraction and digestion with restriction enzymes *Eco*RI and *Hind*III, separation of restriction fragments in agarose gels by electrophoresis, vacuum blotting of DNA fragments onto nylon membranes, and incubation in the presence of a biotinylated cDNA probe prepared from *E. coli* rRNA. Within each outbreak, the isolates were uniform in their banding pattern and a remarkable degree of uniformity of strains studied by SDS–PAGE or ribotyping was observed. Plasmid profiles (Hartstein *et al.*, 1990) and pulse-field gel electrophoresis (PFGE) are being applied for investigation of hospital outbreaks, and studies are in progress. Recently besides chromosomal DNA macro-restriction profiles, polymerase chain reaction (PCR)-mediated fingerprints of *A. baumannii* have been applied in outbreaks of hospital infections (Struelens *et al.*, 1993) and these seem to be promising tools for outbreak delineation and detection of micro-epidemics.

ACINETOBACTER AND ANTIBIOTICS

Evolution of Resistance to Antibiotics in *Acinetobacter* spp.

In early *in vitro* studies, the majority of *Acinetobacter* clinical isolates were susceptible to ampicillin (61–70%), and minocycline (Bergogne-Bérézin and Joly-Guillou, 1985); in 1969, only 3.4% were resistant to carbenicillin and the vast majority of *Acinetobacter* isolates were susceptible to gentamicin (95.8% of strains from medical wards; 87.5% of those from ICUs). Strains of *A. calcoaceticus* var. *anitratus* were significantly more resistant than var. *lwoffi* strains (Bergogne-Bérézin and Joly-Guillou, 1991; Muller-Serieys *et al.*, 1989) and, as a result, a significant change in the isolation frequency of var. *anitratus* (*A. baumannii*)

has been noted, rising from 77.5% of the strains isolated from 1971 to 1980 up to >98% in 1990 (Joly-Guillou *et al.*, 1992a). Other species – *A. lwoffi*, *A. johnsonii*, *A. haemolyticus*, *A. junii* – less frequently involved in nosocomial infections, are more susceptible to most antibacterial agents. High proportions of *A. baumannii* strains have become resistant to antibiotics; *Acinetobacter* strains are resistant to most commonly used antibacterial drugs, including aminopenicillins, ureidopenicillins, cephalosporins of the first (cephalothin) and second (cefamandole) generation (Morohoshi and Saito, 1977; Bergogne-Bérézin and Joly-Guillou, 1991), cephamycins (cefoxitin) (Joly-Guillou *et al.*, 1992a), most aminoglycosides–aminocyclitols (Devaud *et al.*, 1982), chloramphenicol and tetracyclines. Contrasting data are found in the literature for some antibiotics: piperacillin and

TABLE 13.5   EVOLUTION AND CURRENT RESISTANCE TO ANTIBIOTICS OF *ACINETOBACTER* (% RESISTANT)[a]

	Bichat–Claude Bernard University-Hospital								France[b] 1991 %	Germany[c] 1993 (n = 95) %	Spain[d] 1993 (n = 54) %
	1975 %	1980 %	1985 %	1991 %	1992 %[f]	1993 %[f]	1993 %ICU	1994[e] %[f]			
β-Lactams											
Ampicillin	83	94	98	100	–	–	–	–	–	91	98
Carbeni./ticarcillin	16	70	72	77.5	40.4	46	42.9	39.4	44	–	70
Mezlo./piperacillin	–	80	92	88	82.7	94	–	–	–	36	67
Aztreonam	85	93	90	90	–	–	–	–	–	54	98
Imipenem	–	–	0	2	2.3	5	6.9	4.6	0.6	0	0
Cephalos. 2nd gen.	90	95	98	98	–	–	–	–	–	99	–
Cefotaxime	–	55	84.5	95	91.5	98	95	97.4	–	32	69
Ceftazidime	–	19	45.5	92	82.4	91	88	94	76	32	45
Moxalactam	–	90	90	92	–	–	–	–	–	–	–
Aminoglycosides											
Gentamicin	12	81	84	80	74	88	78	77.6	69.5	98	67
Tobramycin	12	22	47	76	58	61	65	66	62	98	50
Netilmicin	–	16	49	85	64.5	79	73	62	44.5	–	34
Amikacin	–	2.5	39	78	68	81	69	61	55	64	28
Kanamycin	17	67	70	89	–	–	–	–	–	–	–
Fluoroquinolones											
Pefloxacin			19	75	75	83	63	73	85	–	–
Ciprofloxacin			18	70	–	–	–	–	80	94	30
Ofloxacin			20	67	–	–	–	–	–	–	28
Norfloxacin			87	95	–	–	–	–	–	–	82

[a] Data for *A. baumannii*.
[b] After Joly-Guillou *et al.* (1992a).
[c] After Seifert *et al.* (1993).
[d] After Vila *et al.* (1993).
[e] Joly-Guillou (unpublished).
[f] Total hospital.
[g] Data from 32 microbiology laboratories.

aminoglycosides were effective in a study of the *in vitro* activity of 25 antibacterial agents (Garcia *et al.*, 1983); aminoglycosides seem no longer active against *A. baumannii* in Germany (Seifert *et al.*, 1993). These differences might be attributable to different patterns of antibiotic usage that exist in Japan (Obana *et al.*, 1985), in Germany (Seifert *et al.*, 1993), in the USA (Garcia *et al.*, 1983) or in France (Joly-Guillou *et al.*, 1992b) (Table 13.5). With some major antibiotics, such as third-generation cephalosporins (cefotaxime, ceftazidime), imipenem, tobramycin and amikacin, the minimal inhibitory concentrations (MICs) have increased between 1980 and 1992; *Acinetobacter* strains initially susceptible to fluoroquinolones have become resistant up to 75–80% to pefloxacin within five years (Table 13.5). Imipenem and rifampicin remain the most active drugs but imipenem resistance in *A. baumannii*, although still limited (0.5–5%), is a threat for the near future; *A. haemolyticus* is highly resistant to rifampicin and aminoglycosides.

Mechanisms of Resistance to β-Lactams

Resistance of *Acinetobacter* to penicillins is due to the presence of TEM-1 and TEM-2 β-lactamases (Devaud *et al.*, 1982; Goldstein *et al.*, 1983) found in representative isolates of epidemic strains that also produced aminoglycoside-modifying enzymes. The genes encoding resistance to β-lactams (encoding as well resistance to aminoglycosides, tetracyclines, chloramphenicol and sulphonamides) have been identified in plasmids (Devaud *et al.*, 1982; Towner, 1991). In a recent study (Joly-Guillou *et al.*, 1988) a TEM-1 type enzyme (p*I* 5.4) was identified in 34% of the strains, while 7% of the strains produced a new β-lactamase of p*I* 6.3, which inactivated ampicillin and carbenicillin, but not methicillin or cloxacillin and was identified as a CARB-5 enzyme (Paul *et al.*, 1989). Inducible cephalosporinase described by Morohoshi and Saito (1977) has been demonstrated in 70% of *Acinetobacter* strains (Joly-Guillou *et al.*, 1988); more recently, chromosomally mediated cephalosporinases (Hood and Amyes, 1989) were designated ACE_1 to ACE_4

enzymes; they inactivate penicillins, first and second-generation cephalosporins and to a variable extent third-generation cephalosporins. They have also contributed to the impressive list of β-lactam-inactivating enzymes in *Acinetobacter* (Table 13.6). A β-lactamase-mediated resistance to imipenem has been observed (Paton *et al.*, 1993) in *Acinetobacter* designated ARI_1. This enzyme has a limited spectrum of inhibitory activities and does not hydrolyse second- and third-generation cephalosporins. Mechanisms of β-lactam resistance other than enzymatic have been proposed in rare studies: diminished outer membrane permeability in relation to decreased production of porin proteins (porins 1 and 2) (Obara and Nakai, 1991) or the presence of only a small number of small-size porins (Sato and Nakae, 1991) were implicated in β-lactam resistance in *Acinetobacter*; penicillin-binding protein (PBP) alterations with diminished affinity of imipenem to PBPs should also be responsible for imipenem resistance (Gehrlein *et al.*, 1991).

Mechanisms of Resistance to Aminoglycosides

Aminoglycosides have been used since the mid-1960s. The emergence of resistance was observed in *Acinetobacter* during the early phase of aminoglycoside therapy when kanamycin and gentamicin were the major antibiotics available. Among the three major mechanisms of resistance – (1) alteration of the target site on the ribosomes; (2) reduced aminoglycoside permeability; (3) inactivation of the aminoglycoside by enzymatic modification – the latter mechanism is by far the most common type of aminoglycoside resistance in *Acinetobacter* spp. A number of studies since 1975 have shown the presence of three types of aminoglycoside-modifying enzymes: acetylating enzymes (acetyltransferases), conferring resistance to kanamycin, tobramycin, dibekacin and sisomycine (AAC(6′)) (Bergogne-Bérézin and Joly-Guillou, 1991; Gomez-Lus *et al.*, 1980); phosphotransferases, which modify kanamycin (APH(3′)I and II) (Devaud *et al.*, 1982), amikacin (APH(3′)IV) (Lambert *et al.*, 1990);

TABLE 13.6 *β*-LACTAMASES IN *ACINETOBACTER* AND OTHER AEROBIC GRAM-NEGATIVE BACILLI

Enzyme type	Characteristics	p*I*	Molecular weight	Bush group	Inhibition by clavulinic acid	Authors
Acinetobacter calcoaceticus var. *anitratus*						
TEM-type (1 and 2)	Plasmid mediated	5.4–5.6	28 000	2c	Yes	Joly-Guillou *et al.* (1988)
Carbenicillinase (CARB-5)	Plasmid mediated	6.3	28 000	1	Yes	Paul *et al.* (1989)
ACE$_1$ to ACE$_4$	Chromosomal	7.3/8.8	640 000 to >1 000 000		No	Hood and Amyes (1989)
Cephalosporinase	Inducible	8	35 000	1	No	Morohoshi and Saito (1977) Joly-Guillou *et al.* (1988)
ARI$_1$	Plasmid mediated Imipenem resistance	6.65	23 000		No	Paton *et al.* (1993)
Flavobacterium meningosepticum						
Oxyimino-cephalosporinase		5.1	30 000	2b		Raimondi *et al.* (1986)
Carbapenemase	Metallo-β-lactamase			3		
Flavobacterium odoratum						
Carbapenemase[a]	Chromosomal	5.8	26 000		No	Sato *et al.* (1985)
Stenotrophomonas maltophilia[b]						
Penicillinase	Metallo-enzyme			3	No	Saino *et al.* (1982)
Cephalosporinase	Chromosomal inducible	8.4	56 000	L2	Yes	Bush (1989)
Carbapenemase[a]	Chromosomal inducible	6.9	118 000 (4 subunits)	L1	No	
Other β-lactamases	Constitutive/inducible	2.7/5.5/8.7/9				
Alcaligenes xylosoxidans						
Chromosomal	Constitutive	7.4	32 000		No	Levesque *et al.* (1983)
Plasmid	Cephalosporinase Constitutive	8.1	36 000			
Alcaligenes denitrificans subsp. *xylosoxidans*						
OXA type		7.7		2d	Yes	Decré *et al.* (1992)
CARB type	Chromosomal[c]	5.7			Yes	
Broad spectrum	Inducible	9.5			Yes	

[a] Chromosomally mediated zinc carbapenemases.
[b] New designation (1994) for *Xanthomonas maltophilia*.
[c] Probably.

kanamycin, butirosin and amikacin (APH(3')VI)
(Bergogne-Bérézin and Joly-Guillou 1991; Lambert *et al.*, 1990; Chopade *et al.*, 1985); *adenyl-*
transferases, which confer resistance to streptomycin and spectinomycin (AAD(2''); AAD(3')),
to streptomycin and gentamicin (AAD(3'')IX)
(Table 13.7). The aminoglycosides are today
variably active against *Acinetobacter* strains and
most studies report 50–80% of isolates resistant to
gentamicin and tobramycin; in Germany, highest
percentages of resistance to aminoglycosides
(98%) were reported recently (Seifert *et al.*,
1993); the resistance rates are generally lower with
netilmicin and amikacin (Table 13.5).

Resistance to Other Antibiotics

Besides resistance to β-lactams, aminoglycosides
and chloramphenicol (by production of a chloramphenicol acetyltransferase), *Acinetobacter* strains
showed a rapid development of resistance to
fluoroquinolones. In 1985 pefloxacin, ciprofloxacin

and ofloxacin inhibited about 80% of strains
(Table 13.5); the frequency of selecting quinolone-
resistant mutants is higher in non-fermenting
organisms than in Enterobacteriaceae and within a
few years the incidence of resistant *Acinetobacter*
strains has risen from 18–20% to 75–80% in
France (Joly-Guillou *et al.*, 1992a) and to 94% in
Germany (Seifert *et al.*, 1993). The mechanisms
of quinolone resistance in *Acinetobacter* are
thought to be either decreased uptake of quinolones (permeability mutants) or mutation at the
DNA gyrase A subunit (*gyrA* mutations): they are
currently under investigation.

Genetic Bases of Resistance

Due to the difficulty in locating antibiotic resistance genes in *Acinetobacter* by conventional
transfer experiments, available data on plasmids
and transposons are limited. However, plasmid-
mediated antibiotic resistance has been demonstrated in several studies (Towner, 1991; Vivian,

TABLE 13.7   AMINOGLYCOSIDE MODIFYING ENZYMES IN *ACINETOBACTER*

Enzymes	Modified substrates	Authors
Phosphotransferases		
APH(3') I	Kanamycin	Gomez-Lus *et al.* (1980)
		Bergogne-Bérézin *et al.* (1991)
APH(3') II	Kanamycin, amikacin	Murray and Moellering (1980)
APH(3') VI	Kanamycin, amikacin	Bergogne-Bérézin and Joly-Guillou (1991)
		Lambert *et al.* (1990)
Adenyltransferases		
AAD(2'')	Streptomycin netilmicin, gentamicin, tobramycin	Murray and Moellering (1980)
AAD(3'')I	Streptomycin Spectinomycin	Shimizu *et al.* (1981)
		Devaud *et al.* (1982)
		Goldstein *et al.* (1983)
AAD(3'') IX	Streptomycin, spectinomycin Gentamicin	Chopade *et al.* (1985)
Acetyltransferases		
AAC(2') I	Gentamicin, netilmicin, tobramycin	Chopade *et al.* (1985)
		Dowding (1979)
AAC(6')	Netilmicin, tobramycin kanamycin, sisomycin amikacin	Bergogne-Bérézin and Joly-Guillou (1991)
		Gomez-Lus *et al.* (1980)
		Murray and Moellering (1980)
AAC(3')	Gentamicin, sisomycin	Devaud *et al.* (1982)
AAC(3) I	Gentamicin, tobramycin	Bergogne-Bérézin and Joly-Guillou (1991)
		Gomez-Lus *et al.* (1980)

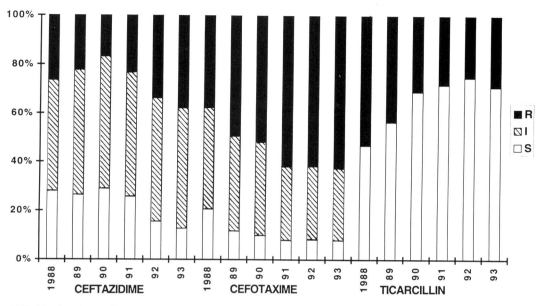

Figure 13.2. Evaluation of β-lactam resistance of *Acinetobacter baumannii* during a six-year surveillance in France. R, resistant; I, intermediate; S, susceptible.

1991). *Acinetobacter* can acquire plasmids from Enterobacteriaceae (Chopade *et al.*, 1985) but the opposite transfer seems to be a rare event (Gomez-Lus *et al.*, 1980; Goldstein *et al.*, 1983). Lambert *et al.* (1990) reported transfer of the aminoglycoside resistance gene by conjugation at frequencies ranging from 10^{-4} to 10^{-8} to other *Acinetobacter* spp. but not to *E. coli*. *Acinetobacter* is often considered as a reservoir of antibiotic resistance plasmids (Towner, 1991; Chopade *et al.*, 1985) and some authors have found antibiotic resistance mediated by non-conjugative plasmids (Shimizu *et al.*, 1981). Many strains of *Acinetobacter* carry multiple plasmids of variable molecular size; indigenous plasmids of less than 23 kb have been found (Gerner-Smidt, 1989) in 75 of 93 strains examined. The determination of plasmid profiles has been used as a genotypic epidemiological marker in *Acinetobacter* infection outbreaks. Transposons conferring antibiotic resistance have been reviewed by Towner (1991) and reports of chromosomally located antibiotic resistance transposons in *Acinetobacter* have shown that they were neither self-transmissible nor associated with

plasmid DNA. Sparse observations of mobilization of transposons are found in the literature: Shimizu *et al.* (1981) mobilized a 5 kb DNA sequence encoding aminoglycoside resistance from a strain isolated in Japan; Devaud *et al.* (1982) mobilized a 24 kb DNA sequence encoding multiple resistance from an *Acinetobacter* strain isolated in an ICU. The occurrence of multi-resistant nosocomial isolates of *Acinetobacter* seems to be related to the presence of transposable DNA sequence encoding resistance to β-lactams, aminoglycosides, tetracyclines and chloramphenicol, as found in endemic hospital strains (Towner, 1991).

Therapeutic Problems

Only a limited number of major antibiotics are still active in the treatment of *Acinetobacter* infections. Very few β-lactams might be used, after a careful *in vitro* susceptibility testing has been carried out: ticarcillin, often combined with sulbactam (the latter being a β-lactamase inhibitor often active by itself against *Acinetobacter*) (Urban *et al.*, 1993); ceftazidime and most often imipenem, which is by far the most active drug in *Acinetobacter* infection. Aminoglycosides can be used in the treatment of *Acinetobacter* infections when combined to still-effective β-lactams such as ticarcillin, ceftazidime or imipenem. Combination therapy is always recommended, associating a β-lactam with an amino-glycoside, or a fluoroquinolone, or rifampicin after *in vitro* susceptibility testing of antibiotics and of their combinations. The addition of β-lactamase inhibitors such as clavulanic acid to ticarcillin, or of sulbactam to a third-generation cephalosporin, may significantly enhance the β-lactam activity, in addition to the intrinsic sulbactam anti-*Acinetobacter* activity. Preventative measures such as surveillance programmes of prevalent organisms in ICUs and control of bacterial contamination of the hospital environment are important measures and can be of help in prevention of *Acinetobacter* infection as well as that of other nosocomial infections.

OTHER AEROBIC GRAM-NEGATIVE BACILLI

INTRODUCTION

Many aerobic Gram-negative bacilli, other than *Pseudomonas* spp. and *Acinetobacter* spp., can be identified as non-fermenters, motile or non-motile organisms, that can or cannot oxidize sugars and that are generally oxidase positive (Figure 13.1). They include three genera that are important in medical bacteriology: *Xanthomonas*, *Flavobacterium* and *Alcaligenes*. They have undergone many changes in taxonomy in recent years: classified for long on a phenotypic basis (morphology, motility, metabolism), the taxonomy of these bacteria has been revised on a genetic basis and the position of some species has been recently reassigned to different genera on the basis of hybridization percentages of DNA−rRNA and DNA−DNA, and G + C contents. The current nomenclature of the species belonging to the three genera described below is shown in Table 13.8 (Bruckner and Colonna, 1993; Pickett *et al.*, 1991). These bacteria are all saprophytic organisms that can be found in water, soil and foodstuffs. In the hospital environment, moist items can be contaminated, such as irrigating fluids, ventilatory equipments, nebulizers and humidifiers, infusion fluids and disinfectants (0.05% chlorhexidine) and these contaminated sources may be responsible for outbreaks of nosocomial infection (Von Gravenitz, 1985).

XANTHOMONAS/ STENOTROPHOMONAS MALTOPHILIA

Taxonomy

The genus *Xanthomonas* (genus II of family I Pseudomonadaceae) as initially identified by Dowson in 1939 and according to *Bergey's Manual* (1984) has evolved recently. Closely related to the genus *Pseudomonas*, it included initially phyto-pathogenic species of which the type species was *X. campestris* (identified by Pammel in 1895). The genus *Xanthomonas* also includes *Xanthomonas maltophilia*, formerly *Pseudomonas maltophilia*, which has been assigned to the genus *Xanthomonas* on the basis of phenotypic and genotypic characters (Swings *et al.*, 1983). The latest designation is *Stenotrophomonas maltophilia* (1994). These bacteria are characterized by the presence of single or a small number of polar flagella (motile bacteria), frequently pigmented colonies (in yellow or yellowish-orange), oxidase-negative reaction, and acidified sugars (except for rhamnose or mannitol). They are generally proteolytic (Figure 13.1 and Table 13.8). *Stenotrophomonas maltophilia* is the most clinically important species of the genus.

Habitat and Pathogenicity of *S. maltophilia*

Isolated from soil, plants, water and raw milk, this ubiquitous bacteria is frequent in the hospital environment and is an emerging opportunistic pathogen (Marshall *et al.*, 1989). It has been isolated frequently from ventilatory equipment (thermal humidifying units) and from moist respirometers as well as from dialysis fluids and antiseptic solutions. In patients *S. maltophilia* can be isolated from multiple sites of nosocomial infections:

TABLE 13.8   CURRENT NOMENCLATURE OF NON-FERMENTATIVE BACILLI[a]

Genus, species, current name	Synonyms	Percentage of strains positive		
		Oxidase	Grown on MacConkey agar	Glucose acidified
Alcaligenes faecalis	*A. odorans* *Pseudomonas odorans*	100	100	0
Alcaligenes piechaudii	*A. faecalis* type I	100	100	0
Alcaligenes xylosoxidans subsp. *denitrificans*	*A. denitrificans*	100	100	0
Alcaligenes xylosoxidans supsp. *xylosoxidans*	*Achromobacter xylosoxidans* IIIa and IIIb	100	100	78
Flavobacterium breve	*Bacillus brevis* *Bacterium canale* *Pseudobacterium brevis*	100	100	100
Flavobacterium indologenes	*F. baiustinum* *F. gleum,* CDC group IIb	96	63	98
Flavobacterium meningosepticum	CDC group IIa	99	92	99
Flavobacterium multivorum	*Sphingobacterium multivorum,* CDC group II k-2	100	100	100
Flavobacterium odoratum	CDC group M-4F	99	96	0
Flavobacterium spiritivorum	*Sphingobacterium spiritivorum,* CDC group II k-3	100	55	100
Flavobacterium thalpophilum	*Sphingobacterium thalpophilum,* CDC group II k-2	100	100	100
Flavobacterium sp. group IIe sp. group IIh sp. group IIi	CDC group IIe CDC group IIh CDC group IIi	100 100 100	0 0 100	100 100 0
Weeksella virosa	*Flavobacterium* IIf	100	10	0
Weeksella zookelcum	*Flavobacterium* IIj	100	2	0
Xanthomonas maltophilia[b]	*Pseudomonas maltophilia*	*Negative*[c]	+	+

[a] Pertinent characteristics: Gram-negative, aerobic, non-fermenters, may or may not oxidize sugars, catalase positive, oxidase generally positive.
[b] *Stenotrophomonas maltophilia*: newer designation (1994).
[c] Or slowly and weakly positive.
After Bruckner and Colonna (1993); Pickett *et al.* (1991).

TABLE 13.9 TESTS FOR IDENTIFICATION OF GRAM-NEGATIVE NON FERMENTATIVE AEROBIC BACILLI (CLINICALLY IMPORTANT SPECIES OF THREE GENERA *XANTHOMONAS*, *FLAVOBACTERIUM*, *ALCALIGENES*)

Feature	*Xanthomonas maltophilia*	*F. breve*	*Flavobacterium group IIb*	*F. meningosepticum*	*F. multivorum*	*F. odoratum*	*A. xylosoxidans subsp. xylosoxidans*	*Alcaligenes faecalis*	*A. piechaudii*
Acidified									
Ethanol	0[a]	0	16	57	0	0	100		
Glucose	+[b]	86	98	99	100	0	78		
Lactose	±	0	0	57	100	0	0		
Maltose	+	86	98	100	100	0	0		
Mannitol	+	0	10	99	0	0	0		
Sucrose		0	14	0	100	0	0		
Xylose	±	0	31	3	100	0	98		
Catalase	+	100	99	100	0	100	95		
Citrate (Simmons)	−	0	3	12	61	0	0		
DNAse	+	100	4	100	0	100	0		
Aesculin, hydrolysed	+	0	70	99	100	0	0	22	0
Gelatin, hydrolysed	+	100	78	91	0	96	0	0	0
Indole	−	100	98	100	0	0	100		
MacConkey agar, growth	−	100	63	92	100	96	100	100	100
Nitrate reduced	±	0	22	0	0	0	100	0	100
Nitrite reduced		0	20	37	0	83	100	100	0
Oxidase	−	100	96	99	100	99	100		
Urease	−	0	42	8	95	100	0	0	0
42 °C, growth	±	0	42	45	0	31	84		

Feature	*A. xylosoxidans subsp. xylosoxidans*	*Alcaligenes faecalis*	*A. piechaudii*
Acidified			
Ethanol	100	100	100
Fructose	78	0	0
Alkalinized			
Acetamide	100	100	100
Allantoin	0	0	0
Histidine	100	100	100
Itaconate	100	0	100
Malonate	100	100	100

[a] Percentage of strains positive.
[b] Sugars acidified by *X. maltophilia* in 48 hours in the presence of concentration <1% of sugar.

respiratory tract, endocarditis, bacteraemia, meningitis and UTI. *Stenotrophomonas maltophilia* can be implicated also in severe cutaneous infections, cellulitis and abscesses: this bacteria produces proteolytic enzymes and other pathogenic extracellular enzymes such as DNAase, RNAase, elastase, lipase, hyaluronidase, mucinase and haemolysin which contribute to the severity of these infections in otherwise immunodepressed patients in ICUs (Marshall *et al.*, 1989; Von Gravenitz, 1985). A high incidence of infection with *S. maltophilia* occurs in patients with cancer, leukaemia or lymphoma, and *S. maltophilia* is increasingly implicated in pulmonary superinfections in cystic fibrosis patients. *Stenotrophomonas maltophilia* is frequently associated with other bacteria at sites of infection but is increasingly isolated as the sole pathogen due to its high natural resistance to most major antibiotics and to the selective pressure exerted by antibiotic treatments in ICUs.

Bacteriological Characteristics of *S. maltophilia*

Unlike other *Xanthomonas* spp. *S.(X.) maltophilia* does not produce pigments, and colonies are weakly yellowish or non-pigmented. Selective media can be used for isolation of *S. maltophilia* from human specimens with the addition of imipenem (10 mg/l) (thanks to the intrinsic resistance of the organism) and/or vancomycin to prevent Gram positives when the specimen is polymicrobial. The oxidase reaction is negative or weakly and slowly positive (Table 13.9). Its main biochemical characteristics are shown in Table 13.9., Four characters are important for identification of *X. maltophilia*: it produces a lysine decarboxylase, hydrolyses aesculin and gelatin, and requires L-methionine for growth (50 mg/l in synthetic mineral broth, as described by Swings *et al.*, 1983). Other characters – indole, urease and ornithine decarboxylase production – are negative.

S. maltophilia susceptibility/resistance to antibiotics

Stenotrophomonas maltophilia is naturally resistant to most antibiotics with chromosomally mediated

mechanisms, as was described for β-lactams (Saino *et al.*, 1984): a poor permeability of the outer membrane of the bacteria and naturally produced inactivating enzymes are generally advocated (Saino *et al.*, 1982, 1984; Von Gravenitz, 1985); many β-lactamases have been described in *S. maltophilia*, as shown in Table 13.6.

β-Lactams *Stenotrophomonas maltophilia* is susceptible only to latamoxef and to combinations of ticarcillin and clavulanic acid or piperacillin plus tazobactam. It is naturally resistant to imipenem and meropenem by production of a carbapenemase.

Aminoglycosides Only few strains are susceptible to gentamicin, neomycin and kanamycin; resistance to aminoglycosides is probably plasmid mediated.

Fluoroquinolones *Stenotrophomonas maltophilia* is poorly susceptible to quinolones; newer agents temafloxacin and sparfloxacin seem to be more active than ciprofloxacin. Resistance to quinolones in *S. maltophilia* is generally associated with resistance to chloramphenicol and to doxycycline in more than 50% of cases. This resistance is associated with alteration of outer membrane proteins (Khardori *et al.*, 1990; Lecso-Bornet *et al.*, 1992) (Table 13.10).

TABLE 13.10 SUSCEPTIBILITY (MG/L) OF 42 STRAINS OF *S. MALTOPHILIA* TO 13 QUINOLONES

	MIC_{50}	MIC_{90}	MIC range	% Susceptible
Nalidixic acid	8	32	8–128	80
Pipemidic acid	64	128	32–256	–
Ciprofloxacin	2	4	0.25–16	3–65
Difloxacin	2	8	0.5–32	2.5
Enoxacin	4	16	2–32	2.5–6.5
Fleroxacin	2	8	1–16	35–50
Lomefloxacin	2	8	1–16	35
Norfloxacin	32	64	8–128	–
Ofloxacin	2	4	0.5–1.6	50–65
Pefloxacin	4	8	2–32	2.5–75
Rosoxacin	8	16	4–32	–
Sparfloxacin	0.25	4	0.25–16	80
Temafloxacin	1	8	0.25–32	35

After Lesco-Bornet *et al.* (1972).

Other antibiotics Clinical strains of *S. maltophilia* are variably susceptible to minocycline, rifampicin and combination trimethoprim–sulphmethoxazole. Nosocomial infections due to *S. maltophilia* require combination therapy including rifampicin plus a fluoroquinolone, or ticarcillin plus clavulanic acid associated with tobramycin or amikacin, or even a trimethoprim–sulphamethoxazole combination.

FLAVOBACTERIUM

DEFINITION: TAXONOMY

The genus *Flavobacterium* is a large group of nonmotile, oxidase-positive (except for *F. odoratum*), Gram-negative, strictly aerobic, non-fermentative bacilli. Species belonging to the genus *Flavobacterium* are listed in Table 13.8. The taxonomy of the genus is evolving (Holmes *et al.*, 1988) and two *Flavobacterium*-like species, designated groups IIf and IIj, have been transferred recently to the genus *Weeksella*, designated *W. virosa* and *W. zookelcum* respectively in the new proposed nomenclature (Table 13.8) (Bruckner and Colonna, 1993). These latter species differ from *Flavobacterium* spp. mainly because they do not metabolize sugars; they are rarely recovered from human specimens and unlike *Flavobacterium* spp. they are very susceptible to most antibiotics.

Epidemiology and Pathogenicity

All *Flavobacterium* spp. are ubiquitous organisms and can be found in the hospital environment. Environmental studies have traced the bacterial source to contaminated water, ice machines and humidifiers. Epidemiological markers used for delineation of outbreaks of *F. meningosepticum* infections were phenotypes of resistance and serology based on the O antigenic type; nine O serovars have been identified: **A** through **H** and **K**. The C serovar is isolated in the Far East whereas serovar **G** predominates in European countries and has been isolated from clinical samples in ICUs (tracheal aspirations, expectorations, sinuses). New typing procedures based on molecular biology are being investigated. *Flavobacterium* can be implicated in various nosocomial infections: *F. meningosepticum*, *F. multivorum* and *Flavobacterium* group IIb are the predominant species isolated in septicaemia, meningitis and endocarditis. Many cases of meningitis due to *F. meningosepticum* have been observed in neonates and, infrequently, in immunocompromised patients. In adults *F. meningosepticum* has been isolated from pneumonia, postoperative bacteraemia and meningitis, usually associated with severe underlying pathologies. Rare cases of community-acquired *F. meningosepticum* meningitis have been cited in the literature (Raimondi *et al.*, 1986).

BACTERIOLOGY

Flavobacteria grow between 5 and 30 °C but the strains isolated from human specimens can grow at up to 37 °C. On nutrient agar they produce colonies of 1–2 mm in diameter, frequently pigmented light yellow, or yellowish-orange due to a non-diffusible pigment. The degree of pigmentation may be more pronounced at lower temperatures (15–20 °C). The metabolism is strictly aerobic and sugars are metabolized by the oxidative pathway (except for *F. odoratum* and *Flavobacterium* spp. group IIi, which do not acidify glucose) (Table 13.8). As shown in Table 13.9, indole-positive species (i.e. *F. breve*, *F. meningosepticum*, *F. indologenes*) are usually strongly proteolytic; aesculin, citrate and urease tests are variably positive (Gilardi, 1985; Pickett *et al.*, 1991). The main features for identification of species are reported in Table 13.9.

Antimicrobial Susceptibility

Flavobacterium strains and particularly those isolated from clinical specimens are resistant to many antibiotics: they are generally resistant to all aminoglycosides (MIC > 16 mg/l), to third-generation cephalosporins, anti-*Pseudomonas* penicillins (mezlocillin, piperacillin, ticarcillin), aztreonam and imipenem, to erythromycin and tetracycline. The most active antibiotics against *F. meningosepticum* are rifampicin, clindamycin (MICs

1–4 mg/l) and ciprofloxacin, which has proven efficacious in treating pneumonia in paediatric patients. Cases of neonatal septicaemia have been treated with clindamycin combined with piperacillin. Other antibiotic combinations have been used in treating *Flavobacterium* infections (Raimondi *et al.*, 1986; Von Gravenitz, 1985). Susceptibility to β-lactams can be recovered by combining β-lactamase inhibitors with β-lactam antibiotics: clavulanic acid combined with mezlocillin, ceftazidime or cefotaxime (MIC modes: 8, 128, 16 mg/l respectively) decreased the MICs significantly (1, 2, 3 mg/l respectively) for *Flavobacterium* strains.

ALCALIGENES

TAXONOMY

An early description of *Bacilllus alcaligenes faecalis* was made by Petruschky in 1896 reporting a Gram-negative motile bacillus isolated from beer and from human stools. Many species have been included in the genus *Alcaligenes* on the basis of DNA–DNA and DNA–rRNA hybridizations and taxonomic changes have occurred: *Achromobacter xylosoxidans* has been transferred to the genus *Alcaligenes* as *A. xylosoxidans* subsp. *xylosoxidans* (Table 13.8). All *Alcaligenes* strains are short rods (0.5–2.6 μm), Gram negative, motile with one to eight peritrichous (non-polar) flagella, usually described as degenerated. They are oxidase positive and catalase positive. *Alcaligenes faecalis*, *A. piechaudii* and *A. xylosoxidans* subsp. *denitrificans* are not saccharolytic. The only saccharolytic species is *A. xylosoxidans* subsp. *xylosoxidans*. Not all *Alcaligenes* spp. possess specific physiological or biochemical characteristics (Tables 13.9 and 13.10) and those most commonly involved in nosocomial infections are *A. faecalis* and *A.X.* subsp. *denitrificans*.

EPIDEMOLOGY AND PATHOGENICITY

Alcaligenes faecalis and *A. denitrificans* can be isolated from various environmental sources such as respirators, haemodialysis systems, intravenous solutions and even disinfectants (Decré *et al.*, 1992; Pickett *et al.*, 1991; Von Gravenitz, 1985). They have occasionally been isolated from a variety of human specimens: blood, faeces, sputum, urine, cerebrospinal fluid, wounds, burns and swabs from throat, eyes and ear discharges. *Alcaligenes* strains do not seem to possess any specific virulence determinants and they are an infrequent cause of hospital-acquired infection in patients with severe underlying disease. Rare cases of peritonitis, pneumonia, bacteraemia or UTI are found in the literature; in many instances the organism is considered as a colonizer and its pathogenic role remains sometimes controversial. Nosocomial outbreaks of patent infections are usually associated with an aqueous source of contamination (Mandell *et al.*, 1987).

BACTERIOLOGY

Identification of *Alcaligenes* spp. is based on the main characters cited above. In addition, alcalinization of a series of substrates (malonate, acetamide, allantoin, histidine, itaconate), gelatin hydrolysis (*A. faecalis* and *A. piechaudii*) and several negative characters (Table 13.9) may help to identify *Alcaligenes* spp. (usually by using commercially available multi-test systems) as well as assimilation tests (carbohydrates) and presence or absence of nitrate and nitrite reductases (Pickett *et al.*, 1991) (Table 13.11).

Antimicrobial Susceptibility

Most strains are resistant to aminoglycosides, chloramphenicol and tetracyclines; they are variably susceptible to trimethoprim–sulphamethoxazole and to newer β-lactams. *Alcaligenes xylosoxidans* subsp. *xylosoxidans* has been shown susceptible to ureidopenicillins, latamoxef, imipenem and some fluoroquinolones (ciprofloxacin, ofloxacin). There have been several reports of multiple β-lactam resistance in *A. xylosoxidans* to broad-spectrum penicillins due to constitutive β-lactamase production: three different types of cephalosporinases and the presence of other β-lactamases have been

TABLE 13.11 IDENTIFICATION TESTS AND ANTIBIOTIC SUSCEPTIBILITIES OF SPECIES AND SUBSPECIES OF *ALCALIGENES* (CDC GROUP VD)

	A. faecalis	A. faecalis var. odorans	A. denitrificans subsp. denitrificans	A. denitrificans subsp. xylosoxidans	A. piechaudii
TTR[a]	+	+	+	+	+
M63 lactate, acetate	+	+	+	+	+
Nitrate reductase	v	–	+	+	+
Nitrite reductase	–	+	+	+	–
M63 xylose, glucose	–	–	–	+	–
Urease	–	–	v	–	–
M63 arginine, maltose, trehalose, inositol, mannitol	–	–	–	–	–
M63 acetamide	–	+	(–)	V	–
Malonate	–	+	–	–	–
Simmons citrate	[+]	+	+	+	+
TDA[a]	–	+	–	–	–
L-phenylalanine DA	–	[–]	–	–	–
Growth at 41 °C	v*	v	–	–	–
Susceptibility to					
cefalothin	+	Not available	Not available	–	Not available
cefotaxime	+	Not available	Not available	–	Not available
imipenem	+	Not available	Not available	+	Not available
ureidopenicillins	+	Not available	Not available	±	Not available
gentamicin	+	Not available	Not available	–	Not available
amikacin	+	Not available	Not available	–	Not available
ciprofloxacin	+	Not available	Not available	±	Not available
nalidixic acid	+	Not available	Not available	–	Not available

[a] TTR, tetrathionate reductase; TDA, L-tryptophan deaminase; M63, mineral defined medium; x, variable.

demonstrated (Decré *et al.*, 1992; Levesque *et al.*, 1983) (Table 13.6). Treatment of infections due to this uncommon opportunistic organism requires combination therapy including expanded spectrum β-lactams (piperacillin, imipenem) and recent fluoroquinolones (ciprofloxacin, sparfloxacin) or trimethoprim–sulphamethoxazole.

REFERENCES

Alexander, M., Rahman, M., Taylor, M. *et al.* (1988) A study of the value of electrophoretic and other techniques for typing *Acinetobacter calcoaceticus*. *Journal of Hospital Infection*, **12**, 273–287.

Andrews, H.J. (1986) *Acinetobacter* bacteriocin typing. *Journal of Hospital Infection*, **7**, 169–175.

Anstey, M.N., Currie, B.J. and Withrall, K.M. (1992) Community-acquired *Acinetobacter* pneumonia in the Northern territory of Australia. *Clinical Investigation and Infectious Diseases*, **14**, 83–91.

Avril, J.L. and Mesnard, R. (1991) Factors influencing the virulence of *Acinetobacter*. In *The Biology of Acinetobacter* (ed. K.J. Towner, E. Bergogne-Bérézin and C.A. Fewson), pp. 77–82. Plenum Press, New York.

Bergey's Manual of Systematic Bacteriology (1984) Vol. 1 (ed. N.R. Krieg and J.G. Holt). Williams & Wilkins, Baltimore.

Bergogne-Bérézin, E. and Joly-Guillou, M.L. (1985) An underestimated nosocomial pathogen, *Acinetobacter calcoaceticus*. *Journal of Antimicrobial Chemotherapy*, **16**, 535–538.

Bergogne-Bérjezin, E. and Joly-Guillou, M.L. (1991) Antibiotic resistance mechanisms in *Acinetobacter*.

In *The Biology of Acinetobacter* (ed. K.J. Towner, E. Bergogne-Bérézin, E. and C.A. Fewson) pp. 83–115. Plenum Press, New York.

Bergogne-Bérézin, E., Joly-Guillou, M.L. and Vieu, J.F. (1987) Epidemiology of nosocomial infections due to *Acinetobacter calcoaceticus*. *Journal of Hospital Infection*, **10**, 105–113.

Bleschemidt, B., Borneleit, P. and Kleber, H.P. (1992) Purification and characterization of an extracellular β-lactamase produced by *Acinetobacter calcoaceticus*. *Journal of General Microbiology*, **138**, 1197–1202.

Bouvet, P.J.M. and Grimont, P.A.D. (1986) Taxonomy of the genus *Acinetobacter* with the recognition of *Acinetobacter baumannii* sp. nov., *Acinetobacter haemolyticus* sp. nov., *Acinetobacter johnsonii* sp. nov., and *Acinetobacter junii* sp. nov. and emended descriptions of *Acinetobacter calcoaceticus* and *Acinetobacter Ilwoffi*. *International Journal of Systematic Bacteriology*, **36**, 228–240.

Bøvre K. and Henriksen, S.D. (1976) Minimal standards for description of new taxa within the genera *Moraxella* and *Acinetobacter*: proposal by the subcommittee on *Moraxella* and allied bacteria. *International Journal of Systematic Bacteriology*, **26**, 92–96.

Brisou, J. and Prévôt, A.R. (1954) Etudes de systématique bactérienne. X–Révision des espèces réunies dans le genre *Achromobacter*. *Annales de l'Institut Pasteur*, **86**, 722.

Bruckner, D.A. and Colonna, P. (1993) Nomenclature for aerobic and facultative bacteria. *Clinical Infectious Diseases*, **16**, 598–605.

Bush, K. (1989). Classification of β-lactamases: groups 1, 2a, 2b and 2b'. *Antimicrobial Agents and Chemotherapy*, **33**, 264–270.

Chopade, B.A., Wise, P.J. and Towner, K.J. (1985) Plasmid transfer and behaviour in *Acinetobacter calcoaceticus* EBF65/65. *Journal of General Microbiology*, **131**, 2805–2811.

Debord, G.G. (1939) Organisms invalidating the diagnosis of gonorrhea by the smear method. *Journal of Bacteriology*, **38**, 119–120.

Decré D., Arlet, G., Danglot, C. *et al.* (1992). A β-lactamase-overproducing strain of *Alcaligenes denitrificans* subsp. *xylosoxydans* isolated from a case of meningitis. *Journal of Antimicrobial Chemotherapy*, **30**, 769–779.

Devaud, M., Kayser, F.H. and Bachi, B. (1982) Transposon-mediated multiple antibiotic resistance in *Acinetobacter* strains. *Antimicrobial Agents and Chemotherapy*, **22**, 323–329.

Dijkshoorn, L., Aucken, H., Gerner-Smidt, P. *et al.* (1993) Correlation of typing methods for *Acinetobacter* isolates from hospital outbreaks. *Journal of Clinical Microbiology*, **31**, 702–705.

Dowding, J.E. (1979) A novel aminoglycoside-modifying enzyme from a clinical isolate of *Acinetobacter*. *Journal of General Microbiology*, **110**, 239–241.

French, G.L., Casewell, M.W., Roncoroni, A.J. *et al.* (1980) A hospital outbreak of antibiotic-resistant *Acinetobacter anitratus*: epidemiology and control. *Journal of Hospital Infection*, **1**, 125–131.

Garcia, I., Fainstein, V., Leblanc, B. *et al.* (1983) *In vitro* activities of new beta-lactam antibiotics against *Acinetobacter* spp. *Antimicrobial Agents and Chemotherapy*, **24**, 297–299.

Gehrlein, M., Leying, H., Cullmann, W. *et al.* (1991) Imipenem resistance in *Acinetobacter baumannii* is due to altered penicillin-binding proteins. *Chemotherapy*, **37**, 405–412.

Gerner-Smidt, P. (1989) Frequency of plasmids in strains of *Acinetobacter calcoaceticus*. *Journal of Hospital Infection*, **14**, 23–28.

Gerner-Smidt, P., Tjernberg, I. and Ursing, J. (1992). Ribotyping of the *Acinetobacter calcoaceticus–Acinetobacter baumannii* complex. *Journal of Clinical Microbiology*, **30**, 2680–2685.

Gilardi, G.L. (1985) Cultural and biochemical aspects for identification of glucose-nonfermenting gram-negative rods. *Non-fermentative Gram-negative Rods: Laboratory Identification and Clinical Aspects* (ed. G.L. Gilardi), pp. 17–84. Marcel Dekker, New York.

Glew, R.H., Moellering, R.C. and Kunz, L.J. (1977) Infections with *Acinetobacter calcoaceticus* (*Herellea vaginicola*): clinical and laboratory studies. *Medicine*, **56**, 79–87.

Goldstein, G.W., Labigne-Roussel, A., Gerbaud, G. *et al.* (1983) Transferable plasmid mediated antibiotic resistance in *Acinetobacter*. *Plasmid*, **10**, 138–147.

Gomez-Lus, R., Larrad L., Rubio-Calvo, M.C. *et al.* (1980) AAC(3) and AAC(6') enzymes produced by R plasmids isolated in general hospital. In *Antibiotic Resistance* (ed. S. Mitsuhashi, L. Rosival and V. Kremery), pp. 295–303. Springer-Verlag, Berlin.

Gradon, J.D., Chapnick, E.K. and Lutwick, L.I. (1992) Infective endocarditis of a native valve due to *Acinetobacter*: case report and review. *Clinical Infectious Diseases*, **14**, 1145–1148.

Grimont, P.A.D. and Bouvet, P.J.M. (1991) Taxonomy of *Acinetobacter*. In *The Biology of Acinetobacter* (ed. K.J. Towner, E. Bergogne-Bérézin and C.A. Fewson), pp. 25–36. Plenum Press, New-York.

Hartstern, A.I., Morthland, V.H., Rourke, J.W., Jr *et al.* (1990) Plasmid DNA finger printing of *Acinetobacter calcoaceticus* subsp. *anitratus* from incubated and mechanically ventilated patients. *Infection Controls and Hospital Epidemiology*, **11**, 531–538.

Holmes, B., Weaver, R.E., Steigerwalt, A.G. *et al.* (1988) A taxonomic study of *Flavobacterium spiritivorum* and *Sphingobacterium mizutaii*: proposal of *Flavobacterium yabuuchiae* sp. nov. and *Flavobacterium mizutaii* comb. nov. *International Journal of Systematic Bacteriology*, **38**, 348–353.

Hood, J. and Amyes, S.G.B. (1989) A novel model for identification and distinction of the β-lactamases of the genus *Acinetobacter*. *Journal of Applied Bacteriology*, **67**, 157–163.

Joly-Guillou, M.L., Vallée, E., Bergogne-Bérézin, E. *et al.* (1988) Distribution of beta-lactamases and phenotype analysis in clinical strains of *Acinetobacter calcoaceticus*. *Journal of Antimicrobial Chemotherapy*, **22**, 597–604.

Joly-Guillou, M.L., Decré, D., Wolff, M. *et al.* (1992a) *Acinetobacter* spp: clinical epidemiology in 89 intensive care units. A retrospective study in France during 1991. *2nd International Conference on the Prevention of Infection (CIPI)*, Nice, 4–5 May 1992. Abstract CJ1.

Joly-Guillou, M.L., Decré, D. and Bergogne-Bérézin, E. (1992b) Infections nosocomiales à *Acinetobacter*: surveillance épidémiologique hospitalière. *Bulletin Epidémiologique Hebdomadaire*, no. 45, 211–212.

Juni, E. (1984) Genus III. *Acinetobacter* Brisou and Prévot 1954, 727[AL] In *Bergey's Manual of Systematic Bacteriology*, Vol. 1 (ed. N.R. Krieg and J.G. Hold), pp. 303–307. Williams & Wilkins, Baltimore.

Khardori, N., Reuben, A., Rosembaum, B. *et al. In vitro* susceptibility of *Xanthomonas* (*Pseudomonas*) *maltophilia* to newer antimicrobial agents. *Antimicrobial Agents and Chemotherapy*, **34**, 1609–1610.

Lambert, T., Gerbaud, G., Bouvet, P. *et al.* (1990) Dissemination of amikacin resistance gene aphA6 in *Acinetobacter* spp. *Antimicrobial Agents and Chemotherapy*, **34**, 1244–1248.

Larson, T. (1984) A decade of nosocomial *Acinetobacter*. *American Journal of Infection Control*, **12**, 14–18.

Lecso-Bornet, M., Pierre, J., Sarkis-Karam, D. *et al.* (1992) Susceptibility of *Xanthomonas maltophilia* to six quinolones and study of outer membrane proteins in resistants selected *in vitro*. *Antimicrobial Agents and Chemotherapy*, **36**, 669–671.

Leonov, Y., Schlaeffer, F., Karpuch, J. *et al.* (1990). Ciprofloxacin in the treatment of nosocomial multiply resistant *Acinetobacter calcoaceticus* bacteremia. *Infection*, **18**, 234–236.

Levesque, R.C., Letarte, R. and Péchère, J.C. (1983) Comparative study of the beta-lactamase activity found in *Achromobacter*. *Canadian Journal of Microbiology*, **29**, 819–826.

Mandell, W.F., Garvey, G.J. and Neu, H.C. (1987) *Achromobacter xylosoxidans* bacteremia. *Reviews of Infectious Diseases*, **9**, 1001–1005.

Marshall, W.F., Keating, M.R., Anhalt, J.P. *et al.* (1989) *Xanthomonas maltophilia*: an emerging nosocomial pathogen. *Mayo Clinic Proceedings*, **64**, 1097–1104.

Morohoshi, T. and Saito, T. (1977) Beta-lactamase and beta-lactam antibiotic resistance in *Acinetobacter anitratus* (syn. *A. calcoaceticus*). *Journal of Antibiotics*, **30**, 969–973.

Muller-Serieys, C., Lesquoy, J.B., Perez, E. *et al.* (1989) Infections nosocomiales à *Acinetobacter*: épidémiologie et difficultés thérapeutiques. *La Presse Médicale*, **18**, 107–110.

Murray, B.E. and Moellering, R.C. (1980) Evidence of plasmid mediated production of aminoglycoside-modifying enzyme not previously described in acinetobacter. *Antimicrobial Agents and Chemotherapy*, **17**, 30–36.

Musa, E.K., Desai, N. and Casewell, M.W. (1990) The survival of *Acinetobacter calcoaceticus* inoculated on fingertips and on formica. *Journal of Hospital Infection*, **15**, 219–227.

Ng, P.C., Herrington, R.A., Beane, C.A. *et al.* (1989) An outbreak of *Acinetobacter* septicaemia in a neonatal intensive care unit. *Journal of Hospital Infection*, **14**, 363–368.

Noble, W.C., Hope, Y.M., Midgley, G. *et al.* (1986) Toewebs as a source of Gram-negative bacilli. *Journal of Hospital Infection*, **8**, 248–256.

Obana, Y., Nishino, T. and Tanino, T. (1985) *In vitro* and *in vivo* activities of antimicrobial agents against *Acinetobacter calcoaceticus*. *Journal of Antimicrobial Chemotherapy*, **15**, 441–448.

Obara, M. and Nakai, T. (1991) Mechanisms of resistance to β-lactam antibiotics in *Acinetobacter calcoaceticus*. *Journal of Antimicrobial Chemotherapy*, **28**, 791–800.

Paton, R., Miles, R.S., Hood, J. *et al.* (1993) ARI 1: β-Lactamase-mediated imipenem resistance in *Acinetobacter baumannii*. *International Journal of Antimicrobial Agents*, **2**, 81–88.

Paul, G., Joly-Guillou, M.L., Bergogne-Bérézin, E. *et al.* (1989) Novel carbenicillin-hydrolyzing beta-lactamase (CARB-5) from *Acinetobacter calcoaceticus* var. *anitratus*. *FEMS Microbiological Letters*, **59**, 45–50.

Pickett, M.J., Hollis, D.G. and Bottone, E.J. (1991) Miscellaneous Gram-negative bacteria. In *Manual of Clinical Microbiology*, 5th edn (ed. A. Balows, W.J. Hausler *et al.*), pp. 410–428. American Society for Microbiology, Washington, DC.

Raimondi, A., Moosdeen, F. and Williams, J.D. (1986) Antibiotic resistance pattern of *Flavobacterium meningosepticum*. *European Journal of Clinical Microbiology*, **5**, 461–463.

Rudin, M.L., Michael, J.R. and Huxley, E.J. (1979) Community-acquired *Acinetobacter* pneumonia. *American Journal of Medicine*, **67**, 39–43.

Saino, Y., Kobayashi, F., Inoue, M. *et al.* (1982) Purification and properties of inducible penicillin β-lactamase isolated from *Pseudomonas maltophilia*. *Antimicrobial Agents and Chemotherapy*, **22**, 654–570.

Saino, Y., Inoue, M. and Mitsuhashi, S. (1984) Purification and properties of an inducible cephalosporinase from *Pseudomonas maltophilia*. GN 12873. *Antimicrobial Agents and Chemotherapy*, **25**, 362–365.

Sato, K. and Nakae, T. (1991) Outer membrane permeability of *Acinetobacter calcoaceticus* and its implication in antibiotic resistance. *Journal of Antimicrobial Chemotherapy*, **28**, 35–45.

Sato, K., Fujii, T., Okamoto, R. *et al.* (1985) Biochemical properties of β-lactamase produced by *Flavobacterium odoratum*. *Antimicrobial Agents and Chemotherapy*, **27**, 612–614.

Schaub, I.G. and Hauber, F.D. (1948) A biochemical and serological study of a group of identical unidentifiable Gram-negative bacilli in human sources. *Journal of Bacteriology*, **56**, 379–385.

Seifert, H., Baginski, R., Schulze, A. *et al.* (1993) Antimicrobial susceptibility of *Acinetobacter* species. *Antimicrobial Agents and Chemotherapy*, **37**, 750–753.

Shimizu, S., Inoue, M. and Mitsuhashi, S. (1981) Enzymatic adenylation of spectinomycin by *Acinetobacter calcoaceticus* subsp. *anitratus*. *Journal of Antibiotics*, **34**, 869–875.

Stone, J.M. and Das, B.C. (1986) Investigation of an outbreak of infection with *Acinetobacter calcoaceticus* in a special care baby unit. *Journal of Hospital Infection*, **7**, 42–48.

Struelens, M.J., Carlier, E., Maes, N. *et al.* (1993) Nosocomial colonization and infection with multiresistant *Acinetobacter baumannii*: outbreak delineation using DNA macrorestriction analysis and PCR-fingerprinting. *Journal of Hospital Infection*, **25**, 15–32.

Swings, J., De Vos, P., Van den Mooter, M. *et al.* (1983) Transfer of *Pseudomonas maltophilia* Hugh 1981 to the genus *Xanthomonas* as *Xanthomonas maltophilia* (Hugh 1981) comb. *International Journal of Systematic Bacteriology*, **33**, 409–413.

Taplin, D., Rebell, G. and Zaias, N. (1963) The human skin as a source of *Mima–Herellea* infections. *Journal of the American Medical Association*, **186**, 952–955.

Towner, K.J. (1991) Plasmid and transposon behaviour in *Acinetobacter*. In *The Biology of Acinetobacter* (ed. K.J. Towner, E. Bergogne-Bérézin and C.A Fewson), pp. 1–24. Plenum Press. New York.

Traub, W.H. (1989) *Acinetobacter baumannii* serotyping for delineation of outbreaks of nosocomial cross-infection. *Journal of Clinical Microbiology*, **27**, 2713–2716.

Urban, C., Go, E., Mariano, N. *et al.* (1993) Effect of sulbactam on infections caused by imipenem-resistant *Acinetobacter calcoaceticus* biotype *anitratus*. *Journal of Infectious Diseases*, **67**, 448–451.

Vieu, J.F., Minck, R. and Bergogne-Bérézin, E. (1979) Bactériophages et lysotypie d'Acinetobacter. *Annales de Microbiologie*, **130A**, 405–406.

Vila, J., Marcos, A., Marco, F. *et al.* (1993) *In vitro* antimicrobial production of β-lactamases, aminoglycoside-modifying enzymes, and chloramphenicol acetyltransferase by and susceptibility of clinical isolates of *Acinetobacter baumannii*. *Antimicrobial Agents and Chemotherapy*, **37**, 138–141.

Vivian, A. (1991) Genetic organisation of *Acinetobacter*. In *The Biology of Acinetobacter* (ed. K.J. Towner, E. Bergogne-Bérézin and C.A. Fewson), pp. 191–200. Plenum Press, New York.

Von Gravenitz, A (1985) Ecology, clinical significance and antimicrobial susceptibility of infrequently encountered glucose-nonfermenting gram-negative rods. In *Non-fermentative Gram-negative Rods: Laboratory Identification and Clinical Aspects* (ed. G.L. Gilardi), pp. 181–232. Marcel Dekker, New York.

14

PSEUDOMONAS AERUGINOSA AND OTHER MEDICALLY IMPORTANT PSEUDOMONADS

Tyrone L. Pitt and Afonso L. Barth

INTRODUCTION

Early Descriptions

In 1850, Sédillot, a French military surgeon, observed the formation of blue pus in the wound dressings of injured soldiers. This was also documented by Fordos in 1860, but it was not until 1882 that Gessard described the organism responsible for the pigmentation, which he named *Bacillus pyocyaneus*. In 1900, Migula adopted the generic name *Pseudomonas* (Greek: *pseudes* = false, *monas* = unit) and called the species *P. pyocyanea*. The epithet *aeruginosa* (Latin: *aeruginosus* = full of copper rust, i.e. green) became widely used and is now the approved species name. The early history of this bacterium is reviewed by Forkner (1960).

Taxonomy

The application of molecular techniques to bacterial classification in recent years has resulted in extensive revision of a number of genera, in particular, *Pseudomonas*. Many clinical microbiologists may be unaware of the nomenclatural changes and their taxonomic basis, and the review of Holmes and Howard (1993) is recommended. Up to 1984, over 100 species were included in the genus *Pseudomonas*. Many of these are plant pathogens and their names reflect their primary hosts. The genus was subdivided into five groups based on rRNA homology. Today, only rRNA group I is recognized as the genus *Pseudomonas* (Table 14.1). It contains the fluorescent species *P. aeruginosa*, *P. putida*, and *P. fluorescens*, as well as the non-fluorescent *P. stutzeri*. Organisms which were previously categorized as rRNA group II, 'the pseudomallei group', have now been transferred to the genus *Burkholderia*. This genus includes *B. cepacia*, *B. mallei*, *B. pseudomallei*, and a number of plant pathogens; rRNA group III is now *Comamonas* and incorporates *C. acidovorans*. Members of groups IV and V require specific growth factors and the most

Principles and Practice of Clinical Bacteriology. Edited by A.M. Emmerson, P.M. Hawkey and S.H. Gillespie
© 1997 John Wiley & Sons Ltd

TABLE 14.1   CLASSIFICATION OF MEDICALLY IMPORTANT PSEUDOMONADS

rRNA homology group		Species	Distinguishing features
I *Pseudomonas*	Fluorescent on King's B agar	*P. aeruginosa* oxidase +	Arginine +, grows at 42 °C not 5 °C
		P. fluorescens oxidase +	Arginine +, Grows at 5 °C not 42 °C
		P. putida oxidase +	Arginine +, Grows at 5 °C
	Non-fluorescent	*P. alcaligenes* oxidase +	Glucose −, motile +
		P. pseudoalcaligenes oxidase +	Glucose −, fructose +
		P. stutzeri oxidase +	NO_3 +, arginine −, maltose +
II *Burkholderia*		*B. cepacia* oxidase +	Arginine −, lysine + R-colistin, gentamicin
		B. pseudomallei oxidase +	Arginine +, lysine −, grows at 42 °C R-colistin, gentamicin
		B. mallei oxidase ±	Arginine +, motile −
		B. pickettii oxidase +	NO_3 +, arginine −
		B. gladioli oxidase −	Lactose −, lysine −
III *Comamonas*		*C. acidovorans* oxidase +	Asaccharolytic
IV *Brevundimonas*		*B. diminuta* oxidase +	NO_3 −, arginine −
		B. vesicularis oxidase +	Aesculin hydrolysis
V *Stenotrophomonas*		*S. maltophilia* oxidase −	Maltose +, DNAase +, R-imipenem, gentamicin

familiar human pathogen is *Stenotrophomonas* (*Xanthomonas*) *maltophilia*.

DESCRIPTION OF ORGANISMS

The diversity of the pseudomonads makes it difficult to consider their properties as a single group. Furthermore, the bulk of the literature pertaining to '*Pseudomonas*' concerns specifically *P. aeruginosa*, and less so *B. cepacia* and *B. pseudomallei*, and is relatively sparse for other species. As a result this chapter will deal with each species independently to avoid generalizations which might be inaccurate.

Cultural Characteristics of *Pseudomonas aeruginosa*

Pigments

Pseudomonas aeruginosa grows well on simple bacteriological media and most strains elaborate the blue phenazine pigment pyocyanin and fluorescein (yellow), which gives the characteristic blue-green coloration to agar cultures. The production of pyocyanin is unique to the species and is enhanced by culture on King's A medium (King *et al.*, 1954), which contains potassium and magnesium salts in sufficient concentration to suppress fluorescein production. The latter, which is also called pyoverdin, is optimally produced on King's B medium, which contains less of these salts, and is visible under ultraviolet illumination. Two other uncommon pigments are pyorubrin, which imparts a 'port wine' hue to cultures on nutrient or King's A agar, and the brownish-black pigment pyomelanin, which is best demonstrated on tyrosine agar. This pigment should not be confused with the brown discoloration of blood agar by some weakly haemolytic strains.

Colonial forms and biochemistry

On agar culture at 37 °C, most isolates form flat diffuse colonies with an irregular edge (type 1), and some are 'coliform' in appearance (type 2). Other colony types are generally rare; they include the dry, 'pepper-corn' (type 3), mucoid (type 4), rugose (type 5) and dwarf colonies characteristic of type 6. *Pseudomonas aeruginosa* produces a strong 'sickly-sweet' odour owing to the formation of trimethylamine.

The bacterium is a Gram-negative rod of variable length, motile by means of a single polar flagellum, molecular oxygen being necessary for motility. Anaerobic growth is possible only in the presence of an alternative terminal electron acceptor such as nitrate; motility tests in Craigie tubes are therefore inappropriate. *Pseudomonas aeruginosa* will grow over a wide range of temperatures (10–44 °C) but growth is optimal around 35 °C. Isolates will not grow at 4 °C, which distinguishes it from the psychrophilic species *P. putida* and *P. fluorescens*, but they will grow over three successive subcultures at 42 °C, while the latter do not.

In keeping with other pseudomonads, most strains can utilize a range of single organic compounds as energy sources. The species metabolizes glucose and other sugars by an oxidative pathway. Acid is formed in peptone–water sugars by young cultures but this is neutralized by alkali released by the breakdown of peptone. Sugar utilization is therefore best demonstrated in an ammonium salts-based medium. All strains produce a cytochrome

oxidase *c* enzyme which is detected in the oxidase test with Kovács' reagent. Other common features of *P. aeruginosa* are reduction of nitrate to nitrogen gas, and the formation of ammonia from arginine.

NORMAL HABITAT

Pseudomonas aeruginosa can be found almost anywhere in the natural environment, and this ubiquity may lie in its ability to adapt to habitats ranging from surface waters to disinfectants. It can multiply in distilled water presumably by the utilization of gaseous dissolved nutrients but is rarely isolated from sea water except from sewage outfalls and polluted river estuaries. It is not associated with disease in fish. The species is present in soil and the rhizosphere and as a result may be frequently recovered from fresh vegetables and plants (Rhame, 1980). In hospitals, sinks, taps and drains are invariably colonized by *P. aeruginosa* and other pseudomonads, but the domestic household environment is rarely contaminated.

Natural carriage by man is infrequent. In healthy subjects outside of hospitals the faecal carriage rates vary between 2% and 10%, but may be higher for vegetarians. However, colonization rates increase markedly with hospital stay and reports of 60%, and above, of patients with *P. aeruginosa* in units are common (Levison, 1977). Faecal colonization appears to be transient in healthy persons and there is a rapid turnover of strain types. *Pseudomonas aeruginosa* dies rapidly on dry healthy skin, but in conditions of superhydration, such as in divers undergoing long-term saturation dives, the frequency of skin colonization is increased and accompanied by infections, particularly otitis externa (Alcock, 1977).

PATHOGENICITY

Virulence-associated Factors

Pseudomonas aeruginosa produces a wide array of factors, some of which have been closely linked with disease-producing potential. Nevertheless, in the absence of impairment of host defences the species has low intrinsic virulence for man and to cause disease must be introduced into the tissues, or systemically, in sufficient numbers to overwhelm the host defences. This feature probably explains some of the conflicting experimental evidence concerning the role of different virulence factors. Various animal models such as the burned-mouse, neutropenic mouse (induced with cyclophosphamide) and the murine corneal scratch model have been used by investigators but have not been universally adopted.

Adherence

Injury to the epithelial mucosa by viral infection or previous colonization by other bacteria predisposes tissue to the attachment of *P. aeruginosa*. Adherence of the organism to respiratory epithelial cells is correlated with the loss of fibronectin from the cell surface and with increased levels of salivary proteases. Three main groups of adhesin molecules have been identified which mediate attachment of *P. aeruginosa* to host tissues and respiratory mucus glycoproteins; they are pili, mucin-binding outer membrane protein and alginate. The contribution of each class of adhesin to attachment of strains to different tissues is difficult to quantify. However, nearly all strains of *P. aeruginosa* produce pili under favourable conditions. These are uni- or bipolar in distribution and are flexible filaments about 2500 nm long (range 100–5000 nm) composed of a protein, pilin, which has a molecular weight of about 18 000 Da. Pili are serologically heterogeneous

TABLE 14.2 PHENOTYPIC PROPERTIES OF STRAINS OF *P. AERUGINOSA* ASSOCIATED WITH CYSTIC FIBROSIS

Production of alginate
Loss of the O-antigenic fraction of LPS
Serum sensitivity
Lack of flagella
Hypersensitivity to β-lactams/increased resistance to
    antibiotics
Low proteolytic activity
Auxotrophy

and contain a region which binds specifically with epithelial cell ceramide receptors. Tang *et al.* (1995) examined the role of piliation in the development and course of acute pulmonary infection in an infant mouse model and showed that piliated strains caused more cases of pneumonia, bacteraemia and mortality than non-piliated strains.

Exotoxin S also functions as an adhesin and is found on the cell surface, where it interacts with glycososphingolipid receptors. The receptor for alginate on respiratory cells is thought to be carbohydrate containing *N*-acetylneuraminic acid, galactose or *N*-acetylglucosamine.

Flagella

The loss of flagella by strains is strongly correlated with a decrease in virulence in the experimental animal. However, flagella can only be considered a significant virulence factor in that they promote chemotaxis and motility during invasion of the tissues. Most strains of *P. aeruginosa* from patients with cystic fibrosis (CF) lack flagella and these isolates are generally resistant to macrophage phagocytosis (Mahenthiralingam *et al.*, 1994).

Lipopolysaccharide

The cell envelope of *P. aeruginosa*, as with other Gram-negative bacteria, is composed of an external unit membrane (outer membrane, OM), a layer of peptidoglycan and an inner cytoplasmic membrane; the latter is mainly composed of phospholipids with randomly intercalated molecules of proteins. The OM is an asymmmetrical bilayer containing phospholipids on the inner side and lipopolysaccharide (LPS), as the major lipidic molecule, on the outer cell surface. The LPS of *P. aeruginosa* consists of three basic units: lipid A, core polysaccharide and O-specific side chain. The lipid A has five or six fatty acids linked to a backbone of diglucosamine phosphate. The core polysaccharide is covalently linked to lipid and contains an unusual sugar, 2-keto-3-deoxyoctanoate, as well as a variety of heptose and hexose residues. The extremity of the oligosaccharide core may be substituted (capped) with a variable number of oligosaccharide units, which is the O-specific region.

The LPS of *P. aeruginosa* has a lower intrinsic toxicity compared with that of Enterobacteriaceae. It plays a major role in protecting the cell from the complement-mediated bactericidal action of normal human serum. Most isolates of *P. aeruginosa* from clinical samples are resistant to serum and the highest frequency of resistance is found in isolates from blood. However, isolates from chronic infection, in particular CF and bronchiectasis, and less frequently persistent urinary tract infection in paraplegics, are often sensitive to serum. LPS-deficient mutants are invariably serum sensitive and avirulent in the experimental animal. Furthermore, antibody to LPS is protective not only in animal models but also in humans. Recent evidence suggests that antibodies specific for O antigens of *P. aeruginosa*, particularly the high-molecular-weight O polysaccharide, can protect against mucosal surface colonization by *P. aeruginosa*, and this is achieved through circulating antibody alone rather than by induction of local IgA antibodies (Pier *et al.*, 1995).

Extracellular polysaccharides

All strains of *P. aeruginosa* elaborate an extracellular slime that aggregates loosely around the cell. More than 50% of the dry weight of slime is composed of polysaccharide, chiefly of the sugars glucose, rhamnose and mannose with galactosamine, glucuronic acid, nucleic acids (20%), and proteins as a minor fraction (Brown *et al.*, 1969). A chemically distinct polysaccharide, alginate, is hyper-produced by mucoid strains of *P. aeruginosa*. This exopolysaccharide is composed of β-1,4-linked D-mannuronic acid and L-gluronic acid, the ratio of which confers the degree of viscosity on the polymer. Mucoid strains are almost exclusively isolated from the sputum of patients with CF and bronchiectasis. A minority (<3%) of strains from other sources exhibit the mucoid characteristic (Doggett, 1969). Alginate production by other species is rare but *Azotobacter*

vinelandii, and some pseudomonads (*P. fluorescens*, *P. putida* and *P. mendocina*) can elaborate the polymer. The consortia of alginate and bacterial cells (microcolonies) is the basis of the biofilm mode of growth and confers to the bacteria protection from the external environment such as complement and antibiotics.

Exotoxins

The lethal toxin of *P. aeruginosa*, exotoxin A (ETA), is produced by approximately 90% of the species and is closely related to diphtheria toxin. Both toxins catalyse the transfer of the ADP-ribosyl moiety of oxidized NAD (NAD$^+$) to elongation factor 2 (EF2). This reaction inactivates EF2, terminates peptide chain elongation and leads to inhibition of protein synthesis and cell death. The toxin is composed of two fragments. Fragment A is of molecular weight 21 000 Da and has enzymic activity; fragment B is 37 000 Da and acts as the binding moiety. ETA is optimally produced in iron-limited conditions and is encoded by a single copy of a structural gene, *toxA*, and regulated by two genes *regA* and *regB* (Wick *et al.*, 1990). It is highly toxic for mammalian cells (LD$_{50}$ for mice <0.01 mg/kg) and enters the cell via a receptor-mediated endocytic pathway; ETA also has activity as a T cell mitogen and interleukin 1 inducer (Nicas and Iglewski, 1986).

Pseudomonas aeruginosa produces another ADP-ribosyl transferase, exotoxin S (ETS); it catalyses the transfer of ADP-ribose from NAD$^+$ to other eukaryotic proteins. ETS is more resistant to heat and is not neutralized by antibodies to ETA; it is also partially destroyed by the reducing agents urea and dithiothreitol, which potentiate ETA activity (Nicas and Iglewski, 1986). Strains lacking only ETS are less virulent than those with ETS activity but the significance of the toxin in virulence is unclear.

Haemolysins

Two distinct haemolysins have been identified in *P. aeruginosa*: a heat-labile phospholipase C (PLC), and a heat-stable rhamnolipid (Vasil, 1986). PLC is believed to be exclusive to the species and is found in almost all strains. It degrades phospholipids containing quaternary ammonium groups such as phosphatidylcholine, the major phospholipid component of lung surfactant. PLC is therefore a potential virulence factor particularly for strains colonizing the human lung. Rhamnolipid also degrades phospholipids due to its detergent action and in high concentrations attracts and lyses leucocytes, and has ciliostatic action (Woods and Vasil, 1994).

Proteases

Most strains of *P. aeruginosa* produce a range of proteolytic enzymes which are active against a variety of substrates such as gelatin, casein, elastin, collagen and fibrin. Three classes of protease have been identified: a general protease, elastase and alkaline protease. They are distinguishable by their optimum pH of activity, substrate specificity and physical properties (Woods and Vasil, 1994). The general protease is lysine specific and has a limited range of activity. Alkaline protease has not been widely studied but has activity against a wider range of substrates and has been implicated in corneal damage in *P. aeruginosa* eye infections. Elastase degrades a number of proteins such as human lung elastin, immunoglobulins, complement factors, basement membrane constituents and mucins. Elastolytic activity is the result of at least two proteins, LasA and LasB, under the control of *lasR*. Elastase production by strains is controlled, at the translational level, by the levels of zinc and iron in the environment (Brumlik and Storey, 1992).

Janda and Bottone (1981) described an association between exoenzyme production and the potential pathogenic role of *P. aeruginosa*. They found that clinical isolates produced significant levels of haemolysin, protease, fibrinolysins and other enzymes, in contrast to strains from the natural environment which were relatively inactive enzymatically. Their results also suggested that elevated protease activities were associated with isolates from systemic disease, and they concluded that the production of these enzymes might play an important role in the dissemination of *P. aeruginosa* from local sites. This finding has not been confirmed by other workers (Mansi *et al.*, 1995).

Cytotoxins

The majority of *P. aeruginosa* organisms produce a leucocidin which was purified by Lutz (1979) and renamed cytotoxin because of its action on other eukaryotic cells. The toxin is localized in the periplasmic space as an inactive form, but is activated by proteases, including an endogenous elastase. Cytotoxin alters the phospholipid composition of the cell membrane, inducing an influx of calcium which leads to loss of the lysosomal content into the cytosol. Leucocidin may be linked to the observed lack of leucocytes during sepsis due to *P. aeruginosa*, and the fall in the granulocyte count in some patients.

Siderophores

In order to obtain iron, an essential requirement for the establishment and maintenance of bacterial infection, *P. aeruginosa* excretes iron chelators such as pyochelin and pyoverdin (Visca *et al.*, 1992). These siderophores play a key role in the growth and virulence of the species in iron-limited conditions. Pyochelin is poorly water soluble and of low molecular weight (325 Da), while pyoverdin (approximately 1500 Da) is highly soluble in water and more active.

Pyocyanin

The phenazine pigment pyocyanin and its colourless precursor 1-hydroxyphenazine are highly toxic for human respiratory epithelial cilia. They induce, at low concentrations, ciliary dyskinesis, and later disrupt the integrity of the epithelial surface (Wilson *et al.*, 1987). Pyocyanin causes a fall in intracellular adenosine $3':5'$-cyclic monophosphate (cyclic AMP) and ciliary beat can be restored by agents such as the β_2-adrenoceptor agonist salmeterol and isoprenaline.

Pyocyanin is bactericidal for a number of species including *Escherichia coli*, *Staphylococcus aureus* and *Mycobacterium smegmatis*. Other activities of pyocyanin include the production of reactive nitrogen intermediates, and promotion of elastase–anti-elastase imbalance by increasing the release of neutrophil elastase and enhancing the oxidative inactivation of α_1-protease inhibitor.

Pseudomonas aeruginosa also produces a specific anti-staphylococcal substance, which is distinct from pyocyanin, pseudomonic acid and a number of other phenazines (Machan *et al.*, 1992).

EPIDEMIOLOGY

Despite the apparent ubiquity of *P. aeruginosa* in the natural environment, the incidence of community-acquired infections in healthy subjects is relatively low. However, in the hospital environment, particularly in immunosuppressed and debilitated patients, the incidence of *P. aeruginosa* infection may be among the highest for all bacterial species. The organism can be isolated from the stools of up to 15% of healthy subjects but this number is sharply increased in hospitalized patients (Stoodley and Thom, 1970), which is possibly linked to ingestion of contaminated food and the use of antibiotics. The salivary carriage rate is similar in hospital patients and normal controls (approximately 5%) but skin colonization in burned patients may reach 80% by the ninth day post burn (Holder, 1977).

Almost any type of hospital equipment or utensil has been implicated as a reservoir for *P. aeruginosa*, including disinfectants, antiseptics, intravenous fluids and eye wash solutions. These sources may serve as foci for the dissemination of the organism in common-source outbreaks and usually are the result of poor sterilization. Widespread contamination of the inanimate ward environment such as sink traps and taps has been cited by many workers as a potential infection hazard particularly for the contamination of the hands of personnel, but not all studies have supported this conclusion (Beck-Sagué *et al.*, 1994).

According to the National Nosocomial Infections Surveillance (USA) data, between 1985 and 1991 *P. aeruginosa* was the fifth most frequent pathogen isolated and accounted for 10% of nosocomial infections. The organism was the most frequent cause of pneumonia (17%), and the third, fifth and eighth most common agent in urinary tract, surgical wounds and bloodstream infections respectively. The proportion of patients with *P. aeruginosa* infections also varied according to whether the patient was in an intensive care unit. This is clearly the case with burn sepsis, in which *P. aeruginosa* was by far the most common, and dangerous, microorganism in the 1960s and 1970s. Today, due to the improvements in burn management and treatment, the number of serious infections caused by *P. aeruginosa* has declined considerably.

INFECTIONS

Skin and Eye

Pseudomonas aeruginosa rarely causes disease in the healthy individual, when it has to be introduced into the tissues in relatively large numbers. Examples are water-associated infections of the skin such as folliculitis and soggy dermatitis of the interdigital spaces, or otitis externa, which are the result of prolonged exposure to usually in excess of 10^6 colony-forming units/(cofu)/ml. Folliculitis due to *P. aeruginosa* is characterized by a diffuse maculopapular or vesiculopustular rash, either resulting from contaminated swimming pools, spas and hot tubs (Schlech *et al.*, 1986). The condition is usually self-limiting but topical treatment and rarely, systemic antibiotics are required.

Pseudomonas aeruginosa is probably the most devastating of bacterial pathogens for the human eye, in particular the cornea, where it produces ulceration or keratitis. Other infections include conjunctivitis, endophthalmitis and orbital cellulitis. The most common sources of the organism are contact lens fluids, ocular medications and mascara which have been become contaminated with *P. aeruginosa* (Zloty and Belin, 1994).

It may also cause an invasive form of otitis externa which does not respond to topical antibiotic therapy. This malignant infection can lead to erosion through the external auditory canal and involvement of cranial nerves, with a mortality of 20%.

Burns

Pseudomonas aeruginosa is a common cause of infections in burns, established through colonization of the burn wound by the patient's own flora or from the environment. Most fatalities (usually arising from septicaemia) are associated with full-thickness burns and there is a strong correlation with the percentage area of the burn (Smith, 1994).

The most commonly used anti-pseudomonal topical agent is silver sulphadiazine, which is most effective when used prophylactically; the addition of cerium increases its antibacterial properties as well as its persistence in the eschar. Topical silver nitrate also reduces mortality in patients with extensive burns, and methylated sulphonamide (mafenide) cream has good burn eschar penetration.

Due to pharmacokinetic changes in burned patients which result in altered intra- and extravascular fluid volumes, albumin-bound antibiotics are rapidly lost. In general, antibiotic doses and schedules are increased to take account of the increased volume of distribution and more rapid renal clearance. Most burn centres combine an aminoglycoside with an extended-spectrum penicillin (piperacillin or ticarcillin) which may act synergistically.

Wounds

Pseudomonas aeruginosa is a common isolate from surgical wounds and its frequency is related to the site and extent of the surgery and the underlying clinical state of the patient. Data from the National Nosocomial Infection Surveillance (NNIS) survey in the USA showed an incidence in surgical wounds of about 7% in ward areas compared with 10% in intensive care patients (Beck-Sagué et al., 1994).

Bone and Joints

Bone and joints can be infected either by direct injection in puncture wounds (rare) or by haemotogenous spread in intravenous drug abusers and diabetic subjects, resulting in chronic osteomyelitis. Removal of the focus as well as the surrounding soft tissue is necessary if antibiotic therapy is to be successful. Septic arthritis is unusual and many patients have a history of drug abuse or a predisposing condition (Mader et al., 1994).

Blood and cerebrospinal fluid

Reports of *P. aeruginosa* bacteraemia are relatively rare in the early literature, but since the 1970s the number of cases recorded has increased dramatically. This is undoubtedly due to the increased susceptibility of the hospitalized population. Frequencies of *P. aeruginosa* bacteraemia today vary from 5% to 20% in a number of studies (Baltch, 1994) and septicaemia is most common in the immunocompromised, in particular granulocytopenic patients and the elderly. Mortality rates for septicaemia can be as high as 60%. A minority of patients exhibit a skin manifestation, ecthyma gangrenosum and, if untreated, necrosis of deep tissue can occur. The primary sources of bacteraemia are the gastrointestinal tract, the respiratory tract and skin. Early treatment is critical, particularly in the immunocompromised, and combination therapy with an aminoglycoside and a β-lactam is usual.

Infection of the central nervous system (CNS) with *P. aeruginosa* is uncommon. Nevertheless, the risk is increased for neonates, those undergoing neurosurgery or transplantation, or those with a chronic underlying condition. *Pseudomonas aeruginosa* may be isolated from a minority of intracranial abscesses but the incidence rises in patients with chronic otitis media and mastoiditis. Ceftazidime is recommended as the drug of choice in CNS infection and should be combined with an aminoglycoside at least for the first week of therapy (Fong and Tompkins, 1985).

Urinary tract

Primary urinary tract infection acquired in the community due to *P. aeruginosa* is rare except in those patients with anatomical abnormalities and spinal cord injuries. The great majority of urinary tract infections are of nosocomial origin and are invariably the consequence of long-term catheterization. Haematogenous spread from a primary focus is uncommon. Paraplegic patients in institutional care are especially at risk and reservoirs of contaminated urine such as drainage bottles and bed pans are probably the major sources for the organism. The infection is usually resolved by the removal of the catheter or other predisposing factor, but prostatic infections in the presence of calculi are exceedingly difficult to treat (see review by Kunin (1994).

RESPIRATORY TRACT AND CYSTIC FIBROSIS

Pseudomonas aeruginosa frequently colonizes the lower respiratory tract of intubated patients, and those with a tracheostomy and exposure to contaminated inhalation equipment. In many without anatomical abnormalities or prolonged immunosuppression, infection is relatively transient and specific treatment is not indicated. Nevertheless, the organism may account for up to 15% of all nosocomial pneumonias in the intensive therapy unit (ITU). The mortality rate for pneumonia with bacteraemia may be 80% greater than the non-bacteraemic form and overall mortality ranges from 30% to 80%.

Pseudomonas aeruginosa commonly infects the lungs of patients with non-CF bronchiectasis and a chronic infected state which is seldom relieved by therapy is established. The isolates from these patients may exhibit some of the features normally associated with CF, such as mucoid alginate production.

Recently, there have been a number of reports of *P. aeruginosa* respiratory infections in AIDS patients (Ali *et al.*, 1995). Most infections appear to be community acquired and the organism is often present in pure culture. Morbidity and mortality are difficult to define accurately as many patients have advanced HIV disease, but mortality may reach 40%. Risk factors identified include advanced HIV immunosuppression, use of systemic *Pneumocystis* prophylaxis and/or broad-spectrum antibiotics, and sinusitis.

Cystic Fibrosis

Until the 1970s, most CF patients who succumbed to bacterial infection were infected with *Staphylococcus aureus*, and *P. aeruginosa* infection was relatively rare. Since that time there has been an inexorable rise in the number of patients who harbour *P. aeruginosa* and today in some centres as many as 90% of all patients are colonized or infected. There is a general acceptance that it has a pathogenic role in chronic lung infection in these patients.

Acquisition

As *P. aeruginosa* is ubiquitous, CF patients may acquire it from a variety of sources in the environment. This is corroborated by the fact that patients are, with the exception of siblings, usually colonized by different strains. The gut does not appear to be the principal source of the organism as respiratory tract colonization most often precedes the recovery of the organism from the faeces of CF patients. There is, however, a reported risk of cross-infection with *P. aeruginosa* among CF patients and this is highest when non-colonized patients come into contact with chronically infected patients in hospitals, CF centres or summer holiday camps (Govan and Nelson, 1992). *Pseudomonas aeruginosa* exhibits 'opportunistic adherence' in that strains adhere more readily to desquamating cells of infected tracheal tissue than to normal mucosa, and the adherence of non-mucoid *P. aeruginosa* is also increased on CF buccal epithelia in comparison with normal subjects.

Antibodies

There is pronounced antibody production by the CF patient in response to the initial colonization by *P. aeruginosa*. This increased humoral response is associated with a poor prognosis. IgA and IgG antibodies are significantly elevated in CF compared with normal subjects, while IgM is not. Precipitating antibodies against *P. aeruginosa* are significantly elevated in at least 30% of patients and these antibodies are always detectable when the mucoid phenotype of *P. aeruginosa* is present in the sputum. Indeed, the rise in precipitins is much more evident with chronically colonized as opposed to intermittently colonized patients.

Pier *et al.* (1987) postulated that the survival of CF patients to adulthood without being colonized by mucoid *P. aeruginosa* was related to the presence of specific serum antibodies against the mucoid exopolysaccharide. These antibodies were termed 'opsonic-killing' and were significantly more common in older CF patients who were not colonized by *P. aeruginosa*. Chronically colonized patients also had high titres of these antibodies but they were not specific for the exopolysaccharide. This suggested that the opsonic-killing antibodies against alginate protected patients against chronic colonization with mucoid *P. aeruginosa*.

An enzyme-linked immunosorbent assay (ELISA) which measures antibody to the lipid A, core oligosaccharide, and O polysaccharide of *P. aeruginosa* LPS has shown that the systemic antibody response is increased to all parts of the molecule (Kronborg *et al.*, 1992). Furthermore, antibodies in sputum are mainly anti-lipid A and anti-O polysaccharide of the IgG and IgA isotypes. The determination of serum antibody by ELISA is of value, particularly in paediatric CF patients, where it may help to detect *P. aeruginosa* infection at an early stage and aid the differentiation between early infection and harmless colonization and to monitor disease progression. In general, positive serum IgG antibody titres do not predate isolation of *P. aeruginosa* from sputum in CF patients but in some are present soon after acquisition of the organism. A positive titre indicates significant exposure to *P. aeruginosa* and may be useful to detect infection in sputum-negative patients and possibly indicate the effect of early treatment. It is paradoxical, however, that CF patients with high titres of antibodies, which supposedly protect against infection, are those who are chronically colonized by *P. aeruginosa*. It is clear, therefore, that elevated antibodies against *P. aeruginosa*, which may protect against septicaemia, are insufficient to eliminate the bacterium from the lungs of CF patients. Once *P. aeruginosa* is established in the CF airways it undergoes a variety of phenotypic modifications in order to adapt and persist in the unique environment of the lung (Table 14.2).

Alginate

Pseudomonas aeruginosa isolated from patients with CF are frequently mucoid due to the abundant production of alginate. Alginate exists as a loose viscous polymer in which the cells are suspended as a microcolony. Most *P. aeruginosa* strains have the genetic capacity to synthesize alginate, and non-mucoid strains produce basal levels of the polymer. A variety of typing methods have confirmed that non-mucoid strains arise from mucoid parent forms, and it has been suggested that non-mucoid isolates may become mucoid when deprived of nutrients (Speert *et al.*, 1990). Increased osmolarity is another factor which has been suggested to lead to mucoid forms.

A cluster of genes has been identified which control the expression of alginate (Govan and Nelson, 1992). In non-mucoid cells, the protein AlgU (product of the *algU* gene) which plays an important role in transcription of alginate biosynthetic genes is repressed by MucA and possibly MucB. In mucoid strains, mutations that inactivate the *mucA* gene relieve AlgU from inhibition, which in turn activates *algD*, and alginate production ensues. It is believed that *P. aeruginosa* mutants with inactivated *mucA* are selected in the CF lung and these alginate hyper-producers establish a biofilm in which there is effective protection against opsonins, phagocytosis, neutrophil attraction and antibiotics. It may also enhance the neutrophil oxidative burst, indicating that the exopolysaccharide functions as both a defensive and offensive virulence factor in CF (Pedersen *et al.*, 1990).

LPS deficiency

Many isolates of *P. aeruginosa* from CF have an altered LPS structure in their cell envelope. This involves loss of all or part of the polysaccharide side chain (O antigen) and results in the absence of a specific O-serotype reaction for the majority of strains (Hancock *et al.*, 1983). By electron microscopy LPS-deficient strains exhibit outer layers characterized by atypical extrusions (lipophilic blebs) from the cell wall. These strains are also invariably serum sensitive, which requires both the action of the classical and alternative complement pathways. Both LPS-deficient and LPS-complete strains can activate complement but only in the deficient form is the terminal complement complex able to anchor stably in the outer membrane. Serum-sensitive strains should not survive in the bloodstream, and this is consistent with the rare finding of septicaemia in CF patients.

Non-motility

Pseudomonas aeruginosa from CF patients often lack flagella and are thus not motile, in contrast to 95% motility for strains from other sources. Non-motile isolates are resistant to phagocytosis by macrophages and this may favour their selection in the CF lung (Mahenthiralingam *et al.*, 1994).

Hypersusceptibility

Paradoxically, 20% of isolates of *P. aeruginosa* from CF patients may be hypersusceptible to the penicillins, even including ampicillin. Irvin *et al.* (1981) found that 12 of 22 patients harboured carbenicillin-hypersusceptible strains (minimal inhibitory concentration (MIC) 1 mg/l) which were indistinguishable from contemporaneous resistant strains. Furthermore, representatives of these strains were uncharacteristically sensitive to tetracycline and trimethoprim, and were usually isolated from patients receiving these antibiotics.

Exoproducts

There is much evidence that during the course of infection with *P. aeruginosa* in CF the production of virulence exoproducts by strains is reduced, probably as a result of selection. Strains from CF patients with severe respiratory disease often produce less exoproducts than isolates from mild disease (particularly DNAase, elastase and haemolysin).

Antibiotics may also affect the expression of virulence factors by *P. aeruginosa*. Sub-MIC concentrations of aminoglycosides are able to protect the epithelium from damage by inhibition of the formation of exotoxin A and elastase, and as little as 1/20 MIC of an antibiotic totally abolishes exoenzyme activity. There was also significantly less histological damage in the lungs of infected rats which received subinhibitory doses of the antibiotics (Grimwood *et al.*, 1988).

Auxotrophy

A number of isolates of *P. aeruginosa* from CF patients are auxotrophic, (i.e., require specific growth factors). The most common requirement is for methionine but other amino acids such as leucine, arginine or ornithine are less commonly required (Barth and Pitt, 1995). Auxotrophic and prototrophic (wild-type) *P. aeruginosa* isolates colonizing the same CF patient invariably constitute an isogenic group and it is most likely that auxotrophs are selected from the prototrophic population during the course of pulmonary infection.

LABORATORY DIAGNOSIS

Media

Pseudomonas aeruginosa grows readily on simple media It is relatively resistant to quaternary ammonium compounds, in particular cetyltrimethyl ammonium chloride (cetrimide) and benzalkonium chloride. Cetrimide resistance has been exploited as a selective feature for the isolation and presumptive identification of the species from clinical specimens and cetrimide-containing media combined with nalidixic acid are commercially available. Irgasan is also selective for *P. aeruginosa*. However, some isolates from CF patients may exhibit hypersensitivity to both compounds and thus fail to grow on these media. Enrichment in acetamide broth has been recommended for the isolation of *P. aeruginosa* from faeces.

Typing Methods

Owing to the ubiquity of *P. aeruginosa* in the natural and hospital environment, it is often necessary to type strains for epidemiological studies. A number of phenotypic and genotypic methods have been described.

Serological typing

Pseudomonas aeruginosa is serologically heterogeneous and is characterized by a number of somatic and flagellar antigen groups. The LPS somatic antigens are similar to enterobacterial LPS in that they are comprised of O-specific polysaccharide side chains radiating from the cell surface linked through a membrane-bound common core oligosaccharide to lipid A deep in the outer membrane. The LPS is unusually rich in phosphorus and amino sugars and is the immunodominant molecule of the cell. Being heat stable, specific antibody may be readily prepared by the intravenous immunization of an animal (rabbit) with a boiled cell suspension; IgM antibody is formed first and IgG levels are maximal within three weeks. A number of O-antigenic schemes for *P. aeruginosa* have been described worldwide and some are country specific, e.g. the schemes of Homma in Japan, and Lányi in Hungary. An international trial in the 1970s resulted in agreement of a scheme of 17 O serotypes in the International Antigenic Typing Scheme (IATS) (Liu *et al.*, 1983). This scheme is based on the original 12 O serotypes of Habs, with five additional types from other authors. The 17 serotypes are not specific. Types O2, O5 and O16 are closely related (Figure 14.1) and can only be separated by the use of absorbed antisera or monoclonal antibodies; these serotypes can be grouped together and referred to as group II (Pitt, 1988). Further cross-reactions are observed between serotypes O7 and O8, and between O13 and O14. Antisera and monoclonal antibodies to the IATS serotypes are available commercially. Three further types, O18 to O20, have been proposed but have not been internationally validated.

Isolates are typed by slide agglutination with live cultures from agar plates or in microtitre trays with

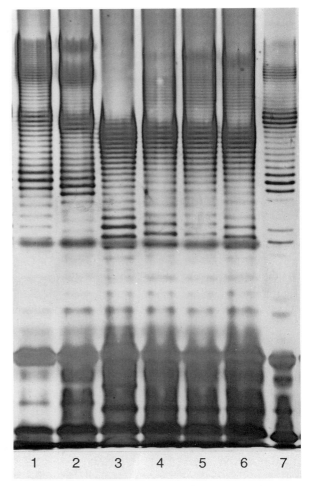

Figure 14.1. Homogeneity of electrophoretic patterns of phenol–water purified lipopolysaccharides from strains of *P. aeruginosa* of serotypes O2, O5 and O16. Note close correspondence of ladder rungs between patterns of strains of the same serotype or subtype. Lane (1) serotype O16, (2) O2(a), (3) O5, (4) O2(b), (5) O2(b), (6) O5, (7) O16.

boiled suspensions. The percentage typeability by O serotyping for most isolates of *P. aeruginosa* (excluding CF patients) is approximately 90% and the reproducibility is high. However, discrimination is poor as two serotypes predominate in clinical material, O6 (20%) and O11 (15%), O11 being particularly frequent in hospital outbreaks.

Serotype O6 can be subdivided into four minor antigens with the use of cross-absorbed antisera or monoclonal antibodies. Other frequent serotypes are O10, O11 (O2, O5, O16) and O4, and together with O6 and O11 account for about two-thirds of clinical strains. Serotypes O15 and O17 are very rare, and type O12 is uncommon but is highly associated with multiresistance to antibiotics (Pitt *et al.*, 1989).

A feature of the type-specific LPS of *P. aeruginosa*, unlike most enterobacterial LPS, is the relatively few oligosaccharide core residues substituted with O-antigenic side chains. Further loss of O side chains, as occurs during chronic infection of the lung of CF patients, results in a loss of serotype specificity which is manifest by polyagglutination of cell suspensions in antisera to unrelated O serotypes. These LPS-defective forms may also be autoagglutinable in saline and cannot be allocated to a serotype. Polyagglutinating and autoagglutinating strains may account for more than 80% of CF isolates, and this is closely correlated with sensitivity of the strain to the bactericidal action of normal human serum (Hancock *et al.*, 1983).

A second LPS molecule is detectable on the surface of *P. aeruginosa* (Lam *et al.*, 1989). This is termed 'common' LPS due to the fact that it is antigenically conserved in all strains. This LPS does not react with O-type specific antibodies and is best visualized in O-LPS-defective strains or by specific binding in immunoblots with a monoclonal antibody.

Various flagellar antigen typing schemes have been proposed for *P. aeruginosa* but have not been widely applied mainly because of diphasic variation leading to the occurrence of antigenically distinct flagellar antigens by cells of the same strain.

Bacteriophage typing

A large number of bacteriophages active against *P. aeruginosa* have been described (Bergan, 1978). Both DNA- and RNA-containing phages for the species have been reported, with $G + C$ mole% ratios of 46–63. The latent time ranges from 35 to 65 minutes, with a burst size of 10–200 phages per cell. The morphology of most DNA phages resembles

T-even phages, and in the Lindberg phage typing set at least eight morphotypes, all with tails, can be identified. The phages of *P. aeruginosa* attach to a number of cell surface receptors including outer membrane proteins and LPS, slime polysaccharide and pili, but phages that adsorb to flagella have not been described. *Pseudomonas aeruginosa* phages are generally resistant to heat (50–60 °C) but are inactivated at 65–70°C, and are stable in a pH range of 6.5–10.0. Three of the 21 Colindale phages are sensitive to chloroform, and six of the phages require calcium for optimum activity. Most strains of *P. aeruginosa* are lysogenic and as many as 10 different lysogenic phages have been detected in a single strain. Nevertheless, more than 80% of clinical isolates are sensitive to the Colindale set. Plaques vary from small (0.5 mm) to large (3–5 mm) and most phages are easily propagated by standard methods. Phage suspensions are used at routine test dilution (RTD – the dilution that just fails to give confluent lysis) to type field strains.

Owing to the lack of reproducibility, a three strong-reaction-difference rule needs to be applied before pairs of isolates of the same O serotype from the same incident of infection can be considered distinct. Phage typing is therefore only of value for the subdivision of strains that have been grouped together by a primary method of relatively low discrimination. Isolates with defective LPS are less sensitive to phages because of the lack of the receptor; mucoid isolates are similarly insensitive due to the inhibition of phage adsorption by exopolysaccharide.

Bacteriocin typing

The bacteriocins of *P. aeruginosa* are collectively known as pyocins. Three types of pyocin particles have been identified, R, F and S, signifying retractile, flexuous and soluble. The R pyocins resemble the tails of contractile phages and are distinguishable morphologically from the F pyocins; S pyocins have no discernible structure, are of low molecular weight and diffuse through agar. The use of standard strains to detect the activity of pyocins expressed by field strains was first described by Gillies and Govan (see Govan, 1978).

In the original scheme pyocins were detected by cross-streaking eight indicator strains across an area of an agar plate that had previously supported the growth of the producer strain. The pattern of growth inhibition of the indicator strains defined the pyocin type of the field strain. Five indicator strains were added subsequently to provide further discrimination between isolates of the frequent types 1, 3, 5 and 10, or untypeable strains. At least 105 primary types and 26 subtype patterns have been published but many other patterns have been identified at a local level. The cross-streaking method of pyocin typing has largely been replaced by a soft agar overlay method (Fyfe *et al.*, 1984) which involves the application of dense suspensions of the producer strains to a shallow agar plate with a multipoint applicator (Figure 14.2). After a short period of incubation, the growth is killed by chloroform vapour and the indicator strain is applied in a thin soft-agar overlay. Following incubation, pyocin activity is shown by the inhibition of the indicator lawn over the inoculum

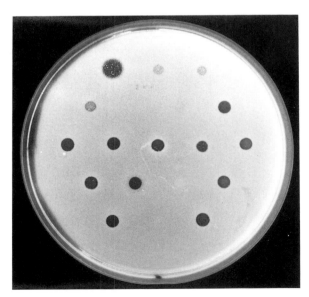

Figure 14.2. Pyocin typing of *P. aeruginosa* by agar overlay method. Clinical isolates are spotted on agar and chloroformed after a short period of incubation. The agar overlay contains a pyocin indicator strain and zones of inhibition are evident after overnight incubation.

spots of the producer strains. The method is considerably more rapid than the traditional one and the differentiation of R and F pyocins from S pyocins on the basis of inhibition zone size allows increased discrimination between strains.

Pyocin typing is reproducible if care is taken over the standardization of inocula, media and incubation temperature. About 90% of clinical strains are typeable and the discriminatory power is similar to O serotyping. Some pyocin types are associated with O serotypes but this does not markedly reduce the ability of pyocin typing to subdivide strains of the same O serotype.

Due to problems of inadequate discrimination and reproducibility, sometimes combined with poor typeability of the phenotypic methods, a range of genotyping methods have been evaluated for the typing of *P. aeruginosa*.

Plasmids

Plasmids are relatively rare in clinical isolates of *P. aeruginosa*. A survey by Poh *et al.* (1988) used two rapid screening methods and reported plasmids ranging from 1.2 to 60 MDa in 15% of isolates examined.

Restriction endonuclease analysis (REA)

DNA fingerprinting of strains of *P. aeruginosa* by REA has been employed for epidemiological studies. Loutit and Tompkins (1991) used conventional agarose electrophoresis to separate DNA fragments generated by digestion of purified chromosomal DNA of isolates from CF patients with the frequent cutting restriction endonucleases *Sal*I and *Sma*I. The discrimination of the method is sufficient to allow the differentiation of strains from different patients, but the large number of fragments generated by these enzymes make resolution between bands difficult.

Rare cutting enzymes, in particular *Dra*I and *Spe*I, have been widely utilized and generate fragments in excess of 50 kb that cannot be resolved without the aid of pulsed-field gel electrophoresis (PFGE). The two PFGE systems that have been applied to typing of *P. aeruginosa* are field-inversion gel electrophoresis (FIGE) and contour-clamped homogeneous electric field (CHEF). Both give comparable resolution but larger fragments (up to 2000 kb) are separated by the CHEF apparatus. Fingerprinting by CHEF analysis of DNA macrorestriction fragments (Figure 14.3) has been used successfully to trace *P. aeruginosa* strains in outbreaks in hospitals and the technique is more discriminatory than ribotyping or exotoxin A gene probe typing (Grundmann *et al.*, 1995). In the latter study 77 distinct CHEF patterns were identified among 81 geographically, temporally and epidemiologically unrelated strains of *P. aeruginosa*. The number of band differences allowed for the definition of distinguishable strains by PFGE is problematic but genomic similarity between 80% and 100% is accepted to denote related strains.

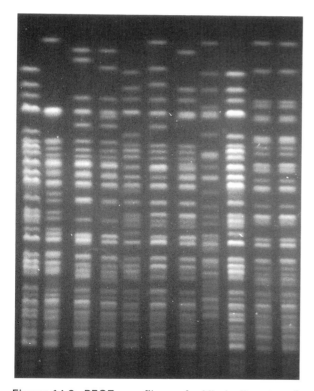

Figure 14.3. PFGE profiles of *XbaI* digests of chromosomal DNA of *P. aeruginosa* from a suspected outbreak of infection.

Gene probes

Stull *et al.* (1988) proposed that the method of indexing variation in rRNA of bacteria be termed ribotyping. Ribotyping has been applied to *P. aeruginosa* epidemiology and its discrimination is dependent on the restriction enzymes used. *PvuII* offers the highest discrimination but is less sensitive than PFGE in distinguishing between strains (Grundmann *et al.*, 1995).

Most *P. aeruginosa* strains possess the exotoxin A (ETA) structural gene. This gene and its variable upstream region, a 741 bp *PstI-NruI* fragment, can be used as a probe for species identification and as a strain marker (Grundmann *et al.*, 1995). The ETA gene and hypervariable region have been inserted into a plasmid, pCMtox, for strain typing and this offers the advantage of higher yield and sensitivity of the probe, and the identification of strains lacking the hypervariable region. Approximately 5% of strains of *P. aeruginosa* are not typeable by the ETA or pCMtox probe. An alternative gene probe for these, and other strains, is a pilin probe, a 1.2 kbp *Hind*III fragment containing the *P. aeruginosa* PAK pilin gene. However, the discriminatory power of this probe is poor and relatively broad strain groups are defined. A similar limitation applies to other gene probes proposed for the typing of the species, such as alginate and elastase genes which are too highly conserved to be useful for the differentiation of strains (Loutit and Tompkins, 1991).

Polymerase chain reaction (PCR)

PCR amplification of specific nucleic acid sequences has been applied to comparative typing of *P. aeruginosa* and both random primed (RAPD), or AP-PCR, and other more specific primers such as the enterobacterial repetitive intergenic consensus (ERIC-PCR) have been used. Both approaches appear to be almost as discriminatory as PFGE and are reasonably reproducible (Lau *et al.*, 1995). Since the PCR method is considerably less labour intensive and more economical, this may become the method of choice for the fingerprinting of strains in the specialist clinical laboratory.

Other methods

A number of other methods have been applied by individuals to the epidemiology of *P. aeruginosa*. They include multi-locus enzyme electrophoresis (MLEE), pyrolysis mass spectrometry (PyMS) and fatty acid analysis, among others. Of these, MLEE is worthy of further mention. In this technique the electrophoretic mobilities of multiple enzymes from isolates are compared. It is based on the concept that different molecular forms of the same enzyme, which may differ in net charge or amino acid sequence, will differ in electrophoretic mobility. This change in form of an enzyme reflects differences in nucleic acid sequence and is best applied to genetic analysis of bacterial population structures. It is a laborious technique and has not been systematically applied to *P. aeruginosa*, but the considerable diversity in the esterases may be worth studying.

ANTIBIOTIC RESISTANCE AND THERAPY

Compared with the Enterobacteriaceae, *P. aeruginosa* is relatively resistant to many antibiotics. However, there are a number of compounds with good to excellent activity against the species. They include the semisynthetic penicillins (e.g. ticarcillin), ureidopenicillins (piperacillin), carboxypenicillins (carbenicillin), third-generation cephalosporins (ceftazidime), carbapenems (imipenem), monobactams (aztreonam), aminoglycosides (gentamicin) and fluoroquinolones (ciprofloxacin). In order to attempt to reduce the emergence of resistant strains, an aminoglycoside is often combined with a β-lactam, third-generation cephalosporin, monobactam or carbapenem.

A recent survey of nearly 2000 isolates of *P. aeruginosa* from British hospitals showed that the great majority of isolates were sensitive to gentamicin, amikacin, azlocillin, ceftazidime, ciprofloxacin, imipenem and meropenem. Resistance was relatively uncommon, with the exception of isolates from patients in intensive care units (Chen *et al.*, 1995). In some parts of southern Europe, southeast Asia and South America, however, resistance rates may be as high as 50% for a number of the compounds listed above.

The mechanisms of resistance to antibiotics include (a) low cell wall permeability conferring intrinsic resistance; (b) the production of extracellular chromosomal and plasmid-mediated β-lactamases, aminoglycoidases and cephalosporinases; (c) an alteration in antibiotic-binding protein sites; and (d) an active efflux mechanism which pumps out antibiotic from the cell. The development of resistance to β-lactams *in vivo* during treatment is often the result of derepression of chromosomal β-lactamase expression. Some antibiotics, in particular cefoxitin, are potent inducers of these enzymes and may select out subpopulations resistant to other cephalosporins such as ceftazidime. Development of resistance during therapy with β-lactam antibiotics may also be due to the modification of the penicillin-binding proteins of *P. aeruginosa*.

The treatment of pulmonary infection in CF patients is a controversial issue. Some problems are intrinsic to the disease, such as the altered pharmacokinetics of antibiotics in these patients, in particular aminoglycosides and cephalosporins. Therefore increased doses of aminoglycosides are recommended. The treatment of acute exacerbations with anti-pseudomonal drugs is not always successful and eradication of *P. aeruginosa* from the sputum is rare. Some physicians favour early and aggressive treatment in order to avoid, or at least delay, establishment of chronic pulmonary infection. In Denmark, patients are admitted to hospital to receive intensive (intravenous and nebulized) therapy at regular intervals regardless of whether or not they are experiencing exacerbations. This approach is claimed to increase survival rates of patients dramatically, even after the onset of chronic infection.

The definition of antibiotic sensitivity or resistance for *P. aeruginosa* from CF is unclear as colonies from the same sputum may give a range of MIC values for different antibiotics. The value of testing discrete colonies versus testing of the mass of the bacterial growth has been increasingly debated. Recent data appear to favour testing multiple morphotypes together as an accurate and cost-effective approach. Nevertheless, the testing of individual morphotypes may be more accurate with resistant strains.

VACCINES

Pseudomonas aeruginosa expresses a number of antigenic surface structures and extracellular products, many of which have been investigated for their potential to induce protective antibodies. They include O polysaccharide, exotoxins A and S, elastase, alkaline protease, alginate, flagella, pili and outer membrane proteins.

The O polysaccharide is the serotype-specific moiety of the LPS of the organism and a limited number of serotypes account for the vast majority of clinical strains. The native LPS is poorly immunogenic and it is best bound to a carrier protein, such as exotoxin A or tetanus toxoid, to stimulate an antibody response in the subject. An alternative approach is the use of high-molecular-weight polysaccharide polymers from culture supernatants which are highly antigenic and free of the toxicity of native LPS.

A number of clinical trials with O polysaccharide-based vaccines have been reported (Cryz, 1994), and the results vary with the type and quality of the preparations. The first whole cell vaccines reduced mortality rates in burn patients when compared with controls but it was not until the heptavalent LPS vaccine, Pseudogen, that large-scale studies in different patient groups were undertaken. The vaccine gave little or no protection to cancer patients against *P. aeruginosa* and was also ineffective in intensive care patients and in cystic fibrosis. Another LPS-based vaccine, PEV-01, entered clinical trials and initial results in burn patients were promising, although this has been questioned on the grounds of poor study design (Cryz, 1994). An octavalent O polysaccharide–toxin A conjugate vaccine, Aerugen Berna, was shown to be safe in volunteers and patient groups and elicited functional anti-LPS and antitoxin A antibodies following immunization. The vaccine has been investigated in bone marrow transplant patients, shock/trauma patients and CF patients.

Native alginate is poorly immunogenic but both the high-molecular-weight polysaccharide moiety, or alginate combined with toxin A, elicit opsonizing antibodies in humans (Garner *et al.*, 1990). It has been shown that the larger the polymer size, the more immunogenic is the alginate vaccine. At a dose of 100 µg of alginate, long-lasting opsonic antibodies are formed in humans which enhance deposition of C3 onto mucoid cells and mediate killing of the challenge strain.

Alternative vaccines that have been proposed for immunization against *P. aeruginosa* include, among others, lectins derived from a strain of *P. aeruginosa*, a common protein antigen shared by *P. aeruginosa* and *Vibrio parahaemolyticus*, and genetically engineered mutants of *P. aeruginosa* which cannot survive at 36 °C.

Despite advances in our knowledge of the pathophysiology of the organism and improvements in diagnosis and treatment, the mortality of *P. aeruginosa* infections probably remains as high today as it was 30 years ago. Normal human serum contains *P. aeruginosa* specific antibody and in the past pools of normal IgG have proved successful for the reduction of septicaemia and mortality of burned patients infected with *P. aeruginosa*. There were therefore great expectations for passive immunotherapy with hyperimmune plasma; however, it was disappointing in clinical use. Many aspects of passive immunotherapy such as the prophylactic value of such preparations, the type of patients most amenable to treatment, the duration of treatment and the most reliable clinical indicators of therapy remain contentious (Cryz, 1994). Both murine and human monoclonal antibodies have been prepared against specific LPS and other antigens of *P. aeruginosa*, including toxin A, and have performed in animal challenge models with varying success (Saravolatz *et al.*, 1991).

OTHER 'PSEUDOMONADS'

Burkholderia cepacia

The species was first described by Burkholder as the agent of slippery skin in onions. Subsequent to this it became known as '*Pseudomonas multivorans*' and 'Pseudomonas kingii' but following the proposal of Palleroni and Holmes the epithet P. cepacia was adopted. However, in 1992, Yabuuchi and others proposed the transfer of seven species of rRNA homology group II, including P. cepacia, to a new genus, Burkholderia (Yabuuchi et al., 1992).

Burkholderia cepacia grows moderately well on nutrient agar at 25–30 °C, and most strains will grow, albeit slowly, at 41 °C but not at 42 °C, or 4 °C. Cultures on blood agar tend to die off after three or four days and survival on agar slants is poor. A variety of non-fluorescent pigments is produced by most strains and range from greyish-white or greenish-yellow to a deep melanin-like brown colour. The species does not produce gas from nitrate but reduces the latter to nitrite only. Other key biochemical reactions are failure to utilize arginine or starch, and formation of acid from galactitol but not from ethanol in ammonium salt-based media. Several selective and differential media have been described for the isolation of B. cepacia from mixed cultures. The most commonly used medium is commercially available and contains crystal violet, bile salts, ticarcillin and polymyxin.

Nosocomial infections

A common feature of infections in man with B. cepacia is the association of infusion of contaminated fluids. Numerous nosocomial outbreaks have been documented involving contamination of antiseptics, infusion fluids, tubing for irrigation and pressure-monitoring devices, but in general outbreaks are rare and can usually be curtailed by the recognition and removal of the source. Infections also tend not to be severe and systemic sepsis is uncommon. Patient-to-patient spread is unusual and prolonged carriage by individuals (with the exception of CF) has not been documented. However, an association between B. cepacia and chronic granulomatous disease has been reported (O'Neil et al., 1986).

Pathogenicity

In the natural plant host B. cepacia exerts its pathological effects through pectolytic enzymes and, in onions, the degree of rot correlates with polygalacturonase activity. Strains from human infections are apparently less pathogenic for plants than those from the natural environment. In animals, B. cepacia is relatively avirulent and lethal doses exceed 1×10^8 cfu/ml, unless the animal is compromised by burn or immunosuppression. Many cellular and extracellular products have been implicated as putative virulence factors and include adhesins, surface hydrophobicity, extracellular polysaccharide, ornithine amine lipids, proteases, lipases, haemolysin and siderophores (Nelson et al., 1994).

Cystic fibrosis

In the mid-1980s reports began to appear of the increased isolation of B. cepacia from CF patients in North American centres, and frequencies as high as 40% were recorded. In the UK the rate seldom exceeded 10% but there was general agreement that there was an increase in the number of patients infected or colonized by the organism. Ribotyping and PFGE typing suggest that B. cepacia is transmitted between patients both in and out of hospitals; however, some strains are more transmissible than others. Strains from the original outbreak in Toronto, Canada, were shown to express peritrichous, giant cable (Cb1)-like pili that bound to CF mucin and respiratory epithelia. This property was later shown by DNA sequencing of the cb1A pilin gene to be shared by isolates from a number of North American CF centres and the Edinburgh centre, and this was indicative of intercontinental spread of an epidemic clone (Sun et al., 1995).

It is not known from which primary environmental sources patients acquire B. cepacia, but contamination of their immediate environment by colonized patients may pose an infectious risk for non-colonized patients. Following acquisition of B. cepacia some patients may exhibit asymptomatic carriage or a gradual but accelerated decline in clinical status. However, a minority are characterized by a rapidly fatal fulminant septicaemia and it is this feature that has prompted various national CF authorities to issue guidelines to patients outlining the risks of different activities for the acquisition of the organism.

Typing methods

A number of typing methods have been described for *B. cepacia*. They include biotyping, serotyping of O and H antigens, bacteriocin production/sensitivity, plasmid profiling, chromosomal DNA analysis and multilocus enzyme electrophoresis (Wilkinson and Pitt, 1995). The methods vary in their discriminatory power, reproducibility and typeability, and therefore a combination of them is recommended. Ribotyping is the method of choice with the enzyme *Eco*RI, and further discrimination can be achieved by PFGE using *Xba*I or *Dra*I digestion.

Antibiotic sensitivity

Burkholderia cepacia has high intrinsic resistance to antimicrobials and is generally resistant to the antibiotics active against *P. aeruginosa*. Nearly all strains are resistant to the aminoglycosides, polymyxin, ticarcillin, azlocillin and imipenem, while variable sensitivity is shown to temocillin, aztreonam, ciprofloxacin and tetracycline. A recent study of isolates from 178 CF patients (Pitt *et al.*, 1996) found that the only agents active against more than two-thirds of the strains were ceftazidime, piperacillin, piperacillin/tazobactam and meropenem. Combinations of two, three or even four agents may show *in vitro* synergy against *B. cepacia*. Resistance to β-lactams is attributed both to β-lactamases and low cell wall permeability, and decreased expression of the major porins leads to elevated resistance to β-lactams and other antibiotics (Wilkinson and Pitt, 1995).

Burkholderia pseudomallei

Burkholderia pseudomallei is the causative agent of melioidosis, which is a glanders-like disease of man and animals. The species has been known by a number of names in the past and was for a long time classified among the genus *Pseudomonas*, but has now been transferred to *Burkholderia*

(Yabuuchi *et al.*, 1992). *Burkholderia pseudomallei* and *B. mallei* formed a distinct group within *Pseudomonas* RNA group II due to their phenotypic similarities, DNA–rRNA homologies, and high G + C molar%; the two species have 92–94% DNA–DNA homologies and identical 16S rRNA sequences.

The organism grows well on nutrient agar at an optimum temperature of 37 °C (range 15–43 °C). Colonial morphology is best observed after 48 hours at 37 °C although growth is visible after 24 hours. Colonies may be smooth and opaque or wrinkled; the latter is enhanced by glycerol. The growth has a characteristic musty odour, and on blood agar there may be weak haemolysis. Variation between rough and smooth colonial forms is frequent and purified colonies may not breed true on subculture. Cells exhibiting bipolar staining are apparently associated with the rough colonial form. The pigmentation of strains is dependent on the culture medium but on nutrient agar many isolates exhibit faint yellow to orange pigments, and others may have a pinkish hue.

Burkholderia pseudomallei is a strict aerobe, but in the presence of nitrates it can grow anaerobically due to the production of a nitrate reductase. It oxidizes glucose and breaks down arginine, and in ammonium salt-based media is dulcitol, lactose, maltose and mannitol positive. Most isolates can be reliably identified by conventional tests as well as in kit systems such as API 20NE which correctly identifies 97.5% of clinical isolates (Dance *et al.*, 1989b). The species is constitutively resistant to gentamicin and colistin, and the former antibiotic is in the selective medium of Ashdown. A latex agglutination test can be used to confirm the presence of the LPS antigen of *B. pseudomallei*, which is conserved throughout the species. *Burkholderia pseudomallei* may be misidentified as *B. mallei*, *B. cepacia*, *P. stutzeri* or *Flavobacterium* spp. *Burkholderia mallei* is not motile, and is arginine and nitrate negative.

Epidemiology

Burkholderia pseudomallei is a free-living saprophyte in soil and water in the areas where melioidosis is endemic between latitudes 20 °N and 20 °S in southeast Asia, particularly Thailand, Malaysia, Singapore and Vietnam, and parts of northern Australia. However, cases of melioidosis have been reported outside of these areas (Dance, 1990). The organism persists in soil during the dry season and spreads through the surface with the rains. Some early medical texts suggest that *B. pseudomallei* is spread by infected rodents but this has never been supported by bacteriological data.

The organism has been recovered from a wide variety of sources within endemic areas but the relationship between environmental contamination and the incidence of melioidosis is unclear. This may be due to lower numbers of *B. pseudomallei* in the soil in regions where the disease is less common. Furthermore, the species is able to survive well in conditions of nutrient depletion and this may be relevant to its persistence in the environment.

Infection is acquired through wounds and skin abrasions and by inhalation and rarely through ingestion. The organism may also enter the body through mucosal membranes of the eye and nose. Venereal spread of melioidosis has been described in humans, and intrauterine and mammary infection in goats. Early workers postulated that an insect vector was involved in the transmission of the organism, but this is now refuted.

Typing methods

Until recently, relatively few methods have been applied to the epidemiological type identification of *B. pseudomallei*. There is little, if any, serological heterogeneity that can be exploited for typing schemes. The immunodominant epitope of the outer membrane, LPS, is structurally and antigenically conserved, and there is minimal variation in outer membrane and cellular proteins. The flagella are antigenic but no H typing scheme has been described. A capsule-like exopolysaccharide has been identified and a monoclonal antibody to it was specific for other strains of *B. pseudomallei* and *B. mallei*.

Ribotyping was the first molecular typing method used for studies of the epidemiology of *B. pseudomallei*. Restriction fragment length poly-

morphism (RFLP) typing using *Eco*RI or *Bam*HI digests of chromosomal DNA probed with rRNA differentiates the species into a number of broad groups and unique type patterns, but the discrimination is inadequate for the definition of distinct strains due to the high frequency of two to three patterns. Ribotypes may be further differentiated by random amplified polymorphic DNA (RAPD) typing and PFGE of total chromosomal DNA digested with *Xba*I.

Pathogenesis and infection

Although a heat-labile lethal toxin has been identified in *B. pseudomallei* there is relatively little known about the pathogenic factors of the organism. Some evidence suggests that *B. pseudomallei* may survive intracellularly within macrophages but this has not been demonstrated unequivocally. All strains have endotoxin and the majority produce extracellular enzymes such as protease, lipase and haemolysins.

A survey in northeastern Thailand (Chaowagul *et al.*, 1989) found diabetes mellitus (32%) and renal disease (27%) to be the major predisposing factors in patients with melioidosis, with compromised immunity accounting for 11% of the remaining patients. In this region melioidosis is widespread and *B. pseudomallei* accounts for about one-fifth of cases and, at the time of the survey, 40% of deaths from community-acquired septicaemia. *Burkholderia pseudomallei* has a specific high-affinity binding site for human insulin and this feature may be related to the predisposing influence of diabetes mellitus for melioidosis.

Melioidosis varies greatly in clinical presentation (Dance, 1990). Patients may be asymptomatic but seropositive, or may have a fulminating rapidly fatal septicaemia. It may also present as a localized infection. A chronic state is established in some patients and relapse may occur after the apparent cure or remission of primary infection.

The definitive diagnosis of melioidosis is made by the isolation of *B. pseudomallei* from tissues or body fluids. In Gram-stained smears the organism may be present in only small numbers and bipolar staining may not be observed. An immuno-fluorescence antibody test, ELISA latex agglutination test and PCR have been used for rapid diagnosis. Serodiagnosis of melioidosis is based on the demonstration of a rising antibody titre to reference strains of *B. pseudomallei*. The indirect haemagglutination assay (IHA) is probably the most widely used but high background titres in non-infected patients from endemic areas reduce its effectiveness. IHA titres of 40–80 in non-infected adults in endemic areas are not unusual but titres of 640 or above are considered strongly indicative or diagnostic of the disease (Dance, 1990). ELISA tests for the detection of both specific IgG and IgM antibody to *B. pseudomallei* have been proposed, with claims of high specificity and sensitivity. The ELISA is comparable in performance with an IgG immuno-fluorescence assay and is more sensitive than the IHA test.

Antibiotic susceptibility and treatment

In general, *B. pseudomallei* is susceptible to imipenem, piperacillin, doxycycline, amoxycillin + clavulanic acid, azlocillin, ceftazidime, ticarcillin + clavulanic acid, ceftriaxone, cefotaxime, aztreonam and chloramphenicol. Aminoglycoside resistance is uniform, although 60% of strains may be sensitive to kanamycin. Sulphamethoxazole and trimethoprim sensitivity tests may be unreliable due to poorly defined endpoints (Dance *et al.*, 1989a). Cefotaxime and ceftriaxone are poorly active *in vivo*. Resistance to ampicillin is mediated by a clavulanate-susceptible β-lactamase, three different mechanisms of β-lactam resistance being identified in *B. pseudomallei* (Godfrey *et al.*, 1991).

The conventional treatment for melioidosis is chloramphenicol, doxycycline and trimethoprim–sulphamethoxazole, in combination. Ceftazidime with or without co-trimoxazole has been shown to halve the mortality of severe melioidosis compared with the conventional regimen, and is the drug of choice for severe infections. Prolonged courses of oral conventional therapy, or amoxycillin–clavulanic acid particularly for children and pregnant women, are recommended to prevent recurrent infection (White *et al.*, 1994).

Stenotrophomonas maltophilia

The work of Swings *et al.* placed strains of the species *Pseudomonas maltophilia* into the genus *Xanthomonas*. However, many strains of the former did not form the bright-yellow colonies of many *Xanthomonas* strains. A new genus was proposed by Palleroni and Bradbury (1993). *Stenotrophomonas* (a unit feeding on few substrates) *maltophilia* forms opaque grey-green yellowish colonies on nutrient agar at 37 °C, and often has a lavender hue on blood agar. It has several polar flagella and gives a variable weak oxidase reaction. Most strains require methionine for growth. Maltose, glucose and xylose are utilized in ammonium salt-based media and nitrate is reduced.

Stenotrophomonas maltophilia is widely distributed in the natural world and has been isolated from various environments (soil, water, milk). After *P. aeruginosa*, it is probably the most frequently isolated pseudomonad in the clinical laboratory. It is an occasional cause of bacteraemia, endocarditis and pneumonia, and has been recovered from a number of other disease states. Nevertheless, the clinical significance of *S. maltophilia* is unclear. Although it can cause severe and fatal infections, in a number of patients, particularly those with wound infections, infection is often trivial and self-limiting. However, mechanically ventilated patients receiving antimicrobials in the ITU and neutropenic patients are at increased risk of *S. maltophilia* infection/colonization. Contamination of monitoring equipment and hands of personnel contributes probably to its spread. The hospital sources from which the organism has been isolated include sinks, nebulizers, transducers, disinfectants, defrost water baths and ice-making machines.

Many typing methods have been applied to epidemiological studies of *S. maltophilia*. O serotyping is poorly discriminatory due to the disproportionate frequencies of three of the 31 types described (Schable *et al.*, 1992), and the technique has not been widely used. Other methods proposed for typing include protein profiles, bacteriocins and pyrolysis mass spectrometry. Ribotyping is highly discriminatory for the species, and PFGE is able to resolve genetically distinct strains. Arbitrarily primed PCR is slightly less discriminatory than PFGE, but offers the advantage of speed and less labour. Typing of isolates from apparent outbreaks usually reveals the presence of multiple strains, with small clusters of patients sharing the same strain. Indeed, the diversity of genotypes identified in *S. maltophilia* incidents argues against clonal spread of resistant hospital strains, and the marked genetic distance between strains may lead to further examination of the homogeneity of the species.

Stenotrophomonas maltophilia is resistant to imipenem due to the production of a zinc dependent carbapenemase which may explain in part its prevalence in intensive care and neutropenic patients. Most strains are sensitive to co-trimoxazole, doxycycline, minocycline, ticarcillin/clavulanic acid, cefotaxime and ceftazidime. Synergy, *in vitro*, has been observed for combinations of co-trimoxazole with a number of agents, including carbenicillin, rifampin and gentamicin (Felegie *et al.*, 1979). There may be significant differences in sensitivity test results of strains after incubation at different temperatures. Strains are more resistant to aminoglycosides at 30 °C and more sensitive to colistin at 37 °C. There is also considerable discrepancy between disc diffusion susceptibility values for strains and broth dilution MICs.

Miscellaneous Species

Pseudomonas fluorescens and *P. putida* are both fluorescent pseudomonads; both grow poorly at 37 °C and most strains will grow at 4 °C. This property contributes to the fact that these species, in particular *P. fluorescens*, are able to multiply in stored blood and blood products and may give rise to fatal reactions when injected intravenously due to the release of endotoxin. They are both of low pathogenicity for man but have been isolated from urine, faeces, sputum and occasionally the blood of immunosuppressed patients. Hospital outbreaks of infection are rare but *P. fluorescens* will often be recovered from hospital sites such as floors and sink traps, in environmental screens.

Burkholderia pickettii is a non-pigmented pseudomonad which grows well at 37 °C, and less so at 41 °C, and which does not attack arginine. It resembles *B. cepacia* biochemically and has been incorporated into the genus *Burkholderia* by Yabuuchi *et al.* (1992). The species is synonymous with the organism earlier described as *P. thomasii*. Most strains are resistant to aminoglycosides and colistin but are generally susceptible to chloramphenicol, co-trimoxazole and cephalosporins. *Burkholderia pickettii* is an occasional cause of infection in hospital patients and has been recovered from the ward environment as well as contaminated antiseptic and disinfectant solutions.

Pseudomonas stutzeri has a characteristic appearance on agar and colonies may grow 'rough', 'smooth' or intermediate even in pure cultures. The rough colonies may be confused with *B. pseudomallei*, and older cultures may appear light brown in colour. The species is actively denitrifying and large volumes of gas are produced in nitrate broth. Most strains will grow at 41 °C. *Pseudomonas stutzeri* has been widely reported from hospital-acquired infections but these are usually self-limiting. Isolates are sensitive to β-lactams, colistin and gentamicin.

Pseudomonas diminuta and *Pseudomonas vesicularis* are closely related species now placed in the genus *Brevundimonas*; they have specific growth requirements and grow slowly on nutrient agar. Both species are occasionally isolated from clinical material and are susceptible to anti-pseudomonal penicillins and aminoglycosides.

REFERENCES

Alcock, S.R. (1977) Acute otitis externa in divers working in the North Sea: a microbiological survey of seven saturation dives. *Journal of Hygiene (Cambridge)*, **78**, 395–409.

Ali, N.J., Kessel, D. and Miller, R.F. (1995) Bronchopulmonary infection with *Pseudomonas aeruginosa* in patients infected with human immunodeficiency virus. *Genitourinary Medicine*, **71**, 73–77.

Baltch, A.L. (1994) *Pseudomonas aeruginosa* bacteremia. In *Pseudomonas aeruginosa Infections and Treatment* (eds A.L. Baltch and R.P. Smith), pp. 73–128. Marcel Dekker, New York.

Barth, A.L. and Pitt, T.L. (1995) Auxotrophic variants of *Pseudomonas aeruginosa* are selected from prototrophic wild-type strains in respiratory infections in cystic fibrosis patients. *Journal of Clinical Microbiology*, **33**, 37–40.

Beck-Sagué, C.M., Banerjee, S.N. and Jarvis, W.R. (1994) Epidemiology and control of *Pseudomonas aeruginosa* in U.S. hospitals. In *Pseudomonas aeruginosa Infections and Treatment* (ed. A.L. Baltch and R.P. Smith), pp. 51–71. Marcel Dekker, New York.

Bergan, T. (1978) Phage typing of *Pseudomonas aeruginosa*. In *Methods in Microbiology*, Vol 10 (ed. T. Bergan and J. Norris), pp. 169–199. Academic Press, London.

Brown, M.R.W., Foster, J.H.S. and Clamp, J.R (1969) Composition of *Pseudomonas aeruginosa* slime. *Biochemical Journal*, **112**, 521–525.

Brumlik, M.J. and Storey, D.G. (1992) Zinc and iron regulate translation of the gene encoding *Pseudomonas aeruginosa* elastase. *Molecular Microbiology*, **6**, 337–344.

Chaowagul, W., White, N.J., Dance, D.A.B. *et al.* (1989) Melioidosis: a major cause of community-acquired septicemia in Northeastern Thailand. *Journal of Infectious Diseases*, **159**, 890–899.

Chen, H.Y., Yuan, M., Ibrahim-Elmagboul, I.B. and Livermore, D.M. (1995) National survey of susceptibility to antimicrobials amongst clinical isolates of *Pseudomonas aeruginosa*. *Journal of Antimicrobial Chemotherapy*, **35**, 521–534.

Cryz, S.J. (1994) Vaccines, immunoglobulins, and monoclonal antibodies for the prevention and treatment of *Pseudomonas aeruginosa* infections. In *Pseudomonas aeruginosa Infections and Treatment* (ed. A.L. Baltch and R.P. Smith), pp. 519–545. Marcel Dekker, New York.

Dance, D.A.B. (1990) Melioidosis. *Reviews in Medical Microbiology*, **1**, 143–150.

Dance, D.A.B., Wuthiekanun, V., Chaowagul, W. and White, N.J. (1989a) The antimicrobial susceptibility of *Pseudomonas pseudomallei*: emergence of resistance in vitro and during treatment. *Journal of Antimicrobial Chemotherapy*, **24**, 295–309.

Dance, D.A.B., Wuthiekanun, V., Naigowit, P. and White, N.J. (1989b) Identification of *Pseudomonas pseudomallei* in clinical practice: use of simple screening tests and API20NE. *Journal of Clinical Pathology*, **42**, 645–648.

Doggett, R.G. (1969) Incidence of mucoid *Pseudomonas aeruginosa* from clinical sources. *Applied Microbiology*, **18**, 936–937.

Felegie, T.P., Yu, V.L., Rumans, L.W. and Yee, R.B. (1979) Susceptibility of *Pseudomonas maltophilia* to antimicrobial agents, singly and in combination. *Antimicrobial Agents and Chemotherapy*, **16**, 833–837.

Fong, I.W. and Tomkins, K.B. (1985) Review of *Pseudomonas aeruginosa* meningitis with special emphasis on treatment with ceftazidime. *Reviews of Infectious Diseases*, **7**, 604–612.

Forkner, C.E. (1960) *Pseudomonas aeruginosa* infections *Modern Medical Monographs*, No. 22, pp. 1–5. Grune & Stratton, New York.

Fyfe, J.A.M., Harris, G. and J.R.W. Govan (1984) Revised pyocin typing method for *Pseudomonas aeruginosa*. *Journal of Clinical Microbiology*, **20**, 47–50.

Garner, C.V., Desjardins, D. and Pier, G.B. (1990) Immunogenic properties of *Pseudomonas aeruginosa* mucoid exopolysaccharide. *Infection and Immunity*, **58**, 1835–1842.

Godfrey, A.J., Wong, S., Dance, D.A.B. *et al.* (1991) *Pseudomonas pseudomallei* resistance to β-lactams. *Antimicrobial Agents and Chemotherapy*, **35**, 1635–1646.

Govan, J.R.W. (1978) Pyocin typing of *Pseudomonas aeruginosa*. In *Methods in Microbiology*, Vol. 10 (eds T. Bergan and J. Norris), pp. 61–91. Academic Press, London.

Govan, J.R.W. and Nelson J.W. (1992) Microbiology of lung infection in cystic fibrosis. *British Medical Bulletin*, **48**, 912–930.

Grimwood, K., To, M., Rabin, H.R. and Woods, D.E. (1988) Inhibition of *Pseudomonas aeruginosa* exoenzyme expression by subinhibitory antibiotic concentrations. *Antimicrobial Agents and Chemotherapy*, **33**, 41–47.

Grundmann, H., Schneider, C., Hartung, D. *et al.* (1995) Discriminatory power of three DNA-based typing techniques for *Pseudomonas aeruginosa*. *Journal of Clinical Microbiology*, **33**, 528–534.

Hancock, R.E.W., Mutharia, L.M., Chan, L. *et al* (1983) *Pseudomonas aeruginosa* isolates from cystic fibrosis: a class of serum sensitive, nontypable strains deficient in lipopolysaccharide O side chains. *Infection and Immunity*, **42**, 170–177.

Holder, I.A. (1977) Epidemiology of *Pseudomonas aeruginosa* in a burns hospital. In *Pseudomonas aeruginosa: Ecological Aspects and Patient Colonization* (ed. V.M. Young), pp. 77–95. Raven Press, New York.

Holmes, B. and Howard, B.J. (1993) Nonfermentative Gram-negative bacteria. In *Clinical and Pathogenic Microbiology*, 2nd edn (eds B.J. Howard, J.F. Keiser, T.F. Smith *et al.*), pp. 337–368. Mosby, St Louis.

Irvin, R.T., Govan, J.R.W., Fyfe, J.A.M and Costerton, J.W. (1981) Heterogeneity of antibiotic resistance in mucoid isolates of *Pseudomonas aeruginosa* obtained from cystic fibrosis patients: role of outer membrane proteins. *Antimicrobial Agents and Chemotherapy*, **19**, 956–1063.

Janda, J.M. and Bottone, E.J. (1981) *Pseudomonas*

aeruginosa enzyme profiling: predictor of invasiveness and as an epidemiological tool. *Journal of Clinical Microbiology*, **14**, 55–60.

King, E.O., Ward, M.K. and Raney, D.A. (1954) Two simple media for the demonstration of pyocyanin and fluorescein. *Journal of Laboratory and Clinical Medicine*, **44**, 301–307.

Kronborg, G., Fomsgaard, A., Galanos, G. *et al.* (1992) Antibody response to lipid A, core, and O-sugars of the *Pseudomonas aeruginosa* lipopolysaccharide in chronically infected cystic fibrosis patients. *Journal of Clinical Microbiology*, **30**, 1848–1855.

Kunin, C.M. (1994) Infections of the urinary tract due to *Pseudomonas aeruginosa*. In *Pseudomonas aeruginosa Infections and Treatment* (ed. A.L. Baltch and R.P. Smith), pp. 237–256. Marcel Dekker, New York.

Lam, M.Y.C., McGroarty, E.J., Kropinski, A.M. *et al.* (1989) Occurrence of a common lipopolysaccharide antigen in standard and clinical strains of *Pseudomonas aeruginosa*. *Journal of Clinical Microbiology*, **27**, 962–967.

Lau, Y.J., Liu, P.Y.F., Hu, B.S. *et al.* (1995) DNA fingerprinting of *Pseudomonas aeruginosa* serotype O11 by enterobacterial repetitive intergenic consensus polymerase chain reaction and pulsed-field gel electrophoresis. *Journal of Hospital Infection*, **31**, 61–66.

Levison, M.E. (1977) Factors influencing colonization of the gastrointestinal tract with *Pseudomonas aeruginosa*. In *Pseudomonas aeruginosa: Ecological Aspects and Patient Colonization* (ed. V.M. Young), pp. 97–109. Raven Press, New York.

Liu, P.V., Matsumoto, H., Kusama, H. and Bergan, T. (1983) Survey of heat-stable, major somatic antigens of *Pseudomonas aeruginosa*. *International Journal of Systematic Bacteriology*, **33**, 256–264.

Loutit, J.S. and Tompkins, L.C. (1991) Restriction enzyme and southern hybridization analysis of *Pseudomonas aeruginosa* strains from patients with cystic fibrosis. *Journal of Clinical Microbiology*, **29**, 2897–2900.

Lutz, F. (1979) Purification of a cytotoxin protein from *Pseudomonas aeruginosa*. *Toxicon*, **17**, 467–475.

Machan, Z., Taylor, G.W., Pitt, T.L. *et al.* (1992) 2-Heptyl-4-hydroxyquinolone *N*-oxide, an antistaphylococcal agent produced by *Pseudomonas aeruginosa*. *Journal of Antimicrobial Chemotherapy*, **30**, 615–623.

Mader, J.T., Vibhagool, A., Mader, J. and Calhoun, J.H. (1994) *Pseudomonas aeruginosa* bone and joint infections. In *Pseudomonas aeruginosa Infections and Treatment* (ed. A.L. Baltch and R.P. Smith), pp. 293–326. Marcel Dekker, New York.

Mahenthiralingam, E., Campbell, M.E. and Speert, D.P. (1994) Nonmotility and phagocytic resistance of *Pseudomonas aeruginosa* isolates from chronically colonized patient; with cystic fibrosis. *Infection and Immunity*, **62**, 596–405.

Mansi, A, Orsi, G.B., Tomao, P. *et al.* (1995) Virulence determinants in human and environmental *Pseudomonas aeruginosa* isolates from hospital wards. *Medical Microbiology Letters*, **4**, 238–246.

Nelson, J.W., Butler, S.L., Kreig, D. and Govan, J.R.W. (1994) Virulence factors of *Burkholderia cepacia*. *FEMS Immunology and Medical Microbiology*, **8**, 89–98.

Nicas, T.I. and Iglewski, B.H. (1986) Toxins and virulence factors of *Pseudomonas aeruginosa*. In *The Bacteria*, Vol. X (ed. T.I. Nicas and B.H Iglewski), pp. 195–213. Academic Press, New York.

O'Neil, K., Herman, J.H., Modlin, J.F. *et al.* (1986) *Pseudomonas cepacia*: an emerging pathogen in chronic granulomatous disease. *Journal of Pediatrics*, **108**, 940–942.

Palleroni, N.J. and Bradbury, J.F. (1993) *Stenotrophomonas*, a new bacterial genus for *Xanthomonas maltophilia* (Hugh 1980) Swings *et al.* 1983. *International Journal of Systematic Bacteriology*, **43**, 606–609.

Pedersen, S.S., Kharazami, A. Espersen, F. and Hoiby, N. (1990) *Pseudomonas aeruginosa* alginate in cystic fibrosis sputum and the inflammatory response. *Infection and Immunity*, **58**, 3363–3368.

Pier, G.B., Saunders, J.M, Ames, P. *et al.* (1987) Opsonophagocytic killing antibody to *Pseudomonas aeruginosa* mucoid exopolysaccharide in older non colonized patients with cystic fibrosis. *New England Journal of Medicine*, **317**, 793–798.

Pier, G.B., Meluleni, L. and Goldberg, J.B. (1995) Clearance of *Pseudomonas aeruginosa* from the murine gastrointestinal tract is effectively mediated by O-antigen specific circulating antibodies. *Infection and Immunity*, **63**, 2818–2825.

Pitt, T.L. (1988) Epidemiological typing of *Pseudomonas aeruginosa*. *European Journal of Clinical Microbiology and Infectious Diseases*, **7**, 238–247.

Pitt, T.L., Livermore, D.M, Pitcher, D. *et al.* (1989) Multiresistant serotype O12 *Pseudomonas aeruginosa*: evidence for a common strain in Europe. *Epidemiology and Infection*, **103**, 565–576.

Pitt, T.L., Kaufmann, M.E., Patel, P.S. *et al.* (1996) Type characterisation and antibiotic susceptibility of *Burkholderia (Pseudomonas) cepacia* isolates from patients with cystic fibrosis in the United Kingdom and the Republic of Ireland. *Journal of Medical Microbiology*, **44**, 203–210.

Poh, C.L., Yap, E.H., Tay, L. and Bergan, T. (1988) Plasmid profiles compared with serotyping and pyocin typing for the epidemiological surveillance of *Pseudomonas aeruginosa*. *Journal of Medical Microbiology*, **25**, 109–114.

Rhame, F.S. (1980) The ecology and epidemiology of *Pseudomonas aeruginosa*. In *Pseudomonas aeruginosa: The Organism, Diseases it Causes, and their Treatment* (ed. L.D. Sabath), pp. 31–51. Hans Huber, Bern.

Saravolatz, L.D., Markowitz, N., Collins, M.S. *et al.* (1991) Safety, pharmacokinetics, and functional activity of human anti-*Pseudomonas aeruginosa* monoclonal antibodies in septic and nonseptic patients. *Journal of Infectious Diseases*, **164**, 803–806.

Schable, B., Rhoden, D.L., Jarvis, W.R. and Miller, J.M. (1992) Prevalence of serotypes of *Xanthomonas maltophilia* from world-wide sources. *Epidemiology and Infection*, **108**, 337–341.

Schlech, W.F., Simonsen, N., Sumarah, R. and Martin, R.S. (1986) Nosocomial outbreak of *Pseudomonas aeruginosa* folliculitis associated with a physiotherapy pool. *Canadian Medical Association Journal*, **134**, 909–913.

Smith, R.P. (1994) Skin and soft tissue infections due to *Pseudomonas aeruginosa*. In *Pseudomonas aeruginosa Infections and Treatment* (ed. A.L. Baltch and R.P. Smith), pp. 327–369. Marcel Dekker, New York.

Speert, D.P., Farmer, S.W., Campbell, M.E. *et al.* (1990) Conversion of *Pseudomonas aeruginosa* to the phenotype characteristic of strains from patients with cystic fibrosis. *Journal of Clinical Microbiology*, **28**, 188–194.

Stoodley, B.J. and Thom, B.T. (1970) Observations on the intestinal carriage of *Pseudomonas aeruginosa*. *Journal of Medical Microbiology*, **3**, 367–375.

Stull, T.L., LiPuma, J.J. and Edlind, T.D. (1988) A broad-spectrum probe for molecular epidemiology of bacteria: ribosomal RNA. *Journal of Infectious Diseases*, **157**, 280–286.

Sun, L., Jiang, R.-Z., Steinbach, S. *et al.* (1995) The emergence of a highly transmissible lineage of cbl^+ *Pseudomonas (Burkholderia) cepacia* causing CF centre epidemics in North America and Britain. *Nature Medicine*, **1**, 661–666.

Tang, H., Kays, M. and Prince, A. (1995) Role of *Pseudomonas aeruginosa* pili in acute pulmonary infection. *Infection and Immunity*, **63**, 1278–1285.

Vasil, M.L. (1986) *Pseudomonas aeruginosa*: Biology, mechanisms of virulence, epidemiology. *Journal of Pediatrics*, **108**, 195–213.

Visca, P., Colotti, G., Serino, L. *et al.* (1992) Metal regulation of siderophore synthesis in *Pseudomonas aeruginosa* and functional effects of siderophore-metal complexes. *Applied Environmental Microbiology*, **58**, 2886–2893.

White, N.J. (1994) Melioidosis. *Zentralblatt für Bakteriologie*, **280**, 439–443.

Wick, M.J., Frank, D.W., Storey, D.J. and Iglewski, B.H. (1990) Identification of *reg*B, a gene required for optimal exotoxin A yields in *Pseudomonas aeruginosa*. *Molecular Microbiology*, **4**, 489–497.

Wilkinson, S.G. and Pitt, T.L. (1995) *Burkholderia (Pseudomonas) cepacia*: surface chemistry and typing methods: pathogenicity and resistance. *Reviews in Medical Microbiology*, **6**, 1–17.

Wilson, R., Pitt, T.L., Taylor, G. *et al.* (1987) Pyocyanin and 1-hydroxyphenazine produced by *Pseudomonas aeruginosa* inhibit the beating of human respiratory cilia *in vivo*. *Journal of Clinical Investigation*, **79**, 221–229.

Woods, D.E. and Vasil, M.L. (1994) Pathogenesis of *Pseudomonas aeruginosa* infections. In *Pseudomonas aeruginosa Infections and Treatments* (ed. A.L. Baltch and R.P. Smith), pp. 21–50. Marcel Dekker, New York.

Yabuuchi, E., Kosako, Y., Oyaizu, H. *et al.* (1992) Proposal of *Burkholderia* gen. nov. and transfer of seven species of the genus *Pseudomonas* homology group II to the new genus, with the type species *Burkholderia cepacia* (Palleroni and Holmes 1981) comb. nov. *Microbiology and Immunology*, **36**, 1251–1275.

Zloty, P. and Belin, M.W. (1994) Ocular infections caused by *Pseudomonas aeruginosa*. In *Pseudomonas aeruginosa Infections and Treatment* (ed. A.L. Baltch and R.P. Smith), pp. 371–399. Marcel Dekker, New York.

15

MISCELLANEOUS GRAM-NEGATIVE BACILLI

W. Frederiksen and W. Mannheim

INTRODUCTION

The species belonging to the genera covered in this chapter are Gram-negative bacilli and are more or less fastidious, often requiring special media for their isolation from clinical specimens and often needing special methods, only available at reference laboratories, for their identification.

DESCRIPTION

All the species considered here are Gram-negative bacilli; they vary in size from very small, short, coccoid, typical for *Pasteurella multocida* and *Francisella tularensis* to the long, slender, somewhat fusiform shape seen in *Capnocytophaga*. Most others may be called small bacilli (Table 15.1). Capsules are seen in *P. multocida* and *F. tularensis*. All lack flagella and do not show 'swimming' movement, but gliding motility is seen in *Capnocytophaga*. This movement is not always evident; it is dependent on age of the culture and on media. In one- to two-day-old cultures on horse blood agar plates with Difco's Bacto blood agar base No. 2 mobility is best demonstrated and seen in wet mounts among cells adhering to the cover-

slip or slide. Dancing and/or somersaulting is seen, and sometimes real gliding. It should be remembered that gliding may be seen directly in wet mounts from spinal fluids or blood cultures.

Taxonomy

The genus *Actinobacillus* contains a number of species with narrow host specificity; most of them are animal pathogens and not seen in man, but two, *A. ureae* and *A. hominis*, are human parasites and occur only in man. *A. actinomycetemcomitans* has been known as a human pathogen since the beginning of the century and was included with *Actinobacillus* for convenience. It does not belong to *Actinobacillus sensu stricto* and should be moved to a separate genus; it does not belong to *Haemophilus*.

The genus *Pasteurella* and especially *P. multocida* has been recognized as an important animal pathogen for many years and only relatively recently has it been recognized as a pathogen in man. In recent years, several newly named *Pasteurella* spp. have become known as 'animal bite wound' (dog, cat) organisms that may cause bite wound infection: *P. dagmatis*, *P. canis* and *P.*

TABLE 15.1 SOME USEFUL FEATURES OF THE TAXA CONSIDERED

	Related to animal contact	Requirement for CO_2 on prim. isolation	Slow growth	Need for NaCl	Cell morphology	Cell organization
Pasteurella						
multocida	+	−	−	−	Coccoid	
canis	+	−	−	−	Small bacilli	
stomatis	+	−	−	−	Small bacilli	
taxon 16	+	−	−	−	Small bacilli	
dagmatis	+	−	−	−	Small bacilli	
aerogenes	+	−	−	−	Small bacilli	
bettyae	−	−	−	−	Small bacilli	
Actinobacillus						
ureae	−	−	−	−	Pleomorph	'Morse code'[a]
hominis	−	−	−	−	Pleomorph	'Morse code'[a]
actinomycetemcomitans	−	+	+	−	Small bacilli	Stars[b]
Haemophilus aphrophilus	−	+	+	−	Small bacilli	Stars[b]
Cardiobacterium	−	+	+	−	Pleomorph	Stars[c]
Eikenella	−	+	+	−	Small bacilli	
Capnocytophaga						
ochracea	−	+	+	−	Fusiform	Gliding
canimorsus	+	+	+	−	Fusiform	Gliding
Francisella						
tularensis	+	−	+	−	Coccoid	
philomiragia	?	−	+	+	Small bacilli	Protoplasts

[a] On Gram strain, actinobacilli appear as morse code-like small chains.
[b] Star-like or 'flower-like' structures are seen in old colonies.
[c] Star-like structures can be seen in wet mounts and in Gram-stained smear.

stomatis (Eiscande and Lion, 1993) '*P.*' taxon 16 of Bisgaard and Mutters (1986) is similar to *P. stomatis* and of similar importance (Eckert *et al.*, 1991) but has no closer genetic affinity to the genus *Pasteurella*.

Several other *Actinobacillus* and *Pasteurella* spp. have occasionally been isolated from man, e.g. from horse bite wounds (*A. lignieresii*, *P. caballi*) or from sputum (*A. lignieresii*). They will not be detailed further, but it should be stressed

that the diagnosis of unusual isolates should be confirmed by a reference laboratory.

The need for V-factor (NAD) has been considered a trait only of the genus *Haemophilus*; this can no longer be sustained, as there are both *Actinobacillus* and *Pasteurella* spp. that require NAD, e.g. *A. pleuropneumoniae* (Pohl *et al.*, 1983) and *P. volantium*, and even strains of *P. multocida* that require NAD have been described (Krause *et al.*, 1987; Mutters *et al.*, 1989). For the purpose of human clinical bacteriology it may still be argued that NAD-requiring strains could be considered to be *Haemophilus*.

The genus *Capnocytophaga* contains species that were known to be difficult to handle and called dysgonic fermenters (DF). Some were considered to be anaerobic and/or carbon dioxide requiring e.g. '*Bacteroides ochraceus*'. A special feature – gliding motility – that may be difficult to demonstrate, seems to reflect their real nature, as the genus *Cytophaga* seems to be the closest relative.

Eikenella corrodens was once combined with *Bacteroides urealyticus* as *Bacteroides corrodens*. Both play a role in synergistic infection arising from the human mouth but should be considered separately.

The genus *Francisella* seems to occur among lagomorphs and rodents and is occasionally transmitted to man in different ways, causing disease; it has caused serious disease in North America, whereas varieties occurring in Eurasia cause more benign diseases. The newly recognized *F. philomiragia* (Hollis *et al.*, 1989) was first considered a *Yersinia*.

The taxonomy of these groups has been hampered by a general lack of definite descriptions because many early investigators neglected the need for good media and thorough characterization of isolated strains. However, extensive characterization with phenotypical methods, along with DNA–DNA hybridization (Mutters *et al.*, 1985), DNA–rRNA hybridization (De Ley *et al.* 1990) and 16S rRNA sequencing (Dewhirst *et al.* 1993) of many strains has led to a classification that is now widely accepted.

The Appendix illustrates the taxonomic affiliations of the organisms mentioned.

HABITAT

Actinobacillus

Actinobacillus actinomycetemcomitans is found in the human mouth, chiefly on the teeth, dental plaque and in the gingival pocket. It can be found also in similar sites in macaque and cynomolgus monkeys, but such strains are probably unrelated

to strains from man (Guthmiller *et al.*, 1993). *Actinobacillus ureae* and *A. hominis* have been isolated only from man. There is no information as to the occurrence in healthy persons, but the presence in the upper respiratory tract of man must be assumed.

Pasteurella

Pasteurella multocida may occur in many different animal species, especially mammals, but also in birds. Occurence in the upper respiratory tract is common in some animals, e.g. dogs and cats, and assumed in many others.

Pasteurella canis, *P. stomatis*, *P. dagmatis* and '*P*'. taxon 16 are normal inhabitants of the mouth and upper respiratory tract of dogs and cats (Ganiere *et al.*, 1993).

Pasteurella aerogenes is known to occur in the pig intestine, but must be assumed to belong also in the mouth of swine, as it is a 'pig bite wound' organism. *Pasteurella bettyae*, known to occur only in man, is isolated mainly from the genital tract. Its occurrence in healthy men and women has not been reported.

Cardiobacterium, Eikenella

Cardiobacterium hominis occurs in the mouth of healthy persons and is probably part of the normal mucosal microflora.

Eikenella corrodens is found in the composite flora of dental plaque and gingival pockets but is probably part of the normal mucosal flora in the human mouth. Similar organisms may be isolated from animals, but it is not known if they really are *E. corrodens*.

Capnocytophaga

Capnocytophaga ochracea belongs to the microflora of human gingival pockets. *Capnocytophaga canimorsus* (and *C. cynodegmi*) are assumed in a similar way to belong to the mouth and dental flora of dogs and maybe cats, as they are transferred to man by bites of dogs and sometimes cats.

Francisella tularensis

Francisella tularensis occurs mainly in rodents and lagomorphs; it may cause devastating disease among these animals, that constitutes an animal reservoir. It can also survive in insect and other arthropod vectors and in running water. The habitat of *F. philomiragia* may be salt water (Wenger *et al.*, 1989).

PATHOGENICITY

Several of the organisms considered in this chapter become pathogenic when they are introduced into tissue through (animal) bites. This applies to several *Pasteurella* spp.: *P. canis*, *P. stomatis*, *P. dagmatis*, '*P*'. taxon 16, and sometimes *Eikenella corrodens*. They have a low potential to invade and to cause generalized infections. Some of the organisms from the human mouth, can become part of a synergistic infection called actinomycosis; this applies to *Actinobacillus actinomycetemcomitans* and *E. corrodens*. The production of toxins that affect leucocytes and probably tissue seems to confer an *A. actinomycetemcomitans* and *C. ochracea* a causal role in the process leading to periodontitis. The pathogenic properties that enable *C. canimorsus* to establish severe generalized infection when introduced through bite wounds are unknown. *Pasteurella multocida* may produce a toxin that is bone destroying and the main cause of atrophic rhinitis in pigs. Toxin-producing strains can be isolated also from man (Donnio *et al.*, 1991), but the role of the toxin is unknown. The capsule that is often found on strains of *P. multocida* is probably of great significance in many severe generalized infections in animals. Its role in human infection is less obvious. Some of the organisms residing in the mouth and on the teeth will enter the blood regularly and sometimes initiate endocarditis, if they are able to adhere to the endocardium. This applies to *A. actinomycetemcomitans* (and *Haemophilus aphrophilus*) and *C. hominis*. The pathogenicity of *F. tularensis* is based on its capsule and its capacity for intracellular growth.

EPIDEMIOLOGY

The majority of the organisms considered here can be divided into human parasites and agents transferred from animals to man, i.e. causing zoonoses.

They are not involved in major disease outbreaks in man; there is no tendency to spread from man to man. It must be assumed that *Pasteurella multocida* can be transferred from animal to man via the airborne route, as *P. multocida* respiratory tract infection in man is seen mainly among the farming population. It seems probable that pigs with atrophic rhinitis may transmit *P. multocida* to their carers. It is not known if atrophic rhinitis may be transferred to pigs from people harbouring toxin-producing *P. multocida* in their airways. Such interactions could be elucidated because epidemiological tools such as biotyping, phage-typing, ribotyping etc. are at hand.

Francisella tularensis can be transmitted from animals to man in a number of ways: by directly handling diseased animals (airborne or direct contact); through biting insects and other arthropods that have fed on ill animals; airborne through dust that contains animal excreta or faeces (hay harvest, sugar-beet harvest); and water-borne, from still or running water contaminated with excreta from diseased animals. This capacity to infect with rather small inocula makes *F. tularensis* one of the organisms renowned to produce laboratory-acquired infections (e.g. a number of Edward Francis's coworkers acquired tularaemia in the lab).

There are probably no sharp geographical limitations to the occurrence of most of the organisms; *P. multocida* airway infections may be connected to the rearing of pigs.

Francisella tularensis occurs only in the Northern Hemisphere, but in two varieties; both occur in North America, but in Europe and Asia in a form producing a less severe disease, *Francisella tularensis* does not seem to occur in Denmark or in the UK.

CLINICAL FEATURES

Among local infections, infected bite wounds dominate. *Pasteurella multocida* has been considered the main culprit, but with improved diagnostic abilities *P. canis*, *P. stomatis*, *P. dagmatis* and '*P*'. taxon 16 are recognized with increasing frequency in wounds inflicted by dogs and cats (Escande and Lion, 1993).

Dog bites occur very often all over the world; it is assumed that only one-tenth of the wounds become infected; cat bites are less common, but relatively more become infected. Cat bites are often more penetrating, but in both instances lesions of underlying structures like bones and joints, tendons and nerves may lead to protracted and sometimes invalidating illness.

Much less common are infected pig bite wounds from which *Pasteurella aerogenes* can be isolated (Lester *et al.*, 1993), and bites inflicted by the big cats (lions, tigers etc.), from which organisms similar to but not identical with recognized *Pasteurella* spp. have been isolated.

From human bite wounds, especially so-called 'clenched fist injuries', *Eikenella corrodens* has been isolated. Such bite wound infections are no less severe than most animal bite wound infections.

The synergistic infection, often called 'actinomycosis', is a pathological process from which *Actinomyces* spp. and one or more 'accompanying' organisms can be isolated. *Actinobacillus actinomycetemcomitans*, *Haemophilus aphrophilus* and *Eikenella corrodens* are commonly found, but other mouth or dental organisms may be found also. Such infections occur mainly in the head and neck region and are related to poor dental hygiene. Infections may also be mediastinal or pleuropulmonary, and sometimes provoked by foreign bodies like dental fragments or tooth picks.

The destructive process of peridontitis is probably multifactorial, but the ability of *Actinobacillus actinomycetemcomitans* and *Capnocytophaga ochracea* to produce toxins that affect leucocytes and other cells is no doubt a contributory factor. Chronic respiratory tract disease may be more or less acutely complicated by bronchopulmonary infection from which *Pasteurella multocida*, *A. ureae* and *A. hominis* may be isolated. The causal role of these organisms in the pathological process

is as confused as that seen with pneumococci and haemophili.

Generalized infections with *Pasteurella* spp. are rare; two to three cases a year of *P. multocida* septicaemia are reported in the UK; they occur mainly in patients with underlying disease, e.g. malignancy or cirrhosis of the liver. Similar cases have been reported especially from France; mortality is high.

Septicaemia with *Capnocytophaga ochracea* is seen mainly in immunocompromised patients. Such infections often run a benign course even if not treated optimally with antibiotics (Bremmelgaard *et al.*, 1986). Chorioamnionitis may be a feature of generalized *Capnocytophaga* infection (Iralu *et al.*, 1993).

The related organism *Capnocytophaga canimorsus* (formerly DF$_2$) is often involved in life-threatening infections arising from dog bites or 'dog exposure' and sometimes from cat bites. The infection may run a fatal course with the same fulminant picture as meningococcal septicaemia, dominated by disseminated intravascular coagulation (Kullberg *et al.*, 1991). About five cases a year of *C. canimorsus* septicaemia are seen now in Denmark. Cases in children are very rare.

Central nervous system infections in the form of meningitis are rarely seen, but both *Pasteurella multocida* and *Actinobacillus ureae* may cause meningitis.

Endocarditis is seen mainly with organisms that enter the bloodstream from the gingiva or teeth and are able to adhere to the cardiac endothelium. *Actinobacillus actinomycetemcomitans* and *Haemophilus aphrophilus* fulfil these criteria; they adhere to glass and show mural colonies and granular growth. It can be assumed that this adhesive capacity is a major reason for their well-known ability to cause endocarditis. They are both also among the main organisms isolated from brain abscesses. Even though the two organisms should be regarded as separate, and can readily be differentiated in the laboratory and may belong to separate genera, they share so many features of habitat, pathogenicity, and phenotypical characteristics in the lab that they should be treated in common. *Eikenella corrodens* shares a number of features with the aforementioned, but is much less commonly seen in endocarditis. *Cardiobacterium hominis* is known only because it can cause endocarditis, although rarely (Wormser and Bottone, 1983).

Francisella tularensis when introduced through an insect bite or other skin lesion will cause a local infection which ulcerates, and a regional lymphadenitis that may suppurate and will show a characteristic granulomatous histological picture. When introduced by the oral or respiratory route, it may cause a feverish disease with pneumonia or possibly a septicaemic disease with no obvious focus.

Francisella philomiragia has been isolated from blood and other body fluids from patients with a fever and pneumonia (Wenger *et al.*, 1989).

DIAGNOSTIC METHODS

Specimens

From open wounds (bite lesions etc.) specimens should be taken with care to avoid contamination with the normal flora of skin and mucous membranes. From closed lesions and lymph nodes, material is best obtained with needle and syringe, perforating normal skin (or mucous membrane) after disinfection. Careful sampling and examination of sputum samples should be undertaken. There is usually no value in examining the mouth or dental flora of patients or biting animals, unless one is prepared to do detailed comparisons between isolates from a pathological process and from the biting animal.

Septicaemia and meningitis should be diagnosed with cultures of blood and spinal fluid in the usual way. Tularaemia suspicion should be confirmed histologically and immunologically and usually not from specimens for culture. No special rules for transport and storage of specimens are needed; Stuart's transport medium can often be used, and stored in a refrigerator, when needed.

In the laboratory, examination of specimens should proceed according to good laboratory practice; in most instances direct microscopy of wet mounts or stained smears will not be diagnostic, but it should be remembered that *Capnocytophaga canimorsus* may be seen directly in spinal fluids and in a smear of periferal blood (Pedersen *et al.*, 1993), and diagnosed via its gliding motility.

Isolation

Blood and/or chocolate agar plates incubated in a moist atmosphere with 5–10% carbon dioxide will support the growth of most of these organisms, colonies appearing after 24–48 hours. One problem is to establish the presence of *Capnocytophaga canimorsus*, which can be grown in most blood cultures systems, but will often not grow on plate media when subcultured from a positive blood bottle. Blood agar plates incubated anaerobically are the best means to secure growth; blood or chocolate agar plates with added cysteine may be useful.

There is no need for selective media, except when studying the possible role played by certain organisms as part of a normal flora.

Growth Requirements

As the majority of these taxa are parasites of warm-blooded animals they grow optimally at 35–37 °C; they grow poorly or not at all at 20–22 °C. Most of these organisms are facultatively anaerobic, but enhanced growth and bigger colonies may be seen when grown aerobically; some may grow best at slightly reduced oxygen tension. *Francisella tularensis* is strictly aerobic.

A moist atmosphere with 5–10% carbon dioxide is recommended for most of the organisms. Carbon dioxide is required for growth of *Actinobacillus actinomycetemcomitans* and *Cardiobacterium hominis*; *Capnocytophaga* has been considered carbon dioxide requiring, but laboratory-adapted cultures are not. Enriched media like blood agar and chocolate agar are suitable for isolation and cultivation of most of the species considered, but *Capnocytophaga* spp. are more exacting, especially *C. canimorsus*, which needs cysteine added to most media. This can be done by placing a disk/strip, incorporating 1% cysteine, on an inoculated plate.

Francisella tularensis will grow best on freshly prepared rabbit blood agar or Columbia sheep blood agar, but usually grows on chocolate agar. However, isolation or cultivation of *F. tularensis* should only be attempted under circumstances where the risk of laboratory infection is contained, i.e. category 3 laboratories, and where the clinical need for a culture is deemed relevant.

The groups considered here have no need for NAD, and usually do not show symbiotic growth; they may, however, grow in symbiosis on non-enriched media with the addition of staphylococci which provide growth-enhancing factors (e.g. pyridoxine or thiamine). Symbiotic growth is typically shown by *Cardiobacterium hominis* and strains of *C. canimorsus* on infusion agar plates.

Actinobacillus actinomycetemcomitans and *Cardiobacterium hominis* need two to three days to produce colonies that are >1 mm. Most organisms produce colonies with no special features, but *Eikenella corrodens* and *Capnocytophaga ochracea* typically corrode the agar, producing colonies punched out in the agar. *Eikenella* colonies seldom reach a size of >1 mm. *Capnocytophaga* colonies may produce a peculiar hue, which together with the corroding and spreading growth and a smell of bitter almond may be diagnostic of *C. ochracea* (Heltberg *et al.*, 1984; Kristiansen *et al.*, 1984). *Capnocytophaga ochracea* has a yellowish pigment that on addition of 15% KOH turns violet.

Eikenella corrodens produces a strong and distinctive smell ('*Haemophilus*-like') which together with corrosion is almost diagnostic. It should be remembered that not all *Eikenella* cultures/colonies will corrode the agar. The indole-positive *Pasteurella* spp. produce a characteristic smell of indole.

A number of these organisms survive only for short periods in plates on shelves or in refrigerators; plates should be kept in jars or bags in the incubator.

Identification

In order to characterize further many of these bacteria, it is important to use media of good quality and to use sufficient inoculum of a living culture. For a number of tests a method with a high sensitivity is mandatory, this applies to tests for indole, urease, NO_3 and NO_2 reduction.

For the purpose of identifying *Pasteurella* and *Actinobacillus*, good fermentation media with bromothymol blue as indicator can be used. A suitable selection of carbohydrate media should be combined with a number of other tests (see Table 15.2), among which indole, urease and ONPG (*O*-nitrophenyl-β-*D*-glalactopyranoside) are cardinal. The Kovacs oxidase test is not reliable for characterization in this area, as strains may turn out positive or negative depending on the medium on which they are grown. The catalase test is useful, as certain taxa are characteristically negative (see Table 15.2). A number of commercial kits have been marketed for use in this area. There are reasons to predict that these rather fastidious organisms may not perform well in certain kits, and several examples are known. However, rapid tests in miniaturized form may well turn out to be suited to characterize fastidious organisms grown on media that support good growth. No such well-tested systems have been published to our knowledge.

Most mucoid strains of *Pasteurella multocida* belong to Carter's serogroup A and produce hyaluronic acid capsules for which a decapsulation test (small colonies around *Staphylococcus aureus* on moist blood agar surfaces) is a good diagnostic tool. In situations where organisms are found in unusual or unexpected situations, or when rare organisms are found, it is advisable to make use of reference laboratories and/or reference cultures. Too many 'interesting observations' are published from less reliable sources.

Capnocytophaga

For the characterization of *Capnocytophaga* ordinary fermentation media are not suitable. Fermentation of carbohydrates is best seen in serum-enriched fermentation media (Brenner *et al.*, 1989). Tests for preformed enzymes can be done 'in house' or with commercial systems using heavy inocula prepared from growth on suitable media (see Table 15.3).

TABLE 15.2   IDENTIFICATION TABLE FOR *PASTEURELLA AND ACTINOBACILLUS*

	Porphyrin	PGUA (β-glucuronidase)	Urease	ONPG (β-galactosidase)	CAMP	Haemolysis	Indole	Nitrate reduction	Nitrite reduction	Lysine decarboxylase	Ornithine decarboxylase	Catalase	Gelatinase	l-Arabinose	d-Xylose	l-Rhamnose	d-Glucose	d-Galactose	d-Mannose	Sucrose	Lactose	Maltose	Cellobiose	Trehalose	Melibiose	Adonitol	Dulcitol	d-Sorbitol	d-Mannitol	Inositol	Salicin	Aesculin	Gas glucose
P. multocida, spp. *multocida*	+	d-	o	d	o	o	+	+	o	o	+	+	o	d	+	o	+	+	+	+	d	d	o	d	o	o	o	+	+	o	o	o	o
P. multocida, septica	+	o	o	o	o	o	+	+	o	o	+	+	o	o	+	o	+	+	+	+	o	d	o	o	o	o	o	o	+	o	o	o	o
P. multocida, gallicida	+	o	o	o	o	o	+	+	o	o	+	+	o	d	+	o	+	+	+	+	o	o	o	d	o	o	o	+	+	o	o	o	o
P. canis 1	+	o	o	o	o	o	+	+	o	o	+	+	o	o	o	o	+	+	+	+	o	o	o	+	o	o	o	o	o	o	o	o	o
P. stomatis	+	o	o	o	o	o	+	+	o	o	+	+	o	o	o	o	+	+	+	+	o	o	o	+	o	o	o	o	o	o	o	o	o
Taxon 16	+	o	+	(+)	o	o	+	+	o	xp	o	+	xp	o	o	o	+	+	+	+	o	+	o	+	o	o	o	o	o	x	o	o	o
P. dagmatis	(+)	o	+	o	o	o	+	+	o	o	o	+	o	o	o	o	+	+	+	+	o	+	o	+	o	o	o	o	o	x	o	o	d+
P. pneumotropica Jawetz	+	o	+	+	o	o	+	+	o	o	+	+	o	o	o	o	+	+	+	+	x	+	o	+	+	o	o	o	o	x	o	o	o
P. pneumotropica Heyl	+	o	+	+	o	o	+	+	o	o	+	+	o	+	+	o	+	+	o	+	x	+	o	o	o	o	o	o	+	x	o	o	o
P. haemolytica	+	d-	o	d	+	+	o	+	d	o	o	+	o	o	+	o	+	+	o	+	d	+	o	+	+	o	o	+	+	x	+	+	o
P. trehalosi	+	o	o	o	+	+	o	+	o	o	o	+	o	o	+	o	+	+	+	+	o	+	+	+	o	o	o	+	+	o	+	+	o
P. bettyae	+	o	o	o	o	o	+	+	d	o	o	o	o	o	o	o	+	o	o	o	o	o	o	o	o	o	o	o	o	o	o	o	+
P. aerogenes	+	o	+	+	o	o	o	+	+	o	d+	+	o	d+	d+	d-	+	+	+	+	x	+	o	+	o	o	o	o	o	d+	o	o	+
A. ureae	+	o	+	o	o	o	o	+	+	o	o	(+)	o	o	o	o	+	o	+	+	o	+	o	o	o	o	o	o	+	o	o	o	o
A. hominis	+	o	+	+	o	o	o	+	+	o	o	+	o	o	+	o	+	o	o	+	x	+	o	+	+	o	o	o	+	o	o	o	o
A. equuli	+	o	+	+	o	o	o	+	+	o	o	d	d	+	+	o	+	+	+	+	+	+	o	o	+	o	o	o	+	o	o	o	o
A. lignieresii	+	o	+	+	o	o	o	+	+	o	o	o	o	o	+	o	+	+	o	+	x	+	o	o	o	o	o	o	+	o	o	o	o
A. pleuropneumoniae	+	o	+	+	+	+	o	+	+	o	o	d	o	o	+	o	+	o	o	+	x	+	+	o	o	o	o	o	+	o	+	+	o
A. capsulatus	+	o	+	+	o	o	o	+	+	o	o	d	o	+	+	o	+	+	+	+	x	+	o	+	+	o	o	+	+	o	o	o	o
A. suis	+	o	+	+	o	+	o	+	+	o	o	o	o	+	+	o	+	+	+	+	+	+	+	+	+	o	o	o	o	o	+	+	o
A. actinomycetemcomitans	+	o	o	o	o	o	o	+	+	o	o	+	o	o	d	o	+	+	d	o	o	o	o	o	o	o	o	o	d+	o	o	o	+
Haemophilus aphrophilus	(+)	o	o	+	o	o	o	+	+	o	o	o	o	o	o	o	+	+	+	+	+	+	o	+	+	o	o	o	o	o	o	o	+

+, >90% of strains positive within 3 days; -, >90% of strains negative within 3 days; d+, majority of strains positive; d-, majority of strains negative; (+), weak reaction; x, late reaction (>3 days).

For some taxa results are based on rather few strains.

TABLE 15.3 IDENTIFICATION TABLE FOR *CARDIOBACTERIUM*, *SUTTONELLA*, EF 4 A, *EIKENELLA* AND *CAPNOCYTOPHAGA*

	Oxidase, Kovacs	Catalase	Urease	ONPG (β-glucuronidase)	Haemolysis	Indole	NO₃ reduction	NO₂ reduction	Lysine decarboxylase	Ornithine decarboxylase	Arginine dihydrolase	Gelatinase	l-Arabinose	d-Xylose	l-Rhamnose	d-Glucose	d-Galactose	d-Mannose	Sucrose	Lactose	Maltose	Cellobiose	Trehalose	Melibiose	Adonitol	Dulcitol	d-Sorbitol	d-Mannitol	Inositol	Salicin	Aesculin hydrolysis	Gas glucose
																				Acid from												
Cardiobacterium hominis	+	0	0	0	0	+	0	+	0	0	0	0	0	0	0	+	0	+	+	0	+	0	0	0	0	0	+	+	0	0	0	0
Suttonella indologenes	+	0	0	0	0	+	0	+	0	0	0	0	0	0	0	+	0	+	+	0	+	0	0	0	0	0	0	0	0	0	0	0
EF 4 a	+	+	0	0	0	0	+	+	0	0	+	d	0	0	0	+	0	0	0	0	0	0	0	0	0	0	0	0	0	0	0	0
Eikenella corrodens	+	0	0	0	0	0	+		d+	+	0	d	0	0	0	0	0	0	0	0	0	0	0	0	0	0	0	0	0	0	0	0
Capnocytophaga																																
C. ochracea	0	0	d−	+	0	0	0	0	0	0	0	d	0	0	d+	+	d+		+	+	+	d	0	0	0	0	0	0	0	0	+	0
C. canimorsus	+	+	0	+	0	0	0	d+	0	0	+	d	0	0	d+	+	d+		0	+	+	+	0	+	0	0	0	0	0	0	d+	0
C. cynodegmi	+	+	0	+	0	0	d−	d+	0	0	0	0	+	+	+	+	d+		+	+	+	+	0	+	0	0	0	0	0	0	+	0
DF 3	0	0	0	0	0	d+	0	0	0	0	0	0	0	+	+	+	+		+	+	+	0	0	0	0	0	0	0	0	0	+	0
Francisella philomiragia	+	(+)	0			0			0	0	0	d+		0		dx			dx	0	dx							0				0

+, >90% of strains positive within 3 days; −, >90% of strains negative within 3 days; d−, majority of strains negative within 3 days; d+, majority of strains positive; (+), weak reaction; x, late reaction (>3 days).
For some taxa results are based on rather few strains.

The differentiation between *Capnocytophaga ochracea*, *C. sputigena* and *C. gingivalis* is often not possible (Speck *et al.*, 1987), and the name *C. ochracea* has been used in this text for all three.

Capnocytophaga canimorsus and *C. cynodegmi* are very similar to each other, and sucrose fermentation seems to be the only test to separate them. However, *C. cynodegmi* is very rarely, if ever, invasive but it may be isolated from dog bite wounds. *Francisella philomiragia* is less fastidious than *F. tularensis*; however, on media without NaCl it will grow not at all (Hollis *et al.*, 1989) or as protoplasts only.

Antimicrobial Susceptibility

For a number of the organisms considered, antimicrobial susceptibility can be determined by standard methods. For *Capnocytophaga*, enriched media and extended incubation time are needed, making evaluation of agar diffusion test results difficult (Bremmelgaard *et al.*, 1989). It is our experience that diffusion tests may be performed on enriched chocolate agar incubated in a moist carbon dioxide atmosphere for two or more days, but breakpoints must be adjusted, precluding routine use of this method. However, a rather uniform susceptibility pattern has been found by several investigators; the different *Capnocytophaga* spp. are susceptible to penicillin G and to ampicillin, third-generation cephalosporins and imipenem, as well as to several quinolones (but not to nalidixic acid) and to erythromycin and clindamycin. They are usually resistant to aztreonam, trimethoprim, colistin, metronidazole and to the aminoglycosides. Strains that produce β-lactamase appear to be rare, although six out of 19 strains recently reported from Canada were β-lactamase producing (Roscoe *et al.*, 1992).

Among *Actinobacillus* and *Pasteurella* susceptibility to penicillin and ampicillin is the rule, although *A. actinomycetemcomitans* and *P. aerogenes* have MIC values about 1 μg/ml. *Pasteurella* strains that produce β-lactamase have often been reported from domestic animals, but are only exceptionally seen in man. Susceptibility to a wide range of antibiotics is the rule, but usually erythromycin is not very active

and all species are clindamycin resistant; also the aminoglycosides give MIC values that preclude treatment with these agents alone. *Eikenella corrodens* is susceptible to a wide range of antibiotics, including β-lactams and quinolones (Goldstein *et al.*, 1986); its susceptibility to penicillin G is, however, intermediate, with MIC values of 1–4 μg/ml, and it is resistant to clindamycin; β-lactamase-producing strains have been described.

Cardiobacterium hominis is highly susceptible to most antibiotics (Miller *et al.*, 1991), including β-lactams and aminoglycosides; quinolones have not been studied systematically; clindamycin resistance has been reported, but not β-lactamase production. *Francisella tularensis* (Scheel *et al.*, 1993) and *F. philomiragia* (Hollis *et al.*, 1989) are resistant to most β-lactam antibiotics, but sensitive to aminoglycosides, tetracycline and chloramphenicol; quinolones seem to offer the lowest MIC values.

MANAGEMENT

For bite wound infections, local treatment including surgery is important. In many cases this will need to be supported by antibiotic treatment, and penicillin G is the drug of choice, with third-generation cephalosporins as alternatives. Early intervention may prevent damage and late sequelae of bones, joints and tendons. Antibiotic treatment in chronic respiratory tract infection is controversial; if considered necessary, penicillin G or ampicillin are drugs of choice for *Pasteurella* and *Actinobacillus*. Septicaemias and meningitis caused by *Actinobacillus*, *Pasteurella* and *Capnocytophaga* should be treated with penicillin G (or ampicillin) in high doses for one to two weeks. Endocarditis caused by *A. actinomycetemcomitans*, *Haemophilus aphrophilus* or *Cardiobacterium* should be treated with ampicillin in high dosage for an extended period, possibly in combination with an aminoglycoside for one to two weeks. Third-generation cephalosporins are second drugs of choice for all these generalized infections. MIC determinations may be indicated, especially in case of endocarditis.

Septicaemias caused by *Capnocytophaga canimorsus* with the threat of disseminated intravascular coagulation should be managed in the same way as meningococcal septicemia, as the clinical situation is exactly the same. Infections with *Francisella* (tularaemia) are usually treated with streptomycin or an other aminoglycoside; tetracyclines and chloramphenicol have been used, but relapses are seen. The quinolones seem to provide good alternatives to streptomycin.

PREVENTION AND CONTROL

Prevention of bite injuries is probably not realistic; many wounds do not become infected, so a general antibiotic prophylaxis is not indicated. However, it seems advisable to give antibiotics prophylactically to splenectomized or immunocompromised persons who are bitten by dogs, cats or other animals, and penicillin G is the drug of choice. Dental and oral hygiene is considered of importance in prevention of endocarditis in patients prone to this. Whether antibiotic prophylaxis as recommended around dental surgery etc. to patients at risk of endocarditis will prevent endocarditis with organisms considered here is not known.

There are no vaccines available as preventive measures against *Pasteurella* infections in man, although several vaccines are used to prevent infection among domestic animals.

APPENDIX: TAXONOMIC AFFILIATION OF THE ORGANISMS CONSIDERED

Proteobacteria subclass	Superfamily of De Ley	Family, genus
Gamma	I	Pasteurellaceae Pohl 1981 *Pasteurella* *Actinobacillus* *Haemophilus*
Gamma	Below I–II	Cardiobacteriaceae Dewhirst *et al.* 1991 *Cardiobacterium* *Suttonella* *Dichelobacter*
Beta	III	Neisseriaceae Prévot 1933 *Neisseria* *Kingella* *Simonsiella* *Eikenella*
	Below I–II	*Francisella*
–	V	*Flavobacterium– Cytophaga* complex *Cytophaga* *Capnocytophaga* *Flavobacterium*

REFERENCES

Bisgaard, M. and Mutters, R. (1986) Characterization of some previously unclassified *Pasteurella* spp. obtained from the oral cavity of dogs and cats and description of a new species tentatively classified with the family Pasteurellaceae Pohl 1981 and provisionally called taxon 16. *Acta Pathologica Microbiologica et Immunologica Scandinavica B*, **94**, 177–184.

Bremmelgaard, A., Kristiansen, J.E., Pers, C. *et al.* (1986) Eight cases of *Capnocytophaga* infections in Denmark. *European Journal of Clinical Microbiology*, **5**, 355–358.

Bremmelgaard, A., Pers, C., Kristiansen, J.E. *et al.* (1989) Susceptibility testing of Danish isolates of *Capnocytophaga* and CDC group DF-2 bacteria. *Acta Pathologica Microbiologica et Immunologica Scandinavica*, **97**, 43–48.

Brenner, D.J., Hollis, D.G., Fanning, G.R. *et al.* (1989) *Capnocytophaga canimorsus* sp. nov. (formerly CDC group DF-2), a cause of septicemia following dog bite, and *C. cynodegmi* sp. nov., a cause of localized wound infection following dog bite. *Journal of Clinical Microbiology*, **27**, 231–235.

De Ley, J., Mannheim, W., Mutters, R. *et al.* (1990) Inter- and intrafamilial similarities of rRNA cistrons of the Pasteurellaceae. *International Journal of Systematic Bacteriology*, **40**, 126–137.

Dewhirst, F.E., Paster, B.J., Olsen, I. *et al.* (1993) Phylogeny of the Pasteurellaceae as determined by comparison of 16S ribosomal ribonucleic acid sequences. *Zentralblatt für Bakteriologie*, **279**, 35–44.

Donnio, P.Y., Avril, J.L., Andre, P.M. *et al.* (1991) Dermonecrotic toxin production by strains of *Pasteurella multocida* isolated from man. *Journal of Medical Microbiology*, **34**, 333–337.

Eckert, F., Stenzel, A., Mutters, R. *et al.* (1991) Some unusual members of the family Pasteurellaceae isolated from human sources: phenotypic features and genomic relationships. *Zentralblatt für Bakteriologie*, **275**, 143–155.

Escande, F. and Lion, C. (1993) Epidemiology of human infections by *Pasteurella* and related groups in France. *Zentralblatt für Bakteriologie*, **279**, 131–139.

Ganiere, J.P., Escande, F., Andre, G. *et al.* (1993) Characterization of *Pasteurella* from gingival scrapings of dogs and cats. *Comparative Immunology, Microbiology and Infectious Diseases*, **16**, 77–85.

Goldstein, E.J.C., Citron, C.M., Vagvolgyi, A.E. *et al.* (1986) Susceptibility of *Eikenella corrodens* to newer and older quinolones. *Antimicrobial Agents and Chemotherapy*, **30**, 172–173.

Guthmiller, J.M., Kolodrubetz, D. and Kraig E. (1993) A panel of probes detects DNA polymorphisms in human and non-human primate isolates of a periodontal pathogen, *Actinobacillus actinomycetemcomitans*. *Microbial Pathogenesis*, **14**, 103–115.

Heltberg, O., Busk, H.E., Bremmelgaard, A. *et al.* (1984) The cultivation and rapid enzyme identification of DF-2. *European Journal of Clinical Microbiology*, **3**, 241–243.

Hollis, D.G., Weaver, R.E., Steigerwalt, A.G. *et al.* (1989) *Francisella philomiragia* comb. nov. (Formerly *Yersinia philomiragia*) and *Francisella tularensis* biogroup novicida (formerly *Francisella novicida*) associated with human disease. *Journal of Clinical Microbiology*, **27**, 1601–1608.

Iralu, J.V., Roberts, D. and Kazanjian, P.H. (1993) Chorioamnionitis caused by *Capnocytophaga*: case report and review. *Clinical Infectious Diseases*, **17**, 457–461.

Krause, T., Bertschinger, H.U., Corboz, L. *et al.* (1987) V-factor dependent strains of *Pasteurella multocida* supsp. *multocida*. *Zentralblatt für Bakteriologie und Hygiene*, A **266** 255–260.

Kristiansen, J.E., Bremmelgaard, A., Busk, H.E. *et al.* (1984) Rapid identification of *Capnocytophaga* isolated from septicemic patients. *European Journal of Clinical Microbiology*, **3**, 236–240.

Kullberg, B.J., Westendorp, R.G.J., Van't Wout, J.W. *et al.* (1991) Purpura fulminans and symmetrical peripheral gangrene caused by *Capnocytophaga canimorsus* (formerly DF-2) septicemia: a complication of dog bite. *Medicine*, **70**, 287–292.

Lester, A., Gerner-Smidt, P., Gahrn-Hansen, B. *et al.* (1993) Phenotypical characters and ribotyping of *Pasteurella aerogenes* from different sources. *Zentralblatt für Bakteriologie*, **279**, 75–82.

Miller, M.A., Mockler, D.F., Hinshaw, R.R. *et al.* (1991) Characterization of *Cardiobacterium hominis*: antibiotic susceptibility, morphological variations, plasmid and membrane analysis. *Current Microbiology*, **23**, 197–205.

Mutters, R., Ihm, P., Pohl, S. *et al.* (1985) Reclassification of the genus *Pasteurella* Trevisan 1887 on the basis of deoxyribonucleic acid homology, with proposals for the new species *Pasteurella dagmatis*, *Pasteurella canis*, *Pasteurella stomatis*, *Pasteurella anatis*, and *Pasteurella langaa*. *International Journal of Systematic Bacteriology*, **35**, 309–322.

Mutters, R., Mannheim, W. and Bisgaard, M. (1989) Taxonomy of the group. In *Pasteurella and Pasteurellosis* (ed. C. Adlam and J.M. Rutter), pp. 3–34. Academic Press, London.

Pedersen, G., Schønheyder, H.C. and Nielsen, L.C. (1993) *Capnocytophaga canimorsus* bacteraemia demonstrated by a positive peripheral blood smear. *Acta Pathologica Microbiologica et Immunologica Scandinavica*, **101**, 572–574.

Pohl, S., Bertschinger, H.U., Frederiksen, W. *et al.* (1983) Transfer of *Haemophilus pleuropneumoniae* and the *Pasteurella haemolytica*-like organism causing porcine necrotic pleuropneumonia to the genus *Actinobacillus* (*Actinobacillus pleuropneumoniae* comb. nov.) on the basis of phenotypic and deoxyribonucleic acid relatedness. *International Journal of Systematic Bacteriology*, **33**, 510–514.

Roscoe, D.L., Zemcov, S.J.V., Thornber, D. *et al.* (1992) Antimicrobial susceptibilities and β-lactamase characterization of *Capnocytophaga* species. *Antimicrobial Agents and Chemotherapy*, **36**, 2197–2200.

Scheel, O., Hoel, T., Sandvik, T. *et al.* (1993) Susceptibility pattern of Scandinavian *Francisella tularensis* isolates with regard to oral and parenteral antimicrobial agents. *Acta Pathologica Microbiologica et Immunologica Scandinavica*, **101**, 33–36.

Speck, H., Kroppenstedt, R.M. and Mannheim, W. (1987) Genomic relationships and species differentiation in the genus *Capnocytophaga*. *Zentralblatt für Bakteriologie und Hygiene A*, **266**, 390–402.

Wenger, J.D., Hollis, D.G., Weaver, R.E. *et al.* (1989) Infection caused by *Francisella philomiragia* (formerly *Yersinia philomiragia*): a newly recognized human pathogen. *Annals of Internal Medicine*, **110**, 888–892.

Wormser, G.P. and Bottone, E.J. (1983) *Cardiobacterium hominis*: review of microbiologic and clinical features. *Reviews of Infectious Diseases*, **5**, 680–691.

SUPPLEMENTARY READING

Bottone, E.J. (ed.) (1983) *Unusual Microorganisms: Gram-negative Fastidious Species*. Marcel Dekker, New York.

(a) Goldstein E.J.C and Gombert, M.E. *Eikenella corrodens*: a new perspective. pp. 1–43.

(b) Forlenza, S. and Newman, M.G. *Capnocytophaga*. pp. 45–66.

(c) Wormser, G.R. and Bottone, E.J. *Cardiobacterium hominis*: review of microbiological and clinical features. pp. 67–86.

Frederiksen, W. (1989) Pasteurellosis of man. In *Pasteurella and Pasteurellosis* (ed. C. Adlan and J.M. Rutter), pp. 303–320. Academic Press, London.

Frederiksen, W. (1993) Ecology and significance of Pasteurellaceae in man: an update. *Zentralblatt für Bakteriologie*, **279**, 27–34.

Kaplan, A.H., Weber, D.J., Oddone, E.Z. *et al.* (1989) Infection due to *Actinobacillus actinomycetem-comitans*: 15 cases and review. *Reviews of Infectious Diseases*, **11**, 46–63.

Kilian, M., Frederiksen, W. and Biberstein, E.L. (eds) (1981) *Haemophilus, Pasteurella* and *Actinobacillus*. Academic Press, London.

Pers, C., Gahrn-Hansen, B. and Frederiksen, W. (1996) *Capnocytophaga canimorsus* in Denmark 1982–1995. A review of 39 cases. *Clinical Infectious Diseases*, **23**, 71–75.

Zambon, J.J. (1985) *Actinobacillus actinomycetem-comitans* in human periodontal disease. *Journal of Clinical Periodontology*, **12**, 1–20.

16

AEROMONAS AND *PLESIOMONAS*

S.E. Millership

INTRODUCTION

Although both genera are at present included within the Vibrionaceae, recent molecular evidence suggests that aeromonads should be in their own family, the Aeromonadaceae, and the plesiomonads within the Enterobacteriaceae (Martinez-Murcia *et al.*, 1992).

DESCRIPTION OF THE ORGANISM

Definition

Members of both genera are Gram-negative straight rods. The aeromonads if motile usually have a single polar flagellum, whereas the plesiomonads have several polar flagella. Both genera are oxidase- and catalase-positive facultative anaerobes. The aeromonads break down carbohydrates with the production of acid or acid and gas, the plesiomonads produce acid only. The optimum temperature of growth for aeromonads is usually quoted as 22–28 °C. Some strains will grow at 5 °C, although others are killed at this temperature. The maximum growth temperature is 40–44 °C. Most isolates of clinical significance will grow readily at 37 °C. Plesiomonads grow between 8 and 40–44 °C, with an optimum of 30–37 °C. The pH range of aeromonads is 5.5–9.0, whereas for plesiomonads it is 5–7.7. Neither genus is salt requiring, and growth is inhibited in 6% salt broth.

Plesiomonas Taxonomy

The name *Plesiomonas* was proposed by Habs and Schubert in 1962 (Schubert, 1984), although such isolates were recognized as a separate group in 1947 when Ferguson and Henderson described strain 'C27'. The C27 organisms were initially assigned to the Enterobacteriaceae. They were then placed in the genus *Pseudomonas* as '*Pseudomonas shigelloides*', and later transferred to *Aeromonas* as *Aeromonas shigelloides* and finally given their own genus *Plesiomonas*. Only one species has been described so far: *Plesiomonas shigelloides*. The species epithet relates to the minority of strains which share a common O antigen with *Shigella sonnei*.

Aeromonas Taxonomy

The genus *Aeromonas* was proposed by Kluvyer and van Neil in 1936 (Popoff, 1984). The taxonomy of the species within *Aeromonas* is unfortunately much more complex. The literature is confused because the same name has been

Principles and Practice of Clinical Bacteriology. Edited by A.M. Emmerson, P.M. Hawkey and S.H. Gillespie

applied to different groups of strains at various times. Thus *A. hydrophila* has variously meant all the mesophilic, motile strains as distinct from psychrophilic non-motile strains known as *A. salmonicida*; mesophilic strains with subspecies *anaerogenes* and *hydrophila* (now usually known as the phenotypes *A. hydrophila* and *A. caviae*) as distinct from *A. sobria*; and most recently hybridization group 1 strains only.

Phenotypic classification

The basis of the taxonomic divisions generally accepted today was a numerical study by Popoff and Veron in 1976. These authors divided the mesophilic, generally motile strains into two main groups known as *A. hydrophila* with subspecies *hydrophila* and *anaerogenes* and *A. sobria*. These are now usually known as *A. hydrophila*, *A. caviae* and *A. sobria* respectively. Psychrophilic, non-motile strains are called *A. salmonicida*. Their preference for growth temperatures below 37 °C means that they are unusual in clinical practice. These divisions, often called phenotypes, may still be the most useful ones for clinical laboratories. Biochemical distinction is relatively simple and there is good correlation between phenotype and production of certain toxins which may be related to pathogenicity, as discussed below. Recently two further distinct phenotypes, *A. veronii* (Hickman-Brenner *et al.*, 1987) and *A. schubertii* (Hickman-Brenner *et al.*, 1988), have been described but are

unusual in clinical practice. Table 16.1 lists readily available tests useful in the discrimination of these phenotypes. Some highly discriminatory tests, such as growth in KCN and elastase production, require reagents which are difficult to obtain or handle and have therefore been omitted.

DNA hybridization

DNA hybridization studies suggest that each of the phenotypes above has more than one genomic species, of which 12 have been described so far. Furthermore phenotypes and genotypes do not completely correspond. An example of this growing confusion is hybridization group 3 which has been named *A. salmonicida* (Janda, 1991). This has two subspecies: one with the psychrophilic, non-motile strains sometimes producing a brown water-soluble pigment of phenotype *A. salmonicida*, and the other mesophilic strains of phenotype *A. hydrophila*. The latter may be distinguished from other strains of this phenotype by the production of acid from sorbitol. It is therefore important to establish exactly what is meant by the term *A. salmonicida*; particular confusion can arise when commercial kits incorporating tests not usually recognized in the differentiation of this species are used.

A similar problem of non-correlation of phenotype with genomic species exists for hybridization groups 8 and 10 (Hickman-Brenner *et al.*, 1987; Janda, 1991). Although described independently and with very different phenotypes they are gene-

TABLE 16.1 TESTS TO DISTINGUISH THE PHENOTYPES OF MESOPHILIC *AEROMONAS* STRAINS

Phenotype	A. caviae	A. hydrophila	A. sobria	A. veronii	A. schubertii
β-Haemolysis	−	+	+	*	*
Lactose fermenter on MacConkey agar	d	−	−	*	*
Moeller's lysine	−	+	+	+	+
Moeller's ornithine	−	−	−	+	−
Aesculin	+	+	−	+	−
Gas from glucose	−	+	+	+	−
Salicin fermentation	+	+	−	+	−
Arabinose fermentation	+	+	−	−	−
Voges–Proskauer	−	+	+	+	d
Gluconate oxidation	−	+	d	*	*

+, typically positive; −, typically negative; d, variable; *, not recorded. Data from Hickman-Brenner *et al.* (1987, 1988); Janda (1991); Barer *et al.* (1986).

tically identical. The rules of taxonomic nomenclature mean that the species name is *A. veronii*. The much better-known species epithet *sobria* is now used to describe a biotype: thus *A. veronii* biotype *sobria*.

Some progress has been made towards biochemical differentiation of genomic species (Abbott *et al.*, 1992; Altwegg *et al.*, 1990). However, very limited numbers of characters, including those in commercial kits, have been used to distinguish some species and the reliability of such differentiation remains to be confirmed. Differentiation of all the known groups using only conventional biochemical tests has been claimed on the basis of an analysis of 133 strains (Abbott *et al.*, 1992), but less than 10 isolates from six of the 12 hybridization groups were examined. Table 16.2 lists the genomic species together with the corresponding phenotype and any readily available biochemical tests proposed for differentiation of genomic species within a phenotype.

A further difficulty is that the correlation between phenotype and hybridization group may

not be as good as is often suggested. One study showed that eight of 26 isolates of phenotype *A. hydrophila* were in fact group 8, not 1–3 as would be expected (Kuijper *et al.*, 1989).

So far most reported clinical studies have used the names of *Aeromonas* spp. in their phenotypic sense. Surveys of mainly faecal isolates support this; 85% of human isolates are represented by only three hybridization groups (HGs). These are HG 1 (phenotype *A. hydrophila*); 4 (*A. caviae*); and 8 (*A. sobria*). Therefore in the rest of this chapter mesophilic *Aeromonas* spp. will be named according to phenotypes *hydrophila*, *caviae*, *sobria*, *veronii* and *schubertii*. The term *A. salmonicida* will be reserved for psychrophilic, non-motile strains.

PATHOGENICITY

Aeromonas

Determination of the factors responsible for human disease has been hampered by lack of

TABLE 16.2   RELATIONSHIP OF GENOTYPE TO PHENOTYPE AMONG *AEROMONAS* SPECIES

Phenospecies	HG	Genospecies	Proposed tests to discriminate genotypes within the phenotype				
			Rham	Sorb	Lact		
Hydrophila	1	hydrophila	d	–	d		
Hydrophila	2	unnamed	d	–	–		
Hydrophila	3	salmonicida	–	d	+		
Salmonicida	3	salmonicida		psychrophilic			
			Cit	Gly	Gas		
Caviae	4	caviae	+	d	–		
Caviae	5	media	+	+	–		
Caviae	6	eucrenophila	–	–	+		
			Amp	Arg	VP	Mann	Suc
Sobria	7	sobria	–	–	–	+	+
Sobria	8/10	veronii	–	+	+	+	+
Sobria	9	jandaei	–	+	+	+	–
Sobria	13	trota	+	+	–	d	d
				Arg	VP		
Veronii	8/10	veronii		–	+		
Veronii	11	veronii		+	–		
Schubertii	12	schubertii					

Rham, D-rhamnose; Sorb, D-sorbitol; Lact, lactose; Cit, citrate; Gly, glycerol; Gas, gas from glucose; Amp, sensitivity to ampicillin; Arg, arginine dihydrolase; VP, Voges–Proskauer; Mann, mannitol; Suc, sucrose.
+, typically positive; –, typically negative; d, variable.
Data from Janda (1991); Abbott *et al.* (1992); Kuijper *et al.* (1989).

suitable animal models. Most animal data suggests that *A. hydrophila* and *A. sobria* are pathogenic whereas *A. caviae* is not. In fish and mice *A. hydrophila* and *A. sobria* are usually more virulent than *A. caviae* although there is considerable strain variation. The 'suicide phenomenon' (Namdari and Bottone, 1988), where strains lose viability in 0.5% glucose broth, has also been associated with enteropathogenicity and virulence in mesophilic strains. However, with one possible exception – the S-layer of *A. salmonicida* – no one factor appears responsible for strain variation in pathogenicity (see below).

Surface array protein

In *A. salmonicida* autoagglutinating strains have a single surface array protein of about 50 kDa (S-layer) (Kay *et al.*, 1981). Spontaneous loss of this layer results in 1000- to 10 000-fold increases in the lethal dose for fish. The layer confers surface hydrophobicity, resistance to complement-mediated lysis and enhances association with phagocytic monocytes. Some strains with S-layers have now been identified among human isolates of *A. hydrophila* (HG 1) and *A. sobria* (HG 8), usually from cases of bacteraemia and meninigitis (Kokka *et al.*, 1991). However, this layer is rather different from that of *A. salmonicida*. Although the overall amino acid composition is similar the molecular weight of the protein is 52–58 kDa and sequence analysis shows no homology at the amino termini. Its properties are also different in that there is no change in surface hydrophobicity and it does not preferentially absorb Congo red, unlike the *A. salmonicida* layer.

Fimbriae

In a strain of *A. hydrophila* two types of fimbriae were described: straight, and curved or flexible (Ho *et al.*, 1990). Straight fimbriae do not have any haemagglutinating activity although sequencing of the first 55 amino acids at the N terminus indicates homology with *Escherichia coli* type I fimbriae. Flexible fimbriae have a molecular weight of only 4000 and are maximally expressed at 22 °C in broth under reduced iron conditions. They agglutinate human type O, guinea-pig, sheep, horse and chicken erythrocytes in the presence of divalent cations maximally at 4 °C.

Agglutination is not inhibited by fucose, mannose or galactose. It was suggested that the latter may be colonization factors whose production is stimulated by exposure to environmental conditions although there is no direct evidence for this.

Lipopolysaccharide

Three major types of lipopolysaccharide (LPS) have been described (Shaw and Hodder, 1978), depending on the oligosaccharide present in the core region. Subsequent taxonomic studies indicated that most chemotype I were HG 2; chemotype II were heterogeneous with a majority of *A. caviae* phenotypes but also the type strain of *A. hydrophila* (HG 1); and chemotype III were *A. sobria* phenotypes. In serogroup 011 (Kokka *et al.*, 1991) strains there is an unusual LPS side-chain structure which appears on sodium dodecyl sulphate–polyacrylamide gel electrophoresis as a small number of silver-staining bands, rather than the ladder pattern more usually seen. This appears to anchor the S-layer possessed by these strains. The strains are usually of the *A. hydrophila* or *A. sobria* phenotype and cause severe invasive disease in humans and animals.

Outer membrane proteins

The outer membrane proteins (OMPs) of certain groups of isolates have been examined (Janda, 1991). *Aeromonas hydrophila* and *A. sobria* strains have heterogeneous profiles, whereas those of *A. caviae* and *A. salmonicida* are more consistent. Iron restriction resulted in the synthesis of new OMPs in *A. hydrophila* and *A. salmonicida* in one study.

Siderophores

Almost all strains of *Aeromonas* so far examined produce siderophores, which in other Gram-negative genera have been associated with the establishment of infection. Among the mesophilic strains, *A. hydrophila* and *A. caviae* and some *A. sobria* produce a new siderophore called amonabactin (Barghouthi *et al.*, 1989), which enhances growth in iron-deficient media.

Complement resistance

Both psychrophilic and mesophilic strains may be resistant to complement-mediated lysis of human, rabbit or fish serum (Janda, 1991). Among mesophiles *A. hydrophila* and *A. sobria* strains are more resistant than *A. caviae*. Serum resistance in one study was associated with a group of aeromonads most virulent in trout (Mittal *et al.*, 1980).

Invasive potential

Attempts at determination of invasive potential have been hampered by the production of the haemolysin (see below) which kills tissue culture cells. However, several studies have suggested that some strains are invasive for HEp-2 cells, and that invasion is strain dependent (Gray *et al.*, 1990). Invasion seems to be associated with *A. hydrophila* and *A. sobria* strains.

Toxins

Much research has concentrated on the extracellular factors produced by the aeromonads, particularly in relation to gastrointestinal disease. In a genus belonging to the Vibrionaceae it would seem reasonable to search for a toxin similar to cholera toxin as a virulence factor in acute gastroenteritis. Since 1974, when accumulation of fluid in rabbit ileal loops caused by strains of *Aeromonas* was described, there have been numerous publications on possible enterotoxins. Multiple extracellular activities can be detected in cultures of mesophilic strains with degradation of complex protein, polysaccharide and lipid-containing molecules. The physiological function of most of these is not known. However, four or five different proteases, two major classes of haemolysin and a

cytotonic enterotoxin have all been postulated to play a role in virulence. The β-haemolysins, producing clear zones of haemolysis on blood agar, have been studied in some detail (Asao *et al.*, 1984; Howard and Buckley, 1985; Potomski *et al.*, 1987a; Garland and Buckley, 1988). Their properties include molecular weight of approximately 50 000 and sensitivity to heat at 56 °C for 10 min. Studies with a single strain designated *A. hydrophila* producing a haemolysin termed 'aerolysin' (Howard and Buckley, 1985; Garland and Buckley, 1988) showed that aerolysin was secreted as a precursor which could be cleaved by trypsin or *Aeromonas* extracellular protease to the active form. This had 250 times the haemolytic activity of the precursor. Aerolysin bound to glycophorin receptors on erythrocytes and aggregated at both 4 and 37 °C. However, formation of 3 nm holes in the erythrocyte membrane and disruption of the membrane only occurred at 37 °C. Active aerolysin was resistant to further proteolysis but was difficult to store because it spontaneously aggregated.

Studies have shown that purified haemolysin preparations are cytotoxic to tissue culture cell lines and enterotoxigenic in rabbits, mice and rats (Asao *et al.*, 1984; Potomski *et al.*, 1987; Millership *et al.*, 1992) (Figure 16.1) Differences in physical, chemical and immunological reactivity suggest that there are several if not multiple β-haemolysins (Brenden and Janda, 1987; Kozaki *et al.*, 1989).

An α-haemolysin has also been described, but this has been much less studied.

There may be another enterotoxigenic factor, but the evidence for this is confusing. Tissue culture activity similar to that of cholera toxin (Ljung *et al.*, 1977; Honda *et al.*, 1985; Potomski *et al.*, 1987b; Schultz and McCardell, 1988) elicited by heating crude *Aeromonas* culture filtrates has been described by several authors (Ljung *et al.*, 1977; Schultz and McCardell, 1988). Reactivity of bacterial culture filtrates with polyclonal anti-cholera toxin has also been found (Potomski *et al.*, 1987b; Schultz and McCardell, 1988). Enterotoxic activity in animals has been attributed to a variety of non-β-haemolysin molecules, but in general

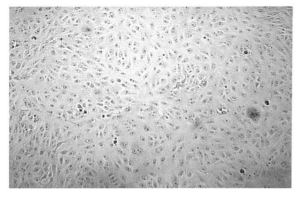

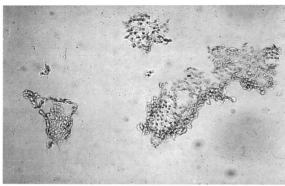

Figure 16.1. Effects of *Aeromonas* haemolysin/ cytotoxin on tissue culture monolayers. (a) Normal vero cell monolayer. (b) After 18 hours incubation with culture filtrate of a strain of *A. sobria* (filtrate prepared from a 14-hour shake culture in tryptone soya broth with 1% yeast extract).

these have been much less well characterized than the haemolysins. It is not clear that tissue culture cytotoxin, immunoreactivity with anti-cholera toxin and enterotoxigenicity represent the activity of the same molecule.

Plesiomonas

Plesiomonas has not attracted the research attention of the aeromonads. Comparatively little is known about potential virulence factors. Unlike the aeromonads, plesiomonads produce few extracellular enzymes. Many authors have been unable to demonstrate enterotoxin-like activity in

rabbit ileal loops, rabbit skin permeability tests, suckling mice or tissue culture (Pitarangsi *et al.*, 1982; Herrington *et al.*, 1987). There have been occasional claims to the contrary (Sanyal *et al.*, 1980), but no potential enterotoxin has been even partially characterized. A large plasmid (>100 MDa) has been described (Herrington *et al.*, 1987), but unlike the shigellae its presence was not associated with invasiveness in tissue culture.

EPIDEMIOLOGY

Natural habitat

Aeromonas

Mesophilic aeromonads are common in raw surface water (Hazen *et al.*, 1978). Much of the work on their ecology has been done in the USA, but scattered reports suggest that they are present worldwide. They occur over a wide range of temperature, pH, turbidity and salinity. Counts tend to rise with a rise in water temperature, and in the deeper more anoxic layers there may be more than 10^5 per gram of mud, and more than 10^5 per litre of surface water. In summer they form the majority of the aerobic heterotrophic flora.

They have also been isolated from drinking water (Burke *et al.*, 1984) in several parts of the world, including India, Australia, Canada, UK and USA even when chlorination produced water of an otherwise bacteriologically acceptable standard. They are more common than is often realized, some studies finding aeromonads in more than 10% of samples. Counts may be greater than 10^5 per litre. Aeromonads have also been found in many foods (Palumbo *et al.*, 1989) such as raw meat and poultry, fresh vegetables, fish and seafood. If enrichment techniques are used *Aeromonas* can be recovered from the faeces of between 2% and 4% of apparently healthy people (Figura *et al.*, 1986).

Unlike the mesophilic aeromonads *A. salmonicida* is not usually cultured from environmental samples. Even at the height of outbreaks of fish infections the bacterium cannot be demonstrated in water. *Aeromonas salmonicida* is taken up by fish within 2 minutes and initial *in vitro* work suggested the organism was short lived outside the host. A later study indicated that it may be present in water in a viable, non-culturable state (Allen-Austin *et al.*, 1984).

Plesiomonas

Much less attention has been paid to the plesiomonads. They have been found in the intestine of fish in Japan and Europe. They have also been found in surface waters in the warm season, numbers declining or becoming undetectable when the temperature drops below 7 °C (Schubert, 1984), which might be expected from the minimum growth temperature. Few studies have been carried out in the UK but in my experience plesiomonads are rare in surface water here.

Plesiomonads have also been found in the gut of other aquatic animals and some mammals such as pigs, dogs and cats. Work in the 1960s suggested that there was no carrier state in man, although this may reflect the difficulty of detection of low numbers of organisms. Studies in Australia (Cooper and Brown, 1968; Holmberg *et al.*, 1986; Kain and Kelly, 1989) and North America have shown that as with the aeromonads there is a high rate of infection with other recognized pathogens (10–30%) in those who have *Plesiomonas* in their faeces.

Aeromonas Infections

The association of soft tissue infections caused by mesophilic *Aeromonas* strains and contact with raw surface water is well known. Apart from this there is little information on the epidemiology of infections outside the gastrointestinal tract.

Many studies have examined the association of *Aeromonas* in the faeces with diarrhoeal disease. In general rates of isolation are higher in those with diarrhoea, especially in small children under two years of age (Gracey *et al.*, 1982), and the very old. Isolation rates are also higher in travellers with diarrhoea than in those without, whereas in the native population isolation rates are the same

whether or not the patient has diarrhoea (Sack *et al.*, 1987). Disease has also been correlated with strains of the toxin-producing phenotypes *A. sobria* and *A. hydrophila* in most studies (Barer *et al.*, 1986) although in some *A. caviae* has been implicated.

No outbreak has yet been definitely documented, although this may reflect the lack of a generally accepted typing system, and there is no animal model, therefore Koch's postulates cannot be fulfilled.

Plesiomonas Infections

In some animals and in man *P. shigelloides* appears to cause diarrhoea. A number of outbreaks in Africa, India and Japan have been attributed to this organism (Schubert, 1984) and sporadic cases occur in many parts of the world, including the UK. Serotyping has shown the same type of a drinking-water source and among individuals with diarrhoea.

CLINICAL FEATURES

Aeromonas

Systemic infections

Given the ubiquitous distribution of the motile aeromonads it is perhaps surprising that more human disease is not recorded. There are many case reports of aeromonads causing systemic disease in a variety of organ systems (von Graevenitz and Altwegg, 1991). Bacteraemia and septicaemia are among the most common, usually in patients with chronic underlying disorders such as leukaemia, solid tumours and liver or renal disease. Ecthyma gangrenosum may occur in association with septicaemia. Another group of reports concerns skin and soft tissue infections, about half of which are associated with presumably contaminated water in, for instance, infections of cuts in divers. Aeromonads have been described as a cause of infections in many sites including meningitis, arthritis, osteomyelitis, peritonitis, cholecystitis, liver abscess, urinary tract infection, endocarditis and eye infections (von Graevenitz and Altwegg, 1991).

Enteric infection

Most recent research interest has concerned the possible role of aeromonads in acute gastroenteritis (Janda, 1991). In the last decade many reports have described an increased incidence of aeromonads from the faeces of patients with diarrhoea (Janda, 1991; Sack et al., 1987). A wide range of symptoms have been ascribed to these organisms. Most authors describe a short-lived syndrome of watery diarrhoea accompanied by mild fever and some vomiting lasting less than a week in the majority of patients, with more prolonged or severe symptoms in a minority. In a case–control study (Gracey et al., 1982) including over 2000 children, 118 with diarrhoea and seven without had Aeromonas spp. in their faeces. Among the symptomatic children 37% had symptoms for more than two weeks, which in four lasted for over three months. A fifth of the children had blood and mucus in the stool which in some led to consideration of a diagnosis of ulcerative colitis.

Experimental infection of human volunteers had inconclusive results (Morgan et al., 1985). Fifty-seven healthy adults were given doses of up to 10^{10} cfu of a strain producing both cytotoxin and enterotoxin. Only two individuals developed mild diarrhoea. There were several difficulties with this study. At the time little was known about adhesive factors relevant in pathogenesis. It was also not possible to check that the excreted strains were the same as that in the initial inoculum. As aeromonads are present in the water supply it may also be that immunity to local strains is present in the adult population. This was suggested by workers studying the aeromonads in Peace Corps volunteers and the local population in Thailand. In the volunteers episodes of traveller's diarrhoea were associated with Aeromonas spp. in the faeces, whereas in the locals no symptoms occurred. These authors suggested that this also explained the study's failure to produce diarrhoea in a rhesus monkey model; aeromonads were frequently isolated from other monkeys in the animal house and the water supply (Pitarangsi et al., 1982).

In spite of numerous studies of the incidence of aeromonads in faeces, reports of an immunological response to infection are very few. One study showed antibody responses to Aeromonas cell envelopes and cytotoxin, and another rises in secretory IgA titres in limited numbers of patients (Janda, 1991). Although strains produce extracellular toxin there is little evidence that this can be detected directly in the faeces, possibly because activity is lost rapidly. A further problem is the frequency of associated bowel disease in patients with diarrhoea who have aeromonads in their faeces. Over 40% (Millership et al., 1986) may have another recognized pathogen or non-infective disease such as cancer or ulcerative colitis. This makes any assessment of the role of aeromonads in causing symptoms very difficult. The reasons for the association have received very little attention: it has been suggested that damage to the gut mucosa from any cause permits colonization of aeromonads present in water or food

Animal infections

Aeromonas salmonicida is an important pathogen of fish, causing furunculosis (a chronic or acute haemorrhagic septicaemia) in salmon and related species. Atypical strains produce a superficial ulcerative form of furunculosis in salmonids, ulcer disease in goldfish and erythrodermatitis in carp.

Plesiomonas

Symptoms attributed to Plesiomonas included diarrhoea and abdominal pain in all of 30 Canadian patients (Kain and Kelly, 1989). This study suggested that Plesiomonas was frequently associated with severe illness. A high proportion had signs of tissue invasion (nearly a third had bloody diarrhoea, a third had fever) and in three-quarters illness lasted more than two weeks (more than four weeks in a third). The majority (71%) of these patients had a history of recent travel. Other authors have described a generally short-lived illness of two to three days duration, the majority of patients experiencing watery diarrhoea and abdominal pain with a minority having vomiting, fever, bloody stools and/or prolonged illness.

DIAGNOSTIC METHODS

Aeromonas

Isolation media

The mesophilic aeromonads grow readily on most media used in the clinical laboratory, including those containing bile. Isolation from normally sterile sites is not difficult. Colonies on blood agar after 18 hours incubation in air are 1–2 mm, circular, convex and entire. They may appear mucoid or rough, and may have a greenish tinge which can be distinguished from *Pseudomonas aeruginosa*. They have a distinct sulphurous odour which increases with the age of the culture. Haemolysis is highly variable, including broad zones of β-haemolysis, double zones of partial clearing or no apparent change in the medium around single colonies. On MacConkey's medium colonies may be lactose or non-lactose fermenting. In the former case colonies often appear oxidase negative, and thus the medium cannot be recommended for the isolation of aeromonads from faeces and other highly contaminated samples. A further problem is that in the presence of a high proportion of lactose-fermenting species even discrete colonies of normally non-lactose-fermenting strains of *Aeromonas* may appear to acidify the medium.

Selective media

Thus enteric media normally employed for the recovery of pathogens are not satisfactory for the isolation of aeromonads from faeces and other heavily contaminated samples. Many different selective agars (von Graevenitz and Bucher, 1983; Kelly *et al.*, 1988), at least 20, have been described. Ampicillin has been used at concentrations of 10, 20 and 30 mg/l in modified formulations for enteric pathogens or blood agar to suppress the growth of Gram-negative flora. Most mesophilic aeromonads have a minimal inhibitory concentration (MIC) to ampicillin of >32 mg/l; however, about 1% of isolates are partially sensitive and a new species, *A. trota* (Janda, 1991), has been described which is fully sensitive. At concentrations of ampicillin below 20 mg/l overgrowth may be a problem.

Indicator media

A variety of carbohydrates, such as trehalose, have been used to detect *Aeromonas* colonies. However, the oxidase reaction cannot be tested directly, thus wasting a day when identifying suspicious colonies. Aeromonads are generally non-xylose fermenters, unlike most members of the Enterobacteriaceae. Xylose has been used to replace lactose in deoxycholate citrate (DCA) medium with some success. This may be a particularly useful medium because heavy suppression of other flora prevents the masking of *Aeromonas* colonies by fermenting colonies.

Formulations with low concentrations (0.1%) of brilliant green were originally described for the detection of plesiomonads. They may also be useful for the aeromonads, especially if carbohydrates are omitted and the plates flooded with oxidase reagent.

CIN (cefsulodin–irgasan–novobiocin) agar has also been used as a selective medium. This was originally designed for *Yersinia* spp., and thus it was hoped that some economy of media could be achieved by using one agar for both bacteria. However, the concentration of cefsulodin (4 mg/l) required for the aeromonads is much less than for *Yersinia* (15 mg/l) (Kelly *et al.*, 1988) and thus increased growth of contaminating flora may be a problem. Some authors found it necessary to combine CIN with another medium for optimal recovery rates, thus eliminating the economic advantage of CIN.

Most research studies have found xylose DCA or ampicillin BA to be most suitable for optimal recovery rates. Unfortunately there are few commercial sources for these media. In every study in which alkaline peptone water (pH. 8.6) has been used isolation rates have been improved two- to four-fold. This may be best incubated on the bench rather than at 37 °C.

However, it has been argued that isolates recovered only from enrichment, and therefore presumably present in low numbers only, are not of clinical significance. It has also been suggested that the usually non-lactose-fermenting strains of *A. hydrophila* and *A. sobria* are those associated with gastroenteritis. Thus it is not clear how useful special selective media and enrichment broths really are in clinical practice, although they are essential for adequate research studies of the incidence of aeromonads in stool samples.

Water samples

These media may be used for isolation from water and environmental samples. It may be necessary to incubate water samples anaerobically, to distinguish aeromonads from other oxidase-positive species commonly present in water.

Aeromonas salmonicida grows on nutrient agar, optimally at about 20 °C. Strains do not usually grow above 35 °C, thus isolates would be unusual in clinical laboratories. After 24 hours colonies are minute, reaching 1 mm at seven days. They are circular, convex, entire and friable. Growth is improved by blood or serum, and haemolysis is apparent on blood agar after two days. Pigment-producing strains show a diffusible melanin-like pigment in air but not anaerobically on media with sufficient tyrosine or phenylalanine.

Identification

Care should be taken to distinguish *Aeromonas* strains from other members of the Vibrionaceae, especially *Vibrio fluvialis*, which is biochemically identical to the mesophilic aeromonads in most respects. In my experience *V. fluvialis* is rare in clinical practice in the UK and isolates identified as *V. fluvialis* with commercial kits are usually aeromonads. Distinction is made by the failure of *Aeromonas* to grow in 6% salt broth and its resistance to a 150 μg disk of vibriostatic agent O/129 (2,4-diamino-6,7-diisopropylpteridine) (Popoff, 1984).

Biochemical differentiation of *Plesiomonas*

from other members of the Vibrionaceae is not difficult. Plesiomonads are ornithine, arginine and lysine decarboxylase positive by Moeller's method, ferment inositol but do not produce gas from glucose (Schubert, 1984). They are sensitive to a 150 μg disc of O/129 but variably resistant to a 10 μg disc. Commercial kits incorporating these organisms in the database are usually satisfactory for identification.

Plesiomonads and mesophilic aeromonads grow on nutrient agar, and most commonly used laboratory media. Growth on TCBS medium is variable. Plesiomonads always appear as non-lactose fermenters, whereas aeromonads may be lactose or non-lactose fermenting on enteric media. On blood agar after 24 hours colonies are circular, convex, entire and 1–4 mm in diameter.

Colonies of *Plesiomonas* are often smaller than those of the Enterobacteriaceae but are otherwise difficult to distinguish from them unless an oxidase test is performed.

Colonies of mesophilic strains of *Aeromonas* often have a brown or green hue, quite different from that of the pseudomonads, which darkens with age. They may also have quite a strong, characteristic odour similar to that of other members of the Vibrionaceae which becomes overpowering if plates are left at room temperature for more than a day or two. Haemolysis is very variable, from a faint clearing of the medium under the colony, to double zones of partial clearing, to a wide zone of complete β-haemolysis. The last is indicative that the isolate is of the *A. hydrophila* or *A. sobria* phenotype. Colonies are typically very moist, may be frankly mucoid or occasionally small and dry. After several subcultures the small dry colonial form may appear in mixed culture with the original form. This change is particularly noticeable when accompanied by a loss of haemolytic activity.

Isolates of *A. salmonicida* phenotype would not normally occur in clinical laboratories. Growth occurs on nutrient agar but may take up to a week at 20 °C to reach 1 mm. Growth is said to be improved by blood or serum. On tryptone soya agar, colonies are visible after 48 hours at 22 °C. They are usually circular, convex and entire.

Several forms including rough and smooth, associated with differences in virulence, have been described. Some strains produce a brown, water-soluble melanin-like pigment on media such as tryptone soya agar with sufficient tyrosine or phenylalanine when incubated in air.

Plesiomonas

Isolation media

Plesiomonas grows on nutrient agar. Colonies on blood agar at 24 hours are 1–2 mm, grey, circular, convex and entire. No pigments are produced. A variety of media have been suggested for enrichment and selective isolation, but none have achieved wide acceptance. Unlike the aeromonads, no selective agents reliably differentiating them from members of the Enterobacteriaceae have been described. Plesiomonads grow on a variety of enteric agars such as MacConkey, *Salmonella–Shigella*, deoxycholate–citrate and cysteine lactose electrolyte-deficient agar as non-lactose-fermenting colonies. However, they are not easy to recover in the presence of large numbers of competing flora on the less inhibitory media. It has also been shown that *Pseudomonas aeruginosa* and *Enterococcus faecium* strains produce substances inhibitory to plesiomonads (Janda, 1987). Inositol bile salts brilliant green agar has been used with some success (von Graevenitz and Bucher, 1983). The concentration of brilliant green, however, is much less than in media for the selection of coliforms or salmonellae and is not very inhibitory to competing flora. Ampicillin-containing media are unlikely to be successful as plesiomonads are not as reliably resistant to this antibiotic as are the aeromonads.

Numerous enrichment media have been described. Alkaline peptone water (pH 8.6) has often been used. It is unlikely to be effective because plesiomonads do not grow above pH 8, which the present author confirmed by artificial inoculation of stool samples. A variety of bile-containing media including broth with bile salts and brilliant green, bile peptone broth, Gram-negative broth, Rappaport broth and tetrathionate broth have

been used. In the individual studies these improved the isolation rates of plesiomonads over direct plating, but none has found wide acceptance.

Antimicrobial Susceptibility

Aeromonas

Mesophilic aeromonads are usually resistant to ampicillin (MIC >128 mg/l), with the exception of the newly described species *A. trota*. They are also resistant to penicillin, carbenicillin and ticarcillin (von Graevenitz and Altwegg, 1991). The mechanisms for this are not fully established. Four β-lactamases among 13 *Aeromonas* isolates have been described on the basis of substrate profiles. Some isolates produced two enzymes. There were two enzymes inhibited by clavulanic acid with imipenem hydrolysing activity, one of which also hydrolysed penicillin, the other penicillin and a cephalosporin. Imipenem hydrolysis was confined to *A. hydrophila*, *A. sobria* and *A. veronii* (Bakken et al., 1988). This carbapenemase activity is of considerable current interest because it is relatively unusual among Gram negatives. The only other species where it is common is *Stenotrophomonas maltophilia*.

Two further enzymes hydrolysing penicillins and cephalosporins but not imipenem were present in *A. caviae*; one was susceptible to clavulanic acid, one was not.

β-lactamases in all but one strain were inducible, which together with the low proportion of strains reported to possess conjugative plasmids suggests that these enzymes are chromosomally mediated, although this has not yet been definitely established. Clavulanic acid did not reduce MICs to the susceptible range, even when the β-lactamase was inactivated by it. One strain had no detectable β-lactamase, yet was still resistant to penicillin and ampicillin, suggesting that aeromonads possess another mechanism of resistance.

Most aeromonads are susceptible to azlocillin, piperacillin, second- and third-generation cephalosporins, aminoglycosides, tetracycline, chloramphenicol, trimethoprim–sulphamethoxazole and the quinolones (von Graevenitz and Altwegg,

1991). Susceptibility may vary with country of origin; a higher proportion of Asian isolates have been reported as resistant to cefamandole and tetracycline.

Plesiomonas

A few studies have examined antibiotic susceptibility. Plesiomonads are generally sensitive to trimethoprim–sulphamethoxazole, tetracycline, chloramphenicol, quinolones and gentamicin (von Graevenitz and Altwegg, 1991). They are variably sensitive to ampicillin, probably because they produce β-lactamase.

Typing Systems

Several typing systems have been suggested for the motile aeromonads (von Graevenitz and Altwegg, 1991), but none has been widely adopted Serotyping with antibodies against O antigens suffers from poor typability. The group is highly heterogeneous and it is difficult to build up a sufficiently large set of antisera. Only 30–70% of strains react with any given set. Haemagglutination and haemagglutination inhibition patterns are poorly reproducible. Phage typing appears more promising; in one study 81% of 96 strains could be divided into 73 phage types (Altwegg et al., 1988). A number of electrophoretic methods, including whole cell proteins, outer membrane proteins, Western blotting, restriction endonuclease analysis and rRNA gene restriction patterns have been tried, again demonstrating the heterogeneity of strains. There is no obvious correlation with taxonomy except for isoenzyme analysis which allows identification to genospecies. All methods indicate a considerable diversity of strains, which with the exception of serogroup O11 have no clear association with virulence. No one method or combination of methods has yet achieved wide acceptance.

A system of phage typing for strains of *A. salmonicida* was described in 1971 (Popoff, 1984). Fourteen types were identified using eight phages. Phages have been recovered from water, sewage and lysogenic isolates.

A typing system for *Plesiomonas* based on O and H serogroups has been described by Japanese workers. There are 107 serovars with 50 O and 17 H antigens (Schubert, 1984; von Graevenitz and Altwegg, 1991).

MANAGEMENT OF INFECTIONS

In general, management of infections caused by aeromonads and plesiomonads does not present particular problems. Standard antibiotic regimens have been used for infections outside the gastrointestinal tract. Several descriptive studies have been reported in which the majority of infections occurred in patients with depressed immunity. Usually two antibiotics, one of which was an aminoglycoside, were used.

Reports of enteric infections often do not mention antibiotic treatment, presumably because many patients have short-lived symptoms which resolve spontaneously. In those whose symptoms are more prolonged most of the antibiotics which appear suitable *in vitro* have been tried, with rapid (two to three days) resolution of symptoms. However, most reports are of small numbers of cases, and few are controlled.

Trimethoprim–sulphamethoxazole and tetracycline have been reported as suitable for *Plesiomonas* enteric infections.

PREVENTION AND CONTROL

There is little evidence for person-to-person spread of the aeromonads or plesiomonads. No special precautions are required.

REFERENCES

Abbott, S.L., Cheung, W.K.W., Kroske-bystrom, S. *et al.* (1992) Identification of *Aeromonas* strains to the genospecies level in the clinical laboratory. *Journal of Clinical Microbiology*, **30**, 1262–1266.

Allen-Austin, D., Austin, B. and Colwell, R.R. (1984) Survival of *Aeromonas salmonicida* in river water. *FEMS Microbiological Letters*, **21**, 143–146.

Altwegg, M., Altwegg-Bissig, R., Demarta, A. *et al.* (1988) Comparison of four typing methods for

Aeromonas species. *Journal of Diarrhoeal Diseases Research*, **6**(2), 88–94.

Altwegg, M., Steigerwalt, A.G., Altwegg-Bissig, R. et al. (1990) Biochemical identification of *Aeromonas* genospecies isolated from humans. *Journal of Clinical Microbiology*, **28**, 258–264.

Asao, T., Kinoshita, Y., Kozaki, S. et al. (1984) Purification and some properties of *Aeromonas hydrophila* hemolysin. *Infection and Immunity*, **46**, 122–127.

Bakken, J.S., Sanders, C.C., Clark, R.B. et al. (1988) β-lactam resistance in *Aeromonas* spp. caused by inducible β-lactamases active against penicillins, cephalosporins, and carbapenems. *Antimicrobial Agents and Chemotherapy*, **32**, 1314–1319.

Barer, M.R., Millership, S.E. and Tabaqchali, S. (1986) Relationship of toxin production to species in the genus *Aeromonas*. *Journal of Medical Microbiology*, **22**, 303–309.

Barghouthi, S., Young, R., Olson, M.O.J. et al. (1989) Amonabactin, a novel tryptophan- or phenylalanine-containing phenolate siderophore in *Aeromonas hydrophila*. *Journal of Bacteriology*, **171**, 1811–1816.

Brenden, R. and Janda, J.M. (1987) Detection, quantitation and stability of the β haemolysin of *Aeromonas* spp. *Journal of Medical Microbiology*, **24**, 247–251.

Burke, V., Robinson, J., Gracey, M. et al. (1984) Isolation of *Aeromonas hydrophila* from a metropolitan water supply: seasonal correlation with clinical isolates. *Applied and Environmental Microbiology*, **48**, 361–366.

Cooper, R.G. and Brown, G.W. (1968) *Plesiomonas shigelloides* in South Australia. *Journal of Clinical Pathology*, **21**, 715–718.

Figura, N., Marri, L., Verdiani, S. et al. (1986) Prevalence, species differentiation and toxigenicity of *Aeromonas* strains in cases of childhood gastroenteritis and controls. *Journal of Clinical Microbiology*, **23**, 595–599.

Garland, W.J. and Buckley, J.T. (1988) The cytolytic toxin aerolysin must aggregate to disrupt erythrocytes, and aggregation is stimulated by human glycophorin. *Infection and Immunity*, **56**, 1249–1253.

Gracey, M., Burke, V. and Robinson, J. (1982) *Aeromonas*-associated gastroenteritis. *Lancet*, **ii**, 1304–1306.

Gray, S.J., Stickler, D.J. and Bryant, T.N. (1990) The incidence of virulence factors in mesophilic *Aeromonas* species isolated from farm animals and their environment. *Epidemiology and Infection*, **105**, 277–294.

Hazen, T.C., Fliermans, C.B., Hirsch, R.P. et al. (1978) Prevalence and distribution of *Aeromonas hydro-*

phila in the United States. *Applied and Environmental Microbiology*, **36**, 731–738.

Herrington, D., Tzipori, S., Robins-Browne, R.M. et al. (1987) In vitro and in vivo pathogenicity of *Plesiomonas shigelloides*. *Infection and Immunity*, **55**, 979–985.

Hickman-Brenner, F.W., MacDonald, K.L., Steigerwalt, A.G. et al. (1987) *Aeromonas veronii*, a new ornithine decarboxylase-positive species that may cause diarrhoea. *Journal of Clinical Microbiology*, **25**, 900–906.

Hickman-Brenner, F.W., Fanning, G.R., Arduino, M.J. et al. (1988) *Aeromonas schubertii*, a new mannitol-negative species found in human clinical specimens. *Journal of Clinical Microbiology*, **26**, 1561–1564.

Ho, A.S.Y., Meitzner, T.A., Smith, A.J. et al. (1990) The pili of *Aeromonas hydrophila*: identification of an environmentally regulated 'mini pilin'. *Journal of Experimental Medicine*, **172**, 795–806.

Holmberg, S.D., Wachsmuth, I.K., Hickman-Brenner, F.W. et al. (1986) *Plesiomonas* enteric infections in the United States. *Annals of Internal Medicine*, **105**, 690–694.

Honda, T., Sato, M., Nishimura, T. et al. (1985) Demonstration of cholera toxin-related factor in cultures of *Aeromonas* species by enzyme-linked immunosorbent assay. *Infection and Immunity*, **50**, 322–323.

Howard, S.P. and Buckley, J.T. (1985) Activation of the hole-forming toxin aerolysin by extracellular processing. *Journal of Bacteriology*, **163**, 336–340.

Janda, J.M. (1987) Effect of acidity and antimicrobial agent-like compounds on viability of *Plesiomonas shigelloides*. *Journal of Clinical Microbiology*, **25**, 1213–1215.

Janda, J.M. (1991) Recent advances in the study of the taxonomy, pathogenicity and infectious syndromes associated with the genus *Aeromonas*. *Clinical Microbiology Reviews*, **4**, 397–410.

Kain, K.C. and Kelly, M.T. (1989) Clinical features, epidemiology and treatment of *Plesiomonas shigelloides* diarrhea. *Journal of Clinical Microbiology*, **27**, 990–1001.

Kay, W.W., Buckley, J.T., Ishiguro, E.E. et al. (1981) Purification and disposition of a surface protein associated with virulence of *Aeromonas salmonicida*. *Journal of Bacteriology*, **147**, 1077–1084.

Kelly, M.T., Stroh, E.M.D. and Jessop, J. (1988) Comparison of blood agar, ampicillin blood agar, MacConkey–Ampicillin–Tween agar, and modified Cefsulodin–Irgasan–Novobiocin agar for isolation of *Aeromonas* spp. from stool specimens. *Journal of Clinical Microbiology*, **26**, 1738–1740.

Kokka, R.P., Janda J.M., Oshiro, L.S. et al. (1991) Biochemical and genetic characterization of autoagglutinating phenotypes of *Aeromonas* species associated with invasive and noninvasive disease. *Journal of Infectious Diseases*, **163**, 890–894.

Kozaki, S., Asao, T., Kamata, Y. *et al.* (1989) Characterization of *Aeromonas sobria* hemolysin by use of monoclonal antibodies against *Aeromonas hydrophila* hemolysins. *Journal of Clinical Microbiology*, **27**, 1782–1786.

Kuijper, E.J., Steigerwalt, A.G., Schoenmakers, B.S.C.I.M. *et al.* (1989) Phenotypic characterization and DNA relatedness in human fecal isolates of *Aeromonas* spp. *Journal of Clinical Microbiology*, **27**, 132–138.

Ljungh, A., Popoff, M. and Wadstrom, T. (1977) *Aeromonas hydrophila* in acute diarrheal disease: detection of enterotoxin and biotyping of strains. *Journal of Clinical Microbiology*, **6**, 96–100.

Martinez-Murcia, A.J., Benlloch, S. and Collins, M.D. (1992) Phylogenetic interrelationships of members of the genera *Aeromonas* and *Pleisiomonas* as determined by 16S ribosomal DNA sequencing; lack of congruence with results of DNA–DNA hybridizations. *International Journal of Systematic Bacteriology*, **42**, 412–421.

Millership, S.E., Barer, M.R. and Tabaqchali, S. (1986) Toxin production by *Aeromonas* spp. from different sources. *Journal of Medical Microbiology*, **22**, 311–314.

Millership, S.E., Barer, M.R., Mulla, R. *et al.* (1992) Enterotoxic effects of *A. sobria* haemolysin in a rat jejunal perfusion system identified by specific neutralisation with monoclonal antibody. *Journal of General Microbiology*, **138**, 261–267.

Mittal, K.R., Lalonde, G., Leblanc, D. *et al.* (1980) *Aeromonas hydrophila* in rainbow trout: relation between virulence and surface characteristics. *Canadian Journal of Microbiology*, **26**, 1501–1503.

Morgan, D.R., Johnson, P.C., DuPont, H.L. *et al.* (1985) Lack of correlation between known virulence properties of *Aeromonas hydrophila* and enteropathogenicity for humans. *Infection and Immunity*, **50**, 62–65.

Namdari, H. and Bottone, E.J. (1988) Correlation of suicide phenomenon in *Aeromonas* species with virulence and pathogenicity. *Journal of Clinical Microbiology*, **26**, 2615–2619.

Palumbo, S.A., Bencivengo, M.M., Corral, F.D. *et al.* (1989) Characterization of the *Aeromonas hydrophila* group isolated from retail foods of animal origin. *Journal of Clinical Microbiology*, **27**, 854–859.

Pitarangsi, C., Echeverria, P., Whitmire, R. *et al.* (1982) Enteropathogenicity of *Aeromonas hydrophila* and *Plesiomonas shigelloides*: prevalence among individuals with and without diarrhea in Thailand. *Infection and Immunity*, **35**, 666–673.

Popoff, M. (1984) *Aeromonas*. In *Bergey's Manual of Determinative Bacteriology*, Vol. 1 (ed. J.G. Holt), pp. 545–548. Williams & Wilkins, Baltimore.

Popoff, M. and Veron, M. (1976) A taxonomic study of *Aeromonas hydrophila–Aeromonas punctata* group. *Journal of General Microbiology*, **94**, 11–22.

Potomski, J., Burke, V., Watson, I. *et al.* (1987a) Purification of cytotoxic enterotoxin of *Aeromonas sobria* by use of monoclonal antibodies. *Journal of Medical Microbiology*, **23**, 171–177.

Potomski, J., Burke, V., Robinson, J. *et al.* (1987b) *Aeromonas* cytotonic enterotoxin cross reactive with cholera toxin. *Journal of Medical Microbiology*, **23**, 179–186.

Sack, R.B., Lanata, C., Kay, B.A. (1987) Epidemiological studies of *Aeromonas*-related diarrheal diseases. *Experientia*, **43**, 364–365.

Sanyal, S.C., Sarswathi, B. and Sharma, P. (1980) Enteropathogenicity of *Plesiomonas shigelloides*. *Journal of Medical Microbiology*, **13**, 401–409.

Schubert, R.H.W. (1984) *Plesiomonas*. In *Bergey's Manual of Determinative Bacteriology*, Vol. 1 (ed. J.G. Holt), pp. 545–548. Williams & Wilkins, Baltimore.

Schultz, A. and McCardell, B. (1988) DNA homology and immunological cross-reactivity between *Aeromonas hydrophila* cytotonic toxin and cholera toxin. *Journal of Clinical Microbiology*, **26**, 57–61.

Shaw, D.H. and Hodder, H.J. (1978) Lipopolysaccharides of the motile aeromonads: core oligosaccharide analysis as an aid to taxonomic classification. *Canadian Journal of Microbiology*, **24**, 864–868.

von Graevenitz, A. and Altwegg, M. (1991) *Aeromonas* and *Plesiomonas*. In *Manual of Clinical Microbiology*, 5th edn (ed. A. Balows), pp. 396–401. American Society for Microbiology, Washington, DC.

von Graevenitz, A. and Bucher, C. (1983) Evaluation of differential and selective media for isolation of *Aeromonas* and *Plesiomonas* spp. from human faeces. *Journal of Clinical Microbiology*, **17**, 16–21.

17a

HELICOBACTER PYLORI

Alan Cockayne

HISTORICAL BACKGROUND

For many decades, the highly acidic nature of the gastric lumen was thought to preclude long-term colonization by bacteria. However, a number of early histological studies had identified spiral bacteria associated with the human gastric mucosa (Goodwin, 1993). Later histological and ultrastructural studies confirmed these earlier findings, but the bacteria could not be isolated from gastric biopsies and since the organisms appeared to be non-invasive they were dismissed as insignificant contaminants. It was not until the early 1980s in Perth, Western Australia, that further histological studies established a possible relationship between bacterial colonization of the gastric mucosa and the presence of gastritis (Goodwin, 1993). The recognition that fortuitous treatment of a single patient with antibiotics resulted in resolution of gastritis provided the first direct evidence of bacterial involvement in gastric pathology (Goodwin, 1993).

The individuals involved in this major observation, Barry Marshall and Richard Warren, in collaboration with other colleagues then attempted to isolate this unusual organism from gastric biopsy specimens. Despite using a variety of culture media and conditions these initial attempts failed principally because the primary incubation period was restricted to 48 hours. Only when primary incubation was extended accidentally to five days over a holiday period were cultures found to be positive, resulting in the isolation of the organism now known as *Helicobacter pylori* on 14 April 1982 (Goodwin, 1993). The link between *H. pylori* infection and gastritis, initially greeted with some scepticism, was subsequently confirmed following self-inoculation studies in human volunteers (Marshall *et al.*, 1985).

Initially, based on gross morphological and cultural similarities, the organism was thought to belong to the genus *Campylobacter* and was therefore named *Campylobacter*-like-organism or CLO. Further studies resulted in the proposal in 1984 that this novel gastric bacterium be named *Campylobacter pyloridis* but this name was subsequently changed to the more grammatically correct *Campylobacter pylori* in 1987 (Marshall and Goodwin, 1987). As additional comparative taxonomic studies were performed, however, it became apparent that this bacterium differed significantly from other members of the genus *Campylobacter*. Both 5S and 16S RNA sequencing studies and analysis of fatty acid profiles placed this organism (and a similar bacterium isolated from the gastric mucosa of the ferret) in a genus distinct from

Principles and Practice of Clinical Bacteriology. Edited by A.M. Emmerson, P.M. Hawkey and S.H. Gillespie
© 1997 John Wiley & Sons Ltd

TABLE 17a.1   *HELICOBACTER* SPECIES AND THEIR HOSTS (AS OF 1996)

Species	Natural hosts	Principal site of infection
pylori	Human, monkey, ?cat	Stomach
mustelae	Ferret	Stomach
felis	Cat, dog	Stomach
nemestrinae	Pig-tailed macaque	Stomach
acinonyx	Cheetah	Stomach
muridarum	Rats, mice	Stomach
canis	Dog	Large intestine
cinaedi	Human, rodents	Large intestine
fennelliae	Human	Large intestine
rappini	Dogs, human, sheep	Liver, stomach, large intestine
heilmanii[a]	Human, ?monkey	Stomach
pamentensis	Birds	Isolated from faeces
pullorum	Human, birds	Large intestine, faeces
hepaticus	Laboratory mice	Liver, intestine
bilis	Laboratory mice	Liver, intestine

[a] Formerly *Gastrospirillum hominis*.
Fox *et al.* (1995).

Campylobacter (Goodwin, 1993; Goodwin *et al.*, 1989). Although these novel gastric bacteria showed some similarity to members of the genus *Wolinella*, overall their distinctive taxonomic properties merited their inclusion in the new genus *Helicobacter* (Goodwin *et al.*, 1989).

Subsequent studies have identified additional *Helicobacter* spp. which have been isolated from man and other animals (Table 17a.1) (Fox *et al.*, 1995). These organisms are morphologically and genetically quite diverse, and inclusion in the genus is based primarily on RNA sequence similarities. It seems likely that additional members of this genus will be isolated in the future.

DESCRIPTION OF *HELICOBACTER PYLORI*

Helicobacter pylori is a Gram-negative, non-sporing bacillus measuring 0.5–1.0 μm in width and 2.5–4.0 μm in length (Goodwin and Armstrong, 1990). This organism stains weakly with conventional Gram stain and better counterstaining is achieved using stains such as carbol fuchsin. In sections of gastric biopsies the organism shows a gently curved spiral morphology but on laboratory subculture frequently grows as straight rods (Figure 17a.1). In older cultures the organism produces coccoid forms (Goodwin and Armstrong,

1990). *Helicobacter pylori* is motile with five or six unipolar flagella which are characteristically sheathed and bear terminal knobs. The organism produces large quantities of a urease enzyme, whose activity can readily be detected using a standard urease broth. Urease activity appears to be conserved among the gastric *Helicobacter* spp. but those such as *H. fennelliae* and *H. cinaedi* isolated from non-gastric sites are urease negative (Goodwin, 1993). *Helicobacter pylori* is also oxidase and catalase positive, and these activities, taken in combination with a positive urease result and Gram stain morphology, allow a rapid presumptive identification.

Helicobacter pylori grows well in media supplemented with whole or lysed blood or serum but will also grow in simpler media containing bovine serum albumin, starch or cyclodextrins (Tompkins, 1993). Agar plates should not be over-dried. Primary isolation may require incubation for four or five days before significant growth is visible, but once subcultured growth is quicker and good yields of organisms can be achieved in two or three days. Bacterial colonies are 2 mm in diameter, entire and translucent on chocolate horse blood agar after three days' incubation. Weak haemolysis is visible on blood agar plates. The organism also grows fairly well in liquid media such as Isosensitest, brain heart infusion or

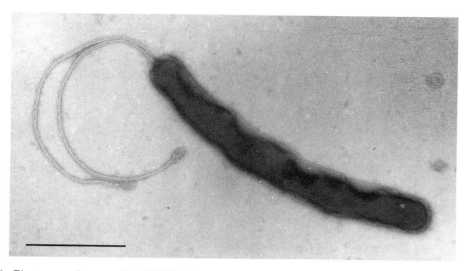

Figure 17a.1. Electron micrograph of *Helicobacter pylori* NCTC 11637 showing polar sheathed flagella with terminal knobs. This micrograph was kindly provided by Dr N. Powell. Scale bar = 1 μm.

Brucella broths supplemented with 5% fetal calf or newborn calf serum.

Helicobacter pylori is generally considered to be microaerobic, and incubation in moist atmospheres of 6% oxygen, 5% carbon dioxide in nitrogen is routinely used though some workers have reported growth of *H. pylori* in air or in 10% carbon dioxide in air (Kosunen and Megraud, 1995).

Early attempts to develop *H. pylori* typing schemes for epidemiological studies (e.g. serotyping) proved disappointing. Restriction fragment length polymorphism (RFLP) and polymerase chain reaction (PCR) analyses of *H. pylori* DNA have subsequently been used (Owen *et al.*, 1994; Taylor *et al.*, 1995) and show a remarkable level of genetic diversity among *H. pylori* isolates. Almost every isolate has a unique DNA fingerprint suggesting a rapid rate of mutation in *H. pylori* and that (unlike many other bacterial pathogens), isolates are non-clonal in origin. Epidemiologically, DNA analysis has been useful in determining the relatedness of *H. pylori* strains isolated from different members of the same family and in assessing recrudescence and reinfection after therapy (Taylor *et al.*, 1995). These studies have also shown that some individuals are

simultaneously infected by more than one strain of *H. pylori* (Owen *et al.*, 1994; Taylor *et al.*, 1995). As a result of this extreme level of strain variability, typing schemes for *H. pylori* are currently limited to the division of isolates into two groups designated type I and type II (Xiang *et al.*, 1995) (see Pathogenesis section).

PATHOGENICITY

Currently, the exact mechanisms by which *H. pylori* infection causes tissue damage are poorly understood. The bacterium is a chronic pathogen and is able to survive in the host despite induction of significant local and systemic humoral and cell-mediated immune responses. It seems likely that cytokines produced following interaction with gastric epithelial cells and leucocytes play a major role in the chronicity of the disease process and may possibly downregulate cell-mediated immunity.

The involvement of *H. pylori* in pathologies of varying severity suggests that some strains of the organism are more virulent than others. Those associated with peptic ulcer disease and gastric cancer – type I strains – share several common features with strains which are more frequently isolated from patients with chronic low-grade gastritis – type II strains (Table 17a.2) – but also produce two additional proteins, the cytotoxin-associated gene product CagA, and the vacuolating cytotoxin VacA, which appear to be associated with enhanced virulence (Xiang et al., 1995).

The CagA⁺ Phenotype

CagA, a protein of 120–140 kDa, is produced by approximately 65% of H. pylori isolates (Xiang et al., 1995; Suerbaum and Wadstrom, 1995). Virtually all strains isolated from peptic ulcer patients produce CagA, compared with only 30–50% of those isolated from patients with non-ulcer dyspepsia. Currently the function of CagA is unknown but it is highly immunogenic and serological studies indicate that a large proportion of H. pylori-infected peptic ulcer and gastric cancer patients have antibodies to this protein, indicating current or previous infection with CagA⁺ strains. Early studies showed that H. pylori strains which make CagA induced higher levels of interleukin 8 (IL-8) production from gastric epithelial cells than CagA⁻ strains (Crabtree et al., 1994). Subsequent studies using isogenic mutants have shown, however, that CagA itself has no direct involvement in IL-8 induction but acts as a marker for the presence of other genes, picA and picB which appear

to be more closely involved with cytokine induction (Tummuru et al., 1995). CagA, picA and picB are located on a large DNA fragment or so-called 'pathogenicity island' – the cagI region – which is unique to type I strains of H. pylori (Tummuru et al., 1995).

The Vacuolating Cytotoxin VacA

Approximately 60% of H. pylori isolates produce VacA, an 87–94 kDa secreted protein which causes vacuolation of a variety of tissue culture cell lines in vitro (Suerbaum and Wadstrom, 1995). The toxin is synthesized as a 139 kDa protoxin which is subsequently cleaved to produce the cytotoxin and a second fragment of approximately 50 kDa which may be involved in secretion of the toxin from the bacterial cell. Virtually all H. pylori strains isolated from peptic ulcer patients produce VacA and the purified toxin causes tissue damage when administered intragastrically to mice (Suerbaum and Wadstrom, 1995). The exact mode of action of VacA on tissue culture cells is unknown but appears to involve stimulation of ATPase activity, and studies have shown that the vacuoles derive from late endosomal compartments. Vacuolation is not frequently seen as a cell response in vivo but the toxin may have additional as yet unidentified effects on cell function. Recent studies indicate the gene

TABLE 17a.2   VIRULENCE FACTORS PRODUCED BY TYPE I AND TYPE II ISOLATES OF H. PYLORI

Virulence factor	Function	Reference
Factors common to type I and II isolates		
Urease	Urea hydrolysis	Suerbaum and Wadstrom (1995)
Flagella	Motility	Suerbaum and Wadstrom (1995)
Adhesins	Adherence	Suerbaum and Wadstrom (1995)
Heat shock protein	Chaperonin	Suerbaum and Wadstrom (1995)
Superoxide dismutase	Protection against free radicals	Spiegelhalder et al. (1993)
Haemolysins	Lysis of red blood cells	Drazek et al. (1995)
Mucinases	Mucin degradation	Smith et al. (1994)
Neutrophil activating protein	Activation of neutrophils	Evans et al. (1995)
Factors specific to type I isolates		
CagA	Unknown – immunodominant antigen	Suerbaum and Wadstrom (1995)
PicA	Transport function, IL-8 induction	Tummuru et al. (1995)
PicB	Transport function, IL-8 induction	Tummuru et al. (1995)
VacA	Vacuolating cytotoxin	Suerbaum and Wadstrom (1995)

encoding the cytotoxin – *vacA* which is present in all *H. pylori* strains – shows mosaicism and is of variable structure in different isolates (Atherton *et al.*, 1995). This appears to correlate with quantitative differences in VacA production between isolates and their ability to induce variable levels of damage in human tissue.

Other Putative Virulence Determinants Shared by Type I and Type II Strains

Urease

All *H. pylori* isolates produce large quantities of a urease (Suerbaum and Wadstrom, 1995). The enzyme has a native molecular weight of approximately 600 kDa and is composed of two subunits – A and B – of 29 and 62 kDa respectively. The enzyme is constitutive and unusually has two pH optima – one at acid pH which probably allows it to function in the highly acidic environment of the gastric lumen. Urease is important as a colonization factor since urease-negative mutants fail to colonize experimental animals (Suerbaum and Wadstrom, 1995). The principal, though not exclusive, function of the urease in colonization is in modulating pH in the immediate vicinity of the bacterium. *Helicobacter pylori* urease acts on urea present in gastric juice, releasing NH_3, which causes a localized increase in pH and protects the bacterium from gastric acid until it is able to penetrate the mucous layer where pH conditions are more favourable. In the absence of urea *H. pylori* is rapidly killed at low pH and, conversely, in the presence of urea it is killed if the pH is allowed to rise above pH 8. Ammonia and its reaction products, the monochloramines, generated by urease activity may also have a direct toxic effect on mammalian cells.

Motility and chemotaxis

Animal studies using *H. pylori* isolates of differing motilities suggest that *H. pylori* motility is an important colonization factor, possibly allowing penetration of the mucous layer (Suerbaum and Wadstrom, 1995). *Helicobacter pylori* also shows chemotaxis towards hog gastric mucin (Logan *et al.*, 1995), a response which may be important during colonization by directing the bacterium to the mucosal surface. Isogenic mutants in *H. pylori* genes involved in motility and chemotaxis have now been constructed and these will allow the relative importance of these two factors to be more accurately assessed in animal models.

Adhesion

Although the majority of *H. pylori* are found associated with the gastric mucous layer, approximately 10% are seen to be a closely adherent to mucosal cells (Noach *et al.*, 1994). Adhesion results in changes in gastric epithelial cell morphology with loss of microvilli. Electron microscopy has detected small numbers of *H. pylori* inside epithelial cells, but *H. pylori* is not generally considered to be an invasive pathogen (Suerbaum and Wadstrom, 1995). Some ultrastructural studies have also detected the formation of structures resembling adhesion pedestals by gastric epithelial cells, but these results have not been confirmed in all studies. A number of protein adhesins of *H. pylori* have been identified and several putative host cell receptors including phosphatidyl ethanolamine, the Lewis *b* blood group antigen, sialic acid, lamimin, collagen and sulphatides have also been detected (Suerbaum and Wadstrom, 1995). At present, the relative importance of these different factors in mediating adhesion of *H. pylori in vivo* have yet to be proved.

Lipopolysaccharide

Helicobacter pylori produces an unusual lipopolysaccharide (LPS) which is relatively non-toxic when compared with those of other Gram-negative bacteria (Suerbaum and Wadstrom, 1995; Nielsen *et al.*, 1994). The fatty acid composition of the lipid A component appears to be unique and accounts for the reduced pyrogenicity. In common with other Gram-negative organisms, repeated laboratory subculture on plates results in production of a rough form of LPS – a phenomenon which can be reversed by growth of *H. pylori* in broth culture. Detailed nuclear magnetic resonance (NMR) studies have shown that *H. pylori* LPS contains sugar sequences defining the Lewis X blood group antigen (Sherburne and Taylor, 1995), a factor which may have immunomodulatory properties.

NORMAL HABITAT

Currently, there are no well-documented reports of common animal or other environmental reservoirs for *H. pylori*. Although *H. pylori* and other closely related gastric *Helicobacter* spp. have been isolated from captive and wild monkeys (Fox, 1995) it seems unlikely that these animals could act as a significant source of infection for the human population. More recently, however, the isolation of *H. pylori* from domestic cats housed in an animal facility raises the possibility of cats as a potential source of human infection (Handt *et al.*, 1994). Other environmental sources, in particular water supplies, have been investigated as possible reservoirs of *H. pylori* infection. *Helicobacter pylori* is able to survive in water for several days and the coccoid form of the organism has been proposed as a survival stage of the life cycle (Goodwin and Armstrong, 1990; Bode *et al.*, 1993). Although this has yet to be proved, studies which detected *H. pylori* DNA in a water supply serving a population where *H. pylori* infection is endemic (Westblom *et al.*, 1993) indicate the potential of untreated drinking water as a source of infection.

The principal habitat of *H. pylori* is as a pathogen of gastric or gastric-type epithelium (e.g. gastric metaplasia in the duodenum) (Axon and Quina, 1994; Blaser, 1990). Although colonized individuals are frequently asymptomatic, histological gastritis is always present, indicating that *H. pylori* is not merely acting as a commensal in this situation.

Several studies have attempted to isolate *H. pylori* from other body sites including the human mouth and faeces (Kosunen and Megrand, 1995; Megraud, 1995). Although *H. pylori* DNA can readily be detected in saliva, gingival scrapings and faeces, culture of the bacterium from such sites has proved difficult due to the richness and complexity of the normal bacterial flora associated with these sites (Kosunen and Megraud, 1995; Megraud, 1995). Reports of successful culture of viable *H. pylori* from gingival scrapings have been published, but this has not been achieved in all studies and may relate to reflux of gastric contents into the mouth (Megraud, 1995). Similarly, although several groups have detected *H. pylori* in human faeces by PCR and successful isolation of the organism from this source has been reported in two studies, several other investigators have failed to isolate viable *H. pylori* from faeces (Megraud, 1995). Detection of *H. pylori* in these extragastric sites is, however, of interest in relation to the possible modes of transmission of the bacterium within the community.

EPIDEMIOLOGY AND DISEASE ASSOCIATIONS

Although *H. pylori* infection occurs worldwide, the prevalence of disease varies markedly between different countries (Eurogast Study Group, 1994; Mendall and Pajares-Garcia, 1995). Seroepidemiological studies have shown that the prevalence of *H. pylori* infection increases with age and is associated with a poor socioeconomic background. For example, up to 90% of the adult population in African countries may be infected, compared with only 10% of white Americans. More detailed studies have been able to show an age cohort effect which would suggest that infection is primarily acquired in childhood (Mendall and Pajares-Garcia, 1995).

Currently, the most likely source of infection appears to be other infected individuals. Since familial · studies show clustering of infection, situations which result in poor hygiene and close physical contact, particularly in childhood (e.g. overcrowding and bed sharing) may provide the situation in which infection is readily transmitted (Mendall and Pajares-Garcia, 1995). Detection of *H. pylori* in the oral cavity and faeces (Megraud, 1995) would support direct oral–oral or possible faecal–oral routes of transmission. Currently, however, the possibility that infection is also associated with exposure to other common environmental sources cannot be totally excluded (Mendall and Pajares-Garcia, 1995).

Although there do not appear to be any major additional risk factors that have been identified in patients with *H. pylori* gastritis, a number of independent genetic and environmental factors have been shown to be important in patients with peptic ulcer disease (Kuipers *et al.*, 1995): non-secretor phenotypes of blood groups predispose to both gastric and duodenal ulceration, whereas blood group A predominates in gastric ulcer and group O in duodenal ulcers. Smoking increases the risk for both types of ulcer and excessive salt intake that for gastric ulcer. The relationship, if any, between these factors and *H. pylori* infection in the pathogenesis of peptic ulcers has yet to be clarified.

Retrospective seroepidemiological studies have indicated a strong correlation between *H. pylori* infection and the development of intestinal and possibly diffuse types of gastric cancer (Forman, 1995), and indicate that *H. pylori*-infected individuals are at least six times more likely to develop gastric cancer than uninfected subjects. Based on these data, it is estimated that *H. pylori* infection may be a significant factor in up to 60% of gastric cancers, and has resulted in the International Agency for Research on Cancer designating *H. pylori* as a recognized carcinogen (International Agency for Research on Cancer, 1994).

Although these studies generally show that populations with high levels of gastric cancer usually have a high prevalence of *H. pylori* infection, local and regional variations in this pattern have been detected. The apparent failure to detect *H. pylori* infection serologically in some cancer patients may result from loss of the organism after development of gastric atrophy and a subsequent fall in antibody titres (Forman, 1995).

It is unlikely that *H. pylori* infection alone is the cause of gastric cancer, but that other host or environmental factors, e.g. increased dietary salt intake and decreased intake of vitamins C and E, will be cofactors. Earlier serological studies did not give an indication of the duration of infection in these patients, but more recent data controlled for age of acquisition of *H. pylori* indicate that

chronic infection over many years is involved in development of this type of disease.

A second type of gastric cancer – MALToma – has also been associated with *H. pylori* infection (Forman, 1995; Parsonnet *et al.*, 1994) and several independent treatment studies have shown that eradication of *H. pylori* leads to rapid regression of the lymphoma (Wotherspoon *et al.*, 1993). The mechanism by which *H. pylori* triggers development of lymphoma is at present unknown.

Recently, a new *Helicobacter* – *H. hepaticus* – has been recognized as a cause of hepatic cancer in laboratory mice (Rice, 1995), an observation which strengthens the link between this group of organisms and oncogenesis.

CLINICAL FEATURES AND PATHOPHYSIOLOGY OF INFECTION

Although originally recognized as a cause of type B chronic active gastritis, *H. pylori* infection is now linked with a spectrum of pathologies of vastly differing severities (Axon and Quinn, 1994; Blaser, 1990). Once acquired, infection if untreated appears to be lifelong, with only 1% of patients undergoing spontaneous clearance of the organism. Most commonly, infection is asymptomatic and there are no long-term sequelae. Although a number of bacterial factors which may be important in determining disease severity have now been identified, it seems likely that it is the combination of bacterial phenotype in association with additional host or environmental factors which dictates the final outcome of *H. pylori* infection.

Pathology is primarily associated with the gastric epithelium (Axon and Quinn, 1994; Blaser, 1990). The distribution of the organism within the stomach and the type of pathology observed may be influenced by age of acquisition, duration of infection and other factors, including therapy. The bacterium may also be isolated from the duodenum, where it is found exclusively in areas of gastric metaplasia – foci of gastric type epithelium produced by duodenal tissue in response to overexposure to gastric acid (Axon and Quinn, 1994; Blaser, 1990).

Immunopathology

The majority of *H. pylori* organisms are found associated with the gastric mucous layer which protects the organism from luminal acid. Around 10% of the organisms are actually adherent to gastric epithelial cells (Noach *et al.*, 1994). *Helicobacter pylori* initially adheres to the tips of microvilli, a process which subsequently results in disruption of gastric epithelial cell morphology, causing loss of microvillus integrity and leading to localized micro-erosions in the mucosal surface (Noach *et al.*, 1994). A reduction in the thickness of the gastric mucous layer and changes in the composition of the mucous have also been reported (Goggin and Northfield, 1993).

Histologically, acute infection is characterized by a marked polymorphonuclear leucocyte infiltration (Blaser, 1990), with chronic infection resulting in variable levels of activity (neutrophilic) and chronicity (lymphocyte infiltration). The extent of inflammation is dependent on the density of bacterial colonization. In children, the cellular infiltrate is primarily lymphocytic, organized as discrete follicles (follicular nodular gastritis).

Acute and chronic *H. pylori* infection results in the induction of localized (IgA) and systemic (IgG) antibody responses (Rathbone *et al.*, 1986), although IgM is only detectable in subjects with acute infection (Sobala *et al.*, 1991). Similar antibody responses can be detected in saliva (Patel *et al.*, 1994), and form the basis of some diagnostic assays. There is marked variation in antigen recognition in infected individuals, reflecting antigenic differences between the infecting strains. Interestingly, many infected patients have antibodies which cross-react with human gastric epithelial tissue (Negrini *et al.*, 1991). This crossreactivity may be stimulated by conserved epitopes on bacterial and mammalian heat shock proteins, and suggests that autoimmune responses may play a role in *H. pylori* gastritis.

Several groups have studied cytokine responses in *H. pylori* infection including IL-1, IL-3, IL-4 IL-6, IL-8, interferon γ and tumour necrosis factor α (Fauchere and Andersen, 1995). Of these, IL-8 has been studied in most detail and elevated levels have been detected in infected tissue. These observations have been confirmed *in vitro* using cultured biopsy material or tissue culture cell lines where enhanced synthesis of IL-8 mRNA and protein have been observed (Crabtree *et al.*, 1994).

IL-8 is a potent chemokine and activator of polymorphonuclear leucocytes (PMNs), attracting these cells to the site of infection, and several studies have shown a close correlation between tissue IL-8 concentrations, polymorph numbers and the extent of gastric tissue damage, suggesting a key role for IL-8 in promoting *H. pylori*-associated pathology. Reactive oxygen metabolites, free radicals and degradative enzymes produced by PMNs may contribute to the observed tissue damage. Other cytokines may downregulate production of specific subsets of T lymphocytes, and modulate the immune response to infection. An active suppression of T cell-mediated responses to *H. pylori* has been suggested as a mechanism to explain the failure of the immune system to eradicate *H. pylori* (Fauchere and Andersen, 1995; Fan *et al.*, 1994).

CLINICAL FEATURES

Acute Infection

Both acute and chronic *H. pylori* infection cause gastric inflammation which is frequently asymptomatic (Blaser, 1990). There are no specific symptoms or signs associated with naturally acquired acute *H. pylori* infection. However, with higher infective doses from volunteer (Marshall *et al.*, 1985) or accidental inoculation studies and iatrogenic transmission (from inadequately sterilized pH-monitoring equipment) acute infection can cause nausea, vomiting, anorexia, epigastric pain and burping.

Acute infection may be associated with a pangastritis and transient hypochlorhydria (Sobala *et al.*, 1991; Kreiss *et al.*, 1995). A factor produced by *H. pylori* which reduces acid synthesis by parietal cells *in vitro* has been identified (Jablonowski *et al.*, 1994).

Chronic Infection

In chronic infection the distribution of inflammation varies between individuals (Kreiss *et al.*, 1995; Levine and Price, 1993). The commonest finding in chronic infection is of a low-grade pangastritis (i.e. infection of the antrum and corpus of the stomach) and it is in this group of patients that gastric ulceration and gastric carcinoma may develop in a small proportion of cases. In contrast, infected patients with chronic active gastritis limited predominantly to the antrum are at increased risk of developing duodenal ulcer.

Long-standing pangastritis is associated with the development of progressive hypochlorhydria (Kreiss *et al.*, 1995).

H. pylori and Peptic Ulcer Disease

Over 75% of patients with gastric ulcers and more than 95% of those with duodenal ulcer are infected with *H. pylori* (Kuipers *et al.*, 1995). Numerous studies have shown that relapse in duodenal ulcer patients is rare in those patients in whom *H. pylori* is eradicated, suggesting a very strong link between *H. pylori* infection and duodenal ulcer (Kuipers *et al.*, 1995). Currently, however, there is no direct experimental evidence confirming a causitive role for *H. pylori* in these conditions. Duodenal ulcer is associated with chronic, predominantly antral gastritis, and occurs in approximately 10% of *H. pylori*-infected individuals (Kuipers *et al.*, 1995). It has been suggested that ulcers are more likely to develop in patients who have more severe gastritis, *H. pylori* in the gastric crypts or bacterial penetration of gastric epithelial cell intracellular junctions. Histologically, it has been shown that ulcers develop at transition sites between antral and corpus epithelia in the stomach and duodenal and gastric-type tissue in the duodenum. Ulceration is thought to be the end result of *H. pylori*-induced ultrastructural damage to the gastric or duodenal epithelium exacerbated by normal or increased acid secretion from gastric parietal cells. This in turn has been shown to be related to decreased levels of antral somatostatin resulting in a loss of the normal inhibitory effect of gastrin release from G cells and leading to an expansion in the parietal cell mass (Kreiss *et al.*, 1995).

H. pylori and Gastric Cancer

In a small proportion of patients, long term infection with *H. pylori* (up to 30–40 years) may result in development of atrophic pangastritis (Kreiss *et al.*, 1995; Levine and Price, 1993). Development of atrophic gastritis is important as it is recognized as an antecedent to gastric cancer and if progressive leads to intestinal metaplasia and dysplasia.

Loss of acid secretory function and overgrowth by other bacteria may account for the difficulty in isolating or detecting *H. pylori* by culture and histology in these patients (Forman, 1995).

DIAGNOSTIC METHODS

Invasive and non-invasive methods used in the detection of *H. pylori* infection are listed in Table 17a.3. The inaccessibility of the gastric and duodenal mucosae has been a major obstacle to diagnosis and research and has led to the development of several non-invasive methods for detecting infection.

Invasive Procedures

Gastric or duodenal biopsies obtained at endoscopy provide a source of tissue for microbiological and histological analysis.

Direct staining techniques

Helicobacter pylori can be detected by direct staining of biopsy smears using modified Gram stain or histologically in fixed tissue sections using a variety of staining methods (Dixon, 1993). Although a skilled histopathologist may be able to detect *H. pylori* by haematoxylin and eosin staining, special stains (e.g. Giemsa and modified Warthin–Starry) must be used to detect low levels of infection.

TABLE 17a.3   INVASIVE AND NON-INVASIVE TESTS USED IN DIAGNOSIS OF *H. PYLORI* INFECTION

Test	Sensitivity	Specificity	Cost[a]	Other comments	Reference
Non-invasive					
ELISA serology	84–95	82–94	+	Local validation needed	Kosunen and Megraud (1995)
Rapid antibody tests	63–75	88–92	+	Rapid preliminary result	Duggan *et al.* (1995)
^{13}C breath test	90–98	99	+ +	Unrestricted use	Atherton and Spiller (1994)
^{14}C breath test	90–98	99	+ +	No set protocol	Atherton and Spiller (1994)
Invasive					
Histology	85–90	93–100	+ + +	Useful reference	Tompkins (1993)
Culture	80–90	95–100	+	Requires experience	Tompkins (1993)
Urease test	85–95	99	+	Rapid result	Tompkins (1993)
Gram stain	91	93–100	+	Rapid result	Tompkins (1993)
PCR	94–96	100	+ +	Very sensitive	Kosunen and Megraud (1995)

[a]+, <5; + +, 5–15; + + +, .15

Culture

Microbiological culture is taken as the gold standard as proof of *H. pylori* infection but may not be as sensitive as histology in all cases. Culture is necessary, however, if antimicrobial sensitivity testing is required. Since colonization of the gastric or duodenal mucosa may be patchy, multiple biopsies from different sites (but especially the antrum) offer the best chance of detection of the bacterium. In addition, since bile reflux or treatment with powerful acid-suppressing drugs (proton pump inhibitors) may cause changes in distribution of *H. pylori* (from the antrum to the corpus of the stomach) and reduce the density of antral colonization, better isolation rates may be achieved by culturing biopsies from both sites (Tompkins, 1993; Kosunen and Megraud, 1995). Since contaminated endoscopes and biopsy forceps have been shown to act as a route of transmission of *H. pylori* infection (Tytgat, 1995), it is important that they are adequately decontaminated between patients.

Biopsies may be transported in saline or bacteriological broth media such as nutrient broth if they can be examined within three to four hours (Tompkins, 1993). If culture is delayed longer, better isolation rates are achieved if transport media such as Portagerm pylori or Stuart's transport medium are used. Transport and storage at 40 °C may also improve isolation rates. If biopsies cannot be processed immediately, they can be suspended in a cryoprotectant and snap frozen in liquid nitrogen for storage at −80 °C for at least six months without significant loss of *H. pylori* viability.

For isolation of *H. pylori* biopsies may simply be vigorously smeared onto agar plates or if quantitative data are required biopsies may first be gently homogenized in broth prior to plating. The remainder of the biopsy can be stored frozen for further study. Frequently *H. pylori* is isolated in large numbers and in pure culture from biopsies. Where contamination with other organisms is a problem, agar incorporating selective antibiotics, e.g. Dent supplement, can be used (Tompkins, 1993).

Rapid urease tests

A rapid indication of the presence of *H. pylori* in biopsies can be made using a rapid urease test directly on the biopsy material (Kosunen and Megraud, 1995). Commercially available CLO tests or cheaper home-made equivalents can be used in the endoscopy clinic and allow rapid decisions about patient management to be made at the time of endoscopy.

Polymerase chain reaction

Recent studies have shown the potential of PCR for detection of *H. pylori* in fresh or fixed gastric biopsies (Kosunen and Megraud, 1995). This technique provides a highly specific and sensitive approach to detection of *H. pylori*. To avoid false positives, it is essential that biopsy forceps are adequately cleaned between different patients (Kosunen and Megraud, 1995).

Non-invasive Techniques

Although endoscopy provides biopsy material for culture and histology and allows other non-*H. pylori*-related pathologies to be detected, expense, restricted availability and associated risks have contributed to the development of additional methods for the detection of *H. pylori* infection. In particular, urea breath tests are now increasingly used in the initial screening of patients and for monitoring the efficacy of anti-*H. pylori* therapy. Endoscopy is now often reserved for further investigation of patients with proven *H. pylori* infection or when initial therapy has proven unsuccessful.

Breath tests

Urea breath tests are based on the principle that *H. pylori* urease will hydrolyse labelled urea to produce water and labelled carbon dioxide which is absorbed into the bloodstream and exhaled in the breath (Atherton and Spiller, 1994). Patients are given a small quantity of $[^{13}C]$- or $[^{14}C]$urea orally, and a sample of exhaled breath is collected 30 minutes later for analysis for the presence of labelled carbon dioxide. Breath tests have been shown to be highly sensitive and specific for *H. pylori* infection. One major advantage over biopsy methods is that breath tests are not affected by the patchy distribution of *H. pylori* in the stomach, which may lead to false negative results at culture or histology. Urea breath tests are relatively inexpensive and can be performed by suitably trained non-medical personnel. The choice of the use of ^{13}C – a naturally occurring element – or ^{14}C is based on a number of factors, including local availability of mass spectrometry or scintillation counting facilities for analysis of breath samples and the expected frequency of testing for individual patients.

Serology

Serology has been used principally for epidemiological studies of the prevalence of *H. pylori* infection (Mendall and Pajares-Garcia, 1995). The potential use of serological responses to particular *H. pylori* antigens as a means of screening prior to endoscopy or commencement of anti-*H. pylori* therapy is now increasingly being considered. Serum IgG is most usually detected, but more recently antibody in saliva has also been used (Patel *et al.*, 1994). This antibody is thought to enter saliva from the general circulation via gingival mucosa.

A large number of commercially available enzyme-linked immunosorbent assay (ELISA)-based assays are available (Kosunen and Megraud, 1995; Schembri *et al.*, 1993). Earlier assays which used crude whole cell or glycine extracts perform reasonably well, but second- and third-generation assays have now been developed employing partially purified or recombinant antigens. Commercial kits may still need local validation to first determine cut-off points for positive and negative reactions in any given population. Quantitative assays can achieve sensitivities and specificities exceeding 95% in the hands of experienced personnel. Antibody titres may take three months or longer to show a significant decrease following successful eradication of *H. pylori*, limiting the use of serology for monitoring the efficacy of treatment at present (Kosunen and Megraud, 1995).

ANTIMICROBIAL SENSITIVITIES

Helicobacter pylori is sensitive to a wide range of antibiotics *in vitro* (Tytgat, 1994). These include the penicillins, macrolides and nitroimidazoles. Two other compounds used in the treatment of *H. pylori* infection – bismuth salts and the proton pump inhibitors lansoprazole and omeprazole – also have anti-*H. pylori* activity *in vitro*.

Frequently, antibiotic sensitivity testing is not performed prior to commencement of treatment, since this requires isolation of the infecting organism from biopsies collected at endoscopy. Although eradication of infection may be achieved in a high percentage of cases without prior testing, the emergence of antibiotic resistance has become a problem in many countries, and the requirement for sensitivity testing has therefore increased. At present there are no internationally agreed standard methods for sensitivity testing for *H. pylori*. Disc diffusion or plate incorporation methods for minimal inhibitor concentration (MIC) and breakpoint determinations have been used extensively (Glupczynski, 1996). MIC_{50}, MIC_{90} and MBC testing has been used, but the relative clinical relevance of these values has yet to be shown. More recently, E tests have been employed for MIC testing of *H. pylori* (Glupczynski *et al.*, 1991). This system is easy to use and has the advantage that resistant variants can be readily detected growing in the zone of inhibition around the antibiotic strip.

Although these methods have failed to detect significant resistance to penicillins, higher variable levels of resistance to the macrolides and nitroimidazoles have been found (Tytgat, 1994; Glupczynski, 1996). For example, stable resistance to metronidazole varies with the population tested. In developing countries where metronidazole is widely used to treat diarrhoeal disease, up to 90% of *H. pylori* isolates may be resistant to metronidazole. In contrast, resistance in the UK is estimated between 10% and 25%. The exact mechanism of metronidazole resistance is at present unclear and reduced drug penetration, decreased nitroreduction and enhanced DNA repair mechanisms have all been proposed. The activity of metronidazole is associated with its reduction, and recent evidence suggests that pyruvate oxidoreductase activity is lower in metronidazole-resistant isolates (Hoffman *et al.*, 1995). Resistance to tetracycline and clarithromycin have also been reported. Clarithromycin resistance, which may be unstable, has been shown to be due to post-transcriptional adenylation and point mutations in *H. pylori* 23S ribosomal RNA which decrease the affinity of the drug for ribosomes (Versavolic *et al.*, 1995).

MANAGEMENT OF INFECTION

The recognition of the role of *H. pylori* infection in the pathogenesis of peptic ulcer disease has revolutionized the treatment of these conditions. The importance of treating ulcers with antibacterials was reinforced in 1994 by a statement from the National Institutes of Health (NIH), who recommended *H. pylori* eradication in all patients with duodenal ulcer disease (NIH, 1994). Earlier approaches to treating ulcers based solely on long-term suppression of acid secretion as the principal mode of treatment have now been replaced by combined one- or two-week therapies employing both acid suppression and antibacterials. Eradication of *H. pylori* using these treatment regimens has resulted in a marked reduction in the relapse of peptic ulcer.

Initial attempts to eradicate *H. pylori* infection using long-term bismuth therapy proved largely unsuccessful because bismuth salts failed to penetrate the gastric pits and only killed *H. pylori* exposed on the surface of the gastric mucosa (Tytgat, 1994). Antibiotic therapy was then introduced, but despite studies showing sensitivity of *H. pylori* to a range of antimicrobials *in vitro* early results using antimicrobial monotherapy and bismuth subcitrate were disappointing. Eradication rates were relatively low and recrudescence of infection was common. In addition, the use of antibiotic monotherapy therapeutically was associated with rapid development of antibiotic resistance (Tytgat, 1994). Low gastric pH, which affects the activity of penicillins, poor penetration of antibiotics through the mucous layer and difficulty in maintaining therapeutic levels of orally administered antibiotics in the stomach, all contribute to therapeutic failure. The possibility that *H. pylori* avoids antibacterials by migrating to so-called 'sanctuary' sites in the stomach has also been proposed.

Triple therapy, using bismuth and two antibacterials – metronidazole, which is active at low pH, and tetracycline in combination – improved eradication rates (Tytgat, 1994). Although achieving better results, the complexity, long duration and associated side effects of this regimen often caused poor patient compliance (which together with primary resistance to metronidazole) resulted in failure to eradicate *H. pylori*. Despite these limitations, triple therapy is still used in some centres, where eradication rates of >90% have been reported. Triple therapy may also be combined with the use of proton pump inhibitors.

Dual therapies (proton pump inhibitors, e.g. omeprazole, and amoxicillin) were developed to overcome problems associated with bismuth-based triple therapy (Tytgat, 1994). However, results were highly variable. Smoking, poor patient compliance and dosing affected efficacy.

Two weeks' treatment with omeprazole and clarithromycin – the most effective antibiotic monotherapy for *H. pylori* infection – has higher eradication rates (75–80% of patients). Omeprazole modifies the pharamacokinetics of clarithromycin *in vivo*, raising concentrations in the gastric mucous and gastric antrum and increasing the plasma half-life (Tytgat, 1994). The efficacy of this regimen is also unaffected by smoking and currently less than 10% of *H. pylori* isolates show primary resistance to clarithromycin.

New therapeutic strategies are still being developed. One-week, low-dose triple therapy with omeprazole, clarithromycin and metronidazole or tinadazole has been reported to achieve eradication in 90–100% of patients in different trials (Kreiss *et al.*, 1995). Amoxicillin can be substituted for the nitroimidazoles.

Currently treatment of *H. pylori* non-ulcer infection is not recommended. Although *H. pylori* treatment in patients with MALToma has resulted in remission in some cases (Wotherspoon *et al.*, 1993), the benefits of treating a *H. pylori*-infected subject at risk of developing gastric cancer has yet to be established in suitably designed clinical trials.

VACCINE DEVELOPMENT

At present there are no vaccines available for prevention of *H. pylori* infection. The development of antibiotic resistance, the high prevalence of *H. pylori* infection in both developed and particularly developing countries and the association of infection with development of gastric cancer have however, provided the impetus for initiation of studies assessing the feasibility of vaccine development (Covacci *et al.*, 1995; Ghiara and Michetti, 1995).

Animal Models of *Helicobacter* Infection

In common with vaccine development programmes for other microbial pathogens, the availability of animal models which mimic *H. pylori* infection and disease symptoms is a prerequisite for vaccine testing. Although such models have been developed, none yet reproduce exactly the spectrum or topography of pathologies seen with *H. pylori* infection in humans (Covacci *et al.*, 1995; Ghiara and Michetti, 1995).

The earliest studies showed that non-human primates, gnotobiotic pigs and beagles could be experimentally infected with *H. pylori*. Although these models show some of the characteristic pathology associated with *H. pylori* gastritis in humans, the expense and restricted availability of such models have limited their use. Attempts to develop small animal models of *H. pylori* infection in rodents such as conventional mice and rats initially failed, though immunodeficient animals could be colonized. More recently, it has been shown that fresh clinical isolates, but not those repeatedly passaged *in vitro*, can infect conventional Balb/c mice (Marchetti *et al.*, 1995). This model again produces some but not all of the pathology associated with *H. pylori* gastritis in humans and may be a promising system in which to test potential vaccine candidates.

In addition to infection models which use *H. pylori*, two other *Helicobacter* spp. have been used extensively for vaccine studies. *Helicobacter felis* readily infects conventional mice, where it induces a chronic non-active gastritis, but unlike *H. pylori* does not adhere to gastric epithelial cells and *H. felis* does not produce CagA or VacA (Covacci *et al.*, 1995; Ghiara and Michetti, 1995). *Helicobacter mustelae* causes gastritis and uniquely for models of *Helicobacter* infection also induces ulcer formation in ferrets (Covacci *et al.*, 1995; Ghiara and Michetti, 1995). This latter model therefore provides a system in which the pathogenesis of ulcer disease and its prevention may be more readily assessed.

Disease models which use crude *H. pylori* extracts or purified subcellular components to induce pathology in the absence of infection have also been developed (Covacci *et al.*, 1995; Ghiara and Michetti, 1995). Antigens from both *H. pylori* and *H. felis* have been used in protection studies in disease models in mice.

Candidate Antigens and Immunization Strategy

Since *H. pylori* is a pathogen of the gastric mucosa, vaccination should ideally stimulate protective local mucosal immune responses. Immunogens which may induce autoimmune reactions or downregulate cell-mediated responses should be avoided if possible. Immunization with purified, preferably recombinant antigens which are conserved across all *H. pylori* strains would therefore appear to be the most promising in terms of vaccine development.

Orally administered *H. pylori* urease or its subunits, given with cholera toxin as an adjuvant, have been shown to protect mice from chronic infection with *H. felis* (Covacci *et al.*, 1995; Ghiara and Michetti, 1995). The immune response generated is complex but anti-urease IgA production appears important in protection and anti-urease IgA given orally to mice is also protective. Worryingly, however, some studies have shown that immunization may itself induce gastritis in the *H. felis* mouse model. Immunization with purified urease and *Escherichia coli* heat-labile toxin (LT) prevented colonization by *H. pylori* in Balb/c mice. *Helicobacter pylori* heat shock protein HspA, administered orally to mice, has recently been shown to protect against *H. felis* infection. The previous observation that *H. pylori* heat shock proteins have been associated with development of autoimmune reactions (Covacci *et al.*, 1995; Ghiara and Michetti, 1995) suggests that the use of these proteins as immunogens has to be viewed with caution.

Although VacA is not produced by all *H. pylori* strains, its association with peptic ulcer disease makes it a potential candidate antigen for vaccine development (Covacci *et al.*, 1995; Ghiara and

Michetti, 1995). Oral administration of purified VacA and *E. coli* LT has been shown to protect mice from subsequent challenge with *H. pylori*. Since VacA seems to be capable of inducing significant damage to gastric mucosal tissue, the use of genetically detoxified VacA as an immunogen would seem to be required for use in humans.

Although these studies indicate the potential for vaccination against *H. pylori* infection, several major areas require further investigation before clinical trials could be undertaken in humans. Antigen selection to avoid induction of gastritis and the development of suitable adjuvants and delivery systems need to be addressed. Decisions about which populations should be vaccinated and when need to be made and the cost implications of large-scale vaccination programmes balanced against those currently associated with *H. pylori* therapies.

Therapeutic Vaccination

Since prophylactic treatment of animals with *H. pylori* antigens has been shown to protect against later bacterial challenge, the possibility of using therapeutic immunization to eradicate established infection has also been addressed (Covacci *et al.*, 1995; Ghiara and Michetti, 1995). Two studies in mice, and a third in ferrets, have shown elimination of *Helicobacter* infection following oral administration of bacterial antigens, raising the possibility of using a similar approach for therapy in humans.

ACKNOWLEDGEMENT

The author would like to thank Dr R.P.H. Logan for his assistance in the preparation of this work.

REFERENCES

Atherton, J.C. and Spiller, R.C. (1994) The urea breath test for *Helicobacter pylori*. *Gut*, **35**, 723–725.

Atherton, J.C., Cao, P., Peek, R.M., Jr *et al.* (1995) Mosaicism in vacuolating cytotoxin alleles of *Helicobacter pylori*: association of specific *vacA* types with cytotoxin production and peptic ulceration. *Journal of Biological Chemistry*, **270**, 17771–17777.

Axon, A.T.R. and Quina, M. (1994) Ten year milestones. *Current Opinion in Gastroenterology*, **10** (Suppl. 1), 1–5.

Blaser, M.J. (1990) *Helicobacter pylori* and the pathogenesis of gastroduodenal inflammation. *Journal of Infectious Diseases*, **161**, 626–633.

Bode, G., Mauch, F. and Malfertheimer, P. (1993) The coccoid forms of *Helicobacter pyori*: criteria for their viability. *Epidemiology and Infection*, **111**, 483–490.

Covacci, A., Chiara, P. and Rappoul, R. (1995) *Helicobacter pylori*: pathogenesis and feasibility of vaccine development. In *Molecular and Clinical Aspects of Bacterial Vaccine Development* (ed. D.A.A. Ala'Aldeen and C.E. Hormaeche), pp. 323–348. Wiley, Chichester.

Crabtree, J.E., Farmery, S.M., Lindley, I.J.D. *et al.* (1994) CagA/cytotoxic strains of *Helicobacter pylori* and interleukin-8 in gastric epithelial cell lines. *Journal of Clinical Pathology*, **47**, 945–950.

Dixon, M. (1993) Histological diagnosis. In *Helicobacter pylori Infection* (ed. T.C. Northfield, M. Mendall and P.M. Goggin), pp. 110–115. Kluwer, Dordrecht.

Drazek, E.S., Dubois, A., Holmes, R.K. *et al.* (1995) Cloning and characterization of hemolytic genes from *Helicobacter pylori*. *Infection and Immunity*, **63**, 4345–4349.

Duggan, A.E., Knifton, A. and Logan, R.P.H. (1995) Validation of two rapid blood tests for *H. pylori*. *Gut*, **37** (Suppl. 1), A58 (abstract).

Eurogast Study Group (1994) Epidemiology of, and risk factors for *Helicobacter pylori* infection among 3194 asymptomatic subjects in 17 populations. *Gut*, **34**, 1672–1676.

Evans, D.J., Jr, Evans, D.G., Takemura, T. *et al.* (1995) Characterization of a *Helicobacter pylori* neutrophil-activating protein. *Infection and Immunity*, **63**, 2213–2220.

Fan, X.J., Chua, A., Shahi, C.N. *et al.* (1994) Gastric T lymphocyte response to *Helicobacter pylori* in patients with *H. pylori* colonisation. *Gut*, **35**, 1379–1384.

Fauchere, J.L. and Andersen, L.F.P. (1995) Immunological aspects. *Current Opinion in Gastroenterology*, **11** (Suppl. 1), 21–24.

Forman, D. (1995) The prevalence of *Helicobacter pylori* infection in gastric cancer. *Alimentary and Pharmacology and Therapeutics*, **9** (Suppl. 2), 71–76.

Fox, J.G. (1995) Non-human reservoirs of *Helicobacter pylori*. *Alimentary and Pharmacology and Therapeutics*, **9** (Suppl. 2), 93–103.

Fox, J.G., Yan, L.L., Dewhirst, F.E. *et al.* (1995) *Helicobacter bilis* sp. nov., a novel *Helicobacter* species isolated from bile, livers and intestines of aged inbred mice. *Journal of Clinical Microbiology*, **33**, 445–454.

Ghiara, P. and Michetti, P. (1995) Development of a vaccine. *Current Opinion in Gastroenterology*, **52–56**, 52–56.

Glupczynski, Y. (1996) Culture of *Helicobacter pylori* from gastric biopsies and antimicrobial sensitivity testing. In *Helicobacter pylori*: *Techniques for Clinical Diagnosis and Basic Research* (ed. A. Lee and F. Megraud), pp. 17–32. Saunders, Philadelphia.

Glupczynski, Y., Labbe, M., Hansen, W. *et al.* (1991) Evaluation of the E test for quantitative antimicrobial sensitivity testing of *Helicobacter pylori*. *Journal of Clinical Microbiology*, **29**, 2072–2075.

Goddard, A. and Logan, R. (1995) One-week-low-dose triple therapy: new standards for *Helicobacter pylori* treatment. *European Journal of Gastroenterology and Hepatology*, **7**, 1–3.

Goggin, P. and Northfield, T. (1993) Mucosal defence. In *Helicobacter pylori Infection* (ed. T.C. Northfield, M. Mendall and P.M. Goggin), pp. 62–74. Kluwer, Dordrecht.

Goodwin, C.S. (1993) Historical and microbiological perspectives. In *Helicobacter pylori Infection* (ed. T.C. Northfield, M. Mendall and P.M. Goggin), pp. 1–10. Kluwer, Dordrecht.

Goodwin, C.S. and Armstrong, G.A. (1990) Microbiological aspects of *Helicobacter pylori* (*Campylobacter pylori*). *European Journal of Clinical Microbiology and Infectious Diseases*, **9**, 1–13.

Goodwin, C.S., Armstrong, G.A., Chilvers, T. *et al.* (1989) Transfer of *Campylobacter pylori* and *Campylobacter mustelae* to *Helicobacter* gen. nov. and *Helicobacter pylori* comb. nov. and *Helicobacter mustelae* comb. nov., respectively. *International Journal of Systematic Bacteriology*, **39**, 397–405.

Handt, L.K., Fox, J.G., Dewhirst, F.E. *et al.* (1994) *Helicobacter pylori* isolated from the domestic cat: public health implications. *Infection and Immunity*, **62**, 2367–2374.

Hoffman, P.S., Goodwin, A., Johnsen, J. and Veldhuyzen van Zanten, S. (1995) Metabolic pathways in metronidazole sensitive and resistant strains of *Helicobacter pylori*. *Gut*, **37** (Suppl. 1), A66 (abstract).

International Agency for Research on Cancer (1994) *Schistosomes, Liver Flukes and Helicobacter pylori*, Vol. 61, pp. 177–241. IARC, Lyon, 177–241.

Jablonowski, H., Hengels, K.J., Kraemer, N. *et al.* (1994) Effects of *Helicobacter pylori* on histamine and carbachol stimulated acid secretion by human parietal cells. *Gut*, **35**, 755–757.

Kosunen, T.U. and Megraud, F. (1995) Diagnosis of *Helicobacter pylori*. *Current Opinion in Gastroenterology*, **11** (Suppl. 1), 5–10.

Kreiss, C., Blum, A.L. and Malfertheimer, P. (1995) Peptic ulcer pathogenesis. *Current Opinion in Gastroenterology*, **11**, (Suppl. 1), 25–31.

Kuipers, E.J., Thijs, J.C. and Festen, P.M. (1995) The prevalence of *Helicobacter pylori* in peptic ulcer disease. *Alimentary and Pharmacology and Therapeutics*, **9**, (Suppl. 2), 59–69.

Levine, T. and Price, A. (1993) The precancer – cancer sequence. In *Helicobacter pylori Infection* (ed. T.C. Northfield, M. Mendall and P.M. Goggin), pp. 88–98. Kluwer, Dordrecht.

Logan, R.P.H., Cockayne, A., Hawkey, C.J. and Borriello, S.P. (1995) Chemotactic response to mucus and acid by *Helicobacter pylori*. *Gut*, **37** (Suppl. 1), A64 (abstract).

Marchetti, M., Arico, B., Burroni, D. *et al.* (1995) Development of a mouse model of *Helicobacter pylori* infection that mimics human disease. *Science*, **267**, 1655–1658.

Marshall, B.J. and Goodwin, C.S. (1987) Revised nomenclature of *Campylobacter pyloridis*. *International Journal of Systematic Bacteriology*, **37**, 68.

Marshall, B.J., Armstrong, J.A., McGechie, D.B. and Glancy, R.J. (1985) Attempt to fulfil Koch's postulates for pyloric *Campylobacter*. *Medical Journal of Australia*, **142**, 436–439.

Megraud, F. (1995) Transmission of *Helicobacter pylori*: faecal–oral versus oral–oral. *Alimentary and Pharmacological Therapy*, **9**.(Suppl. 2), 85–92.

Mendall, M.A. and Pajares-Garcia, J. (1995) Epidemiology and transmission of *Helicobacter pylori*. *Current Opinion in Gastroenterology*, **11** (Suppl. 1), 1–4.

Negrini, R., Lisato, L., Zanelli, I. *et al.*, (1991) *Helicobacter pylori* infection induces antibodies cross-reacting with gastroduodenal tissues. *Gastroenterology*, **101**, 437–445.

Nielsen, H., Birkholz, S., Andersen, L.P. and Moran, A.P. (1994) Neutrophil activation by *Helicobacter pylori* lipopolysaccharides. *Journal of Infectious Diseases*, **170**, 135–139.

NIH Consensus Development Panel on *Helicobacter pylori* in peptic ulcer disease (1994), *Journal of the American Medical Association*, **272**, 65–69.

Noach, L.A., Rolf, T.M. and Tytgat, G.N.J. (1994) Electron microscopic study of association between *Helicobacter pylori* and gastric and duodenal mucosa. *Journal of Clinical Pathology*, **47**, 699–704.

Owen, R.J., Bickley, J., Hurtando, A. *et al.* (1994) Comparison of PCR-based restriction length polymorphism analysis of urease genes with *rRNA* gene profiling for monitoring *Helicobacter pylori* infections in patients on triple therapy. *Journal of Clinical Microbiology*, **32**, 1203–1210.

Parsonnet, J., Hansen, S., Rodriquez, L. *et al.* (1994) *Helicobacter pylori* infection and gastric lymphoma. *New England Journal of Medicine*, **330**, 1267–1271.

Patel, P., Mendall, M.A., Khulusi, S. *et al.* (1994) Salivary antibodies to *Helicobacter pylori*: screening dyspeptic patients before endoscopy. *Lancet*, **344**, 511–512.

Rathbone, B.J., Wyatt, J.I., Worsley, B.W. *et al.* (1986) Systemic and local antibody responses to gastric *Campylobacter pyloridis* in non-ulcer patients. *Gut*, **27**, 642–647.

Rice, J.M. (1995) *Helicobacter hepaticus*, a recently recognised bacterial pathogen, associated with chronic hepatitis and hepatocellular neoplasia in laboratory mice. *Emerging Infectious Diseases*, **1**, 129–131.

Schembri, M.A., Lin, S.K. and Lambert, J.R. (1993) Comparison of commercial diagnostic tests for *Helicobacter pylori* antibodies. *Journal of Clinical Microbiology*, **31**, 2621–2624.

Sherburne, R. and Taylor, D.E. (1995) *Helicobacter pylori* expresses a complex surface carbohydrate, Lewis X. *Infection and Immunity*, **63**, 4564–4568.

Smith, A.W., Chahal, B. and French, G.L. (1994) The human gastric pathogen *Helicobacter pylori* has a gene encoding an enzyme first classified as a mucinase in *Vibrio cholerae*. *Molecular Microbiology*, **13**, 153–160.

Sobala, G.M., Crabtree, J.E., Dixon, M.F. *et al.* (1991) Acute *Helicobacter pylori* infection: clinical features, local systemic immune response and gastric juice ascorbic acid concentrations. *Gut*, **32**, 1415–1418.

Spiegelhalder, C., Gerstenecker, B., Kersten, A. *et al.* (1993) Purification of *Helicobacter pylori* superoxide dismutase and cloning and sequencing of the gene. *Infection and Immunity*, **61**, 5315–5325.

Suerbaum, S. and Wadstrom, T. (1995) Bacterial pathogenic factors. *Current Opinion in Gastroenterology*, **11** (Suppl. 1), 11–15.

Taylor, N.S., Fox, J.G., Akopyants, N.S. *et al.* (1995) Long-term colonization with single and multiple strains of. *Helicobacter pylori* assessed by DNA fingerprinting. *Journal of Clinical Microbiology*, **33**, 918–923.

Tompkins, D. (1993) Microbiological tests. In *Helicobacter pylori Infection* (ed. T.C. Northfield, M. Mendall and P.M. Goggin) pp. 116–126. Kluwer, Dordrecht.

Tummuru, M.K.R., Sharma, S.A. and Blaser, M.J. (1995) *Helicobacter pylori picB*, a homologue of the *Bordetella pertussis* secretion protein, is required for induction of IL-8 in gastric epithelial cells. *Molecular Microbiology*, **18**, 867–876.

Tytgat, G.N.J. (1994) Treatments that impact favourably upon the eradication of *Helicobacter pylori* and ulcer recurrence. *Alimentary and Pharmacological Therapy*, **8**, 359–368.

Tytgat, G.N.J. (1995) Endoscopic transmission of *Helicobacter pylori*. *Alimentary and Pharmacological Therapy*, **9** (Suppl. 2), 105–110.

Versavolic, J., Kibler, K., Small, S. *et al.* (1995) Molecular basis of clarythromycin resistance in *Helicobacter pylori*. *Gastroenterology*, **108**, A250 (abstract).

Westblom, T., Fritz, S., Phadnis, S. *et al.* (1993) PCR analysis of Peruvian sewage water: support for fecal–oral spread of *Helicobacter pylori*. *Acta Gastro-enterologica Belgica*, **56** (Suppl.), abstract 47.

Wotherspoon, A.C., Doglioni, C., Diss, T.C. *et al.* (1993) Regression of primary low-grade B-cell lymphoma of mucosa-associated lymphoid tissue type after eradication of *Helicobacter pylori*. *Lancet*, **342**, 575–577.

Xiang, Z., Censini, S., Bayeli, P.F. *et al.* (1995) Analysis of expression of CagA and VacA virulence factors in 43 strains of *Helicobacter pylori* reveals that clinical isolates can be divided into two major types and that CagA is not necessary for expression of the vacuolating cytotoxin. *Infection and Immunity*, **63**, 94–98.

17b

CAMPYLOBACTER AND *ARCOBACTER*

J.L. Penner and S.D. Mills

INTRODUCTION

The family Campylobacteraceae includes two genera, *Campylobacter* and *Arcobacter*. The new family was proposed in 1991 as an outcome of phylogenetic studies that questioned the existing taxonomy of groups of Gram-negative spiral-shaped bacteria (Vandamme and De Ley, 1991). The revised scheme is a welcome development as classification has been a source of debate and confusion since the 1970s when serious attention first focused on these groups (Butzler *et al.*, 1973; Dekeyser *et al.*, 1972; Skirrow 1977). A number of important taxonomic issues were resolved through studies that exploited DNA–rRNA hybridization, DNA–DNA hybridization and 16S rRNA sequencing. It was found that *Campylobacter* and *Arcobacter*, although different, are nevertheless sufficiently related to be included in the same family, whereas the genus *Helicobacter* is too unrelated to *Campylobacter* and *Arcobacter* to be included. Phenotypic characteristics by which the species of *Campylobacter* and *Arcobacter* can be differentiated were also identified, providing support for this latest in taxonomy (Thompson *et al.*, 1988; Vandamme *et al.*, 1991, 1992b). The species currently in the two genera are of importance not only to medical and veter-

inary science, but some species are also of interest to investigators in the field of dental pathology. Four species have been assigned to the genus *Arcobacter*: two that have been transferred from the genus *Campylobacter* and two recently described species that have been implicated in disease production in humans and animals.

Although the revisions have provided a timely and much-needed clarification of the physiological and genetic relationships among members of the family, there is marked diversity among the species with respect to natural habitats, potential for disease production and procedures for isolation and culturing in the laboratory. Habitats may occur in the oral cavity of the human, the intestinal tracts of either humans or animals or of both, the genital tracts of cattle and, in the case of one species, the sediments in salt marshes. The varieties of diseases caused include diarrhoea, bacteremia, septic abortion, infertility and possibly diseases of human teeth. Considerable variation also exists among the species in the temperature, the atmospheric conditions and the composition of the medium for their optimum isolation and culturing in the laboratory. Paradoxically, the diversity is not mirrored in a spectrum of discriminating phenotypic characteristics by which the genera and species can be differentiated

Principles and Practice of Clinical Bacteriology. Edited by A.M. Emmerson, P.M. Hawkey and S.H. Gillespie
© 1997 John Wiley & Sons Ltd

readily and, therefore, identification and classification continue to remain a challenging problem for the clinical laboratory.

PROPERTIES OF THE FAMILY CAMPYLOBACTERACEAE

Eleven species are recognized which are curved, S-shaped or spiral Gram-negative rods. Two species, *C. showae* and *C. rectus*, produce only straight rods. Campylobacteria may stain poorly with Gram counterstains other than carbol or basic fuchsin. The cells vary in length from 0.5 μm to 8 μm and in width from 0.2 μm to 0.9 μm. All the species have a darting type of motility produced by the action of unsheathed flagella. There may be a single polar flagellum or bipolar flagella in all species except *C. showae*, which has a cluster of two to five flagella at one end. Spores are not produced but spherical coccal forms have been observed in some species in older cultures or under unfavorable growth conditions.

A characteristic common to all Campylobacteraceae is their ability to grow under microaerophilic conditions. None of the species ferment or oxidize carbohydrates and all species utilize organic amino acids as sources of carbon. All species of the family except *A. nitrofigilis* are either commensals or pathogens of humans or animals. *Arcobacter nitrofigilis* is unique in the family in its ability to fix nitrogen and in its association with the roots of halophytic plants. A list of the species is provided in Table 17b.1.

The genus *Campylobacter*

Bacteria of the genus *Campylobacter* remain largely unfamiliar to the general public although their importance to human health is as great, or greater, than the well-known *Salmonella*, *Shigella*

TABLE 17b.1   CLASSIFICATION OF CAMPYLOBACTERACEAE

Genus *Campylobacter*
Group 1. Thermophilic enteropathogenic species
   C. jejuni subsp. *jejuni*
   C. jejuni subsp. *doylei*
   C. coli
   C. lari
   C. upsaliensis
   C. helveticus

Group 2. Animal pathogens and commensals that may infect humans
   C. fetus subsp. *fetus*
   C. fetus subsp. *venerealis*
   C. hyointestinalis
   C. sputorum biovar sputorum
   C. sputorum biovar bubulus
   C. sputorum biovar fecalis
   C. mucosalis

Group 3. Species associated with periodontal disease
   C. concisus
   C. curvus
   C. rectus
   C. showae

Genus *Arcobacter*
   A. nitrofigilis
   A. cryaerophilus
   A. butzleri
   A. skirrowii

Note: The type species of genus *Campylobacter* and genus *Arcobacter* are *C. fetus* subsp. *fetus* and *A. nitrofigilis*.

and verotoxin-producing *Escherichia coli*. The earliest report that campylobacteria were responsible for human illness was by King, who referred to them as 'related vibrios' to distinguish them from species of *Vibrio*, e.g. *V. cholerae* (King, 1957, 1962). It took more than a decade before the association of these organisms with human diarrhoea was convincingly demonstrated (Dekeyser *et al.*, 1972; Butzler *et al.*, 1973); However, it was not until a medium was designed for isolating the organisms routinely that widespread interest in the bacteria emerged and their true significance to human health was established (Skirrow, 1977). The phylogenetic studies undertaken in recent years have played a dominant role in clarifying the taxonomic relationships between *Campylobacter* and related organisms. The important changes in taxonomy were the creation of two new genera, *Arcobacter* and *Helicobacter*, to which species were transferred from the genus *Campylobacter*. However, four new species have recently been assigned to *Campylobacter* to produce the present list of 13. These can be conveniently separated into three groups on the basis of phenotypic characteristics (Table 17b.1). The first and most important group to human health consists of five thermophilic enteropathogenic species. In this group are *C. jejuni*, with two subspecies, *C. coli*, *C. lari*, *C. upsaliensis* and *C. helveticus*. A second group includes four species well known to veterinary microbiologists because of their frequent occurrence as pathogens or commensals in farm livestock, although some species have been shown to be pathogenic for humans. Included are *Campylobacter fetus*, with two subspecies, *C. hyointestinalis*, *C. sputorum* with three biovars and *C. mucosalis*. A third group, found in human periodontal disease, consists of *C. concisus* and three recent additions to the genus: *C. curvus*, *C. rectus* and *C. showae*.

Genetics and Pathogenicity

Genetic analysis of *Campylobacter* spp. had to await the development of molecular techniques specific for these organisms. DNA has been successfully introduced into *C. jejuni* subsp. *jejuni* by natural transformation, electrotransformation or conjugation (Taylor, 1992a). However, not all strains appeared to be competent and plasmid DNA transformed with low frequency regardless of the technique. Several shuttle vector series are now available for *Campylobacter* genes and these can be used for cloning, expression systems, sequence analysis and for site-specific mutagenesis (Taylor *et al.*, 1992a; Yao *et al.*, 1993). These vectors were not functional for genes from *C. hyointestinalis* and so a separate vector has been developed (Waterman *et al.*, 1993).

Genes cloned from various *Campylobacter* spp. now number over 20 and most of these are listed along with the method used to obtain them in a recent review (Taylor, 1992a). The chromosomal genes which have been stably expressed in *E. coli* include amino acid biosynthesis genes, ribosomal RNA genes and transfer RNA genes. One of the genes (*flbA*) involved in flagellar biogenesis in *C. jejuni* subsp. *jejuni* was cloned although expression in *E. coli* was not detected (Miller *et al.*, 1993). All of these genes are general housekeeping genes and appear to be highly conserved across species boundaries.

Flagellar genes

Several attempts have been made to clone toxin genes as well as membrane proteins from *C. jejuni* subsp. *jejuni* but none of these efforts has resulted in stable, entire clones (Calva *et al.*, 1989; Taylor, 1992a). The only virulence-related genes that have been cloned from *C. jejuni* subsp. *jejuni* are related to flagella biosynthesis; however, no expression of gene products in *E. coli* has ever been detected. Both *C. jejuni* subsp. *jejuni* and *C. coli* produce two flagellin genes, *flaA* and *flaB*, which have strong sequence homology but differ in their regulatory mechanisms (Guerry *et al.*, 1992; Taylor, 1992a). Although both protein products are present in flagella, mutations in the *flaA* gene induce the synthesis of truncated flagella which result in only partial motility, whereas *flaB* mutations do not alter the length of the flagella or the motility of the cell. The presence of two flagellin genes in *Campylobacter* may enable cells harboring a defective *flaA* gene to restore full motility by a recombination which has been demonstrated (Wassenaar *et al.*, 1985).

Phase variation

Phase variation in *Campylobacter* spp. occurs relatively frequently *in vitro* and the transition from aflagellate to flagellate has also been observed *in vivo* by passage through the rabbit intestine (Caldwell *et al.*, 1985). The genetic mechanism for this is unknown but may involve turning off or on of the expression of the *flaA* gene. *Campylobacter* spp. are also able reversibly to express flagella of different antigenic specificities and, at least in some cases, this corresponds to the production of multiple flagellins and to a DNA rearrangement (Guerry *et al.*, 1992). A recombination event within the hypervariable sequences in the internal region of the *fla* genes may account for this rearrangement but the exact mechanism is unknown.

Surface problems

Virulence-related surface layer proteins (S proteins) from *C. fetus* have been cloned (*sapA* genes) and will express in *E. coli* (Blaser and Gotschlich, 1990). It was shown that wild-type and S⁻ mutants possessed several *sapA* homologs but that only the mutants lacked expression sequences (Tummuru and Blaser, 1993). Comparison of *sapA* sequences from a pair of variant strains suggested that antigenic variation had occurred as a result of site-specific recombination of unique coding regions. The occurrence of Guillain-Barré syndrome (GBS) following infection with *C. jejuni* (in particular serotype 0:19) has provoked much interest. It has been found that lipopolysaccharides extracted from *C. jejuni* have core oligosaccharides with terminal structures resembling human gangliosides G_{M1} and G_{D1a} (Aspinall *et al.*, 1994). The difficulties that have been experienced during the cloning of *Campylobacter* genes are numerous and include both the failure to express the gene in *E. coli* and the instability of the genes in this host. The possible reasons for this

may include differences in methylation between species, differences in promoter sequences used, the high A–T content of *Campylobacter* DNA, and/or the lack of accessory proteins which might enable expression. As well, *C. hyointestinalis* was shown to have a restriction barrier against DNA from other *Campylobacter* spp. (Waterman *et al.*, 1993).

Considerable effort has been made to construct a physical map of the *C. jejuni* subsp. *jejuni* and *C. coli* chromosomes using the technique of pulsed-field gel electrophoresis (Taylor, 1992a). It appears that the genome of campylobacteria is a single circular molecule of approximately 1.7–1.8 Mbase, which is only one-third of the size of the *E. coli* chromosome. This is consistent with the small size of these organisms, their fastidious nature and their biochemical inertness. To date, 24 genes have been assigned a place on this genetic map (Kim *et al.*, 1993). A recent advance has been the cloning of the gene for hippurate hydrolysis (benzoyl glycine aminohydrolase) in *C. jejuni* (Hani and Chan, 1995). Since the gene was shown to be absent from other *Campylobacter* spp. it is now possible to produce a species-specific diagnostic probe that would be more sensitive than the biochemical test for hippurate hydrolysis.

Thermophilic Enteropathogenic Campylobacteria: Clinical Significance, Occurrence and Epidemiology

Thermophilic enteropathogenic species, with few exceptions, are isolated from the intestinal tracts of humans and/or animals at 42–43 °C. *Campylobacter jejuni* subsp. *jejuni* is recognized as the most important cause of *Campylobacter* enteritis (campylobacteriosis) in humans occurring in 89–93% of the cases. *Campylobacter coli* is most closely related to *C. jejuni* and is the cause of 7–10% of the human cases, while *C. lari* is the cause of only 0.1–0.2% (Healing *et al.*, 1992). The frequency of infections in the human population due to these three species is difficult to estimate precisely but incidences ranging from 6–7 per 100 000 to 87 per 100 000 have been reported in the USA and the UK (Skirrow and

Blaser, 1992). Most infections are due to sporadic cases: a UK national case–control study showed that exposure to raw meat, a pet with diarrhoea and drinking untreated water were all significantly associated with such cases (Adak *et al.*, 1995), family outbreaks and larger community outbreaks arising from contaminated food, water or unpasteurized milk. The bacteria have also been implicated in travellers' diarrhoea. In developing countries it is the paediatric population in which the largest number of cases occur. Incidences as high as 40 000 per 100 000 have been reported and most of these occur in children two years old or younger. The adult population in the underdeveloped world is much less affected, presumably owing to the development of immunity during childhood exposure. Isolates of these three thermophilic species are rarely recovered from healthy humans in developed countries but they can be obtained almost as frequently from healthy children as from children with diarrhoea in underdeveloped countries (Taylor, 1992b).

The campylobacteriosis produced in humans by these three thermophilic species varies from a mild short-term diarrhoea of two days to a severe form that may last a week or longer. The diarrhoea is watery and may contain blood. Vomiting only occurs in a small percentage of cases. The diarrhoea may be accompanied by severe pain, leading to suspicions of acute appendicitis, cholecystitis or peritonitis. Complications are infrequent but include septicaemia, reactive arthritis, GBS erythema nodosum and meningitis.

C. jejuni *subsp.* jejuni

In addition to its role as a major cause of human enteritis, *C. jejuni* subsp. *jejuni* also causes diarrhoea in cattle and has been isolated from dogs, cats and non-human primates with diarrhoea. The species has also been implicated as the cause of mastitis in cattle and abortion in sheep. In chickens, turkeys, pigeons, crows and gulls and other wild birds the species constitutes part of normal intestinal flora. Other sources of isolates include hamsters, flies and mushrooms. Since there are such a large number of potential contributors

to the contamination of natural waters it is not surprising that large outbreaks have been traced to unchlorinated water supplies. Unpasteurized milk has also been implicated in a number of milkborne outbreaks. However, the majority of the human cases can be traced to poultry, particularly to the consumption of chickens that have been incompletely cooked or to cookware, utensils and cutting boards that have been contaminated during the preparation of the chicken. These cases are, for the most part, sporadic but they constitute the majority of the human cases. Transmission of the organisms from cats and dogs has been reported to be the cause of sporadic cases, usually limited to a small number of associated individuals often in the same family (Tauxe, 1992).

Through epidemiological investigations it has been confirmed that campylobacteriosis is a zoonotic disease. Tracing of the infections to animal sources has been accomplished mostly through the use of serotyping systems. These systems are used mainly by reference laboratories (Penner, 1988). One system distinguishes strains on the basis of differences in specificities in thermostable antigens that are known to be lipopolysaccharide (Penner system) and the other employs differences in thermolabile antigens to distinguish between strains (Lior system). Other techniques to distinguish strains include plasmid profile determinations, phage typing, analysis of proteins from outer membranes, multilocus enzyme electrophoresis and ribotyping. The molecular techniques are generally too complex for routine use and future research needs to be directed toward simplification. The use of polymerase chain reaction (PCR) to amplify the *flaA* gene encoding flagellin and restriction fragment length polymorphism (RFLP) analysis of the amplimer is a promising method for typing *C. jejuni* (Birkenhead *et al.*, 1993). The work of the reference laboratories would also be considerably facilitated when commercially produced serotyping antisera for both serotyping systems become available.

C. jejuni *subsp.* doylei

The subspecies *C. jejuni* subsp. *doylei*, has been proposed for groups of bacteria isolated from fecal samples of paediatric patients with diarrhoea in Australia and South Africa and from gastric biopsies of adults in West Germany and the UK (Steele and Owen, 1988). These bacteria, previously referred to as atypical *C. jejuni* or as GCLO-2, grow optimally at 35–37 °C and poorly or not at all at 42 °C. They do not reduce nitrate to nitrite and approximately 20% do not produce catalase. The isolates are susceptible to cephalothin and generally also to nalidixic acid. Because of their preference for a growth temperature of 35–37 °C and their susceptibility to cephalothin they are not likely to be isolated with procedures used routinely for *C. jejuni* subsp. *jejuni* and other thermophiles.

The bacteria produce non-haemolytic, pinpoint colonies after incubation of five to six days at 37 °C. In this respect and in their inability to reduce nitrate or grow at 42 °C they resemble *Helicobacter fennelliae* (formerly *C. fennelliae*), with which they may be confused. Unlike *C. jejuni* subsp. *doylei*, however, the colonies of *H. fennelliae* have a distinct bleach-like odour and a tendency to swarm (Tenover and Fennell, 1992). A clinical significance of *C. jejuni* subsp. *doylei* isolates has not yet been demonstrated.

C. coli

Campylobacter coli is a significant cause of human enteritis but its incidence is much lower than that of *C. jejuni* subsp. *jejuni*. This may be due to under-reporting as some *C. coli* strains are inhibited by the antibiotics in the isolation media (Tenover and Fennell, 1992). Moreover, the incidence is variable from one area to the next as it is known that a higher proportion of the cases of human enteritis in developing countries are caused by *C. coli* (Skirrow and Blaser, 1992). *Campylobacter coli* is well known as the species that is most frequently found in healthy pigs but it also occurs in the intestines of cattle, sheep and chickens. Many strains of this species can be serotyped on the basis of their thermostable and thermolabile antigens. Although most strains of the species are susceptible to nalidixic acid, recent reports have drawn attention to the development of resistance to this antibiotic. In such cases they

may be misclassified as *C. lari*, which are characteristically resistant to nalidixic acid.

C. lari

Organisms of this species were first isolated from seagulls and referred to as nalidixic acid-resistant thermophilic *Campylobacter* (NARTC). They have also been obtained from other species of birds and from dogs, monkeys and sheep (Tenover and Fennell, 1992). The species is also a cause of human enteritis but relative to *C. jejuni* subsp. *jejuni* such cases are rare. Some strains of the species are capable of producing urease, a characteristic not shared by any other species of the genus. The ability to grow anaerobically in 0.1% trimethylamine-*N*-oxide hydrochloride is a key distinguishing feature and permits its differentiation from other species of the thermophilic enteropathogenic group of the genus.

C. upsaliensis

In studies to investigate transmission of campylobacteria from dogs to humans a number of strains were isolated from dogs that differed from the typical thermophilic enteropathogenic species in negative or weak reactions when tested for catalase production. They were known as the catalase-negative or weak (CNW) group of strains before it was recognized that they were representatives of a new species. This species, named *C. upsaliensis*, consists of strains that are generally more susceptible to antibiotics and have a wider diversity in their susceptibilities than have the other members of the thermophilic group. For effective isolation the filtration technique and media without antibiotics are recommended. Adoption of these measures has permitted the isolation of *C. upsaliensis* from patients with gastroenteritis and bacteremia, providing a convincing line of evidence that they are causes of diarrhoea in humans (Goossens and Butzler, 1992). The finding of identical isolates from a patient with diarrhoea and from his diarrhoeic dog has confirmed earlier suspicions that *C. upsaliensis* is a cause of zoonotic infections.

Isolates of *C. upsaliensis* are readily different-iated from other thermophilic species by a negative or weak reaction for catalase, and by their inability to hydrolyse hippurate or grow anaerobically in 0.1% trimethylamine *N*-oxide hydrochloride.

Campylobacter upsaliensis isolates are also susceptible to both cephalothin and nalidixic acid. They resemble most closely *C. helveticus* strains, from which they can be differentiated by their positive reactions for reduction of selenite and growth on potato starch.

C. helveticus

The most recently defined species of the ther-mophilic enteropathogenic group is *C. helveticus*. It was discovered during studies on the detection of *C. upsaliensis* in cats and dogs with gastroen-teritis (Stanley *et al.*, 1992). The species reflects the phenotypic characteristics of *C. upsaliensis* but has a homology level of only 35% in DNA–DNA hybridizations and less homology with other species of the thermophilic group. Its differentiation from *C. upsaliensis* is based on its inability to reduce selenite or grow on potato starch. It is differentiated from the other ther-mophilic species by its lack of catalase production. On blood agar *C. helveticus* produces smooth, flat colonies with a characteristic blue-green hue and a watery spreading appearance.

Approximately half of the campylobacteria isolated from cats belong to *C. helveticus* and the species is present in both healthy cats and in cats with gastroenteritis, but only 2% of the campylo-bacteria isolated from dogs belong to this species. At this time there is no information on the occur-rence of *C. helveticus* in humans or on its significance as a pathogen in household pets.

Laboratory Diagnosis

Procedures for isolating campylobacteria

Bacteria of the genus *Campylobacter* have a characteristic cell morphology and a darting type of motility that permits their identification by direct examination of broth suspensions of faeces. However, *C. jejuni* subsp. *jejuni* cannot be distin-guished from *C. coli* by this procedure and the test is considerably less sensitive than isolation by culture.

A method used in early studies to isolate cam-pylobacteria from faeces employed filtration. The supernatant from a saline suspension of faeces is drawn up in a syringe and then forced through a 0.65 μm filter. The filtered fluid which contains the campylobacteria because they are able to pass through the filter is inoculated on a solid isolation medium (Dekeyser *et al.*, 1972). Although the method is effective, it is cumbersome and has been replaced by direct plating on a selective isolation medium, the first of which was described in 1977 (Skirrow, 1977). The Skirrow medium consists of a blood agar base in which is incorporated lysed horse blood, vancomycin, trimethoprim and polymyxin B. Blood contains catalase, peroxidase and superoxide dismutase which are believed to remove toxic oxygen derivatives that inhibit campylobacteria, while the three antibiotics inhibit the growth of other enteric bacteria. The Skirrow medium is immensely successful in isolating *C. jejuni* subsp. *jejuni* but some faecal flora are not inhibited and some species of *Campylobacter* are inhibited. This has prompted investigations of other media formu-lations to overcome these problems. Different cephalosporins have been examined for their inhibi-tion of faecal bacteria, and amphotericin B and cycloheximide have been used to inhibit yeasts. Activated charcoal has been discovered to serve as a replacement for blood in isolation media, and blood-free media containing charcoal are now in use. Such media are generally less expensive and have an advantage in areas of the world where regular supplies of sterile horse or sheep blood are not readily available. One blood-free selective medium developed to replace blood with charcoal is referred to as modified charcoal cefoperazone deoxycholate agar (CCDA medium). It also contains ferrous sulfate and sodium pyruvate to enhance aerotoler-ance and growth of the bacteria (Hutchinson and Bolton, 1984).

A novel method of filtering faecal suspensions that does not require the use of a syringe has recently been gaining acceptance in clinical laboratories. To a membrane filter (0.4 μm or 0.65 μm pore size) placed on a solid base medium with blood are applied six to eight drops of faecal suspension. The filter is removed and discarded 30 minutes after the application of the suspension. Only about 10% of the campylobacteria in the sample pass through the filter to produce colonies, thereby limiting detectability of these organisms in faeces to those samples with more than 10^5 colony-forming units per gram (Goossens and Butzler, 1992) but the method is particularly useful for strains that are susceptible to the antibiotics in isolation media. Some authors advocate that both inoculation on a selective medium and filtration on a non-selective medium be performed to enhance recovery of the thermophilic species. There is evidence that *C. upsaliensis* isolations would be increased significantly if both methods were routinely used.

To isolate *Campylobacter* spp. from water, milk or food, pre-enrichment steps are recommended. Enrichment is usually unnecessary for fresh stool samples but should be considered for samples that have been stored or maintained in transport media. A number of enrichment media have been described and tested but agreement is lacking on the choice of an enrichment medium. Those that have been examined include Campy-thio broth, alkaline peptone water, Doyle and Roman enrichment broth, Lovett's enrichment broth and the Preston semi-solid enrichment medium. It should be noted that these media have been tested primarily for improving isolation of *C. jejuni* and their efficacy for other species remains largely unknown (Goossens and Butzler, 1992; Tenover and Fennell, 1992).

Since campylobacteria are microaerophils it is essential that they be cultured in an atmosphere with reduced oxygen concentration. The recommended gaseous mixture is 5% oxygen, 10% carbon dioxide and 85% nitrogen. The most convenient method of achieving such an atmosphere is with commercially available gas-generating envelopes that are activated in the anaerobic jars. Hydrogen has been shown to enhance growth of some species and to be essential for microaerobic growth of *C. mucosalis*, *C. concisus*, *C. curvus*, *C. rectus* and *C. showae* (Goossens and Butzler, 1992). Gas-generating envelopes that produce an atmosphere of approximately 10% hydrogen, 10% carbon dioxide and 80% nitrogen are available but it should be noted that the hydrogen may be hazardous (Tenover and Fennell, 1992). A less practical method of producing microaerophilic conditions consist of evacuating the air from the anaerobic jars and replacing it with a gas mixture of hydrogen, carbon dioxide and nitrogen. Another method of reducing the oxygen consists of burning a candle in the jar but since this reduces the oxygen concentration to only about 17% the method is not suitable for optimum recovery of most campylobacteria. A commercially available supplement consisting of equal concentrations of ferrous sulfate, sodium metabisulfite and sodium pyruvate may be incorporated in the isolation medium to enhance aerotolerance and growth. The use of this supplement is recommended by many workers and is particularly important in laboratories that use the burning candle to reduce the concentration of oxygen.   '

Most laboratories incubate plates at 42 °C when most campylobacteria, apart from *C. fetus*, will grow. However, campylobacteria and arcobacteria grow well at 37 °C when some selective media, such as CCDA, are still selective. It has been suggested that culture should be made at both 37 °C and 42 °C or repeated at 37 °C, if negative at 42 °C (Nachamkin, 1995).

Identification

A well-recognized difficulty in identifying campylobacteria is the lack of tests that are effective discriminators of the species. The phenotype tests that are used in the clinical laboratory include only a small number of biochemical tests and a few tests of tolerance to different temperatures and to agents that inhibit growth. Authors generally agree that tests for oxidase, catalase, hippuricase, urease, indoxyl acetate hydrolysis, nitrate and nitrite reductases, hydrogen sulfide production, susceptibility to nalidixic acid and cephalothin, and growth at 15 °C, 25 °C and 42 °C, are the most reliable for differentiation. Less reproducible are tests for tolerance to 1% glycine, 3.5% sodium chloride and 0.1% trimethylamine *N*-oxide. Although confusion because of the different habitats occupied by *Campylobacter* spp. and *Helicobacter* spp. is unlikely, the former have been reported as always being sensitive to polymyxin B, whereas the latter are rarely sensitive (Burnens and Nicolet, 1993).

The experienced worker may be aided by slight differences in colony morphology on isolation media. Colonies produced by *C. jejuni* subsp. *jejuni* are grey, moist, flat and spreading after 42 hours of incubation at 42 °C. They are often found to spread along the lines of inoculation. *Campylobacter coli* colonies tend to be creamy-grey, moist and more discrete than those of *C. jejuni* subsp. *jejuni*. Colonies of *C. lari* are generally grey and discrete but more variable, resembling either *C. jejuni* subsp. *jejuni* or *C. coli* colonies. A list of the reactions by which the thermophilic species may be differentiated are shown in Table 17b.2.

Non-conventional tests for identifying *C. jejuni* subsp. *jejuni* and *C. coli* and some of the other enteropathogenic species that are less frequently isolated, such as *C. upsaliensis*, have been developed. These include radioactive and non-

radioactive DNA probes and latex agglutination tests. Both types of DNA probes are either species specific or they identify strains of both *C. jejuni* subsp. *jejuni* and *C. coli*. In the latex agglutination tests, now commercially available, a specific antibody is affixed to latex particles which agglutinate in the presence of cells or extracts from cultures of *C. jejuni* subsp. *jejuni* or *C. coli*. The high levels of specificity of the novel tests is an important advantage that may be the factor governing their eventual adoption by clinical laboratories for routine use.

Antibiotic Susceptibility

Antibiotic resistance genes, usually carried on plasmids, have been cloned and will express in *E. coli*. The tetracycline resistance gene (*tetO*) appears to be closely related to the *tetM* gene found in *Streptococcus* sp. (Taylor, 1984, 1992a) and both protein products function as GTPase proteins (Grewel *et al.*, 1993). The chloramphenicol resistance determinant (*cat*) is closely related to genes found among *Clostridium* spp. and specifies a chloramphenicol transferase (Taylor, 1984, 1992a). Kanamycin resistance is due to the production of 3'-*O*-aminoglycoside phosphotransferase, which is encoded by three different genes:

TABLE 17b.2 CHARACTERISTICS FOR DIFFERENTIATING THERMOPHILIC ENTEROPATHOGENIC SPECIES OF *CAMPYLOBACTER*

Phenotypic characteristics	*C. jejuni* subsp. *jejuni*	*C. jejuni* subsp. *doylei*	*C. coli*	*C. lari*	*C. upsaliensis*	*C. helveticus*
Catalase	+	v	+	+	−/w	−
Nitrate reduction	+	−	+	+	+	+
Hippurate hydrolysis	+	+	−	−	−	−
Indoxyl acetate hydrolysis	+	+	+	−	+	+
Growth at 42 °C	+	+w	+	+	+	+
Growth at 25 °C	−	−	−	−	−	−
Anaerobic growth with trimethylamine *N*-oxide	−	−	−	+	−	−
Susceptibility to nalidixic acid (30 µg disk)	S	S	S	R	S	S
Cephalothin (30 µg disk)	R	S	R	R	S	S

Test reactions: +, positive; −, negative; w, weak; v, variable reactions; S, susceptible; R, resistant. For some tests occasional strains may give results other than those indicated.
Sources of data include Goossens and Butzler (1992), Stanley *et al.* (1992), Steele and Owen (1988) and Tenover and Fennell (1992).

aphA-1, which is chromosomally mediated and found among the Enterobacteriaceae, *aphA*-3, which is found in Gram-positive cocci, and *aphA*-7 which is thought to be indigenous to *Campylobacter* (Taylor, 1992a).

Resistance to fluoroquinolones arises from a mutation in *gyrA* (position 86 threonine) and this can arise from both human and veterinary use of fluoroquinolones (Piddock, 1995).

Treatment

Treatment of *Campylobacter* infections has been confined to those with prolonged serious symptoms in which severe physiological disturbance may occur, immunocompromised persons and infection in pregnancy in which the fetus may be affected (Allos and Blaser, 1995). Erythromycin has been used for more than 15 years for the treatment of *Campylobacter* enteritis with low toxicity, cost and resistance rates. Fluoroquinolones, such as ciprofloxacin, have been demonstrated to be effective and are increasingly used, but increasing resistance rates may change this trend.

Prevention

As infection with *Campylobacter* spp. is a zoonosis, control is largely directed against removing the source of infection. The consumption of unchlorinated water is a well-recognized source. Contamination of drinking water for poultry may be a significant source of intestinal colonization in poultry flocks and control measures can lead to reduced carriage (Healing *et al.*, 1992). Adequate cooking of poultry is probably the single most important control measure. Pasteurization of milk is also important, as is protection of doorstep bottles of milk from pecking by birds (Healing *et al.*, 1992).

ANIMAL PATHOGENS AND COMMENSAL CAMPYLOBACTERIA THAT MAY CAUSE OPPORTUNISTIC INFECTIONS IN HUMANS

The four species within this group (*C. fetus*, *C. hyointestinalis*, *C. sputorum* and *C. mucosalis*) are, with the exception of *C. sputorum* biovar *sputorum*, either pathogens or commensals of farm animals. Human infections are uncommon and those that have been reported are usually opportunistic in predisposed patients. There is considerable diversity among the species in their habitats, pathogenicity, atmospheric conditions for growth and biochemical reactions (Table 17b.3) although genetic analysis has shown them to be a closely related group (Vandamme *et al.*, 1991; Thompson *et al.*, 1988).

C. fetus

Bacteria now classified as *C. fetus* have been known since 1913, when they were believed to belong to the genus *Vibrio* (Tenover and Fennell, 1992). Currently, the species consists of two groups classified as *C. fetus* subsp. *fetus* and *C. fetus* subsp. *venerealis*. The assignment of the two groups to the taxonomic status of subspecies is based more on convenience than on differences that can be demonstrated by either DNA hybridization or phenotypic characteristics that are used to identify and classify campylobacteria. The subspecies are, however, quite distinct in their habitats and in the sites of the host where they produce infections. The major habitat of *C. fetus* subsp. *fetus* is the intestinal tract of cattle and sheep, and isolations of the organisms from healthy animals are not uncommon. It is believed that the bacteria are acquired from food or water that has been contaminated with bacteria from faeces, aborted fetuses or from vaginal discharges of infected animals. After colonization of the intestine the organisms spread via the bloodstream to the placenta, for which they have a high affinity, and multiply in the developing fetus, which is then generally aborted.

The normal habitat of *C. fetus* subsp. *venerealis* is the prepuce of the asymptomatic bull; venereal transmission of organisms can cause a chronic inflammation of the cow genital tract and infertility. The disease is known as bovine genital campylobacteriosis (formerly bovine vibriosis) and is important in the cattle industry.

TABLE 17b.3   DIFFERENTIATION OF *C. FETUS, C. HYOINTESTINALIS, C. SPUTORUM* AND *C. MUCOSALIS*

Phenotypic characteristics	C. fetus subsp. fetus	C. fetus subsp. venerealis	C. hyointestinalis	C. sputorum biovar sputorum	C. sputorum biovar bubulus	C. sputorum biovar fecalis	C. mucosalis
Catalase	+	+	+	−	−	+	−
Nitrite reduction	−	−	−	+	+	+	+
Growth at 42 °C	v	−	+	+	+	+	+
Growth at 25 °C	+	+	+	−	−	−	+
H₂S production	−	−	+	+	+	+	+
Hydrogen requirement	−	−	−	−	−	−	+
Growth in 1% glycine	+	−	+	+	+	+	+
Growth in 3.5% NaCl	−	−	−	−	+	−	−
Susceptibility to:							
Nalidixic acid (30 µg disk)	R	R	R	S	R	R	R
Cephalothin (30 µg disk)	S	S	S	S	S	S	S

Test reactions: +, positive; −, negative; v, variable reactions; S, susceptible; R, resistant. Sources of data include Goossens and Butzler (1992), Gebhart *et al.* (1985), Roop *et al.* (1985) and Tenover and Fennell (1992).

Human infections caused by *C. fetus* subsp. *fetus* are rare and usually occur in immunocompromised or debilitated patients. Complications arising from septicaemia include meningitis, salpingitis, endocarditis, infection of the fetus and abortion. *Campylobacter fetus* subsp. *fetus* has also been isolated from the human intestinal tract and the premise that it is a cause of human diarrhoea is gaining support. Some of the intestinal isolates have been recovered at 42 °C but most strains of the species cannot tolerate this temperature and are also susceptible to cephalothin, the most common selective agent for culture. Since many, if not most, of the *C. fetus* subsp. *fetus* strains would not be isolated, an accurate determination of the incidence of this subspecies in human diarrhoea is not available.

To optimize recovery of these campylobacteria and ascertain their incidence in human infection from stools it is recommended that the filtration technique be used, along with antibiotic-free media, and that incubation be carried out under microaerophilic conditions at 35–37 °C. Campylobacteria, which are smaller than most enteric bacteria, pass through the filters and produce colonies, while the larger enteric bacteria are excluded.

The involvement of *C. fetus* subsp. *venerealis* in human disease is even much less frequent than is *C. fetus* subsp. *fetus*. Only two cases of human

infections have been reported and both patients were compromised and suffered complications, one with meningitis and the other with hepatitis (Garcia *et al.*, 1983).

C. hyointestinalis

A group of bacteria isolated from pigs with proliferative ileitis (Gebhart *et al.*, 1983) was confirmed to be a separate species and was named *C. hyointestinalis* (Gebhart *et al.*, 1985). Although bacteria of this species and bacteria belonging to *C. coli* and *C. mucosalis* are readily isolated from porcine intestines they have not been shown to have a direct effect in the development of this intestinal disease. From recent work it appears that such porcine diseases may be caused by intracellular *Campylobacter*-like organisms that cannot be cultured (Gebhart *et al.*, 1991; McOrist *et al.*, 1989). However, it is interesting to note that *C. hyointestinalis* and *C. mucosalis* occur far more frequently in piglets with intestinal lesions than in healthy animals, but the basis for this observation is not clear.

Campylobacter hyointestinalis has also been isolated from the intestines of the hamster and from the faeces of humans (Gebhart *et al.*, 1985). Isolates obtained from a homosexual male (Fennell *et al.*, 1986) first implicated the species as another aetiological agent of human diarrhoea. In subsequent studies isolates from both male and female patients with diarrhoea have been reported (Edmond *et al.*, 1987) but isolates have also been obtained from asymptomatic individuals (Salama *et al.*, 1992) and the suggestion has been raised that *C. hyointestinalis* may be an opportunistic enteropathogen in humans (Minet *et al.*, 1988).

Campylobacter hyointestinalis is most closely related to *C. fetus* subsp. *fetus* (Vandamme *et al.*, 1991) and the two species possess a number of the same phenotypic characteristics, including colony morphology, production of catalase, reduction of nitrate but not nitrite, growth in 1% glycine, susceptibility to cephalothin and resistance to nalidixic acid. In contrast to *C. fetus*, *C. hyointestinalis* grows optimally at 35–37 °C, less well at 42 °C and not at all at 25 °C. The colonies are yellow, and do not swarm on moist media or show haemolysis (Gebhart *et al.*, 1985). The species is differentiated from *C. fetus* by its production of hydrogen sulfide in triple sugar iron medium and by its growth in trimethylamine *N*-oxide hydrochloride under anaerobic conditions.

The number of reports of isolations of *C. hyointestinalis* from humans has not increased substantially since the first report of a human isolate (Fennell *et al.*, 1986) and thus its frequency as a pathogen or commensal in the human population remains uncertain. The lack of isolations has been attributed to the isolation procedure in the clinical laboratory, which is primarily designed for thermophilic enteropathogenic species. Recovery of *C. hyointestinalis* is therefore often unsuccessful because the bacteria do not grow optimally at 42–43 °C and they may be susceptible to selective antibiotics.

C. sputorum

The species consists of three biovars (biotypes): *C. sputorum* biovar *sputorum*, *C. sputorum* biovar *bubulus* and *C. sputorum* biovar *fecalis*. The biovars can be differentiated on the basis of their habitats and simple biochemical tests. Although there are reports of an isolate of *C. sputorum* biovar sputorum from a human leg abscess and another isolate from the faeces of an infant with

diarrhoea the organisms of this biovar are believed to be commensals because they can be isolated from the oral cavity and faeces of healthy humans (Karmali and Skirrow, 1984). Isolates of *C. sputorum* biovar *bubulus* have been isolated from healthy cattle, in which they are found in the preputial cavity of the male and in the vagina of the female, but a pathogenic role has not been established and the organisms are believed to be commensals. *C. sputorum* biovar *fecalis* was originally believed to represent a separate species and was first classified as *Vibrio fecalis*, but it was shown to constitute a separate biogroup within the species *C. sputorum* in DNA relatedness studies (Roop *et al.*, 1985). Organisms of this biovar have been isolated from sheep faeces, bovine semen and the bovine vagina, but evidence for a pathogenic role has not been forthcoming.

The morphology of the bacterial cells of the three biovars is characteristic of the genus except that the cells are not as tightly coiled as are those of *C. jejuni* subsp. *jejuni* (Tenover and Fennell, 1992). Isolates of each of the biovars grow microerophically at 42 °C but prefer 37 °C. They do not grow at 25 °C. The colonies are small (1–2.5 mm in diameter), grey in colour and do not swarm on moist agar. Some show low levels of α-haemolysis. The isolates reduce nitrate and nitrite, produce hydrogen sulfide in triple sugar iron medium and are susceptible to cephalothin. Tests for differentiating among the biovars are few. *Campylobacter sputorum* biovar *sputorum* is the only biovar likely to be encountered in specimens from human sources. It differs from the other two biovars in its susceptibility to nalidixic acid and from *C. sputorum* biovar *fecalis* in a negative test for catalase. *Campylobacter sputorum* biovar *bubulus* is the only one of the three biovars that can grown in 3.5% sodium chloride and, although somewhat of an unreliable test, it has been used to differentiate this biovar from the other two.

C. mucosalis

Campylobacter mucosalis (formerly classified as *C. sputorum* subsp. *mucosalis*) is of interest primarily to veterinarians because of its occurrence in the intestinal mucosa of pigs with intestinal adenomatosis and proliferative haemorrhagic enteropathy (Roop *et al.*, 1985). The species can also be isolated from the intestinal contents and the oral cavities of healthy pigs but a role in the aetiology of these porcine diseases has not been demonstrated. Human infections are unknown except for one case of an immunocompromised patient with symptoms of pneumonia from whom a blood isolate of *C. mucosalis* was cultured (Söderström *et al.*, 1991). The fever resolved with a 10-day course of erythromycin and netilmicin, indicating that the isolate was the cause of the illness. This suggests that *C. mucosalis* may be a rare opportunistic agent of infections in humans but determination of the true frequency in the human population will require microbiology laboratories to implement procedures more appropriate for its isolation.

Organisms of *C. mucosalis* are short, curved, and spiral shaped with a single polar flagellum. Coccoid bodies and filamentous forms may occur in older cultures. The bacteria are capable of growth at temperatures from 25 °C to 42 °C. The colonies are noted for their yellowish colour, best seen when the colony is spread on white paper.

Hydrogen is necessary for microaerophilic growth, a requirement that permits differentiation from *C. fetus*, *C. hyointestinalis*, *C. sputorum* and species of the thermophilic enteropathogenic group. The four species associated with periodontal diseases in humans (see below) also require hydrogen for microaerophilic growth but they can be differentiated from *C. mucosalis* on the basis of their inability to grow at 25 °C.

Campylobacter Species Associated with Periodontal Disease

Four species are included in this group: *C. concisus*, *C. rectus*, *C. curvus* and *C. showae*. With few exceptions, strains of these species have been isolated from the oral cavities of apparently healthy humans or from humans with periodontal disease but a role in the production of this disease has not been established. Of the four species, only *C. concisus* has been isolated from non-oral sites in humans. It has been obtained from faeces of humans with diarrhoea, leading some authors to conclude that it is a cause of this illness. Such isolates could not be recovered with the use of

TABLE 17b.4 CHARACTERISTICS FOR DIFFERENTIATING *C. CONCISUS*, *C. RECTUS*, *C. CURVUS* AND *C. SHOWAE*

Characteristic	C. concisus	C. rectus	C. curvus	C. showae
Catalase activity	−	−	−	+
Indoxyl acetate	−	+	+	+
Growth at 42 °C	+	W	+	+
Growth at 25 °C	−	−	−	−
Growth in presence of:				
3.5% Nacl	−	−	−	−
1% glycine	+	+	+	v
0.05% NaF	+	−	−	+
H$_2$ requirement	+	+	+	+
H$_2$S production	+	+	+	+
Urease activity	−	−	−	−
Nitrite reduction	+	+	+	+
Susceptibility to:				
Nalidixic acid	R	S	R	R
Cephalothin	R	S	S	S
Number of flagella	1	1	1	2–5
Cell morphology:				
Helical curved	+	−	+	−
rod shaped	−	+	−	+

Test reactions: +, positive; −, negative; v, variable; w, weak reactions. Sources of data include Etoh *et al.* (1993), Goossens and Butzler (1992) and Tanner *et al.* (1981, 1984).

selective media containing antibiotics but they were recoverable by the filtration method. The blood, oesophagus, stomach and duodenum are other sites from which the organisms have been isolated (Goossens and Butzler, 1992).

Two species, *C. concisus* and *C. rectus*, were described as a result of a taxonomic study on bacteria associated with periodontal disease (Tanner *et al.*, 1981). *Campylobacter concisus* consists of bacteria typical of the genus *Campylobacter* in morphology and microaerophilicity, but another group was reported to consist of anaerobic, straight unbranched cells with rounded ends. The latter group, now known as *C. rectus*, was first assigned to the genus *Wolinella* with the specific name '*recta*'. *Campylobacter curvus* was initially also placed in the genus *Wolinella* with the specific name '*curva*' to reflect the shape of the cells. However, the bacteria of both groups have been shown to be true microaerophils and not anaerobes (Han *et al.*, 1991). By DNA–rRNA hybridization and immunotyping they were also shown to be more closely related to the genus *Campylobacter* than to the type species of the genus *Wolinella* (Vandamme *et al.*, 1991). With corrections in the spelling of the epithets the two species were therefore transferred to the genus *Campylobacter* (Vandamme *et al.*, 1991).

DNA–DNA hybridization tests, 16S rRNA sequence data and biochemical reactions typical of campylobacteria supported the proposal for creating a new species, *C. showae*, for another group of strains isolated from dental plaque and human gingival crevices of apparently healthy adults (Etoh *et al.*, 1993). The species differs from others of the genus in having rod-shaped bacteria with two to five flagella at one end of the cell. It is differentiated from *C. concisus*, *C. rectus* and *C. curvus* in its ability to produce catalase. Additional characteristics for differentiating these species are shown in Table 17b.4.

THE GENUS *ARCOBACTER*

The genus *Arcobacter* was created to include two species, *A. nitrofigilis* and *A. cryaerophilus*, that were formerly in the genus *Campylobacter*, but the genus *Arcobacter* has been expanded to include two new species: *A. butzleri* and *A. skirrowii* (Vandame *et al.*, 1991, 1992b). In many respects the bacteria resemble campylobacteria but have a number of phenotypic traits that warrant their placement in a separate genus. The name *Arcobacter* was selected to suggest a bow shape but, like campylobacteria, they are usually curved, S-shaped or helical cells. There is considerable diversity among the four *Arcobacter* spp. in the range of temperatures and atmospheric conditions under which they can grow, but all species are capable of growing aerobically at 30 °C, anaerobically at 35–37 °C and microaerophically, with or without hydrogen, at 25–30 °C. Optimal growth occurs under microaerophilic conditions with oxygen concentrations of 3–10%. *Arcobacter nitrofigilis* and *A. craerophilus* are capable of growth at 15 °C or at lower temperatures but only the occasional strain of *A. cryaerophilus* grows at 42 °C, in contrast to 67% of *A. butzleri* and 33% of *A. skirrowii* strains that grow at this temperature.

All strains of the genus produce oxidase, hydrolyse indoxyl acetate and catalase, but isolates of *A. butzleri* characteristically exhibit a weak catalase reaction. Virtually all strains of *A. nitrofigilis*, *A. butzleri* and *A. skirrowii* and 70% of the *A. cryaerophilus* strains have DNAase activity. All strains are resistant to the pteridine vibriostatic agent 0/129. Tests for nitrite reduction and hippurate hydrolysis are negative and hydrogen sulfide is not produced in either the triple sugar iron medium or in the rapid test for hydrogen sulfide production, but some strains of *A. nitrofigilis* and *A. butzleri* produce hydrogen sulfide from cysteine.

Considerable diversity exists among the four species and among the strains of each species in their reactions to a number of tolerance tests. Although such tests permit the characterization of individual strains they are generally unsatisfactory for species identification and classification. Some, but not all, of the tolerance tests that have been advocated include tests for growth in sodium chloride (in concentrations ranging from 1.0% to 3.5%), growth in bile (1.0%), in triphenyltetrazolium chloride (0.04–0.1%), sodium selenite

(0.1%), cadmium chloride (2.5 μg and 2.0 μg disks), glucose (8%), brilliant green (0.001–0.003%) and in glycine (1.0%). Of the selective media that have been examined, only the use of MacConkey agar has value as a differentiating test because it separates *A. butzleri* strains, which grow on the medium, from *A. skirrowii* strains, which do not. Virtually all *Arcobacter* strains (92–100%) are susceptible to nalidixic acid (30 μg disks) but there is much diversity among the species in susceptibility to cephalothin (30 μg disks).

A very effective but not often used tool in taxonomy exploits gas–liquid chromatography (GLC) for determining the profiles of cellular fatty acids (Lambert *et al.*, 1987). Each species of *Arcobacter* has a unique profile providing a phenotypic characterization that is consistent with the groupings produced from the results of DNA–rRNA and DNA–DNA hybridizations (Vandamme *et al.*, 1992b). From a practical standpoint, however, the clinical microbiologist does not generally have immediate access to GLC apparatus or to facilities for genetic analysis and must rely on conventional phenotypic characters

that can be readily demonstrated. Because such species-specific characters are limited in the genus *Arcobacter,* difficulties may be encountered in achieving correct identifications.

Some of the more useful characteristics in identification are shown in Table 17b.5. Key characteristics for identifying strains of *A. nitrofigilis* include tolerance to glycine and sodium chloride, production of a water-soluble brown pigment from tryptophan and production of urease and nitrogenase enzymes. *Arcobacter nitrofigilis* strains are the least tolerant of the arcobacteria to glycine but are the most tolerant to NaCl. It has been reported that some strains can grow in a concentration of NaCl as high as 7.0% (McClung *et al.*, 1983). The production of brown pigment from tryptophan is also unique to *A. nitrofigilis* and the production of urease by strains belonging to other species of *Arcobacter* has not been reported (McClung *et al.*, 1983). *Arcobacter nitrofigilis* is capable of nitrogen fixation and a test for nitrogenase is critical for a complete identification, but the test is not routinely provided in the clinical laboratory (Hardy *et al.*, 1968).

TABLE 17b.5   CHARACTERISTICS FOR DIFFERENTIATING SPECIES OF GENUS *ARCOBACTER*

Characteristics	Species of genus *Arcobacter*			
	A. nitrofigilis	*A. cryaerophilus*	*A. butzleri*	*A. skirrowii*
Catalase	+	+	+w	+
Nitrate reduction	+	v	+	+
DNase	+	v	v	+
Nitrogenase	+	–	–	–
Urease	+	–	–	–
Growth on MacConkey agar	v	v	+	–
Growth at 37 °C	–	+	+	+
Growth at 42 °C	–	v	v	v
Growth on or in the presence of:				
3.5% NaCl	+	–	v	v
1% glycine	–	v	v	–
1% bile	–	v	v	–
8% glucose	+	+	+	v
Production of brown pigment from tryptophan	+	–	–	–
Alpha haemolysis	–	–	–	v

Symbols: +, 90% or more positive; –, 90% or more negative; v, 11–89% positive; w, weak. Data compiled from Kiehlbauch *et al.* (1991), McClung *et al.* (1983), Neill *et al.* (1985) and Vandamme *et al.* (1991, 1992b).

Another criterion for differentiating the species of *Arcobacter* is colony appearance (Vandamme *et al.*, 1992b). On charcoal medium white colonies are produced by *A. nitrofigilis*, beige to yellow colonies by *A. cryaerophilus*, white to beige by *A. butzleri* and greyish colonies by *A. skirrowii*. Although only a small number of *A. butzleri* strains have become available for study, a characteristic of the species that appears to be of discriminating value is the weak catalase reaction. But in general the genus reflects the problem encountered in the genus *Campylobacter*, that differentiation of the species to produce sharp, clearly defined divisions is not readily accomplished through the use of routinely applicable tests for phenotypic characteristics. Therefore a judicious consideration of a number of characteristics regarded as variable and common to two or more species must be taken into account for identification.

The data in Table 17b.5 are compiled from results obtained in the small number of studies that have been reported. In some cases, there are discrepancies between different workers presumably through use of different sets of small numbers of strains. As interest in the genus grows, more strains will be isolated and a more effective system for identification and classification can be expected as discriminating characteristics will be more rigorously assessed.

SPECIES OF THE GENUS *ARCOBACTER*

A. nitrofigilis

Arcobacter nitrofigilis is the type species of the genus (Vandamme *et al.*, 1991) but it comprises the most unique group in the genus. The bacteria are microaerophilic, nitrogen fixing and associated with the roots of a halophytic plant, *Spartina alterniflora*, which has as its habitat the sediments of salt marshes where the oxygen content is at reduced levels (McClung and Patriquin, 1980). It is not surprising, therefore, that in the laboratory it is capable of growth at low temperatures and in media with high concentrations of sodium

chloride. The observation that cells suspended in distilled water undergo rapid lysis suggests that viability is dependent on the presence of salt. Bacteria of this species are thus unlikely to be isolated in clinical laboratories that set the temperature for isolation at 37 °C or 42 °C. There is no known significance with respect to disease production in humans or animals.

A. cryaerophilus

During investigations of spiral-shaped organisms from aborted bovine fetuses an unusual group of strains was isolated on *Leptospira* medium under microaerophilic conditions at 30 °C. On subculture the bacteria were culturable under aerobic, anaerobic and microaerophilic conditions (Ellis *et al.*, 1977). The requirement for the two-step isolation procedure and the ability to grow in air at low temperatures are unique attributes of the strains. They were first assigned to a newly created species in the genus *Campylobacter* with the epithet '*cryaerophila*' to reflect both their characteristic growth at low temperatures and their aerotolerance, although it was recognized that the group displayed considerable heterogeneity and that, as a group, they were more distantly related to *Campylobacter* spp. than were the *Campylobacter* spp. to each other (Neill *et al.*, 1985). DNA–rRNA hybridization experiments showed that they clustered along with *C. nitrofigilis* in a separate group that did not include any of the other *Campylobacter* spp. (Vandamme *et al.*, 1991). The relationships were confirmed by DNA–DNA hybridization and were in agreement with the 16S rRNA homology groups determined by others (Thompson *et al.*, 1988). In accordance with these results, the species (accompanied by a correction of the spelling of the epithet, was transferred along with *C. nitrofigilis* to the newly described genus *Arcobacter* (Vandamme *et al.*, 1991).

Early collection of *A. cryaerophilus* isolates originated mostly from bovine, ovine and porcine fetal tissue but a significance in pathogenesis of animal diseases has not been established. In a collection of *A. cryaerophilus* strains made at the

Centers for Disease Control (CDC) in Atlanta, Georgia, two isolates were from human blood cultures and one from the stool of a patient with severe gastroenteritis (Kiehlbauch *et al.*, 1991). Although no medical significance has been linked to these human isolates it does suggest that with adoption by clinical laboratories of appropriate isolation techniques the occurrence of *A. cryaerophilus* in human specimens could be shown to be much higher than is now suspected.

A. butzleri

Through a study of aerotolerant spiral-shaped bacteria at the CDC a group of strains was discovered on the basis of DNA–DNA hybridizations to be distinct from bacteria now classified as *A. cryaerophilus*. A new species was proposed with the epithet '*butzleri*' and assigned to the genus *Campylobacter*, although the authors recognized that the new species would be placed in genus *Arcobacter* when the proposal for the new genus was accepted (Kiehlbauch *et al.*, 1991).

The first indication that *A. butzleri* strains were associated with human enteritis was through the report of a faecal isolate from a patient who experienced diarrhoea and abdominal pain. The isolate was identified as *C. cryaerophilus* (Tee *et al.*, 1988) but in subsequent investigations at the CDC it was confirmed that it belonged to *A. butzleri* (Kiehlbauch *et al.*, 1991). Of the 63 other *A. butzleri* strains under investigation at the CDC approximately 75% were also from human cases of diarrhoea (Kiehlbauch *et al.*, 1991). Evidence for a pathogenic role for *A. butzleri* mounted with the report of an outbreak of abdominal cramps without diarrhoea in a nursery and primary school in Italy (Vandamme *et al.*, 1992a). Fourteen isolates of *A. butzleri* from this outbreak were demonstrated to be epidemiologically linked through the application of PCR-mediated DNA fingerprinting (Vandamme *et al.*, 1993). *Arcobacter butzleri* is found not only in humans but also in a variety of animals. Among the CDC isolates 10 were from non-human primates, three from porcine tissue samples, one from a bovine stomach, and one from an ostrich yolk sac (Kiehlbauch *et al.*, 1991). Seven *A. butzleri* strains have also been recovered from infant monkeys in a nursery facility (Russell *et al.*, 1992).

Authors with experience in investigating arcobacteria, particularly *A. butzleri*, stress the importance of improving the isolation procedure. *Arcobacter butzleri* is not often isolated with media and cultural conditions appropriate for *C. jejuni* subsp. *jejuni*. Further investigations are advocated to identify the most efficient isolation medium, the optimum temperature for incubation and the optimum atmospheric conditions for incubation. The filtration method for recovering isolates should also be evaluated as an alternative procedure for isolation.

A. skirrowii

This species is the most recent addition to the genus *Arcobacter*. It was described for a group of aerotolerant strains that were initially believed to belong to *A. cryaerophilus* (Vandamme *et al.*, 1992b). The organisms were obtained from preputial fluids of bulls, aborted fetuses of sheep, cattle and pigs, and from cow and sheep feces. Only 18 strains have been studied and a role in pathogenesis remains to be established.

REFERENCES

Adak, G.K., Cowden, J.M., Nicholas, S. and Evan, H.S. (1995) The PHLS national case control study of primary indigenous sporadic cases of campylobacter infection. *Epidemiology and Infection*, **115**, 15–22.

Allos, B.M. and Blaser, M.J. (1995) *Campylobacter jejuni* and the expanding spectrum of related infections. *Clinical Infectious Diseases*, **20**, 1092–1101.

Aspinall, G.O., Fugimoto, G.O., McDonald, A.E. *et al.* (1994) Lipopolysaccharides from *Campylobacter jejuni* associated with Guillain– Barré syndrome patients mimic human gangliosides in structure. *Infection and Immunity*, **62**, 2122–2125.

Birkenhead, D., Hawkey, P.M., Heritage, J. *et al.* (1993) PCR for the detection and typing of campylobacters. *Letters in Applied Microbiology*, **17**, 235–237.

Blaser, M.J. and Gotschlich, E.C. (1990) Surface array protein of *Campylobacter* fetus: cloning and gene structure. *Journal of Biological Chemistry*, **265**, 14529–14535.

Burnens, A.P. and Nicolet, J. (1993) Three supplementary diagnostic tests for *Campylobacter* species and related organisms. *Journal of Clinical Microbiology*, **31**, 708–710.

Butzler, J.-P., Dekeyser, P., Detrain, M. and DeHaen, F. (1973) Related vibrios in stools. *Journal of Pediatrics*, **82**, 493–495.

Caldwell, M.B., Guerry, P., Lee, E.C. *et al.* (1985) Reversible expression of flagella in *Campylobacter jejuni*. *Infection and Immunity*, **50**, 941–943.

Calva, E., Torres, J., Vazquez, M. *et al.* (1989) *Campylobacter jejuni* chromosomal sequences that hybridize to *Vibrio cholerae* and *Escherichia coli* LT enterotoxin genes. *Gene*, **75**, 243–251.

Dekeyser, P., Goussuins-Detrain, M., Butzler, J.-P. and Sternon, J. (1972) Acute enteritis due to related *Vibrio*: first positive stool cultures. *Journal of Infectious Diseases*, **125**, 390–393.

Edmonds, P., Patton, C.M., Griffen, P.M. *et al.* (1987) *Campylobacter hyointestinalis* associated with human gastrointestinal disease in the United States. *Journal of Clinical Microbiology*, **25**, 685–691.

Ellis, W.A., Neill, S.D., O'Brien, J.J. *et al.* (1977) Isolation of Spirillum/vibrio-like organisms from bovine fetuses. *Veterinary Record*, **100**, 451–452.

Etoh, Y., Dewhirst, F.E., Paster, B.J. *et al.* (1993) *Campylobacter showae* sp. nov. isolated from the human oral cavity, *International Journal of Systematic Bacteiology*, **43**, 631–639.

Fennell, C.L., Rompalo, A.M., Totten, P.M. *et al.* (1986) Isolation of '*Campylobacter hyointestinalis*' from a human. *Journal of Clinical Microbiology*, **24**, 146–148.

Garcia, M.M., Eaglesome, M.D. and Rigby, C. (1983) Campylobacters important in veterinary medicine. *Veterinary Bulletin*, **53**, 793–818.

Gebhart, C.J., Ward, G.E., Chang, K. and Kurtz, H.J. (1983) *Campylobacter hyointestinalis* (new species) isolated from swine with lesions of proliferative ileitis. *American Journal of Veterinary Research*, **44**, 361–367.

Gebhart, C.J., Edmonds, P., Ward, E.G. *et al.* (1985) '*Campylobacter hyointestinalis*' sp. nov.: a new species of *Campylobacter* found in the intestines of pigs and other animals. *Journal of Clinical Microbiology*, **21**, 715–720.

Gebhart, C.J., Lin, G.-F., McOrist, S.M. *et al.* (1991) Cloned DNA probes specific for the intracellular *Campylobacter*-like organisms of porcine proliferative enteritis. *Journal of Clinical Microbiology*, **29**, 1011–1015.

Goossens, H. and Butzler, J.-P. (1992) Isolation and identification of *Campylobacter* spp. In *Campylobacter jejuni. Current Status and Future Trends* (ed. I. Nachamkin, M.J. Blaser and L.S. Tompkins), Ch.

11. American Society for Microbiology, Washington, DC.

Grewel, J., Manarathu, E.K. and Taylor, D.E. (1993) Effect of mutational alteration of *asn*-128 in the putative GTP-binding domain of tetracyline resistance determinant *tet*(O) from *Campylobacter jejuni*. *Antimicrobial Agents and Chemotherapy*, **37**, 2645–2649.

Guerry, P., Alm, R.A., Power, M.E. and Trust, T.J. (1992) Molecular and structural analysis of *Campylobacter* flagellin. In *Campylobacter jejuni: Current Status and Future Trends* (ed. I. Nachamkin, M.J. Blaser and L. Tompkins), pp. 267–281. *Proceedings of the NIH Symposium on Campylobacters*, ASM Publications, Washington, DC.

Han, Y.-H., Smibert, R.M. and Krieg, N.R. (1991) *Wolinella recta*, *Wolinella curva*, *Bacteroides ureolyticus* and *Bacteroides gracilis* are microaerophils, not anaerobes. *International Journal of Bacteriology*, **41**, 218–222.

Hani, E.K. and Chan, V.L. (1995) Expression and characterization of *Campylobacter jejuni* benzoylglycine aminohydrolase (hippuricase) gene in *Escherichia coli*. *Journal of Bacteriology*, **177**, 2396–2402.

Hardy, R.W.F., Holsten, R.D., Jackson, E.K. and Burns, R.C. (1968) The acetylene–ethylene assay for nitrogen fixation: laboratory and field evaluation. *Plant Physiology*, **43**, 1185–1207.

Healing, T.D., Greenwood, M.H. and Pearson, A.D. (1992) Campylobacters and enteritis. *Reviews in Medical Microbiology*, **3**, 159–167.

Hutchinson, D.N. and Bolton, F.J. (1984) Improved blood free selective medium for the isolation of *Campylobacter jejuni* from faecal specimens. *Journal of Clinical Pathology*, **37**, 956–957.

Karmali, M.A., and Skirrow, M.B. (1984) Taxonomy of the genus *Campylobacter*. In *Campylobacter Infection in Man and Animals* (ed. J.-P. Butzler), pp. 1–20. CRC Publications, Boca Raton, Florida.

Kiehlbauch, J.A., Brenner, D.J., Nicholson, M.A. *et al.* (1991) *Campylobacter butzleri* sp. nov. isolated from humans and animals with diarrhoeal illness. *Journal of Clinical Microbiology*, **29**, 375–385.

Kim, N.W., Lombardi, R., Bingham, H. *et al.* (1993) Fine mapping of the three rRNA operons on the updated genomic map of *Campylobacter jejuni* TGH9011 (ATCC 43431) *Journal of Bacteriology*, **175**, 7468–7470.

King, E.O. (1957) Human infections with *Vibrio fetus* and a closely related vibrio. *Journal of Infectious Diseases*, **101**, 119–128.

King, E.O. (1962) The laboratory recognition of *Vibrio fetus* and a closely related *Vibrio* isolated from cases of human vibriosis. *Annals of the New York Academy of Sciences*, **98**, 700–711.

Lambert, M.A., Patton, C.M., Barrett, T.M. and Moss, C.M. (1987) Differentiation of *Campylobacter* and *Campylobacter*-like organisms by cellular fatty acid composition. *Journal of Clinical Microbiology*, **25**, 700–713.

McClung, C.R. and Patriquin, D.G. (1980) Isolation of nitrogen-fixing *Campylobacter* species from the roots of *Spartina alterniflora* Loisel. *Canadian Journal of Microbiology*, **26**, 881–886.

McClung, C.R., Patriquin, D.G. and Davis, R.E. (1983) *Campylobacter nitrofigilis* sp. nov., a nitrogen-fixing bacterium associated with roots of *Spartina alterniflora*. *International Journal of Systematic Bacteriology*, **33**, 605–612.

McOrist, S., Boid, R. and Lawson, G.H.K. (1989) Antigenic analysis of *Campylobacter* species and an intracellular *Campylobacter*-like organism associated with porcine proliferative enteropathies. *Infection and Immunity*, **57**, 957–962.

Miller, S., Pesci, E.C. and Pickett, C.L. (1993) A *Campylobacter jejuni* homolog of the LcrD/FlbF family of proteins is necessary for flagellar biogenesis. *Infection and Immunity*, **61**, 2930–2936.

Minet, J., Grosbois, B. and Megraud, F. (1988) *Campylobacter hyointestinalis*: an opportunistic enteropathogen. *Journal of Clinical Microbiology*, **26**, 2659–2660.

Nachamkin, I. (1995) *Campylobacter* and *Arcobacter*. In *Manual of Clinical Microbiology*, 6th edn (ed. P.R. Murray), Ch. 37. Washington, DC.

Neill, S.D., Campbell, J.N., O'Brien, J.J. et al. (1985) Taxonomic position of *Campylobacter cryaerophila* sp. nov. *International Journal of Systematic Bacteriology*, **35**, 342–356.

Penner, J.L. (1988) The genus *Campylobacter*: a decade of progress. *Clinical Microbiology Reviews*, **1**, 157–172.

Piddock, L.J.V. (1995) Quinolone resistance and *Campylobacter* spp. *Journal of Antimicrobial Chemotherapy*, **36**, 891–898.

Roop, R.M., Smibert, R.M., Johnson, J.L. and Krieg, N.R. (1985) *Campylobacter mucosalis* (Lawson, Leaver, Pettigrew, and Rowland, 1981) comb. nov.: emended description. *International Journal of Systematic Bacteriology*, **35**, 189–192.

Russell, R.G., Kiehlbauch, J.A., Gebhart, C.J. and DeTolla, L.J. (1992) Uncommon *Campylobacter* species in infant *Macaca nemestrina* monkeys housed in a nursery. *Journal of Clinical Microbiology*, **30**, 3024–3027.

Salama, S.M., Tabor, H., Richter, M. and Taylor, D.E. (1992) Pulse-field gel electrophoresis for epidemiologic studies of *Campylobacter hyointestinalis*. *Journal of Clinical Microbiology*, **30**, 1982–1984.

Skirrow, M.B. (1977) Campylobacter enteritis: a 'new' disease. *British Medical Journal*, **ii**, 9–11.

Skirrow, M.B. and Blaser, M.J. (1992) Clinical and epidemiologic considerations. In *Campylobacter jejuni. Current Status and Future Trends* (ed. I. Nachamkin, M.J. Blaser and L.S. Tompkins), pp. 3–8. American Society for Microbiology, Washington, DC.

Söderström, C., Schalén, C. and Walder, M. (1991) Septicaemia caused by unusual *Campylobacter* species (*C. laridis* and *C. mucosalis*) *Scandinavian Journal of Infectious Diseases*, **23**, 369–371.

Stanley, J., Burnens, A.P., Linton, D. et al. (1992) *Campylobacter helveticus* sp. nov., a new thermophilic species from domestic animals: characterization and cloning of a species-specific DNA probe. *Journal of General Microbiology*, **138**, 2293–2303.

Steele, T.W. and Owen, R.J. (1988) *Campylobacter jejuni* subsp. *doylei* subsp. nov., a subspecies of nitrate-negative campylobacters isolated from human clinical specimens. *International Journal of Systematic Bacteriology*, **38**, 316–318.

Tanner, A.C.R., Badger, S., Lai, C.-H. et al. (1981) *Wolinella* gen nov., *Wolinella succinogenes* (*Vibrio succinogenes* Wolin et al.) comb. nov., and description of *Bacteroides gracilis* sp. nov., *Wolinella recta* sp. nov., *Campylobacter concisus* sp. nov., and *Eikenella corrodens* from humans with peridontal disease. *International Journal of Systematic Bacteriology*, **31**, 432–445.

Tanner, A.C.R., Listgarten, M.A. and Ebersole, J.L. (1984) *Wolinella curva* sp. nov., '*Vibro succinogenes*' of human origin. *International Journal of Systmatic Bacteriology*, **34**, 275–282.

Tauxe, R.V. (1992) Epidemiology of *Campylobacter jejuni* infections in the United States and other industrialized nations. In *Campylobacter jejuni. Current Status and Future Trends* (ed. I. Nachamkin, M.J. Blaser and L.S. Tompkins), Ch. 2. American Society for Microbiology, Washington, DC.

Taylor, D.E. (1984) Plasmids from *Campylobacter*. In *Campylobacter* infection in man and animals (ed. J.-P. Butzler), pp. 87–96. CRC Publications, Florida.

Taylor, D.E. (1992a) Genetics of *Campylobacter* and *Helicobacter*. *Annual Reviews in Microbiology*, **46**, 35–64.

Taylor, D.N. (1992b) *Campylobacter* infections in developing countries. In *Campylobacter jejuni: Current Status and Future Trends* (ed. I. Nachamkin, M.J. Blaser and L.S. Tompkins), pp. 20–30. American Society for Microbiology, Washington, DC.

Tee, W., Baird, K., Dyall-Smith, M. and Dwyer, B. (1988) *Campylobacter cryaerophila* isolated from a human. *Journal of Clinical Microbiology*, **26**, 2469–2473.

Tenover, F.C. and Fennell, C.L. (1992) The genera *Campylobacter* and *Helicobacter*. In *A Handbook on* the *Biology of Bacteria: Ecophysiology, Isolation, Identification, Application* (ed. A. Balows, H.G. Truper, M. Dworkin *et al.*), pp. 3488–3511. Springer-Verlag, New York.

Thompson III, L.M., Smibert, R.M., Johnson, J.L. and Krieg, N.R. (1988) Phylogenetic study of the genus *Campylobacter. International Journal of Systematic Bacteriology*, **38**, 190–200.

Tummuru, M.K.R. and Blaser, M.J. (1993) Rearrangement of *sap*A homologs with conserved and variable regions in *Campylobacter fetus. Proceedings of the National Academy of Sciences USA*, **90**, 7265–7269.

Vandamme, P. and De Ley, J. (1991) Proposal for a new family, Campylobacteraceae. *International Journal of Systematic Bacteriology*, **41**, 451–455.

Vandamme, P., Falsen, E., Rossau, R. *et al.* (1991) Revision of *Campylobacter, Helicobacter* and *Wolinella* taxonomy: emendation of generic descriptions and proposal of *Arcobacter* gen. nov. *International Journal of Systematic Bacteriology*, **41**, 88–103.

Vandamme, P., Pugina, P., Benzi, G. *et al.* (1992a) Outbreak of recurrent abdominal cramps associated with *Arcobacter butzleri* in an Italian School. *Journal of Clinical Microbiology*, **30**, 2335–2337.

Vandamme, P., Vancanneyt, M., Pot, B. *et al.* (1992b) Polyphasic taxonomic study of the emended genus *Arcobacter* with *Arcobacter butzleri* comb. nov. and *Arcobacter skirrowii* sp. nov., an aerotolerant bacterium isolated from veterinary specimens. *International Journal of Systematic Bacteriology*, **42**, 344–356.

Vandamme, P., Giesendorf, B.A.J., VanBelkum, A. *et al.* (1993) Discrimination of epidemic and sporadic isolates of *Arcobacter butzleri* by polymerase chain reaction-mediated DNA finger printing. *Journal of Clinical Microbiology*, **31**, 3317–3319.

Wassenaar, T.M., Fry, B.N. and van der Zeijst, B.A. (1995) Variation of the flagellin gene locus of *Campylobacter jejuni* by recombination and horizontal gene transfer. *Microbiology*, **141**, 95–101.

Waterman, S.R., Hackett, J. and Manning, P.A. (1993) Isolation of a restriction-less mutant and development of a shuttle vector for the genetic analysis of *Campylobacter hyointestinalis. Gene*, **125**, 19–24.

Yao, R., Alm, R., Trust, T.J. and Guerry, P. (1993) Construction of new *Campylobacter* cloning vectors and a new mutational *cat* cassette. *Gene*, **130**, 127–130.

18

ANAEROBIC COCCI

J.S. Brazier

INTRODUCTION

History

Since 1893, when Veillon first described anaerobic cocci in cases of Ludwig's angina, Bartholin's abscess and various other soft-tissue infections, their presence in a broad array of human sepsis has been recognized. Over a century later, however, despite advances in the isolation and identification of these organisms, and in their overall classification, very little progress in understanding their pathogenic potential in human sepsis has been made.

In man, the anaerobic cocci are members of the commensal microflora of the mucous membranes of the oropharnygeal, intestinal and genitourinary tracts; they are also present in the dermis of the skin. Trauma, intercurrent infection or underlying pathology may precipitate their access to the bloodstream, from where they may lodge in normally sterile body sites, setting up foci of infection.

Like many other human endogenous anaerobic bacteria, they are predominantly opportunist pathogens, often present in polymicrobial infections with other obligate or facultative anaerobes. In such infections it is generally difficult to discern which organisms are the primary pathogens at a given site, and which are merely found 'at the scene of the crime'.

It has become common practice for clinical diagnostic laboratories not to identify anaerobes accurately, especially those in mixed infections. This is due in part to the the limited resources of laboratories and the 'panacea-like' chemotherapeutic effect of metronidazole. The anaerobic cocci suffer more than most in this respect, since often they are present in mixed infections only; they are commonly reported in a descriptive form as 'anaerobic cocci' or misleadingly as 'anaerobic streptococci', and are seldom identified even to genus level. Because they are not routinely identified they may become unrecognized, because they are unrecognized they go unreported; thus, a downward spiral of interest and awareness as to their true significance in clinical sepsis is perpetuated. Although the anaerobic cocci are not particularly virulent, they are found in pure culture in some infections. Anaerobic cocci have attracted far less detailed study than other non-sporing anaerobes such as *Bacteroides fragilis*. A deeper understanding of their taxonomy and characteristics should improve the understanding of the role in human sepsis of this unique group of organisms.

Principles and Practice of Clinical Bacteriology. Edited by A.M. Emmerson, P.M. Hawkey and S.H. Gillespie

TAXONOMY

The anaerobic cocci comprise eight genera which, mainly for reasons of convenience rather than necessity, are usually considered together in textbooks on clinical microbiology.

Gram-positive anaerobic cocci (GPAC) include the genera *Coprococcus*, *Ruminococcus*, *Sarcina*, *Peptococcus* and *Peptostreptococcus*, of which only the latter is commonly isolated from human clinical material. The Gram-negative anaerobic cocci (GNAC) consist of *Veillonella*, *Acidaminococcus* and *Megasphaera*, of which only *Veillonella* may be commonly present in clinical material.

Gram-positive Anaerobic Cocci

Peptococci and peptostreptococci

After reports in the literature describing GPAC in various clinical infections, Prevot (1933) commenced to classify them. He described three groups – A, B and C – based on their ability or inability to produce gas and foul odour. Colebrook and Hare (1933) grouped the 'anaerobic streptococci' according to colonial morphology on blood agar and gas production, recognizing four types, A.–D. Stone (1940) studied 26 strains of 'anaerobic streptococci' for antigens which might allow a classification based on serogrouping, without success. Foubert and Douglas (1948) studied 52 strains of 'anaerobic micrococci'. The latter researchers included them in the genus *Micrococcus* and described three new species: *M. prevotii*, *M. saccharolyticus* and *M. variabilis*. Later classification of the GPAC relied on morphological features such as the tendency to form chains or clumps when stained and viewed under the microscope.

Some of these were assigned to the classification of Hare *et al.* (1952), who studied 99 strains of GPAC from human origin. They studied gas formation and fermentation reactions and defined six groups, designated I–VI. Of the 99 strains studied, 92 could be placed into this classification scheme. They also concluded that colonial and cellular morphology was of little value in classifying GPAC. This classification was later extended to 10 groups by Thomas and Hare (1954), and the Hare groups still form the basis of taxonomical studies on GPAC to the present day.

The name *Peptostreptococcus* (Greek: the digesting streptococcus) was assigned to the chain-forming group and *Peptococcus* (Greek: the digesting coccus) to the clumping group. Lambert and Armfield (1979) described a method of differentiating between these genera using gas–liquid chromatography (GLC) of cell wall fatty acids and metabolic end products. A simpler method based on sensitivity or resistance to a 5 μg novobiocin disk was described by Wren *et al.* (1977a). Attempts at differentiating between these two genera was made redundant, however, after Ezaki *et al.* (1983) analysed the DNA G + C% content of the two genera. They showed that the type species of the peptostreptococci, *Peptostreptococcus anaerobius*, has a G + C content of 33 mol%, a value similar to those species defined as belonging to the genus *Peptococcus*, e.g. *P. magnus*, *P. indolicus*, *P. prevotii* and *P. asaccharolyticus* (29–34 mol% G + C). Only one peptococcus (*P. niger*) warranted the status of a separate genus, having a G + C content of 51 mol%. All other species previously classified as peptococci are now included in the genus *Peptostreptococcus*. Although this classification has been generally accepted, Huss *et al.* (1984) analysed the murein content in cell walls of peptostreptococci and found a diversity of murein types within the same species. Table 18.1 lists the 14 currently recognized species of peptostreptococci and their synonyms.

Murdoch *et al.* (1988a, 1988b) performed studies on clinical isolates and reference strains of GPAC using preformed enzyme substrates. They concluded that this method was good for the routine identification of *Peptostreptococcus anaerobius*, *Ps. asaccharolyticus*, *Ps. indolicus*, *Ps. magnus* and *Ps. micros*, but reported a heterogeneity among the butyric acid-producing group which includes *Ps. prevotii*, and Hare group III, and suggested further taxonomical investigations would prove fruitful.

TABLE 18.1 CURRENT CLASSIFICATION OF THE GENUS *PEPTOSTREPTOCOCCUS*

Species	Synonym
Peptostreptococcus anaerobius	
Peptostreptococcus asaccharolyticus	*Peptococcus asaccharolyticus*
Peptostreptococcus barnesae	
Peptostreptococcus heliotrinreducens	
Peptostreptococcus hydrogenalis	
Peptostreptococcus indolicus	*Peptococcus indolicus*
Peptostreptococcus lacrimalis	
Peptostreptococcus lactolyticus	
Peptostreptococcus magnus	*Peptococcus magnus*
Peptostreptococcus micros	*Peptococcus glycinophilus*
Peptostreptococcus prevotii	*Peptococcus prevotii*
Peptostreptococcus productus	
Peptostreptococcus tetradius	*Gaffyka anaerobia*
Peptostreptococcus vaginalis	

Studies currently in progress in Cardiff, UK indicate that the current taxonomy is incomplete and that there are probably at least three new species of peptostreptococci awaiting description.

Other 'anaerobic' Gram-positive cocci

Various classifications, including that of Hare, have encompassed microaerophilic or capnophilic cocci, which has confused the situation. Some members of the genus *Streptococcus* and *Staphylococcus* are preferentially anaerobic when first isolated from clinical material and initially may be mistaken for peptostreptococci. Indeed, the organisms previously known as *Peptostreptococcus intermedius* and *Peptostreptococcus parvulus* have both been transferred to the genes *Streptococcus*, and *Peptococcus saccharolyticus* to the genus *Staphylococcus*. Watt and Jack (1977) attempted a working definition of anaerobic cocci as those which fail to grow in 10% carbon dioxide in air after seven days incubation. They noted that this group were sensitive to a 5 μg metronidazole disk, but those that grew in carbon dioxide were resistant. This simple and quicker test has therefore become an easy way to recognize this group.

An example is *Staphylococcus saccharolyticus*, which grows poorly or not at all in air, and produces catalase on media containing haemin or blood. It is coagulase negative, sensitive to novobiocin but resitant to metronidazole. It usually ferments glucose with the production of acetic acid as the major end product.

Microaerophilic streptococci such as the 'milleri group' of *Streptococcus anginosus*, *S. intermedius* and *S. constellatus* may appear as anaerobic on primary culture. They are also resistant to metronidazole and become aerotolerant upon serial subculture. They are also strongly saccharolytic, unlike most true anaerobic cocci, and are best identified by methods suitable for streptococci rather than anaerobes (see page 7). *Streptococcus morbillorum* is now considered to be a member of the genus *Gemella* (Kilpper-Balz and Schleiffer, 1981), although this organism is aerotolerant after primary isolation. *Streptococcus pleomorphus* and *S. hansenii* are obligately anaerobic but their taxonomic position remains in doubt.

Sarcina

The genus *Sarcina* consists of GPAC that form large clumps or 'packets' due to cellular replication occurring consecutively in three perpendicular planes. Spores may also be formed. *Sarcina* spp. metabolize glucose to form carbon dioxide, hydrogen, ethanol and acetic acid end products. Two species have been described – *S. ventriculi* and *S. maxima* – of which only the former has ever been isolated from human material. It is believed to be carried in the gut particularly by vegetarians and has been isolated from faeces, gall-bladder and diseased stomach contents. It is rarely, if ever, found in other diseased sites or in pure culture.

Coprococci *and* ruminococci

Coprococcus spp. and *Ruminococcus* sp. are predominantly commensals of the human and bovine intestinal tracts. Ruminococci and coprococci are not thought to play a role in any human or animal infections, and as such receive little attention in clinical textbooks such as this. They do, however, play an important role in the rumen ecosystem.

The Gram-negative Anaerobic Cocci

The first description of Gram-negative cocci in a human infection was by Veillon and Zuber (1898). They called their isolate *Staphylococcus parvulus*. Three years later, Lewkowicz described an identical organism which he called *Micrococcus gazogenes alcalescens anaerobius*. Hall and Howitt (1925) described GNAC in saliva which they concluded was the same organism described by Lewkowicz, but renamed it *M. gazogenes*. Because of its apparent failure to retain the Gram stain it was later placed in the genus *Veillonella* by Prevot (1933). Rogosa (1965) described seven groups of veillonellae based on a serological typing method of whole cell agglutination using rabbit antiserum. Two species were recognized: *V. parvula* and *V. alcalescens*; differentiation was based on the catalase reaction. Each of the seven serological groups species was assigned as a subspecies. These seven subspecies were elevated to full species status by Mays *et al.* (1982), who performed DNA–DNA hybridization studies. The specific epithets were mainly attributed to the commonest source of each strain; i.e. *V. ratti* is

found in the oral cavity of rats, *V. criceti* in the mouth of hamsters, *V. caviae* in guinea-pigs, and *V. rodentium* in various rodents. The species found in humans were designated *V. atypica*, *V. parvula* and *V. dispar*.

Acidaminococcus

The genus *Acidaminococcus* consists of one species, *A. fermentans*. The cocci are approximately 1.0 μm in diameter, occurring in pairs. It is non-motile, oxidase, catalase and nitrate negative and, despite its name, is asaccharolytic. Amino acids, particularly glutamate, are its main energy source, with the formation of acetic and butyric acids. The G + C content is 56 mol%. It has been isolated from the faeces of man and pigs, and is rarely found in human infective processes.

Megasphaera

The genus *Megasphaera* also consists of one species, *M. elsdenii*. As its name suggests, it forms large cocci of 2.4–2.6 μm diameter in pairs or short chains. It is non-motile, catalase and nitrate negative. It ferments glucose, producing caproic acid as the major metabolite, with smaller amounts of acetic, butyric, valeric acids and their iso-acids. The G + C content is 54 mol% and it is found in the rumen of cattle and sheep and in the intestine of man. It is rarely found in human infections.

GENERAL DESCRIPTIONS OF THE ORGANISMS

Gram-positive Anaerobic Cocci

The cocci range in diameter from 0.4–2.0 μm and may be in clumps, diplococci, short or long chains or a mixture of both forms. *Peptostreptococcus* spp. are obligately anaerobic, with a G + C ratio of 29–34 mol%, and may be found as part of the normal microflora of the human oral cavity, skin, and gastrointestinal and female genital tracts. *Peptococcus* spp. produce catalase and dark pigmented colonies, with a DNA G + C ratio of 50 mol%, and is part of the normal flora of the vagina. Neither genus produces spores or exhibits motility.

Peptostreptococci and peptococci survive moderate exposure to air as they are not exquisitely sensitive to oxygen. Ten per cent carbon dioxide enhances the growth of many strains. Both genera are usually sensitive to metronidazole, a test which aids differentiation from anaerobic members of the genera *Streptococcus* and *Staphylococcus*.

Gram-negative Cocci

Veillonella are commonly found in the oral cavities of man and other mammals, most notably rodents. In man they have been demonstrated in high numbers in saliva and on the surface of the tongue, where they have been shown to adhere particularly well to the epithelial cells on this surface.

Veillonella are small cocci less than 1 μm in diameter occurring in pairs, clusters or short chains. They are non-sporing and non-motile; some species produce catalase but all reduce nitrate to nitrite. Oxidase and urease are not produced. Colonies on blood agar are non-haemolytic, circular, grey-white and fairly featureless. After 48 hours they are 1–2 mm across. Non-saccharolytic except for fructose fermentation by one species, metabolic end products are acetic and propionic acids.

PATHOGENICITY

Compared with other anaerobes, such as clostridia and the Bacteroidaceae, the anaerobic cocci have been neglected regarding studies of their virulence mechanisms. Little is known about their pathogenic role, especially in mixed infections. Even when isolated in pure culture from blood, for example, their significance may be questioned. Virulence factors of GPAC and veillonellae are poorly elucidated. Many strains of GPAC can produce enzymes with pathogenic potential such as coagulase, urease or hyaluronidase, as well as a range of proteolytic enzymes. Krepel *et al.* (1992) reported that the proteolytic enzymes produced by strains of *Peptostreptococcus magnus* may have

an important effect on the pathogenesis of certain soft tissue infections. Brook and Walker (1984) demonstrated the ability of anaerobic cocci to synergize with other organisms. In a mouse animal model they showed that the presence of injected anaerobic cocci significantly increased the size and severity of an abscess, compared with a control mouse in which the cocci were omitted from the microbial insult.

The lipopolysaccharide in the cell wall of *Veillonella* is an endotoxin that can elicit fever in experimental animals, but despite this it would seem they are not particularly virulent pathogens. *Peptostreptococcus magnus* has been shown to possess a cell wall protein (L) which has a high affinity to human immunoglobulin (Ig) light chains (DeChateau *et al.*, 1993) – evidence perhaps that the human immune system copes well with GPAC.

CLINICAL FEATURES

Apart from a synergistic gangrene where GPAC and *Staphylococcus aureus* combine to cause a progressive gangrenous skin condition (Meleney, 1931), anaerobic cocci are not associated with any specific infective process *per se*. They may be present in inflammatory processes involving any body site – often those in close proximity to the sites they inhabit as commensals. Several studies have shown the high incidence of GPAC in clinical material.

Incidence in Human Infections

Holland *et al.* (1977) reported on a study of 826 clinical specimens obtained over a 14-year period, from which anaerobes were isolated from 58.5%. GPAC accounted for 40% of the total anaerobic isolates. In the same year, Wren *et al.* (1977b) analysed the anaerobic isolates from clinical material over a 14-month period. Peptostreptococci and peptococci accounted for one-third of the total number of 1392 anaerobic isolates obtained; this was second only in total to the *Bacteroides*. *Peptostreptococcus magnus* was the most common, accounting for 20% of the total cocci and 6.1% of the total anaerobes isolated. The GPAC accounted for 24.1% of the anaerobic isolates from abdominal sites and 39.3% of strains from superficial wounds.

Gynaecological Infections

GPAC are recognized as significant pathogens in infections involving the female genital tract, e.g. septic abortion, puerperal sepsis, endometritis and tubo-ovarian abscess. They also play a prominant role in cases of postoperative wound infections after gynaecological surgery. Species normally inhabiting the vagina include *Peptostreptococcus magnus*, *Ps. asaccharolyticus*, *Ps. anaerobius* and *Ps. prevotii*. As early as 1926 Schwarz and Dieckman studied postpartum endometritis in 165 women and reported *Ps. anaerobius* in 28% of cases and 'anaerobic streptococci' in a further 13%.

Infections of Head and Chest Region

Infections of the brain, head and neck region commonly involve the anaerobic cocci which occupy the linings of the oropharynx comprising mainly *Peptostreptococcus anaerobius*, *Ps. magnus* and *Ps. prevotii*. Infections involving these organisms include chronic otitis media, sinusitis, brain abscess and periodontitis. Brain abscesses and meningitis are believed to result from GPAC gaining access to the central nervous system from either rhinogenic, otogenic or odontogenic origin. These same organisms can also gain access to the lower respiratory tract by aspiration, causing pneumonitis, empyaema and lung abscess. Although *Veillonella* spp. are believed to outnumber the Gram-positive anaerobic cocci in the mouth, especially on the tongue and in saliva, they are less frequently isolated from infections of the head and neck, which indicates that they have lower virulence.

Abdominal Infections

Intra-abdominal infections with GPAC may result from faecal contamination of the peritoneum resulting from appendicitis, diverticular disease,

surgical/accidental trauma, or malignancy. These infections are predominantly mixed with other obligate and facultative anaerobes. Liver abscess may also result from GPAC from this source.

Infections of Bones and Joints

Infections of bone or joints involving GPAC are predominantly due to *Peptostreptococcus magnus*. Bourgault *et al.* (1980) reported on a survey of 222 patients from whom *Ps. magnus* was isolated. Thirty-two cases (14%) involved bone or joint infections in which *Ps. magnus* was isolated in pure culture, particularly when a foreign body such as an orthopaedic prosthesis was present. Hall *et al.* (1983) reported on 40 patients with osteomyelitis from whom 60% of the 92 anaerobic isolates were GPAC; 30% of these were identified as *P. magnus*.

Bacteraemia

The incidence of bacteraemia due to anaerobic cocci varies greatly between centres. A recent report on the incidence and clinical significance of anaerobic bacteraemias in America listed peptostreptococci as the second most frequently isolated anaerobes, present in 23% of positive cases (Peraino *et al.*, 1993). An earlier report listed anaerobic cocci in 4% of anaerobic bacteraemias (Rosenblatt, 1985). In England and Wales figures reported to the Communicable Disease Surveillance Centre for 1992 list 1337 anaerobic bacteraemias of which 137 (10.2%) were due to anaerobic cocci, placing them third behind *Bacteroides* and clostridia.

LABORATORY DIAGNOSIS

Rapid Methods

The laboratory diagnosis of infections involving anaerobic cocci relies essentially on traditional bacteriological methods. As yet, there are no commercially available kits aimed specifically at the rapid diagnosis of GPAC or *Veillonella* infections. As for other anaerobic infections, though, direct gas–liquid chromatographical analysis of clinical material (exudate or blood culture) can detect volatile metabolites indicative of obligate anaerobes. However, as some of the GPAC produce only acetic acid they would not be differentiated from facultative bacteria such as staphylococci by this method. The commonest isolate, *Peptostreptococcus anaerobius*, and the butyric acid group (*Ps. prevotii*, *Ps. asaccharolyticus* etc.), however, do lend themselves to rapid diagnosis by this method (see Figure 18.1).

Cultural Methods

Methods suitable for the culture of other fastidious non-spore-forming anaerobes are generally sufficient for the isolation of anaerobic cocci from clinical material. Compared with other anaerobes, however, relatively little work has been performed with regard to selective media aimed specifically at this group. Selective agents for other non-spore-forming anaerobes such as neomycin sulphate (70 mg/l) may be used for GPAC and *Veillonella* quite successfully. Wren (1978), however, found the combination of naladixic acid and Tween to be superior at recovering anaerobic cocci from clinical material. This medium, however, will not be suitable for Gram-negative anaerobes; therefore another plate will be needed. Other agents used in combination include bicomycin–neomycin (Watt

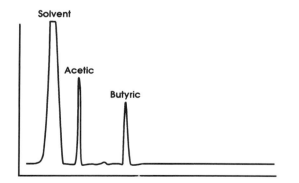

Figure 18.1. Volatile fatty acid analysis by GLC of a blood culture containing *Peptostreptococcus asaccharolyticus*.

and Brown, 1983), and neomycin–phenylethyl alcohol. Apart from selective agents certain growth factors for anaerobic cocci are known. *Veillonella* spp. for example, benefit from sodium pyruvate and nitrate in the medium, and arginine is a growth factor for some species of peptostreptococci. As for other obligate anaerobes, the use of a 5 μg metronidazole disk placed in the streaked-out inoculum facilitates their easy recognition in mixed culture.

Identification

Beginning with Gram staining (See Figure 18.2), anaerobic cocci can be grouped into presumptive genera. Equivocal Gram variables can be checked by the potassium hydroxide slide test (Halebian *et al.*, 1981). Those that produce 'strings' after emulsification in 3% KOH are Gram negative. A nitrate reduction test differentiates the veillonellae from *Acidaminococcus* and *Megasphaera*, whilst the production of a dark-pigmented colony splits peptococci from peptostreptococci.

Many of the anaerobic cocci are asaccharolytic and inert in many of the traditional biochemical tests applied to other anaerobes. Kits that rely largely on sugar fermentation tests are therefore unhelpful in distinguishing between the species. A more productive approach is the study of pre-formed proteolytic enzyme profiles as tested by commercially available identification kits such as the API ATB 32A (Murdoch *et al.*, 1990). Even this approach, however, frequently needs supplementing with analysis of volatile fatty acid (VFA) end products of metabolism by gas–liquid chromatography (GLC) to attain speciation. Using this data, peptostreptococci can be split into three main groups: those that produce acetic acid only or no major acids, those that produce major butyric acid, and those that produce isovaleric and/or isocaproic acids.

Because VFA analysis by GLC is not routinely available in most diagnostic microbiology laboratories, the successful identification of this group is not always straightforward; a few simple tests, however, can lead to a presumptive species identification.

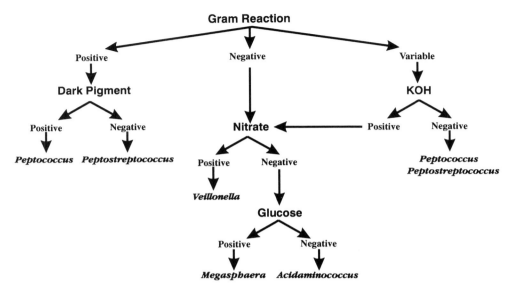

Figure 18.2. First-stage table for identification of anaerobic cocci to genus level. KOH, 3% potassium hydroxide slide test for formation of 'strings'; Nitrate, reduction of nitrate to nitrite; Glucose, fermentation of glucose with acid production; Dark Pigment, formation of dark colonies on blood agar after prolonged incubation.

Presumptive methods of identifying common species of peptostreptococci

Colonies of all species of peptostreptococci on blood agar are non-haemolytic, sensitive to metronidazole and tend to be rather deficient in distinguishing features to aid recognition of the species. Colonial descriptions of each species are unhelpful. There are relatively few simple phenotypic tests with which to easily and confidently differentiate between species. Figure 18.3 is a dichotomous key enabling presumptive speciation of peptostreptococci and listed below are 'thumbnail sketches' in note form of the species most commonly isolated from clinical specimens and some clues to their recognition.

Peptostreptococcus anaerobius

The species is coccobacillary, often in chains, and can sometimes be mistaken for a short rod such as *Eubacterium*; it is easily over-decolorized, and thus may appear as a Gram-variable coccobacillus (See Figure 18.4). It is sensitive to liquoid (sodium polyanethol sulphonate) (Graves *et al.*, 1974) at a concentration of 1000 μg gives a large zone of sensitivity compared with no zone with other species, or a very small zone with *Ps. prevotii*. *Ps. anaerobius* colonies have a characteristic odour reminiscent of new plasticine; typical API 32A profile = 04000300; it produces isovaleric and/or isocaproic acids.

Peptostreptococcus asaccharolyticus

This species is easily over-decolorized; it forms clusters, short chains and pairs (see Figure 18.5); it is indole positive with the spot indole reagent (*p*-dimethylaminocinnamaldehyde). Colonies have a musty odour; typical API 32A profile = 00006101; it produces butyric acid.

Peptostreptococcus prevotii

This species is strongly staining; it forms clumps and short chains. A few strains produce indole; it is urease positive, catalase variable, and there is no obvious colonial odour. There is a wide variation

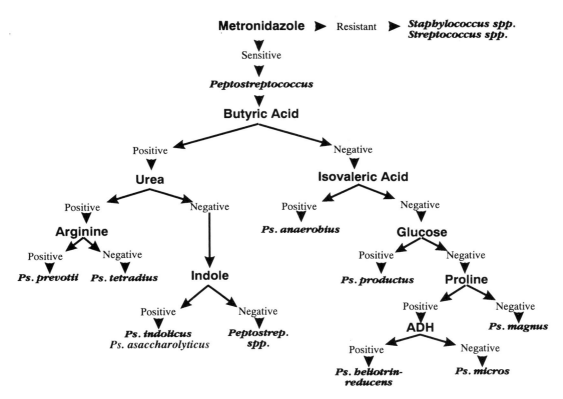

Figure 18.3. Second-stage table for identification of Gram-positive anaerobic cocci. Metronidazole, sensitivity to 5 μg disk; Butyric/Isovaleric Acid, metabolic end product determined by GLC; Urea, hydrolysis of urea; Indole, production from tryptophan-containing media; Glucose, fermentation of glucose with acid production; Arginine/Proline/ADH, preformed enzyme substrates.

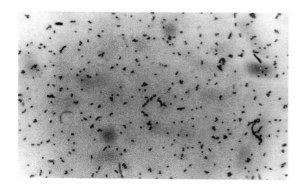

Figure 18.4. *Peptostreptococcus anaerobius.*

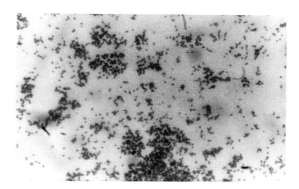

Figure 18.5. *Peptostreptococcus asaccharolyticus.*

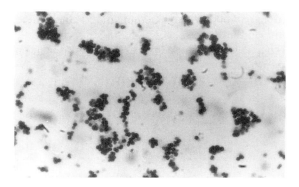

Figure 18.6. *Peptostreptococcus magnus*.

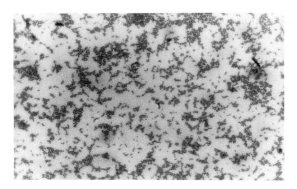

Figure 18.7. *Peptostreptococcus micros*.

of possible profiles in API 32A; it produces butyric acid.

Peptostreptococcus magnus

This species is a large coccus; it is Gram variable, and occurs in large clumps and clusters of twos, threes and fours (see Figure 18.6); it is catalase variable and indole negative; typical API 32A profile = 00004564. It produces acetic acid only.

Peptostreptococcus micros

This species is a small coccus which occurs in short chains and clusters (see Figure 18.7). It is catalase negative and indole negative; it is a slow grower, with a 'fish-paste' colonial odour; typical API 32A profile = 00004777. It produces acetic acid only.

Colonies of GPAC on blood agar may also be recognized by their ability to fluoresce under long-wave (365 nm) ultraviolet (UV) light. The ability of 55 strains of GPAC colonies to fluoresce under UV on Fastidious Anaerobe Agar incorporating 6% horse blood was studied by Brazier (1989). He reported a yellow fluorescence as a variable property of 55 strains representing six species of peptostreptococci. Fluorescence was most common in *Ps. prevotii*, *Ps. asaccharolyticus* and *Ps. anaerobius* with 6/6, 5/5 and 7/8 strains positive respectively (Table 18.2). Some strains of *Ps. magnus* and *Ps. micros* also produced a pinkish fluorescence. Combined with Gram staining and sensitivity to a metronidazole disk placed in the streaked-out inoculum, it was shown that this method is useful in picking out colonies of GPAC in primary mixed culture. Although some species have names suggesting their size, i.e. *Ps. magnus* (large) and *Ps. micros* (small), this property is subject to variation depending on the growth conditions and media composition. It should not be

TABLE 18.2   ABILITY OF 55 STRAINS OF *PEPTOSTREPTOCOCCUS* SPP. TO FLUORESCE ON FASTIDIOUS ANAEROBE BLOOD AGAR UNDER U.V. (365 NM) ILLUMINATION

Species	No. examined	No. positive	Colour
Peptostreptococcus anaerobius	8	7	Yellow
Peptostreptococcus asaccharolyticus	5	5	Yellow
Peptostreptococcus indolicus	4	1	Yellow
Peptostreptococcus magnus	21	12	(7 yellow, 5 pink)
Peptostreptococcus micros	11	8	(5 Yellow, 3 Pink)
Peptostreptococcus prevotii	6	6	Yellow
Total	55	39	

relied upon too heavily as an aid to identification, particularly by the inexperienced.

In the final analysis, the definitive identification of anaerobic cocci requires analysis of metabolic end products by GLC combined with details of morphology, basic biochemical reactions and preformed enzyme profile by API 32A.

Methods for identification of Veillonella species

Phenotypic tests useful for the speciation of veillonellas are very limited. All species produce acetic and propionic acids; therefore GLC has no intraspecific discriminatory value. Figure 18.8 is a simple key to identification based on catalase, fructose fermentation and origin of strain.

Colonies of *Veillonella parvula* and *V. alcalescens* on blood agar were reported by Chow *et al.* (1975) as being capable of a red fluorescence under long-wave UV light. The authors suggested this method would be a simple way of recognizing *Veillonella* spp. in mixed culture. This phenomenon, however, was regarded with some scepticism in the UK, since it could not be reproduced. Brazier and Riley (1988) investigated this further, testing seven species of veillonellae on a range of agar bases in the presence of either sheep or horse blood. They demonstrated the effete nature of the fluorescence which was shown to be due to a porphyrin pigment that faded rapidly upon exposure to the air. Except for one species (*V. criceti*, which is found only in hamsters), fluorescence only occurred on brain–heart infusion-based media (commonly used in the USA but not in the UK), and was unaffected by the type of blood used. This explained the lack of fluorescence in the UK and proved why this test has little value for recognizing veillonellas in mixed primary culture.

Antimicrobial Susceptibility

Widespread resistance to antimicrobials does not appear to be a problem for either the Gram-positive or Gram-negative anaerobic cocci. All β-lactam agents inhibit over 95% of strains of peptostreptococci (Wexler, 1991), and penicillin G remains the drug of choice. Metronidazole is very highly active against peptostreptococci. Goldstein *et al.* (1978) reported 88% of strains susceptible to 0.5 mg/l, and 97% of strains susceptible to 2 mg/l metronidazole. Other highly active antibiotics include chloramphenicol and imipenem, but over 10% of strains are resistant to 64 mg/l of clindamycin (Sutter and Finegold, 1976). Tetra-

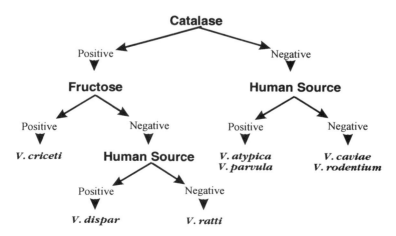

Figure 18.8. Second-stage table for identification of *Veillonella* spp. Catalase, liberation of bubbles from hydrogen peroxide; Fructose, fermentation of fructose with acid production; Human Source, isolate from human clinical specimen.

cycline and erythromycin activity remains unpredictable, with 52% of strains being resistant to 4 mg/l.

Veillonella spp. susceptibilities have received little attention but were studied by Rogosa (1974), who reported susceptibilities of <1 mg/l to chloramphenicol, tetracyclines and polymixin B. Sutter and Finegold (1976) reported MIC 50 and MIC 90 values to metronidazole as <1.0/<1.0 mg/l, tetracycline 0.5/32 mg/l, and erythromycin <2.0/8.0 mg/l. Aminoglycosides and vancomycin have poor activity *in vitro*.

MANAGEMENT PREVENTION AND CONTROL OF INFECTION

The clinical management of sepsis involving anaerobic cocci does not differ in principle from the management of infections involving other non-spore-forming anaerobes. Surgical drainage of abscess formation is usually performed and is very beneficial, as is the empirical administration of systemic antibiotics such as metronidazole and/or penicillin. Therapy can be altered if indicated after laboratory results become available. Some confusion may arise with the applicability of metronidazole if incomplete identification of GPAC or no susceptibility testing has occurred. Since infections with anaerobic cocci are endogenous there are no specific infection control procedures that apply to infections with these organisms other than the correct disposal of infected dressings etc.

CONCLUSION

The anaerobic cocci are a loose association of a heterogeneous group of organisms which continue to be under-studied and probably under-recognized in clinical laboratories. If the general level of interest can be raised, so will our understanding, to the ultimate benefit of both patients and microbiologists alike. This will take time; it is just as Alfred Lord Tennyson said:

> Science moves, but slowly slowly,
> Creeping on from point to point.

ACKNOWLEDGEMENTS

I am grateful to Dr J.T. Magee for his help with the design and preparation of the figures.

REFERENCES

Bourgault, A.M., Rosenblatt, J.E. and Fitzgerald, R.H. (1980) *Peptococcus magnus*: a significant human pathogen. *Annals of Internal Medicine*, **93**, 244–248.

Brazier, J.S. (1989) Studies of ultra-violet fluorescence of anaerobic bacteria. PhD thesis, Council for National Academic Awards, UK.

Brazier, J.S. and Riley, T.V. (1988) UV red fluorescence of *Veillonella* spp. *Journal of Clinical Microbiology*, **26**, 383–384.

Brook, I. and Walker, R.I. (1984) Pathogenicity of anaerobic Gram positive cocci. *Infection and Immunity*, **45**, 320–324.

Chow, A.W., Patten, V. and Guze, L.B. (1975) Rapid screening of *Veillonella* by ultraviolet fluorescence. *Journal of Clinical Microbiology*, **2**, 546–548.

Colebrook, L. and Hare, R. (1933) The anaerobic streptococci associated with puerperal fever. *Journal of Obstetrics and Gynaecology of the British Empire*, **40**, 609–629.

De Chateau, M., Wilson, B.H.K., Erntell, M. *et al.* (1993) On the interaction between protein L and immunoglobulins of various mammalian species. *Scandinavian Journal of Immunology*, **37**(4), 399–405.

Ezaki, T., Yamamoto, N., Ninomiya, K. *et al.* (1983) Transfer of *Peptococcus indolicus*, *Peptococcus asaccharolyticus*, *Peptococcus prevotii*, and *Peptococcus magnus* to the genus *Peptostreptococcus* and proposal of *Peptostreptococcus tetradius* sp. *nov*. *International Journal of Systematic Bacteriology*, **33**, 683–698.

Foubert, E.L. and Douglas, H.C. (1948) Studies on the anaerobic micrococci. *Journal of Bacteriology*, **56**, 25–34.

Goldstein, E.J., Sutter, V.L. and Finegold, S.M. (1978) Comparative susceptibilities of anaerobic bacteria to metronidazole, ornidazole and SC-28538. *Antimicrobial Agents and Chemotherapy*, **14**, 609–612.

Graves, M.H., Morello, J.A. and Kocka, F.E. (1974) Sodium polyanetholsulfonate sensitivity of anaerobic cocci. *Applied Microbiology*, **27**, 1131–1133.

Halebian, S., Harris, B., Finegold, S.M. *et al.* (1981) Rapid method that aids in distinguishing Gram positive from Gram negative anaerobic bacteria. *Journal of Clinical Microbiology*, **13**, 444–448.

Hall, B.B., Fitzgerald, R.H. and Rosenblatt, J.E. (1983) Anaerobic osteomyelitis. *Journal of Bone and Joint Surgery of America*, **65**, 30–35.

Hall, I.C. and Howitt, B. (1925) Bacterial factors in pyorrhea alveolaris. IV. *Micrococcus gazogenes*, a minute Gram negative, non sporulating anaerobe prevalent in human saliva. *Journal of Infectious Diseases*, **37**, 112–125.

Hare, R., Wildy, P., Billett, F.S. *et al.* (1952) The anaerobic cocci: gas formation, fermentation reactions, sensitivity to antibiotics and sulphonamides. Classification. *Journal of Hygiene*, **50**, 295–319.

Holland, J.W., Hill, E.O. and Altemeier, W.A. (1977) Numbers and types of anaerobic bacteria isolated from clinical specimens since 1960. *Journal of Clinical Microbiology*, **5**, 20–25.

Huss, V.A.R., Festl, H. and Schleifer, R.H. (1984) Nucleic acid hybridization studies and deoyribonucleic acid base compositions of anaerobic Gram positive cocci. *International Journal of Systematic Bacteriology*, **34**, 95–101.

Kilpper-Balz, R. and Schleifer, R.H. (1981) Transfer of *Peptococcus saccharolyticus* (Foubert and Douglas) to the genus *Staphylococcus*: *Staphylococcus saccharolyticus* (Foubert and Douglas) comb. nov. *Zentralblatt für Bakteriologie, Parasitenkunde, Infections Krankheiten und Hygiene Abteilung*, **2**, 324–331.

Krepel, C.J., Gohr, C.M., Walker, A.P. *et al.* (1992) Enzymatically active *Peptostreptococcus magnus*: association with site of infection. *Journal of Clinical Microbiology*, **30**, 2330–2334.

Lambert, M.A.S. and Armfield, A.Y. (1979) Differentiation of *Peptococcus* and *Peptostreptococcus* by gas–liquid chromatography of cellular fatty acids and metabolic products. *Journal of Clinical Microbiology*, **10**, 464–476.

Mays, T.D., Holdeman, W.E.C., Rogosa, M. *et al.* (1982) Taxonomy of the genus *Veillonella* (Prevot). *International Journal of Systematic Bacteriology*, **32**, 28–36.

Meleney, F.L. (1931) Bacterial synergism in disease process with a confirmation of the synergistic bacterial aetiology of a certain type of progressive gangrene of the stomach wall. *Annals of Surgery*, **19**, 961–968.

Murdoch, D.A., Mitchelmore, I.J. and Tabaqchali, S. (1988a) Identification of Gram positive anaerobic cocci by use of systems for detecting pre-formed enzymes. *Journal of Medical Microbiology*, **25**, 289–293.

Murdoch, D.A., Mitchelmore, I.J., Nash, R.A. *et al.* (1988b) Preformed enzyme profiles of reference strains of Gram positive anaerobic cocci. *Journal of Medical Microbiology*, **27**, 65–70.

Murdoch, D.A., Wilks, M., Mitchelmore, I.J. *et al.*

(1990) Identification of Gram positive anaerobic cocci by gas–liquid chromatography and pre-formed enzyme profile using a commercial kit, ATB 32A. In *Clinical and Molecular Aspects of Anaerobes* (ed. S.P. Borriello), pp. 285–291. Wrightson Biomedical, Petersfield, UK.

Peraino, V.A., Cross, S.A. and Goldstein, E.J.C. (1993) Incidence and clinical significance of anaerobic bacteremia in a community hospital. *Clinical Infectious Diseases*, 16 (Suppl. 4), S288–291.

Prevot, A.R. (1933) Etudes de systematique bacterienne. I. Lois generales. II Cocci anaerobies. *Annales des Science Naturelles Botanique*, **15**, 23–260.

Rogosa, M. (1965) The genus *Veillonella*. IV. Serological groupings and genus and species emendations. *Journal of Bacteriology*, **90**, 704–707.

Rogosa, M. (1974) Genus 1. *Veillonella*. In *Bergey's Manual of Determinative Bacteriology*, 8th edn (ed. Buchan and Gibbons), pp. 446–447. Williams and Wilkins, Baltimore.

Rosenblatt, J.E. (1985) Anaerobic cocci. In *Manual of Clinical Microbiology*, 4th edn (ed. E.H. Lennette, A. Balows, W.J. Hausler *et al.*), pp. 445–449. American Society for Microbiology, Washington, DC.

Schwarz, D. and Dieckman, W.J. (1926) Anaerobic streptococci: their role in puerperal infection. *Southern Medical Journal*, **19**, 470–479.

Stone, M.L. (1940) Studies on the anaerobic streptococcus. I. Certain biochemical and immunological properties of anaerobic streptococci. *Journal of Bacteriology*, **39**, 559–582.

Sutter, V.L. and Finegold, S.M. (1976) Susceptibility of anaerobic bacteria to 23 antimicrobial agents. *Antimicrobial Agents and Chemotherapy*, **10**, 736–752.

Thomas, C.G.A. and Hare, R. (1954) The classification of anaerobic cocci and their isolation in normal human beings and pathological processes. *Journal of Clinical Pathology*, **7**, 300–304.

Veillon, M.A. (1893) Sur un microcoque anaerobie trouve dans des suppurations fetides. *Comptes Rendus Société de Biologie*, **5**, 807–809.

Veillon, M.A. and Zuber, M.M. (1898) Recherches sur quelques microbes strictement anaerobies et leur role en pathologie. *Archives de Medicine, Experimental Anatomy and Pathology*, **10**, 517–545.

Watt, B. and Brown, F.V. (1983) A selective agent for anaerobic cocci. *Journal of Clinical Pathology*, **36**, 605–606.

Watt, B. and Jack, E.P. (1977) What are anaerobic cocci? *Journal of Medical Microbiology*, **10**, 461–468.

Wexler, H.M. (1991) Susceptibility testing of anaerobic bacteria: myth, magic, or method? *Clinical Microbiology Reviews*, **4**, 470–484.

Wren, M.W.D. (1978) A new selective medium for the isolation of non-sporing anaerobic bacteria from clinical specimens. *Medical Laboratory Sciences*, **35**, 371–378.

Wren. M.W.D., Eldon, C.P. and Dakin, G.H. (1977a) Novobiocin and the differentiation of peptococci and peptostreptococci. *Journal of Clinical Pathology*, **30**, 620–622.

Wren, M.W.D., Baldwin, A.W.F., Eldon, C.P. *et al.* (1977b) The anaerobic culture of clinical specimens: a 14-month study. *Journal of Medical Microbiology*, **10**, 49–61.

19a

THE CLOSTRIDIA

David M. Lyerly and Stephen D. Allen

INTRODUCTION

The clostridia represent a diverse group of Gram-positive sporulating bacteria that are rod shaped and that require anaerobic conditions for growth. The group includes organisms that produce organic solvents such as acetone and butanol (e.g. *Clostridium acetobutylicum*), organisms that convert nitrogen into ammonia by nitrogen fixation (e.g. *C. pasteurianum*), and organisms that cause disease and are medically important because they are pathogenic for humans and animals. The purpose of this chapter is to discuss the major human clostridial diseases, including tetanus, botulism, antibiotic-associated diarrhoea and pseudomembranous colitis, gas gangrene, *C. perfringens*-induced food poisoning, and enteritis necroticans (e.g. 'Pig-Bel') (Table 19a.1).

The medically important clostridia are well known for the variety of toxins that they produce. It is the production of these toxins that leads to the distinctive clinical features of the diseases they cause. Of more than 85 species of clostridia described in *Bergey's Manual*, at least 20 produce toxins. The clinical features of tetanus and botulism, for example, result from the production of neurotoxins that are among the most lethal substances known to humans. It has been estimated that as little as 100 ng of either toxin is sufficient to kill an adult. These two diseases have been recognized for many years. Tetanus was originally described in some of the ancient Greek literature whereas botulism became recognized following several outbreaks in the late 1800s after the ingestion of contaminated meats and vegetables. The incidence of botulism is very low. Tetanus, on the other hand, continues to represent a major problem in underdeveloped countries. It has been estimated that more than a million persons die from tetanus each year, with half of these being infants. This alarming number of cases is especially unfortunate when one considers the fact that this terrible disease can be effectively prevented by vaccination.

Gas gangrene became prominent during World War I because of the high incidence of the disease. The gas gangrene clostridia include *C. perfringens*, *C. septicum*, *C. novyi*, *C. histolyticum* and *C. sordellii* as the major members, all of which produce potent tissue-damaging and lethal toxins. In addition to its role in gas gangrene, *C. perfringens* represents a major source of food poisoning because of an enterotoxin that it produces. Fortunately, *C. perfringens* food poisoning is self-limiting and of short duration. Only rarely does it develop into a life-threatening condition.

Principles and Practice of Clinical Bacteriology. Edited by A.M. Emmerson, P.M. Hawkey and S.H. Gillespie

TABLE 19a.1   HUMAN DISEASES CAUSED BY THE CLOSTRIDIA

Disease	Species
Gas gangrene	*C. perfringens*
	C. septicum
	C. novyi type A
	C. sordellii
	C. histolyticum
Tetanus	*C. tetani*
Classical botulism	*C. botulinum* types A, B, E, F
Infant botulism	*C. botulinum* types A, B
Food poisoning	*C. perfringens* type A
Pig-Bel	*C. perfringens* type C
Pseudomembranous colitis and antibiotic-associated diarrhoea	*C. difficile*

The identification of *C. difficile* as the cause of pseudomembranous colitis and antibiotic-associated diarrhoea was demonstrated in the late 1970s, making this organism a fairly 'new' pathogen. *Clostridium difficile* disease, which occurs most typically as a nosocomial disease in elderly patients treated with antibiotics, represents an excellent example of an opportunistic pathogen that causes disease once the normal protective flora of the gut has been altered. The disease has reached epidemic proportions in some medical centres.

DESCRIPTION OF THE GENUS

The clostridia are considered to be obligate anaerobes generally. However, they exhibit a wide range in the amount of oxygen that they tolerate. *Clostridium perfringens*, for example, is fairly aerotolerant and exhibits growth at oxygen tensions of up to 70–80 mmHg. This organism can be exposed to air for several days without any adverse effect on subculturing and viability. *Clostridium tetani*, on the other hand, is much less tolerant and will not grow well unless the oxygen tension is <2 mmHg. Exposure of this organism to air for more than an hour will drastically reduce the viability of the culture. Other clostridia tend to be more moderate in the amount of oxygen that they tolerate. Included in this group are species such as *C. septicum* and *C. difficile*. Many of the toxin producers such as *C. botulinum*, *C. difficile*, *C. sordellii*, *C. septicum* and *C. perfringens* grow

effectively and produce high levels of toxin under conditions that do not include strict anaerobic atmospheres. For the isolation of clostridia from clinical specimens, however, it is important to use high-quality anaerobic media and proper anaerobic methodology.

Although the clostridia are spore-forming anaerobes by definition, this definition has led to some taxonomic confusion because some clostridia are poor spore-formers whereas others form spores readily (Allen and Baron, 1991). The absence of spores in cultures of Gram-positive anaerobic bacilli may suggest a *Eubacterium* species instead of a *Clostridium* species. Not only do different clostridial species exhibit differences in spore formation, but spore production may vary significantly within a given species. Some isolates of *C. difficile*, for example, are much better spore-formers than other isolates. Heating at 80 °C for 15 minutes or alcohol shock in a 50% mixture of specimen with absolute ethanol for one hour is often necessary to induce the formation of spores (Allen and Baron, 1991). The spores in clostridia typically distend the shape of the cell. On occasion, it becomes necessary to differentiate between aerotolerant clostridia, such as *C. tertium*, *C. histolyticum*, or *C. carnis*, and *Bacillus* spp., the other genus of spore-forming rods encountered clinically. These genera differ in that *Clostridium* spp. tend not to produce spores on aerobically incubated solid media, and by definition do not degrade 3% hydrogen peroxide (catalase not produced). On the other hand, *Bacillus* spp. form spores aerobically and usually show strong catalase activity (Allen and Baron, 1991).

On solid media, the clostridia tend to give irregular-shaped colonies. Further differentiation sometimes can be made using blood agar. Some types of *C. perfringens*, for example, produce distinctive patterns of hemolysis (α or β) that aid in identification. The hemolytic activity varies depending on the type of blood incorporated into the agar. For example, >99% of clinically isolated *C. perfringens* produce a double zone of hemolysis on sheep blood agar. The clostridia are distinguished by their saccharolytic and proteolytic activities (Table 19a.2) and by their characteristic volatile fatty acid profiles. For additional information useful for characterization of clostridia, including details on volatile fatty acid profiles, the reader is referred to the Anaerobe Laboratory Manual (Holdeman *et al.*, 1977) or the chapter on clostridia by Allen and Baron (1991).

Tetanus

Microbiology

Clostridium tetani is an obligate anaerobe. Although it will grow in anaerobe jars, it is important that proper anaerobic technique is followed. The organism also grows well in anaerobic chambers in atmospheres of 85% nitrogen–10% hydrogen–5% carbon dioxide. Endospores are terminal and give the organism a drumstick appearance. The organism possesses peritrichous flagella and grows well at 37 °C but poorly at 25 °C. *Clostridium tetani* is Gram positive in young cultures but tends to become Gram negative in older cultures. On blood agar, narrow zones of β-hemolysis may be present. The organism is non-saccharolytic, non-proteolytic on egg yolk agar, does not digest milk or meat, is indole positive and gelatinase positive, although the hydrolysis of gelatin occurs slowly. The major products by gas–liquid chromatography are acetic and butyric acids and butanol, along with small amounts of propionic acid. *Clostridium tetani* is related to *C. cochlearium* culturally and biochemically, but the two species are clearly distinguished by DNA homology studies. The organism is prevalent in the soil and in faeces from animals (especially horses) and humans, although there is some variation in the recovery of the spores from human faeces. In a study carried out in Japan, *C. tetani* and/or its toxin were recovered from 10% of soil samples when just 1 mg of soil was analysed (Ebisawa *et al.*, 1986).

Pathogenesis

Clostridium tetani produces a neurotoxin (*tetanospasmin*) that causes the clinical features of tetanus. The clinical findings associated with tetanus result from the growth of the organism in tissue and occur following the production and release of the neurotoxin through autolysis. Tetanus develops following the infection of tissue through contamination of a wound. The widespread nature of the tetanus spore in the soil and faeces of humans and animals makes this a potential threat to persons not properly vaccinated. Neonatal tetanus occurs following the contamination of the umbilical stump. The clinical condition develops once the toxin blocks the inhibitory synapses of the central

TABLE 19a.2   SACCHAROLYTIC AND PROTEOLYTIC ACTIVITIES OF THE CLOSTRIDIA

Saccharolytic and proteolytic	Saccharolytic and non-proteolytic	Proteolytic and non-saccharolytic	Non-saccharolytic and non-proteolytic
C. sordellii	C. barati	C. histolyticum	C. malenominatum
C. botulinum types A, B, F	C. butyricum	C. botulinum type G	
C. perfringens	C. clostridioforme	C. tetani	
C. difficile	C. innocuum		
C. chauvoei	C. novyi types A, B		
C. septicum	C. haemolyticum		
	C. botulinum types B, C, D, E, F		

and peripheral nervous systems. The toxin accomplishes this inhibition by preventing the release of γ-aminobutyric acid (GABA) and glycine, which are inhibitory mediators.

Tetanospasmin is produced as a single polypeptide chain with a molecular weight of about 150 000. The toxin subsequently is cleaved by an intrinsic protease, resulting in 50 000 and 100 000 molecular weight fragments held together by a disulfide bond. The heavy chain represents the portion that binds to neuronal cells whereas the light chain blocks the release of the neurotransmitter. Antibodies against a fragment (referred to as fragment C) that comprises about one-third of the molecule at the COOH- terminus completely block the action of the toxin. The portion of the gene encoding the light chain of tetanus toxin has been sequenced and some similarities of this gene with the gene encoding the botulinum toxin have been identified. Both toxins contain the sequence -H-E-x-x-H-, which represents a zinc binding site, and it has been shown that tetanus toxin contains one atom of zinc bound to the light chain. These findings possibly explain why both of the toxins are inactivated by zinc chelating agents.

Once the toxin is released from the bacterial cell, the current view of many researchers is that it probably binds to a receptor at the neuromuscular membrane. Although it has been established that the toxin can bind to G_{T1b} and other gangliosides, questions have been raised casting doubt on the likelihood that these serve as the peripheral nerve cell receptors. Once bound, the toxin is believed to be internalized by receptor-mediated endocytosis. However, the exact mechanism of release from its membrane receptor and data on the precise details of toxin internalization into the neuron are lacking. What has been definitely established is that retrograde intra-axonal transport of the toxin takes place. Tetanus toxin can be transported experimentally through motor neurons, sensory neurons, and adrenergic neurons.

There are two main clinical forms of tetanus: localized and generalized. In localized tetanus, an extremity with a contaminated wound develops painful spasticity in a few muscles innervated by a certain segment in the spinal cord. In this case,

tetanospasmin is transported intra-axonally through peripheral motor neurons to the spinal cord and the toxin is believed to act on the spinal cord half-segment(s) that innervate(s) the spastic muscles. In generalized tetanus, relatively larger amounts of tetanospasmin may spread widely via the lymphatics and blood to myoneural junctions all over the body, resulting in retrograde intra-axonal spread to the cranial nerve nuclei as well as to nerve cells within the cord. The symptoms and signs of tetanus do not occur until the toxin (or a fragment of it) is translocated across the synapse and reaches the presynaptic terminals of motor neurons within the central nervous system. Accordingly, a fragment of the toxin appears to act on a membrane or cytoplasmic component, resulting in a breakdown of the synaptic process. Both tetanospasmin and botulinum type B neurotoxin have endopeptidase activity and cleave synaptobrevin, which is an integral membrane protein of small synaptic vesicles believed to be involved in the control of neurotransmitter release (Schiavo et al., 1992a, 1992b). These findings provide a mechanism for the actions of these neurotoxins at the molecular level. They are substantiated by the finding that specific inhibitors of zinc endopeptidases prevent intoxication by either toxin.

A block in release of the neurotransmitters glycine and GABA, which are used by group 1A inhibitory afferent motor neurons, causes uninhibited firing of motor nerve transmissions to muscles resulting in spastic contractions of both agonist and antagonist muscles that are characteristic of tetanus. In addition, a loss of inhibition of sympathetic nerves may be involved in severe cases, resulting in hypertension, elevated heart rate, arrhythmias, diaphoresis, hyperthermia, laryngeal spasm, urinary retention and other problems.

Clostridium tetani also produces an oxygen-labile hemolysin called tetanolysin. Tetanolysin is related to the oxygen-labile hemolysins produced by a number of other organisms, including streptolysin O, perfringolysin O (θ-toxin), cereolysin, and lysteriolysin. These oxygen-labile hemolysins act on the mammalian cell membrane and are inhibited by cholesterol. A role for tetanolysin in disease has not been established.

Epidemiology

In the USA, the frequency of tetanus is very low due to the extensive vaccination programme with tetanus toxoid. The reported incidence, for example, decreased from 560 cases in 1947 to 53 cases in 1983, and in 1985 only 70 cases were reported to the Centers for Disease Control (1986, 1991). In 1986–1989, there were 48–64 cases reported each year, and in 1989–1990 53 cases and 64 cases, respectively, were reported from 34 states. This results in an incidence of approximately 0.02 per 100 000 population and represents a decline of >90% since the late 1940s. Most of the cases that have been reported occurred in older persons (>60 years of age) who were not vaccinated or inadequately vaccinated.

The disease occurs almost exclusively in persons who are not vaccinated or who are inadequately vaccinated with tetanus toxoid. Of the 513 reported cases in 1982 through 1989, 95% of those cases involved persons who were 20 years of age or older and not properly vaccinated (Furste, 1987). In developing countries, the incidence is much higher. There are between 500 000 and 1 000 000 cases per year of neonatal tetanus with a mortality rate of 85% or higher. In addition, there are estimated to be a similar number of cases of non-neonatal tetanus with a mortality rate of about 50%.

Clinical features

Localized tetanus occurs rarely and involves an extremity in relation to a wound and is relatively benign (Finegold and George, 1989). Another unusual form, called *cephalic tetanus*, is associated with infection of the head. It is characterized by cranial nerve dysfunction (e.g., facial paralysis, dysphagia) following a short incubation period. Tetanus usually occurs as a generalized disease characterized by spastic paralysis. In the early stage, the jaw muscles are involved. This results in trismus with difficulty in opening the mouth ('lockjaw') and in swallowing. Facial muscle spasm results in a characteristic distorted grin that is referred to as risus sardonicus. Eventually, other muscles become contracted, resulting in opisthotonos, a term used to describe spastic paralysis in which the head and heels are bent backward towards each other, lower extremities are extended, the body is bowed forward, and the upper extremities are adducted over the chest with clenched fists, tightness of the abdomen and back. Any sudden sound or bright light can cause generalized convulsions. The muscle spasms may begin near the site of the initial infection and progress to generalized tetanus. Neonatal tetanus, which occurs because of infection of the umbilical stump often related to the practice in some countries/cultures of applying cattle dung to this site, develops similarly.

Diagnosis

The diagnosis of tetanus is based on the clinical picture. The Council of State and Territorial Epidemiologists and the CDC adopted the following clinical definition for tetanus: 'acute onset of hypertonia and/or painful muscular contractions (usually of the muscles of the jaw and neck) and generalized muscle spasms without other apparent medical cause (as reported by a health professional)'. This definition was placed into effect essentially because of the lack of suitable diagnostic methods for the disease. In early stages, it is important to distinguish the disease from other disorders such as meningitis and encephalitis, rabies, and certain types of poisoning such as strychnine poisoning. Also, in some instances, the wound or site of infection may not be obvious and the physician must be aware of this possibility. The organism may be isolated from the infected wound, but this usually is not done because the clinical picture of tetanus is easily recognized. Neutralization tests can be performed in mice in which culture filtrates or cultures mixed either with buffer or tetanus antitoxin are injected (Holdeman et al., 1977). These usually are not done or else they are performed primarily as confirmatory tests.

Treatment and management

Once the diagnosis of tetanus is determined, tetanus immune globulin (TIG) should be administered intramuscularly in an effort to neutralize toxin that is not already bound to neural tissue (Finegold and George, 1989). The optimal dose for adults has not been established, but usually ranges from 500 to 10 000 units. It has been suggested that 10 000 units should be more than adequate in severe cases, while a dose of 3000 units may be used in less severe cases. For neonatal tetanus, a dose of 250 units intramuscularly is believed to be appropriate (Finegold and George, 1989). TIG (human) can be obtained from Cutter Biological and Massachusetts Public Health Biologic Labs, USA, and other major reference centres. Analgesics are administered to the patient to relieve the pain. In addition, sedatives such as phenobarbitol can be used in mild cases of the disease but pentothal may be required for more severe cases. Muscle relaxant drugs such diazepam (Valium) are used by some physicians in an attempt to promote muscle relaxation, sedate the patient, control spasms, and prevent convulsions. Diazepam is known to enhance GABA-ergic central nervous system inhibition by increasing affinity of the transmitter at the GABA receptor (Finegold and George, 1989). Antibiotics such as penicillin or metronidazole are active against *C. tetani in vitro* but they will not be highly effective in treating tetanus because the toxin has already been produced and is present in the circulatory system. However, certain antibiotics are effective against secondary complications of tetanus such as the onset of pneumonia and for that reason they may be administered. A human monoclonal antibody that neutralizes tetanus toxin has been developed and shown to protect animals *in vivo* (Simpson *et al.*, 1990). However, it has not been evaluated in humans. For further information on treatment, the review by Groleau (1992) or the text by Finegold and George (1989) is recommended.

Prevention

The disease in the USA and in other industrialized countries has dropped significantly over the past five decades because of an effective immunization campaign. Unfortunately, this has not been the case in less developed countries. The lack of an effective vaccination program and the ubiquitous presence of tetanus spores in the soil means that this disease will continue to be a major problem in these countries. This is unfortunate because proper immunization is highly effective (almost 100%). The current recommendations for the vaccination of individuals over seven years of age who have not previously been vaccinated consist of a primary series of three vaccinations at least four weeks apart, with the third dose given six weeks after the second vaccination (Groleau, 1992). Primary vaccination with tetanus toxoid provides protection for at least 10 years in most adults and a booster dose quickly elicits protective antibodies in vaccinated persons. Adults in whom 10 years have elapsed since the primary series or booster should receive a booster vaccination. The vaccination schedule for children consists of a diphtheria, tetanus, and pertussis (DTP) vaccine given at two, four, six, and 15 months of age followed by a booster dose between the ages of four and six years. The need for vaccination in persons with wounds needs to be based on the previous vaccination history and the condition of the wound. The toxoid is available in both an adsorbed form and a fluid form.

Botulism

Microbiology

The *C. botulinum* group represents a major taxonomical problem because it is comprised of a collection of organisms with a wide range of phenotypic properties. There are seven distinct types, designated A to G, based on the type of neurotoxin that they produce. Types A, B, and F are proteolytic and are highly related to *C. sporogenes*. Organisms in this group are positive for lipase on egg yolk, indole negative, and they ferment glucose. Their metabolic products include major amounts of acetic and butyric acids, and smaller amounts of propionic, isobutyric, and isovaleric acids, along with propyl, isobutyl, butyl, and isoamyl alcohols. There also are some organisms in the type B and type F groups, along with type E, that are non-proteolytic. These organisms are highly related to *C. novyi*. They ferment glucose and sucrose, are indole negative, and they are positive for lipase on egg yolk agar. They produce acetic and butyric acids as their end products. Types C and D organisms are related to *C. subterminale*, and are non-proteolytic, indole-negative, and positive for lipase on egg yolk agar. They produce major amounts of acetic, propionic, and butyric acids. The type G organisms are proteolytic, non-saccharolytic, indole negative, and negative on egg yolk agar. They produce major amounts of acetic acid with lower amounts of isobutyric, butyric, isovaleric, and lactic acids. The name *C. argentinense* has been proposed for the type G group. Two clostridia, *C. subterminale* and *C. hastiforme*, are very closely related to the organisms in this group. Interestingly, two other clostridia have been found to produce neurotoxins that are related to those of *C. botulinum*. Some isolates of *C. barati* produce a type F neurotoxin whereas an isolate of *C. butyricum* has been shown to produce a type E neurotoxin.

Bacteriophages and plasmids have been found in types A to F organisms, suggesting that the production of neurotoxin may be plasmid or phage mediated. A direct correlation, however, has only been demonstrated in the type C and D organisms. Organisms in these groups that are cured of their phage do not produce toxin. Upon phage reinfection, a conversion from toxin negative to toxin positive occurs. Type G organisms that produce toxin carry a 81 MDa plasmid. Growth at 44 °C causes a loss of the plasmid along with a conversion from toxin positive to toxin negative, suggesting that the toxin genes may be plasmid associated.

Pathogenesis

Botulism is characterized by a descending flaccid paralysis caused by the neurotoxin produced by *C. botulinum*. The spores are ubiquitous in nature and often contaminate various types of foods such as vegetables, fruits, meat products and fish. There are several types of botulism. In adults, *food-borne botulism* results when improperly stored or undercooked food that is contaminated with preformed neurotoxin is eaten. Under the appropriate conditions, the spores germinate and grow in the food, resulting in the production of neurotoxin. A second type of botulism, *wound botulism*, occurs following the infection of a wound with *C. botulinum* spores. The organism grows in the infected tissue and releases toxin locally which then disseminates via the circulation. A third type of botulism is *infant botulism*. In this instance, spores are ingested, germinate in the intestine, and produce toxin *in vivo*. The toxin is subsequently absorbed and spread via the circulation. The minimum infective dose in infant botulism has been estimated to be as low as 10–100 spores (Finegold and George, 1989).

The clinical manifestations of botulism are caused by the neurotoxin. The botulinum toxins are classified into groups A to G (A, B, C or C1, D, E, F, G), based on their distinctive antigenic properties. Antibodies against type A neurotoxin, for example, are specific for the type A toxin and neutralize only the type A toxin. All of the botulism neurotoxins are similar in size and have a molecular weight of about 150 000. However, the type C1 neurotoxin exists as a larger molecule in culture filtrates because of the association of the neurotoxin with a non-toxic protein that has hemagglutinating activity. This type of aggregate probably occurs with some of the other *C. botulinum* neurotoxins, thus accounting for some of the discrepancies in the literature regarding size.

Once the toxins are produced, they are cleaved by an intrinsic protease, resulting in a 50 000 and a 100 000 molecular weight fragment held together by a disulfide bond. The heavy chain represents the portion that recognizes and binds to neuronal cells. The light chain contains the activity that blocks the release of acetylcholine, the neurotransmitter. The portion of the gene encoding the light chain has been sequenced and some similarities of this gene with the gene encoding the tetanus toxin (tetanospasmin) have been identified, as mentioned previously. Both toxins contain the amino acid sequence -H-E-x-x-H-, which represents a zinc binding site. Like tetanospasmin, botulinum toxin is inactivated by zinc chelating agents.

The toxin enters the circulation and eventually binds to receptors on the peripheral nerve endings. The toxin is believed to enter cells by a receptor-mediated process, and after processing the toxin acts by inhibiting the release of acetylcholine. Like tetanus toxin, botulinum type B neurotoxin has been shown to have endopeptidase activity and cleave synaptobrevin, which is an integral membrane protein of small synaptic vesicles (Schiavo et al., 1992a, 1992b). It has been suggested that this activity may inhibit the release of the neurotransmitter, providing a molecular model for the mechanism. The inhibition of the release of acetylcholine at the neuromuscular junction, in turn, prevents the muscle from responding to nerve impulses, leading to the flaccid paralysis seen in severe cases of the disease.

In addition to neurotoxin, type C and D strains produce a binary toxin referred to as C2 toxin. This toxin consists of two protein components that are not linked but that are both needed for the expression of toxic activity (Aktories, 1990). The larger of the two components is referred to as the heavy chain component and has a molecular weight of about 100 000. This component is believed to bind to the target cell. The small component is the light chain component and has a molecular weight of about 50 000. This component has mono-(ADP-ribosyl)transferase activity and catalyzes the transfer of the ADP-ribosyl moiety of NAD onto the Arg^{177} residue of monomeric actin (Figure 19a.1). *Clostridium perfringens* and *C. spiroforme* also produce binary toxins with ADP-ribosylating activity and, like C2, they ribosylate actin (Simpson et al., 1987; Stiles and Wilkins, 1986). The binary toxins of *C. perfringens* and *C. spiroforme*, both of which are referred to as iota toxin, are related antigenically to each other but not to C2 toxin. They also are slightly smaller than the C2 toxin. C2 acts on β/γ-non-muscle actin and γ-smooth muscle actin but not skeletal muscle actin, cardiac actin, or α-smooth muscle actin. The iota toxins from both *C. perfringens* and *C. spiroforme*, on the other hand, act on all of these actin molecules. The ADP-ribosylation results in the inhibition of the polymerization of actin at the barbed end of actin which represents the rapidly growing end.

All of the binary toxins are cytotoxins that cause tissue cultured mammalian cells to round up, indicating an affect on the cytoskeletal system. In addition, they are lethal and they cause a fluid response when injected into ligated intestinal loops. The role of the C2 toxin and the iota toxins in disease is not known. None of these toxins is completely responsible for disease findings that occur in experimental animals infected with these organisms and their role in human disease has not been firmly established. At this time, more is known about their action at the molecular level than their roles in disease. A single isolate of another species, *C. difficile*, has been identified that produces a light chain with ADP-ribosylating activity which antigenically cross-reacts with the light chains of iota toxin from *C. perfringens* and *C. spiroforme* (Popoff et al., 1988) However, this isolate does not produce the heavy chain, and the light chain by itself is not toxic to tissue cultured cells or animals.

Some type C and type D organisms produce another ADP-ribosylating enzyme referred to as C3 exotransferase (Rosener et al., 1987). This enzyme modifies the rho subfamily of proteins. These are ras-related low molecular weight GTP-binding proteins that are believed to play an important role in the organization of the cytoskeletal system. The C3 exotransferase enzyme is not related to either the neurotoxin or binary toxin C2 of *C. botulinum* and its role in disease has not been determined.

Epidemiology

The CDC have maintained records on the number of reported cases of botulism since 1950. Between the years of 1950 and 1985, there were 396 outbreaks of food-borne botulism involving 916 cases. The mortality rate in persons with the disease has declined over the past several decades due to better and earlier health care, and the current rate is about 10%. Most of the cases in humans result from types A and B, and in most instances home-canned vegetables are believed to have been the source of contamination. There have been several type E outbreaks in Alaska and

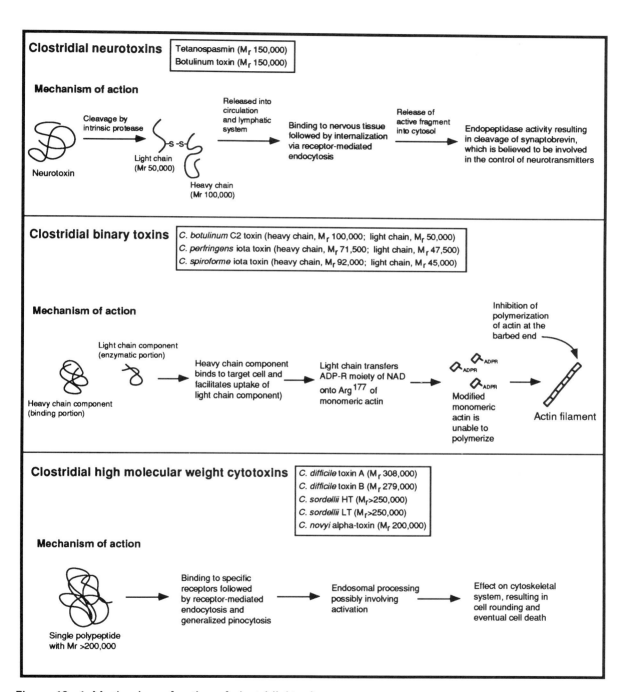

Figure 19a.1. Mechanism of action of clostridial toxins.

these have been associated with home-processed fish or meat from marine animals. Other outbreaks have been attributed to potato salad, commercial pot pies, sauteed onions immersed in margarine, mushrooms, peppers, meat stews, and hazelnut yogurt. Type F is the least common botulism of humans. Types C and D are causes of botulism in birds and mammals, but do not cause botulism in humans. Most of the incidents have involved only one or a few persons. There have been, however, several large outbreaks since 1977 involving restaurants. In Michigan, an outbreak involving 59 persons was attributed to type B botulism and in 1978 there were outbreaks in New Mexico and Colorado involving 34 and seven persons, respectively. More recently, there was an outbreak involving 28 persons in Illinois in 1983. The symptoms in these persons ranged from blurry vision to severe paralysis. In 1992, a family outbreak of botulism type E was attributed to salt-cured fish. Type A botulism tends to be more severe whereas type E botulism develops more rapidly (Woodruff et al., 1992). The number of reported cases of wound botulism is less than food-borne botulism. Between 1973 and 1985, only 21 cases of wound botulism were reported to the CDC (MacDonald et al., 1986).

Infant botulism in the USA has only been reported in infants of one year or less. As of 1988, close to 700 cases were reported to the CDC. Most US cases reported east of the Mississippi have been type B; the majority of cases from western states have been type A. The disease has been reported from other countries as well, and in most instances the causative organism has been identified as type A or type B. There has been a case of type F infant botulism reported, and two cases in which a toxin that had properties of both type B and type F neurotoxin (referred to as B/F) was noted. In addition, certain strains of C. barati and C. butyricum producing type F and type E neurotoxins, respectively, have been implicated in infant botulism (Hall et al., 1985; McCroskey et al., 1986; Aureli et al., 1986; Gimenez et al., 1992). In infant botulism, there is strong evidence that the gastrointestinal tract becomes colonized with C. botulinum acquired in the form of spores

ingested from environmental sources (e.g. food, soil, dust). The spores germinate within the infant gut and the organism produces toxin in vivo. Honey contaminated with type A or type B spores has been identified as the contaminated food in several instances, and at this time it is advised that honey and corn syrups not be given to infants although these foods are perfectly suitable for older children and adults. There has been some speculation that infant botulism may be responsible for some cases of sudden infant death. However, other studies in the USA, Germany, and Canada on sudden infant death syndrome have failed to demonstrate any significant correlation with the presence of toxigenic strains of C. botulinum (Hatheway, 1990; Gurwith et al., 1981).

Clinical features

The symptoms of botulism may begin to develop within 6 hours after ingesting the toxin. In most patients, the latent period is longer and symptoms usually begin 12–36 hours after ingestion. In some instances, the onset may not occur for one to two weeks. There are several features that are useful in distinguishing botulism poisoning from other diseases and disorders such as myasthenia gravis, atypical Guillain-Barré syndrome, tick paralysis, chemical poisoning, and poliomyelitis that are associated with paralysis. Botulism is characterized by symmetrical descending flaccid paralysis, beginning with cranial nerves. This often results in blurry vision, difficulty in swallowing, and slurring of speech in the early stages of the disease. The central nervous system usually remains functional and there is very little, if any, fever. Sensation usually remains intact. These clinical features are characteristic of all types (food-borne, wound, and infant) of botulism. Food-borne botulism may be accompanied by nausea and vomiting whereas infant botulism is often accompanied by constipation.

Diagnosis

The initial diagnosis of botulism is based on the clinical features. Confirmation of the diagnosis of classic food-borne botulism is based on the presence of neurotoxin in the patient's faeces and serum, the recovery of *C. botulinum* from the stool specimen, and supporting epidemiological evidence such as the identification of suspected foods that are contaminated with the organism. The presence of neurotoxin is usually determined by injecting samples into mice and determining if the toxicity is neutralized by specific toxin-type antitoxin (Holdeman *et al.*, 1977; CDC, 1979). The determination of toxin and isolation of the organism should be done by persons experienced with the procedures. In the USA, all suspected cases should be reported to the appropriate public health department. There have been enzyme immunoassays (EIAs) developed for the detection of botulinum toxin and they are reported to be very sensitive. However, additional evaluations are needed. Currently, the mouse assay, which detects about 6 pg of toxin, is used as a confirmatory test.

The diagnosis of infant botulism may be suspected in infants who have constipation (often the first sign), listlessness, difficulty in sucking and swallowing, an altered cry, hypotonia, and generalized muscle weakness. The infant may eventually appear 'floppy', lose head control, and develop ptosis, a flaccid facial expression and dysphagia. The isolation and identification of *C. botulinum* from the faeces of an infant with clinical signs consistent with botulism is considered diagnostic (Finegold and George, 1989; Hatheway, 1992); the organism is rarely, if ever, present in the 'normal' faecal flora of healthy infants. Although botulinal toxin can be demonstrated in the infant's faeces, along with the organism, botulinal toxin is rarely ever detected in the infant's serum.

Treatment and management

The primary therapy for botulism consists of supportive care, especially respiratory therapy, since death may result from the paralysis of the respiratory muscles. It is very important that cases of botulism be reported to the proper health authorities to identify other persons at risk. Most cases occur following ingestion of home-preserved meats, fish, and vegetables. The complications that typically occur in patients with botulism include pneumonia and other types of secondary infections. The recovery period typically requires several months and a long convalescent period. A multivalent antitoxin against types A, B, and E, which are the types most commonly associated with adult botulism, is available from state health departments and the CDC etc., but requests must be accompanied by consultation. It is important that the antitoxin be given as soon as possible since it functions by blocking the binding of the toxin to its target receptor. Once the toxin has bound to the receptor, the antitoxin is not protective. Currently, the CDC recommends that two vials be administered to the patient as soon as possible after the initial symptoms have appeared. One is given intravenously and the other is injected intramuscularly. The antitoxin that is used is produced in horses and as a result, hypersensitivity may occur as a side effect. Therefore, it is recommended that an initial skin test be preformed to determine if the patient is allergic to the antitoxin. If the patient exhibits hypersensitivity, the antitoxin should not be given. The value of antibiotics for the treatment of food-borne botulism is not clear. Some physicians treat adult patients with penicillin in order to decrease carriage of *C. botulinum* in the intestinal tract and prevent further toxin production by *C. botulinum* within the bowel. However, antibiotics such as penicillin may be useful in the treatment of wound botulism since they help to eliminate the organism and remove the source of the toxin. Nonspecific supportive measures (especially respiratory care and nutritional care) are relied upon in the management of patients with infant botulism. There is a risk of anaphylaxis with the currently available equine botulinal antitoxin; however, a human-derived antitoxin is being investigated. Antibiotics have been tried in the treatment of infant botulism but are not effective, and may even prolong the illness related to release of toxin within the gut from cells of *C. botulinum* exposed to antibiotics (Finegold and George, 1989).

Prevention

The neurotoxins of *C. botulinum* are inactivated by heating at 80 °C for 30 minutes. Spores are destroyed by heating at 121 °C for several minutes. Many preserved foods are not subjected to these conditions, either because of inadequate facilities or because these conditions affect the quality of the food. Proper processing and storage of foods must be done when food is preserved. The production of toxin is inhibited below pH 4.6 and foods that are acidic are less likely to be contaminated with toxin during preservation. However, many fruits and vegetables are preserved only by pasteurization, and yeast and spores of other bacteria may grow sufficiently to raise the pH of the food. Many meats are preserved by the addition of salt and nitrate with a concomitant decrease in pH to <5.0. Occasionally, however, the pH is not sufficiently lowered. Any increase in the pH may allow contaminating *C. botulinum* spores to vegetate and produce toxin. Most cases (>90%) of botulism have occurred following the ingestion of home-preserved foods. Commercial products in restaurants have an excellent safety record.

Pseudomembranous Colitis and Antibiotic-associated Diarrhoea

Microbiology

Clostridium difficile is a Gram-positive sporeformer that becomes Gram variable in older stationary cultures. The production of spores by this organism is not associated with toxin production. Many clinical laboratories isolate the organism from faecal specimens as an aid in the diagnosis of *C. difficile* disease and the recovery of spores can be improved by alcohol or heat shock procedures. Some strains produce thin capsules and structures that resemble fimbriae but an association of these structures with virulence has not been demonstrated. The organism will grow in media that is reduced but not held under strict anaerobic conditions. For clinical isolation, however, it is important that anaerobic conditions be used for optimal recovery. Colonies of *C. difficile* fluoresce when grown on some types of agar, especially agar supplemented with blood, and several unusual metabolites, including isocaproic acid and *p*-cresol,

are produced. These unusual properties are useful in the presumptive identification of *C. difficile* but some of the other clostridia and other anaerobes exhibit similar properties; thus, these characteristics are not unique to *C. difficile*. In addition to producing isocaproic acid, the organism produces high levels of acetic, isobutyric, and butyric acid. The selective medium most commonly used for the isolation of the organism is cycloserine–cefoxitin–fructose agar, developed by George *et al.* (1979). This medium serves as both a selective and differential medium and detects as few as 2000 organisms in a total count of 6×10^{10} bacteria per gram of wet faeces.

Pathogenesis

Clostridium difficile produces two large protein toxins, A and B. Toxin A, which is the largest bacterial toxin known, has a molecular weight of 308 000. Toxin B is slightly smaller and has a molecular weight of 269 000. Both are produced as single polypeptides. Both of the toxins are cytotoxic for mammalian cells, although toxin B is much more potent against most cell lines. The cytotoxic activity occurs as a rounding of the cells and is similar to the cell rounding observed with the ADP-ribosylating binary toxins of *C. botulinum*, *C. perfringens*, and *C. sordellii*. However, toxins A and B are not related to the binary toxins and they do not have ADP-ribosylating activity. Both toxin A and toxin B are lethal; about 50 ng of either toxin is sufficient to kill a mouse. In addition to its cytotoxic and lethal activities, toxin A is enterotoxic and agglutinates rabbit erythrocytes. Toxin B does not have these activities. Toxin A is believed to be the primary toxin in the pathogenesis of *C. difficile* disease because of its potent enterotoxic activity. This toxin is as potent as cholera toxin in eliciting fluid but, unlike cholera toxin, toxin A causes extensive tissue damage. The toxin binds to galactose residues containing the core structure $Gal\beta1–4GlcNAc$ (Krivan *et al.*, 1986) and is internalized by receptor-mediated endocytosis and generalized pinocytosis. After endosomal processing, the toxin possibly acts on an intracellular target. The initial tissue damage by toxin A possibly exposes target mucosal areas to toxin B, which then exerts its toxic activity. Both of the toxins possibly disseminate from the intestinal tract and act distally on other target organs.

Toxigenic strains of *C. difficile* vary in the level of toxin they produce. Highly toxigenic strains produce high levels of both toxins. Weakly toxigenic strains, which may produce 100 000-fold less toxin than the highly toxigenic strains, produce low amounts of both toxins. Non-toxigenic strains do not produce either toxin. One strain has been described that initially was reported to produce only toxin B (Lyerly *et al.*, 1992). It was subsequently shown, however, that this strain also carries the front portion of the toxin A gene. Whether this portion is expressed is not known. Toxin B from this unusual strain is more cytotoxic than toxin B from other strains and it is weakly enterotoxic.

The genes for toxins A and B have been sequenced and exhibit an overall homology of about 45% (Dove *et al.*, 1990; Barroso *et al.*, 1990). There are several highly conserved features identified from the sequencing data. Both toxins contain a complex series of contiguous repeating units at the COOH terminus. In toxin A, these serve as the binding portion of the toxin that recognizes the receptor, and they likely serve a related function in toxin B. Both toxins share four conserved cysteine residues, a hydrophobic region located near the midpoint of each toxin, and a putative ATP-binding site. The exact function of these conserved features is not known. However, they suggest that toxins A and B possibly arose by gene duplication.

Clostridium sordellii produces two large toxins, toxin HT (haemorrhagic toxin) and toxin LT (lethal toxin), that are highly related to the toxins of *C. difficile* (Martinez and Wilkins, 1992). Toxin HT is highly related antigenically to toxin A and, like toxin A, is enterotoxic and agglutinates rabbit erythrocytes. Toxin LT, on the other hand, is very similar to toxin B in its antigenic structure. Interestingly, toxin LT is about 10 times more lethal than toxin B but at least 1000 times less cytotoxic. The cross-reaction and cross-neutralization of the toxins of *C. sordellii* led to the discovery of *C. difficile* as the cause of pseudomembranous colitis and antibiotic-associated diarrhoea. Unlike *C. difficile*, *C. sordellii* is not an intestinal pathogen. Its primary role as a pathogen is in wound infections in animals.

Clostridium novyi produces a large cytotoxin, α-toxin, that causes the same type of rounding as the toxins of *C. sordellii* and *C. difficile* (Ball *et al.*, 1993). The α-toxin does not cross-react with toxins A and B or toxins HT and LT. Like *C. sordellii*, *C. novyi* is primarily a wound pathogen. The large cytotoxins from these species represent a novel class of high molecular weight cytotoxins that share several features (Table 19a.3). Toxins A and B of *C. difficile* are the best-studied toxins in this group because of their involvement in pseudomembranous colitis and antibiotic-associated diarrhoea.

Epidemiology

Clostridium difficile-associated disease occurs most often in the elderly population. Older persons who receive antibiotic therapy in a hospital setting comprise the population at highest risk. There have been a number of typing methods, including serotyping by agglutination, restriction endonuclease mapping, protein profiles, bacteriophage typing, and plasmid and bacteriocin typing, developed for *C. difficile* because of its role as a major nosocomial pathogen. Of these, serotyping, restriction endonuclease mapping, and protein profiles have been the most useful because some strains do not contain plasmids or are not sensitive to bacteriophages or bacteriocins. All of these methods have been used to demonstrate the fact that *C. difficile* is prevalent in hospitals and is spread from patient to patient, usually by health care workers. The organism is a major problem because it persists in the environment and because of the huge numbers of spores shed by infected patients. The organism can be isolated from bookshelves, curtains, and floors in the rooms of infected patients. The longer a patient is hospitalized, the higher the risk of developing *C. difficile* disease. This is illustrated by the finding that only a very low percentage (<3%) of healthy persons carry *C. difficile*. Upon admission to a

TABLE 19a.3 COMPARISON OF THE BIOLOGICAL ACTIVITIES OF THE CLASS OF HIGH MOLECULAR WEIGHT CYTOTOXINS OF *C. DIFFICILE, C. SORDELLII,* AND *C. NOVYI*

Toxin	Molecular weight	Cytotoxic dose	Lethal dose in mice	Enterotoxic dose in rabbit ileal loops	Hemagglutinating activity
C. difficile toxin A	308 000	10 ng	50 ng	1 μg	1 μg/ml (temperature-dependent)
C. difficile toxin B	279 000	1 pg	50 ng	Negative	Negative
C. sordellii toxin HT	>250 000	100 ng	50–100 ng	10 μg	1 μg/ml (temperature-dependent)
C. sordellii toxin LT	>250 000	1 ng	5 ng	Negative	Negative
C. novyi α-toxin	200 000	100 pg	5 ng	Negative	Negative

hospital, many of these persons become carriers, and in one study about 40% of the carriers eventually developed the disease (MacFarland *et al.*, 1991).

Up to 50% of infants have *C. difficile* and toxin in their faecal specimens but they do not show any significant illness. Infants that are debilitated in some manner and that require extensive antibiotic therapy may develop the disease but this occurs only rarely. The presence of *C. difficile* in infants may account for the spread of the organism in a hospital setting, although there is some evidence suggesting that infants tend to be colonized with strains that are distinct from those that cause disease in adults (Pantosti *et al.*, 1988; Toma *et al.*, 1988). *Clostridium difficile* disease occurs in AIDS patients. This is not unexpected because many AIDS patients are receiving drugs that alter the normal protective flora.

Clinical features

Any antibiotic or drug that disrupts the normal integrity of the gastrointestinal tract can predispose a patient to *C. difficile* disease. The clinical criteria, as defined by Gerding and Brazier (1993), include (1) diarrhoea in which no other cause has been established, (2) loose or unformed stools that take the shape of the container, (3) three or more bowel movements per day, (4) duration of at least two days, and (5) a prior history of antibiotic or antineoplastic agents in the preceding four to six weeks. Some patients may experience abdominal pain and fever. A positive response to vancomycin

or metronidazole is considered by some to be confirmatory evidence but these antibiotics are not specific for *C. difficile*. Although *C. difficile* probably causes most cases of pseudomembranous colitis, it is believed to cause only about 20–25% of the cases of antibiotic-associated diarrhoea.

The onset of *C. difficile* disease may begin several days after starting antibiotic therapy or it may be delayed in its onset and not begin until up to two months following therapy. Diarrhoea and cramping usually represent the first symptoms. These may be accompanied by fever and chills in severe cases. Occasionally there may be bleeding. In the severe stages, pseudomembranes appearing as small whitish-yellow plaques on the colonic mucosa may be observed by sigmoidoscopy. Pseudomembranes are composed of inflammatory cells, necrotic cells, and debris. Histologically, the tips of the microvilli are eroded. The disease is localized to the colon in most cases.

Diagnosis

Clinically, the presence of pseudomembranes is considered diagnostic for pseudomembranous colitis. Because of improvements in detection systems, the disease may be identified before pseudomembranes appear. There are four methods currently used as aids in the diagnosis of *C. difficile* disease. These are (1) isolation of the organism, (2) latex agglutination, (3) tissue culture assay, and (4) EIA. A description of these methods is shown in Table 19a.4. The isolation of the organism is done using the selective

TABLE 19a.4   METHODS AND TESTS FOR THE DETECTION OF *CLOSTRIDIUM DIFFICILE* AND ITS TOXINS

Method	Protein detected	Advantages	Limitations	Available tests and sources
Culturing	Organism	Highly sensitive Low cost	Efficiency varies from lab to lab Does not distinguish toxigenic and non-toxigenic isolates	Selective media (cycloserine–cefoxitin supplement and CCFA media) available from a variety of sources
Latex Agglutination	Glutamate dehydrogenase	Rapid Simple	Not extremely sensitive Does distinguish toxigenic and non-toxigenic isolates	Meritec *C. difficile* (Meridian Diagnostics, Inc.) CDT (Becton Dickinson)
EIA	Glutamate dehydrogenase	Rapid Simple	More sensitive than latex Does distinguish toxigenic and non-toxigenic isolates	ImmunoCard *C. difficile* (Meridian Diagnostics, Inc.)
Tissue culture	Toxin B	Sensitive Specific Adaptable	Requires 24–48 hours Toxin B can be inactivated, resulting in false negatives	*C. difficile* Toxititer (Bartels Immunodiagnostics, Inc.) *C. difficile* Toxin/Antitoxin Kit (TechLab, Inc.)
EIA	Toxin A Toxins A and B	Rapid Sensitive Simple	May have higher percentage of indeterminant readings	Premier (Meridian Diagnostics, Inc.) Toxin A EIA (Bartels Immunodiagnostics, Inc.) VIDAS-CDA (Vitek Systems) Tox-A Test (TechLab, Inc.) Toxin A Test (Becton Dickinson) Cytoclone A + B (Cambridge Biotech)

cycloserine–cefoxitin–fructose agar (George *et al.*, 1979) or it can be done using an alcohol or heat-shock spore selection procedure (Allen and Baron, 1991). The isolation of the organism, however, does not distinguish between non-toxigenic and toxigenic strains. Non-toxigenic isolates form spores, persist in hospitals, and are spread from patient to patient as well as toxigenic isolates. Therefore, it can be important to distinguish between toxigenic and non-toxigenic isolates using a toxin test. The isolation and recovery rates of the organism from clinical specimens are affected by the quality of media and the experience of the technologist. Nonetheless, isolation of *C. difficile* is required for epidemiologic typing of isolates in suspected outbreaks, and has the advantages over other methods of relatively high sensitivity and low cost.

The latex test was initially marketed as a test for toxin A. However, it has since been determined that the test detects glutamate dehydrogenase instead of toxin A. Glutamate dehydrogenase, which is a metabolic enzyme, has no relationship to either toxin A or toxin B and it is produced in similar levels by both toxigenic and non-toxigenic strains. Thus, the latex test does not confirm the presence of toxin. There have been reports of high false positivity rates with this procedure. Although it probably is best suited in a hospital setting as a screen with positive specimens being tested further using a toxin assay, its low sensitivity precludes reliance on negative latex test results because of its high rate of falsely negative test results; thus, negative test results should be confirmed by using another method (e.g., cytotoxin, culture for toxigenic organism, or EIA for toxin A).

The tissue culture test and new EIAs that are now available are specific for *C. difficile* toxin. The tissue culture test represents the 'gold standard' because of its high sensitivity. It detects as little as 1 pg of toxin B and it is well suited for use in clinical laboratories that routinely perform tissue culture assays. The drawbacks to the test are the time required for test results (i.e. most positives are detected overnight, but negatives cannot be reported until at least 48 hours of incubation) and lack of standardization. If too much specimen is used in the assay, non-specific rounding of the tissue culture cells may occur and may be misinterpreted as a true positive reaction. The EIAs represent the newest testing method for *C. difficile* toxin. There are several that are specific for toxin A and one that is specific for both toxins. They are rapid (<3 hours) and sensitive. Overall, the EIAs exhibit a correlation of >85% (depending on the test used) with the tissue culture assay.

Treatment and management

In many instances, *C. difficile* disease may be self-limiting and the patient may improve if the inciting agent is stopped. If a patient appears to be improving, additional therapy may not be necessary. This approach depends on the condition of the patient and supportive measures may be necessary to correct any fluid loss. The most common method of treating *C. difficile* disease, once the clinical criteria have been met, is the oral administration of vancomycin or metronidazole. Vancomycin is poorly adsorbed in the intestine and high concentrations can be achieved. As a result, it is very effective. The typical dose of vancomycin is 125–500 mg every 6 hours. The lower dose usually is effective unless the patient is critically ill. Most studies on metronidazole have been done on patients who are not critically ill, and in these patients it is very effective. In critically ill patients with pseudomembranous colitis, vancomycin is considered by some to be the drug of choice. The overuse of vancomycin, however, has raised concern over the development of vancomycin-resistant enterococci.

Anion-exchange resins such as cholestyramine and colestipol have been used to treat mild cases of *C. difficile* disease. These resins bind the toxin without exposing the microflora to additional antibiotics. Another promising treatment that currently is being investigated is the administration of *Saccharomyces boulardii*, which is a non-pathogenic yeast used as a probiotic to treat persons with gastrointestinal illness. The yeast has been used successfully in several instances to treat persons that have relapsed. The exact mechanism for protection by this yeast in patients with *C.*

difficile disease is not clear. The yeast capsules are available in Europe but they have not been approved for use in the USA.

Prevention

Clostridium difficile is spread from patient to patient and a major mode of transmission is the health care worker. There is little threat to the worker but there are certain precautions that minimize the spread of the organism. Vinyl disposable gloves, laboratory coats, and proper hand-washing procedures are highly recommended. All items should be cleaned and disinfected, and patients should be isolated with enteric precautions. Disposable or protected sheath rectal thermometers are recommended and commodes and endoscopes should be cleaned properly. Cleaning the rooms of *C. difficile* patients using sporicidal agents and disinfectants may be helpful, but their efficacy should be monitored. Programs should be implemented to reduce the use of unnecessary antibiotics. The treatment of asymptomatic carriers with antibiotics has been suggested as a way to lower the spread and development of the disease, but this practice is questionable and is not recommended.

Gas Gangrene

Microbiology

The clostridia most commonly associated with gas gangrene include *C. perfringens*, *C. septicum*, *C. novyi*, *C. histolyticum*, and *C. sordellii*, with *C. perfringens* being the most common. Other clostridia also may be associated with wound infections but those listed above are the ones most commonly associated with clostridial myonecrosis. A description of these clostridia is presented in Table 19a.5. These organisms vary in their spore production *in vitro*. Few spores are seen in cultures of *C. perfringens* and *C. histolyticum* whereas they are more commonly observed in cultures of *C. septicum* or *C. sordellii*. The organisms exhibit different haemolytic activity and specificity based on the type of red cell employed. The haemolytic activity results from the action of their toxins (see 'Pathogenesis' below). Some of the organisms in this group are fairly aerotolerant. *Clostridium histolyticum*, for example, is aerotolerant and *C. perfringens* may be, but it is strongly recommended, however, that good anaerobic techniques be used for recovering these organisms from clinical specimens.

Pathogenesis

The clostridia involved in gas gangrene, especially *C. perfringens*, produce a variety of toxins that cause tissue damage (Table 19a.6). In clostridial myonecrosis, which occurs following contamination of a wound infection by clostridial spores, the spores germinate and begin to grow in a reduced environment. The growth is followed by the production of toxins which cause extensive tissue

TABLE 19a.5 DESCRIPTION OF THE MAJOR SPECIES INVOLVED IN CLOSTRIDIAL MYONECROSIS

Species	Description	Egg yolk reaction (lecithinase activity)	Major volatile fatty acids
C. perfringens	Large boxcar-shaped, spores uncommon in tissue lesions; double zone hemolysis	Positive	Acetic and butyric acids
C. novyi	Discrete colonies	Positive	Acetic, propionic, and butyric acids
C. histolyticum	Atypical pleomorphic shapes	Negative	Acetic acid
C. septicum	Large bacillus; pleomorphic forms common; may swarm	Negative	Acetic and butyric acids
C. sordellii	Spores common; highly related to *C. bifermentans*	Positive	Acetic, isobutyric, and isovaleric acids

TABLE 19a.6   TOXINS OF THE GAS GANGRENE CLOSTRIDIA

Species	Toxin	Characterization
C. chauvoeii and C. septicum	α-Toxin β-Toxin γ-Toxin δ-Toxin	Oxygen-stable haemolysin with necrotic and lethal activity Deoxyribonuclease Hyaluronidase Oxygen-stable haemolysin
C. histolyticum	α-Toxin β-Antigen γ-Antigen δ-Antigen	Lethal and necrotic toxin that is related to C. septicum α-toxin Collagenase Thiol-activated protease Protease
C. novyi	α-Toxin β-Toxin γ-Toxin δ-Antigen ε-Antigen	Lethal and necrotizing Phospholipase C Phospholipase C Oxygen-labile haemolysin Lipase

Type A: α-toxin, γ-toxin, δ-antigen, ε-antigen
Type B: α-toxin, β-toxin
Type C: no toxin
Type D: β-toxin (type D is also referred to as *C. hemolyticum*)

C. perfringens	α-Toxin β-Toxin ι-Toxin Enterotoxin	Phospholipase C that is lethal and necrotizing Lethal and necrotizing Lethal and necrotizing toxin with ADP-ribosylating activity Lethal and emetic protein found in sporulating cells

Type A: α-toxin
Type B: α-toxin, β-toxin, ε-toxin
Type C: α-toxin, β-toxin
Type D: α-toxin, ε-toxin
Type E: α-toxin, ι-toxin

C. sordellii	α-Toxin Toxin HT Toxin LT	Phospholipase C related to the α-toxin of C. perfringens Haemorrhagic toxin related to toxin A of C. difficile Lethal toxin related to toxin B of C. difficile

damage and necrosis, further reducing the supply of oxygen to the infected tissue. This, in turn, leads to continued tissue destruction that can rapidly become life threatening if treatment is not initiated.

Clostridium perfringens produces more toxins than any other pathogen. The primary toxins that cause tissue destruction in myonecrosis and that are used for typing purposes are α-, β-, ε-, and τ-toxin. All of these toxins are distinct proteins that do not cross-react immunologically. α-Toxin, which was the first toxin to be identified as an enzyme, is phospholipase C, which hydrolyzes the cleavage of phosphatidylcholine to phosphoryl-choline and 1,2-diglyceride. It is lethal, necrotic,

and haemolytic, and is produced by all types of *C. perfringens*, although the levels of α-toxin vary between the different types. α-Toxin is a zinc metalloenzyme with a molecular weight of 42 500. The gene has been cloned and sequenced (Tittall *et al.*, 1989). α-Toxin is regarded as the most important toxin in clostridial myonecrosis caused by *C. perfringens* or by mixed infections containing *C. perfringens*. β-Toxin and ε-toxin are lethal and necrotizing, and are sensitive to oxidation. These toxins have not been studied in as much detail as α- and τ-toxin. The τ-toxin is a binary toxin that ADP-ribosylates actin. Component A (M_r 47 500) of τ-toxin is the enzyme that has the ADP-ribosylating activity and component

B (M_r 71 500) is believed to be the binding portion. The toxin causes cell-rounding of tissue cultured mammalian cells, is enterotoxic in ligated ileal loops, and lethal when injected into mice. It is highly related immunologically to τ-toxin of *C. spiroforme* and exhibits the same type of cytotoxic and enterotoxic activity as τ-toxin of *C. spiroforme* and C2 toxin of *C. botulinum*.

The α-toxin of *C. novyi* is the major toxin produced by this organism. The toxin is large, cytotoxic, and highly lethal, and in this regard it mimics the high molecular weight cytotoxins of *C. difficile* and *C. sordellii* (see Table 19.3). *Clostridium novyi* is a wound pathogen and is not associated with gastrointestinal disease. *Clostridium septicum* typically has been associated with gas gangrene over many decades but recently it has become associated with gas gangrene in patients with neoplastic diseases, especially leukaemia/lymphomas, adenocarcinomas of the colon, and other solid tumour malignancies (Kornbluth *et al.*, 1989). In patients with *C. septicum* bacteraemia, the portal of entry is often the large bowel, whether or not the patient has underlying malignancy. The α-toxin is the lethal factor produced by this organism It has an M_r of 48 000, is haemolytic, and does not cross-react with toxins of the other clostridia (Ballard *et al.*, 1992). *Clostridium sordellii* produces two large cytotoxins that are related to the toxins of *C. difficile* (see Table 19.3). These toxins are tissue damaging and lethal and they play a role in disease once the organism infects a wound. In addition, the organism produces other factors, including phospholipase, protease, haemolysins, and sialidase, and these factors likely play a role in disease. *Clostridium histolyticum* produces an α-toxin that has been reported to be related to the α-toxin of *C. septicum*. It also is lethal and necrotizing. In addition to α-toxin, *C. histolyticum* produces tissue-damaging proteases (β-, γ-, and δ-toxins) that probably are involved in the necrosis that occurs in gas gangrene.

Epidemiology

Gas gangrene is associated with wound infections. The disease has been most typically associated with war casualties, although it does occur in civilians. Injuries or wounds that result in contamination to the muscle tissue, especially to the large muscle groups, represent the major predisposing factor. Compound fractures, for example, may result in the introduction of spores directly to the muscle mass. The histotoxic clostridia are ubiquitous in soil and water, and are part of the indigenous intestinal microbiota of humans and other animals. Thus, the source of the organism may be soil (exogenous) or the patient's own intestinal tract (endogenous). *Clostridium perfringens* is the most prevalent organism in these cases, with it being associated with >80% of the cases, followed by *C. novyi* and *C. septicum* in frequency. *Clostridium perfringens* types A and C are human pathogens whereas types B, D, and E cause disease primarily in animals such as sheep, goats, and rabbits. Of the four types of *C. novyi*, only type A is implicated in human disease.

Clinical features

One of the first symptoms commonly associated with clostridial myonecrosis is the acute onset of pain in the region associated with a wound. The onset may occur in less than 10 hours, but typically the incubation period usually is less than three days. There is extensive pain and swelling, and the skin becomes very tense and white with some blue or black discoloration. The amount of exudate and odour is variable and there may be gas (crepitance on palpation) within the affected tissue. A toxaemia ensues, resulting in rapid and serious systemic changes. In some instances, clostridial cellulitis may occur due to less virulent clostridia and this condition usually is not life threatening. In clostridial myonecrosis, there is a marked change to the muscle tissue. Initially, the blood supply to the muscle decreases, resulting in a change in muscle colour. In severe cases, the muscle may even become liquefied (i.e., liquefactive necrosis). The major muscle masses may be particularly involved because of the nature of the infection. The clostridial species involved may affect the incubation period. Infection with *C. perfringens*, for example, is rapid and clinical features may develop within 10–48 hours. The incubation period with *C. septicum*, on the other hand, may be two to three days, and with *C. novyi* it may be five to six days.

Diagnosis

The diagnosis of clostridial myonecrosis is based on a combination of clinical findings, the presence of dead muscle (gas gangrene) and information derived from microbiological examination(s). A number of clinical findings suggest this diagnosis. The sudden onset of severe pain in the area of a wound that steadily increases in severity and spreads as the infection spreads often is one of the first clues. At this time, the skin over the affected area appears tight because of prominent, local oedema, is cooler than normal, tender on palpation, and pale, often marbled, bluish-purple. The wound may show a thin, frothy haemorrhagic exudate. There may be crepitance owing to the presence of gas in the tissue, but the absence of gas does not rule out clostridial myonecrosis, nor is its presence diagnostic for this condition only. The skin later develops a bronzed appearance, and bullae filled with dark sanguinolent fluid which may discharge on the skin surface, along with patches of necrotic, sloughed skin are seen. A peculiar, sweetish or perhaps 'mousy' odour, but usually not an acrid odour, may be noticed by the physician. The patient may be alert and quite anxious about the seriousness of his/her condition, toxic, the temperature may be only moderately elevated (e.g. 100 °F), and there is tachycardia. Later findings include haemolytic anemia, hypotension, renal failure, shock, and other findings consistent with fulminant septicaemia. In confirming a clinical diagnosis of suspected gas gangrene, a close working relationship between the clinician and the clinical microbiology laboratory is often of urgent importance. The direct microscopic examination of Gram-stained smears of aspirated material from a myonecrotic lesion may reveal a necrotic background without inflammatory cells and morphologic forms of bacteria revealing clostridia (e.g. large, boxcar-shaped Gram-positive rods). Other conditions that might be considered in the differen-

tial diagnosis of clostridial myonecrosis, including anaerobic cellulitis, polymicrobic mixed aerobic–anaerobic gas-forming infections, streptococcal fasciitis, and synergistic necrotizing cellulitis, may show muscle cell outlines, polymorphonuclear leukocytes and mixed morphologic forms of bacteria. The detection of *Clostridium* spp. in a wound culture is not diagnostic because these organisms may be isolated from many wounds that are considered non-infected because of the absence of any significant clinical features. On the other hand, when the clinical setting and Gram-stained smears suggest clostridial infection (e.g. myonecrosis), cultures of involved tissues and blood cultures aid in confirming the clinical diagnosis and identifying the species involved. Several excellent references are available for further details (Finegold and George, 1989; Bartlett, 1990; MacLennan, 1962). The term gas gangrene, which often is used interchangeably with clostridial myonecrosis, may be misleading because in many instances no gas is present. The disease can become irreversible and life threatening in a period of only a few hours. Therefore, it is imperative to distinguish myonecrosis from clostridial cellulitis and other related diseases.

Treatment and management

Treatment involves surgical débridement of all infected tissue. This must be done early and extensively, and surgical exploration should be done if there is the possibility of clinical myonecrosis. Often, the affected limbs must be amputated to preserve life. Antibiotic therapy with penicillin G should be initiated since these organisms are sensitive to the action of this class of antibiotics. The value of hyperbaric oxygen is not clear although it may be used in very severe cases in which there are no other alternatives. In uterine clostridial myonecrosis, hysterectomy usually is necessary to save the life of the patient.

Prevention

The ubiquity of clostridial spores and the lack of appropriate vaccines make this disease very difficult to prevent. In addition, the wide range of toxins produced by this group of organisms makes the production of vaccines unlikely in the near future. Fortunately, the incidence of this disease is very low in the civilian population and the incidence of the disease in wars since World War I has been significantly lower than the high incidence reported in that war.

Clostridium perfringens Food Poisoning

Microbiology

Some of the phenotypic properties of *C. perfringens* are described in the section above. Food poisoning caused by this organism results from the production of a spore-associated enterotoxin. Another important feature is its ability to grow rapidly over a wide range of temperatures (room temperature to 50 °C) and to produce spores under these conditions. Under optimal conditions in chopped meat media, the generation time of *C. perfringens* may be as short as eight minutes. The vegetative cells are not destroyed unless the temperature is above 50 °C. Studies on the enterotoxin of *C. perfringens* have progressed more rapidly since the development of media that improves spore formation, thus yielding higher levels of enterotoxin. The medium, which was developed by Duncan and Strong (1968), contains yeast extract (0.4%), proteose peptone (1.5%), soluble starch (0.4%), sodium thioglycolate (0.1%), and $Na_2HPO_4.7H_2O$ (1.0%).

Pathogenesis

Food poisoning by *C. perfringens* occurs because of the production of an enterotoxin. The toxin is a single polypeptide with a molecular weight of about 35 000. The toxin is not heat stable and is rapidly inactivated at 60 °C, distinguishing it from the enterotoxins of *Staphylococcus aureus*. The toxin is directly associated with sporulation and is believed to be produced once the organism begins to sporulate in the intestine. The enterotoxin may actually be a structural component of the spore coat. Once the enterotoxin is produced and released, it acts by stimulating the loss of fluid and electrolytes from the intestinal mucosa. This loss is believed to result from the mucosal damage caused by the toxin. The enterotoxin affects a variety of tissue cultured mammalian cells. The initial step in the intoxication process is the binding of the toxin to a proteinaceous receptor. The toxin, or a toxic fragment, then is inserted into the membrane, resulting in extensive changes to the permeability of the cell. These changes eventually result in cell death.

Epidemiology

In results published in the USA by the CDC, *C. perfringens* was found to account for approximately 5–10% of the outbreaks in which the causative agent was identified (MacDonald and Griffin, 1985; Shandera *et al.*, 1983) and was third behind *Salmonella* and *Staphylococcus aureus* as a leading bacterial cause of food poisoning. In many instances of food poisoning outbreaks, the aetiological agent is never identified and many persons suspect that the incidence of *C. perfringens* food poisoning is considerably higher (Shandera *et al.*, 1983). Meat or meat products, including beef and poultry, are usually the contaminated food. Most outbreaks have been associated with commercial food services for restaurants and institutions. Interestingly, the peak incidence usually is in the spring or autumn instead of the summer as would be expected because of the association with improperly heated food.

Clinical features

Food poisoning associated with *C. perfringens* is mild and self-limiting, frequently with an incubation period of 8–12 hours following the ingestion of contaminated food. Most patients exhibit diarrhoea and complain of abdominal cramping. Some patients will exhibit nausea and vomiting. Because of the short duration of the disease, most patients do not seek treatment. Characteristic clues include short incubation time (8 to 12 hours), suspected meat source, diarrhoea and cramping, and short duration of illness.

Diagnosis

Because of the short duration of the disease, the diagnosis usually is made after recovery and serves primarily as confirmatory evidence. Typically, a diagnosis may be considered confirmed if there are $>10^5$ of *C. perfringens* per gram of suspected food, $>10^6$ *C. perfringens* per gram of faeces, and demonstration that the organisms recovered from the suspected food and faeces of the patients are the same type. The specimens should be collected and stored at 4 °C as soon as possible. An alternative to this approach is to test the clinical specimen for enterotoxin. There are several different assays for the detection of enterotoxin such as an animal model, tissue culture assay, and passive reversed haemagglutination. However, these methods either are not sensitive or rapid enough or they exhibit background problems. An EIA has been described that detects the enterotoxin at a level of 1 ng/ml within several hours. This is sufficiently sensitive to detect the toxin in faeces of suspected persons since infected patients typically have 0.5–16 µg per gram of faeces. Because of its sensitivity and rapid turn-around time, the EIA may be suitable as a diagnostic test. The test is now under commercial development.

Treatment and management

Because this disease is mild and almost always self-limiting, antibiotic therapy is not recommended. However, it is important that the patient receive plenty of fluids and seek medical attention if complications arise. The number of deaths reported following *C. perfringens* food poisoning is very low and have occurred only in elderly persons who were debilitated. Isolation of patients is not necessary since the disease is not transmissible from person to person.

Prevention

The disease results from the contamination of foods, primarily meats, and it is important that meats be properly cooked to destroy the spores. Foods should be refrigerated to minimize the growth of the organism and rewarmed meats should be heated to >75 °C internally to destroy the bacteria. Any suspected cases should be reported to the local public health authorities in order to identify and remove any contaminated food and to correct any improper food preparation methods that may result in additional contamination.

Enteritis Necroticans (Pig-Bel)

Microbiology

Enteritis necroticans is caused by *C. perfringens* ('*C. welchii*') type C, which produces α- and β-toxin. Both toxins are believed to be involved in the disease although the β-toxin may be more important. The organism responsible for the disease causes enterotoxemia in farm animals, and it has been suggested that Pig-Bel represents a zoonosis.

Pathogenesis

The disease develops primarily because of the consumption of improperly cooked pork. In the Highlands of Papua New Guinea, it is common practice to cook a hog or slabs of pork between layers of fruit, bread, and leaves at low temperatures (approximately 70–80 °C). The large slabs of pork, which are not thoroughly cooked, are contaminated even further by handling the meat in dirty environments. The contaminated meats are ingested and the organism grows in the intestinal tract, releasing α- and β-toxins which are lethal and necrotizing. Interestingly, these toxins are rapidly destroyed by endogenous proteases, including trypsin, and it has been suggested that the production and destruction of the toxins plays a key role in the pathogenesis of the disease. It has been suggested that a combination of the following factors is necessary for the disease to develop: (1) presence of *C. perfringens* type C, (2) consumption of nutrients for rapid growth of the organism, (3) low trypsin secretion, and (4) presence of trypsin inhibitors in the diet or from parasites (Lawrence and Cooke, 1980).

Epidemiology

Pig-Bel has been studied in detail in the Highlands of Papua New Guinea where it is a common cause of death in children older than one year of age. The annual incidence has been estimated at 48.3 per 10 000 in the adult population and 33.6 per 10 000 in children under the age of 15 years. The organism has been isolated from human and pig faeces as well as from soil samples in villages in which it is prevalent. The disease also occurs in other parts of Southeast Asia, parts of China and Africa, and other areas of the world. As expected, the incidence rises when pig feasting activities begin. The epidemiology of the disease can be followed based on pork consumption.

Clinical features

Pig-Bel may develop in several different forms. In the acute stage, the disease may be fulminating and result in the death of the patient within 24 hours. Children who develop acute Pig-Bel have severe upper abdominal pain that begins within several days after a high-protein meal, usually pork. There may be mild diarrhoea, constipation, and vomiting. The intake of food may cause intestinal pain, even though the child may be hungry. Alternatively, the disease may occur as a milder form that is difficult to distinguish from gastroenteritis. In this case, the patient usually recovers with proper management. Some patients who have past histories of either the acute disease or a milder form in conjunction with malnutrition occasionally develop sudden intestinal obstruction referred to as chronic Pig-Bel.

Diagnosis

The diagnosis typically is based on patient history and clinical features. The pain associated with the disease may be similar to that associated with ascariasis. Other differential diagnoses may include typhoid and paratyphoid fever, appendicitis, and bowel obstructions. Patients with Pig-Bel may develop elevated antibody levels against the organism and its toxins, but this type of analysis is not performed routinely.

Treatment and management

The primary decisions in the treatment of Pig-Bel are when to operate and when to start intravenous feeding. Operating early in the disease lowers the mortality rate but involves some children who would recover with proper medical management. Delaying the surgery may exacerbate the disease. Children with Pig-Bel often have protein malnutrition, which slows wound healing and increases the morbidity and mortality. Guidelines for the treatment of mild and severe Pig-Bel have been established and are described in detail elsewhere (Finegold and George, 1989).

Prevention

Vaccination against *C. perfringens* using β-toxoid protects against Pig-Bel. In one study, the annual incidence decreased from 33 cases per 10 000 to four cases per 10 000. Other studies have shown similar decreases in the incidence. It is now recommended that β-toxoid be administered to children in high-risk areas at four, six, and 12 months and that boosters be given to increase the immunity.

FURTHER READING

Allen, S.D., and Baron, E.J. (1991) *Clostridium*. In *Manual of Clinical Microbiology*, 5th edn (ed. A. Balows, W.J. Hausler Jr, K.L. Herrman *et al.*), pp. 505–521. American Society for Microbiology, Washington, DC.

Borriello, S.P. (1985) *Clostridia in Gastrointestinal Disease*. CRC Press, Boca Raton, FL.

Finegold, S.M. and George, W.L. (1989) *Anaerobic Infections in Humans*. Academic Press, San Diego, CA.

Hatheway, C.L. (1990) The toxigenic clostridia. *Clinical Microbiology Reviews*, **3**, 66–98.

Holdeman, L.V., Cato, E.P. and Moore, W.E.C. (1977) *Anaerobe Laboratory Manual*, 4th edn. Virginia Polytechnic Institute and State University, Blacksburg, VA.

Levett, P.N. (1991) *Anaerobic Microbiology: A Practical Approach*. IRL Press, New York.

McClane, B.A., Hann, P.C. and Wnek, A.P. (1988) *Clostridium perfringens* enterotoxin. *Microbial Pathogenesis*, **4**, 317–323.

Rolfe, R.D. and Finegold, S.M. (1988) *Clostridium difficile: Its Role in Intestinal Disease*. Academic Press, New York.

Schanta, E.J. and Johnson, E.A. (1992) Properties and use of botulinum toxin and other microbial neurotoxins in medicine. *Microbiological Reviews*, **56**, 80–99.

Willis, A.T. and Phillips, K.D. (1988) *Anaerobic Infections: Clinical and Laboratory Practice*. Public Health Laboratory Service, Spire Litho, Salisbury, UK.

REFERENCES

Aktories, K. (1990) Clostridal ADP-ribosyltransferases: modification of low molecular weight GTP-binding proteins and of actin by clostridial toxins. *Medical Microbiology and Immunology*, **179**, 123–126.

Allen, S.D. and Baron, E.J. (1991) *Clostridium*. In *Manual of Clinical Microbiology*, 5th edn (ed. A. Balows, W.J. Hawler, K.L. Herrman *et al.*), pp. 505–521. American Society for Microbiology, Washington, DC.

Aureli, P., Fenicia, L., Pasolini, B. *et al.* (1986) Two cases of type E infant botulism caused by neurotoxigenic *Clostridium butyricum* in Italy. *Journal of Infectious Disease*, **154**, 201–206.

Ball, D.W., Van Tassell, R.L., Roberts, M.D. *et al.* (1993) Purification and characterization of alpha-toxin produced by *Clostridium novyi* type A. *Infection and Immunity*, **61**, 2912–2918.

Ballard, J., Bryant, A., Stevens, D. *et al.* (1992) Purification and characterization of the lethal toxin (alpha-toxin) of *Clostridium septicum*. *Infection and Immunity*, **60**, 784–790.

Barroso, L.A., Wang, S.-Z., Phelps, C.J. *et al.* (1990) Nucleotide sequence of *Clostridium difficile* toxin B gene. *Nucleic Acids Research*, **18**, 4004.

Bartlett, J.G. (1990) Gas gangrene (other *Clostridium*-associated diseases). In *Principles and Practice of Infectious Diseases*, 3rd edn (ed. G.L. Mandell, R.G. Douglas Jr and J.E. Bennett), pp. 1850–1860. Churchill Livingstone, Edinburgh.

Cato, E.P., George, W.L. and Finegold, S.M. (1986) Genus *Clostridum* Prazmowski 1880, 23^AL. In *Bergey's Manual of Systematic Bacteriology, Vol. 2* (ed. P.H.A. Sneath, N.S. Mair, M.E. Sharpe and G.E. Holt), pp. 1141–1200. Williams and Wilkins, Baltimore.

CDC (1979) *Botulism in the United States, 1899–1977. Handbook for Epidemiologists, Clinicians, and Laboratory Workers*. Centers for Disease Control, Atlanta, GA.

CDC, Public Health Service, US Department of Health, Education, and Welfare (1986) Notifiable diseases of low frequency, United States. *Morbidity and Mortality Weekly Report*, **34**, 774.

CDC (1991) Summary of notifiable disease, United States, 1990. *Morbidity and Mortality Weekly Report*, **39**, 55–61.

Dove, C.H., Wang, S.-Z., Price, S.B. *et al.* (1990) Molecular characterization of the *Clostridium difficile* toxin A gene. *Infection and Immunity*, **58**, 480–488.

Duncan, C.L. and Strong, D.H. (1968) Improved medium for sporulation of *Clostridium perfringens*. *Applied Microbiology*, **16**, 82–89.

Ebisawa, I., Takayanagi, M., Kurata, M. *et al.* (1986) Density and distribution of *Clostridium tetani* in the soil. *Japanese Journal of Experimental Medicine*, **56**, 69–74.

Finegold, S.M. and George, W.L. (1989) *Anaerobic Infections in Humans*. Academic Press, San Diego, CA.

Furste, W. (1987) Seventh international conference on tetanus, Copanello (Catanzaro), Italy, Sept. 10–15, 1984. *Journal of Trauma*, **27**, 99–103.

Gerding, D. and Brazier, J.S. (1993) Optimal methods for identifying *Clostridium difficile* infections. *Clinical Infectious Diseases* **16**, S439–S442.

Gimenez, J.A., Gimenez, M.A. and Dasgupta, B.R. (1992) Characterization of the neurotoxin isolated from a *Clostridium barati* strain implicated in infant botulism. *Infection and Immunity*, **60**, 518–522.

George, W.L., Sutter, V.L., Citron, D. *et al.* (1979) Selective and differential medium for isolation of *Clostridium difficile*. *Journal of Clinical Microbiology*, **9**, 214–219.

Groleau, G. (1992) Tetanus. *Emergency Clinics of North America*, **10**, 351–360.

Gurwith, M.J., Langston, C. and Citron, D.M. (1981) Toxin-producing bacteria in infants. *American Journal of Diseases of Children*, **135**, 1104–1106.

Hall, J.D., McCroskey, L.M., Pincomb, B.J. *et al.* (1985) Isolation of an organism resembling *Clostridium barati* which produces type F botulinal toxin from an infant with botulism. *Journal of Clinical Microbiology*, **21**, 654–655.

Hatheway, C.L. (1990) The toxigenic clostridia. *Clinical Microbiology Reviews*, **3**, 66–98.

Hatheway, C.L. (1992) *Clostridium botulinum*. In *Infectious Diseases* (ed. S.L. Gorbach, J.G. Bartlett and N.R. Blacklow), pp. 1583–1587. Saunders, Philadelphia.

Holdeman, L.V, Cato, E.P. and Moore, W.E.C. (1977) *Anaerobe Laboratory Manual*, 4th edn. Virginia Polytechnic Institute and State University, Blacksburg, VA.

Kornbluth, A.A., Danzig, J.B. and Bernstein, L.H. (1989) *Clostridium septicum* infection and associated malignancy: report of 2 cases and review of the literature. *Medicine* (Baltimore), **68**, 30–37.

Krivan, H.C., Clark, G.F., Smith, D.F. and Wilkins, T.D. (1986) Cell surface binding site for *Clostridium difficile* enterotoxin: evidence for a glycoconjugate containing the sequence Galα1-3Galβ1-4GlcNAc. *Infection and Immunity* **53**, 573–581.

Lawrence, G., and Cooke, R. (1980) Experimental pigbel: the production and pathology of necrotising enteritis due to *Clostridium welchii* type C in the guinea-pig. *British Journal of Experimental Pathology*, **61**, 261.

Lyerly, D.M., Barroso, L.A., Wilkins, T.D. *et al.* (1992) Characterization of a toxin A-negative, toxin B-positive strain of *Clostridium difficile*. *Infection and Immunity*, **60**, 4633–4639.

MacDonald, K.L. and Griffin, P.M. (1985) Foodborne disease outbreaks, Annual summary, 1982. *Morbidity and Mortality Weekly Report*, **35**, 7SS–16SS.

MacDonald, K.L., Cohen, M.L. and Blake, P.A. (1986) The changing epidemiology of adult botulism in the United States. *American Journal of Epidemiology*, **124**, 794–799.

MacLennan, J.D. (1962) The histotoxic clostridial diseases of man. *Bacteriological Review*, **26**, 177–275.

Martinez, R.D. and Wilkins, T.D. (1992) Comparison of *Clostridium sordellii* toxins HT and LT with toxins A and B of *C. difficile*. *Journal of Medical Microbiology*, **36**, 30–36.

McCroskey, L.M., Hatheway, C.L., Fenicia, L. *et al.* (1986) Characterization of an organism that produces type E botulinal toxin but which resembles *Clostridium butyricum* from the faeces of an infant with type E botulism. *Journal of Clinical Microbiology*, **23**, 201–202.

McFarland, L.V., Mulligan, M.E., Kwok, R.Y.Y. *et al.* (1991) Nosocomial acquisition of *Clostridium difficile* infection. *New England Journal of Medicine*, **320**, 204–210.

Pantosti, A., Cerquetti, M. and Gianfrilli, P.M. (1988) Electrophoretic characterization of *Clostridium difficile* strains isolated from antibiotic-associated colitis and other conditions. *Journal of Clinical Microbiology*, **26**, 540–543.

Popoff, M.R., Rubin, E.J., Gill, D.M. *et al.* (1988) Actin-specific ADP-ribosyltransferase produced by a *Clostridium difficile* strain. *Infection and Immunity*, **56**, 2299–2306.

Rosener, S., Chatwal, G.S. and Aktories, K. (1987) Botulinum ADP-ribosyltransferase C3 but not botulinum neurotoxins C1 and D ADP-ribosylates low molecular mass GTP-binding proteins. *Federation of the European Biochemical Society Letters*, **224**, 38–42.

Schiavo, G., Poulain, B., Rossetto, O. *et al.* (1992a) Tetanus toxin is a zinc protein and its inhibition of neurotransmitter release and protease activity depend on zinc. *EMBO Journal*, **11**, 3577–3583.

Schiavo, G., Benfenati, F., Poulain, B. *et al.* (1992b) Tetanus and botulinum-B neurotoxins block neurotransmitter release by proteolytic cleavage of synaptobrevin. *Nature*, **359**, 832–834.

Shandera, W.X., Tacket, C.O. and Blake, P.A. (1983) Food poisoning due to *Clostridium perfringens* in the United States. *Journal of Infectious Disease*, **147**, 167–170.

Simpson, L.L., Stiles, B.G., Zepeda, H.H. *et al.* (1987) Molecular basis for the pathological actions of *Clostridium perfringens* iota toxin. *Infection and Immunity*, **55**, 118–122.

Simpson, L.L., Lake, P. and Kozaki, S. (1990) Isolation and characterization of a novel human monoclonal antibody that neutralizes tetanus toxin. *Journal of Pharmacology and Experimental Therapy*, **254**, 98–103.

Stiles, B.G. and Wilkins, T.D. (1986) Purification and characterization of *Clostridium perfringens* iota toxin: dependence on two nonlinked proteins for biological activity. *Infection and Immunity*, **5**, 683–688.

Titball, R.W., Hunter, S., Martin, K. *et al.* (1989) Molecular cloning and nucleotide sequence of the alpha-toxin (phospholipase C) of *Clostridium perfringens*. *Infection and Immunity*, **57**, 367–376.

Toma, S., Lesiak, G., Majus, M. *et al.* (1988) Serotyping of *Clostridium difficile*. *Journal of Clinical Microbiology*, **26**, 426–428.

Woodruff, B.A., Griffin, P.M., McCroskey, L.M. *et al.* (1992) Clinical and laboratory comparison of botulism from toxin types A, B, and E in the United States, 1975–1988. *Journal of Infectious Disease*, **166**, 1281–1286.

19b

ACTINOMYCES

J.S. Brazier and V. Hall

HISTORICAL INTRODUCTION

Early Descriptions

The filamentous organisms that were eventually to become known as *Actinomyces* first came to the attention of microbiologists in the late 1870s when several reports of fungal-like masses in lesions of cattle and lacrimal concretions of man were published. In 1877 Bollinger described the first case of actinomycosis in cattle, followed two years later by Harz's classic description of a 'ray fungus' seen in stained preparations from cases of 'lumpy jaw' in cattle (Harz, 1879). Although Harz did not culture the organism, he named it *Actinomyces bovis*, the name being derived from its origin and appearance (*aktino* = ray, *myces* = fungus). Israel (1878) recognized a similar organism in human postmortem material, and Bujwid (1889) claimed to be the first to have cultured the organism from a case of human actinomycosis.

Despite these earlier reports, it was the paper by Wolff and Israel (1891) which became known as the classic description of the organism now classified as *Actinomyces israelii*. Other workers compared isolates from human and bovine sources and, considering them to be morphologically identical, coined the name '*Streptothrix*', believing this to be a more taxonomically correct term. Cohn (1875), however, preferred the name '*Leptothrix*' to describe filamentous and/or branching organisms; both of these outdated terms have somehow managed to persist over many decades particularly amongst workers in other branches of pathology.

Wright (1905) clarified the differences between *Actinomyces* and the aerobic filamentous genus of *Nocardia* which had hitherto been confused by some workers. Until 1940 the causative agent of both human and bovine actinomycosis was believed to be *A. bovis*. Erikson (1940) suggested that *A. israelii* was a distinct species associated specifically with human disease, whereas *A. bovis* was only found in cattle. This viewpoint was not universally accepted, however, until it was verified by Thompson in 1950. At this stage there was still some debate as to whether *Actinomyces* were fungi or bacteria. It was not until 1962 that Cummins produced evidence that they were true bacteria, and that they were distinct from other branching genera. He also showed that many other species within the genus could be identified.

Principles and Practice of Clinical Bacteriology. Edited by A.M. Emmerson, P.M. Hawkey and S.H. Gillespie
© 1997 John Wiley & Sons Ltd

DESCRIPTION OF THE GENUS
ACTINOMYCES

Definition

Actinomyces are Gram-positive non-spore-forming facultatively anaerobic bacilli which may exhibit true branching. They are non-motile, non-acid fast and conidia are not produced. Some species are catalase positive; nitrate reduction is variable; indole is not produced. Metabolism is fermentative, and end products include acetic, lactic and succinic acids but not propionic acid. Cell wall peptidoglycan contains lysine and may contain aspartic acid or ornithine but not diaminopimelic acid or glycine. Various sugars occur in the cell wall but not arabinose or xylose. The G + C ratio is 57–69 mol%.

Classification

The genus name *Actinomyces* was proposed by Breed and Cohn (1919) and was ratified by a Judicial Commission a year later by Winslow *et al.* (1920). At that time the classification of Buchanan (1918) placed the genus *Actinomyces* in the order Actinomycetales, family Actinomycetaceae. Other members of the family included *Actinobacillus*, *Leptotrichia* and *Nocardia*. This classification was clearly unsatisfactory, since it grouped Gram positives with Gram negatives and aerobes with anaerobes. It was later modified by Waksman and Henrici (1943), who reduced the family Actinomycetaceae to include only *Actinomyces* and *Nocardia*, and moved the other aerobic filamentous bacteria to the family Streptomycetaceae. The eighth edition of *Bergey's Manual of Determinative Bacteriology* (Sneath *et al.*, 1986) removed *Nocardia* and classified Actinomycetaceae into five genera: *Actinomyces*, *Arachnia*, *Bifidobacterium*, *Bacterionema* and *Rothia*. Despite the attentions of Schaal and Schofield (1984) the Family Actinomycetaceae remained a heterogeneous group.

The development of chemotaxonomic methods has allowed some clarification of the taxonomy of the genus *Actinomyces* and related taxa. At genus level the determination of cell wall peptidoglycan, carbohydrate constituents and DNA base-pair compositions, together with end products of glucose metabolism, form the standard criteria for inclusion in the genus. On such a basis, Reddy *et al.* (1982) proposed the transfer of *Corynebacterium pyogenes* (Glage) Eberson to the genus *Actinomyces* as *A. pyogenes* (Glage).

At species level DNA homology studies and polyacrylamide gel electrophoresis have aided the development of the taxonomy, and serological typing has been applied extensively for delineation of both species and subspecies. Antigenic variations have been demonstrated by fluorescent antibody, immunodiffusion and cell wall agglutination procedures. Of these, direct or indirect fluorescent antibody techniques have been used most widely. The direct method was first employed by Slack *et al.* (1961) and later revised to demonstrate serogroups corresponding to the then recognized species of *Actinomyces*. They established two serotypes within each serogroup and suggested the existence of others. Strain-variable cross-reactions were noted both between species and serotypes but these were usually eliminated by dilution or absorption of the antiserum. Other workers, including Gerencser (1979), Schofield and Schaal (1981) and Schaal and Gatzer (1985) generally supported these findings and further delineated the serological relationships of members of the genus.

The species *A. naeslundii* and *A. viscosus* are closely related and, amongst others, Fillery *et al.* (1978) concluded that they formed separate serotypes of one species rather than separate species. However, in their comprehensive numerical taxonomic study, Schofield and Schaal (1981) demonstrated differential characteristics between these species and between their serotypes as defined by the indirect immunofluorescence method of Schaal and Pulverer (1973). Johnson *et al.* (1990) further clarified the taxonomy of the genus in their comparative study of strains of *Actinomyces* from human periodontal flora, and from other habitats wherein genetic relatedness was determined by DNA hybridization. The species status of strains of *A. israelii* serotype 1,

A. meyeri, *A. odontolyticus* serotypes 1 and 2, *A. bovis* and *A. hordeovulneris* were confirmed. *Actinomyces israelii* serotype 2 was found to be both genetically and phenotypically distinct from other species and serotypes including *A. israelii* serotype 1 and therefore was recognized as a separate species, namely, *A. gerencseriae*. Similarly, distinct strains isolated from human gingival crevices and the previously designated 'Actinomyces DO8' were named as *A. georgiae*. Within the *A. naeslundii*/*A. viscosus* complex strains of *A. naeslundii* serotype 1 were found to be genetically distinct from other species and distantly related to strains of *A. naeslundii* serotypes 2 and 3, *A. viscosus* serotype 2 and 'Actinomyces serotype NV' which formed a closely related group. These subdivisions were designated as *A. naeslundii* genospecies 1 and 2 respectively. Strains of 'Actinomyces serotype WVU963' were more distantly related and were considered to form a third genospecies. However, as there were no reliable phenotypic tests to differentiate these genospecies, no taxonomic changes were proposed. *Actinomyces viscosus* serotype 1 was also distantly related to the proposed *A. naeslundii* genospecies.

From samples of dental plaque of dairy cattle Dent and Williams isolated strains of *Actinomyces* which were found to be closely related to, but phenotypically distinct from, *A. naeslundii* and *A. viscosus*. On the basis of polyacrylamide electrophoresis patterns, cell wall carbohydrate constituents, DNA–DNA homologies and DNA mean base compositions, these isolates were delineated and named as *A. denticolens* (Dent and Williams, 1984a), *A. howellii* (Dent and Williams, 1984b) and *A. slackii* (Dent and Williams, 1986).

The developing nature of the taxonomy of the genus *Actinomyces* has resulted in differences in the species listed according to the textbook consulted. Table 19b.1 lists the currently recognized members of the genus *Actinomyces* along with former synonyms, their usual host and pathogenicity.

Recently Funke *et al.* (1994) have proposed the assignment of human-derived CDC group 1 and CDC group 1-like coryneform bacteria to the genus *Actinomyces*: as *A. neuii* subsp. *neuii* sp. nov., subsp. nov., and *A. neuii* subsp. *anitratus* subsp. nov. respectively. These proposals are supported by analysis of 16S rRNA gene sequences, other molecular findings and phenotypic tests.

TABLE 19b.1 LIST OF CURRENT TAXA OF *ACTINOMYCES*, THEIR NORMAL HABITAT AND PATHOGENIC POTENTIAL

Species (synonyms)	Main host	Pathogenicity
A. bovis (*A. bovis* Harz)	Cow	+
A. denticolens	Cow	?
A. georgiae (*Actinomyces* DO8)	Man	–
A. gerencseriae (*A. israelii* serotype II)	Man	+
A. hordeovulneris	Dog	+
A. howellii	Cow	–
A. israelii (*Streptothrix israeli*)	Man	+
A. meyeri (*Actinobacterium meyeri*)	Man	+
A. naeslundii	Man and animals	+
A. odontolyticus	Man	+
A. pyogenes (*Corynebacterium pyogenes*)	Animals[a] and man	+
A. slackii	Cow	–
A. viscosus (*Odontomyces viscosus*)	Man	+

[a] Various domestic and farm animals.

The taxonomic positions of two former species included in the genus, namely *A. humiferus* and *A. suis*, is currently uncertain and are awaiting reclassification. Similarly, other former members of the genus which have been satisfactorily reclassified include '*A. eriksonii*' (*Bifidobacterium dentium*) and '*A. propionicus*' (*Propionibacterium propionicum*).

Morphology

Bacilli are straight or curved and less than 1 μm in width. Length varies from short (coccoid) rods through a diphtheroid-like morphology, to long filaments 50 μm or more in length. The diphtheroid-like rods may occur in V, Y or palisade arrangements, may have clubbed ends, and Gram staining is usually deep and uniform. Filamentous forms are usually slender, may be straight or wavy, and frequently demonstrate true branching. Irregular staining is common and the resultant beaded filaments may be mistaken for chains of streptococci by the inexperienced. Micro-colonies composed of profusions of branching filaments forming dense, deeply staining masses with irregular fringes may be present, particularly in direct smears of clinical material where they are a useful diagnostic pointer.

Most species of *Actinomyces* demonstrate both short and filamentous bacilli but in *A. bovis*, diphtheroids predominate and *A. meyeri* is generally coccobacillary to diphtheroidal.

Colonial Morphology and Growth Characteristics

The morphology of mature colonies varies considerably between and within each species and can be classified broadly as rough and smooth types. Colonies of both types reach 0.5–2.0 mm in diameter after 7–14 days under optimal conditions. Rough colonies are classically described as 'molar-tooth', 'breadcrumb' or 'raspberry-like' because of their heaped-up irregular shape, with or without a central depression. They may be soft and friable or hard, making them difficult to emulsify in saline. Pitting of the agar is a common feature, and colonies may be tightly adherent to its surface. Smooth colonies are convex to domed with entire edge and are soft and non-adherent. *Actinomyces viscosus* is named after its viscous colonies. Overall, species recognition by colonial morphology is limited, as there may be considerable variation in colony type within a species. However, in general, *A. israelii* and *A. hordeovulneris* produce predominantly rough colonies; *A. naeslundii*, rough or smooth colonies; *A. bovis*, *A. gerencseriae*, *A. odontolyticus* and *A. viscosus*, predominantly smooth colonies; and *A. howelli*, *A. meyeri* and *A. pyogenes*, entirely smooth colonies. Colonies of most species are white to grey-white or cream, but most strains of *A. odontolyticus* produce a dark-red pigment on blood-containing media. This develops in 2–10 days anaerobic incubation and may be enhanced when plates are exposed to air for 30 minutes at room temperature. Strains of *A. denticolens* may show a pink pigment, and the authors have also observed a pink coloration in some strains of *A. israelii*, *A. naeslundii* and *A. viscosus* grown on Fastidious Anaerobe Agar (LabM) with 5% horse blood (authors' unpublished observation).

β-Haemolysis is always seen in strains of *A. pyogenes*. Other species show little or no haemolysis. Browning (chocolatizing) of blood-containing agar may occur, particularly with strains of *A. naeslundii* and *A. odontolyticus*.

All species grow under anaerobic conditions, optimally at 35–37 °C, and growth is enhanced by carbon dioxide and serum. Colonies may be visible in as little as 48 hours or may take 7–14 days to develop. On initial isolation, strains of *A. naeslundii*, *A. viscosus*, *A. pyogenes*, *A. georgiae* and *A. slackii* grow well aerobically without additional carbon dioxide. *Actinomyces bovis* and *A. meyeri* grow poorly in 5% carbon dioxide and do not grow in air. Aerotolerance of strains of *A. israelii*, *A. gerencseriae*, *A. odontolyticus* and *A. denticolens* is variable. Upon repeated subculture all species become increasingly aerotolerant, and the growth rate increases to produce macroscopically visible colonies in 24–48 hours. Thus growth in air is not a reliable aid to identification of stored attenuated strains.

PATHOGENICITY

Actinomyces are endogenous commensals that may cause disease if the normal host–parasite relationship is disturbed. They are incapable of invading an intact mucous membrane and therefore require a traumatized surface to initiate disease. This may occur as a result of accidental or surgical trauma, primary bacterial or viral infection, or an underlying malignancy.

Little is understood about the mechanism by which *Actinomyces* establish infection in humans; no virulence factors such as toxins have been demonstrated, although the advanced stage of the disease in man is degenerative with destruction of tissue and bone. Actinomycotic lesions invariably contain a mixed bacterial population. Holm (1950, 1951) investigated 600 closed lesions and noted that 0/600 contained a pure growth of *Actinomyces* spp. Thoracic and pulmonary lesions often contained *Actinobacillus actinomycetemcomitans* and a 'corroding bacillus' (*Eikenella corrodens*), and abdominal lesions frequently included coliforms. This alludes to the role of accompanying organisms in the synergic nature of actinomycosis. *Actinobacillus actinomycetemcomitans* has been shown to produce a leucotoxin which could explain the virulent nature of such synergy. In turn, the formation of granules by *A. israelii* is thought to afford some physical protection against the host response to other bacteria in the lesion.

The immune response to actinomycotic infections is mediated via both a cellular and a humoral response, although the exact role played by antibodies is unclear. There is also some evidence that there may be a degree of immunosuppression of the cell-mediated response in some patients.

NORMAL HABITAT

Actinomyces are found predominantly as part of the commensal microflora of the oral cavities of man and dentate mammals. Within the oral cavity of man they may be found occupying several niches such as the subgingival plaque in peridontal pockets, dental plaque, carious teeth, saliva and tonsillar crypts. Counts performed on dental calculus of volunteers with no overt signs of disease revealed a total of 1.9×10^7 particles per gram wet weight, consisting of 6.32×10^6 *A. israelii*, 5.37×10^6 *A. naeslundii*, 1.75×10^6 *A. viscosus* and 0.1×10^6 *A. odontolyticus*. In a comparable group of patients with periodontal disease the respective counts were 14.01×10^6 *A. israelii*, 2.38×10^6 *A. naeslundii*, 4.39×10^6 *A. viscosus* and 1.26×10^6 *A. odontolyticus* (Collins *et al.*, 1973).

The mucous membrane lining of the female genital tract is also inhabited by *Actinomyces* spp., although these are in lower numbers than in the mouth. Smears of the cervix and vagina have shown *A. israelii*, *A. naeslundii* and *A. viscosus* (Schaal and Pulverer, 1984). *Actinomyces* spp. can also be isolated from the faeces of healthy individuals, probably as transients from the mouth. Some species of *Actinomyces* appear host species specific. *Actinomyces bovis*, for example, has never been isolated from a human source, and is associated with bovine actinomycosis. A study of the plaque of healthy cattle (Slack and Gerencser, 1975) found no trace of *A. bovis*. They did find strains that were eventually to be assigned to two new species, namely, *A. denticolens* and *A. howellii*. Later, Dent and Williams (1986) described *A. slackii*, also from the dental plaque of healthy dairy cattle. The agent of canine actinomycosis, *A. hordeovulneris*, is believed to be associated with the awns of the foxtail plant (*Hordeum* spp.). This barbed structure may become embedded in the coat of the dog as it passes through the undergrowth, causing trauma which then acts as a focus for infection with this organism. This condition is particularly common in California which has an abundance of foxtails (Buchanan *et al.*, 1984).

CLINICAL FEATURES

Members of the genus *Actinomyces* are involved in two major disease processes of man: namely, periodontal disease and actinomycosis. These two conditions differ markedly in their occurrence. Periodontitis (gingivitis in the early stage) is an extremely common condition in adults in Western civilization, while actinomycosis affects only between 1 : 40 000 and 1 : 83 000 per head of population per year. Various species of *Actinomyces* may be involved in actinomycotic lesions; in the study by Schaal and Pulverer (1984) 1002 clinical isolates collected from cervicofacial lesions over a 10-year period consisted of nine different species. Not surprisingly, *A. israelii* was the commonest, present in 82% of cases. The remainder consisted mainly of *A. naeslundii* and *A. viscosus*, and one non-actinomyces, *Propionibacterium propionicum*.

Periodontal Disease

Periodontitis is a complex disease process involving an array of host factors and anaerobic bacteria. *Actinomyces* form a part of the complex microflora of the human oral cavity and plays an important role in the initiation of both the disease processes of periodontitis and caries. To maintain a stable position in the oral ecological niche, organisms must first adhere to the various surfaces involved; *A. naeslundii* and *A. viscosus* synthesize extracellular polymers which assist in their adherence to the enamel tooth surface. After establishing themselves and multiplying on the tooth surface they provide a filamentous mesh which augments the attachment of other bacteria and hence fosters the development of plaque. Filamentous mouth bacteria are not thought to be the sole prime causes of enamel decay. However, germ-free animals fed on a regimen of a carbohydrate-rich diet and live *Actinomyces* developed severe periodontal lesions, thus demonstrating their importance in this condition. *A. viscosus* has been implicated as a prime cause of gingivitis, and whole cells or cell walls of this organism have been shown to induce neutrophil lysozyme production which results in damage to the hard and soft tissues supporting the teeth.

Human Actinomycosis

Classical actinomycosis is described as a progressive, chronic inflammatory disease with suppuration, often leading to sinus formation in the advanced stages of disease. In the pre-antibiotic era the disease ran a very protracted course which could be fatal. In 1938 Cope reported 902 fatalities in England in the period 1916–1935. There were 525 fatalities due to actinomycosis reported in the USA between 1949 and 1965 (Slack and Gerencser, 1975). The disease has a worldwide distribution.

Various studies have shown that actinomycosis is more common in males than in females at a ratio of between 2 : 1 and 4 : 1. The anatomical distribution of disease in man is approximately 60% cervico-orofacial, 20% abdominal, 15% thoracic and 5% in other body sites, mainly in the pelvic area of females (See Figure 19b.1).

Cervico-orofacial Actinomycosis

This is by far the commonest presentation of disease and is typified by an indurated swelling in the area of the lower jaw, which develops into sinus tracts that drain a thin discharge containing small yellow particles (sulphur granules). These are seen predominantly in association with infections due to *A. israelii* rather than infections due to other *Actinomyces* spp. Disease is commonly associated with patients having generally poor oral hygiene and neglected dental care. There may be existing periodontal disease and rampant caries which indicates the portal of entry.

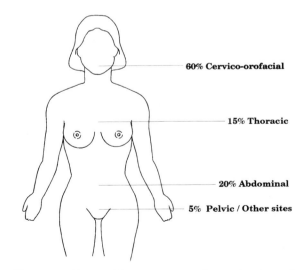

Figure 19b.1. Distribution of actinomycotic disease in humans.

Actinomycosis may be preceded by either accidental or surgical trauma to the oral cavity and usually follows either of two courses. It may present as a painless enlarging swelling usually on the lower border of the mandible, or as a more widespread painful mass in the parotid area of the neck. Other sites infected in this region may include the palate, tongue, salivary glands, lacrimal duct, orbit and larynx. *Actinomyces* spp. have also been reported in the brain and spinal cord tissue, either as a direct extension of cervicofacial actinomycosis (Fetter *et al.*, 1967) or as part of the mixed flora commonly found in otogenic or odontogenic brain abscesses (Ariza *et al.*, 1986). A recent detailed report of the anaerobes isolated from otogenic brain abscesses found *A. meyeri* in two of three cases, and *A. odontolyticus* in one of three (Brazier *et al.*, 1994).

Lacrimal canaliculitis or 'ocular actinomycosis' was one of the earliest forms of the disease to be described. Although there is evidence that true *Actinomyces* spp. may be involved in this condition, there is mounting evidence that the majority of cases are caused by *Propionibacterium propionicum*, formerly known as *Arachnia propionica*. Pine and Hardin (1959) described the isolation of an *Actinomyces*-like organism that produced propionic acid from a case of canaliculitis; but as the taxonomy at that time was unclear, they still believed it belonged to the genus *Actinomyces*. Seal *et al.* (1981) described a case of lacrimal canaliculitis due to *P. propionicum* in a 14-year-old boy. They stated that this organism may often be involved in chronic eye infections that do not resolve with topical antibiotics, as this organism is usually resistant to eye drops containing gentamicin, neomycin or chloramphenicol. Brazier and Hall (1993) reviewed 18 cases of lacrimal canaliculitis in which this organism was the aetiological agent rather than true *Actinomyces*. Further analysis of patient details revealed a significant age/sex propensity for this condition in females in their later years (mean 61 years).

Abdominal Actinomycosis

The clinical features of abdominal actinomycosis are complex. Symptoms include fever, leucocytosis and a chronic localized inflammation often without a draining sinus. It is therefore often difficult to diagnose in the early stages, mimicking other conditions such as carcinoma, appendicitis or Crohn's disease, depending on the area of localized inflammation. In the later stages of disease, however, the classic draining sinuses usually appear, making the diagnosis more straightforward. Abdominal actinomycosis may be preceded by an acute perforative gastrointestinal disease such as appendicitis or trauma (surgical or accidental). Putman *et al.* (1950) reported that 72% of 122 cases were preceded by a perforated appendix several weeks or months previous to the onset of symptoms.

Thoracic Actinomycosis

This form of disease may result from aspiration of *Actinomyces* spp. from the upper respiratory tract, via haematogenous spread, or via invasion of the thoracic cavity by a primary abdominal or cervical lesion. The initial focus of infection may be in the bronchial tree or in the lung parenchyma. Diseased tissue spreads to produce multiple abscesses, eventually crossing the chest wall to form the draining sinuses characteristic of actinomycotic disease. The main symptoms are chest pains, fever, productive cough and weight loss – symptoms that may easily be mistaken for tuberculosis, especially in the early stages. Two distinguishing features are that the sputum usually does not contain blood and may contain sulphur granules.

Pelvic or Genital Actinomycosis

Genital actinomycosis is associated with use of intrauterine contraceptive devices (IUCDs) since there is a higher incidence of actinomycotic disease in this group of women. However, even amongst IUCD wearers infection is relatively uncommon. It has been estimated that in approximately 50 million patient years of IUCD use there have been only 500 cases reported in the literature (Persson, 1987). In this form of disease, the mucous membranes of the female genital tract may be compromised by the fitting of such a foreign body, allowing ascending infection from the vagina. Symptoms are variable but often include pain, pyrexia, weight loss and leucocytosis. It can present as a tubo-ovarian abscess or have endometrial or uterine involvement. Pathological investigations may reveal features associated with malignancy such as fibrosis and invasion.

The first case associated with the use of an IUCD was described in 1926, although carriage of *Actinomyces* in the female genital tract was not recognized until 1976 when Gupta *et al.* (1976) demonstrated 'actinomyces-like organisms' (ALOs) in Papanicolaou-stained cervicovaginal smears from women with IUCDs. Subsequent studies confirmed a carriage rate of between 1% and 20% in this group of women. The predominant pathogen is *A. israelii* but this organism has been reported as part of the normal genital flora of healthy women both with and without IUCDs. There is no evidence that women with Papanicolaou smears positive for ALOs are at greater risk of developing genital actinomycosis, and clinicians should guard against the unnecessary removal of IUCDs based solely on this evidence.

Other Sites

Occasionally species of *Actinomyces* may be involved in cases of osteomyelitis, endocarditis and bacteraemia. However, the majority of putative *Actinomyces* isolates referred to the Public Health Laboratory Service (PHLS) Anaerobe Reference Unit from blood cultures are identified as *Propionibacterium* spp. and most of these are *P. acnes.*

LABORATORY DIAGNOSIS

As the disease is no longer common in the modern world, actinomycosis may easily be misdiagnosed, particularly in its early stages. Symptoms may mimic other conditions such as carcinoma, tuberculosis or actinomycetoma, and histological investigations alone may not always correctly diagnose the aetiology. Bacteriological examination of the lesion is generally regarded as the definitive method of diagnosis of actinomycosis. Samples of aspirated pus, sinus discharge, biopsy material or fine-needle aspirations are suitable specimens for examination but care should be taken to minimize contamination of the sample with commensal bacteria from mucocutaneous surfaces.

Infections involving *A. israelii* are often associated with the presence of small (<1 mm), hard, yellow particles; these are the so-called 'sulphur granules' of classical actinomycosis. They may either be scanty, requiring careful macroscopic examination of the specimen, or so numerous that the discharge resembles the consistency of semolina. Although not regarded as entirely pathognomonic for actinomycotic infection, their presence is strongly indicative and specimens from likely sites (jaw, neck) should be examined for their presence. If found, they should be picked out and crushed on a glass slide prior to staining by Gram's method. The presence of filamentous, branching or beaded rods is highly suggestive of actinomycotic infection. Remaining granules should be washed in sterile distilled water prior to culture on appropriate media and prolonged anaerobic incubation. This selective enrichment step is very important since the distribution of colony-forming units of *Actinomyces* in clinical material is not homogeneous. In the absence of sulphur granules, Gram-stained smears of exudate should be carefully scrutinized for characteristic filaments.

Isolation Media

The ubiquitous presence of other bacteria in clinical material from cases of actinomycosis and the relatively slow growth of *Actinomyces* spp. necessitates the use of selective media for their isolation. Several semi-selective agars have been formulated, including the CNAC-20 medium of Ellen and Balcerzak-Raczkowski (1975) which incorporated cadmium sulphate (20 μg/ml) as the selective agent for *A. naeslundii* and *A. viscosus* from dental plaque. Kornman and Loesche (1978) increased the selectivity of this medium by the addition of metronidazole (10 μg/ml) in a gelatin-based agar. Zylber and Jordan (1982) developed a complex medium containing cadmium sulphate, sodium fluoride, neutral acriflavin, potassium tellurite and basic fuchsin in a blood-based medium. However, these formulations have limited value for clinical specimens as cadmium sulphate is inhibitory to some species, including *A. israelii*. Traynor *et al.* (1981) described a medium incorporating metronidazole (2.5 μg/ml), primarily for the isolation of *Actinomyces* from clinical material. They reported an 86% isolation rate of ALOs from women who had positive cervical stained smears for this condition. This selective medium, however, was still not optimal since many facultative anaerobes could still outgrow any *Actinomyces* present.

Some unpublished work performed in the PHLS Anaerobe Reference Unit used nalidixic acid (30 μg/ml) in combination with metronidazole (10 μg/ml) in both blood agar and selective broth formulations. This combination of selective agents, which is now available commercially (Lab M Ltd, Bury, UK), inhibits obligate anaerobes and facultative Gram-negative organisms, while allowing the growth of various *Actinomyces* spp. There is still competition from Gram positives such as lactobacilli, bifidobacteria and streptococci, however, and good spreading technique combined with the use of a 50 μg metronidazole disk is required for the successful isolation of *Actinomyces* spp.

Plates should be incubated anaerobically at 35–37 °C for up to 14 days. If an anaerobic chamber is used, plates should be examined within the chamber after 48 hours incubation and daily thereafter. If an anaerobic jar is used, it should not

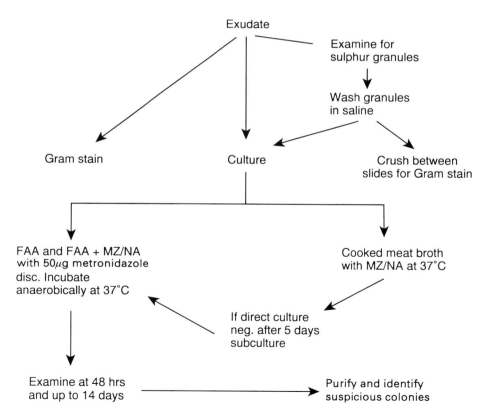

Figure 19b.2. Procedure for isolation of *Actinomyces* from clinical material. FAA, Fastidious Anaerobe Agar; Mz/NA, metronidazole 10 mg/l, nalidixic acid 30 mg/l.

be opened before seven days incubation. Suspicious colonies should be selected for confirmation of cellular morphology by Gram staining prior to subculture to non-selective fastidious anaerobe agar for purity and to blood agar plates incubated in air and in air plus 5% carbon dioxide to assess oxygen requirement. Examination of plates under low-power light microscopy may aid recognition and purification of suspicious colonies. Repeated subcultures may be necessary before purity is achieved. Figure 19b.2 shows a suggested flow chart for the isolation of *Actinomyces* from clinical material.

Identification of Actinomyces Species

The identification of anaerobic Gram-positive non-sporing rods is notoriously difficult for routine laboratories. The classical cellular morphology of *A. israelii* (i.e. long branching filaments) is not a consistent feature among other members of the genus, and other species may easily be mistaken for bifidobacteria, propionibacteria, lactobacilli, corynebacteria or even streptococci. Evidence of this came to light in a survey of 82 referrals of putative *Actinomyces* to the PHLS Anaerobe Reference Unit which revealed only 54% actually belonged to the genus *Actinomyces*. The remaining 46% belonged to various other genera; 65% were *Propionibacterium* spp., 21% were *Bifidobacterium* spp., 11% were *Lactobacillus* spp., and the remainder consisted of a miscellany of aerobic Gram-positive bacilli. The most common organism mistaken for *Actinomyces*, *Propionibacterium acnes*, can be presumptively identified by positive indole and catalase tests. Accurate identification to genus level is greatly dependent on gas–liquid chromatography for analysis of the end products of metabolism (see Table 19b.2). *Actinomyces* spp. differ from other anaerobic non-sporing Gram-positive rods in producing moderate amounts of the volatile acetic acid with no propionic acid, and moderate to major amounts of the non-volatile lactic and succinic acids.

Identification of *Actinomyces* to species level by conventional tests is frequently problematic. Difficulties may be encountered in the following

TABLE 19b.2 DIFFERENTIATION OF ANAEROBIC GRAM-POSITIVE NON-SPORING BACILLI TO GENUS LEVEL

Sensitive to 5 μg disk of metronidazole
Eubacterium (*Clostridium*[a], *Peptostreptococcus*[b])

Resistant to 5 μg disk of metronidazole
Growth generally better in air than anaerobically
Possible *Rothia*, *Nocardia*, *Corynebacterium*, *Arcanobacterium*, (*Streptococcus*[b])

Growth generally better anaerobically
Major volatile and non-volatile fatty acid products analysed by gas–liquid chromatography:

Propionic acid	= *Propionibacterium*
Lactic and succinic acid	= *Actinomyces*
Acetic and lactic acid	= *Bifidobacterium*
Lactic acid	= *Lactobacillus*

[a] May present in nonsporing bacillary form.
[b] Strains with aberrant cellular morphology.

areas: discrepancies in the stated reactions between various published schemes; lack of discriminatory tests; and technical problems in test performance. Discrepancies between schemes may arise through the use of different methodologies. Some test results, urease for example, are very method dependent for this group of organisms. The absence of some currently recognized species from older schemes adds further inconsistencies. A particular example is the recognition of *A. gerencseriae*, formerly *A. israelii* serovar 2, as a distinct species. *Actinomyces gerencseriae* is differentiated from *A. israelii* by its inability to ferment arabinose; thus, in schemes grouping the two species as *A. israelii*, this reaction may be listed as variable. The percentages of positive reactions listed vary considerably with the range and number of strains tested as few reactions are 100% positive or negative for any *Actinomyces* species and few tests are truly discriminatory. Therefore, whilst individual reactions may point to a presumptive identification (see Figure 19b.3), in the authors' experience confirmation of identity is often best derived from a consensus of phenotypic reactions combined with colonial morphology (see Table 19b.3). Technical difficulties may arise from the slow rate of growth, nutritional requirements and the non-homogeneous growth produced by some species in broths. These problems are overcome if the 'sugar-plate' method

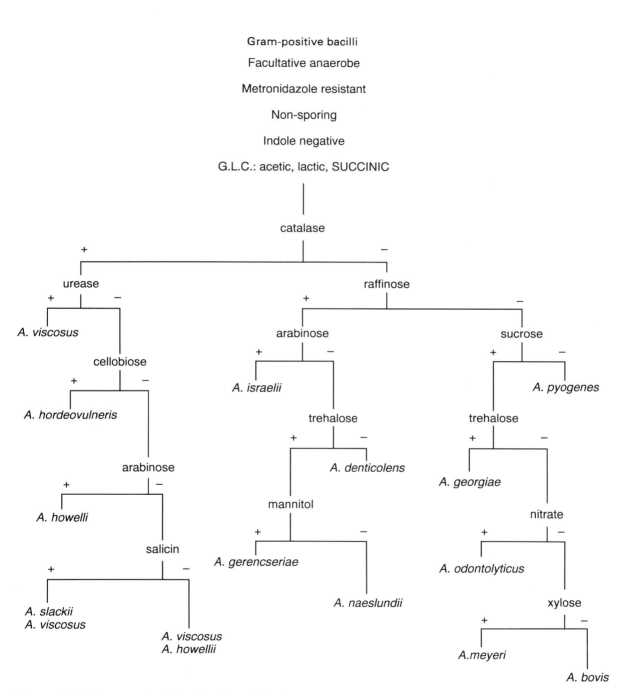

Figure 19b.3. Presumptive identification of *Actinomyces* spp.

TABLE 19b.3   PHENOTYPIC REACTIONS OF *ACTINOMYCES* SPECIES

Reaction	1	2	3	4	5	6	7	8	9	10	11	12	13
Growth O_2	−	±	+	±	ND	ND	±	−	+	±	+	+	+
Growth $O_2 + CO_2$	±	+	+	±	+	+	±	±	+	+	+	+	+
$AnO_2 + CO_2$	+	+	+	+	+	+	+	+	+	+	+	+	+
Pigment	−	p/−	−	−	−	−	−/p	−	−/p	r/−	−	−	−/p
Nitrate reduction	−	+	∓	∓	−	ND	±	−	+	+	∓	ND	±
Catalase	−	−	−	−	W	+	−	−	−	−	−	+	+
Urease	−	ND	−	−	−	ND	−	∓	±	−	−	ND	±
Indole	−	−	−	−	−	−	−	−	−	−	−	−	−
Aesculin hydr.	±	+	ND	+	+	ND	+	−	+	±	−	−	±
Starch hydr.	+	ND	ND	±	ND	ND	−	−	±	±	±	ND	±
Amygdalin	−	∓	ND	ND	ND	−	+	±	±	−	−	−	−
Arabinose	−	−	ND	−	−	±	+	±	−	±	±	−	−
Cellobiose	−	∓	ND	+	+	−	+	−	±	−	±	−	+
Glucose	+	+	+	+	+	+	+	+	+	+	+	+	+
Mannitol	−	±	ND	+	−	−	±	−	−	−	−	−	−
Raffinose	−	+	−	+	±	+	+	−	+	−	−	+	+
Ribose	−	±	ND	+	−	−	+	+	±	±	+	−	±
Salicin	−	+	ND	+	ND	−	+	−	±	±	−	+	±
Sucrose	+	+	ND	+	ND	+	+	+	+	+	−	±	+
Trehalose	−	−	+	+	+	±	+	−	+	−	±	±	±
Xylose	−	−	ND	+	+	±	+	+	−	±	±	−	−

1, *A. bovis*; 2, *A. denticolens*, 3, *A. georgiae*; 4, *A. gerencseriae*; 5, *A. hordeovulneris*; 6, *A. howellii*; 7, *A. israelii*; 8, *A. meyeri*; 9, *A. naeslundii*; 10, *A. odontolyticus*; 11, *A. pyogenes*; 12, *A. slackii*; 13, *A. viscosus*.
+, 90–100% strains positive; ±, 50–90% strains positive; ∓, 10–50% strains positive; −, 0–10% strains positive.
w, weak reaction; ND, no data available; p, pink pigment; r, red pigment.

of Phillips (1976) is employed for carbohydrate fermentation tests. This solid agar method enables easy confirmation of the purity and viability of the inoculum and is well controlled, allowing faith in the results. It is the authors' experience that the currently available commercial identification kits generally perform poorly with this group of organisms, probably due to poor database compilation which, in turn, is compounded by the taxonomical uncertainties mentioned above. Technical difficulties may also be experienced in obtaining a sufficiently heavy and homogeneous suspension for inoculation of kits.

Serological methods employing either direct or indirect fluorescent antibody staining have been employed successfully to identify *Actinomyces* to species level in both pure culture and in clinical material. Amongst others, Spence *et al.* (1978) used fluorescein isothiocyanate (FITC)-labelled specific antisera to confirm the identity of ALOs seen in cervical smears as *A. israelii*. However, these techniques are generally restricted to a few specialist centres as antisera are not widely avail-

able. Suitable methodologies have been published by Gerencser (1979) and by Schaal and Gatzer (1985).

ANTIMICROBIAL SUSCEPTIBILITY AND TREATMENT

In common with many other suppurative infections, an integral part of the treatment of human actinomycosis is surgical drainage of the lesion and removal of all infected tissue. In the pre-antibiotic era compounds such as iodides, arsenicals and copper sulphate were tried as therapeutic agents, without much documented success. Sulphonamides were probably the first antimicrobial agents to have a real therapeutic effect. Poulton in 1937 reported on a case of abdominal actinomycosis that was successfully treated with sulphonamides, and a year later Walker (1938) confirmed this finding. With the dawn of penicillin in the 1940s, expectations for an alternative treatment were high, especially after Abraham *et al.* (1941) reported that *A. bovis* was sensitive to penicillin *in vitro*. Florey and Florey (1943) treated two patients suffering from actinomycosis with 400 000 units of penicillin but neither responded. Subsequent experiences of other workers led to an understanding of the main problems of treating this disease with antibiotics, i.e. the need for high dosage and prolonged treatment (several months) due to the inefficient penetration of drugs into actinomycotic lesions. Although the penicillins have remained extremely active against *Actinomyces* spp., and to this day still remain the drug of choice in the treatment of human actinomycosis, many other drugs are active *in vitro* (Lerner, 1974), offering alternatives for penicillin-allergic patients. Tetracycline is usually considered as the next-best choice for treatment although a six-month course may be necessary. It is apposite to mention here that metronidazole has virtually no activity against the genus despite the anaerobic nature of most species; however, owing to the mixed nature of most infections involving *Actinomyces* a short course of this agent may be appropriate especially in periodontal disease. Susceptibility testing of *Actinomyces* is fraught with technical difficulties due to the slow growth of some species (*A. israelii*) and the granular nature of growth in broth culture. Species remain exquisitely sensitive to a wide range of antibiotics in *in vitro* tests. Very large zones of inhibition are attained on disk testing, thus limiting the number of tests to two or three per plate. Probably the best results are obtained by the agar dilution method, although preliminary results at the Anaerobe Reference Unit using the E-Test method (AB Biodisk Ltd, Sweden) are highly promising.

REFERENCES

Abraham, E.P., Chain, E., Fletcher, C.M. *et al.* (1941) Further observations on penicillin. *Lancet*, **241**, 177–188.

Ariza, J., Casanova, A., Fernandez Viladrich, J. *et al.* (1986) Etiological agent and primary source of infection in 42 cases of focal intracranial suppuration. *Journal of Clinical Microbiology*, **24**, 899–902.

Bollinger, O. (1877) Ueber eine neu pilzkrankheit beim rinde. *Zentralbl Med Wiss*, **15**, 481–485.

Brazier, J.S. and Hall, V. (1993) *Propionibacterium propionicum* and infections of the lacrimal apparatus. *Clinical Infectious Diseases*, **17**, 892–893.

Brazier, J.S., Hall, V., Carbarns, N.J.B. *et al.* (1994) Detailed anaerobic bacteriology of three otogenic brain abscesses. *Medical Microbiology Letters*, **3**, 228–234.

Breed, R.S. and Cohn, H.J. (1919) The nomenclature of the Actinomycetaceae. *Journal of Bacteriology*, **4**, 585–602.

Buchanan, A.M., Scott, J.L., Gerencser, M.A. *et al.* (1984) *Actinomyces hordeovulneris* sp. nov., an agent of canine actinomycosis. *International Journal of Systematic Bacteriology*, **34**, 439–443.

Buchanan, R.E. (1918) Studies in the classification and nomenclature of the bacteria. VIII. The subgroups and genera of the Actinomycetales. *Journal of Bacteriology*, **3**, 403–460.

Bujwid, O. (1889) Ueber die Reinkultur des Actinomyces. *Zentralblatt für Bakteriologie* **6**, 630–633.

Cohn, F. (1875) Untersuchungen uber bacterien II. *Beitrage zur biologie der pflangen III*, 141–207.

Collins, P.A., Gerencser, M.A. and Slack, J.M. (1973) Enumeration and identification of Actinomycetaceae in human dental calculus using the fluorescent antibody technique. *Archives of Oral Biology*, **18**, 145–153.

Cope, V.Z. (1938) *Actinomycosis*. Oxford University Press, London.

Cummins, C.S. (1962) Chemical composition and antigenic structure of cell walls of *Corynebacterium*, *Mycobacterium*, *Nocardia*, *Actinomyces* and *Arthrobacter*. *Journal of General Microbiology*, **28**, 35–50.

Dent, V.E. and Williams, R.A.D. (1984a) *Actinomyces denticolens* Dent and Williams sp. nov: a new species from the dental plaque of cattle. *Journal of Applied Bacteriology*, **56**, 183–192.

Dent, V.E. and Williams, R.A.D. (1984b) *Actinomyces howellii*, a new species from dental plaque of dairy cattle. *International Journal of Systematic Bacteriology*, **34**, 316–320.

Dent, V.E. and Williams, R.A.D. (1986) *Actinomyces slackii* sp. now. from dental plaque of dairy cattle. *International Journal of Systematic Bacteriology*, **36**, 392–395.

Ellen, R.P. and Balcerzak-Raczkowski, I.B. (1975) Differential medium for detecting dental plaque bacteria resembling *Actinomyces naeslundii*. *Journal of Clinical Microbiology*, **2**, 305–310.

Erickson D. (1940) Pathogenic anaerobic organisms of the *Actinomyces* group. *Medical Research Council Special Report Series*, **240**, 1–63.

Fetter, B.F., Klintworth, G.K. and Hendry, W.S. (1967) *Mycoses of the Central Nervous System*. Williams & Wilkins, Baltimore.

Fillery, E.D., Bowden, G.H. and Hardie, J.M. (1978) A comparison of strains of bacteria designated *Actinomyces viscosus* and *Actinomyces naeslundii*. *Caries Research*, **12**, 299–312.

Florey, M.E. and Florey, H.W. (1943) General and local administration of penicillin. *Lancet*, **244**, 387–397.

Funke, G., Stubbs, S., von Graevenitz, A. *et al.* (1994) Assignment of human-derived CDC group 1 coryneform bacteria and CDC 1-like coryneform bacteria to the genus *Actinomyces* as *Actinomyces neuii* subsp. *neuii* sp. nov., subsp. nov., and *Actinomyces neuii* subsp. *anitratus* subsp. nov. *International Journal of Systematic Bacteriology*, **44**, 167–171.

Gerencser, M.A. (1979) The application of fluorescent antibody techniques to the identification of *Actinomyces* and *Arachnia*. In *Methods in Microbiology* (ed. T. Bergan and J.R. Norris), pp. 287–321. Academic Press, London.

Gupta, P.K., Hollander, D.H. and Frost, J.K. (1976) Actinomycetes in cervico-vaginal smears: an association with IUD usage. *Acta Cytologica*, **20**, 295–297.

Harz, C.O. (1879) *Actinomyces bovis* ein neuer schimmel in dem geweben des rindes. *Jahrebericht der K. Central Thieraznei Schule in Munchen für 1877–1878*, **5**, 125–140.

Holm, P. (1950) Studies on the aetiology of human actinomycosis. I. The 'other microbes' of actinomycosis and their importance. *Acta Pathologica et Microbiologica Scandinavica*, **27**, 736–751.

Holm, P. (1951) Studies on the aetiology of human actinomycosis. II. Do the 'other microbes' of actinomycosis possess virulence? *Acta Pathologica et Microbiologica Scandinavica*, **28**, 391–406.

Israel, J. (1878) Neue beobachtungen auf dem gebiete der mykosen des menschen. *Arch Pathol Anat Physiol Klin Med*, **74**, 15–53.

Johnson, J.L., Moore, L.V.H., Kaneko, B. *et al.* (1990) *Actinomyces georgiae* sp. nov., *Actinomyces gerencseriae* sp. nov., designation of two genospecies of *Actinomyces naeslundii*, and inclusion of *A. naeslundii* serotypes II and III and *Actinomyces viscosus* serotype II in *A. naeslundii* genospecies 2. *International Journal of Systematic Bacteriology*, **40**, 273–86.

Kornman, K.S. and Loesche, W.J. (1978) New medium for isolation of *Actinomyces viscosus* and *Actinomyces naeslundii* from dental plaque. *Journal of Clinical Microbiology*, **7**, 514–518.

Lerner, P.I. (1974) Susceptibility of pathogenic actinomycetes to antimicrobial compounds. *Antimicrobial Agents and Chemotherapy*, **5**, 302–309.

Persson, E. (1987) Genital actinomycosis and *Actinomyces israelii* in the female genital tract. *Advances in Contraception*, **3**, 115–123.

Phillips, K.D. (1976) A simple and sensitive technique for determining the fermentation reactions of nonsporing anaerobes. *Journal of Applied Bacteriology*, **41**, 325–328.

Pine, L. and Hardin, H. (1959) *Actinomyces israelii*, a cause of lacrimal canaliculitis in man. *Journal of Bacteriology*, **78**, 164–170.

Poulton, E.P. (1937) Discussion on the treatment of bacterial diseases with substances related to sulphanilamide. *Proceedings of the Royal Society of Medicine*, **31**, 164.

Putman, H.C., Dockerty, M.C. and Waugh, J.M. (1950) Abdominal actinomycosis: an analysis of 122 cases. *Surgery*, **28**, 781–800.

Reddy, C.A., Cornell, C.P. and Fraga, A.M. (1982) Transfer of *Corynebacterium pyogenes* (Glage) Eberson to the genus *Actinomyces pyogenes* (Glage) comb. nov. *International Journal of Systematic Bacteriology*, **32**, 419–429.

Schaal, K.P. and Gatzer, R. (1985) Serological and numerical phenotypic classification of clinically significant fermentative actinomycetes. In *Filamentous Microorganisms: Biomedical Aspects* (ed. T. Arai). Japan Scientific Societies Press, Tokyo.

Schaal, K.P. and Pulverer, G. (1973) Fluoreszenserologische differenzierung von fakultativ anaeroben Aktinomyzeten. *Zentralblatt für Bakteriologie*, **225**, 424–430.

Schaal, K.P. and Pulverer, G. (1984) Epidemiologic, etiologic, diagnostic, and therapeutic aspects of endogenous actinomycotic infections. In *Biological, Biochemical and Biomedical Aspects of Actinomycetes*, (ed. L. Ortiz-Ortiz, L.F. Bojalil and V. Yakeloff), pp. 13–32. Academic Press, London.

Schaal, K.P. and Schofield, G.M. (1984) Classification and identification of clinically significant Actinomycetaceae. In *Biological, Biochemical and Biomedical Aspects of Actinomycetes* (ed. L. Ortiz-Ortiz, L.F. Bojalil and V. Yakeloff), pp. 505–520. Academic Press, London.

Schofield, G.M. and Schaal, K.P. (1981) A numerical taxonomic study of members of the Actinomycetaceae and related taxa. *Journal of General Microbiology*, **127**, 237–259.

Seal, D.V., McGill, J., Flanagan, D. *et al.* (1981) Lacrimal canaliculitis due to *Arachnia* (*Actinomyces*) *propionica*. *British Journal of Ophthalmology*, **65**, 10–13.

Slack, J.M. and Gerencser, M.A. (1975) *Actinomyces, Filamentous Bacteria. Biology and Pathogenicity*. Burgess, Minneapolis.

Slack, J.M., Winger, A. and Moore, D.W. (1961) Serological grouping of *Actinomyces* by means of fluorescent antibodies. *Journal of Bacteriology*, **82**, 54–65.

Sneath, P.H.A., Mair, N.S., Sharpe, M.E. *et al.* (eds)

(1986) *Bergey's Manual of Systematic Bacteriology.* Williams & Wilkins, Baltimore.

Spence, M.R., Gupta, P.K., Frost, J.K. *et al.* (1978) Cytologic detection and clinical significance of *Actinomyces israelii* in women using intrauterine contraceptive devices. *American Journal of Obstetrics and Gynecology*, **131**, 295–298.

Thompson, L. (1950) Isolation and comparison of *Actinomyces* from human and bovine infections. *Proceedings of Staff Meetings of the Mayo Clinic*, **25**, 81–86.

Traynor, R.M., Parratt, D., Duguid, H.L.D. *et al.* (1981) Isolation of actinomycetes from cervical specimens. *Journal of Clinical Pathology*, **34**, 914–916.

Waksman, S.A. and Henrici, A.T. (1943) The nomenclature and classification of the Actinomycetes. *Journal of Bacteriology*, **46**, 337–341.

Walker, O. (1938) Sulphanilamide in the treatment of actinomycosis. *Lancet*, **i**, 1219–1220.

Winslow, C.E.A., Broadhurst, J., Buchanan, R.E. *et al.* (1920) The families and genera of bacteria. *Journal of Bacteriology*, **5**, 191–229.

Wolff, M. and Israel, J. (1891) Ueber reincultur des *Actinomyces* und seine uebertragbarkeit auf Thiere. *Arch Pathol Anat Physiol Klin Med*, **126**, 11–59.

Wright, J.H. (1905) The biology of the microorganism of actinomycosis. *Journal of Medical Research*, **8**, 349–404.

Zylber, L.J. and Jordan, H.V. (1982) Development of a selective medium for detection and enumeration of *Actinomyces viscosus* and *Actinomyces naeslundii* in dental plaque. *Journal of Clinical Microbiology*, **15**, 253–259.

20

GRAM-NEGATIVE NON-SPORE-FORMING ANAEROBES AND *MOBILUNCUS*

B.I. Duerden

HISTORICAL INTRODUCTION

Gram-negative non-sporing anaerobic bacilli form the family Bacteroidaceae. They are a major component of the normal microbial flora of mucosal surfaces of man and the whole range of animals from invertebrates such as termites to primates, and are also important pathogens, usually in infections related to those colonized mucosal sites. Their contribution to human infection was first recognized in a report of pulmonary gangrene and appendicitis by Veillon and Zuber from the Institute Pasteur in 1898 although organisms now classified as *Fusobacterium necrophorum* had already been shown to cause calf 'diphtheria' (by Loeffler in 1884), liver abscesses in cattle and facial necrosis in rabbits. Pasteur himself had introduced the term anaerobe for microorganisms that would grow only in the absence of free oxygen in 1861. Before 1900, the role of non-sporing anaerobes in suppurative diseases of the middle ear, mastoid and sinuses, pulmonary gangrene and genital tract infection was established by the group of researchers at the Faculté de Medicin de Paris. However, with a few notable exceptions, non-sporing anaerobes were largely ignored in mainstream medical microbiology for most of the twentieth century, until the 'anaerobic renaissance' of the 1970s when improved laboratory methods for reliable routine anaerobic microbiology became more widely available. The findings of the early workers were then rediscovered and the widespread role of these organisms in infections of the abdomen, perineum and genitalia, mouth and respiratory tract, and compromised soft tissues at other sites became more generally recognized (Finegold, 1994).

Development of Taxonomy

Veillon and Zuber named their isolates *Bacillus fragilis*, *Bacillus fusiformis*, etc., and the current classification dates from 1919 when Castellani and Chalmers proposed the name *Bacteroides* for all obligately anaerobic, non-sporing bacilli; this definition was modified to exclude Gram-positive organisms by Weiss and Rettger in 1937. Knorr (1922) introduced the name *Fusobacterium* for the spindle-shaped Gram-negative anaerobes. Despite a variety of subsequent proposals for new genus names, all of which were subsequently deemed to be invalid, these two genera were the basis of the

Principles and Practice of Clinical Bacteriology. Edited by A.M. Emmerson, P.M. Hawkey and S.H. Gillespie
© 1997 John Wiley & Sons Ltd

TABLE 20.1   CHEMOTAXONOMIC CHARACTERS OF THE MAIN GENERA OF BACTEROIDACEAE

Character	Bacteroides	Bilophila	Prevotella	Porphyromonas	Fusobacterium	'B'. ureolyticus
Major products	Acetate, succinate	Acetate, succinate	Acetate, succinate,	Butyrate	Butyrate	Acetate, propionate
Dehyrogenases	G-6-PDH, 6-PGDH, MDH, GDH	...	MDH, GDH	MDH, GDH	GDA	...
DNA G + C (mol%)	40–48	39–40	40–50	48–54	28–32	28
Peptidoglycan diamino acid	meso-DAP	...	DAP	DAP, lysine	DAP, lanthionine	...
Fatty acids	Straight saturated ante iso- and iso-methyl branched		Straight saturated ante iso- and iso-methyl branched	isomethyl branched	Straight chain, monounsaturated	...
Quinones	MK-10, -11		MK-10, -11, -13	MK-9	–	...
Sphingolipids	+	...	–	–	–	...
Urease	–	+	–	–	–	+

G-6-PDH, glucose-6-phosphate dehydrogenase; 6-PGDH, 6-phosphogluconate dehydrogenase; MDH, malate dehydrogenase; GDH, glutamate dehydrogenase; DAP, diaminopimelic acid.

classification presented in the eighth (1974) edition of *Bergey's Manual of Determinative Bacteriology*, with the addition of the single-species genus *Leptotrichia* (*L. buccalis*) for fusiform organisms that produce lactic acid rather than butyric acid as their major metabolic product (Holdeman and Moore, 1974). The genus *Bacteroides* contained five groups of species: (1) *B. fragilis*, divided into five subspecies; (2) bile-sensitive non-pigmented species such as *B. oralis*; (3) *B. melaninogenicus* including all strains that produced black or brown pigmented colonies on lysed blood agar and divided into three subspecies; (4) non-saccharolytic non-pigmented species; and (5) other, unrelated saccharolytic species. This was the starting point for the rapid growth of clinical and taxonomic studies with Gram-negative anaerobes (Duerden, 1983).

The subspecies of *Bacteroides fragilis* were given species status and several new species were added to this fragilis group of intestinal *Bacteroides*, and as other species have been removed to new genera, it is now proposed that the genus *Bacteroides sensu stricto* should encompass only those species of the 'fragilis' group. It was also recognized that a single species *B. melaninogenicus*, which had been described by Oliver and Wherry in 1921, could not include organisms as diverse as the saccharolytic subspecies *intermedius* and *melaninogenicus* and the non-saccharolytic but highly proteolytic subspecies *asaccharolyticus*. *B. asaccharolyticus* was first separated as a distinct species and then assigned to a new genus, *Porphyromonas*, together with related isolates from diseases of the mouth, *P. gingivalis* and *P. endodontalis*; further new species of human and animal origin have been added recently. The saccharolytic pigmented species were shown to share many properties with the group 2 non-pigmented organisms that were mostly of oral or genital tract origin. These became the melaninogenicus–oralis group and were then assigned to a new genus as *Prevotella* spp. The other '*Bacteroides*' spp. that do not belong to these three main genera of human isolates have mostly been assigned to various new genera although a few remain with the inappropriate name '*Bacteroides*' while awaiting reclassification. With the exception of '*B.*' *ureolyticus* and *Bilophila wadsworthia*, these are of little concern in medical microbiology.

The genus *Fusobacterium* is now defined in biochemical and genetic terms as encompassing Gram-negative non-sporing anaerobes with DNA G + C content of 32–33 mol% that produce butyric and propionic acids as major metabolic products. Many that conform with this description do not exhibit the classical fusiform appearance. The more significant members of the genus in human disease are *F. necrophorum* and *F. nucleatum*.

The early taxonomic studies on the Bacteroidaceae were based upon conventional cultural and biochemical tests, which were difficult to perform reliably and to interpret in anaerobic growth conditions. The use of gas–liquid chromatography (GLC), introduced into this area of work in the late 1960s, was a significant advance in showing the possession of distinct metabolic pathways giving reproducible patterns of fatty acid end products. However, the significant advances since 1980 have been based upon a combination of chemotaxonomy and genetic analysis (Shah and Gharbia, 1991). The chemotaxonomic characters of the main genera are shown in Table 20.1.

DESCRIPTION OF THE ORGANISMS

General Properties

All members of the family Bacteroidaceae are obligately anaerobic, Gram-negative bacilli, although many are highly pleomorphic and microscopic appearances range from coccobacillary to long filamentous forms. Their susceptibility to oxygen varies; some, such as *Bacteroides fragilis*, can remain viable (subcultivable) after exposure to oxygen for many hours after growth on agar media, whereas some others cannot withstand exposure for more than a few minutes. Most of those of concern in medical microbiology are at the more tolerant end of this spectrum and can be manipulated on the open bench, although speed of regrowth and percentage viability are generally better if bacteria are handled in an anaerobic cabinet without exposure to air. Anaerobic conditions for growth are provided by incubation in anaerobic jars or cabinets, or other small-scale culture systems that exclude air and have a chemical system for removing traces of oxygen. The most commonly used gas mixture is hydrogen 10%, carbon dioxide 10%, nitrogen 80% for cabinets, or jars that incorporate a paladium catalyst to ensure the removal of remaining oxygen by reaction with the hydrogen. The species assigned to the main genera of Bacteroidaceae are listed in Table 20.2.

Bacteroides

Bacteroides fragilis and other members of the genus *Bacteroides sensu stricto* are indistinguishable by microscopy or by colonial appearance. They are small, moderately pleomorphic, non-motile Gram-negative bacilli; coccobacilli are common but long filaments are rare. They grow well on conventional laboratory media containing blood to form circular, low convex, smooth, shiny, translucent or semi-opaque grey colonies, 1–3 mm in diameter, that are often moist or frankly mucoid after incubation for 24–28 hours.

Most strains are non-haemolytic, but a few are slightly haemolytic and a small proportion are distinctly β-haemolytic. They are strongly saccharolytic organisms, producing acid from a range of carbohydrates, and moderately proteolytic. The main end products of metabolism detected by GLC are acetic and succinic acids, with smaller amounts of various other acids but not *n*-butyric or lactic acids. Growth is generally stimulated by whole bile and isolates are tolerant of the bile salt sodium taurocholate, but inhibited by sodium deoxycholate. *Bacteroides splanchnicus* is an intestinal bacteroides that differs from the other true *Bacteroides* spp. in producing propionic and *n*-butyric acids and in genetic and chemotaxonomic characters; it probably represents a distinct genus.

Prevotella

The various species of *Prevotella* cannot be distinguished by cell morphology. Most are short pleomorphic Gram-negative bacilli, often with many coccobacillary forms. They are divided into pigmented and non-pigmented groups by the ability of some to assimilate haemoglobin from blood in the medium, converting it to protohaemin

TABLE 20.2   BACTEROIDACEAE OF CLINICAL SIGNIFICANCE

Bacteroides	Prevotella	Porphyromonas	Fusobacterium
B. fragilis	Pr. melaninogenica[a]	P. asaccharolytica	F. necrophorum
B. distasonis	Pr. denticola[a]	P. gingivalis	F. nucleatum
B. ovatus	Pr. loescheii[a]	P. endodontalis	F. varium
B. thetaiotaomicron	Pr. intermedia[a]	P. macacae	F. mortiferum
B. vulgatus	Pr. nigrescens[a]	P. levii	F. naviforme
B. uniformis	Pr. corporis[a]	P. salivosus	F. pseudonecrophorum
B. eggerthii			F. russii
B. caccae	Pr. buccae		F. ulcerans
B. merdae	Pr. oris		
B. stercoris	Pr. buccalis		
	Pr. oralis		
('B.' splanchnicus)			
	Pr. veroralis		
	Pr. heparinolytica		
	Pr. oulora		
Bilophila	Pr. zoogleoformans		
wadsworthia	Pr. bivia		
	Pr. disiens		
'B.' ureolyticus			

[a] Black- or brown-pigmented *Prevotella* spp.

which accumulates in the cells, making the colonies dark brown or black after incubation for several days. Most pigmented strains are haemolytic and pigmentation depends upon lysis of the red cells in the medium and develops most rapidly on lysed blood agar. Pigmentation can vary from almost black to pale brown. Colonies of the non-pigmented species are indistinguishable from each other and very similar to those of the *Bacteroides* spp.: 1–2 mm in diameter, circular, shiny, convex and light buff or grey coloured; most are non-haemolytic. *Prevotella* spp. are moderately to strongly saccharolytic. All produce acid from glucose and various other carbohydrates and, like *Bacteroides* spp., their major metabolic products are acetic and succinic acids; *n*-butyric acid is not produced. Most species are moderately to strongly proteolytic. They are inhibited by bile and by bile salts.

Porphyromonas

Formerly known as the asaccharolytic *Bacteroides melaninogenicus* strains, *Porphyromonas* spp. are similar to pigmented *Prevotella* spp. in microscopic and colony morphology. They are small, mainly coccobacillary organisms with few long filaments. Growth is slower than with *Bacteroides* spp. and some *Prevotella* spp.; small colonies may be visible after incubation for 24 hours but many do not appear until 48 hours when they are <1 mm in diameter, smooth, shiny and grey. Dark brown or black pigmentation develops after three to seven days on blood agar, more rapidly on lysed blood agar. After four to five days, they are 1–2 mm in diameter and haemolytic – lysis of the cells being essential for pigmentation. Most strains have a characteristically strong, putrid smell, even more noticeable than that of other non-sporing anaerobes. They do not produce acid from glucose or other carbohydrates but their metabolism, as with all anaerobes, is fermentative. The major metabolic end product is *n*-butyric acid. Like *Prevotella* spp., *Porphyromonas* spp. are inhibited by bile or bile salts. They are vigorously proteolytic and this is considered to be a factor in their virulence.

Fusobacterium

Fusobacteria are anaerobic Gram-negative bacilli of varied size and morphology. Classical fusobacteria, such as *F. nucleatum*, are fairly long (4–6 μm), regular bacilli with tapered or pointed ends. Spheroplasts and spindle forms are common. Others (e.g. some strains of *F. necrophorum*) are pleomorphic with a mixture of long, filamentous organisms with rounded ends and many short or even coccobacillary forms and numerous spheroplasts and L-forms. Yet others are mostly coccobacillary. Colonial appearance is also varied, but most fusobacteria produce moderate to large colonies, 1–3 mm in diameter, generally with an irregular or dentate edge. They vary from translucent to granular and opaque. Their metabolism varies; carbohydrates are fermented only feebly or not at all but most species are proteolytic and the more virulent species such as *F. necrophorum* produce a range of enzymes that can break down tissue components (see below). The major metabolic products of fusobacteria, which help define the genus, are *n*-butyric and propionic acids, the latter produced by deamination of threonine. The G + C content of fusobacteria is low at 32–33 mol% and these and *Leptotrichia* are phylogenetically distinct from the other genera of Bacteroidaceae.

Leptotrichia

The species *L. buccalis* may be synonymous with the original fusiform organism described by Vincent. It has typical, long fusobacterial cells, 5–15 μm long, many with pointed ends. Its colonies are lobate or convoluted, opaque and grey/yellow in colour. Unlike the fusobacteria, it produces acid from several sugars and the only major metabolic product is lactic acid, with a small amount of acetic acid; *n*-butyric acid is not produced.

Bilophila

The single species *B. wadsworthia* is a slow-growing, small Gram-negative bacillus that is stimulated by bile and requires pyruvate for growth. It has no genetic homology with *Bacteroides* spp., is asaccharolytic and urease positive.

'Bacteroides' ureolyticus

This slender Gram-negative anaerobe typically forms pitting colonies on agar media (hence its former name *B. corrodens*). It is asaccharolytic, strongly proteolytic and urease positive. Its G + C content of 28 mol% clearly sets it apart from the other genera of Bacteroidaceae.

Growth Conditions

As well as requiring anaerobic conditions, most Gram-negative anaerobic bacilli require enriched media for growth; none grows readily on minimal media or unsupplemented nutrient agar. Most require a source of haemin for synthesis of the menaquinones that are essential components of their anaerobic electron transport systems. Some *Prevotella* and *Porphyromonas* spp. also require menadione (vitamin K). Media for optimal growth comprise a rich nutrient base, e.g. Fastidious Anaerobe Agar (Lab M), Columbia agar base (Oxoid), Brucella agar or Wilkins Chalgren agar, with 5–10% blood plus haemin and menadione. *Bacteroides* spp. and some of the more vigorous *Prevotella* spp. produce reasonable growth after 24 hours, but other species grow more slowly and require undisturbed anaerobic incubation for 48–72 hours, or even longer, for recognizable growth (Moore and Moore, 1977; Summanen *et al.*, 1993).

NORMAL HUMAN FLORA

All the Bacteroidaceae associated with man are part of the normal microbial flora of the gastrointestinal, oral or genitourinary mucosae, where they form a major part of the complex and interdependent ecosystems. However, the species found at the three sites are quite distinct and each species appears to have a distinct ecological niche (Drasar and Duerden, 1991).

Gastrointestinal Tract

This is the normal habitat of all the species of *Bacteroides sensu stricto* (*B. fragilis* group). They are one of the predominant groups of organisms in the faecal and colonic flora, having populations of c. 10^{12} cfu/g wet weight of faeces and outnumbering the facultative enterobacteria by at least 1000 : 1. Not all species are equally common. The main components of the normal flora are *B. vulgatus*, *B. distasonis*, *B. thetaiotaomicron* and *B. uniformis*, whereas the principal pathogen in gut-associated sepsis, *B. fragilis* (c. 75% of isolates from abdominal infections), accounts for fewer than 10% of faecal isolates of *Bacteroides*, although it may be more prevalent at the mucosal surface of the colon than in the lumen. *Bilophila wadsworthia* is also a common but not dominant member of the faecal flora. The gastrointestinal tract is probably also the normal habitat of *Porphyromonas asaccharolytica* and *'B.' ureolyticus*, but these are present only in small numbers.

Genitourinary Tract

Gram-negative anaerobes are part of the normal flora of the vagina although present in relatively small numbers (c. 10^6 cfu/g of secretions) and outnumbered by Gram-positive species such as lactobacilli. Most isolates belong to the genus *Prevotella*, principally *P. bivia* and *P. disiens*, which are uncommon elsewhere in the body; the pigmented species *P. melaninogenica* is also present, but in smaller numbers and less frequently.

Mouth

The oral flora has long been recognized as a source of a wide range of Gram-negative anaerobic species. The main habitat for these organisms in the mouth is the gingival crevice where both *Prevotella* and *Fusobacterium* spp. make a major contribution to the complex flora. The most commonly reported isolates are *P. melaninogenica*, *P. oralis* (and other non-pigmented *Prevotella* spp. characterized only recently) and fusobacteria, mainly *Fusobacterium nucleatum. Prevotella intermedia* is also isolated from the normal gingival flora but, like *Bacteroides fragilis* in the colon, represented a much smaller proportion of the total count of *Prevotella* spp. than do other species. *Porphyromonas gingivalis* is rarely isolated from healthy gingivae.

PATHOGENICITY

A wide range of Bacteroidaceae have been isolated at one time or another from infections of man but a high proportion of these infections are caused by only a few, more virulent species. Three main features are common to most of these infections: (1) the source of infection is the endogenous flora of the patient's own gastrointestinal, oropharyngeal or genitourinary mucosa; (2) alterations of the host tissue, e.g. trauma and/or hypoxia, provide suitable conditions for the development of secondary opportunist anaerobic infections; and (3) the infections are generally polymicrobial, often involving mixtures of several anaerobic and facultative species acting synergically to cause damage. The initiation of infection generally depends on host factors, but even in such opportunist situations some species show particular pathogenic potential not evident for the majority of related species from the same normal habitat. Thus, most species have some pathogenic capability but the majority of serious anaerobic infections are caused by the small number of more virulent species (Duerden, 1994).

The types of infection generally associated with Gram-negative anaerobes are listed in Table 20.3. The species most commonly isolated and considered to be significant pathogens in these situations are: *Bacteroides fragilis* in abdominal infections; *Prevotella intermedia, Porphyromonas gingivalis,* and *Fusobacterium nucleatum* in periodontal disease and other infections related to the mouth; *Porphyromonas asaccharolytica* and *'B.' ureolyticus* in superficial necrotizing infections; and *F. necrophorum* in the invasive disease necrobacillosis. *Fusobacterium necrophorum* has more of the characteristics of a virulent primary pathogen than other anaerobic species; typically it

causes severe purulent tonsillitis with pseudomembrane formation and lymph node involvement, septicaemia, and metastatic abscess formation. It may be fatal even for a previously healthy person.

To establish an infection, bacteria must attach to target cells (generally mucosal or epithelial cells), invade the tissues, establish themselves by multiplying at the site of infection and avoiding elimination by the host's defence mechanisms, and cause damage both to local tissues and, in systemic infections, to the whole patient. The more virulent Gram-negative anaerobes exhibit virulence factors that help elicit these stages of infection.

Adhesion

Bacteroides fragilis shows a particularly pronounced ability to adhere to epithelial cells and to cause haemagglutination. It produces fimbriae and a capsule, both of which may be involved in attachment. The capsule is important in adhesion to mucosal epithelial cells and peritoneal mesothelium and also protects against phagocytosis and induces abscess formation. *Bacteroides fragilis*

TABLE 20.3 BACTEROIDACEAE ISOLATED FROM THE NORMAL FLORA AND FROM INFECTIONS

Normal flora	Infections
Faeces	Abdominal
B. vulgatus	B. fragilis
B. distasonis	Bil. wadsworthia
B. thetaiotaomicron	B. thetaiotaomicron
B. uniformis	
Vagina	Genitourinary
Pr. disiens	B. fragilis
Pr. bivia	Prevotella spp.
Pr. melaninogenica	P. asaccharolytica
	'B.' ureolyticus
Mouth	Head and neck
Pr. melaninogenica	P. gingivalis
Pr. intermedia	Pr. intermedia
Pr. ovalis	F. nucleatum
F. nucleatum	F. necrophorum
	Superficial
	P. asaccharolytica
	'B.' ureolyticus
	B. fragilis
	F. ulcerans

also adheres to fibronectin and laminin, but this varies amongst strains. Mucosal adhesion may increase the proportion of *B. fragilis* organisms present at the mucosal surface, thereby enhancing the likelihood of infection once the mucosa is breached. Periodontal pathogens also exhibit adhesive properties. *Fusobacterium nucleatum*, *Porphyromonas gingivalis* and *Prevotella intermedia* adhere to crevicular epithelium and cause haemagglutination. Another aspect of adhesion that may be important in polymicrobial infections is the ability of bacterial species to coaggregate. These coaggregates may be important in creating appropriate conditions for the symbiotic metabolism and pathogenic interaction characteristic of anaerobic infections. This feature is manifest by oral *Prevotella* and *Porphyromonas* spp. together with streptococci, actinomyces and other oral species.

Invasion

Most anaerobic pathogens are not primarily invasive. Initiation of infection depends on initial damage due to trauma, hypoxia, neoplasia or some other alteration to provide the route of entry for the anaerobes. *Fusobacterium necrophorum* is an exception to this rule.

Establishing Infection

Once the initial damage has allowed the anaerobes to penetrate the tissues, they must establish a focus of infection by multiplying and avoiding elimination by the host's defence mechanisms. Most anaerobic infections are polymicrobial and the metabolic interdependency of the bacterial mixtures involved (both anaerobic and facultative species) is important to their establishment in the tissues, to the satisfaction of their nutritional requirements, and to the expression of their synergic pathogenicity; thus the virulence of anaerobic species is a reflection of their ability to exploit a compromised host environment. Tissue damage and necrosis, a reduction in blood supply leading to hypoxia, and the presence of a blood clot or foreign body or substance (especially $CaCl_2$) create conditions appropriate for anaerobic growth.

The capacity of facultative species such as *Escherichia coli* to consume oxygen may help create reduced conditions favourable to the growth of anaerobes. Gram-negative anaerobes require several growth factors and nutrients produced by damaged host tissues or by other bacteria acting in synergy; e.g., *Bacteroides fragilis* uses haemoglobin and haemaglobin–haptoglobin complexes as sources of iron and of the porphyrin component and can use the haem-binding protein from *E. coli* to overcome iron-limiting conditions. It also produces heparinase and condroitin sulphatase, which hydrolyse heparin and condroitin sulphate, allowing their use as nutrients. Similarly, *Porphyromonas gingivalis* lyses erythrocytes by the action of its cysteine proteinase, gingivain, to release haem, and demetalates protohaem to protoporphyrin, providing for its iron needs. Hydrolytic enzymes, neuraminidase and proteases produced by *Porphyromonas gingivalis*, *Porphyromonas asaccharolytica*, *Prevotella intermedia* and *Prevotella denticola* release nutrients from growth factors for these species themselves and for other members of the polymicrobial ecosystems.

Immune Evasion

The host response to anaerobic infection includes phagocytosis and opsonization and killing by serum immunoglobulin and complement. The virulent species of Gram-negative anaerobes have various means of avoiding and resisting these defence mechanisms. *Bacteroides fragilis* and some black-pigmented, Gram-negative anaerobes produce a capsule. The polysaccharide capsule of *B. fragilis* promotes adhesion, provides protection against phagocytosis, and provokes abscess formation. *Bacteroides fragilis* also inhibits macrophage migration and impairs the phagocytosis of other species involved in the polymicrobial infections. The capsular material and the depletion of serum opsonins by *B. fragilis* contribute to this synergic protection but succinic and other short-chain fatty acid metabolic products have also been shown to inhibit chemotaxis, phagocytosis and intracellular killing by phagocytic cells. *Porphyromonas gingivalis* also produces a capsule that protects against phagocytosis and intracellular killing and generates metabolic products that compete with chemotactic peptides, heat-labile opsonins, and complement components to block chemotactic receptors on polymorphs.

Several virulent anaerobic species generate products that inhibit or destroy the humoral components of the host's defences. The lipopolysaccharide of *Bacteroides fragilis* has little endotoxic activity but reduces the opsonic activity of complement. The black-pigmented species produce proteolytic enzymes active against immunoglobulins and complement and most anaerobic bacteria produce soluble metabolites that are leukotoxic, inhibit chemotaxis and damage mucosal cells.

Tissue Damage

Once infection is established, several virulence factors appear to act in combination to produce damage that is manifest as tissue necrosis and abscess formation. Some products of anaerobic metabolism are toxic to mammalian cells: volatile fatty acids, sulphur compounds (e.g. H_2S) and amines.

Extracellular enzymes

Most pathogenic anaerobes also produce extracellular enzymes that hydrolyse tissue components and are thought to play a significant role in pathogenesis. *Bacteroides fragilis*, *Porphyromonas gingivalis*, *Porphyromonas asaccharolytica*, *Prevotella intermedia*, *Prevotella melaninogenica* and *Prevotella denticola* produce hyaluronidase, condroitin sulphatase, heparinase and a range of enzymes that hydrolyse carbohydrates. All of these enzymes play dual roles, causing tissue damage and providing nutrients for the infecting microorganisms. *Fusobacterium necrophorum* produces both a lipase that damages cell membranes and a haemolysin.

Proteolysis

Proteolytic activity is associated with the strongly proteolytic *Porphyromonas* spp. and some *Prevotella* spp. Proteases are thought to be important in the destruction of gingival tissue and of the collagen bridges in the gingival crevice in periodontal disease and may be important in the contribution of *Porphyromonas asaccharolytica* and '*B.*' *ureolyticus* to tissue damage in ulcerative and gangrenous lesions such as genital and perineal ulcers, decubitus and varicose lesions and diabetic gangrene.

Lipopolysaccharide

The lipopolysaccharide (LPS) of most Gram-negative anaerobes exhibits much less endotoxic activity than the LPS of enterobacteria and that of *Bacteroides fragilis* may even inhibit enterobacterial endotoxic activity. LPS from *Bacteroides*, *Porphyromonas* and *Prevotella* spp. contains ketodeoxyoctonate (KDO) but it is in a form detectable only after acid extraction and this is related to its reduced toxicity. However, the LPS of *Porphyromonas gingivalis* appears to play a significant role in the pathogenesis of peridontal disease, in which (like the LPS of *B. fragilis*) it reduces the opsonic activity of serum, stimulates gingival inflammation, increases the secretion of collagenase from host cells and reduces collagen formation, and induces localized bone resorption around the tooth root. These effects are attributable to the release of biologically active agents, including the cytokines interleukin 1 (IL-1) and tumour necrosis factor (TNF) from host cells.

Fusobacterium necrophorum is an exception to the general rule that the LPS from Gram-negative anaerobes is less toxic; its LPS contains classical KDO and displays endotoxic activity similar to that of enterobacterial LPS, particularly during the septicaemic phase of necrobacillosis.

CLINICAL FEATURES OF ANAEROBIC INFECTIONS

Infections with Gram-negative anaerobes are principally endogenous in source and related to the body sites where these microorganisms are part of the normal flora. Several features are typical of most anaerobic infections: they are necrotizing or gangrenous conditions in tissues rendered suscept-ible by trauma, reduced blood supply and poor oxygenation, often in the presence of a foreign body or blood clot, and producing copious amounts of foul-smelling pus; thrombophlebitis of sur-rounding blood vessels is common, enhancing the anaerobic conditions. The characteristic smell of anaerobic infections is caused by the volatile end products of anaerobic metabolism. Infections are rarely 'pure', i.e. monobacterial. Anaerobic species are usually present in association with other anaerobic or facultative species in synergic mixtures (see above), but the anaerobes appear to be the principal causes of tissue damage and abscess formation in these mixed infections. From a clinical perspective, infections may be divided into five broad groups: (1) those derived from the gastrointestinal tract; (2) genitourinary infections in men and women; (3) infections of the head and neck related to the oral flora; (4) infections of other soft tissues; (5) bacteraemia (Finegold and George, 1989; Duerden, 1990).

Gut-associated Infections

Bacteroides spp. represent a large proportion of the normal flora of the lower intestinal tract and are the main cause of serious sepsis associated with surgery, injury, perforation or other underlying abnormality of the large intestine. *Bacteroides* spp. are the main components of the flora of postoperative abdominal wound infections, perito-nitis and intra-abdominal abscesses (appendix, diverticular or paracolic, pelvic, subphrenic etc.). *Bacteroides fragilis* is the most common species isolated from these infections, representing about 75% of the *Bacteroides* isolates in contrast to less than 10% of *Bacteroides* isolates from the faecal flora. Thus, *B. fragilis* clearly appears to have particular pathogenic potential and a much greater capacity to cause infection than the other *Bacteroides* spp., as described in the previous section. Amongst the remaining 25% of isolates, *B. thetaiotao-micron* is the most common, with smaller numbers of *B. distasonis* and *B. vulgatus*. The species other than *B. fragilis* are usually found in mixtures of multiple anaerobic species, often representing

gross faecal soiling of the tissues. *Bilophila wadsworthia* is associated with gangrenous appendicitis and other intra-abdominal sepsis.

Gram-negative anaerobes are predominant compo-nents of the mixed flora of perianal, pilonidal and perineal abscesses. *Bacteroides fragilis* is again the commonest species isolated, but *P. asaccharo-lytica* and '*B.*' *ureolyticus* appear more frequently in these infections than in abdominal infections, as they do in other superficial soft tissue infections such as sebaceous abscesses and decubitus or diabetic ulcers (see below).

Liver abscesses form a specific clinical group of intra-abdominal abscesses. They are generally poly-microbial and anaerobes, particularly *Bacteroides* spp. and anaerobic cocci, often predominate. The route of infection is usually via the portal venous system and the common underlying causes are colorectal malignancy, ulcerative colitis, Crohn's disease and other intraperitoneal abscesses. The commonest species isolated is, again, *B. fragilis*, and *Bacteroides* bacteraemia is a well-recognized complication. Anaerobes are responsible for only a minority of biliary tract infections, being restricted mainly to obstructive empyema of the gall-bladder.

Genitourinary Infections

Gram-negative anaerobes are significant pathogens in a wide range of infections of the genitourinary tract in both men and women. In men, the infec-tions are principally ulcers and abscesses of the external genitalia and perineum, but in women there are also infections of the vagina and of the uterus and deep pelvic tissues.

In local abscesses associated with the secretory glands in women, e.g. Bartholin's and Skein's abscesses, obstruction of the ducts leads to a build-up of secretions and infection with a mixed bacterial flora, predominantly anaerobic, that is similar to the flora of sebaceous cysts and pilonidal abscesses; *Porphyromonas asaccharolytica* is a common and important isolate. Anaerobes are also frequent isolates from genital ulcers, a common problem in both men and women. They are prob-ably not primary causes (genital herpes or trauma are common primary diagnoses) but whatever the cause of the initial damage, anaerobes form a major part of the flora of established ulcers and contribute to the progressive tissue damage. The term genital ulceration covers a range of superficial necrotizing conditions, from erosive balanitis/balanoposthitis in men and superficial labial ulceration in women, through deep, spreading ulcers, typically with undermined edges, to the more severe forms of synergic gangrene. In all groups, regardless of initiating factors, anaerobic bacteria are the predominant cultivable flora once the superficial debris is removed. Gram-negative anaerobes are not normally present on the external genitalia but are the commonest isolates from infected ulcers. Although *Bacteroides* spp. may be present in some cases, the commonest apparently significant isolates are the asaccharolytic and strongly proteolytic *Porphyromonas asaccharolytica* and '*B.*' *ureolyticus* which have a particular association with superficial necrotizing and ulcerative lesions at various body sites. *Prevotella* spp., principally *Prevotella intermedia* (which appears to be the most virulent of the *Prevotella* spp.), are also common isolates, being less common than *Porphyromonas asaccharolytica* in men but about equally common in women, in whom *Prevotella* spp. are part of the normal vaginal flora.

Vaginal discharge is a common complaint of women attending genitourinary medicine clinics, and anaerobes are involved in the majority of cases. The commonest condition is anaerobic (bacterial) vaginosis in which a disturbance of the normal vaginal microflora with loss of the predominant lactobacilli and their replacement by increased numbers of Gram-negative anaerobes results in a discharge with an offensive, fishy smell. With the proliferation of *Prevotella* spp. *Gardnerella vaginalis* and *Mobiluncus* spp., the vaginal pH rises, the lactate concentration falls and the amounts of succinate, acetate, propionate and butyrate increase, together with volatile amines that cause the smell. These same metabolites may induce the excessive secretion from the vaginal mucosa but the factors that initiate the condition, other than its clear association with sexual activity and a relationship with the presence

of seminal fluid in the vagina, are still not clear. The other main causes of vaginal discharge – gonorrhoea, *Chlamydia* and *Trichomonas* infection – also cause a major disturbance of the normal flora with significant increases in the numbers of Gram-negative anaerobes.

Ascending infections of the uterus and pelvis with vaginal anaerobes (mainly *Prevotella* spp.) or with *Bacteroides fragilis* or *Porphyromonas asaccharolytica* are the cause of serious gynaecological sepsis. Some of these infections are the classical infective complications of pregnancy, parturition or abortion such as postpartum or postabortal uterine infections in which retained products of conception provide ideal conditions for anaerobes to proliferate. With the control of streptococcal puerperal infection, anaerobes have become the commonest cause of postpartum sepsis. The same microorganisms also contribute to deep pelvic infections unrelated to pregnancy – endometritis, parametritis, tubo-ovarian and pelvic abscesses, generally grouped together as pelvic inflammatory disease – and wound infections and abscesses complicating gynaecological surgery. Laboratory confirmation of the cause of pelvic sepsis is difficult without surgical exploration; laparoscopy does not provide adequate samples for bacteriological culture but evidence from cases that have required open surgery supports the role of anaerobes in these infections. In gynaecological surgery, the underlying pathology has often resulted in colonization of the usually sterile deep sites and the incidence of wound infection, before antibiotic prophylaxis was routine, was about 20% and most were anaerobic, with both the vaginal *Prevotella* spp. and *B. fragilis* being common isolates.

Infections with Oral Anaerobes

The Gram-negative anaerobes that are part of the normal flora of the gingival crevice cause suppurative infections of the gingiva and immediate surrounding tissues related to dental problems, but can also cause various abscesses and soft tissue infections throughout the head, neck and chest.

Gingivitis and periodontal disease are probably the commonest anaerobic infections, if not the commonest of all infections worldwide, and are the most important cause of tooth loss. Acute ulcerative gingivitis (also known as Vincent's angina, Plaut–Vincent's infection, or trench mouth) was one of the first anaerobic infections of man to be recognized. It is associated with poor oral hygiene, malnutrition and general debility and is now seen as a complication of AIDS. Clinically, there is pain, haemorrhage, inflammation and destruction of gum tissue, and a foul odour. Spirochaetes and fusiform organisms are seen readily in stained films of the exudate and they may play a role in the disease, but the oral Gram-negative anaerobes, principally *Prevotella* and *Porphyromonas* spp., are also present in large numbers and may be more important in the pathogenesis of the condition. In other forms of periodontal disease, *Porphyromonas gingivalis* and *Prevotella intermedia* have been implicated as significant pathogens in rapidly progressive disease. *Fusobacterium nucleatum* and non-pigmented *Prevotella* spp. are also present in large numbers in periodontal disease and may have a pathogenic role.

The oral anaerobes are also important in dental abscesses, root canal infections (a particular association of *Porphyromonas endodontalis*) and soft tissue abscesses, e.g. buccal and pharyngeal abscesses. In the normal healthy state, these anaerobes do not colonize other sites in the head and neck, and do not cause acute primary infections of the throat, middle ear, mastoid or sinuses. However, when pre-existing damage or prolonged infection leads to the development of chronic otitis media, mastoiditis or sinusitis, these compromised air passages become infected with a mixture of oral streptococci and anaerobes such as *Prevotella* spp. These anaerobes are also the commonest cause of brain abscess, especially those originating from chronic otitis media, mastoiditis or sinusitis; cholesteotoma is an important predisposing factor. Infection spreads by direct extension, often with localized osteomyelitis and thrombosis of the lateral sinus. Dental infection may also give rise to brain abscess either by direct extension or by haematogenous spread. Similarly, the oral anaerobes can cause lung abscesses as a result of aspiration of organisms from the mouth when there is already some abnormality such as obstruction due to a malignant tumour or an inhaled foreign body.

Fusobacterium necrophorum differs from almost all other Gram-negative anaerobes in being a primary pathogen capable of causing disease in previously healthy people. Classically, the infection (necrobacillosis, or Lemmiere's disease) begins as a suppurative tonsillitis with pus formation and a pseudomembrane, which spreads to involve the local lymph nodes in the neck and from there to invade the bloodstream, causing septicaemia and disseminating the organisms widely in the tissues to form multiple soft tissue abscesses at many sites in the body (liver, lung, kidney, etc.).

Superficial Soft Tissue Infections

As well as infections related to the normal carriage sites of Gram-negative anaerobes, another group of soft tissue infections occurs at sites not immediately adjacent to the mucosae but in tissue damaged by trauma or hypoxia, or where secretory glands become blocked. These infections include sebaceous and pilonidal abscesses, breast abscesses in non-lactating women, and infection secondary to inadequate perfusion and oxygenation of the skin and subcutaneous tissues – decubitus and varicose ulcers, diabetic gangrene, etc. Although a wide range of anaerobes and facultative species can be isolated from these lesions, there is a particular association between progressively destructive infections and the presence of *Porphyromonas asaccharolytica* and/or '*B.*' *ureolyticus*. There is a specific association of *Fusobacterium ulcerans* with tropical ulcers – deep eroding ulcers, usually of the lower limb, occurring across many tropical regions.

Bacteraemia

Primary bacteraemia with Gram-negative anaerobes is extremely rare. It is an integral part of necrobacillosis in which *Fusobacterium necrophorum* invades the bloodstream as part of the spread of infection from the primary site in the throat. In most other cases, the bacteraemia is secondary to localized infections at some site in the body, e.g. intra-abdominal abscess, pelvic sepsis, and may be the first indication of some serious underlying condition such as a brain abscess. Bacteraemia with a *Bacteroides* spp. may be the first indication of a malignant tumour of the colon, rectum or cervix. The commonest anaerobic species isolated from blood cultures is *B. fragilis*. Mortality and morbidity of *Bacteroides* bacteraemia depends generally upon the underlying cause.

LABORATORY DIAGNOSIS

The site and nature of the infection (e.g. an abdominal abscess or a necrotizing or gangrenous ulcer) may give a clear indication that anaerobes are likely to be involved, and the presence of a foul-smelling exudate or pus is the strongest clinical indication of an anaerobic infection. The diagnosis is confirmed by careful anaerobic culture methods and the identification of the isolates obtained. Because these infections are often associated with sites that have a complex normal bacterial flora (often including the organisms that may be the putative pathogens), and because anaerobes are, by their nature, more or less susceptible to exposure to oxygen, care is needed in specimen collection and transport to try to ensure that the organisms sought do not die in transit to the laboratory and that any cultures obtained represent the flora at the infected site and not contamination from the normal mucosal flora (Summanen *et al.*, 1993; Drasar and Duerden, 1991).

Specimens

The most reliable specimens are pus or exudate from the depths of an open lesion or from a closed lesion. Specimens such as sputum collected from sites with a normal mucosal flora are not suitable for anaerobic culture. Swabs used traditionally to sample wounds and exudate are not ideal for anaerobes that suffer from desiccation and exposure to oxygen, as well as being entrapped in the interstices of the swab. Whenever possible, pus should be aspirated into a sterile container and delivered promptly to the laboratory.

Transport

Direct plating of a sample at the patient's bedside and immediate anaerobic incubation are likely to give the best results, but this is an unattainable ideal in most clinical situations. If pus, or a piece of necrotic tissue obtained by biopsy, is the specimen, it should be transported to the laboratory without delay in a sterile container. Sealed containers with an oxygen-free atmosphere, or from which oxygen can be removed by a simple chemical reaction, are available for optimal transport of such specimens. Pus is generally regarded as its own best transport medium. If there is no alternative to the use of swabs, these should be placed in semi-solid anaerobic transport medium to prevent both desiccation and the toxic effects of oxygen.

Direct Microscopy

Direct microscopy of pus samples may be helpful in some cases; most of the Gram-negative anaerobes are small, pleomorphic organisms that are difficult to see in direct smears. The most useful immediate examination is direct gas–liquid chromatography (GLC) to detect the presence of the volatile fatty acid products of anaerobic metabolism. This will not, generally, give any indication of the specific identity of the anaerobes present, but the demonstration of a mixture of short-chain fatty acids confirms the presence of anaerobic bacteria. Techniques have been developed in some research laboratories for the direct detection of specific pathogenic anaerobes (*Bacteroides fragilis*, *Porphyromonas asaccharolytica*, *Porphyromonas gingivalis*, *Prevotella intermedia*) by DNA probes and by polymerase chain reaction (PCR) technology, but these are not yet available for routine use in diagnostic laboratories. One of the main drawbacks to these approaches is that the laboratory is often trying to determine whether any of a range of species is present, not seeking one particular pathogen.

Isolation

Anaerobic atmosphere

Isolation of Gram-negative anaerobes is by anaerobic culture on selective and non-selective media. Anaerobic culture conditions can be provided in sealed anaerobic chambers equipped with air locks and functioning as anaerobic incubators as well as workstations, or in anaerobic jars. The anaerobic atmosphere generally used in cabinets is nitrogen 80%, hydrogen 10% and carbon dioxide 10% as the growth of many anaerobes is stimulated by carbon dioxide. The same gas mixture can be used in jars operated by an evacuation and refill system and equipped with room temperature-active catalysts to remove any remaining oxygen. Alternatively, jars can be used with sachets that generate hydrogen and carbon dioxide when water is added and depend upon the hydrogen to remove all the oxygen from the jar with the help of the catalyst. There are many variations on the basic anaerobic jar methodology but all must be carefully controlled to ensure that as much as possible of the oxygen is removed and that air cannot leak back into the system.

Many anaerobes grow more slowly than most common aerobic pathogens and anaerobic cultures must be incubated for at least 48 hours undisturbed and for an overall minimum of 72–96 hours. However, some of the more virulent anaerobes (e.g. *Clostridium perfringens* and *Bacteroides fragilis*) produce acceptable growth in 24 hours and most laboratories would not wish to delay the diagnosis by 24 hours. If the use of duplicate sets of plates (one for examination after 24 hours and the other to remain undisturbed for 72–96 hours) is considered too extravagant of resources, a useful compromise is for the one set of plates to be examined quickly after 24 hours and then reincubated after as little exposure as possible for another undisturbed 48–72 hours. This difficulty is overcome by the use of anaerobic cabinets in which the initial examination can be done without removing the plates from the anaerobic atmosphere.

Media

Various media have been recommended for the optimal growth of Gram-negative anaerobes. All comprise a rich nutrient base with added blood. *Bacteroides fragilis* grows well on most formulations of blood agar, but better growth of a wider range of more fastidious species needs more specially enriched media. Most species grow more quickly and produce larger colonies on media such as Fastidious Anaerobe Agar, Brucella agar or BM medium with ingredients such as proteose peptone, trypticase and yeast extract. Menadione and haemin enhance the growth of some species, especially of *Prevotella*; other demanding strains such as '*B.' ureolyticus* require formate and fumarate for good growth and *Bilophila wadsworthia* has an absolute requirement for pyruvate. The use of lysed blood assists in the early recognition of pigment production.

As anaerobic bacteria are generally present in mixed infections, their isolation is aided by the use of selective media containing antibiotics inactive against anaerobes. Aminoglycosides have been widely used for many years. The neomycin blood agar developed for the selective isolation of clostridia is too inhibitory for many Gram-negative anaerobes and kanamycin (75 mg/l) gives better results. An alternative that may be preferred is the use of nalidixic acid (10 mg/l). When it is desirable to eliminate Gram-positive bacteria, the addition of vancomycin 2.5 mg/l provides a medium highly selective for *Bacteroides* spp. Selective media should never be used without parallel non-selective cultures and growth on the selective media generally requires extended incubation.

Identification of Gram-negative Anaerobes

Detailed identification to species level of all isolates of Gram-negative anaerobes is beyond the scope of most diagnostic laboratories and would require excessive commitment of resources. However, they are significant pathogens and certain species either show greater virulence than most of their group (e.g. *Bacteroides fragilis*) or are associated with particular types of infection (e.g. *Fusobacterium necrophorum*, *Porphyromonas gingivalis*, *Porphyromonas asaccharolytica*). It is important that primary diagnostic laboratories can at least determine the presence of the main pathogens and identify other significant isolates at least to genus level, for more detailed study in a reference or research laboratory when appropriate.

Preliminary allocation of isolates to the main genera can be made by a relatively simple set of tests based upon colonial and microscopic morphology, growth in the presence of bile (20% in broth or agar medium) or sodium taurocholate (disc tolerance test), disc resistance tests with antibiotics (neomycin 1 mg, kanamycin 1 mg, penicillin 1 or 2 units, rifampicin 15 μg, colistin 10 μg, and

TABLE 20.4   PRELIMINARY IDENTIFICATION OF BACTEROIDACEAE

	Bacteroides	*Bilophila*	*Prevotella*	*Porphyromonas*	*Fusobacterium*	*Leptotrichia*	*'B.' ureolyticus*
Growth in bile (20%)	+	+	−	−	±	±	−
Tolerance of taurocholate	+	+	−	−	±	±	−
Antibiotic disc resistance tests							
Neomycin (1 mg)	R	S	S	S	S	S	S
Kanamycin (1 mg)	R	S	R	R	S	S	S
Penicillin (1–2 units)	R	R	S/R	S/R	S	S	S
Rifampicin (15 μg)	S	S	S	S	R/S	S	R
Colistin (10 μg)	R	S	S/R	R	S	R	S
Vancomycin (5 μg)	R	R	R	S	R	S	R
Urease	−	+	−	−	−	−	+
GLC	Ac, Su	Ac, Su	Ac, Su	n-Bu	n-Bu	Pro, Lac	Ac, Pro

TABLE 20.5   IDENTIFICATION OF *BACTEROIDES* SPP.

	B. fragilis	*B. vulgatus*	*B. distasonis*	*B. merdae*	*B. caccae*	*B. ovatus*	*B. thetaiotaomicron*	*B. eggerthii*	*B. uniformis*	*B. stercoris*	*(B. splanchnicus)*
Indole	−	−	−	−	−	+	+	+	+	+	+
Aesculin hydrolysis	+	−(+)	+	+	+	+	+	+	+	+	+
Fermentation of											
glucose	+	+	+	+	+	+	+	+	+	+	+
lactose	+	+	+	+	+	+	+	+	+	+	−
sucrose	+	+	+	+	+	+	+	−	+	+	−
rhamnose	−	+	±	+	+	+	+	+	−	+	−
trehalose	−	−	+	+	+	+	+	−	−	−	−
mannitol	−	−	−	−	−	+	−	−	−	−	−
arabinose	−	+	−	−	+	+	+	+	+	−	+
salicin	−	−	+	+	−	+	+	+	−	−	+
xylan	−	−	−	−	−	+	−	+	±	±	−
α-Fucosidase	+	+	−	−	+	+	+	−	+	±	+

vancomycin 5 μg), catalase and urease production (Table 20.4), supported by GLC if available.

More detailed identification depends upon sets of biochemical tests with carbohydrate and other substrates and detection of particular enzyme activities. Some of these can be performed with commercial kits (especially the enzymes tests) and these can be useful for the identification of the more common species isolated from clinical specimens. However, most of these systems suffer from the attempt by most manufacturers to produce a single kit for the whole range of anaerobes – Gram-positive and Gram-negative, cocci and bacilli. Tables 20.5–20.8 give sets of tests that enable the identification of most clinically significant Gram-negative anaerobes. The media and methods for performing these tests are varied and details may be found in manuals or monographs devoted specifically to anaerobic microbiology: the *Wadsworth Anaerobic Bacteriology Manual* (Summanen *et al.*, 1993), the *Virginia Polytechnic Institute Anaerobe Laboratory Manual* (Moore and Moore, 1991) or *Anaerobes in Human Disease* (Wrenn, 1991).

Antibiotic Susceptibility of Gram-negative Anaerobes

Approaches to susceptibility testing of Gram-negative anaerobes have been debated amongst microbiologists and infectious disease physicians for many years. A major consideration is whether susceptibility testing should be, as for most aerobes, concentrated in the primary laboratories doing individual susceptibility tests on clinical isolates from their patients, or whether strains should be collected for batch testing in recognized specialist centres while individual clinical treatment is based upon accumulated data generated by that batch testing. For aerobes, laboratories test their significant isolates and clinicians expect prompt susceptibility data on their own patients' organisms. This has not been the case with anaerobes because of three perceptions: (1) anaerobic investigations are slower – initial culture may take several days and susceptibility tests at least two days more, so that individual results are irrelevant to patient management; (2) methods for susceptibility testing of anaerobes are unreliable,

TABLE 20.6 IDENTIFICATION OF *PREVOTELLA* SPP.

	Pr. buccae	*Pr. oris*	*Pr. zoogleoformans*	*Pr. heparinolytica*	*Pr. oralis*	*Pr. veroralis*	*Pr. buccalis*	*Pr. oulora*	*Pr. bivia*	*Pr. disiens*	*Pr. melaninogenica*	*Pr. denticola*	*Pr. loescheii*	*Pr. intermedia*	*Pr. nigrescens*	*Pr. corporis*
Pigment	−	−	−	−	−	−	−	−	−	−	+	+	+	+	+	+
Indole	−	−	−	+	−	−	−	−	−	−	+	−	−	+	+	−
Aesculin hydrolysis	+	+	+	+	+	+	+	±	−	−	−	+	±	−	−	−
Hippurate hydrolysis	−	−	−	−	−	−	+	−	+	+	...	...	...	...	...	...
α-Fucosidase	−	+	+	+	+	+	+	−	+	−	+	+	+	+	+	−
Fermentation of																
glucose	+	+	+	+	+	+	+	+	+	+	+	+	+	+	+	+
sucrose	+	+	+	+	+	+	+	+	−	−	+	+	+	+	+	−
lactose	+	+	+	+	+	+	+	+	+	−	+	+	+	−	−	−
xylose	+	+	+	+	−	−	−	−	−	−	−	−	−	−	−	−
arabinose	+	+	+	+	−	−	+	−	−	−	−	−	−	−	−	−
cellobiose	+	+	+	+	+	+	+	−	−	−	−	−	+	−	−	−
salicin	+	+	+	+	+	−	−	−	−	−	−	−	−	−	−	−
xylan	+	−	−	−	−	−	−	−	−	−	...	...	...	...	...	...
inulin	+	−	+	±	−	+	±	−	−	−	...	...	...	...	...	...

[a]The only phenotypic distinguishing test is multi-focus enzyme electrophoresis for glutamate and malate dehydrogenases; *Pr. nigrescens* has slower mobilities with both enzymes.

TABLE 20.7 IDENTIFICATION OF HUMAN STRAINS OF *PORPHYROMONAS* SPP.

	P. asaccharolytica	*P. gingivalis*	*P. endodontalis*
Pigment	+	+	+
Indole	+	+	+
Trypsin-like activity	−	+	−
Phenylacetic acid production	−	+	−
α-Fucosidase	+	−	−

especially when done on an individual basis, and batch testing in specialist centres gives more reliable results; (3) the susceptibility of anaerobes is predictable, so that clinical treatment can be based upon the batch data with confidence.

These premises were the basis for susceptibility testing of anaerobes having been neglected in primary laboratories and concentrated in specialist centres that receive clinical isolates from a wide range of sources. However, there is an increasing view from clinicians and microbiologists that the same standard of laboratory data is required in anaerobic infections as in aerobic infections. Testing of individual isolates is supported by four changed perceptions: (1) antibiotic susceptibility in anaerobes is variable and patterns differ in different places and at different times; (2) modern laboratory methodology should enable the prompt isolation of the more common anaerobic pathogens; (3) methods for susceptibility testing of anaerobes are available that can be used in primary laboratories; (4) – the most important reason – patients managed with access to accurate and specific laboratory data on their own anaerobic isolates recover more rapidly, with fewer complications.

Both approaches are necessary. Primary laboratories need to develop adequate susceptibility tests on anaerobes for first-choice agents while reference laboratories should enhance their activities in collecting strains from a wide range of sources and batch testing to provide the best general advice for clinicians in choosing empirical therapy and devising antibiotic policies.

Methods

The selection of methods for susceptibility testing of anaerobes has been a major difficulty. The two basic methodologies for rapidly growing, relatively non-fastidious aerobes – disc susceptibility tests on solid media and breakpoint determination in liquid or solid media – are not readily adaptable to anaerobic work, are difficult to standardize and do not give reliably reproducible results with

TABLE 20.8 IDENTIFICATION OF *FUSOBACTERIUM* SPP.

	F. nucleatum	*F. necrophorum*	*F. pseudonecrophorum*	*F. russii/alocis/sulci*	*F. naviforme*	*F. mortiferum*	*F. varium*	*F. gonidiaformans*	*F. ulcerans*
Indole	+	+	+	−	+	−	±	+	−
Lipase	−	+	−	−	−	−	±	−	−
Aesculin hydrolysis	−	−	−	−	−	+	−	−	−
Propionate from									
lactate	−	+	+	−	±	−	−	−	−
threonine	+	+	+	−	−	+	+	+	+

anaerobes. Anaerobes tend to grow more slowly than many common aerobes and the balance between antimicrobial effect, bacterial growth and antibiotic degradation varies much more, affecting disk susceptibility methods in particular. Many anaerobes need more enriched media than are used for susceptibility testing of aerobes; they are more difficult to standardize and there are interactions between media components and the antibiotics. The presence of fermentable nutrients often results in a very significant drop in pH in the test medium which can have a major impact on the results obtained with pH-sensitive antibiotics. Similarly, many anaerobes require carbon dioxide for growth and all standard anaerobic gas mixtures contain carbon dioxide, which again lowers the pH. Many anaerobes do not grow well from small inocula and semi-confluent growth is difficult to achieve. A further practical difficulty arises because the MICs of several agents for anaerobes cluster near the recommended breakpoints for the agents, so that minor variations in method and inevitable margins of error in any technique can give variable results in terms of clinical interpretation and recommendations. Therefore, disk susceptibility tests for anaerobes have been regarded as unreliable for other than the fast-growing anaerobes. Recommended methods in the past have been based upon agar dilution with multi-point inoculation or broth micro-dilution or macro-dilution methods. Some of these have not been entirely satisfactory and are not appropriate for testing individual clinical isolates, hence the methodology has exerted pressure in favour of batch testing in reference laboratories. A more recent alternative, the E test (AB Biodisc, Denmark), offers the possibility of reliable susceptibility testing with MIC determination for individual isolates. A plastic strip coated with an antibiotic gradient on one side and with an MIC interpretation scale on the other is placed on a seeded plate as in disc susceptibility testing. After incubation, the edge of the zone of inhibition reaches the scale at a point equivalent to the MIC. This shares some of the disadvantages of disc methods but experience has shown it to be generally reliable for a wide range of anaerobes (Summanen et al., 1993; Wexler, 1993; Duerden, 1995).

MANAGEMENT OF ANAEROBIC INFECTIONS

Antibiotic Susceptibility

The susceptibility of Gram-negative anaerobes varies considerably both between and within the major genera. Metronidazole has been the mainstay of therapy and prophylaxis for 20 years and it is reassuring that resistance amongst all Gram-negative anaerobes remains rare (<1%), so that it remains the drug of choice for many of these infections.

Bacteroides *spp.*

Isolates of *B. fragilis* and other *Bacteroides* spp. are resistant to benzylpenicillin and ampicillin/amoxycillin due to β-lactamase production; in almost all cases this resistance is overcome by the use of a combination of ampicillin/amoxycillin with the β-lactamase inhibitors clavulanate or tazobactam. *Bacteroides* spp. are also resistant to many other β-lactam agents. Cefoxitin has been widely used in the USA for anaerobic infections because it has greater activity against *Bacteroides* spp. than most β-lactam agents, but results of susceptibility tests are variable, with up to 40% of isolates giving MIC values around or above the recommended breakpoint of 32 mg/l. Almost all isolates in the UK are currently susceptible to imipenem, but resistance due to production of a metallo-β-lactamase does occur and may become a more significant problem in the future. With inhibitors of protein synthesis, many strains are resistant to erythromycin and tetracycline but most are susceptible to clindamycin. Like the *Bacteroides* spp., *Bilophila wadsworthia* produces a β-lactamase and is resistant to most β-lactam agents.

Porphyromonas *and* Prevotella

Although the genera are generally more susceptible to antimicrobial agents than the *Bacteroides* spp., results are still unpredictable. In the past, they were considered to be generally penicillin sensitive, but one-third or more of clinical isolates, especially of *Prevotella* spp., are resistant due to β-lactamase production. Thus they are susceptible to amoxycillin/ampicillin and clavulanate combinations. Most are susceptible to cefoxitin and highly susceptible to imipenem. They are generally susceptible to erythromycin and clindamycin but up to half of clinical isolates are resistant to tetracycline.

Fusobacterium

The susceptibility of *Fusobacterium* spp. is more predictable, and most isolates are highly susceptible to a wide range of agents, including penicillin and all the β-lactam agents and clindamycin, but a few strains are resistant to erythromycin and tetracycline.

Therapeutic Approach

Because of the multi-factorial nature of infection with Gram-negative anaerobes (described above) (mixed infections, tissue necrosis, inadequate blood supply/oxygenation, patient already compromised by underlying disease) the management of these infections requires a combination of approaches. Antibiotic treatment is important but is rarely effective if used alone. The choice is generally between metronidazole, a β-lactam agent such as amoxycillin–clavulanate or imipenem, or clindamycin, but the recognition of the presence of aerobic or facultative organisms may need to be addressed either by adding an agent effective against, e.g. *E. coli*, to the metronidazole or choosing an agent effective against both, e.g. imipenem.

It is axiomatic in medical microbiology that antibiotics alone are ineffective as treatment for abscesses and many of the anaerobic infections have a component of tissue necrosis and abscess formation. Débridement of necrotic tissue and drainage of pus is essential to the effective management of these infections. An interesting exception is disseminated *Fusobacterium necrophorum* infection with metastatic abscess formation; this responds well to treatment with penicillin or other antibiotics alone.

Many of the patients who develop anaerobic infections are seriously ill, e.g. peritonitis following major abdominal surgery, and there may be a developing sepsis syndrome due to the anaerobes or to other components of the mixed infection. These patients clearly need intensive supportive therapy for respiratory and circulatory functions.

CONTROL AND PREVENTION

As most infections with Gram-negative anaerobes are endogenous, cross-infection is not a significant problem with these patients, although isolation may be appropriate because of the severity of the infection and, on some occasions, because of the intense malodour created by the anaerobes, which can be embarrassing and distressing to the patient and unpleasant and disturbing for others.

Prevention of these infections depends upon prophylactic measures that can be taken to avoid creating the conditions that allow anaerobes to become established. Most of these measures relate to surgical practice in abdominal, gynaecological or orofacial surgery – i.e. in areas where anaerobes predominate in the normal flora. Prevention of postoperative anaerobic infection in these situations depends upon good surgical practice, reduction in the bacterial challenge and the use of appropriate prophylactic antibiotics. Surgical skill goes a long way towards preventing anaerobic infections by not leaving non-viable tissue or foreign bodies at the operation site, ensuring adequate perfusion and oxygenation of the tissues that are left, preventing leakage from the viscus or the accumulation of fluid, and closing off any potential spaces where infection can develop. Thus, the 'soil' is not conducive to anaerobic infection. The bacterial challenge can be reduced in part by physical removal of the normal flora. This is particularly important in the use of laxatives, enemas, or even colonic irrigation to reduce the volume of faeces in the colon before abdominal surgery. The final prophylactic measure is the use of prophylactic antibiotics, which have made a major impact in reducing the incidence of postoperative infection during the last two decades. Since the advent of specific prophylaxis encompassing anaerobic organisms, the incidence of postoperative infection in abdominal and gynaecological surgery has fallen dramatically, e.g. from 35% to 5–10% for major colonic surgery, 20% to <5% for appendicectomy, 25% to 5% for hysterectomy. The aim of prophylaxis is to have high levels of appropriate antibiotics in the tissues at the time of the operation to prevent any implanted organisms becoming established. Prophylaxis in this way is not designed to destroy the bacteria in their normal habitat, e.g. in the gastrointestinal lumen. The choice of agent must include effective anti-anaerobe activity – usually by including metronidazole or amoxycillin/clavulanate – plus activity against other organisms likely to be present. Thus, in abdominal surgery, an aminoglycoside (e.g. gentamicin) or a cephalosporin (e.g. cefuroxime or cefotaxime) may be added to the metronidazole. In some circumstances amoxycillin-clavulanate may fulfil both functions. For effective prophylaxis and to avoid disturbing the normal flora or selecting resistant strains before surgery, the first dose should be given by intravenous injection at induction of anaesthesia. For some operations this will be sufficient. In some regimens, a second dose 6–8 hours later, after completion of the operation, is thought advisable, and if the operation is prolonged a second dose 4 hours after the first and then a third, postoperative dose may be the most effective approach. The whole period of prophylaxis should not need to be more than 24 hours. If infection is already present at operation and more prolonged use of antibiotics is clinically necessary, this becomes a therapeutic course for established infection and not a prophylactic measure (Keighley, 1992; Willis, 1991).

MOBILUNCUS

The genus *Mobiluncus* represents a group of slender, curved, rapidly motile, Gram-variable anaerobic rods found in the vagina and associated with *Gardnerella vaginalis* and *Prevotella* spp. in bacterial (anaerobic) vaginosis. Its taxonomic relationships are unclear but it is probably not a member of the Bacteroidaceae, as first suggested, and has a G + C content of 52–56 mol%. Two morphologically distinct types of *Mobiluncus* are recognized and represent two separate species. *Mobiluncus curtisii* strains have short Gram-positive or Gram-variable cells and are much more active in biochemical tests – they hydrolyse arginine and hippurate, reduce nitrate and produce β-galactonidase. *Mobiluncus mulieris* gives negative reactions in these tests and has much longer cells that appear Gram negative. However, both have a cell wall that is essentially of Gram-positive structure, but the peptidoglycan layer is thin, probably resulting in the variable staining pattern. Both species grow well anaerobically but will grow in 5% oxygen and growth is enhanced by carbon dioxide. Their role in disease is not clear. They may be present in large numbers in vaginosis and were described in vaginal discharge by Curtis in 1915. They are always present along with other potential pathogens and may have a synergic role (Spiegel, 1987).

REFERENCES

Drasar, B.S. and Duerden, B.I. (1991) Anaerobes in the normal flora of man. In *Anaerobes in Human Disease* (ed. B.I. Duerden and B.S. Drasar), pp. 162–179. Edward Arnold, London.

Duerden, B.I. (1983) The Bacteroidaceae: *Bacteroides*, *Fusobacterium*, and *Leptotrichia*. In *Topley and Wilson's Principles of Bacteriology, Virology and Immunity* (ed. G.S. Wilson, A.A. Miles and M.T. Parker), pp. 114–136, 7th edn, Vol. 2. Edward Arnold, London.

Duerden, B.I. (1990) Infections due to Gram-negative anaerobic bacilli. In *Topley and Wilson's Principles of Bacteriology, Virology and Immunity*, 8th edn, Vol. 3 (ed. M.T. Parker and L.H. Collier), pp. 287–305. Edward Arnold, London.

Duerden, B.I. (1994) Virulence factors in anaerobes. *Clinical Infectious Diseases*, **18** (Suppl. 4), S253–S259.

Duerden, B.I. (1995) The role of the Reference Laboratory in susceptibility testing of anaerobes and a survey of isolates referred from laboratories in England and Wales in 1993–1994. *Clinical Infectious Diseases*, **20** (Suppl. 2), S180–S186.

Finegold, S.M. (1994) Review of early research on anaerobes. *Clinical Infectious Diseases* **18**, (Suppl. 4), S249–S249.

Finegold, S.M. and George, L.W. (1989) *Anaerobic Infections in Humans*. Academic Press, San Diego.

Holdeman, L.V. and Moore, W.E.C. (1974) Gram-negative anaerobic bacteria. In *Bergey's Manual of Determinative Bacteriology* (ed. R.E. Buchanan and N.E. Gibbons), 8th edn, pp. 231. Williams & Williams, Baltimore.

Keighley, M.R.B. (1992) Anaerobes in abdominal surgery. In *Medical and Environmental Aspects of Anaerobes* (ed. B.I. Duerden, J.S. Brazier, S.V. Seddon *et al.*), pp. 24–30. Wrighton Biomedical Publishing, Petersfield, UK.

Moore, L.V.H. and Moore, W.E.C. (1977) *VPI Anaerobe Laboratory Manual*, 4th edn. Virginia Polytechnic Institute and State University, Blacksburg. Updates 1987, 1991.

Shah, H.N. and Gharbia, S.E. (1991) *Bacteroides* and *Fusobacterium* classification and relationship to other bacteria. In *Anaerobes in Human Diseases* (ed. B.I. Duerden and B.S. Drasar), pp. 62–84. Edward Arnold, London.

Spiegel, C.A. (1987) New developments in the etiology and pathogenesis of bacterial vaginosis. *Advances in Experimental Biology*, **224**, 127–134.

Summanen, P., Baron, E.J., Citron, D.M. *et al.* (1993) *Wadsworth Anaerobic Bacteriology Manual*, 5th edn. Star Publishing, Belmont.

Wexler, H.M. (1993) Susceptibility testing of anaerobic bacteria: the state of the art. *Clinical Infectious Diseases*, **16** (Suppl. 4), S328–S333.

Willis, A.T. (1991) Abdominal sepsis. In *Anaerobes in Human Disease* (ed. B.I. Duerden and B.S. Drasar), pp. 197–223. Edward Arnold, London.

Wren, M.W.D. (1991) Laboratory diagnosis of anaerobic infections. In *Anaerobes in Human Disease* (ed. B.I. Duerden and B.S. Drasar), pp. 180–196. Edward Arnold, London.

21

TREPONEMES

Helen H.Y. Wong and Charles W. Penn

INTRODUCTION

Treponemes are spiral bacteria widely distributed as commensals or pathogens of animals. Of greatest clinical importance to humans is *Treponema pallidum* in which subspecies *pallidum* causes syphilis, while *T. pallidum* subsp. *pertenue* is isolated from skin eruptions of yaws, a non-venereal treponematosis in children living in warm, humid countries. In spite of the recent low incidence of new syphilis cases in the UK, the disease remains important because of social and behavioural changes following the HIV epidemic. Its incidence is now increasing rapidly in the USA, and treponematoses are major diseases on a world scale.

HISTORY

Syphilis rivalled plague as a scourge of Europe in the late fifteenth century. Syphilis broke out after Columbus returned from the West Indies, and flourished in the aftermath of the siege of Naples. The origin of the disease may never be known – the 'Columbus theory', that it was imported from the New World, is one of several.

The name syphilis derives from the name of an infected shepherd boy in a poem by Fracastorius (1483–1553), a pioneer of scientific epidemiology. At that time syphilis in Europe was an acute, virulent disease, killing up to 25% of those infected (Sell and Norris, 1983) – a very different disease from untreated syphilis in recent times. John Hunter inoculated himself in 1767 with some 'matter of gonorrhoea' which, unknown to him, also contained syphilis organisms. Although he wrongly concluded that gonorrhoeal material caused his chancre, he was able to clarify the progression of syphilis and showed how best to treat the disease with mercury, with which he treated himself.

In 1905, Schaudinn and Hoffman discovered the syphilis spirochaete by microscopy in syphilitic lesions. Landsteiner demonstrated *T. pallidum* by dark-ground microscopy in 1906, and Wasserman detected antilipoidal antibodies associated with the disease using a complement fixation test. 1907 saw the arrival of a revolutionary treatment: Ehrlich's magic bullet – arsenical aniline derivative No. 606, known commercially as Salvarsan. Compared with mercury, Salvarsan cured syphilis more efficiently, with far fewer side effects. An effective and safe treatment came only with the introduction of penicillin.

The importance of syphilis, both socially and medically, during the past five centuries has been

Principles and Practice of Clinical Bacteriology. Edited by A.M. Emmerson, P.M. Hawkey and S.H. Gillespie
© 1997 John Wiley & Sons Ltd

immense. Because of its ability to achieve vertical transmission, syphilis was uniquely feared, in ignorance of any scientific understanding, as a phenomenon of inheritance of a state of moral corruption. The medical importance of the disease resulted in part from the potential of the organism to affect almost every system in the body and to mimic a wide range of other diseases as 'the great imitator'.

DESCRIPTION OF THE ORGANISM

In the following sections we shall refer only to the type species of the genus *T. pallidum*. The only other treponeme species which is of likely clinical importance is *T. denticola*, implicated in periodontal disease, but lack of space precludes its detailed coverage here.

Morphology

Being 0.1–0.15 μm wide (and about 10 μm long) *T. pallidum* is one of the most slender spirochaetes, and is difficult to stain and observe by bright-field microscopy, hence the name '*pallidum*'. Morphological features (Strugnell *et al.*, 1990) are the size and spiral form, useful in diagnostic microscopy (Figures 21.1 and 21.2), and the tip organelle and longitudinal in-line insertion of the axial endoflagella (Figure 21.2). *Treponema pallidum* usually has three endoflagella inserted at each end, and they interdigitate and overlap at the central part of the organism. There are cytoplasmic filaments beneath the cytoplasmic membrane, parallel to the endoflagella. The outer membrane appears to be a typical bilayered lipid structure.

Physiology and Cultivation

Treponema pallidum has never been cultivated axenically *in vitro*, but has been co-cultivated with a rabbit testis-derived cell line (Fieldsteel *et al.*, 1982). It remains necessary to obtain the organism by infection of rabbits for use in research and as diagnostic antigen, although recombinant antigens also are now becoming available. The organism appears extremely fastidious, and its optimal

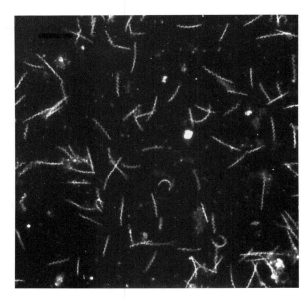

Figure 21.1. Dark-ground light micrograph of a suspension of *Treponema pallidum* obtained from infected rabbit testis. Note between 5 and 10 turns to the spiral of each organism. Bar represents 10 μm. (Taken in part from *Topley and Wilson's Principles of Bacteriology, Virology and Immunity*, 8th edn, 1990, with permission from Edward Arnold.)

survival (shown by its motility) under strictly anaerobic conditions *in vitro* suggested that it was an anaerobe. However it is now known to be microaerophilic. Its lability on exposure to air may be caused by sensitivity to reactive products of molecular oxygen. The organism is killed rapidly by desiccation, surfactants etc. Animal infection experiments suggest a generation time of 33 hours during infection.

The bulk of experimental data on the organism has been obtained using the Nichols strain isolated in the USA in 1913. Modern isolates are very similar antigenically and genetically to the Nichols strain. Cultivation in rabbits involves inoculation of 0.5–1.0 ml of a suspension of *T. pallidum*, containing 10^5 to 10^7 viable treponemes, into the rabbit testis. About 10 days later the testis becomes hardened and enlarged. The animal is killed, the testes removed and chopped into small fragments which are shaken gently at 37 °C in air in

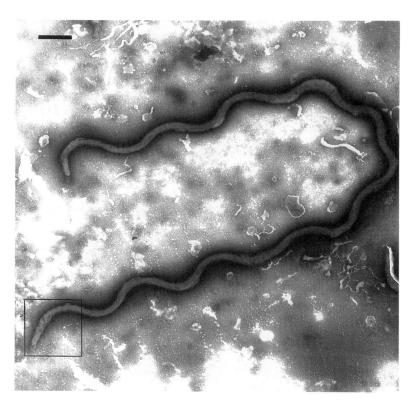

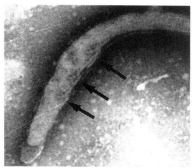

Figure 21.2. Electron micrograph of negatively stained *Treponema pallidum*. Inset: note tip structure and in-line insertion (arrows) of three endoflagella at each end of the organism. Bar represents 0.5 μm. (Taken in part from *Topley and Wilson's Principles of Bacteriology, Virology and Immunity*, 8th edn, 1990, with permission from Edward Arnold.)

20–30 ml of Hanks' balanced salt solution buffered with 20 mM HEPES, and with 2 mM dithiothreitol to lower the redox potential. Over a period of hours, with several changes of medium to control the pH, up to 10^{10} treponemes can be harvested in the supernatant from each testis.

Phylogeny

The syphilis agent *T. pallidum* is classified in one genus of the family Spirochaetaceae, which also includes the pathogenic genera *Borrelia* and *Leptospira* (see pages 691 and 677). All spirochaetes are

are characterized by spiral morphology, motility and the periplasmic location of their flagella. Molecular phylogeny based on 16S rRNA sequences shows that these organisms form a relatively homogeneous group, distinct from other eubacterial branches. Sequence comparisons also show that the species most closely related to *T. pallidum* are the oral organisms *T. denticola* and *T. phagedenis* (Paster *et al.*, 1991). Antigenic cross-reactions between spirochaetes are not uncommon.

Molecular Biology and Antigenicity

While it is clear from the strong antibody response in infected humans that components of the organism are strongly antigenic, the organisms appears not to have surface-exposed antigens in its intact, native state. This seems to be due to an unusually sparse content of surface-exposed proteins in the outer membrane (Penn *et al.*, 1985; Cox *et al.*,

1992). It appears also that lipopolysaccharide may be absent from the outer membrane. Nevertheless several strongly antigenic proteins have been identified. Among these are the endoflagella which contain both 'conventional' flagellins (Fla B) homologous with those of other bacteria in the flagellar core, and an unusual flagellar sheath protein Fla A. Several prominent and antigenically dominant lipoproteins associated with the cell surface but in general not surface-exposed and possibly attached to the cytoplasmic membrane are also important antigens. They include a particularly prominent protein of 45 kDa, and other lipoproteins of 42.5, 39.5, 35.5, 30–38, 24–30, 17 and 15 kDa (Norris, 1993) (see Table 21.1). The reason for the abundance of lipoproteins is not yet clear, and it may relate to the lack of exposure of antigen on the treponemal surface – an aspect of the biology of *T. pallidum* which is currently receiving detailed study (Radolf, 1994).

TABLE 21.1   MAJOR ANTIGENS OF *TREPONEMA PALLIDUM*

Designation[a]	Mol. wt	Description and comments
TpN83	82 000	Major component of cytoplasmic filaments or fibronectin binding protein
TpN60	59 000	Homologue of Hsp60 or GroEL heat shock protein. Cross-reactive antigen
TpN47	45 000	Lipoprotein. The most abundant polypeptide and dominant antigen
TpN44.5 (TmpA)	42 000	Lipoprotein. Also abundant. Recombinant form purified and tested successfully as a diagnostic reagent
TpN41	39 500	Lipoprotein. Homologue of the MglB periplasmic sugar-binding protein of *E. coli*
TpN37	37 000	FlaA flagellin. Abundant, dominant antigen. Member of class of unique spirochaetal flagellar 'sheath' proteins
TpN35	35 500	Lipoprotein. Less abundant and antigenically dominant than TpN47, 44.5
TpN34.5 TpN33 TpN30	34 500 } 33 000 } 32 000 }	FlaB flagellins, homologues of other bacterial flagellins. Form flagellar core
TpN29–35 (TpD)	30–38 000	Lipoprotein, moderately antigenic. Diffuse molecular weight forms smear on electrophoresis
TpN24–28 (TpE)	24–30 000	Lipoprotein, similar properties to TpN29–35
TpN19 (TpF1, 4D[b])	19 000	Subunit of a large, heat-labile complex which in recombinant *E. coli* is a ring structure. In yaws strains, homologue TyF1 usually differs in one base of the sequence
TpN17	17 000	Lipoprotein, strongly antigenic
TpN15	15 000	Lipoprotein, strongly antigenic

[a] TpN designations are those of Norris *et al.* (1993). Names in parentheses were mainly given by van Embden *et al.* (1983).
[b] Designation of Walfield *et al.* (1982).

While the study of antigens of *T. pallidum* by conventional approaches has been hampered because it could not be cultured, modern molecular biological approaches have been very informative. Monoclonal antibody technology has permitted the recognition of individual protein antigens by immunoblotting. Gene cloning has enabled characterization of most of the major antigens by gene sequencing. Summary information on major genetically cloned protein antigens is presented in Table 21.1.

Pathogenicity

The pathogenesis of syphilis is complex and very poorly understood.

Immune Regulation

Experimental work in rabbit and guinea-pig models has largely been responsible for increased understanding of the immune response in treponemal infection. Treponemal infection in humans, however, is a chronic disease in which the organism evades the host immune response. This aspect of the disease is not reproduced in animal models.

Both cellular and humoral arms of host immunity are required for clearance of treponemes. Baker-Zander and Lukehart (1992) demonstrated *in vivo* killing of phagocytosed treponemes in macrophages, and killing was enhanced (by 90%) when the treponemes were opsonized. Experimental data indicate the following scenario.

Wandering macrophages at the site of infection are the first cells to combat the infection. A delayed-type hypersensitivity reaction causes cell infiltration, contributing to the primary chancre. With the help of dendritic cells, antigen is presented to the T helper cells which respond by production of interferon γ, a macrophage-activating factor, and thus the cycle of cell activity heightens to make clearance of treponemes more effective. The T helper cells also activate an antibody response in B cells. Anti-treponemal IgM appears first, followed by IgG and IgA. The IgG binds to antigenic epitopes, if present, on the treponemal surface, rendering it susceptible to macrophage killing. However, at some point, prostaglandin E_2

(PGE_2) production from macrophages begins to downregulate macrophage activity, and also selects for a Th1 to Th2 switch. The antibody production phase takes over between days 9 and 14 post infection, and lasts 90 days and beyond.

Some treponemes which escape phagocytosis may disseminate and multiply slowly in other tissues, their growth constantly checked by the high lever of antibodies. It is when the balance of this host immune regulation tips favourably towards the survival of the treponemes that reactivation in a much more destructive manner occurs, as highlighted in the case of HIV coinfection. The Th2 activity therefore provides a more stable and longer-lasting protection for the host (Fitzgerald *et al.*, 1992). Antibodies appear as early as the first week after infection, and IgG production does not stop for many decades. Two categories of antibodies are produced: those reactive to lipoidal antigens, and those reactive to polypeptide antigens of the treponemes.

Anti-lipoidal antibodies

The most important is anti-cardiolipin, which may be both IgG and IgM. It is unclear whether the response is directed against the treponemal outer membrane lipid, or to tissue breakdown products which include cardiolipin. Anti-lipoidal antibodies are important serological markers in the diagnosis and treatment of infection, being detectable in the first three to five weeks and declining significantly as infection subsides naturally or due to antibiotic intervention.

Anti-treponemal IgM

Anti-treponemal IgM is a feature of active infection, and is the first antibody to be produced. The level is at its highest in the secondary stage of syphilis, but declines after treatment. The rate of antibody clearance depends on the stage of disease: within four weeks if treated in the primary stage, three to nine months if treated in the secondary stage.

Detection of anti-treponemal IgM is a valuable tool in the diagnosis of congenital syphilis. The large molecules cannot cross the placenta, and any IgM detected in the neonate is likely to be fetal in origin.

Anti-treponemal IgG

Production of IgG closely follows that of IgM and the level peaks at four weeks after primary infection. Unlike that of IgM, the anti-treponemal IgG level is maintained at a low level after treatment and is detectable by the FTA-abs and TPHA tests many years after the infection has been successfully treated. Wicher *et al.* (1991) have demonstrated that in human treponemal disease the pathogen-specific antibodies produced at all stages are exclusively of the IgG isotype. The value of traditional laboratory testing for IgM is therefore currently debatable. However, although specificity is now in doubt, the increase in IgM level in active infection and in congenital syphilis continues to provide valuable information in serodiagnosis.

EPIDEMIOLOGY

The onset of the HIV epidemic in the 1980s changed the epidemiology of syphilis infection in Western society, as incidence fell in the high-risk group of homosexual men. Incidence is now increasing in other groups. A new high-risk group heterosexually associated with promiscuity and 'crack house' cocaine abuse now exists, particularly in the USA, with increased incidence of congenital syphilis (Wasserheit, 1994). New York city witnessed a 500% rise in incidence of congenital syphilis between 1986 and 1988. The UK has shown a steady 100 cases of congenital syphilis per year since 1983. In Zambia, up to 1% of infants born in one hospital had signs of congenital syphilis and 40% of stillbirths were attributable to the disease (Rawstron *et al.*, 1993). In the USA, adult cases rose from 10 000 in 1956 to 50 000 in 1990, with the highest number of affected heterosexuals since 1949. Syphilis is also increasing elsewhere (deSchryver and Meheus, 1990). In Africa, a staggering figure of >350 new cases per 100 000 population per year has emerged. New South Wales in Australia recorded a 90% drop in syphilis infection between 1981 and 1989, but in 1990 there was a 340% rise in males and a 540% rise in females (Blackhouse *et al.*, 1991). In England and Wales, new cases reported were 1305 in 1990, compared with 4069 in 1980, but may now increase as in the USA and Australia. Whereas homosexuals have changed their sexual behaviour and are practising safe sex, the same is not true among the new high-risk groups.

In HIV-infected individuals, healing of primary lesions may be delayed (Hutchinson *et al.*, 1994). Immunodeficiency in HIV patients with previously treated syphilis has been shown to facilitate reinfection, and late manifestations of syphilis have increased in HIV cases. The ulcerative nature of syphilis also appears to increase the risk for acquisition of HIV.

Between 1952 and 1969, WHO and UNICEF coordinated a yaws treatment and control programme in endemic areas with an aim to eradicate endemic treponematoses. To a large extent their work was successful, but lack of sustained effort has led to resurgence in endemic foci, including Western and Central Africa, Southeast Asia and the Western Pacific. A minimum of 300 cases of yaws per 100 000 individuals were reported by Noordhoek *et al.* (1991) in a survey in West Sumatra in Indonesia.

CLINICAL FEATURES

Syphilis

The classic features of primary, secondary, latent and tertiary syphilis have been well described.

Primary syphilis

This usually manifests as a chancre which develops at the site of entry, e.g. genitalia, rectum, of the organism to the body two to four weeks after infection. Pathogenesis does not involve adhesion to or colonization of mucosal epithelia; rather treponemes directly invade the tissues, often through skin abrasions. Thus the location of penile chancres is often consistent with localized trauma during intercourse. The motility of *T. pallidum* probably mediates initial invasion of tissues and dissemination, during which the organism may penetrate between endothelial cells. Regional lymph nodes become enlarged.

Organisms multiply and accumulate in the primary chancre. The chancre consists of accumulated interstitial fluid, containing numerous extracellular treponemes, and an infiltrate of mononuclear cells, macrophages and lymphocytes, more characteristic of chronic than acute inflammation. Thus there is an element of host response in chancre formation, but no treponemal toxin or other mediator has been found. The lesion is painless, in line with the absence of acute inflammation. The chancre ultimately may become haemorrhagic and ulcerate, and slowly resolves, presumably as a result of localized host immune responses and macrophage activity. By this time there is a vigorous antibody response to the infection.

Secondary lesions

These develop weeks or months later and are generally disseminated and variable in form, most often comprising a widespread, symmetrical, non-itchy, maculopapular rash on the trunk, hands or feet, or condylomata or mucous patches. There is often generalized lymphadenopathy. The lesions presumably form at sites where the organisms have lodged and multiplied after dissemination from the primary lesions, away from the accumulation of immune cells which cleared organisms from the primary site. Localization at body surfaces may result from reduced temperatures of these tissues; the organism probably has an optimum of $1-2\,°C$ below body temperature. Like primary chancres, secondary lesions are self-limiting and resolve spontaneously; these include snail-track ulcers in the mouth. The patient is potentially infectious during the primary and secondary stages. Again, the mechanism and involvement of immune responses in clearance are not well studied.

Latent and tertiary disease

In about one-third of untreated cases, there is no further infection after secondary lesions disappear. In the majority, however, persistent, asymptomatic *latent* infection follows, and may persist for many years. It is not known where organisms are sequestered. Latency may persist indefinitely. In about one-third of all those infected and not treated, *tertiary* disease eventually occurs. This appears to be primarily the result of a localized host cellular immune response, and treponemes are sparse. The lesions may occur in a wide variety of organs, and may be destructive and life threatening, especially in central nervous system or cardiovascular tissues. Gummas may occur in skin, bones and joints.

A special case of syphilis infection, of great historical importance but now fortunately rare, is *congenital* syphilis. At its most destructive, leading to birth malformations, this results generally from exposure of the fetus to active infection in the mother during the first half of pregnancy and is characterized by massive invasion by spirochaetes of nearly all body tissues.

Yaws, Pinta, Endemic Syphilis

The exact relationship between venereal and non-venereal infections with *T. pallidum* subspp., and between the agents of syphilis and the non-venereal treponematoses, remains unclear.

Laboratory analysis still has not demonstrated significant differences between *T. pallidum* subsp. *pallidum* and subsp. *pertenue*, the yaws agent which is the only other subspecies to be examined at a molecular level. The only reported difference between them is in the DNA sequence of a gene which encodes the '4D' or TpN19 antigen, which in most isolates examined differs by one base between the subspecies. *Treponema carateum*, agent of pinta, remains classified as a separate species because it has not yet been isolated for laboratory studies and subspecies designation cannot be justified.

Yaws, like syphilis, is a chronic infection and likely to involve broadly similar pathogenic processes, albeit modified by the different circumstances of non-venereal infection in childhood and the immunological status of the host. No unique pathogenic attributes of the yaws subspecies are known.

Oral Treponemes and Intestinal Spirochaetes

The oral treponemes *T. denticola* and *T. phagedenis*, the latter including the Reiter treponeme, are phylogenetically close to *T. pallidum*, but they differ fundamentally in genomic and biological properties. The G + C content in the DNA is 38% for *T. denticola* compared with 52% for *T. pallidum*, and barely any genomic DNA hybridization occurs between species. Thus while all are classified in the genus *Treponema*, they are more distantly related to each other than, for example, the distinct genera *Shigella* and *Escherichia*.

Oral spirochaetes share some so-called 'pathogen-specific' antigenic components with the 'pathogenic' *T. pallidum* group (Riviere *et al.*, 1991), leading to the hypothesis that similar pathogenic attributes may exist in members of the oral spirochaete flora which are strongly associated with periodontal disease.

It is now clear that intestinal spirochaetes are also quite diverse, and while it seems likely that these organisms may be pathogenic in some circumstances, much remains to be learned of their biology.

LABORATORY DIAGNOSIS

The diagnosis of a treponemal infection is based on a combination of clinical examination, clinical history, and serological findings with or without the support of dark-ground microscopy (Public Health Service, 1962).

Microscopy

Many genitourinary medicine departments have a dark-ground microscope set up for detection of spirochaetes in suspected chancres. This provides a rapid and direct diagnosis of syphilis but experienced personnel are needed to assess the characteristic morphology and motility of *T. pallidum* (see Figure 21.2). False negative results may be seen in patients with lesions resolving either naturally or because of antibiotic treatment.

A dried and fixed smear from the lesion may also be examined by direct immunofluorescence with polyclonal antiserum in the laboratory. A fluorescein isothiocyanate (FITC)-labelled mouse monoclonal antibody produced against the 37 kDa antigen of *T. pallidum* street strain DAL-1 as described by Ito *et al.* (1992) was equally sensitive.

Treponemal Serology

Antibody testing is adaptable for mass screening as well as providing a pretreatment baseline antibody level for follow-up purposes. Both non-treponemal tests and treponemal tests are widely used for detection of antibodies. Neither is able to distinguish between syphilis and yaws, but the combination provides valuable information on antibody status in screening programmes targeting the antenatal population, genitourinary medicine clinic patients and blood donors.

Non-treponemal tests

The antigen used contains 0.03% cardiolipin, stabilized in an emulsion of standard sensitivity by the addition of 0.9% cholesterol and 0.21% lecithin. The Venereal Disease Research Laboratory (VDRL) slide test requires sera heated at 56 °C for 30 minutes, freshly prepared antigen, and a microscope for reading.

Addition of eidetic acid and choline chloride has enabled the use of unheated serum for field use. The life of the antigen suspension is also thus much prolonged. Several non-treponemal testing kits benefit from this convenient modification. The USR (Untreated Serum Reagin) test is also a microscopic test, but the RPR-Card test, the RST (Reagin Serum Test) and the TRUST (Toluidine Red Untreated Serum Test) may be visualized macroscopically with the aid of carbon, Sudan black and toluidine red respectively. These tests are very simple to perform. All reactive samples must be titrated. A titre of >1 : 8 has a high predictive value for active infection if other treponemal tests are also positive. They are also extremely good markers for treatment efficacy or disease reactivation as the titres drop rapidly, e.g. four-fold within three months if the treatment is successful. Sensitivity is low in primary and late syphilis;

biological false positives (BFP) may be found in patients with autoimmune disease, in chronic infections, in the elderly and in pregnant women.

Treponemal tests

The TPHA detects antitreponemal IgG in sera (Rathlev, 1967). Specificity is enhanced by a sorbent incorporated into the diluent which removes group antibody against non-pathogenic treponemes. Sheep and fowl red cells are used in various commercial kits. Fowl cell kits have the advantage of a shorter settling time due to the heavier nucleated red cells. The test is simple, sensitive, highly reproducible, and lends itself to semi-automation.

EIA (enzyme immunoassay) tests for detection of anti-treponemal IgG or IgG and IgM are also gaining popularity as screening tests, mostly used on their own rather than in combination (Young *et al.*, 1991). These tests are highly sensitive and specific, and like RPR/TPHA screening could be automated. Kits now available commercially vary in the use of solid-phase, antibody capture or plain antigen coating, and amplification of enzyme/ substrate signals.

Confirmatory Tests

FTA–abs test

This is an indirect microimmunofluorescence test for detection of anti-treponemal IgG, usually performed in reference laboratories, although it is also available in kit form; a fluorescence microscope and trained personnel are required (Hunter, 1975). It is the most sensitive serological test for detection of early primary syphilis. The specificity is fractionally higher than TPHA and EIA–IgG tests. False positives may occur where excess antibodies against indigenous non-pathogenic treponemes exist. Because IgG is continuously produced in small quantities even after adequate treatment, the FTA–abs test cannot be used for monitoring disease activity.

FTA–abs IgM test

If a specific anti-human IgM–FITC conjugate is used in the FTA test, anti-treponemal IgM in an active infection can be demonstrated. This test is useful for assessment of activity of infection and

TABLE 21.2   BRIEF GUIDE TO THE INTERPRETATION OF SCREENING TESTS (WASLEY AND WONG, 1988)

Non-treponemal (reagin) tests	Treponemal tests, TPHA or EIA	Interpretation and action
Non-reactive	Negative	1. In the absence of clinical symptoms: no treponemal antibodies found 2. Confirm with FTA–abs test if early infection suspected
Reactive	Negative	1. Possible BFP, titre unlikely to be above 1:8, confirm with FTA–abs test 2. Non-treponemal tests may be reactive before TPHA or EIA IgG response, confirm with FTA–abs test, and retest after one week
Non-reactive	Positive	1. Past treponemal infection (cannot distinguish yaws or syphilis) 2. In follow-up patients, a four-fold decrease in reagin titre in three months indicates successful treatment 3. In absence of relevant clinical history, confirm with FTA–abs test
Reactive	Positive	1. Strongly suggestive of active treponemal infection, especially if reagin titre is >1:8. Confirm with FTA–abs and IgM tests 2. In follow-up patients: four-fold decrease in reagin titre indicates successful treatment 3. Sero-fast reagin titre may coincide with past treated treponemal disease 4. In absence of symptoms, confirm with FTA–abs test for latent or late congenital syphilis 5. BFP in some patients may coincide with past treated treponemal infection

treatment success, and is the most useful test for detecting the presence of congenital infection in neonates. However, the test suffers from interference by rheumatoid factor, and a 19S–IgM version gives a more conclusive result.

Captia-Syphilis-M test (Microgen)

This is a good alternative to the FTA–abs IgM test as this EIA test utilizes a capture technique to minimize the effect of rheumatoid factor. This test is slightly more sensitive for IgM detection than the FTA–IgM test, and it remains positive for up to two years after adequate treatment.

Treponema pallidum immobilization test (TPI)

This test is based on the ability of syphilitic serum to immobilize and kill living *T. pallidum* in the presence of complement. It is the most specific treponemal serology test, but is now obsolete because of the need to cultivate live treponemes.

TmpA–EIA

This is a new commercially available kit for highly specific and sensitive testing of anti-treponemal antibodies. The main component of the antigen is a 42 kDa recombinant antigen, treponemal membrane protein TmpA (TpN 44.5) (see Table 21.1). Reactivity to this test declines rapidly after antibiotic administration, and it could be used for monitoring treatment.

Laboratory Examination of Cerebrospinal Fluid for Neurosyphilis

Diagnosis of neurosyphilis has always been problematical. Parameters to be studied include detection of inflammatory processes, production of intrathecal globulins, presence of antibodies against treponemes in blood and cerebrospinal fluid (CSF), or even the detection of treponemes in CSF.

A reactive CSF VRDL test is still the only standard test recognized by the Centers for Disease Control (CDC), Atlanta, for serological confirmation of neurosyphilis, but up to 40% may be missed. A negative CSF FTA–abs test has high negative predictive value, but a positive result may merely indicate blood–brain barrier transudation of IgG. The TPHA index and ITPA index may be used to clarify the source of IgG as intrathecal or otherwise:

$$\text{TPHA index} = \frac{\text{CSF TPHA titre}}{\text{Albumin quotient}}$$

$$\text{ITPA index} = \frac{\text{TPHA titre in CSF}}{\text{Total mg IgG in CSF}} \div$$

$$\frac{\text{TPHA IgG titre in serum}}{\text{Total mg IgG in serum}}$$

RIT (rabbit infectivity test)

This test can detect as few as 10 live treponemes in a specimen. However, 15–30% of patients with a positive RIT do not show any CSF abnormality.

PCR (polymerase chain reaction)

This is a promising diagnostic tool for neurosyphilis, particularly in HIV patients who may have abnormal serology patterns. The amplified DNA may be specifically identified by DNA probe. At least 65 organisms in 0.5 ml CSF may be needed to demonstrate a positive PCR, so sensitivity may need to be improved (Hay *et al.*, 1990).

DNA technology

This represents a modern approach to the detection of treponemal infection (Wicher *et al.*, 1992). PCR is no longer a novelty in routine laboratories, and is increasingly favoured for demonstrating treponemal DNA in CSF and blood. Choice of primers, determining the particular DNA sequence to be amplified, may be crucial, for example using primers specific for the gene encoding the 19 kDa protein TpF1 (TpN19, Norris, 1993). Hybridization of the amplified DNA with specific TyF1 and TpF1 antigen DNA probes is at last showing promise for differentiating syphilis and yaws infections.

TABLE 21.3 AN ABBREVIATED WHO RECOMMENDED SCHEDULE OF PENICILLIN TREATMENT

	Benzathine Penicillin	Procaine Penicillin
Early syphilis	Single dose: 2.4 mega units intramuscularly	600 000 units intramuscularly for 10 days
Late syphilis	2.4 mega-units weekly for three weeks	600 000 units intramuscularly daily for 15 days
Congenital syphilis		50 000 units/kg body weight intramuscularly daily for 10 days.

TREATMENT

Penicillin is still the preferred antibiotic for treatment of all stages of syphilis. Current WHO recommendations are summarized in Table 21.3.

The treatment of neurosyphilis is not well studied but one of the established treatments which is effective in stopping disease progression is intramuscular injection of 1.8 or 2.4 mega-units of aqueous procaine penicillin for 21 days.

In case of penicillin allergy alternative antibiotics such as ceftriaxone and doxycycline are used. Ceftriaxone is used at 250 mg daily for 10 days in early syphilis or 1 g daily for 14 days in neurosyphilis. Doxycycline may be used at 200 mg daily for 20 days for early syphilis (see review by Goldmeier and Hay, 1993, for update on treatment).

Zidovudine, however, is not found to eradicate syphilis from HIV-positive syphilitic patients and this group should be treated as for neurosyphilis patients.

PREVENTION AND CONTROL

The control of treponematoses relies on demographic data and accurate, efficient testing. Cost-effective measures must include screening policies in low- or high-risk groups.

Screening of blood donors does not merely rule out current or past treponematosis. As syphilis is associated with other sexually transmitted diseases including HIV, a negative serology adds confidence to the quality of the blood.

The recent increase in congenital syphilis in some countries has highlighted the cost-effectiveness of antenatal screening. CDC recommends testing at first trimester and at delivery. Where the incidence of syphilis is high, and in women of high-risk groups, third-trimester blood is also tested. If abnormality is seen in this group, the non-treponemal test may be performed with diluted serum to rule out a prozone phenomenon due to a high antibody level.

In 1989, the CDC published a new case definition for diagnosis of congenital syphilis. Presumptive and confirmed cases are redefined based on physical examination, radiology of long bone, history of mother's serology and treatment, and laboratory findings on the neonatal blood. Others suggest that no infant should be discharged until the maternal serology is known. Asymptomatic neonates with reactive serology must be followed up at one, two, three, six and 12 months to establish the elimination of maternal antibodies. Those with stable or rising titres should be treated. Infants with reactive CSF VDRL must be treated appropriately and lumbar puncture repeated every six months until negative serology is obtained. Failure to resolve to negative serology suggests treatment failure and retreatment may be necessary (Zenker and Berman, 1991). Deficient cellular immunity in HIV patients may cause several abnormalities in the diagnosis of syphilis. These include highly reactive VDRL and negative FTA–abs test in an active infection, unusually rapid progression to neurosyphilis, and treatment failure after therapy due to persistence of *T. pallidum* in the central nervous system. It is widely felt that in HIV patients, and others with secondary syphilis or latent syphilis, CSF should be examined to assist the choice of chemotherapy.

In tropical areas where yaws is resurgent, control depends on local surveillance. Where local laboratory facilities are not available, blood collected and dried on paper disks is useful for mass screening. Where there is >10% infection rate, the whole population may be treated with a full course of penicillin. At 5–10% infection rates, only the children need to be treated. Mass penicillin treatment may, however, cause emergence of resistant strains in other organisms, creating a need for more expensive antibiotics in poor rural countries. Management is complicated as the incidence of syphilis may surge as endemic treponematosis is brought under control.

To limit disease transmission, early diagnosis and treatment are complemented by patient counselling, contact tracing and education, as well as legislation (Public Health Papers, 1977). A more open attitude towards sex in the early 1980s was in part instrumental in halting spread of syphilis amongst male homosexuals. The different high-risk group emerging now requires a modified approach. Apart from free diagnosis and treatment, counselling to drug addicts, prostitutes and immigrants appears effective in encouraging condom use and regular check-up. In the USA legislation requires repeaters (those infected with sexually transmitted disease at least three times) to report to specified clinics for weekly or monthly examination. Prostitutes must comply with treatment until cure before taking up new clients. Some countries require syphilis serology clearance before marriage, immigration or recruitment to certain occupations. Syphilis is a notifiable disease and new cases must be reported to health authorities by clinics or laboratories.

Treponematoses are primarily social and public health problems. Whilst immunization is still not an option in preventing treponemal infection, medical practice and scientific research can at best relieve short-term suffering. It is necessary for governments to address the issue at root and channel resources to combat drug addiction, poor education and poverty.

REFERENCES

Baker-Zander, S.A. and Lukehart, S.A. (1992) Macrophage mediated killing of opsonised *Treponema pallidum*. *Journal of Infectious Diseases*, **165**, 69–74.

Baldry, P. (1976) *The Battle Against Bacteria: A Fresh Look*. Cambridge University Press, Cambridge, UK.

Blackhouse, J.L., Nesteroff, S.I. and Papoutsakis, G. (1991) Early syphilis: cases from New South Wales detected at ICPMR, Westmead Hospital 1980–1990. *Communicable Disease Intelligence*, **15**, 210–212.

Cox, D.L., Chang, P., McDowall, A.W. *et al.* (1992) The outer membrane, not a coat of host proteins, limits antigenicity of virulent *Treponema pallidum*. *Infection and Immunity*, **60**, 1076–1083.

De Schryver, A. and Meheus, A. (1990) Epidemiology of sexually transmitted diseases: the global picture. *Bulletin of the World Health Organization*, **68**, 639–654.

Fieldsteel, A.H., Cox, D.L. and Moeckli, R.A. (1982) Further studies on replication of virulent *Treponema pallidum* in tissue culture of Sf1Ep cells. *Infection and Immunity*, **35**, 449–455.

Fitzgerald, T.L. (1992) Minireview. The Th1/Th2 like switch in syphilitic infection: is it detrimental? *Infection and Immunity*, **60**, 3475–3479.

Goldmeier, D. and Hay, P. (1993) A review and update on adult syphilis, with particular reference to its treatment. *International Journal of Sexually Transmitted Diseases and AIDS*, **4**, 70–82.

Hay, P.E., Clarke, J.R., Taylor-Robinson, D. *et al.* (1990) Detection of treponemal DNA in the CSF of patients with syphilis and HIV infection using the polymerase chain reaction. *Genitourinary Medicine*, **66**, 428–432.

Hunter, E.F. (1975) The fluorescent treponemal antibody–absorption (FTA–abs) test for syphilis. *Critical Review of Clinical Laboratory Science*, **5**, 315–330.

Hutchison, C.M., Hook, E.W., Shepherd, M. *et al.* (1994) Altered clinical presentation of early syphilis in patients with human immunodeficiency virus infection. *Annals of Internal Medicine*, **121**, 94–99.

Ito, F., Hunter, E.F., George, R.W. *et al.* (1992) Specific immunofluorescent staining of pathogenic treponemes with a monoclonal antibody. *Journal of Clinical Microbiology*, **30**, 831–838.

Lukehart, S.A. (1991) Syphilis: issues for the 1990s. *Clinical Microbiological Newsletter*, **13**, 117–120.

Noordhoek, G.T., Engelkens, H.J.H., Judanarso, J. *et al.* (1991) Yaws in West Sumatra, Indonesia: clinical manifestation, serological findings and characterisation of new *Treponema* isolates using DNA probes. *European Journal of Clinical Microbiology and Infectious Disease*, **10**, 12–19.

Norris, S.J. and the *Treponema pallidum* polypeptide research group (1993) Polypeptides of *Treponema pallidum*: progress towards understanding of their structural, functional and immunologic roles. *Microbiological Reviews*, **57**, 750–779.

Paster, B.J., Dewhirst, F.E., Weisburg, W.G. *et al.* (1991) Phylogenetic analysis of the spirochetes. *Journal of Bacteriology*, **173**, 6101–6109.

Penn, C.W., Bailey, M.J. and Cockayne, A. (1985) The outer membrane of *Treponema pallidum*: biological significance and biochemical properties. *Journal of General Microbiology*, **131**, 2349–2357.

Public Health Papers (**65**) (1977) Social and health aspects of sexually transmitted diseases: principles of control measures, WHO Geneva.

Public Health Service (1962) *Laboratory Procedures for Modern Syphilis Serology*. US Department of Health, Education and Welfare.

Radolf, J.D. (1994) Immune evasion by *Treponema pallidum* and *Borrelia burgdorferi*: ultrastructural and molecular correlates. *Trends in Microbiology*, **2**, 307–311.

Rathlev, T. (1967) Haemagglutination test utilising pathogenic *Treponema pallidum* for the sero-diagnosis of syphilis. *British Journal of Venereal Diseases*, **43**, 181–185.

Rawstron, S.A., Bromberg, K. and Hammerschlag, M.R. (1993) STD in children: syphilis and gonorrhoea. *Genitourinary Medicine*, **69**, 66–75.

Riviere, G.R., Wagoner, M.A., Baker-Zander, S.A. *et al.* (1991) Identification of spirochetes related to *Treponema pallidum* in necrotizing gingivitis and chronic periodontitis. *New England Journal of Medicine*, **325**, 539–543.

Sell, S. and Norris, S.J. (1983) The biology, pathology and immunology of syphilis. *International Review of Experimental Pathology*, **24**, 204–276.

Strugnell, R., Cockayne, A. and Penn, C.W. (1990) Molecular and antigenic analysis of treponemes. *Critical Review in Microbiology*, **17**, 231–250.

van Embden, J.D.A., van der Donk, H.J., van Eijk, R.V. *et al.* (1983) Molecular cloning and expression of *Treponema pallidum* antigens in *Escherichia coli*. *Infection and Immunity*, **42**, 187–196.

Walfield, A.M., Hanff, P.A. and Lovett, M.A. (1982) Expression of *Treponema pallidum* antigens in *Escherichia coli*. *Science*, **216**, 522–523.

Wasley, G.D. and Wong, H.H.Y. (1988) *Syphilis Serology: Principles and Practice*. Oxford Medical Publications, Oxford.

Wasserheit, J.N. (1994) Effect of changes in human ecology and behaviour on patterns of sexually transmitted diseases, including human immunodeficiency virus infection. *Proceedings of the National Academy of Sciences of the USA*, **91**, 2430–2435.

Wicher, K., Noordhoek, G.T., Abbruscato, F. and Wicher, V. (1992) Detection of *Treponema pallidum* in early syphilis by DNA amplification. *Journal of Clinical Microbiology*, **30**, 497–500.

Wicher, V., Zabek, J. and Wicher K. (1991) Pathogen-specific humoral response in *Treponema pallidum* infected humans, rabbits and guinea pigs. *Journal of Infectious Diseases*, **163**, 830–836.

Young, H., Moyes, A., McMillan, A. *et al.* (1991) Enzyme immunoassay for anti-treponemal IgG: screening or confirmatory tests? *Journal of Clinical Pathology*, **45**, 37–41.

Zenker, P.N. and Berman S.M. (1991) Congenital syphilis: trends and recommendations for evaluation and management. *Pediatric Infectious Diseases* **10**, 516–522.

22a

LEPTOSPIROSIS

P. N. Levett

INTRODUCTION

Leptospirosis is a zoonosis caused by infection with *Leptospira interrogans*. The most severe manifestation of leptospirosis is the syndrome of multi-organ infection known as Weil's disease, first described by Adolf Weil in Heidelberg in 1886. Weil described an infectious disease with jaundice and nephritis. Earlier descriptions of diseases that were probably leptospirosis were reviewed recently (Faine, 1994). The aetiology of leptospirosis was demonstrated independently in 1915 by Inada and Ido, who detected both spirochaetes and specific antibodies, in the blood of Japanese miners with infectious jaundice and by Uhlenhuth and Fromme, who detected spirochaetes in the blood of German soldiers afflicted by 'French disease' while in the trenches (Gsell, 1984). The importance of occupation as a risk factor was recognized early and the role of the rat as a source of human infection was discovered in 1917, whereas the potential for leptospiral disease in dogs and in livestock was not recognized until the 1930s and 1940s.

CLASSIFICATION

Definition

Leptospires are tightly coiled spirochaetes, usually 0.1 μm $\times$ 6–20 μm, but occasional cultures may contain much longer cells. The cells have pointed ends, either or both of which are usually bent into a distinctive hook (Figure 22a.1). Morphologically all leptospires are indistinguishable. They have Gram-negative cell wall structure and may be stained using carbol fuchsin counterstain (Faine, 1994).

Leptospires are obligate aerobes with an optimum growth temperature of 28–30 °C. They grow in simple media enriched with vitamins (vitamins B2 and B12 are growth factors), long-chain fatty acids and ammonium salts (Johnson and Faine, 1984). Growth of leptospires is often slow on first isolation and cultures are retained for up to 13 weeks before being discarded, but pure subcultures in liquid media usually grow within 10–14 days.

Species

Traditionally the genus has been divided into two

Principles and Practice of Clinical Bacteriology. Edited by A.M. Emmerson, P.M. Hawkey and S.H. Gillespie
© 1997 John Wiley & Sons Ltd

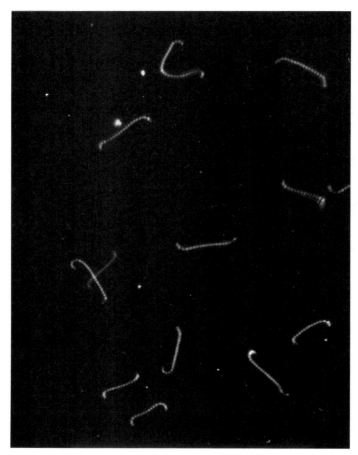

Figure 22a.1. Leptospires viewed by dark-field microscopy (magnification approx. ×1300). (Reproduced with permission from Faine, 1994.)

species: *L. interrogans*, comprising all pathogenic strains, and *L. biflexa*, containing the saprophytic strains isolated from the environment (Johnson and Faine, 1984). *Leptospira biflexa* can be differentiated from *L. interrogans* by the growth of the former at 13 °C, and growth in the presence of 8-azaguanine (225 μg/ml) and by the failure of *L. biflexa* to form spherical cells in 1M NaCl.

Serovars

Both *L. interrogans* and *L. biflexa* are divided into numerous serovars by agglutination and cross-agglutinin adsorption (Johnson and Faine, 1984; Kmety and Dikken, 1993). Antigenically related serovars are grouped into serogroups. Over 60 serovars of *L. biflexa* were recorded by Johnson and Faine (1984). Within the species *L. interrogans* are recognized over 200 serovars, which are organized into 23 serogroups (Kmety and Dikken, 1993). Further serovars have been isolated but have yet to be validly published. The serogroups of *L. interrogans* and some common serovars are shown in Table 22a.1.

Molecular Classification

The phenotypic classification of leptospires has been replaced by a genotypic one, in which 10 species of *Leptospira* were defined by DNA hybridization studies (Yasuda *et al.*, 1987). The 10 genospecies do not correspond to the previous two (*L. interrogans* and *L. biflexa*) and indeed pathogenic and non-pathogenic serovars occur within the same species (Table 22a.2). A further genospecies, *L. kirschneri*, was added by Ramadass *et al.* (1992). While the reclassification of leptospires on genotypic grounds is taxonomically correct, it is incompatible with the system of serogroups which has served clinicians and epidemiologists well for many years. A major

problem with the genotypic classification is that it is based currently upon examination of only a few hundred strains. Many serovars studied have been represented by only single reference strains, and as more strains are studied, it is probable that the number of species will increase further. At present neither serogroup nor serovar reliably

TABLE 22a.1 SEROGROUPS AND SOME SEROVARS OF *LEPTOSPIRA INTERROGANS*

Serogroup	Serovars
Icterohaemorrhagiae	*icterohaemorrhagiae*
	copenhageni
	lai
	zimbabwe
Hebdomadis	*hebdomadis*
	jules
	kremastos
Autumnalis	*autumnalis*
	fortbragg
	weerasinghe
Pyrogenes	*pyrogenes*
Bataviae	*bataviae*
Grippotyphosa	*grippotyphosa*
	canalzonae
	ratnapura
Canicola	*canicola*
Australis	*australis*
	lora
	bratislava
Pomona	*pomona*
Javanica	*javanica*
Sejroe	*sejroe*
	saxkoebing
	hardjo
Cynopteri	*cynopteri*
Djasiman	*djasiman*
Sarmin	*sarmin*
Mini	*mini*
	georgia
Tarassovi	*tarassovi*
Ballum	*ballum*
	arborea
Celledoni	*celledoni*
Louisiana	*louisiana*
	lanka
Panama	*panama*
	mangus
Ranarum	*ranarum*
Manhao	*manhao*
Shermani	*shermani*

TABLE 22a.2 GENOSPECIES OF *LEPTOSPIRA* AND DISTRIBUTION OF SEROGROUPS

Species	Includes some serovars of serogroup
L. interrogans	Icterohaemorrhagiae[a]
	Canicola
	Pomona[a]
	Australis[a]
	Autumnalis[a]
	Pyrogenesa[a]
	Grippotyphosa[a]
	Djasiman
	Hebdomadis[a]
	Sejroe[a]
	Bataviae
L. noguchii	Panama
	Autumnalis[a]
	Pyrogenes[a]
	Louisiana
L. weilii	Celledoni
	Icterohaemorrhagiae[a]
	Sarmin
L. santarosai	Shermanii
	Hebdomadis[a]
	Tarassovi[a]
L. borgpetersenii	Javanica
	Ballum
	Hebdomadis[a]
	Sejroe[a]
	Tarassovi[a]
	Mini
L. meyeri[c]	Ranarum
	Semaranga[a,b]
L. wolbachii[c]	Codice[b]
L. inadai	Serovar *lyme*
L. biflexa[c]	Semaranga[a,b]
L. parva[c]	Serovar *parva*[b]
L. kirschneri	Grippotyphosa[a]
	Autumnalis[a]
	Cynopteri
	Hebdomadis[a]
	Australis[a]
	Pomona[a]

[a] Serovars of these serogroups are found within two or more genospecies.
[b] Serogroups Semaranga and Codice comprise non-pathogenic leptospires, as does serovar *Parva*.
[c] *L. wolbachii*, *L. biflexa* and *L. parva* are species which consist currently of non-pathogenic strains only. *L. meyeri* consists of both pathogenic strains and non-pathogenic strains.

predicts the species of *Leptospira*. DNA hybridization is available in relatively few research laboratories and it is certainly necessary for clinical microbiologists to retain the serological classification of pathogenic leptospires for the foreseeable future.

EPIDEMIOLOGY

Geographical Distribution

Leptospirosis is probably the most widespread zoonosis in the world. The source of infection in humans is usually either direct or indirect contact with the urine of an infected animal. The incidence is very much higher in warm-climate countries than in the temperate regions. This is due mainly to longer survival of leptospires in damp soil with high humidity at ambient temperatures of 25°–30°C, and at a slightly alkaline pH. However, contributing factors include greater opportunities for exposure of the human population to infected animals, whether livestock, domestic pets, wild or feral animals.

Routes of Transmission

The usual portal of entry is intact skin or conjunctiva, or through abrasions or cuts in the skin. Water-borne transmission has been documented; point contamination of water supplies has resulted in several outbreaks of leptospirosis. Inhalation of water or aerosols also may result in infection via the respiratory tract.

Life Cycle

Animals, including man, can be divided into maintenance hosts or accidental (incidental) hosts. A maintenance host is a species in which infection is endemic, usually transferred from animal to animal by direct contact. Other animals (such as man) may become infected by indirect contact with the maintenance host. The most important maintenance hosts are rodents, which may transfer infection to domestic farm animals, dogs and man. The extent to which infection is transmitted depends upon many factors, which include climate, population densities, and the degree of contact between maintenance and accidental hosts. Different rodent species may be reservoirs of distinct serovars, but rats are generally maintenance hosts for serovars *copenhageni* or *ballum*. Domestic animals are also maintenance hosts; dairy cattle may harbour *hardjo* and *pomona*, pigs *pomona*, *tarassovi* or *bratislava*, and dogs usually *canicola*. Distinct variations in maintenance hosts and serovars occur throughout the world.

Occupational Exposure

Occupation is a significant risk factor for humans. Direct contact with infected animals accounts for most infections in farmers, veterinarians, abattoir workers and meat inspectors, while indirect contact is important for sewer workers, miners, soldiers, septic tank cleaners, fish-farmers, rice field workers and sugar-cane cutters. There is a significant risk associated with recreational exposures occurring in water-sports, including fresh-water fishing.

Epidemiological Patterns

Faine (1994) defined three epidemiological patterns of leptospirosis. Group I involves temperate climate farming of cattle and pigs. Here there are few serovars involved and human infection is almost invariably by direct contact. Control by immunization of animals and/or humans is potentially possible. Tropical wet areas represent group II, within which there are many more serovars infecting humans and animals, and larger numbers of reservoir species, including rodents, farm animals and dogs. Human exposure is not limited by occupation. Control of rodent populations, drainage of wet areas and occupational hygiene are all necessary for prevention of human leptospirosis. Group III comprises rodent-borne infection in the urban environment. While this is of lesser significance throughout most of the world, it is potentially more important when the urban infrastructure is disrupted by war or by natural disasters.

CLINICAL FEATURES

Leptospirosis has been described as a 'zoonosis of protean manifestations' (Peter, 1982). The spectrum of symptoms is extremely broad; the classical syndrome of Weil's disease represents only the most severe presentation. Formerly it was considered that distinct clinical syndromes were associated with specific serogroups. However, more intense study over the past 30 years has led to this hypothesis being questioned. An explanation for many of the observed associations may be found in the ecology of the maintenance animal hosts in a geographical region. A region with a richly varied fauna will support a greater variety of serogroups than will a region with few animal hosts. In humans, severe leptospirosis is frequently, but not invariably, caused by serovars of the Icterohaemorrhagiae serogroup. The specific serovars involved depend largely on the geographical location and the ecology of local maintenance hosts. Thus, in Europe *copenhageni* and *icterohaemorrhagiae* are usually responsible, while in Southeast Asia serovar *lai* is common.

Natural History

The clinical presentation of leptospirosis is biphasic (Figure 22a.2), the acute, or septicaemic, phase lasting about a week, and being followed by the immune phase, characterized by antibody production and excretion of leptospires in the urine (Turner, 1967; Pritchard, 1990). Most of the complications of leptospirosis are associated with localization of leptospires within the tissues during the immune phase, and thus occur during the second week of the illness.

The great majority of infections are either subclinical or of very mild severity and will probably not be brought to medical attention. A smaller proportion of infections, but the overwhelming majority of the recognized cases, will present with a febrile illness of sudden onset, the symptoms of which include chills, headache, myalgia, abdominal pain, conjunctival suffusion and less often a skin rash (Table 22a.3).

TABLE 22a.3 SYMPTOMS ON ADMISSION IN 88 PATIENTS WITH SEVERE LEPTOSPIROSIS (EDWARDS *ET AL.*, 1990) AND 150 ANICTERIC PATIENTS (BERMAN *ET AL.*, 1973)

Symptom	Prevalence in leptospirosis (%)	
	Severe	Anicteric
Jaundice	95	1.5
Fever	85	97
Anorexia	85	–
Headache	76	98
Conjunctival suffusion	54	42
Vomiting	50	33
Myalgia	49	79
Abdominal pain	43	28
Nausea	37	41
Dehydration	37	–
Cough	32	20
Hepatomegaly	27	15
Lymphadenopathy	21	21
Diarrhoea	14	29
Rash	2	7

Anicteric leptospirosis

This anicteric syndrome usually lasts for about a week, and its resolution coincides with the appearance of antibodies. The fever may be biphasic and may recur after a remission of three to four days. The headache is often intense, resembling that which occurs in dengue, with retro-orbital pain and photophobia. Aseptic meningitis may be found in ≤25% of all leptospirosis cases, and may account for a significant minority of all causes of aseptic meningitis. Mortality is almost nil in anicteric leptospirosis.

The differential diagnosis must include common viral infections, such as influenza, and in the tropics, dengue, in addition to the bacterial causes of PUO (pyrexia of uncertain origin), such as typhoid. Turner (1967) provided a comprehensive list of other conditions that may be mimicked by leptospirosis, including encephalitis, poliomyelitis, rickettsiosis, glandular fever, brucellosis, malaria, viral hepatitis and pneumonitis.

Icteric leptospirosis

Icteric leptospirosis is a much more severe disease, in which the clinical course is often very rapidly

682

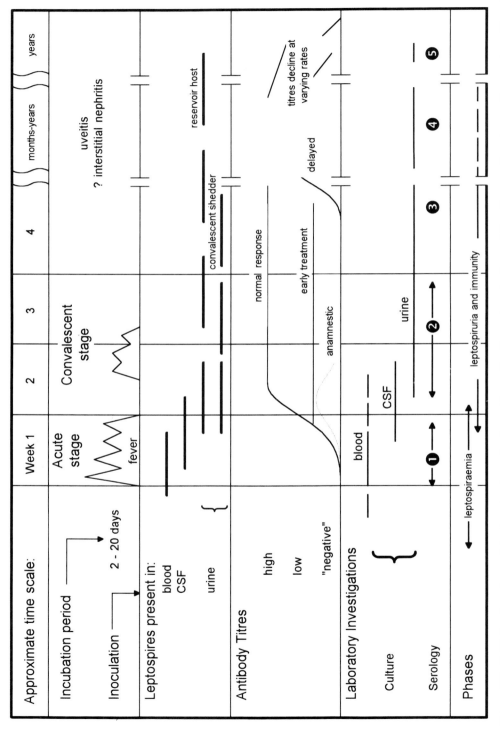

Figure 22a.2. Biphasic nature of leptospirosis and relevant investigations at each stage of the disease. Specimens for serology ❶ and ❷ are acute specimens, ❸ is a convalescent sample which may facilitate detection of a delayed immune response, and ❹ and ❺ are follow-up samples which can provide epidemiological information, such as the presumptive infecting serogroup. (Redrawn with permission from Turner, L.H., *British Medical Journal*, 1969 i, 231–235.)

progressive. Severe cases often present late in the course of the disease, and this contributes to the high mortality rate, which ranges between 5% and 15%. Between 5% and 10% of all patients with leptospirosis have the icteric form of the disease (Heath *et al.*, 1965). In a series of 88 patients with severe leptospirosis confirmed by laboratory investigation, reported by Edwards *et al.* (1990), jaundice was the most common symptom (Table 22a.3), followed by fever, anorexia and headache. Conjunctival suffusion was apparent in over half the patients, but a rash was noted in only 2%.

The jaundice occurring in leptospirosis is not associated with hepatocellular necrosis and liver function returns to normal after recovery. Serum bilirubin concentration may be high; in the series reported by Edwards *et al.* (1990) the mean bilirubin concentration was 138 μmol/l and more than five weeks were required for the concentration to fall to within normal limits. There were moderate rises in transaminase concentrations and minor elevation of the alkaline phosphatase concentration usually occurs.

Complications

The complications of severe leptospirosis emphasize the multi-systemic nature of the disease. Leptospirosis is a common cause of acute renal failure (ARF), which occurs in 16–40% of cases (Ramachandran *et al.*, 1976; Winearls *et al.*, 1984; Edwards *et al.*, 1990). A distinction may be made between patients with prerenal azotaemia (non-ARF) and those with ARF. Plasma creatinine concentrations often exceed 600 μmol/l in patients with ARF, while those with prerenal azotaemia have significantly lower levels (Nicholson *et al.*, 1989). Selection of patients requiring dialysis urgently may be based upon a urine : plasma urea ratio of <7 and a urine : plasma osmolar ratio of <1.2. Patients with higher ratios have prerenal azotaemia and should be rehydrated; decisions regarding dialysis can be delayed for up to 72 hours (Nicholson *et al.*, 1989).

Thrombocytopenia (platelet count $<100 \times 10^9/l$) occurs in $\geqslant 50\%$ of cases and is a significant predictor for the development of ARF (Edwards *et al.*, 1982). However, thrombocytopenia in leptospirosis is transient and does not result from disseminated intravascular coagulation (Edwards *et al.*, 1986). Adult respiratory distress syndrome (Ramachandran and Perera, 1977) is another common complication. Serum amylase levels are often raised significantly, but pancreatitis is not a common finding (Edwards and Everard, 1991).

Rare complications include cerebrovascular accidents (Lessa and Cortes, 1981; Forwell *et al.*, 1984), rhabdomyolysis (Solbrig *et al.*, 1987), pulmonary haemorrhage and Guillain–Barré syndrome. Anterior uveitis, usually bilateral, occurs after recovery from the acute illness in a minority of cases (Barkay and Garzozi, 1984). Uveitis may present weeks, months, or occasionally years after the acute stage. The incidence of ocular complications is variable, but this probably reflects the long time-scale over which they may occur. In the USA the incidence was estimated at 3% (Heath *et al.*, 1965). Late-onset uveitis may result from an autoimmune reaction to subsequent exposure (Faine, 1994).

Mortality

Fatality in severe leptospirosis often follows cardiac arrest, resulting from the development of interstitial myocarditis, pericarditis and arrhythmias (Ramachandran and Perera, 1977; Lee *et al.*, 1986). These complications occur in $\leqslant 30\%$ of patients, and are more common in older patients.

Leptospirosis during pregnancy has been shown to cause fetal infection and death, but only a handful of cases have been reported (Faine *et al.*, 1984).

LABORATORY DIAGNOSIS

Leptospiral diagnosis depends heavily upon serological detection of specific antibodies, but the available assays can be both tedious to perform and difficult to interpret, since many pathogenic serovars exhibit considerable serological cross-reaction. A definitive identification of the infecting serovar is possible only if an isolate is obtained from blood, urine, cerebrospinal fluid (CSF) or other specimen during the acute illness. The selection of appropriate specimens is dependent on the stage of the disease, and therefore an adequate history is essential, with particular attention to the duration of symptoms.

Microscopy

Blood, urine, CSF and other specimens may be examined directly by dark-ground microscopy. However, the sensitivity of microscopy is relatively low. Using a double centrifugation method Wolff (1954) was able to detect leptospires in the blood of only 32% of culture-positive patients. Specificity of microscopy may also be low, since many artifacts may be mistaken for leptospires.

Histopathology

Detection by histology depends upon the demonstration of spirochaetes by silver-staining, using stains such as the modified Warthin–Starry. This approach is not specific for leptospires and should be confirmed by another method.

Specific demonstration of leptospires in tissues can be achieved by immunofluorescence staining (Ellis et al., 1982). Pooled antisera to a range of serogroups conjugated to fluorescein are used to stain frozen sections of tissues such as brain, liver, kidneys, heart and pancreas obtained at autopsy. Placentas from aborting animals can be examined by the same method. Leptospires undergo lysis relatively rapidly and the optimum time for autopsy is within 24 hours of death. Interpretation of IF staining requires great expertise since intact leptospires are seldom seen and both artifacts and high levels of background staining occur.

Culture

Media

Leptospires grow in simple media, to which either serum or albumin and Tween are added (Faine, 1994). Numerous media containing serum have been described and these were reviewed by Turner (1970). Such media include those of Fletcher,

Korthof, Stuart and Ellinghausen. Pooled rabbit serum, rich in vitamin B12, is usually employed.

The most widely used medium for isolation of human leptospires is EMJH, based on the medium developed by Ellinghausen and McCullough (1965) and its modification by Johnson and Harris (1967). This is a serum-free medium, containing Tween 80 and bovine serum albumin fraction V. 5-Fluorouracil (5-FU) may be added to inhibit growth of contaminants (Johnson and Rogers, 1964). EMJH and EMJH + 5-FU are dispensed in 10 ml volumes in universal bottles with septate caps.

Inoculation

During the first (leptospiraemic) phase of the disease, cultures of blood in EMJH are made at the patient's bedside, by injecting one drop of blood into the bottle. Specimens which may be contaminated, such as urine, or contaminated cultures, may be filtered using a 0.22 μm filter before inoculation.

Incubation

Cultures are incubated at 28–30 °C in an aerobic atmosphere. Low-power ($\times 100$–200) dark-ground microscopy is used to examine cultures twice weekly for six weeks, and then weekly for up to 13 weeks before cultures are discarded. Positive cultures are subcultured to duplicate bottles of fresh EMJH medium for growth for identification and for storage.

Molecular typing

Restriction endonuclease analysis (REA) has been used to differentiate genotypes within antigenically homogeneous serovars. Thus, within serovar hardjo, two genotypes, hardjobovis and hardjoprajitno, are recognized. However, the complex patterns produced by REA can be difficult to interpret. Restriction fragment length polymorphism (RFLP) analysis of DNA (ribotyping) is simpler to interpret and has given similar results to REA. Pulsed-field gel electrophoresis (PFGE) following digestion of whole chromosomal DNA by *Not*1 also yields results which distinguish individual serovars. However, the technical complexity of PFGE may limit its wider application.

More recently, polymerase chain reaction (PCR)-based methods have been applied to the typing of leptospires, including RAPD, AP–PCR, PCR–REA, PCR–MRSP and LSSP–PCR (Perolat *et al.*, 1994; Savio *et al.*, 1994). These approaches generate mixtures of products which can be separated by electrophoresis and which may allow serogroup or serovar identification, as well as strain differentiation, thereby facilitating epidemiological investigations. Of particular significance is the potential for some methods (such as PCR–REA and LSSP–PCR), which retain the use of specific primers, to be applied directly to DNA derived from clinical material, without the necessity of first isolating leptospires in culture.

Serology

Serology is the usual means of diagnosis in most cases of leptospirosis. However, antibodies do not appear in the blood until the end of the first week of the disease (Figure 22a.1) and the diagnosis is, thus, often retrospective.

Microscopic agglutination test

The reference method for serological diagnosis of leptospirosis is the microscopic agglutination test (MAT or LMAT), performed on paired sera, usually taken a minimum of three days apart. Patients' sera are reacted with live antigen suspensions of leptospiral serovars. The range of antigens used should include all serogroups and all locally common serovars. After incubation the serum/antigen mixtures are examined microscopically for agglutination and the titres are determined.

The MAT is a complex test to control, perform and interpret. Live cultures of all the serovars must be maintained. Interpretation of the MAT is complicated by the high degree of cross-reaction that occurs between different serogroups, especially in acute-phase samples. This is to some extent predictable, thus patients often have similar

titres to all serovars of an individual serogroup, but 'paradoxical' reactions, in which the highest titres are detected to a serogroup unrelated to the infecting one, are also common.

Acute infection is suggested by a single titre of ⩾800, and confirmed by a four-fold or greater rise in titre between paired sera. Titres following acute infection may be extremely high (⩾25 600) and may take months, or even years, to fall to low levels. Often, it becomes possible to distinguish a predominant serogroup only months after infection, as cross-reacting titres decline at different rates. It is important, therefore, to examine several sera taken at monthly intervals after the acute disease, in order to determine the infecting serogroup.

Some patients are found to have serological evidence of previous infection with a different leptospiral serovar. In these cases, serological diagnosis is complicated further by the 'anamnestic response', in which the first rise in antibody titre is usually directed against the infecting serovar from the previous exposure. Only later does it become possible to identify the serovar or serogroup responsible for the current infection, as the titre of specific antibody rises. Paradoxical reactions also occur in patients who have such infections, and interpretation of serology is even further complicated.

Formalized, freeze-dried antigens have been used in the MAT, in order to overcome some of the difficulties associated with the use of live antigens. Titres obtained with these antigens appear to be somewhat lower, and more cross-reactions are detected. However, for laboratories without the staff or expertise to maintain live antigens, such lyophilized antigens may represent a good alternative.

Other Serological Tests

Because of the complexity of the MAT, rapid screening tests for leptospiral antibodies have been developed as an aid to presumptive diagnosis. Such tests are genus specific and the methods used have included complement fixation, slide agglutination, counter-immunoelectrophoresis (CIE), enzyme-linked immunosorbent assay (ELISA), indirect haemagglutination (IHA) and microcapsule agglutination (MCA). Many methods have been described but relatively few have found widespread use in diagnostic laboratories.

Slide agglutination test

The simplest of the methods remaining in use is the macroscopic slide agglutination test (Galton *et al.*, 1958; Mazzonelli *et al.*, 1974). Formalin-killed suspensions of leptospires are mixed with patient's serum and then rotated for 4 minutes. Agglutination is scored on a scale of 0–4. A prozone phenomenon has been observed and negative sera should be diluted 1 : 5 and retested. Several antigens are used, including common pathogenic serogroups of *L. interrogans* (such as Icterohaemorrhagiae, Autumnalis, Australis, Ballum and Canicola) and the non-pathogenic Patoc strain of *L. biflexa*.

A positive slide agglutination test indicates the presence in serum of genus-specific leptospiral agglutinins. The presence of such antibodies indicates exposure to leptospires but is not necessarily diagnostic of current infection. However, a reaction with all antigens tested is more strongly suggestive of infection than a reaction with one or two antigens only. The slide test may be negative early in the course of acute infection; indeed it may never become positive if the patient dies of fulminating leptospirosis. A reaction in the slide test with one or more antigens indicates the need for further, more specific investigations. However, a patient in whom there is a strong clinical suspicion of leptospirosis should be investigated further regardless of the slide agglutination result.

In areas where leptospirosis is common (as in tropical countries) the slide agglutination test has a low specificity because of the high prevalence of antibodies in the population. Moreover the slide test is quite often negative in patients who have antibodies detectable by ELISA.

Enzyme-linked immunosorbent assay

Several methods for the use of ELISA have been described. Antigens used have included single serovars such as Icterohaemorrhagiae or Copenhageni or combinations of serovars. The Patoc strain of *L. biflexa* has also been employed, in order to give a genus-specific ELISA. Titres vary slightly depending upon the antigen and the infecting serovar, but an IgM titre of $\geqslant 80$ suggests a current or recent infection, while a similar or higher IgG titre on its own indicates past infection. In acute infection, IgM titres often rise much higher ($\geqslant 1280$ is quite common). Lower titres (<80) may be non-specific and a second specimen is required to detect a rise in titre. A high IgM titre also indicates the necessity for a convalescent specimen to be taken 10–14 days after the acute sample. In either case a four-fold or greater rise in titre of IgM or IgG is considered diagnostic.

Other serological tests

The indirect haemagglutination assay (IHA) uses human type O erythrocytes sensitized with ethanol-extracted antigen from *L. biflexa* Patoc. A titre of $\geqslant 100$ indicates active or recent leptospirosis. A one-point microcapsule agglutination (MCA) test uses a synthetic polymer sensitized with a mixture of serovars; antibodies may be detectable by MCA slightly earlier than by ELISA (Seki *et al.*, 1987). Both IHA and MCA tests are available commercially.

Molecular Methods of Diagnosis

Polymerase chain reaction

Several primer sets have been described for use in PCR (Van Eys *et al.*, 1989; Gravekamp *et al.*, 1991, 1993; Hookey, 1992; Mérien *et al.*, 1992), together with specific DNA probes. PCR has been found useful in confirming a diagnosis of leptospirosis, particularly in severe disease, when patients may die before seroconversion occurs (Figure 22a.3). Blood, urine, CSF, dialysate fluid and postmortem tissues have all been used as sources of leptospiral DNA (Brown *et al.*, 1995). Prolonged excretion of leptospires in urine has been demonstrated by PCR (Bal *et al.*, 1994).

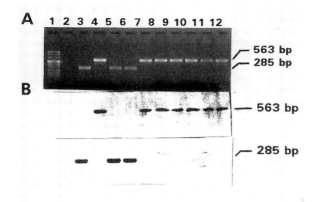

Figure 22a.3. Agarose gel electrophoresis (A) and Southern blot (B) analyses of PCR-amplified DNA extracted from serum and urine samples and amplified with primers G1/G2 (285 bp product) or B64-I/B64-II (563 bp product). Lane 1: molecular weight marker VIII (Boehringer Mannheim); 2: water blank; 3: DNA from serovar *copenhageni* amplified with G1/G2; 4: DNA from serovar *bim* amplified with B64-I/B64-II; 5 and 6: DNA from samples amplified with G1/G2; 7–12: DNA from samples amplified with B64-I/B64-II. Southern blot hybridization at 55 °C with DIG-tailed oligonucleotide probes. (Reproduced with permission from Brown, P.D. *et al.*, *Journal of Medical Microbiology*, 1995, **43**, 110–114).

MANAGEMENT

Treatment of leptospirosis is dependent upon the severity and duration of symptoms at the time of presentation. Patients with mild, flu-like symptoms require only symptomatic treatment, but should be cautioned to seek further medical help if they become jaundiced. Patients who present with more severe anicteric leptospirosis will require hospital admission and close observation. If the headache is particularly severe a lumbar puncture usually produces a dramatic improvement.

Icteric Leptospirosis

The management of icteric leptospirosis requires admission of the patient to the intensive care unit (ICU) initially. Patients with prerenal azotaemia can be rehydrated for the first two to three days while their renal function is observed, but patients in acute renal failure require dialysis as a matter of urgency. This is accomplished satisfactorily by peritoneal dialysis (Grell *et al.*, 1971). Cardiac monitoring is also desirable during the first few days after admission.

Antibiotics

The role of antibiotics in the management of leptospirosis is still contentious, despite numerous reports of their use. However, few well-designed and controlled studies have been reported. A major difficulty in assessing the efficacy of antibiotic treatment results from the late presentation of many patients with severe disease, after the leptospires have localized in the tissues.

Doxycycline (100 mg b.d.s. for seven days) was shown to reduce the duration and severity of illness in anicteric leptospirosis by an average of two days (McClain *et al.*, 1984). Patients with severe disease were excluded from this study.

Two randomized studies of penicillin produced conflicting results. One study included 42 patients with severe leptospirosis, of whom 19 were jaundiced (Watt *et al.*, 1988). No patients required dialysis and there were no deaths. Intravenous penicillin was given at a dosage of 6 MUnits/day for seven days and was found to halve the duration of fever. A second study included 79 patients with icteric leptospirosis, of whom four died (Edwards *et al.*, 1988). Patients in the treatment group received intravenous penicillin at a dosage of 8 MUnits/day for five days. No difference was observed between treatment and control groups in outcome or duration of the illness.

One consistent finding of these studies has been the prevention of leptospiruria or a significant reduction in its duration by antibiotic therapy (McClain *et al.*, 1984; Edwards *et al.*, 1988; Watt *et al.*, 1988). This finding alone is sufficient justification for antibiotic use, but any antibiotic treatment should be started as early as possible, and should be regarded as an adjunct to other therapeutic approaches.

CONTROL

Control and prevention of leptospirosis in humans are inextricably linked with the control of animal reservoirs. The most efficient approaches to control in a given geographical location depend upon the epidemiological pattern present, as discussed by Faine (1994). The epidemiology of leptospirosis may be altered markedly by changing agricultural and cultural practices. The necessity for continued surveillance of human and veterinary leptospirosis should be emphasized.

Immunity to leptospirosis results from the humoral response to lipopolysaccharide. Protective antibody is detectable by serology using the MAT. Immunity is serovar specific, with some serogroup cross-reaction. Thus vaccines must be prepared using locally prevalent serovars. Modern vaccines are killed suspensions of whole cells grown in protein-free medium. Usually two doses are given, followed by annual booster injections.

Immunization of animals may be practised in countries with a group I epidemiological pattern (see above), both for economic reasons and to prevent infection of humans. Cattle are often immunized against serovars Hardjo and Pomona, while pigs may be immunized against Pomona, Tarassovi and Bratislava. Canine vaccines usually include Icterohaemorrhagiae and Canicola. Vaccines are used in some subjects at high risk of acquiring leptospirosis. Widespread human use of vaccines has been restricted to China, Japan and some other Southeast Asian countries, and has been effective in controlling epidemics, particularly in rice-field workers.

ACKNOWLEDGEMENTS

I wish to thank my colleagues Dr C.N. Edwards, G.D. Nicholson and Dr C.O.R. Everard, for their helpful comments, and the staff and students of the Barbados Leptospira Laboratory for their support.

REFERENCES

Bal, A.E., Gravekamp, C., Hartskeerl, R.A. *et al.* (1994) Detection of leptospires in urine by PCR for early diagnosis of leptospirosis. *Journal of Clinical Microbiology*, **32**, 1894–1898.

Barkay, S. and Garzozi, H. (1984) Leptospirosis and uveitis. *Annals of Ophthalmology*, **16**, 164–168.

Berman, S.J., Tsai, C.C., Holmes, K.K. *et al.* (1973) Sporadic anicteric leptospirosis in South Vietnam. *Annals of Internal Medicine*, **79**, 167–173.

Brown, P.D., Gravekamp, C., Carrington, D.G. *et al.* (1995) Evaluation of the polymerase chain reaction for early diagnosis of leptospirosis. *Journal of Medical Microbiology*, **43**, 110–114.

Edwards, C.N and Everard, C.O.R. (1991) Hyperamylasemia and pancreatitis in leptospirosis. *American Journal of Gastroenterology*, **86**, 1665–1668.

Edwards, C.N., Nicholson, G.D. and Everard, C.O.R. (1982) Thrombocytopenia in leptospirosis. *American Journal of Tropical Medicine and Hygiene*, **31**, 827–829.

Edwards, C.N., Nicholson, G.D., Hassell, T.A. *et al.* (1986) Thrombocytopenia in leptospirosis: the absence of evidence for disseminated intravascular coagulation. *American Journal of Tropical Medicine and Hygiene*, **35**, 352–354.

Edwards, C.N., Nicholson, G.D., Hassell, T.A. *et al.* (1988) Penicillin therapy in icteric leptospirosis. *American Journal of Tropical Medicine and Hygiene*, **39**, 388–390.

Edwards, C.N., Nicholson, G.D., Hassell, T.A. *et al.* (1990) Leptospirosis in Barbados: a clinical study. *West Indian Medical Journal*, **39**, 27–34.

Ellinghausen, H.C. and McCullough, W.G. (1965) Nutrition of *Leptospira pomona* and growth of 13 other serotypes: fractionation of oleic albumin complex and a medium of bovine albumin and polysorbate 80. *American Journal of Veterinary Research* **26**, 45–51.

Ellis, W.A., O'Brien, J.J., Neill, S.D. *et al.* (1982) Bovine leptospirosis: microbiological and serological findings in aborted fetuses. *Veterinary Record*, **110**, 147–150.

Faine, S. (1994) *Leptospira and Leptospirosis*. CRC Press, Boca Raton, FL.

Faine, S., Adler, B., Christopher, W. *et al.* (1984) Fatal congenital human leptospirosis. *Zentralblatt für Bakteriologie, Mikrobiologie und Hygiene series A*, **257**, 548.

Forwell, M.A., Redding, P.J., Brodie, M.J. *et al.* (1984) Leptospirosis complicated by fatal intracerebral haemorrhage. *British Medical Journal*, **289**, 1583.

Galton, M.M., Powers, D.K., Hall, A.M. *et al.* (1958) A rapid microscopic-slide screening test for the serodiagnosis of leptospirosis. *American Journal of Veterinary Research*, **19**, 505–512.

Gravekamp, C., van de Kemp, H., Carrington, D. *et al.* (1991) Detection of leptospiral DNA by PCR in serum from patients with *copenhageni* infections. In

Leptospirosis (ed. Y. Kobayashi), pp. 151–164. University of Tokyo Press, Tokyo.

Gravekamp, C., van de Kemp, H., Franzen, M. *et al.* (1993) Detection of seven species of pathogenic leptospires by PCR using two sets of primers. *Journal of General Microbiology*, **139**, 1691–1700.

Grell G., Ho-Ping-Kong, H., Ragbeer, M.M.S. *et al.* (1971) Peritoneal dialysis in severe leptospiral renal failure. *West Indian Medical Journal*, **20**, 76–82.

Gsell, O. (1984) The history of leptospirosis: 100 years. *Zentralblatt für Bakteriologie, Mikrobiologie und Hygiene series A*, **257**, 473–478.

Heath, C.W., Alexander, A.D. and Galton, M.M. (1965) Leptospirosis in the United States. *New England Journal of Medicine*, **273**, 857–864, 915–922.

Hookey, J.V. (1992) Detection of Leptospiraceae by amplification of 16S ribosomal DNA. *FEMS Microbiology Letters*, **90**, 267–274.

Johnson, R.C. and Faine, S. (1984) *Leptospira*. In *Bergey's Manual of Systematic Bacteriology*, Vol. 1 (ed. N.R. Krieg and J.G. Holt), pp. 62–67. Williams & Wilkins, Baltimore.

Johnson, R.C. and Harris, V.G. (1967) Differentiation of pathogenic and saprophytic leptospires. I. Growth at low temperatures. *Journal of Bacteriology*, **94**, 27–31.

Johnson, R.C. and Rogers, P. (1964) 5-Fluorouracil as a selective agent for growth of leptospirae. *Journal of Bacteriology*, **87**, 422–426.

Kmety, E. and Dikken, H. (1993) *Classification of the Species* Leptospira interrogans *and History of its Serovars*. University Press Groningen, Groningen.

Lee, M.G., Char, G., Dianzumba, S. *et al.* (1986) Cardiac involvement in severe leptospirosis. *West Indian Medical Journal*, **35**, 295–300.

Lessa, I. and Cortes, E. (1981) Cerebrovascular accident as a complication of leptospirosis. *Lancet*, **ii**, 1113.

Mazzonelli, J., Dorta de Mazzonelli, G. and Mailloux, M. (1974) Possibilité de diagnostique sérologique macroscopique des leptospires à l'aide d'un antigène unique. *Médecine et Maladies Infectieuses*, **4**, 253–254.

McClain, J.B.L., Ballou, W.R., Harrison, S.M. *et al.* (1984) Doxycycline therapy for leptospirosis. *Annals of Internal Medicine*, **100**, 696–698.

Mérien, F., Amouriaux, P., Perolat, P. *et al.* (1992) Polymerase chain reaction for detection of *Leptospira* spp. in clinical samples. *Journal of Clinical Microbiology*, **30**, 2219–2224.

Nicholson, G.D., Edwards, C.N., Hassell, T.A. *et al.* (1989) Urinary diagnostic indices in the management of leptospirosis. *West Indian Medical Journal*, **38**, 33–38.

Perolat, P., Mérien, F., Ellis, W.A. *et al.* (1994) Characterization of *Leptospira* isolates from serovar hardjo by ribotyping, arbitrarily primed PCR, and mapped restriction site polymorphisms. *Journal of Clinical Microbiology*, **32**, 1949–1957.

Peter, G. (1982) Leptospirosis: a zoonosis of protean manifestations. *Pediatric Infectious Disease Journal*, **1**, 282–288.

Pritchard, D.G. (1990) Spirochaetal and leptospiral diseases. In *Topley & Wilson's Principles of Bacteriology, Virology and Immunity*, 8th edn (ed. M.T. Parker and L.H. Collier), pp. 605–640. Edward Arnold, London.

Ralph, D., McClelland, M., Welsh, J. *et al.* (1993) *Leptospira* species categorized by arbitrarily primed polymerase chain reaction (PCR) and by mapped restriction polymorphisms in PCR amplified rRNA genes. *Journal of Bacteriology*, **175**, 973–981.

Ramachandran, S. and Perera, M.V.F. (1977) Cardiac and pulmonary involvement in leptospirosis. *Transactions of the Royal Society for Tropical Medicine and Hygiene*, **71**, 56–59.

Ramachandran, S., Rajapakse, C.N.A., Perera, M.V.F. *et al.* (1976) Patterns of acute renal failure in leptospirosis. *Journal of Tropical Medicine and Hygiene*, **79**, 158–160.

Ramadass, P., Jarvis, B.D.W., Corner, R.J. *et al.* (1992) Genetic characterization of pathogenic *Leptospira* species by DNA hybridization. *International Journal of Systematic Bacteriology*, **42**, 215–219.

Savio, M.L., Rossi, C., Fusi, P. *et al.* (1994) Detection and identification of *Leptospira interrogans* serovars by PCR coupled with restriction endonuclease analysis of amplified DNA. *Journal of Clinical Microbiology*, **32**, 935–941.

Seki, M., Sato, T., Arimitsu, Y. *et al.* (1987) One-point method for serological diagnosis of leptospirosis: a microcapsule agglutination test. *Epidemiology and Infection*, **99**, 399–405.

Solbrig, M.V., Sher, J.H. and Kula, R.W. (1987) Rhabdomyolysis in leptospirosis (Weil's disease). *Journal of Infectious Diseases*, **156**, 692–693.

Turner, L.H. (1967) Leptospirosis I. *Transactions of the Royal Society for Tropical Medicine and Hygiene*, **61**, 842–855.

Turner, L.H. (1970) Leptospirosis III. Maintenance, isolation and demonstration of leptospires. *Transactions of the Royal Society for Tropical Medicine and Hygiene*, **64**, 623–646.

Van Eys, G.J.J.M., Gravekamp, C., Gerritsen, M.J. *et al.* (1989) Detection of leptospires in urine by polymerase chain reaction. *Journal of Clinical Microbiology*, **27**, 2258–2262.

Watt, G., Padre, L.P., Tuazon, M.L. *et al.* (1988) Placebo-controlled trial of intravenous penicillin for severe and late leptospirosis. *Lancet*, **i**, 433–435.

Winearls, C.G., Chan, L., Coghlan, J.D. *et al.* (1984) Acute renal failure due to leptospirosis: clinical features and outcome in six cases. *Quarterly Journal of Medicine*, **53**, 487–495.

Wolff, J.W. (1954) *The Laboratory Diagnosis of Leptospirosis*. C.C. Thomas, Springfield, IL.

Yasuda, P.H., Steigerwalt, A.G., Sulzer, K.R. *et al.* (1987) Deoxyribonucleic acid relatedness between serogroups and serovars in the family Leptospiraceae with proposals for seven new *Leptospira* species. *International Journal of Systematic Bacteriology*, **37**, 407–415.

22b

BORRELIA BURGDORFERI

Raymond J. Dattwyler and Benjamin J. Luft

HISTORY

Infection with *Borrelia burgdorferi* is associated with a wide array of clinical manifestations. The hallmark of infection with this pathogen is erythema migrans (EM), an annular erythematous skin lesion that usually appears at the site of the tick bite. The most commonly used term for the illnesses caused by *B. burgdorferi* is 'Lyme disease'. This nomenclature originated in 1976 when Allen Steere and his colleagues noted an association between EM and a cluster of patients with knee arthritis in Old Lyme, Connecticut (Steere *et al.*, 1977). Initially they referred to this new illness as 'Lyme arthritis', but when it became apparent that the heart and nervous system could be involved, the name was changed to Lyme disease. Although any reference to Lyme disease in the literature is a recent phenomenon (<20 years), this is not a new disease. Most of the clinical features of what we now call Lyme disease, including its infectious nature, were described in the early and middle parts of the the twentieth century. EM was described by Afzelius in 1909 and the correlation between the presence of an EM and the consequent development of a range of neurological disorders was appreciated by several European investigators. In the 1930s, Hellerstrom linked EM with the development of meningitis, and in the early 1940s Bannwarth associated EM with a syndrome consisting of painful radiculopathy, limb pain and cerebrospinal fluid (CSF) pleocytosis. An association between EM, musculoskeletal complaints, and the following dermatological conditions – acrodermatitis chronicum atrophicans (ACA), lymphadenosis benigna cutis and lymphocytoma – was established in Europe by the 1940s. The first suggestion that this was a spirochetal infection came in 1948 when Lenhoff, a Swedish pathologist, observed spirochete-like structures in skin biopsies from EM lesions. With the advent of the antibiotic era, penicillin and tetracycline began to be used with success in the treatment of EM.

The first well-documented case of EM in the USA was reported by Scrimenti in 1970. Mast and Burrows reported a cluster of cases of EM in southeastern Connecticut in 1976. The first isolate of this disease-causing spirochete only occurred in 1981 when Burgdorfer and his colleagues demonstrated a new spirochete in *Ixodes* ticks collected on Shelter Island, New York (Burgdorfer *et al.*, 1982).

Principles and Practice of Clinical Bacteriology. Edited by A.M. Emmerson, P.M. Hawkey and S.H. Gillespie

EPIDEMIOLOGY

Transmission

Lyme disease is the most common vector-borne infectious disease in North America and Europe. *Ixodes* ticks, the principal vectors of *B. burgdorferi*, primarily acquire *B. burgdorferi* by feeding on infected mammals. Generally, spirochetes are carried in the tick's midgut diverticula and, to a lesser degree, systemically. For infected ticks, feeding causes an increase in the rate of spirochetal cell division in the tick's midgut diverticula and transmission may occur either by regurgitation of part of the midgut contents or via the tick's saliva once the spirochete burden has increased (Benach *et al.*, 1987). Although there is evidence to indicate transovarial passage of the organism to small numbers of filial ticks, the low prevalence of transovarial infection indicates that this phenomenon is of limited importance in the natural cycle (Bosler, 1993).

Vectors

Ixode ticks are three-stage ticks. Although all three stages of the tick can be found on various host species, not all animals are equally favoured. In general, each successive stage typically opts to feed on larger animals. Larval ticks feed preferentially on small rodents. In North America, the white-footed mouse, *Peromyscus leucopus*, is a preferred host; nymphs feed on medium-sized animals such as raccoons and squirrels as well as the mouse, and adult *Ixodes* feed mainly on larger mammals (Bosler, 1993). All stages will feed on humans (Basler *et al.*, 1983).

In Europe, and Central and Northern Asia, *B. burgdorferi* is transmitted by *Ixodes ricinus* and *Ixodes persulcatus*, respectively. Cases of Lyme disease are reported widely in Europe from Great Britain to the Ural Mountains, Asia, China and Japan. Three regions in the USA (coastal areas in the northeast, from Maryland to Massachusetts; the midwest, Wisconsin and Minnesota; and the far west, northern California, southern Oregon and western Nevada) account for the overwhelming majority of cases in North America (Steere *et al.*, 1979). These geographic areas correspond to the distribution of the primary tick vectors of Lyme disease in America: *Ixodes scapularis* in the east and midwest, and *Ixodes pacificus* in the West.

Human Infection

Surveillance of Lyme disease cases has been continuing since 1982. Currently, case reporting is mandatory in 46 states of the USA. The Centers for Disease Control and Prevention (CDC) adopted a case definition for Lyme disease in 1991 and state health departments submit weekly reports to them for publication in *Morbidity and Mortality Weekly Reports*. From these data, we find that Lyme disease affects children and adults of all age groups and sexes. There may be clustering of cases, and cases often occur near wooded areas or after exposure to wooded areas; outdoor workers may be at higher risk than indoor workers (Bowen *et al.*, 1983). Onset of illness is more common in the summer months but cases are reported throughout the year. These epidemiological characteristics are compatible with an illness caused by an infectious agent transmitted by an arthropod vector.

THE ORGANISM

Description

Borrelia burgdorferi belongs to the family Spirochaetaceae, genus *Borrelia*. Measuring approximately $10-30$ μm in length and $0.18-0.25$ μm in width, this motile, loosely coiled spirochete has a flexible helix structure. *Borrelia burgdorferi* possesses both outer cell and cytoplasmic membranes. Between these membranes there are $7-11$ flagella inserted at the ends of the spirochete (Hovind-Hougen, 1984).

At present three genospecies of *B. burgdorferi* – *B. burgdorferi* sensu stricto, *B. garinii* and *B. afzellii* – have been isolated from humans and shown to be pathogenic for man (Baranton *et al.*, 1992; Marconi and Garon, 1992). Although these three are the only ones formally named, the genetic variability of the *B. burgdorferi* species complex is huge. There are at least nine geno-species in this species complex and an unknown number of subspecies (Guy Baranton, personal communication). The other genospecies have been isolated only from either *Ixodes* ticks or mammals, other than man. In the USA, *B. burgdorferi sensu stricto* and three of the unnamed genospecies have been found in nature, whereas in Europe all three pathogenic species and two of the unnamed geno-species are circulating in a natural zoonotic cycle. *Borrelia burgdorferi sensu stricto* is the only known species to exist in both North America and Europe, suggesting recent migration. Only one genospecies is circulating in Japan. It is not yet known whether or not some of these unnamed genospecies are also pathogenic for humans. Further research into this is necessary.

Antigenic Structure

Like most bacteria *B. burgdorferi* expresses a large number of proteins. Two of the most antigenic proteins, flagellen with a molecular weight of 41 kDa and an associated 93 kDa protein, are sheathed by the outer membrane whose proteins are comparatively less immunogenic (Colman and Benach, 1989; Volkman *et al.*, 1991).

In most strains of *B. burgdorferi*, the major outer surface proteins (Osps) are plasmid encoded. Outer surface proteins A through F have been described and others may be defined in the future. However, the first three proteins OspA, OspB and OspC, are the best characterized and appear to be the most important. OspA and OspB are encoded on a 49 kb linear plasmid (Barbour and Garon, 1988) and OspC is encoded on a 28 kb circular plasmid. Organisms carrying the 49 kb linear plasmid quantitatively produce large amounts of OspA and OspB when cultured. When injected into humans or animals, these Osps produce a good humoral response. However, in natural infection, immune response to OspA and OspB develops only in a minority of patients and pri-marily later in the course of infection. Whether this represents diminished expression of these two Osps in early infection is not known. In contrast, the response to OspC tends to occur very early in the course of the infection and may diminish over time, which suggests that this protein is expressed initially.

Population Genetics

An understanding of the demographic and evolu-tionary structure of the *B. burgdorferi* species complex is important for a complete understanding of various clinical manifestations, as well as the development of effective strategies for laboratory diagnosis, disease prevention and control. Two chromosomal genes and the *ospA* gene have been sequenced (Dykhuizen *et al.*, 1993) from a num-ber of genospecies, isolated in the USA and in Europe, from both humans and ticks. A compari-son of the three gene trees shows that there has been no horizontal transfer of chromosomal genes and very little plasmid transfer within or between genospecies of the *B. burgdorferi* species com-plex. This organism evolves by differentiation of lineages (asexually) and is consequently composed of an array of clones. Thus gene trees represent clone trees and can be used to deduce population properties such as migration rate, origin and effective population size.

The distribution of genospecies suggests that the organism has had limited migration. All of 26 isolates from ticks collected at two sites in the Netherlands were *B. afzelii*, as were 57 of 58 isolates from skin of patients with EM or ACA (Van Dam *et al.*, 1988). Interestingly, the 58th isolate could not be identified as a member of any of the three known pathogenic genospecies. So even with limited migration, multiple pathogenic genotypes may exist within an area and under-estimation of unnamed genospecies which are not yet known to be pathogenic is unwise. From a locality near Millbrook, New York, all of the isolates belonged to the genospecies 25015, while isolates from ticks near this area were all *B. burg-dorferi sensu stricto* (Anderson *et al.*, 1988). Each local population appears to be comprised of a single genospecies. This information is extremely important for the development of vaccine candi-dates for Lyme disease.

Although Lyme disease has been reported from

46 states in the USA the three main foci of disease are the northeast coast, the Mississippi valley in Minnesota and Wisconsin, and northern California. The genospecies commonly found in these areas is *B. burgdorferi sensu stricto*. This genospecies is found elsewhere in the USA so there is not a perfect correlation between the presence of this genospecies and foci of disease. Genetic sequence analysis of *B. burgdorferi sensu stricto* isolates from these three endemic areas suggests that there may be considerable migration within the USA since some of the California isolates are more closely related to New York isolates than to isolates form other regions in California (Corporale *et al.*, in press). Seemingly contradictory data indicates that clones of the *B. burgdorferi* species complex are both highly mobile and yet very localized.

CLINICAL MANIFESTATIONS

Lyme disease is a progressive infectious disease with a wide array of clinical manifestations. Infection begins locally in the skin after *B. burgdorferi* is inoculated by a feeding tick. In the majority of individuals, the initial sign of infection is the development of EM, an annular erythematous skin lesion that is characteristic of this illness (Luft and Dattwyler, 1989). Hematogenous dissemination with seeding of multiple organs occurs early (Luft *et al.*, 1992). Even at this early phase of infection the clinical expression of the disease is highly variable. Some individuals are relatively asymptomatic, while others develop fever, arthralgias, myalgias, conjunctivitis, meningismus or multifocal EM lesions, and still others develop more dramatic signs of infection, including acute meningitis, myocarditis with or without conduction block abnormalities, hepatitis, myositis, or frank arthritis. The reason for the wide array of clinical manifestations is unknown, but may be related to strain variation. Between the time of acute dissemination and the onset of the manifestations of chronic disease, there is usually a disease-free interval in which the infection remains latent. Up to 50% of infected individuals will go on to develop manifestations of late

disease if not treated in the acute phase of the infection.

Symptom developments

Some authors have divided this illness into three distinct stages: stage 1, erythema migrans or flu-like illness; stage 2, neurological or cardiac involvement; stage 3, arthritis. Although this scheme is straightforward, it may be misleading since it is apparent that for many patients the infection disseminates early, with multiple organs and tissues becoming involved. Initially, after the tick bite, approximately 50–60% of infected patients will develop the characteristic EM (Luft and Dattwyler, 1989). The infectious load at this stage is fairly high and hematogenous spread may occur very quickly. This can produce a range of acute clinical manifestations, including multifocal EM lesions, fever, conjunctivitis, meningism, headache, arthralgias and myalgias. Associated with dissemination, other systemic manifestations may develop acutely or subacutely, including meningitis, myocarditis with or without heart block, hepatitis, myositis and, less commonly, arthritis. In the chronic phase of the illness, localized inflammatory processes may occur in one or more organ systems, particularly the nervous and the musculoskeletal systems. For this reason, it is preferable to classify this infectious disease according to the evidence of localized skin infection in contrast to a disseminated infection and, if there is dissemination, whether or not there is evidence of central nervous system (CNS) involvement. Furthermore, it may be important to know the chronicity of the infection since the pathogenesis of the disease and the response to therapy may be different in patients with acute versus chronic disease.

Coincident Infections

It is significant to note that other zoonotic diseases transmitted by *Ixodes* ticks may occur concomitantly with *B. burgdorferi*. For instance, in a report of a fatal case of babesiosis, the autopsy revealed significant histopathological evidence of a fulminant myocarditis due to *B. burgdorferi* (Marcus *et al.*, 1985). Patients diagnosed with babesiosis often have a positive serology to *B. burgdorferi* (Benach *et al.*, 1985). Additionally, a high prevalence of infection in nymphal ticks with either *B. burgdorferi* or *Babesia microti* has been reported during the early summer months (Piesman *et al.*, 1986, 1987a, 1987b). Another example is the relationship between *B. burgdorferi* and flavivirus. Russian investigators (Putkonen *et al.*, 1962) have reported a relationship between tick-borne encephalitis due to flaviviruses and EM. Since Lyme borreliosis can be associated with a meningitis or meningoencephalitis, it is not clear whether these particular cases of tick-borne encephalitis associated with EM are due to a dual infection of *B. burgdorferi* and flavivirus or solely to infection with *B. burgdorferi* (Kristoferitsch *et al.*, 1986). Furthermore, Lyme borreliosis should be considered in all patients suspected of arboviral encephalitis (Edlinger *et al.*, 1985; Rodhain and Edlinger, 1987).

Skin

Erythema migrans

In approximately 50–60% of cases, the first indicator of *B. burgdorferi* infection is EM (Luft and Dattwyler, 1989). EM is an expanding, annular erythematous rash that fades in the center, although atypical variants include scaling, vesicular, purpuric and persistent homogeneous erythema which can often be accentuated with heat. The rash occurs between three days and four months after a tick bite and typically occurs at the site of the tick bite. However, in more than half of all cases, the patient is totally unaware of a tick bite primarily because nymphal ticks are so small and the bite is often painless that they escape detection. The lesions may be associated with mild local pruritus or dysesthesias (Weber and Neubert, 1986; Asbrink and Hovmark, 1988), but are seldom painful. The lesions can be located anywhere; however, the thigh, groin, axilla and face (for children) are especially common sites. Constitutional symptoms can vary from absent to mild and transitory, including malaise, fatigue, headache, fever, chills and regional lymphadenopathy, or these constitutional signs and symptoms can be debilitating, and may be associated with profound fatigue, lethargy, mild encephalopathy, meningeal irritation, migratory musculoskeletal pain, hepatitis, generalized lymphadenopathy or splenomegaly. These symptoms, especially the fatigue, can persist for months. Severe constitutional symptoms are most likely to represent evidence of a spirochaetaemia. Although one report in the USA found an incidence of 50% of patients presenting with multiple EM, reports from Europe as well as anecdotal reports from the USA suggest an incidence in the range of 8–10%. These lesions may appear similar to the original lesion, but are generally smaller, migrate less, lack the indurated center and are not associated with a tick bite. In those patients who experience multiple lesions, the constitutional symptoms, including meningism, tend to be more severe. The skin lesions will clear spontaneously, often within weeks to months, but can persist for up to a year. If inadequately treated, EM can relapse. Furthermore, patients with EM are susceptible to reinfection, and thereby to recurrent episodes of rash. *Borrelia burgdorferi* has been isolated from both primary and secondary lesions (Berger *et al.*, 1992).

Lymphocytoma

Borrelia lymphocytoma, which is characterized by a dense lymphocytic infiltrate in the dermis or subcutaneous tissue, has been associated with borrelial infection (Hovmark *et al.*, 1986). These solitary, bluish-red nodules have a predilection for occurring in the ear lobes of children and on the nipple areas of adults. These lesions may occur concurrently with the acute infection of the site of the tick bite, or may occur months later, in an area not geographically associated with the bite. The lymphocytoma may occur with other manifestations of infection such as meningitis, choroiditis, arthritis or acrodermatitis atrophicans (Asbrink and Hovmark, 1988). Clinically, it may be indistinguishable from breast malignancy. Histopathologically, it may be difficult to differentiate the lymphocytoma from lymphoma. *Borrelia burgdorferi* has been isolated from lymphocytoma in only one instance (Asbrink and Hovmark, 1985).

Acrodermatitis chronicum atrophicans (ACA)

ACA is a chronic and insidious skin infection occurring predominantly in females and the elderly (Asbrink and Hovmark, 1988). It has been described throughout Northern, Central and Eastern Europe, but has rarely been reported in the USA. Cases of greater than 10 years duration between the time of onset and eventual diagnosis have been reported in the literature (Asbrink and Hovmark, 1985). The skin lesion usually manifests itself on the distal extremities, typically sparing the face, palms and soles; the trunk, however, may be the site of initial disease. The knees and olecranon areas also are susceptible to this process. The inflammation may subsequently spread to other extremities, and to the torso. Those areas of inflammation may be multicentric, with normal areas of skin separating them. The skin lesions are characterized as red violaceous to bluish-red discolored areas with a doughy consistency. The erythematous component of the lesion may be variable, and swelling of the soft tissue with relatively normal-looking skin may be present. Eventually, the lesions may become atrophic or sclerotic, and may be indistinguishable from localized scleroderma (morphea) or lichen sclerosis atrophicus. Interestingly, EM has been reported to occur prior to, or concomitantly with, the ACA. The EM occurs in the same extremity as the ACA (Asbrink et al., 1986).

Concomitant with the ACA, neurological (Hopf, 1975; Kristoferitsch et al., 1988) and rheumatological (Herzer et al., 1986) evidence of B. burgdorferi infection may be present. These abnormalities frequently occur in the same extremity as the skin lesion. In approximately one-third of patients, there is evidence of a polyneuropathy. Patients complain of paraesthesias, hyperaesthesias, weakness and muscle cramps. On neurological examination, sensory abnormalities tend to predominate, although paralysis or paresis may be present. There have been reports of profound fatigue and weight loss associated with ACA. As well, there is evidence of

central nervous system involvement. Patients with ACA also may have severe rheumatological involvement, with subluxation of the small joints of the hands and feet, arthritis of the large joints and periosteal thickening of the bones. Bursitis, epicondylitis and tendonitis have also been reported to occur with ACA. At times it may be difficult to differentiate between the pain of arthritis and the significant neuritis associated with this disease process.

Joints

Within days to years after infection with B. burgdorferi, a majority of untreated patients develop rheumatological manifestations of disease (Steere, 1986). Arthritis may occur in both patients who have had EM or those who were asymptomatic at the time of initial infection. During the acute infection, patients often complain of arthralgias and myalgias without frank arthritis. However, if the infection is allowed to proceed untreated, more than 50% of patients will ultimately develop a mono- or oligoarticular relapsing arthritis (Bowen et al., 1984). In children, Lyme disease is frequently mistaken for juvenile rheumatoid arthritis (Sagransky, 1986). In particular, children may have acute and severe episodes of synovitis and frank arthritis accompanied by high fever. If joint involvement occurs early in the illness, the usual pattern is one of migratory musculoskeletal pain in joints, tendons, bursae, muscle or bone. Frequently, there is no joint swelling. The pain typically affects one or two sites at a time, and usually lasts from a few hours to several days in a specific location. However, frank arthritis, with intermittent attacks of mono- or oligoarticular arthritis with pain and joint swelling, occurs primarily in large joints, especially in the knee. Affected knees are usually much more swollen than painful; they are frequently hot to the touch, and seldom red. Early in the course of the arthritis, Baker's cysts sometimes form and rupture. Although large joints, including the knees, shoulders, hips and elbows are most commonly affected, small joints and the temporomandibular joint have been reported to be involved (Harris, 1988). A few patients have had symmetrical polyarthritis. Attacks of arthritis usually last from weeks to months, and frequently recur for several years with symptom-free periods lasting from days to months. Fatigue is common with active joint involvement late in the illness. Fever or other systemic symptoms are unusual.

In approximately 10% of patients with arthritis, involvement in large joints becomes chronic, and cartilage and bone are eroded, resulting in permanent joint disability (Lawson and Steere, 1985). Synovial biopsies show a markedly inflamed synovium surface with deposits of fibrin, villous hypertrophy, and vascular proliferation (Duray and Steere, 1988). There is also a heavy infiltration of mononuclear cells, some of which form lymphoid follicles, including plasma cells which are presumed to be capable of producing antibody locally. These patients may be recalcitrant to medical therapy and synovectomy may be necessary (McLaughlin *et al.*, 1986). Endarteritis obliterans of small vessels is characteristic. In Lyme disease, the joint fluid white blood cell counts vary between 500 and 100 000. The predominant cell is a polymorphonuclear leukocyte. The glucose level is usually two-thirds of that found in the serum.

Nervous System

The full scope of neurological involvement in *B. burgdorferi* infection remains incompletely defined. All the neurological syndromes associated with *B. burgdorferi* infection can occur without previous EM (Reik *et al.*, 1986). Although there is a large amount of speculation about how the nervous system is affected by this infection, reasonable evidence for a causal relationship has been established only for a few disorders. This lack of proof is mainly due to the inability to explicitly define this disease microbiologically. Until better diagnostic assays are developed, this area will remain controversial. The simple demonstration of an immune response to *B. burgdorferi* does not by itself prove anything more than that an individual has been exposed to the spirochaete. It is clear, however, that Lyme borreliosis is associated with both acute and chronic neurological abnormalities, affecting both the central and peripheral nervous systems.

Clinical data supports the hypothesis that, in most individuals, *B. burgdorferi* invades the nervous system early in the course of the infection. The most compelling evidence for this is the frequency of complaints referable to the nervous system in patients with EM. In one series of 314 patients with EM, 80% of the patients had malaise, fatigue and lethargy; 64% had headache; and 48% complained of a stiff neck (Steere *et al.*, 1983). Additional evidence of the early invasion of the nervous system is shown by the finding that approximately 12–15% of patients develop one or more of these three acute disorders – meningitis, cranial neuritis or painful radiculitis – within the first three months after infection (Pachner and Steere, 1985). Interestingly, the headache and stiff neck reported by most patients with EM are frequently indistinguishable from those reported by patients with meningitis. The distinguishing feature for patients who develop meningitis is the presence of CSF abnormalities, a mild pleocytosis largely consisting of polymorphonuclear leukocytes or mononuclear cells, a modest elevation of CSF protein, and a normal CSF glucose. Papilloedema and increased CSF pressure can occur, resulting in a syndrome indistinguishable from pseudotumor cerebri (Raucher *et al.*, 1985). Acute meningitis may represent the most acute and dramatic nervous system manifestation of this infectious process.

The CNS abnormalities form a spectrum. Although acute meningitis is the most dramatic manifestation of CNS infection, a mild encephalopathy is the most frequently observed CNS symptom. Malaise, severe fatigue and lethargy are commonly associated with disseminated *B. burgdorferi* infection; however, unlike most other fatigue states, depression is not a major factor in late neuroborreliosis. Rather, this severe fatigue may simply be an indication of chronic CNS infection and, in many cases, the most recognizable symptom of a mild chronic encephalopathy of months to years duration (Bensch *et al.*, 1987). It is usually associated with quantifiable deficits in short-term memory and cognition. CSF reveals a persistent mononuclear pleocytosis. Local antibody production against *B. burgdorferi* and magnetic resonance imaging (MRI) abnormalities have been observed in the more severely affected patients. In the absence of local antibody production, the diagnosis of *B. burgdorferi* CNS infection is highly questionable. Localized CNS processes have been associated with *B. burgdorferi* infection (Broderick *et al.*, 1987). These may present as acute myelitis (Rousseau *et al.*, 1986), localized encephalitis (Feder *et al.*, 1988) or cerebellar ataxia.

Meningopolyneuritis

Meningopolyneuritis (Garin–Bujadoux, Bannwarth's syndrome) is the most dramatic of the peripheral nervous system abnormalities (Henriksson *et al.*, 1986). It is usually characterized by intense radicular pain, paresthaesias or hyperesthaesias. The peripheral neuropathy shows no relationship to the region of tick bite or erythema. The neuritis may be distributed asymmetrically, resembling polyneuritis multiplex. Associated with the neuritis is paresis of the extremities which may be severe. The CSF may reveal a lymphocytic pleocytosis. Concomitant encephalitis and myelitis occur in over 20% of patients. In these patients, long-term sequelae such as spastic paraparesis and neurogenic bladder persist after appropriate therapy. Meningopolyneuritis represents the most severe and obvious example of a widespread peripheral nerve disorder commonly observed in disseminated *B. burgdorferi* infection (Wokke *et al.*, 1987). Sensitive neurophysiological techniques reveal that more than 40% of patients with late disease have demonstrable abnormalities (Halperin *et al.*, 1987). Many of these patients complain of bilateral paraesthesias and hyperesthaesias. In both meningoradiculitis and in the more common peripheral polyneuropathy, sural nerve biopsies reveal a perivascular mononuclear cell infiltrate. The unifying feature of all of these abnormalities is that each is primarily an axonopathy, probably due to vasculopathy.

Cranial neuropathies

Cranial neuropathies are commonly associated with this infection. These may occur with or without evidence of meningitis. Seventh nerve, both unilateral and bilateral (Clark *et al.*, 1985), involvement is by far the most frequent, occurring in up to 10% of patients with this infection. Involvement of other cranial nerves have been reported, but causal relationships have not been established. Still, it is likely that this infection can affect other cranial nerves than the seventh. Abnormalities of the second, third, fourth, fifth, sixth and eighth, optic nerve and the recurrent laryngeal nerve have been reported with some frequency. These cranial nerve abnormalities can occur alone or with other evidence of a polyneuritis. Optic disk oedema can occur as a result of optic neuritis or increased intracranial pressure. Pupillary changes can occur, including the development of a Robertson pupil (Schechter, 1986).

Cardiac Disorders

Cardiac involvement, which appears to be less common than either musculoskeletal or neurological involvement, has been reported in 8–10% of patients with *B. burgdorferi* infection (Steere *et al.*, 1980). The most commonly described abnormality has been with varying degrees of atrioventricular (A–V) block, with the degree of block fluctuating rapidly. A–V block, generally associated with early infection, usually tends to be high grade, often with normal QRS complexes. Syncope can occur. Third-degree block can persist, but the A–V block is usually self-limited.

Other cardiac manifestations have been associated with this infection, including both myocarditis and pericarditis. Diffuse T wave changes (flattening or inversions) and ST segment depression also are frequently observed. The incidence of left ventricular dysfunction in this infection has not been well studied. In one report of 12 patients with cardiac involvement who underwent radionuclide angiocardiograms, four had left ventricular dysfunction (Ponsonnaille *et al.*, 1986). In addition, Lyme myocarditis may be detected by gallium scan (Rienzo *et al.*, 1987). Congestive heart failure has been reported in connection with myocarditis, but it is rare. When left ventricular dysfunction occurs, it usually does not compromise cardiac function; however, rarely it may be clinically occult and fatal (Marcus *et al.*, 1985).

Pericarditis occurs rarely with *B. burgdorferi* infection, and the true incidence is unknown. Arrhythmias have been reported in Lyme borreliosis, but a cause-and-effect relationship between infection and the arrhythmia has not been established. We have observed ventricular arrhythmias, including multifocal premature ventricular contraction, disappear after appropriate intravenous therapy for *B. burgdorferi*. The full range of cardiac abnormalities awaits further study.

Other Organ Systems

B. burgdorferi will localize to other organ systems. Hepatic abnormalities have occurred in both acute and chronic Lyme borreliosis. These abnormalities may occur soon after the onset of EM, and are associated with hepatic tendencies. Mild to moderate portal tract inflammation to moderate liver cell derangement that simulates acute viral hepatitis has occurred in early Lyme disease. In addition, severe hepatitis has been reported in one patient as a late complication of this disease. In this patient, the liver biopsy showed marked ballooning of the hepatocytes, and the organism was demonstrable by silver stain (Goellner *et al.*, 1988). Other lymphoid organs, such as the spleen and lymph nodes, can be involved. In these patients, there may be fever and prominent lymphadenopathy. Tubulointerstitial nephritis associated with chronic infection of the skin has been reported (Aberer *et al.*, 1987).

Cases of myositis, panniculitis, osteomyelitis, uveitis and pneumonitis due to *B. burgdorferi* have been reported (Atlas *et al.*, 1988; Kramer *et al.*, 1986; Jacobs *et al.*, 1986; Steere *et al.*, 1985; Kirsch *et al.*, 1988). Histopathologically, few spirochaetes are demonstrable along with infiltration of lymphocytes, plasma cells and macrophages. The patient with pneumonitis ultimately died of respiratory failure and *B. burgdorferi* was demonstrated in lymph nodes.

DIAGNOSIS

Until the discovery of the causative agent in 1982, the clinical diagnosis of Lyme borreliosis was based solely on the recognition of EM, either historically or by direct observation. Diagnosis has since improved; however, a number of important problems remain. The paramount difficulties lie in isolating *B. burgdorferi* from the infected host and in the lack of a uniform case definition in the face of a continued dependence on a clinical diagnosis. Unlike most bacterial infections, where the diagnosis of active infection is based on the demonstration of the causative organism, via isolation by culture or by observation in clinical material, the diagnosis of *B. burgdorferi* infection is largely dependent upon indirect means. In the absence of EM, the demonstration of an immune response to *B. burgdorferi* in an appropriate clinical setting forms the basis on which most diagnoses are made. Obviously, this is suboptimal. At present, the direct isolation of *B. burgdorferi* is the most specific, but least sensitive, means of diagnosis (Benach *et al.*, 1983).

Microscopy

Borrelia burgdorferi, a loosely coiled spirochaete which is approximately 200 μm wide and 10–30 μm long, is difficult to visualize under bright-field conditions, but is readily visible in phase contrast or dark field. The organism is Gram negative and can also be stained with acridine orange, Giemsa, or by fluorescent antibody technique. Silver stains, either Warthin–Starry or a modified Dieterle strain, have proved to be successful in identifying spirochaetes in fixed, paraffin-embedded tissue. In general, skin biopsy has been the most successful in identifying the pathogen. Spirochaetes have been observed in other tissues, such as the myocardium, synovium and the nervous system, but the yields from them have been very poor. It is unlikely that the direct observation of spirochaetes in infected tissue will ever prove to be a reliable diagnostic technique because of the low numbers of spirochaetes in infected tissues. Better results may be obtained in the future with the use of DNA probes or DNA amplification techniques.

Cultural Methods

Borrelia burgdorferi has been successfully cultured in Barbour–Stoener–Kelly media from skin, CSF, blood and joints (Preac-Mursic *et al.*, 1984). However, the yields have been very low. Steere *et al.* (1984) cultured large volumes of blood from 65 patients and only isolated *B. burgdorferi* in two individuals. The highest yields have been obtained from cultures of skin biopsies of EM lesions; reported success rates have varied from 6% to 45%. Culture techniques have been most successful for samples obtained during the early acute phase of the disease.

Immunological Tests

Immune response

In order to understand the difficulties involved in the interpretation of the serological tests for Lyme disease, it is important to understand the kinetics of the immune response to this organism. Infected individuals develop an early and vigorous T cell response to *B. burgdorferi* (Dattwyler *et al.*, 1988); the B cell response evolves more slowly, frequently over the course of months. IgM responses against individual antigens appear first, followed by IgG responses. Within three to four weeks after the onset of infection, a rise in IgM against one or more spirochaetal antigens can be detected in most individuals. The IgM response usually peaks after six to eight weeks and then gradually declines. Early in the course of infection, the IgM response is mainly directed against a 41 kDa flagella-associated antigen (Luft *et al.*, 1992) and outer surface protein C (OspC). However, epitopes on this 41 kDa antigen are cross-reactive with epitopes found on flagella of other borrelias and treponemes. Recently, areas of the 41 kDa antigen of *B. burgdorferi* have been shown to have a high degree of homology to the 33 kDa protein of *Treponema pallidum* (Luft *et al.*, 1989). Antibodies against this 41 kDa antigen can be found in the serum of most normal individuals, and antibodies against this antigen are not specific. Antibody response to the 60 kDa antigen also does not seem to be specific. Humoral responses to other antigens gradually develop as the disease progresses. Although there are antigenic differences between some strains of *B. burgdorferi*, especially between North America and Europe, antibodies against one or more of the major protein antigens (OspC, 31, 34, 60 or 66 kDa) develop as the infection continues. The humoral response to the higher molecular antigens develops first, followed by a response to the lower molecular antigens, the 31 and 34 kDa antigens in particular.

The cause of this observed evolution of the humoral response has not been delineated. Whether the spirochaete expresses different antigens during the course of infection has not been proved, but this possibility is compatible with what has been observed. Craft *et al.* (1986) found that, in untreated patients, specific IgM antibodies to the 34 kDa OspB antigen developed later in the course of infection. This could explain also why IgM titres may remain elevated late in the course of the infection. Specific IgG and IgA responses gradually increase during the second and third months of infection and, once established, may remain detectable for years. However, as in syphilis, prompt antimicrobial therapy aborts the development of a mature humoral response (Steere *et al.*, 1983). Thus, patients treated before they develop a mature humoral response often lack diagnostic levels of *Borrelia*-specific antibodies.

Choice of test

Currently available serological assays using whole *B. burgdorferi* preparations are not sufficiently sensitive to detect the early rise in antibodies above the background of cross-reactive antibodies. Thus, the serodiagnosis by either indirect immunofluorescence assay (IFA) or enzyme-linked immunosorbent assay (ELISA) in the first few weeks of infection is not dependable. Between 50% and 60% of patients with EM will not have diagnostic antibody titres. Immunoblots can detect antibodies against *B. burgdorferi*, but specificity is the problem. Using highly sensitive Western blots, it has been the author's experience more than 50%

of a control population of individuals with no history of tick bite or EM and a negative specific ELISA will have IgG anti-41 kDa antibody. Additionally, some of these individuals have antibodies against other spirochaetal antigens, including the 60 kDa common antigen. This phenomenon has been noted by others, and is likely to contribute to the high backgrounds seen in IFA tests (often as high as 1 : 128 in normal control sera).

Immunofluorescence

IFA and ELISA are the two most commonly used methods for the detection of antibodies to *B. burgdorferi*. The IFA is performed using whole fixed *B. burgdorferi* and the ELISA generally utilizes crude fractions of sonicated spirochaetes. The negative cut-off for each of these assays differs markedly between laboratories. Neither assay has been standardized, and results vary widely among laboratories. The majority of laboratories use negative cut-offs between 1 : 64 and 1 : 256 for IFA. Unfortunately, differences of two dilutions or more for the same sample have not been uncommon in many laboratories. Attempts at improving the IFA by absorbing patient serum with *Treponema phagedenis* or other spirochaetes have not been successful. Generally, absorption decreases antibody titers to both *T. phagedenis* and to *B. burgdorferi*, and the slight gain in specificity is not worth the loss of sensitivity.

ELISA

ELISAs are more sensitive than IFAs and offer the advantage of having the capability of screening large numbers of patient samples more easily. The negative cut-off for the ELISA is determined statistically. Most laboratories use absorbances of 2.5 to 3 standard deviations above the mean for a group of normal, healthy controls. When carefully performed, the IFA can be as useful as the ELISA for the detection of antibodies against *B. burgdorferi* in the peripheral blood. However, when screening CSF, the sensitivity of the ELISA is an advantage. No matter which assay is used, the results of the assay should be put into the context of the clinical setting. Patients with negative results are unlikely to have *B. burgdorferi* infection. Even for patients with high positive values, the results alone do not indicate a cause-and-effect relationship between the patient's clinical findings and *B. burgdorferi* infection.

Cross-reactions

High titres of antibodies against *B. burgdorferi* are found in the serum of patients with other spirochaetal infections such as syphilis, yaws, pinta and relapsing fever (Magnarelli *et al.*, 1987). Although anti-cardiolipin antibodies have been reported in Lyme borreliosis, the quantity of these antibodies is very low. In patients with syphilis, the reagent antibody assays like the Venereal Disease Research Laboratory Test (VDRL) are positive, while in Lyme borreliosis it is almost invariably negative. Treponemal tests like the fluorescent treponemal antibody absorption test can be positive in Lyme borreliosis patients.

Interpretation

Some individuals lack diagnostic levels of specific antibody in their serum, yet have neurological involvement and diagnostic levels of antibody in their CSF (Stiernstedt *et al.*, 1988; Dattwyles *et al.*, 1988). One possible explanation for this observation is that although commonly used oral antibiotics such as tetracycline or penicillin can effectively eradicate the bulk of *B. burgdorferi*, neither low-dose tetracycline nor low-dose penicillin penetrates the CNS in concentrations sufficient to kill all of the spirochaetes (Dattwyler *et al.*, 1988). Thus, *B. burgdorferi* reaching this immunologically privileged site may remain viable and induce a local immune response. The demonstration of intrathecal production of anti-*B. burgdorferi* antibody may be another specific method to demonstrate CNS involvement. By using the following formula:

$$\frac{\text{Anti-}B.\ burgdorferi\ \text{titer CSF} \times \text{Serum IgG concentration}}{\text{Anti-}B.\ burgdorferi\ \text{titer serum} \times \text{CSF IgG concentration}}$$

it is possible to determine whether the amount of anti-*B. burgdorferi* antibody in the CSF is elevated disproportionately to that found in the serum. If the ratio is greater than 1, localized production of anti-*Borrelia* antibodies has occurred.

The failure of early antimicrobial therapy to completely eradicate the infection, and the subsequent development of late Lyme borreliosis, is especially difficult to diagnose in patients who fail to develop a mature antibody response (Dattwyler *et al.*, 1988). However, specific T cell and/or local humoral responses may be demonstrable in patients who lack diagnostic levels of circulating anti-*B. burgdorferi* antibodies. In contradiction, individuals who have already developed a mature anti-*Borrelia* IgG response will often remain seropositive after successful antibiotic therapy. In these patients, a reduction in specific antibody levels can be observed with time, but their absolute levels may remain above normal. Consequently, the presence or absence of circulating anti-*Borrelia* antibodies following antibiotic therapy is not a reliable indicator of cure.

A strong and specific cellular immune response to *B. burgdorferi* develops early in the course of the infection, frequently preceding the development of a measurable antibody response. This cellular immune response, once developed, is long lasting.

TREATMENT

There is currently no consensus on the optimal therapy for *B. burgdorferi* infection. To understand why this is true, a number of issues must be considered:

(1) Although a number of *in vitro* sensitivity studies have been performed, they have not been carried out in a standardized manner and their relationship to *in vitro* efficacy has not been established.

(2) In a similar manner to *Treponema pallidum*, *B. burgdorferi* is killed *in vitro* only after prolonged incubation with antibiotics. This has been misinterpreted by some to conclude that prolonged courses or antibiotics are required.

(3) Most individuals with Lyme disease will spontaneously remit, even without treatment.

(4) The diagnosis of Lyme disease is not usually made microbiologically, but is essentially a clinical diagnosis.

(5) Assessments of the response to treatment are based primarily on clinical grounds, and not on microbiological criteria.

(6) The mechanisms producing persistent signs and symptoms are not well defined and may be due to a number of factors, such as continued infection, permanent tissue damage or to some undefined immune mechanism.

(7) There have been few randomized prospective studies on the treatment of Lyme disease.

Thus, any suggestions as to the efficacy of treatment in this infection should be taken with reservation.

Most studies of the treatment of Lyme disease, both erythema migrans and late disease have been small, open studies (Hollstrom, 1951; Steere *et al.*, 1983; Preac Mursic *et al.*, 1987; Dattwyler *et al.*, 1990; Berger, 1988; Nadelman *et al.*, 1992). Although useful in developing some indication of what may be efficacious in the treatment of *B. burgdorferi* infection, these trials should be viewed more as preliminary, and not as definitive studies. Despite this, it has been demonstrated that Lyme disease is an antibiotic-responsive illness. Studies on the treatment of patients with EM show that β-lactams and tetracylines are effective against *B. burgdorferi*. However, it is not clear which antibiotic or antibiotic regimen is optimal. Early studies were designed in the absence of *in vitro* sensitivity data and most studies on the treatment of EM have not taken into account that *B. burgdorferi* can spread haematogenously early in the course of disease (Hollstrom, 1951; Steere *et al.*, 1983). Patients with both local infection – single-lesion EM without constitutional signs or symptoms – are patients with clear evidence of dissemination – multiple EM – have often been lumped together in treatment studies.

What is lacking, but clearly needed, are large well-controlled double-blind trials to define the treatment of EM. Yet, despite this lack of truly definitive studies tetracyclines (doxycycline or minocycline) and amoxicillin have an established place in the treatment of this infection. Further amoxycillin 500 mg t.i.d., doxycycline 100 mg b.i.d. or minocycline 100 mg b.i.d. is the first-line treatment for patients with EM. These regimens provide sustained serum levels and adequate tissue penetration for all but active CNS infection.

Intravenous penicillin and ceftriaxone are the most widely used antibiotics for the treatment of CNS infection (Rahn and Malawista, 1991; Kristoferitsch et al., 1987; Dattwyler et al., 1987). Although there are several instances in which acute CNS infection has progressed despite penicillin therapy (Pal et al., 1988; Dattwyler et al., 1988), acute meningitis or meningoencephalitis due to B. burgdorferi is usually very responsive to high-dose penicillin therapy. Meningopolyradiculitis (Bannwarth's syndrome) is more difficult to treat, with as many as 50% of patients continuing to have severe neurological signs, such as spastic paraparesis, after treatment. Similarly, approximately 50% or more of patients with arthritis secondary to B. burgdorferi fail to respond to intravenous penicillin therapy. Treatment of ACA with penicillin is successful in about 50% of patients, with a similar percentage experiencing continued, extracutaneous manifestations (Rahn and Malawista, 1991).

Ceftriaxone and other third-generation cephlosporins may be superior to penicillin in the treatment of late Lyme borreliosis (Dattwyler et al., 1987, 1988; Pal et al., 1988). However, larger long-term studies are required to determine the precise role of this and other third-generation cephalosporins in the treatment of this infection. Even though ceftriaxone appears to be promising, it is still associated with a failure rate of greater than 10%. Currently, patients with disseminated infection and significant organ involvement, especially CNS manifestations, are treated with 14–28 days of ceftriaxone, 2 g once a day. Some physicians, especially in the USA, use longer courses, but there is no study which has demonstrated that a prolonged course of antibiotics provides addition benefit.

PREVENTION

For all tick-borne diseases, advice regarding prevention and removal of ticks is the same. Avoidance of tick bites is the key to prevention of disease. In the laboratory, however, development of a vaccine for Lyme disease is advancing. To date, a vaccine developed using the recombinant OspA from strain N40, a B. burgdorferi sensu stricto strain, does not appear to protect against infection by the other genospecies (Fikrig et al., 1992). It is not yet clear how many different recombinant OspA's would be required to create a useful vaccine. While the discovery of the large degree of divergence within these species increases the difficulty of vaccine development, the strict clonality indicates that an effective vaccine will remain useful for a long time (Dykhuizer et al., 1993). The geographical differences could mean that vaccines need to be targeted for particular regions of North America or the world, recognizing that a general worldwide vaccine may not be effective or may be too costly to produce. It is evident that heterogeneity and population dynamics within this species complex are necessary for rational development of an effective vaccine against Lyme disease.

REFERENCES

Aberer, E., Neumann, R. and Lubec, G. (1987) Acrodermatitis chronica atrophicans in association with lichen sclerosus et atrophicans: tubulo-interstitial nephritis and urinary excretion of spirochete-like organisms. *Acta Dermato-Venereologica*, **67**, 62–65.

Anderson, J., Magnarelli, L.A. and McAnince, J.B. (1988) New *Borrelia burgdorferi* antigenic variant isolated from *Ixodes dammini* from Upstate New York. *Journal of Clinical Microbiology*, **26**, 2209–2212.

Asbrink, E. and Hovmark, A. (1985) Successful cultivation of spirochetes from skin lesions of patients with erythema chronicum migrans Afzelius and acrodermatitis chronica atrophicans. *Acta Pathologica Microbiologica et Immunologica Scandinavica Sect. B*, **93**, 161–163.

Asbrink, E. and Hovmark, A. (1988) Early and late cutaneous manifestations in *Ixodes*-borne borreliosis (erythema migrans borreliosis, Lyme borreliosis).

Annals of the New York Academy of Sciences, **539**, 4–15.

Asbrink, E., Hovmark, A. and Olsson I. (1986) Clinical manifestations of acrodermatitis chronica atrophicans in 50 Swedish patients. *Zentralblatt für Bakteriologie, Mikrobiologie und Hygiene*, **263**, 253–261.

Atlas, E., Novak, S., Duray, P.H. *et al.* (1988) Lyme myositis: muscle invasion by *Borrella burgdorferi*. *Annals of Internal Medicine*, **109**, 245–246.

Baranton, G., Postic, D., Saint Girons, I. *et al.* (1992) Delineation of *Borrelia burgdorferi* sensu stricto, *Borrelia garnii* and Sp. Nov. VS461 associated with Lyme borreliosis. *International Journal of Systematic Bacteriology*, **42**, 378–383.

Barbour, A.G. and Garon, C.F. (1988) The genes encoding major surface proteins of *B. burgdorferi* are located on a plasmid. *Annals of the New York Academy of Sciences*, **539**, 144–154.

Benach, J.L., Bosler, E.M., Hanrahan, J.P. *et al.* (1983) Spirochetes isolated from the blood of two patients with Lyme disease. *New England Journal of Medicine*, **308**, 740–742.

Benach, J.L., Coleman, J., Habicht, G.S. *et al.* (1985) Serological evidence for simultaneous occurrences of Lyme disease and babesiosis. *Journal of Infectious Diseases*, **152**, 473–477.

Benach, J.L., Coleman, J.L., Skinner, R.A. *et al.* (1987) Adult *Ixodes scapularus* on rabbits: a hypothesis for the development and transmission of *Borrelia burgdorferi*. *Journal of Infectious Diseases*, **155**, 1300–1306.

Bensch, J., Olsen, P. and Hagberg, L. (1987) Destructive chronic borrelia meningoencephalitis in a child untreated for 15 years. *Scandinavian Journal of Infectious Diseases*, **19**, 697–700.

Berger, W. (1988) Treatment of erythema chronicum migrans of Lyme disease. *Annals of the New York Academy of Sciences*, **539**, 346–351.

Berger, B.W., Johnson, R.C., Kodner, C. *et al.* (1992) Cultivation of *Borrelia burgdorferi* from erythema migrans lesions and perilesional skin. *Journal of Clinical Microbiology*, **30**, 359.

Bosler, E.M. (1993) Tick vectors and hosts. In Lyme disease (ed. P.K. Coyle), pp. 18–26. Mosby Year Book, Boston, MA.

Bosler, E.M., Coleman, J., Benach, J.L. *et al.* (1983) Natural distribution of the *Ixodes scapularus* spirochete. *Science*, **220**, 321–322.

Bowen, S.G. (1983) A focus of Lyme disease in Monmouth County, New Jersey. *American Journal of Epidemiology*, **120**, 387.

Bowen, G.S., Griffin, M., Hayne, C. *et al.* (1984) Clinical manifestations and descriptive epidemiology of Lyme disease in New Jersey, 1978 to 1982.

Journal of the American Medical Association, **251**, 2236–2240.

Broderick, J.P., Sandok, B. and Mertz, L.E. (1987) Focal encephalitis in a young woman 6 years after the onset of Lyme disease: tertiary Lyme disease? *Mayo Clinic Proceedings*, **62**, 313–316.

Burgdorfer, W., Barbour, A.G., Hayes, S. *et al.* (1982) Lyme disease: a tick-borne spirochetosis? *Science*, **216**, 1317–1319.

Clark, J.R., Carlson, R., Sasaki, C.T. *et al.* (1985) Facial paralysis in Lyme disease. *Laryngoscope*, **95**, 1341–1345.

Coleman, J.L. and Benach, J.L. (1989) Identification and characterization if an endoflagellar antigen of *Borrelia burgdorferi*. *Journal of Clinical Investigation*, **84**, 322.

Corporale, D.A. and Kocher, T.D. (in press) *Molecular Biology and Evolution*.

Craft, J.E., Fisher, D.K., Shimamoto, G.T. *et al.* (1986) Antigens of *Borrelia burgdorferi* recognized during Lyme disease: appearance of an immunoglobulin in response and expansion of immunoglobulin G response late in the illness. *Journal of Clinical Investigation*, **78**, 934.

Dattwyler, R.J., Halperin, J.J., Pass, H. *et al.* (1987) Ceftriaxone as effective therapy in refractory Lyme disease. *Journal of Infectious Diseases*, **155**, 1322–1325.

Dattwyler, R.J., Halperin, J.J., Volkman, D.J. *et al.* (1988) Treatment of late Lyme borreliosis: randomized comparison of ceftriaxone and penicillin. *Lancet*, **ii**, 1191–1195.

Dattwyler, R.J., Volkman, D.J., Luft, B.J. *et al.* (1988) Seronegative Lyme disease: dissociation of specific T- and B-lymphocyte responses to *Borrelia burgdorferi*. *New England Journal of Medicine*, **319**, 1441–1446.

Dattwyler, R.J., Volkman, D.J., Halperin, J.J. *et al.* (1988) Specific immune responses in Lyme borreliosis: characterization of T cell and B cell responses to *Borrelia burgdorferi*. *Annals of the New York Academy of Sciences*, **539**, 93–102.

Dattwyler, R.J., Volkman, D.J., Conaty, S.M. *et al.* (1990) Treatment of early Lyme borreliosis, a randomized trial comparing amoxicillin plus probenecid to doxycycline in patients with erythema migrans. *Lancet*, **336**, 1404–1407.

Duray, P.H. and Steere, A.C. (1988) Clinical pathologic correlations of Lyme disease by stage. *Annals of the New York Academy of Sciences*, **539**, 65–79.

Dykhuizen, D., Polin, D., Dunn, J.J. *et al.* (1993) *Borrelia burgdorferi* is clonal: implications for taxonomy and vaccine development. *Proceedings of the National Academy of Sciences of the USA*, **90**, 10163–10167.

Edlinger, E., Rodhain, F. and Perez, C. (1985) Lyme

disease in patients previously suspected of arbovirus infection. *Lancet*, **ii**, 93.

Feder, H.M. Jr, Zalneraitis, E. and Reik, L., Jr (1988) Lyme disease: acute focal meningoencephalitis in a child. *Pediatrics*, **82**, 931–934.

Fikrig, E., Barthold, S.W. Kantor, P.S. *et al.* (1992) *Borrelia burgdorferi* strain 25015: characterization of outer surface protein A and vaccination against infection. *Journal of Immunology*, **148**, 2256–2260.

Goellner, M.H., Agger, W., Burgess, J.H. *et al.* (1988) Hepatitis due to recurrent Lyme disease. *Annals of Internal Medicine*, **108**, 707–708.

Halperin, J.J., Little, B.W., Coyle, P.K. *et al.* (1987) Lyme disease: cause of a treatable peripheral neuropathy. *Neurology*, **37**, 1700–1706.

Harris, R.J. (1988) Lyme disease involving the temporomandibular joint. *Journal of Oral and Maxillofacial Surgery*, **46**, 78–79.

Henriksson, A., Link, H., Cruz, M. *et al.* (1986) Immunoglobulin abnormalities in CSF and blood over the course of lymphocytic meningoradiculitis (Bannwarth's syndrome). *Annals of Neurology*, **20**, 337–345.

Herzer, P., Wilske, B., Preac-Mursic, V. *et al.* (1986) Lyme arthritis: clinical features, serological, and radiographic findings of cases in Germany. *Klinische Wochenschrift*, **64**, 206–215.

Hollstrom, E. (1952) Successful treatment of erythema migrans Afzelius. *Acta Dermato-Venereologica*, **31**, 325–332.

Hopf, H.C. (1975) Peripheral neuropathy in acrodermatitis chronica atrophicans (Herxheimer). *Journal of Neurology, Neurosurgery and Psychiatry*, **38**, 452–458.

Hovind-Hougen, K. (1984) Ultrastructure of spirochetes isolated from *Ixodes ricinus* and *Ixodes dammini*. *Yale Journal of Biology and Medicine*, **93**, 543–548.

Hovmark, A., Asbrink, E. and Olsson, I. (1986) The spirochetal etiology of lymphadenosis benigna cutis solitaria. *Acta Dermato-Venereologica*, **66**, 479–484.

Jacobs, J.C., Stevens, M. and Duray, P.H. (1986) Lyme disease simulating septic arthritis (letter). *Journal of the American Medical Association*, **256**, 1138–1139.

Kirsch, M., Ruben, F.L., Steere, A.C. *et al.* (1988) Fatal adult respiratory distress syndrome in a patient with Lyme disease. *Journal of the American Medical Association*, **259**, 2737–2739.

Kramer, N., Rickert, R.R., Brodkin, R.H. *et al.* (1986) Septal panniculitis as a manifestation of Lyme disease. *American Journal of Medicines*, **81**, 149–152.

Kristoferitsch, W., Stanek, G. and Kunz, C. (1986) Double infection with early summer meningoencephalitis virus and *Borrelia burgdorferi*. *Deutsche Medizinische Wochenschrift*, **111**, 861–864.

Kristoferitsch, W., Baumhackl, V., Sluga, E. *et al.* (1987) High-dose penicillin therapy in meningopolyradiculitis Garin–Bujadoux–Bannworth: clinical and cerebrospinal fluid data. *Zentralblatt für Bakteriologie, Mikrobiologie und Hygiene A*, **263**, 357–364.

Kristoferitsch, W., Sluga, E., Graf, M. *et al.* (1988) Neuropathy associated with acrodermatitis chronica atrophicans: clinical and morphological features. *Annals of the New York Academy of Sciences*, **539**, 35–45.

Lawson, J.P. and Steere, A.C. (1985) Lyme arthritis: radiologic findings. *Radiology*, **154**, 37–43.

Luft, B.J. and Dattwyler R.J. (1989) Lyme borreliosis: problems in diagnosis and treatment. *Current Clinical Topics in Infectious Diseases*, **11**, 56–81.

Luft, B.J., Jiang, W., Munoz, P. *et al.* (1989) Biochemical and immunological characterization of the surface proteins of *Borrelia burgdorferi*. *Infection and Immunity*, **57**, 3637–3645.

Luft, B.J., Bosler, E.M. and Dattwyler, R.J. (1992) Diagnosis of Lyme borreliosis. In *Molecular and Immunologic Approaches*, pp. 317–324. Cold Spring Harbor Press, Cold Spring Harbor.

Luft, B.J., Steinman, C.R., Schubach, W.H. *et al* (1992) Invasion of the central nervous system by *Borrelia burgdorferi* in acute disseminated infection. *Journal of the American Medical Association*, **267**, 1364–1367.

Magnarelli, L.A., Anderson, J.F. and Johnson, R.C. (1987) Cross-reactivity in serological tests for Lyme disease and other spirochetal infection.s *Journal of Infectious Diseases*, **156**, 183–188.

Marconi, R.T. and Garon, C. (1992) Phylogenetic analysis of the genus *Borrelia*: a comparison of North American and European isolates of *Borrelia burgdorferi*. *Journal of Bacteriology*, **174**, 241–244.

Marcus, L.C., Steere, A.C. and Duray, P.H. (1985) Fatal pancarditis in a patient with coexistent Lyme disease and Babesiosis. *Annals of Internal Medicine*, **103**, 374–376.

Mast, W.E. and Burrows, W.M. (1976) Erythema chronicum migrans in the United States. *Journal of the American Medical Association*, **236**, 859.

McLaughlin, T.P., Zeme, L., Fisher, R.L. *et al.* (1986) Chronic arthritis of the knee in Lyme disease: review of the literature and report of two cases treated by synovectomy. *Journal of Bone and Joint Surgery*, **68**, 1057–1061.

Nadelman, R.B., Luger, S.W., Frank, E. *et al.* (1992) Comparison of cefuroxime axetil and doxycycline in the treatment of early Lyme disease. *Annals of Internal Medicine*, **117**, 273–280.

Pachner, A.R. and Steere, A. (1985) The triad of neuro-logic manifestations of Lyme disease: meningitis, cranial neuritis, and radiculoneuritis. *Neurology*, **35**, 47–53.

Pal, G.S., Baker, J.T. and Wright, D.J. (1988) Penicillin-resistant *Borrelia* encephalitis responding to cetotaxime (letter). *Lancet*, **i**, 50.

Piesman, J., Mather, T., Donahue, J.G. *et al.* (1986) Comparative prevalence of *Babesia microti* and *Borrelia burgdorferi* in four populations of *Ixodes scapularus* in eastern Massachusetts. *Acta Tropica*, **43**, 263–270.

Piesman, J., Mather, T., Dammin, G.J. *et al.* (1987a) Seasonal variation of transmission risk of Lyme disease and human babesiosis. *American Journal of Epidemiology*, **126**, 1187–1189.

Piesman, J., Hicks, T., Sinsky, R.J. *et al.* (1987b) Simultaneous transmission of *Borrelia burgdorferi* and *Babesia microti* by individual nymphal *Ixodes scapularus* ticks. *Journal of Clinical Microbiology*, **25**, 2012–2013.

Ponsonnaille, J., Citron, B., Karsenty, B. *et al.* (1986) Acute myocarditis in Lyme's syndrome: value of myocardial scintigraphy with gallium 67. *Archives des Maladies du Coeur*, **79**, 1946–1950.

Preac-Mursic, V., Wilske, B., Schierz, G. *et al.* (1984) Repeated isolation of spirochetes from the cerebro-spinal fluid of a patient with meningoradiculitis Bannwarth. *European Journal of Clinical Micro-biology*, **3**, 564–565.

Preac Mursic, V., Wilske, B., Schferz, G. *et al.* (1987) In vitro and in vivo susceptibility of *Borrelia burg-dorfen*. *European Journal of Clinical Microbiology*, **6**, 424–426.

Putkonen, T., Mustakallio, K. and Salmineu, A. (1962) Erythema chronicum migrans with meningitis: a rare coincidence of two tick-borne diseases? *Derma-tologica*, **125**, 184–188.

Rahn, D.W. and Malawista, S.E. (1991) Lyme disease: recommendations for diagnosis and treatment. *Annals of Internal Medicine*, **114**, 472–481.

Raucher, H.S., Kaufman, D.M., Goldfarb, J. *et al.* (1985) Pseudotumor cerebri and Lyme disease: a new association. *Journal of Pediatrics*, **107**, 931–933.

Reik, L., Jr, Burgdorfer, W. and Donaldson, J.O. (1986) Neurologic abnormalities in Lyme disease without erythema chronicum migrans. *American Journal of Medicine*, **81**, 73–78.

Rienzo, R.J., Morel, D.E., Prager, D. *et al.* (1987) Gallium avid Lyme myocarditis. *Clinical Nuclear Medicine*, **12**, 475–476.

Rodhain, F. and Edlinger, E. (1987) Serodiagnostic of erythema chronicum migrans (Lyme disease) in cases initially suspected as caused by arboviruses.

Zentralblatt für Bakteriologie, Mikrobiologie und Hygiene A, **263**, 425–426.

Rousseau, J.J., Lust, C., Zangerle, P.F. *et al.* (1986) Acute transverse myelitis as presenting neurological feature of Lyme disease (letter). *Lancet*, **221**, 1222–1223.

Sagransky, D.M. (1986) Lyme disease masquerading as juvenile rheumatoid arthritis. *New Jersey Medicine*, **83**, 451–452.

Schechter, S.L. (1986) Lyme disease associated with optic neuropathy. *American Journal of Medicine*, **81**, 143–145.

Scrimenti, R.J. (1970) Erythema chronicum migrans. *Archives of Dermatology*, **236**, 859–860.

Steere, A.A.C. (1986) Lyme disease. *New England Journal of Medicine*, **321**, 586.

Steere, A.C. and Malwista S. (1979) Cases of Lyme disease in the United States: locations correlated with the distribution of *Ixodes scapularus*. *Annals of Internal Medicine*, **91**, 730–733.

Steere, A.C., Malawista, S.E., Snydman, D.R. *et al.* (1977) Lyme arthritis: an epidemic of oligoarticular arthritis in children and adults in three Connecticut communities. *Arthritis and Rheumatism*, **20**, 7–17.

Steere, A.C., Batsford, W.B., Wienber, M. *et al.* (1980) Lyme carditis: cardiac abnormalities of Lyme disease. *Annals of Internal Medicine*, **93**, 8.

Steere, A.C., Grodziki, R.L., Kornblatt, A.N. *et al.* (1983) The spirochetal etiology of Lyme disease. *New England Journal of Medicine*, **308**, 733–740.

Steere, A.C., Hutchinson, G.J., Craft, J. *et al.* (1983) The early clinical manifestations of Lyme disease. *Annals of Internal Medicine*, **99**, 76–82.

Steere, A., Hutchinson, G.J., Rahn, D.W. *et al.* (1983) Treatment of the early manifestations of Lyme disease. *Annals of Internal Medicine*, **99**, 22–27.

Steere, A.C., Grodzicki, R.L., Craft, J.E. *et al.* (1984) Recovery of Lyme disease spirochetes from patients. *Yale Journal of Biology and Medicine*, **57**, 557–560.

Steere, A.C., Duray, P.H., Kauffmann, D.J.H. *et al.* (1985) Unilateral blindness caused by infection with the Lyme disease spirochete, *Borrelia burgdorferi*. *Annals of Internal Medicine*, **103**, 382–384.

Stiernstedt, G., Gustafsson, R., Karlsson, M. *et al.* (1988) Clinical manifestations and diagnosis of neuroborreliosis. *Annals of the New York Academy of Sciences*, **539**, 46–55.

Van Dam, Kuiper, H., Vos, K. *et al.* (1991) Differential genospecies of *Borrelia burgdorferi* are associated with distinct clinical manifestations of Lyme diseases. *Clinical Infectious Diseases*, **123**, 603–606.

Volkman, D.J., Luft, B.J., Gorevic, P.D. *et al.* (1991) Characterization of an immunoreactive 93 kDa core protein of *Borrelia burgdorferi* with a human IgG monoclonal antibody. *Journal of Immunology*, **146**, 3177.

Weber, K. and Neubert, U. (1986) Clinical features of early erythema migrans disease and related disorders. *Zentralblatt für Bakteriologie und Hygiene A*, **263**, 209–228.

Wokke, J.H., de Koning, J., Stanek, G. *et al.* (1987) Chronic muscle weakness caused by *Borrelia burgdorferi* meningoradiculitis. *Annals of Neurology*, **22**, 389–392.

23

MYCOPLASMAS

Christiane C. Bébéar

INTRODUCTION

Mycoplasmas are ubiquitous microorganisms which have been known as animal pathogens since the end of the nineteenth century. They are members of the class Mollicutes (*mollis cutis*, Latin: soft skin) and the smallest prokaryotes able to multiply autonomously. Even though the term mycoplasma only applies, taxonomically, to the genus *Mycoplasma*, it is still commonly used to indicate these organisms as a whole. It will be used in this chapter to designate any of the organisms in the class *Mollicutes*.

The first *Mycoplasma* was isolated in 1898, by Nocard and Roux. It was *M. mycoides* subsp. *mycoides*, the cause of contagious bovine pleuropneumonia. The first recorded case of a human *Mycoplasma* infection, an abscess of the Bartholin gland, was described in 1937 by Dienes and Edsall. The species isolated was probably *M. hominis*. In 1954, Shepard isolated mycoplasmas from the urogenital tract. These mycoplasmas produced particularly small colonies. They were called T strain, indicating tiny colonies, and are now known as ureaplasmas. It was only in 1962 that Chanock, Hayflick and Barile succeeded in culturing *M. pneumoniae*, the cause of primary atypical pneumonia, in an acellular medium. They

then identified the Eaton agent, which had been cultured on chick embryo, as a *Mycoplasma*. Among the potential human pathogens, *M. genitalium* was discovered in 1981 (Taylor-Robinson, 1995a). Recently, two species of mycoplasmas were found in HIV-seropositive patients: *M. fermentans*, known elsewhere since 1952, and *M. penetrans* (Wang *et al.*, 1993).

CLASSIFICATION AND PHYLOGENY

Mycoplasmas are completely lacking a cell wall. They belong to the class Mollicutes. This class consists of four orders, Mycoplasmatales, Entomoplasmatales, Acholeplasmatales and Anaeroplasmatales, which are distinguished on the basis of their natural habitat, their sterol requirements and a certain number of other properties (Tully *et al.*, 1993).

The species isolated from humans belong mainly to the order Mycoplasmatales, family Mycoplasmataceae, that includes two genera: *Mycoplasma* and *Ureaplasma*. Facultatively anaerobic, they require sterols for growth. Their principal energy sources are sugars and arginine or urea in the case of *Ureaplasma*. Thirteen of the 85 known *Mycoplasma* spp. and one of the five *Ureaplasma* spp., *U. urealyticum*, have been isolated from humans.

Principles and Practice of Clinical Bacteriology. Edited by A.M. Emmerson, P.M. Hawkey and S.H. Gillespie
© 1997 John Wiley & Sons Ltd

The rest are of animal origin. *Acholeplasma laidlawii*, the type species of the order Acholeplasmatales, has been described occasionally in humans. This order is distinguished by its ability to produce its own sterols. The Entomoplasmatales are mycoplasmas isolated from insects and plants. The order contains the *Entomoplasma*, *Mesoplasma* and *Spiroplasma* (mycoplasmas with a helical morphology) genera.

Phylogenetically, mycoplasmas are very simple microorganisms. In spite of their small size, they are highly evolved bacteria coming from anaerobic Gram-positive ancestors (clostridia) containing a low level of G + C. Mycoplasmas probably evolved from these ancestors by successive reduction in the genome and loss of the cell wall. The closest bacterial species to this phylogenetic branch are *Clostridium innocuum* and *C. ramosum*.

HABITAT

Mycoplasmas are ubiquitous microorganisms. In nature, flowers and plant surfaces constitute an important reservoir. Insects act as vectors and can also suffer from specific mycoplasma-caused diseases. Mycoplasmas are also found in animals, especially animals in intensive production facilities and laboratory animals, and humans.

The 15 species found in humans are indicated in Table 23.1. Mycoplasmas can be grouped by the site where they are usually isolated in immunocompetent subjects: the respiratory and genital tracts. Most of the mycoplasmas isolated from the oropharynx are simple commensals (*M. salivarium*, *M. orale*, *M. buccale*, *M. faucium*, *M. lipophilum*, *A. laidlawii*). Only *M. pneumoniae* colonizes the lower respiratory tract and possesses certain pathogenic capacity.

Seven species can be considered genital mycoplasmas. Two of these, *U. urealyticum* and *M. hominis*, are part of the genital commensal flora of a great number of people (Taylor-Robinson, 1989). Frequency of colonization varies with age, hormonal factors, race, socioeconomic level and sexual activity. It is difficult to evaluate the rate of colonization in the general population, although it is known to be higher in women than in men. It may be as high as 50% vaginally in women for *U. urealyticum*, while *M. hominis* is probably less

TABLE 23.1 MAIN CHARACTERISTICS OF MYCOPLASMAS ISOLATED FROM HUMANS

	Pathogenicity	Isolation rate by culture	Metabolism of		
			Glucose	Arginine	Urea
Respiratory tract					
M. pneumoniae	+	Rare	+	−	−
M. salivarium	−	Frequent	−	+	−
M. orale	−	Frequent	−	+	−
M. buccale	−	Rare	−	+	−
M. faucium	−	Rare	−	+	−
M. lipophilum	−	Rare	−	+	−
A. laidlawii	−	Very rare	+	−	−
Genital tract					
U. urealyticum	+	Frequent	−	−	+
M. hominis	+	*frequent*	−	+	−
M. genitalium	+	Very rare	+	−	−
M. fermentans	?	Very rare	+	+	−
M. penetrans	?	Very rare	+	+	−
M. spermatophilum	?	Very rare	−	+	−
M. primatum	−	Rare	−	+	−
Other site					
M. pirum	?	Very rare	+	+	−

than 15%. Both species are responsible for human infections (Krause *et al.*, 1992). The role of the other species (*M. genitalium*, *M. fermentans* and *M. penetrans*) is much less well known because they are rarely detected by culture. *Mycoplasma spermatophilum* and *M. primatum* have been detected on an exceptional basis. The natural habitat of *M. pirum* is unknown.

Mycoplasmas are frequent contaminants of cell cultures, particularly continuous cell lines. Five species (*M. hyorhinis*, *M. orale*, *M. fermentans*, *M. arginini* and *A. laidlawii*) are responsible for about 95% of contaminations. Their frequency and the possible consequences for the use of these cells necessitate regular surveillance by those who use cell lines in their research.

DESCRIPTION OF THE ORGANISMS

Morphology and Structure

Mycoplasmas are very small organisms (0.2–0.3 μm). When examined by dark-field or phase-contrast microscopy, they appear to be pleomorphic, coccoid or filamentous, depending on the species and culture conditions. Spiroplasmas are helical in shape. They are not stained by Gram stain and only weakly stained by Giemsa stain.

Electron microscopy shows that certain species, *M. pneumoniae*, *M. genitalium*, *M. penetrans* and certain animal mycoplasmas, have a specialized terminal structure. This slender extremity plays an important role in the adhesion of mycoplasmas to different substrates and in their mobility using a gliding movement.

Mycoplasmas have no cell wall and differ from L-forms by the absence of precursors of peptidoglycan and binding proteins for penicillins. All of the species of the genera *Mycoplasma* and *Ureaplasma* possess a cytoplasmic membrane containing cholesterol.

The genome of mycoplasmas varies in size, from 580 kbp in *M. genitalium*, which was completely sequenced in 1995, to 2200 kbp in *Spiroplasma citri*. The G + C content ranges from 23% to 41%. With the exception of acholeplasmas, they use the codon UGA to code for tryptophan. They possess one or two rRNA operons and their number of tRNAs is reduced.

Nutritional Requirements

Because of the small size of their genome, mycoplasmas have a very limited capacity to synthesize their component parts. This renders them rather fastidious. In order to grow, they require nucleic acid precursors (yeast extract) and the cholesterol contained in serum (except for acholeplasmas and mesoplasmas).

The optimum atmospheric conditions are equally variable. *Mycoplasma pneumoniae* and *M. genitalium* are aerobic but their growth is stimulated in the presence of 5% carbon dioxide. *Mycoplasma hominis* and *U. urealyticum* are indifferent but grow better on agar media in an atmosphere of 95% nitrogen plus 5% carbon dioxide. *Mycoplasma fermentans* and *M. penetrans* grow better under anaerobic conditions. The optimum temperature for growth is approximately 36–38 °C.

In broth culture, the generation time varies from 1 hour for *U. urealyticum* to 6 hours for *M. pneumoniae* and more for *M. genitalium*. Broth cultures do not usually become cloudy. On agar media, colonies are slow growing. Because they are extremely small, they must be observed with the help of low-power magnification. The appearance of the colonies is variable but takes on a characteristic 'fried-egg' aspect because the organisms penetrate deeply into the agar in the central region of the colony (see Figure 23.1.). Colonies of *U. urealyticum* are very small and irregular (see Figure 23.2.).

Biochemical Characteristics

Species of mycoplasmas isolated from humans can be grouped as glucose fermenters (*M. pneumoniae*, *M. genitalium*, *M. fermentans* and *M. penetrans*) and non-fermenters. Non-fermenters draw their energy from the hydrolysis of arginine by the metabolic pathway of arginine dihydrolase. *Mycoplasma fermentans* and *M. penetrans* use both arginine and glucose. The source of energy of *U.*

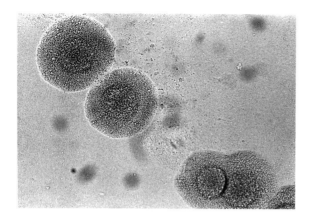

Figure 23.1. Colonies of *M. hominis*.

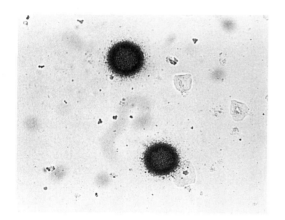

Figure 23.2. Colonies of *U. urealyticum*.

urealyticum most certainly involves the degradation of urea (Table 23.1).

Mycoplasma pneumoniae is able to reduce 2,3,5-triphenyltetrazolium chloride. Haemadsorption and haemagglutination of guinea-pig or chicken erythrocytes and production of peroxides which confer haemolytic abilities are also found in this species. These characteristics are used to identify mycoplasmas of human origin.

Antigenic Structure

Membrane antigens probably play an essential role in the host response to infection. *Mycoplasma*

pneumoniae possesses a glycolipid which is not completely specific and can be found in diverse tissues, microorganisms, plants and several membrane bound-proteins playing a role in adhesion. The P1 protein (170 kDa), found on the narrow extremity, is the major cytadhesin but other proteins also take part (P30 and HMW (high molecular weight) 1–5). Although variability of cytadhesin P1 has been described, *M. pneumoniae* is a very homogeneous species. *Mycoplasma hominis* is much more heterogeneous. There are at least seven serovars. Fourteen serovars corresponding to two different biovars are known for *U. urealyticum*. An additional level of antigenic variability, related to variations in the size of antigen proteins, has been described for several species of mycoplasmas, *U. urealyticum* in particular (Zheng *et al.*, 1995).

PATHOGENESIS

Mycoplasma pneumoniae

The pathogenesis of infection with *M. pneumoniae* has been studied using different models, organ cultures and experimental animal models, hamsters inoculated intranasally and chimpanzees. In these animal models, *M. pneumoniae* colonizes the respiratory epithelium diffusely and provokes lesions comparable histopathologically to those observed in humans (perivascular and peribronchiolar infiltration of mononuclear cells).

Two mechanisms contribute to the pathogenesis of *M. pneumoniae* infections: adhesion of *M. pneumoniae* to the respiratory epithelium, followed by localized cellular lesions and immunopathological disorders which can lead to lesions elsewhere. *Mycoplasma pneumoniae* can adhere to a number of substrates: glass, plastic, red blood cells and respiratory epithelial cells. *In vivo*, this adhesion permits the organism to escape the ciliary movement and come into close contact with the cell membrane. This role is confirmed by the loss of pathogenicity for hamsters of nonadherent strains. Adhesion, which takes place at the narrow extremity of the terminal structure, is structure, is mediated by several proteins, including P1, the principal cytadhesin involved. The host cells have receptors containing sialic acid. The adhesion blocks ciliary action and cause cellular alterations due to the production of peroxides and superoxides by *M. pneumoniae*.

Immunopathological mechanisms are suspected to be involved in some of the lesions provoked by *M. pneumoniae*. The histological appearance of these lesions, the presence of lesions at a distance, from which mycoplasmas are rarely isolated (cutaneous lesions and synovial fluid) and the presence of autoantibodies argue in favour of this hypothesis.

Genital Mycoplasmas

The pathogenesis of genital mycoplasmas is less well known. Various models of genital infections have been developed using different animals. In mice, establishment of *M. hominis* and *U. urealyticum* in the vagina is improved by treating the animals with hormones. Extension of the infection toward the upper genital tract has been observed. In male chimpanzees, intraurethral inoculation of *U. urealyticum* or *M. genitalium* leads to a local leucocyte reaction followed sometimes by dissemination in the blood for *M. genitalium*. Upper genital tract infections (salpingitis and parametritis) have been provoked after inoculation of female monkeys with *M. genitalium* (Taylor-Robinson, 1995a).

The adhesion process has been described for the three species *U. urealyticum*, *M. hominis* and *M. genitalium*. The latter organism possesses an adhesin, MgPa, which is very similar to P1 of *M. pneumoniae*.

Diverse enzymatic activities (urease and IgA1 protease for *U. urealyticum*, phospholipase for *U. urealyticum* and *M. hominis*) and the production of certain metabolites explain, in part, their pathogenicity. *Mycoplasma hominis* and *M. genitalium* are capable of penetrating into the host cell (Jensen *et al.*, 1994). It is not known if certain biovars or serovars of *U. urealyticum* and *M. hominis* have a particular pathogenicity capability.

CLINICAL FEATURES

Respiratory Infections

Mycoplasma pneumoniae

This is the mycoplasma most often concerned. It causes acute respiratory infections, most frequently in children from four years of age to young adults. The infection is endemic in the population, with epidemic peaks every four or five years. A surge occurred in Europe in the 1990s. Although more frequent in cold weather, there is not a clear seasonal trend in frequency. This infection is not very contagious. The persistence of *M. pneumoniae* in the respiratory tract contributes to the endemic nature of the disease (Foy, 1993). In hypogammaglobulinaemic subjects, the infection can persist for a long time. Other than during epidemics, when it can be found in the oropharynx of healthy subjects, *M. pneumoniae* is not usually found among the commensal flora of the respiratory tract.

Infection often starts as a simple tracheobronchitis. *Mycoplasma pneumoniae* is the second most common cause of community-acquired pneumonia after *Streptococcus pneumoniae* and is probably responsible for 15–20% of X-ray-proven cases of pneumonia (Foy, 1993). In its characteristic form, this disease develops as a primary atypical pneumonia with a progressive installation, fever, involvement of the upper respiratory tract, dry cough and marked radiological lesions. It evolves slowly and progressively. The disease is ordinarily mild. Respiratory symptoms alone do not distinguish *M. pneumoniae* from other causes of atypical pneumonia. Association with other symptoms can be a better indication: cutaneous lesions (Stevens–Johnson syndrome, multiform erythaemia), otitis media, pharyngitis, neurological involvement (meningitis, meningoencephalitis), haemolytic anaemia due to the presence of cold haemagglutinins, coagulation problems, arthritis, myocarditis, pericarditis, involvement of the pancreas, digestive tract and kidneys. These complications may occur alone and therefore be difficult to associate with their actual causal agent.

Other mycoplasmas

In adults, these are all commensal organisms with the possible exception of *M. fermentans*. A certain number of cases of fulminant infections with a syndrome of respiratory distress with or without systemic involvement have been reported in subjects previously in good health (Lo *et al.*, 1993). Five of six of the published cases have been fatal in spite of the administration of erythromycin. The only pathogen identified from lesions post mortem was *M. fermentans*, which is resistant to erythromycin. In experimental animal models, it has been shown that *M. fermentans* can produce cellular lesions (Stadtländer *et al.*, 1993) and penetrate into respiratory epithelial cells (Taylor-Robinson *et al.*, 1993). *M. fermentans* may be a little-known cause of respiratory infections.

Urogenital Tract Infections

Ureaplasma urealyticum *and* Mycoplasma hominis

It is difficult to determine the actual pathogenic capacity of these organisms because they are commonly found as commensals in the lower genital tract and because specimens from the upper genital tract are rarely obtained.

In men, *U. urealyticum* is responsible for non-gonococcal, non-chlamydial urethritis (NGU). It is probably responsible for 15–20% of cases. Its role was confirmed by several different criteria: comparison of the rate of isolation from NGU patients with the rate of isolation from a control population, inoculation of experimental animals and humans, serological studies, and therapeutic trials with antibiotics active against mycoplasmas but not against *Chlamydia*. It can also be responsible for epididymitis. Its role in prostatitis is controversial. *Mycoplasma hominis* probably does not play a role in the occurrence of urethritis.

In women, *U. urealyticum* may be responsible for some urethral syndromes (Stamm *et al.*, 1983). *Myoplasma hominis* and, to a lesser degree, *U. urealyticum*, are among the organisms that proliferate during the course of bacterial vaginosis

and can reach a high level of concentration ($\geqslant 10^5$ for *M. hominis*) (Taylor-Robinson, 1995b). This high concentration can lead to invasion of the upper genital tract and cause a salpingitis. *Mycoplasma hominis* has been isolated from the endometrium and the fallopian tubes in about 10% of women presenting with salpingitis observed by laparoscopy. Isolation was also accompanied by a serological response. Nevertheless, the multi-bacterial nature of these infections makes it difficult to determine the exact role of *M hominis*.

Ureaplasma urealyticum and *M. hominis* are responsible for infections related to pregnancy, chorioamnionitis and postpartum septicaemia which can lead to neonatal infection (Neman-Simha *et al.*, 1992). It is important correctly to diagnose these infections early because of the changes necessary in therapy. Neonatal infections such as pneumopathy, meningitis and septicaemia affect highly hypotrophic premature infants (Waites *et al.*, 1988; Cassell *et al.*, 1993).

Ureaplasma urealyticum is suspected to be the cause of certain cases of sterility, repeated spontaneous abortion, and low birth weight in infants. This remains to be proved.

Ureaplasma urealyticum possesses a strong urease activity. When inoculated into laboratory rats, it causes struvite bladder stones. Ureaplasmas have been found more often in the urine and stones of patients with infection-type stones than in patients with metabolic-type stones (Grenabo *et al.*, 1988). The exact role of ureaplasmas is not known but there may be a causal association. *Mycoplasma hominis* has been isolated from the upper urinary tract of patients presenting with pyelonephritis. It has also been occasionally found in extraurogenital specimens (skin, bone, brain).

Mycoplasma genitalium

First isolated from urethral swabs from homosexuals, it is difficult to evaluate its pathogenicity because it is extremely fastidious. The use of polymerase chain reaction (PCR) has shown that it is most certainly the cause of acute NGU because it has been found in 15–20% of symptomatic patients compared with 6% of subjects without urethritis (Horner *et al.*, 1993; Jensen *et al.*, 1993). On the basis of serological arguments, it is suspected to be the cause of salpingitis (Møller *et al.*, 1984). It has been isolated, in association with *M. pneumoniae*, from throat swabs and synovial fluid.

Mycoplasmas and Immunodepression

The status of the immune system of the host determines the outcome of mycoplasma diseases. Septic arthritis caused by *M. pneumoniae* and *U. urealyticum* has been described in hypogamma-globulinaemic subjects (Furr *et al.*, 1994). Septicaemia caused by *M. hominis* has been described in subjects under immunosuppressive treatment.

A possible role of three species, *M. fermentans*, *M. penetrans* and *M. pirum*, in the course of HIV infection has recently been called into question. The principal arguments for this role come from *in vitro* studies showing an interaction between mycoplasmas and HIV (Lemaître *et al.*, 1992) and from the fact that mycoplasmas have been isolated from the urogenital tract (*M. penetrans*) and deep tissues or blood of HIV-infected patients (*M. fermentans*) (Bébéar *et al.*, 1993a; Katseni *et al.*, 1993). For the moment, no conclusion can be drawn on this subject.

LABORATORY DIAGNOSTICS

Specimens

Whatever the sampling method used, it must collect cells to which mycoplasmas have adhered. Different types of sampling methods can be used for the respiratory tract. Sputum specimens are not very useful because they contain too many con-taminants. Throat swabs and nasopharyngeal aspirations for young children can be used because of the diffuse nature of the infection. Bronchial brushing and bronchoalveolar lavages can also be taken.

Genital mycoplasmas can be cultured from urethral swabs, first-void urine, semen, prostatic secretions, cervicovaginal swabs, endometrial biopsies, tubal brushing, amniotic fluid, placenta, endotracheal samples, etc. Other samples can be used for culture: cerebrospinal fluid, blood, synovial fluid or biopsies, and mucocutaneous samples. The classic media used for blood culture contain anti-coagulants which act as inhibitors for the growth of mycoplasmas.

Transport

As soon as specimens are taken, the swabs must be placed in the appropriate transport medium in order to avoid drying. Different media can be used for transport and storage: culture medium with or without substrate, and sucrose phosphate transport medium (2SP) containing 5% fetal bovine serum, without antibiotics, are likely to be used for selection of both mycoplasmas and *Chlamydia*; commercial transport media.

All samples must be transmitted to the labora-tory as soon as possible. If they cannot be cultured immediately, they should be stored at +4 °C for a maximum of 48 hours and beyond that at −70 °C or in liquid nitrogen.

Culture

Culture of mycoplasmas is relatively simple for certain species such as *U. urealyticum* and *M. hominis*, more delicate for *M. pneumoniae*, and very fastidious and rarely successful for *M. geni-talium*, *M. fermentans*, *M. pirum* and *M. penetrans*.

Culture media

The culture media used are complex and rendered selective by the addition of a β-lactam antibiotic (penicillin or ampicillin) and sometimes poly-myxin. Thallium acetate can act as an inhibitor for some species of mycoplasmas and should, there-fore, be avoided.

For the culture of *M. pneumoniae*, the medium frequently used is a modified Hayflick medium containing heart infusion broth supplemented with 10% (v/v) freshly prepared yeast extract (25% wt/vol.) and 20% horse serum (Freundt,

1983). SP-4 medium is more complex and contains fetal bovine serum (Tully *et al.*, 1979). A number of species of mycoplasmas grow better in this medium. Liquid media contain glucose (0.5%) and phenol red (0.002%). The pH ranges from 7.5 to 7.8.

Ureaplasma urealyticum is cultured at pH 6.0, on a medium based on trypticase soya, enriched with yeast extract, horse serum, cysteine and urea. The liquid medium contains the pH indicator phenol red (Shepard, 1983).

Mycoplasma hominis grows on modified Hayflick medium and SP-4 medium (initial pH around 7.2). The broth form of the two media does not change colour during culture unless the medium contains arginine (1%) instead of glucose. *Mycoplasma hominis* also grows on the medium at pH 6.0 designed for the culture of *U. urealyticum*.

SP-4 medium is the best adapted for the growth of fastidious species. It is enriched with glucose for *M. genitalium* and with glucose and sometimes arginine for *M. fermentans*, *M. penetrans* and *M. pirum*.

Whatever the species sought, it is better to use both liquid and agar media (initially or after subculture). Broth cultures should be serially diluted 1:10 from 10^{-1} to 10^{-4}, in order to eliminate any possible inhibitors present in the tissue and for quantitative evaluation. Agar media should be dot inoculated. Liquid specimens (bronchoalveolar lavage, urine) should be centrifuged before plating. Given the fastidious nature of mycoplasmas, quality control of the culture media is essential.

Detection of growth

In liquid media containing glucose, growth of fermenting species (particularly *M. pneumoniae*), is detected by a change in colour of the pH indicator. Growth of *U. urealyticum* produces an alkalinization of the liquid medium containing urea, as does the growth of *M. hominis* and other such species on broth media containing arginine (Table 23.1). The colour change occurs after 18–24 hours for *U. urealyticum*, 48 hours for *M. hominis*, 6–20 days for *M. pneumoniae* and even longer for more fastidious species.

After specimens have been plated and incubated under appropriate conditions for the particular species sought, colonies must be observed under magnification. The appearance varies from species to species. *Mycoplasma pneumoniae* is often granular, while colonies of *M. hominis* are small (200–300 μm) and fried-egg shaped. Colonies of *U. urealyticum* are irregular and very small (15–30 μm). Colonies grown on solid media containing urea and manganous sulphate or calcium chloride are black, which makes them easier to see and more difficult to confuse with artefacts such as crystals in the medium. These colonies can be observed directly after culture of the specimen on agar, or as a control, after subculture of liquid media which have changed colour.

Identification

Mycoplasma pneumoniae is identified on the basis of certain biochemical properties (fermentation of glucose, lack of arginine hydrolysis), haemadsorption or haemagglutination of guinea-pig or chicken erythrocytes (absent in commensal respiratory mycoplasmas), and haemolysis. Antigenic identification, the reference method, is difficult without commercially available immune serum. Several different techniques can be used: agar growth inhibition, epifluorescence or immunoperoxidase techniques. The latter two permit direct identification of colonies on agar and therefore the detection of a mixture of species. It is, however, difficult to separate *M. pneumoniae* and *M. genitalium* using antigenic identification in that they present closely related antigens and similar biochemical properties. Amplification of genetic material from culture by PCR is an excellent alternative method of identification.

Identification of *U. urealyticum* and *M. hominis* is relatively simple. The change of a colour indicator and the physical appearance of colonies are the principal methods. It is necessary to verify this identification because a colour change can be caused by the presence of other bacteria or cells. Antigenic identification is rarely performed and separation of serovars is not current practice. The two biovars of *U. urealyticum* can be identified by PCR (Robertson *et al.*, 1993).

Different commercial kits have been proposed for the detection of *U. urealyticum* and *M. hominis* from genital swabs. They give satisfactory results if identification is verified by the physical appearance of colonies on agar.

Interpretation

Isolation of *M. pneumoniae* from a patient with a respiratory infection is an important indicator because this organism is not part of the commensal flora.

Isolation of *U. urealyticum* or *M. hominis* poses a more delicate problem of interpretation. Isolation from normally sterile specimens is significant, but for other specimens where they can be present as commensals it is useful to make a quantitative evaluation. The criteria proposed as significant for NGU are as follows: 10^4 colour-changing units (CCU)/ml for a urethral swab and 10^3 CCU/ml for first void urine. The presence of *U. urealyticum* in cervicovaginal swabs is difficult to interpret because of its natural frequency. *Mycoplasma hominis* can be found in high numbers ($\geqslant 10^4$ CCU/ml) during vaginosis. Its presence can also suggest an infection higher up in the genital tract. In this case, clinical signs and associated bacteriological elements must be taken into account. The presence of mycoplasmas in peripheral neonatal specimens can be due to simple contamination. Isolation from endotracheal specimens is more significant.

Rapid Techniques

These techniques are useful for mycoplasmas which are difficult and time consuming to culture. The presence of viable organisms is not necessary.

Antigenic detection

Techniques for detection of antigens have, for the most part, been developed for *M. pneumoniae*. Different techniques (immunoblot, enzyme-linked immunosorbent assay (ELISA)) using monoclonal or polyclonal antibodies have been proposed (Harris *et al.*, 1988; Kok *et al.*, 1988). The level of detection capability of these techniques is not very sensitive (about 10^5 colony-forming units (CFU)/ml), which limits their usefulness.

Molecular hybridization

Different types of probes have been described. Here again, the sensitivity of detection is insufficient (10^4 to 10^5 CFU).

Thus the principal interest is of amplification by PCR. This technique has been described for most of the species potentially pathogenic for humans. For *M. pneumoniae*, different systems have been proposed, including amplification of a random sequence (Bernet *et al.*, 1989) of the 16S rDNA, and the gene for adhesin (de Barbeyrac *et al.*, 1993). This form of detection is very sensitive (10–100 organisms from a clinical specimen) and very specific. It can be used for clinical diagnosis but presently does not exist in the form of commercial kit.

The PCR technique is practically the only method for detection of *M. genitalium* (Palmer *et al.*, 1991; de Barbeyrac *et al.*, 1993), and remains the best method for detection of *M. fermentans* (Wang *et al.*, 1992), *M. penetrans* and *M. pirum*. It is potentially interesting for the detection of *U. urealyticum* (Blanchard *et al.*, 1993) and *M. hominis* from specimens where the organism is not viable (Table 23.2). This technique is also used to detect mycoplasmal contamination of cell cultures (Teyssou *et al.*, 1993).

Serology

Mycoplasma pneumoniae

Because of their simplicity, serological tests are very often used to diagnose *M. pneumoniae* infections (Jacobs, 1993). Their drawback is that they only allow retrospective diagnosis. The presence of cold haemagglutinins (significant at $\geqslant 1/64$) is neither constant nor specific. Demonstration of a significant increase (four-fold) in the specific antibody titre between two successive tests, or a

TABLE 23.2   LABORATORY METHODS RECOMMENDED FOR THE CURRENT INVESTIGATION OF MYCOPLASMA INFECTIONS

	Culture	PCR	Serology
M. pneumoniae	+[a]	+	+
U. urealyticum	+	−[b]	−
M. hominis	+	−[b]	−
M. genitalium	−	+	−

[a] Requires long time for results.
[b] Not useful routinely.

high level of antibody detected by a single or late test, is an important element in diagnosis.

The complement fixation reaction makes use of antibodies directed against a glycolipid antigen. It is valid as long as certain criteria of interpretation are strictly adhered to (seroconversion or a titre of at least 1/64). Nevertheless, it is not very sensitive and cross-reactions have been reported during neurological or pancreatic illness.

Other techniques are available: agglutination of sensitized latex particles or gelatin, microimmuno-fluorescence and, above all, ELISA, which also allows the detection of IgM. These techniques are probably more sensitive that complement fixation. Nevertheless, the problem of specificity remains, particularly the problem of cross-reactions with *M. genitalium*. The use of purified P1 protein as antigen would probably improve the specificity.

Genital mycoplasmas

A number of techniques have been developed for detection of antibodies during *U. urealyticum* or *M. hominis* infection: metabolic inhibition and ELISA. The results of these tests are difficult to interpret because of the lack of information concerning the level of immunity found in the general population. Given the present state of knowledge, serological tests, although theoretically useful, are not recommended in current practice.

Presently, there is no commercialized kit for the detection of antibodies against *M. genitalium*. Efforts to develop such a technique have been blocked by the problem of antigens in common with *M. pneumoniae*.

Antimicrobial Susceptibility

Mycoplasmas have natural characteristics which explain their intrinsic resistance to certain antibiotics. Because they lack peptidoglycan, they are insensitive to all antibiotics which prevent its biosynthesis, in particular, the β-lactam antibiotics. They are resistant to rifampin owing to the weak affinity of their RNA polymerase for this antibiotic. They are also resistant to polymyxins. The families of antibiotics potentially useful are tetracyclines, macrolides and related compounds, and fluoroquinolones.

Study methods

The nutritional and cultural requirements of mycoplasmas are rather distant from the standard conditions recommended for bacteria. The small size of the colonies means that agar diffusion methods cannot be used. Only dilution method can be used.

Studies of minimal inhibitory concentrations (MIC) can be done in broth or agar media. Agar media are recommended for mycoplasmas which produce colonies easily observed with a binocular microscope (practically all the species of the genus *Mycoplasma*), while broth media are recommended for *U. urealyticum*. Initial inoculum should be quantified and contain 10^4 to 10^5 CCU for *Mycoplasma* spp. and 10^3 to 10^4 CCU for *U. urealyticum*. After a period of incubation appropriate for the species, the results should be read when growth becomes visible on the control medium containing no antibiotics. The MIC is the lowest concentration of antibiotic inhibiting the growth of colonies or a colour change of the pH indicator.

There are several kits available for testing antibiotic sensitivity of genital mycoplasmas, *U. urealyticum* and *M. hominis*. These kits should be used after isolation of the organism and not directly on the original specimen. Two concentrations of antibiotic are generally studied. The strain is classed as sensitive, intermediate or resistant. The results obtained with these kits are satisfactory.

Bactericidal activity of antibiotics against mycoplasmas is rarely studied. After the MIC has been determined, several techniques can be employed to determine the minimum bactericidal concentration (MBC): simple passage on medium without antibiotics, and replacement of the medium containing antibiotics by fresh medium after filtration or centrifugation.

In vitro activity

A relationship has never been shown between acquired resistance and a plasmid. The different species of mycoplasmas vary in their sensitivity to antibiotics (Renaudin et al., 1992; Roberts et al., 1992). The MIC values for some of the most common species are given in Table 23.3.

Tetracyclines

Tetracyclines are highly active against all species of mycoplasmas. No case of acquired resistance to tetracyclines has been reported for M. pneumoniae or M. genitalium. Acquired resistance has been reported for U. urealyticum and M. hominis (about 3.5% of strains isolated in France

– this figure is higher in other countries). Resistance is due to the presence of the tet(M) determinant, widely found among genital bacteria (Roberts, 1992). This determinant is part of a conjugative transposon located on the chromosome in mycoplasmas, and coding for a protein which protects the ribosome from the action of tetracyclines. It leads to cross-resistance to tetracycline, doxycycline and minocycline. A new class of derivative, the glycylines, has been shown to be active against strains of M. hominis carrying the tet(M) determinant.

Macrolides and related compounds

Large differences are found between species. Some natural resistances exist for macrolides and lincosamides.

Mycoplasma hominis and M. fermentans are consistently resistant to erythromycin and macrolides with a 14-atom lactonic macrocyclic ring (roxithromycin, clarithromycin, dirithromycin, flurithromycin) and are, on the other hand, sensitive to josamycin and midecamycin (Table 23.3).

TABLE 23.3   MIC OF VARIOUS ANTIBIOTICS AGAINST DIFFERENT MYCOPLASMAS

Antibiotics	MIC range (mg/l)				
	M. pneumoniae	U. urealyticum	M. hominis	M. fermentans	M. genitalium
Doxycycline	0.01–0.02	0.02–1[a]	0.02–0.05[a]	0.13–0.26	≤0.01–0.05
Minocycline	0.01–0.02	0.02–1[a]	0.02–1[a]	ND[b]	≤0.01–0.02
Erythromycin	0.03–0.06	0.5–4	≥128	32–64	≤0.01
Roxithromycin	≤0.01	0.1–2	>16	ND	≤0.01
Clarithromycin	0.05	0.02–0.2	16–≥128	16–64	≤0.01
Azithromycin	≤0.01	0.5–4	4–64	ND	≤0.01
Josamycin	≤0.01–0.02	0.1–1	0.05–0.1	0.2	0.02
Lincomycin	4–8	8–256	0.2–1	0.15–0.2	1–8
Clindamycin	1–2	0.5–16	0.02–0.05	0.14–0.23	0.2–1
Pristinamycin	0.02–0.05	0.1–1	0.1–0.5	0.02–0.05	≤0.01–0.02
Pefloxacin	2	0.5–8	0.5–2	ND	ND
Ciprofloxacin	1	1–16	0.1–1	0.02–016	2
Ofloxacin	0.05–1	0.2–2	0.2–2	0.1–0.2	1–2
Sparfloxacin	0.1	0.1–0.5	≤0.01	≤0.01–0.05	0.05–0.1
Chloramphenicol	4	0.4–3.1	0.5–0.8	3–3.3	0.5–4
Gentamicin	3.2–6.4	3.1–25	3.2–6.4	15.6	ND

[a] Strains susceptible to tetracyclines.
[b] ND, not done.

Azithromycin has little activity. *Mycoplasma hominis* and *M. fermentans* are both sensitive to lincosamides.

Mycoplasma pneumoniae and *M. genitalium* are very sensitive to macrolides, and a little less so to lincosamides (Renaudin *et al.*, 1992). Acquired resistance to macrolides, lincomycin and strepto-gramin B has been described on a rare basis in *M. pneumoniae*. The frequency of this resistance is probably very low.

The MICs of macrolides with regard to *U. urealyticum* are generally higher than that noted for sensitive mycoplasmas. These organisms are often classified as intermediate with regard to these antibiotics. When interpreting these MIC, the fact that the cultural conditions used, i.e. pH 6.0, reduce the activity of macrolides must be taken into account. Clarithromycin gives the lowest MIC. Strains of *U. urealyticum* highly resistant to macrolides have been described.

Pathogenic mycoplasmas, in general, are very sensitive to pristinamycin (Bébéar *et al.*, 1993b) and RP 59500.

Quinolones and other products

Mycoplasmas and ureaplasmas are naturally resistant to nalidixic acid. Like the Gram-positive bacteria to which they are phylogenetically related, they are more sensitive to fluoroquinolones. The more recent compounds are the most active. Sparfloxacin gives very low MICs (Kenny *et al.*, 1991). The fluoro-quinolones are the only antibiotics with a potentially bactericidal effect on mycoplasmas.

Other families of antibiotics are rarely used for the treatment of *Mycoplasma* infections. The aminosides, like the fluoroquinolones, are some-times used for the prevention and treatment of cell cultures contaminated by mycoplasmas. Cases of acquired resistance have been reported.

TREATMENT

Mycoplasma pneumoniae Infection

Because of the lack of simple, rapid detection methods, suspected *M. pneumoniae* infections are treated before they can be confirmed (Bébéar *et al.*, 1993b). Macrolides are usually prescribed for patients of all ages. For adults, fluoroquinolones, which are active *in vitro*, are an interesting alter-native but the number of documented studies is still rather low. The antibiotic treatment can shorten the course of the disease.

Different types of vaccines against *M. pneumoniae* have been tested. None are presently available. The most promising will probably contain the antigenic fraction of purified P1 protein.

Genital Mycoplasma Infection

The choice of antibiotic to treat genital myco-plasma infections must take into account the specific species isolated, any other microorganisms isolated in association and the physical circums-tances of the development of the disease.

In adults, the treatment of these infections is the same as for *Chlamydia*, with which they are sometimes associated. Tetracyclines are the anti-biotics of first choice. There have been some cases of therapeutic failure related to resistance *in vitro*. The fluoroquinolones are certainly interesting. When these antibiotics are contraindicated (pregnancy, neonatal infections), macrolides are considered first. The activity must be tested *in vitro*. It is sometimes necessary to treat neonates with tetra-cycline, for example when the strain involved is resistant to erythromycin. These cases are rare.

The length and method of administration of the treatment depend on the location of the infection. Because most active antibiotics have a bacteriostatic effect on mycoplasmas, the course of treatment must be sufficiently long. Clinical and biological criteria come into play to confirm the efficacy of treatment. Clearing of mycoplasmas is a valid criterion for sites which are normally sterile, but it is no long reliable for sites where mycoplasmas can be found naturally. It must, nevertheless, be said that even though treatment of *Mycoplasma* infections is relatively simple in otherwise healthy subjects, it is much more complicated in immunodepressed subjects. It is then essential to verify eradication of the organism, which can be difficult.

REFERENCES

Bébéar, C., de Barbeyrac, B., Clerc, M.T. et al. (1993a) Mycoplasmas in HIV-1 seropositive patients. *Lancet*, **341**, 758–759.

Bébéar, C., Dupon, M., Renaudin, H. et al. (1993b) Potential improvements in therapeutic options for mycoplasmal respiratory infections. *Clinical Infectious Diseases*, **17** (Suppl., 1), 202–207.

Bernet, C., Garret, M., de Barbeyrac, B. et al. (1989) Detection of *Mycoplasma pneumoniae* by using the polymerase chain reaction. *Journal of Clinical Microbiology*, **27**, 2492–2496.

Blanchard, A., Hentschel, J., Duffy, L. et al. (1993) Detection of *Ureaplasma urealyticum* by polymerase chain reaction in the urogenital tract of adults, in amniotic fluid, and in the respiratory tract of newborns. *Clinical Infectious Diseases*, **17** (Suppl. 1), 148–153.

Cassell, G.H., Waites, K.B., Watson, H.L. et al. (1993) *Ureaplasma urealyticum* intrauterine infection: role in prematurity and disease in newborns. *Clinical Microbiology Review*, **6**, 69–87.

de Barbeyrac, B., Bernet-Poggi, C., Fébrer, F. et al. (1993) Detection of *Mycoplasma pneumoniae* and *Mycoplasma genitalium* by polymerase chain reaction in clinical samples. *Clinical Infectious Diseases*, **17** (Suppl. 1), 83–89.

Foy, H.M. (1993) Infections caused by *Mycoplasma pneumoniae* and possible carrier state in different populations of patients. *Clinical Infectious Diseases*, **17** (Suppl. 1), 37–46.

Freundt, E.A. (1983) Culture media for classic mycoplasmas. In *Methods in Mycoplasmology*, Vol. 1 (ed. S. Razin and J.G. Tully), pp. 127–135. Academic Press, New York.

Furr, P.M., Taylor-Robinson, D. and Webster, D.B. (1994) Mycoplasmas and ureaplasmas in patients with hypogammaglobulinaemia and their role in arthritis: microbiological observations over 20 years. *Annals of the Rheumatic Diseases*, **53**, 183–187.

Grenabo, L., Hedelin, H. and Pettersson, S. (1988) Urinary infection stones caused by *Ureaplasma urealyticum*: a review. *Scandinavian Journal of Infectious Diseases*, **53** (Suppl.), 46–49.

Harris, R, Marmion, B.P., Varkanis, G. et al., (1988) Laboratory diagnosis of *Mycoplasma pneumoniae* infection. II. Comparison of methods for direct detection of specific antigens or nucleic acid sequences in respiratory exudates. *Epidemiology and Infection*, **101**, 685–694.

Horner, P.J., Gilroy, C.B., Thomas, B.J. et al. (1993) Association of *Mycoplasma genitalium* with acute non-gonococcal urethritis. *Lancet*, **342**, 582–585.

Jacobs, E. (1993) Serological diagnosis of *Mycoplasma pneumoniae* infections: a critical review of current procedures. *Clinical Infectious Diseases*, **17** (Suppl. 1), 79–82.

Jensen, J.S., Orsum, R, Dohn, B. et al. (1993) *Mycoplasma genitalium*: a cause of male urethritis? *Genitourinary Medicine*, **69**, 265–269.

Jensen, J.S., Blom, J. and Lind, K (1994) Intracellular location of *Mycoplasma genitalium* in cultivated Vero cells as demonstrated by electron microscopy. *International Journal of Experimental Pathology*, **75**, 91–98.

Katseni, V.L., Gilroy, C.B., Ryait, B.K. et al. (1993) *Mycoplasma fermentans* in individuals seropositive and seronegative for HIV-1. *Lancet*, **341**, 271–273.

Kenny, G.E. and Cartwright, F.D. (1991) Susceptibilities of *Mycoplasma hominis* and *Ureaplasma urealyticum* to two new quinolones, sparfloxacin and Win 57273. *Antimicrobial Agents and Chemotherapy*, **35**, 1515–1516.

Kok, T.W., Varkanis, G, Marmion, B.P. et al. (1988) Laboratory diagnosis of *Mycoplasma pneumoniae* infection. I. Direct detection of antigen in respiratory exudates by enzyme immunoassay. *Epidemiology and Infection*, **101**, 669–684.

Krause, D.C. and Taylor Robinson, D. (1992) Mycoplasma which infect humans. In *Mycoplasmas, Molecular Biology and Pathogenesis* (ed. J. Maniloff, R.N. McElhaney, L.R. Finch et al.), pp. 417–444. American Society for Microbiology, Washington, DC.

Lemaître, M., Henin, Y., Destouesse, F. et al. (1992) Role of mycoplasma infection in the cytopathic effect induced by human immunodeficiency virus type I in infected cell lines. *Infection and Immunity*, **60**, 742–748.

Lo, S.C., Wear D.J., Green S.L. et al. (1993) Adult respiratory distress syndrome with or without systemic disease associated with infections due to *Mycoplasma fermentans*. *Clinical Infectious Diseases*, **17** (Suppl. 1), 259–263.

Møller, B.R, Taylor-Robinson, D. and Furr, P.M. (1984) Serologic evidence implicating *Mycoplasma genitalium* in pelvic inflammatory disease. *Lancet*, **i**, 1102–1103.

Neman-Simha, V., Renaudin, H., de Barbeyrac, B. et al., (1992) Isolation of genital mycoplasmas from blood of febrile obstetrical–gynecologic patients and neonates. *Scandinavian Journal of Infectious Diseases*, **24**, 317–321.

Palmer, H.M., Gilroy, C.B., Furr, P.M. et al. (1991) Development and evaluation of the polymerase chain reaction to detect *Mycoplasma genitalium*. *FEMS Microbiology Letters*, **61**, 199–203.

Renaudin, H., Tully, J.G. and Bébéar, C. (1992) In vitro susceptibility of *Mycoplasma genitalium* to antibiotics. *Antimicrobial Agents and Chemotherapy*, **36**, 870–872.

Roberts, M.C. (1992) Antibiotic resistance. In *Mycoplasmas: Molecular Biology and Pathogenesis* (ed. J. Maniloff, R.N., McElhaney, L.R. Finch *et al.*), pp. 870–872. American Society for Microbiology, Washington, DC.

Robertson, J.A., Vekris, A., Bébéar, C. *et al.* (1993) Polymerase chain reaction using 16S rRNA gene sequences distinguishes the two biovars of *Ureaplasma urealyticum*. *Journal of Clinical Microbiology*, **31**, 824–830.

Shepard, M.C. (1983) Culture media for ureaplasmas. In *Methods in Mycoplasmology*, Vol. 1 (ed. S. Razin and J.G. Tully), pp. 137–146. Academic Press, New York.

Stadtländer, C.T.K.H., Watson, H.L., Simecka, J.W. *et al.* (1993) Cytopathogenicity of *Mycoplasma fermentans* (including strain *incognitus*). *Clinical Infectious Diseases*, **17** (Suppl. 1), 289–301.

Stamm, W.E., Running, K, Hale, J. *et al.* (1983) Etiologic role of *Mycoplasma hominis* and *Ureaplasma urealyticum* in women with the acute urethral syndrome. *Sexually Transmitted Diseases*, **10** (Suppl.), 318–322.

Taylor-Robinson, D. (1989) Genital mycoplasma infections. *Clinics in Laboratory Medicine*, **3**, 501–523.

Taylor-Robinson, D. (1995a) The history and role of *Mycoplasma genitalium* in sexually transmitted diseases. *Genitourinary Medicine*, **71**, 1–8.

Taylor-Robinson, D. (1995b) *Mycoplasma* and *Ureaplasma*. In *Manual of Clinical Microbiology* (ed. P.R. Murray, E.J. Baron, M.A. Pfaller *et al.*), pp. 652–662. American Society for Microbiology, Washington DC.

Taylor-Robinson, D., Sarathchandra, P. and Furr, P.M. (1993) *Mycoplasma fermentans* – HeLa cell interactions. *Clinical Infectious Diseases*, **17** (Suppl. 1), 302–304.

Teyssou, R, Poutiers, F., Saillard, C. *et al.* (1993) Detection of mollicute contamination in cell cultures by 16S rDNA amplification. *Molecular and Cellular Probes*, **7**, 209–216.

Tully, J.G., Rose, D.L., Whitcomb, R.F. *et al.* (1979) Enhanced isolation of *Mycoplasma pneumoniae* from throat washings with a newly modified culture medium. *Journal of Infectious Diseases*, **139**, 478–482.

Tully, J.G., Bové, J.M., Laigret, F. *et al.* (1993) Revised taxonomy of the class Mollicutes: proposed elevation of a monophyletic cluster of arthropod-associated Mollicutes to ordinal rank (Entomoplasmatales ord. nov.) with provision for familial rank to separate species with nonhelical morphology (Entomoplasmataceae fam nov.) from helical species (Spiroplasmataceae), and emended descriptions of the order Mycoplasmatales, family Mycoplasmataceae. *International Journal of Systematic Bacteriology*, **43**, 378–385.

Waites, K.B., Rudd, P.T., Crouse, D.T. *et al.* (1988) Chronic *Ureaplasma urealyticum* and *Mycoplasma hominis* infections of central nervous system in preterm infants. *Lancet*, **i**, 17–21.

Wang, R.Y.H., Wu, W.S., Dawson, M.S. *et al.* (1992) Selective detection of *Mycoplasma fermentans* by polymerase chain reaction and by using a nucleotide sequence within the insertion sequence-like element. *Journal of Clinical Microbiology*, **30**, 245–248.

Wang, R.Y.H., Shih, J.W.K, Weiss, S.H. *et al.* (1993) *Mycoplasma penetrans* infection in male homosexuals with AIDS: high seroprevalence and association with Kaposi's sarcoma. *Clinical Infectious Diseases*, **17**, 724–729.

Zheng X., Teng, L.J., Watson H.R. *et al.* (1995) Small repeating units within the *Ureaplasma urealyticum* MB antigen gene encode serovar specificity and are associated with antigen size variation. *Infection and Immunity*, **63**, 891–898.

24

CHLAMYDIAL INFECTIONS

T.J. Blanchard and D.C.W. Mabey

HISTORY

Trachoma was first recorded in 1500 BC in the Egyptian Ebers papyrus, and was recognized in Roman and medieval writings as a cause of blindness. Soon after Albert Neisser discovered the gonococcus in 1879 it became apparent that this organism could not be isolated from a significant proportion of patients with urethritis or neonatal ophthalmia. The inclusion bodies characteristic of chlamydial infection were first described by Halberstaedter and von Prowazek in 1907, in conjunctival scrapings from orang-utans infected with trachomatous material from patients (Halberstaedter and von Prowazek, 1907). In the following years similar inclusions were identified in conjunctival cells from patients with trachoma, infants with non-gonococcal ophthalmia and cervical cells from their mothers, and in urethral scrapings from men with non-gonococcal urethritis. The first isolation of *Chlamydia psittaci* (in laboratory animals) was made by S.P. Bedson in 1930. *Chlamydia trachomatis* was first grown in the laboratory in Peking by T'ang and colleagues using fertile hen's eggs in 1957. The less laborious and more sensitive cell culture isolation of *C. trachomatis* was introduced by Gordon and Quan in 1965.

DESCRIPTION OF THE ORGANISM

Chlamydial Classification

The genus *Chlamydia* has been divided into four species: *C. trachomatis*, *C. pneumoniae*, *C. psittaci* and *C. pecorum*. *Chlamydia trachomatis* and *C. pneumoniae* are solely human pathogens, whereas *C. psittaci* is predominantly a pathogen of other mammals and avian species and occasionally humans. *Chlamydia pecorum* is a pathogen of sheep and cattle. Chlamydial classification is outlined in Table 24.1.

Chlamydia trachomatis

Chlamydia trachomatis growing inside cells can be distinguished from *C. psittaci* by the presence of glycogen within intracellular inclusions. *Chlamydia trachomatis* is subdivided into strains causing human infections and the mouse pneumonitis agent (often used in laboratory studies of chlamydial infection). Recent DNA sequence studies of major outer membrane protein (MOMP) have confirmed the evolutionary significance of this classification (Zhang *et al.*, 1993). *Chlamydia trachomatis* causes ocular, urogenital and neonatal infections. Serotyping has allowed the discrimination of 18 different

Principles and Practice of Clinical Bacteriology. Edited by A.M. Emmerson, P.M. Hawkey and S.H. Gillespie
© 1997 John Wiley & Sons Ltd

TABLE 24.1 CLASSIFICATION OF CHLAMYDIAE

Chlamydial species/ serotype	Host	Morphology	Clinical association
Chlamydia trachomatis serovars A–C	Human	Intracellular inclusions containing EB and RB; glycogen present	Trachoma
Chlamydia trachomatis serovars D–K	Human	Intracellular inclusions containing EB and RB; glycogen present	Genital tract disease Neonatal disease (pneumonia, ophthalmia)
Chlamydia trachomatis serovars L1–L3	Human	Intracellular inclusions containing EB and RB; glycogen present	Lymphogranuloma venereum
Chlamydia psittaci	Avian, mammalian, others	Intracellular inclusions containing EB and RB; glycogen absent	Ornithosis Abortion
Chlamydia pneumoniae	Human	Intracellular inclusions containing EB and RB; glycogen absent. EB have pear-shaped morphology	Respiratory disease
Chlamydia pecorum	Cattle, sheep	Intracellular inclusions containing EB and RB; glycogen absent	No human disease

serovars of *C. trachomatis* affecting humans (Wang and Grayston, 1991). The serotypic antigenic determinants are localized to the MOMP, correlating with changes in the amino acid sequences of the surface-exposed variable segments I and II (Yuan *et al.*, 1989). These different serovars correlate with the clinical manifestations of infection: serovars A, B, Ba and C are associated with ocular disease, serovars D–K are associated with urogenital disease which may be transmitted to neonates, and the serovars L1–L3 give rise to lymphogranuloma venereum affecting pelvic organs and the draining lymph nodes. Serovars A–C and D–K are very similar in their biological properties, differing principally in their sites of infection. Although serovars D–K have a predilection for the genital tract, ocular infections can occur ('paratrachoma'), often in the context of a coexisting urogenital infection. Serovars A–C and D–K usually infect epithelial surfaces only, whereas serovars L1–L3 are more invasive, usually involving regional lymph nodes and with the potential to spread to other organs. The greater pathogenicity of L

serovars is reflected by enhanced infectivity and growth in tissue culture when compared with other *C. trachomatis* serovars. Experimental studies of genital tract infection in mice suggested there may be serovar-specific variation in pathogenicity within the group of serovars D–K, but this variation has not been confirmed in human infection (Ito *et al.*, 1990).

Chlamydia psittaci

Chlamydia psittaci infects a wide range of hosts, including humans, birds, sheep, cows, pigs, koalas, the African clawed toad and turtles. *Chlamydia psittaci* is a diverse group of organisms from which at least 11 types can be distinguished using microimmunofluorescence and polymerase chain reaction PCR amplification of MOMP (Herring, 1993). It is only a matter of time before *C. psittaci* is subdivided into further species.

Human infection with *C. psittaci* of avian or animal origin causes ornithosis. The disease is a zoonosis, and person-to-person transmission is very rare (Byron *et al.*, 1979). Strictly speaking the term psittacosis should be reserved for chlamydial infections acquired from psittacines (parrots or related birds). There is occasional transmission of the enzootic ovine abortion agent to pregnant women, resulting in severe systemic illness and fetal loss (Helm *et al.*, 1989). *Chlamydia psittaci* is of considerable veterinary importance, causing significant economic losses particularly in sheep farming (enzootic ovine abortion agent and a separate strain causing polyarthritis) and occasional large-scale outbreaks in poultry farming. *Chlamydia pecorum* is not a human pathogen, but causes pneumonia, polyarthritis, encephalomyelitis and diarrhoea in sheep. *Chlamydia pecorum* appears most closely related to non-avian strains of *C. psittaci*, but has a distinctive protein and DNA composition (Fukushi and Hirai, 1992).

Chlamydia pneumoniae

Chlamydia pneumoniae was initially identified as a novel chlamydial serotype (TWAR) isolated from a human ocular infection, and classified as a strain of *C. psittaci* (Kuo *et al.*, 1986). In the 1980s it became apparent that this new strain was a common cause of pharyngitis and community acquired pneumonia. *Chlamydia pneumoniae* is quite distinct from *C. psittaci*, having a characteristic pear-shaped elementary body (EB) on electron microscopy and lacking an animal reservoir. There has been preliminary evidence of antigenic variation within the species *C. pneumoniae* (Black *et al.*, 1991), and morphological variants lacking pear-shaped EB have been described. In contrast, DNA sequencing of MOMP failed to reveal any variation in geographically diverse isolates (Gaydos *et al.*, 1992). Overall, it appears that *C. pneumoniae* represents a much more homogeneous species than *C. trachomatis* or *C. psittaci*. There is one report of an equine chlamydia which is very closely related but not identical to human isolates of *C. pneumoniae*.

Structure

The genus *Chlamydia* contains three species that cause human disease: *C. trachomatis*, *C. pneumoniae* and *C. psittaci*. Chlamydiae are bacteria which are unable to synthesize ATP since they lack enzymes of the cytochrome oxidase pathway, and are, therefore, 'energy parasites' that can only replicate within a eukaryotic host cell. The chlamydiae are also dependent on the host for the biosynthesis of some amino acids and possibly some lipids as well. They have a unique life-cycle of an infectious EB alternating with the non-infectious but metabolically active reticulate body (RB) (Figure 24.1). The EB is a metabolically inert, spore-like structure with a rigid cell wall some 0.3 μm in diameter. The rigidity of the cell wall is conferred by extensive disulphide bonding within the 40 kDa cysteine-rich MOMP, which makes up 60% of the cell wall (Barron, 1988). The cell wall contains no peptidoglycan, although the inner and outer membrane structure is similar to Gram-negative bacteria. The EBs bind to the host cell membrane using a ligand which resembles the glycosaminoglycan heparin. Monoclonal antibodies to MOMP will inhibit this process, suggesting a role for MOMP in adhesion as well. The EBs are actively endocytosed by a poorly defined mechanism which involves phosphorylation of host cytoplasmic proteins. The endocytic vesicle does not fuse with

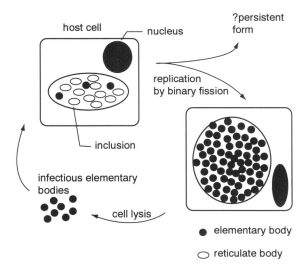

Figure 24.1. Diagram of chlamydial replication cycle.

lysosomes. Within 10 hours the EBs differentiate into the larger (0.8–1 μm) RBs which undergo replication by binary fission. 20–30 hours after entry into the cell a new generation of EBs matures within an enlarged endocytic vesicle (inclusion body) to be released by lysis over the next 18 hours.

Major Antigens

The molecular biology and genetics of chlamydiae are relatively poorly understood, not least because the organism cannot be grown without cell culture and is not readily amenable to genetic manipulation. A few important components have been well characterized, the most important of which is MOMP. MOMP and lipopolysaccharide are immunodominant components of chlamydiae. MOMP, unlike lipopolysaccharide, appears to be immuno-accessible on the surface of the EB. MOMP contains epitopes which are genus, species and serovar specific. The MOMP genes of many chlamydial isolates have been sequenced, revealing a common pattern of five highly conserved regions interspersed with four short variable sequences (VS). Serovar-specific and neutralizing epitopes are located in VS I and VS II. Immunogold electron microscopy studies suggest that MOMP is folded in such a way that VS I and VS II are surface exposed, although the precise three-dimensional structure is unknown. The sequences of several other cysteine-rich outer membrane proteins are known, but these appear to be of less immunological importance.

PATHOGENESIS

Host immunity is responsible for the pathogenesis of many of the clinical features of chlamydial infection. Although chlamydiae are obligate intracellular parasites with a cytolytic effect *in vitro*, there is little evidence of a direct toxic effect *in vivo*. Only a small proportion of the cells of an infected tissue will contain inclusions, although the adjacent cellular infiltrate of B and T cells is often florid. The formation of lymphoid follicles is typical of chlamydial infection, whatever the site,

and these follicles contain typical germinal centres. In contrast the late stages of chlamydial disease are mainly fibrotic with much less cellular infiltrate, as seen in scarring trachoma or fallopian tubes damaged by pelvic inflammatory disease. The immune cells present in these late lesions are predominantly T cells.

Immune damage is thought to be the consequence of a chronically active immune state with the production of fibrogenic cytokines. This is probably caused by a combination of repeated reinfections and possibly persistent infection. Although there is immune activation it may be ineffective in eliminating chlamydial infection. One mechanism which might explain this phenomenon would be a persistent Th2 immune response in the face of infection by an obligate intracellular parasite which would be best eliminated by a Th1 response. Demonstrating the nature of the immune response and correlating this with disease outcome is an area of active research.

There is good evidence from animal models that reinfection provokes a much more vigorous inflammatory response than primary infection, whether the infection is ocular or genital. It has also been convincingly shown that exposure of a previously infected animal to chlamydial heat shock protein 60 (hsp60) will also provoke a vigorous inflammatory response. This observation may be of fundamental importance, because organisms in cell culture exposed to immune cytokines (e.g. interferon γ) tend to continue to express hsp60 whilst reducing expression of MOMP. Such stressed organisms adopt a large and unusual phenotype and stop replicating *in vitro*. It is tempting to speculate that such changes permit persistent infection *in vivo* with chronic immune stimulation.

CLINICAL FEATURES

An important feature of chlamydial disease is the prevalence of asymptomatic infection, especially in the genital tract. Although *C. psittaci* usually causes overt disease in humans, asymptomatic disease in the natural avian or animal reservoir is not uncommon. The disease syndromes are summarized in Table 24.2.

TABLE 24.2 CLINICAL FEATURES OF CHLAMYDIAL INFECTION

Chlamydial species/strain	Clinical features
Chlamydia trachomatis serovars A–C	Asymptomatic, follicular conjunctivitis, inflammatory conjunctivitis, scarring trachoma, entropion and trichiasis, corneal opacity
Chlamydia trachomatis serovars D–K	Asymptomatic, cervicitis, salpingitis and infertility, Fitz-Hugh–Curtis syndrome, urethritis, epididymo-orchitis, paratrachoma, Reiter's syndrome, neonatal infection: conjunctivitis, pneumonia
Chlamydia trachomatis serovars L1–L3	Lymphogranuloma venereum, genital ulcer or papule, proctitis, inguinal adenopathy/buboes, pelvic/inguinal fistulae and sinuses, fever and systemic features, stricture of urethra or rectum, lymphoedema of genitals.
Chlamydia psittaci (avian strains)	Headache, unproductive cough, fever, arthralgia and myalgia, hepatosplenomegaly & hilar adenopathy, exposure to birds Rare: hepatitis, endocarditis, myocarditis, disseminated intravascular coagulation, toxic confusional state, Stevens–Johnson syndrome
Chlamydia psittaci (ovine strains)	Abortion and systemic illness Exposure to lambing ewes
Chlamydia pneumoniae	Asymptomatic, community acquired pneumonia and pharyngitis, bronchitis, sinusitis, otitis media Rare: endocarditis, myocarditis, erythema nodosum, encephalitis, Guillain–Barré syndrome

Genital Tract Infections

Genital tract infection is often asymptomatic, especially in women (up to 70%). Symptomatic infection is usually manifest as urethritis in males; epididymitis and paratrachoma occur occasionally. Men are more prone to subsequent reactive arthritis and full-blown Reiter's syndrome than women. Women may present with urethritis, but asymptomatic cervicitis is more common. Ascending infection results in salpingitis (pelvic inflammatory disease); this may be severe and symptomatic with systemic disturbance or pass unnoticed. The late sequelae of tubal infertility and predisposition to ectopic pregnancy often occur without a recognized episode of pelvic inflammatory disease.

Epidemiology

Chlamydia trachomatis serotypes D–K are common genital pathogens, and serotypes D, E and F are most commonly found. It has been estimated that in the USA in 1990 there was approximately 4 million cases of chlamydial infection per year, costing the country nearly $2.5 billion annually (Washington *et al.*, 1987). Reported cases of chlamydial infection in the USA rose from 3.2 per 100 000 in 1984 to 182.6 per 100 000 in 1992 according to Centers for Disease Control (CDC) statistics. This reflects improved case finding following the introduction of screening programmes. The prevalence of genital tract infection with *C. trachomatis* peaks with sexual activity in the late teens and early twenties, and is associated with risk factors such as multiple sexual partners, coexisting sexually transmitted disease and cervical ectopy. In groups such as American and European college or university students asymptomatic infections occur in 7–10% of men and women, rising to 50% of men with a clinical diagnosis of non-specific urethritis. As many as 12.3% of asymptomatic sexually active adolescent males in Philadelphia were found to harbour *C. trachomatis* when screened by culture. In a London inner city practice 9% of women were found to have chlamydial infection when assessed by immunofluorescence examination of a specimen obtained routinely (Oakeshott *et al.*, 1992). As might be expected, those attending sexually transmitted disease (STD) clinics have a higher prevalence of chlamydial infection, with proportionately more heterosexual than homosexual males affected. A two-year quantitative survey of specimens collected from STD clinics in London processed by direct immunofluorescence revealed a 15–16% positive rate overall for men and women; EBs were detected most often in men with nongonococcal urethritis (40%), neonates with conjunctivitis (30%) and contacts of chlamydiae-positive patients (25%) and least often in 'prostatitis' (2.9%) and patients tested to determine the success of treatment (2.7%) (Thomas *et al.*, 1990). Chlamydial infection is the commonest bacterial sexually transmitted disease in the developed world, easily outstripping the prevalence of other bacterial STDs. Chlamydial infection is the commonest bacterial STD in non-industrialized countries and coinfection is particularly frequent. In an urban setting in West Africa a prevalence of 18% was observed in postpartum women aged under 21 using direct immunofluorescence and culture (Leclerc *et al.*, 1988). There is no evidence of any significant difference in presentation or severity of disease between the various genital serotypes of *C. trachomatis*.

Chlamydial infection of the genital tract has been implicated as a risk factor for the heterosexual transmission of HIV by several studies from Africa (Laga *et al.*, 1993; Plummer *et al.*, 1991). The mechanism by which HIV transmission is enhanced is unclear, but may relate to ulceration of cervical columnar epithelium in conjunction with local lymphocytic infiltration, or chlamydial infection may simply be acting as a marker for cervical ectopy.

Cervicitis

Cervicitis is the commonest manifestation of chlamydial infection in women. The majority of chlamydial infections of women are asymptomatic, although they are often associated with cervicitis on clinical examination (Masse *et al.*, 1991). It is important to recognize and treat patients with chlamydial cervicitis or at high risk of chlamydial cervicitis because of the risk of subsequent ascending infection and as a public health measure (in concert with contact tracing measures). Risk factors for chlamydial cervicitis include young (<25) single heterosexual women with multiple partners or a new partner, a sexual partner with known chlamydial disease (highly predictive), oral contraceptive usage and new intermenstrual bleeding in women taking oral contraceptives, absence of barrier contraceptive use, known gonorrhoea or previous chlamydial infection (Masse *et al.*, 1991). Cervicitis is associated with purulent or mucopurulent discharge, and is often only apparent on direct inspection of the cervix. Inspection of the cervix may reveal cervical ectopy. Cervical ectopy is associated with oral contraceptive use and is probably an independent risk factor for the acquisition of chlamydial cervicitis. Clinical findings and cervical smear are insufficient to make a diagnosis of chlamydial cervicitis, so laboratory confirmation should be obtained.

Chlamydial infection plays no direct role in bacterial vaginosis, but in about 13% of women with bacterial vaginosis there is coexistent chlamydial cervicitis (Bleker *et al.*, 1989). Bartholinitis is usually caused by various enterobacteria and *Neisseria gonorrhoeae*; very occasionally *C. trachomatis* has been identified as a cause (Bleker *et al.*, 1990).

Pelvic inflammatory disease

Chlamydial cervicitis may progress to endometritis which later involves the fallopian tubes. Further spread to the peritoneum may occur, resulting in perihepatitis (known as Fitz-Hugh–Curtis syndrome), which may mimic gall-bladder disease clinically. The characteristic clinical presentation of chlamydial pelvic inflammatory disease (PID) is one of pelvic pain, fever and leukorrhoea in a sexually active woman. Examination will reveal lower abdominal tenderness and possibly swelling of adnexal structures; there may be cervical discharge and excitation. A tubo-ovarian abscess may be visualized on ultrasound examination. Laparoscopy may be necessary to confirm the diagnosis and exclude surgical pathology (e.g.appendicitis or ectopic pregnancy). Infection with *Neisseria gonorrhoeae* and *C. trachomatis* often coexist. The proportion of cases due to *N. gonorrhoeae* versus those due to *C. trachomatis* will depend on the exact population studied and the assiduousness of the microbiological investigation. An American series showed that 60% of women with laparoscopically verified salpingitis had *C. trachomatis* detectable by PCR of cervical swabs (Witkin *et al.*, 1993). Ascending infection is more common after cervical trauma due, for example, to termination of pregnancy or insertion of an intrauterine device. Although the symptoms of chlamydial PID are usually less severe than those of gonococcal disease, sequelae are common and may be more severe as chlamydial salpingitis leads to chronic inflammation and scarring of the fallopian tubes, resulting in secondary infertility and increased risk of ectopic pregnancy (Cates and Wasserheit, 1991). It is difficult to demonstrate active chlamydial infection in patients presenting with tubal infertility, although approximately 80% will have antibodies present in sera compared with approximately 20% of women with non-tubal infertility (Osser *et al.*, 1989). Chlamydial salpingitis leading to tubal obstruction is frequently asymptomatic, emphasizing the importance of identifying and treating chlamydial cervicitis before ascending infection occurs. The appearance of normal fallopian tubes on laparoscopy does not exclude chlamydial infection (Stacey *et al.*, 1990).

Perihepatitis

Perihepatitis was first described by Fitz-Hugh and Curtis in the context of gonococcal infection but it is now apparent that *C. trachomatis* is the main cause. It occurs in young sexually active women, presenting with fever, right upper quadrant abdominal pain and tenderness. It is usually thought to occur as an ascending infection traversing the fallopian tubes into the peritoneum, but it has infrequently occurred following tubal ligation and also in men (Lopez Zeno *et al.*, 1985). The diagnosis may be confirmed by isolation of *C. trachomatis* from the cervix in most cases;

laparoscopy should not be necessary if there is a prompt response to macrolide antibiotics following a clinical diagnosis. Perihepatitis may occur without overt evidence of salpingitis. There have been case reports of perisplenitis, perinephritis and even chronic ascites in association with *C. trachomatis* infection (Gatt and Jantet, 1987).

Urethritis

Urethritis is the commonest presentation of sexually transmitted chlamydial infection in men. Chlamydial urethritis does occur in women, but is usually asymptomatic. Urethritis presents with symptoms of dysuria, itching and urethral discharge. The incubation period ranges from two days to more than four weeks, with 50% of men symptomatic within four days of exposure. A sexual history should be taken to facilitate contact tracing and determine the risk of other sexually transmitted diseases. Clinical examination is generally unremarkable, it may be possible to demonstrate the presence of urethral discharge. Close examination of the genitalia and related lymph nodes is necessary to exclude coexisting venereal disease. Urethral discharge is usually scanty or can only be demonstrated by milking the urethra. Clinical features are unreliable means of establishing a diagnosis of chlamydial urethritis even under optimal circumstances; laboratory tests are essential (Lefevre *et al.*, 1991). A urethral swab should be taken to detect chlamydial infection and the other infectious agents causing urethritis, including *Neisseria gonorrhoeae*, *Ureaplasma urealyticum*, *Trichomonas vaginalis*, and rarely herpes simplex virus or *Treponema pallidum*. *Chlamydia trachomatis* can be isolated from the urethra of 20–50% of men with nongonococcal urethritis and it is also an important cause of postgonococcal urethritis (Oriel and Ridgway, 1983). It is possible, but not proven, that *C. trachomatis* is a cause of chronic urethritis and urethral stricture.

Epididymitis

Chlamydia trachomatis is the commonest cause of acute epididymitis in young men, *Neisseria gonorrhoeae* accounting for most of the remainder (Oriel, 1992). In men over 35 epididymitis is usually caused by urinary tract pathogens, although *C. trachomatis* may still be found in about one in 10 patients (Krieger, 1984; De Jong *et al.*, 1988). Chlamydial epididymitis is rarely associated with underlying abnormality of the genitourinary tract, in contrast to epididymo-orchitis of other causes. The clinical presentation is of unilateral scrotal pain in a young man, accompanied by fever, local swelling and tenderness. Examination reveals a tender indurated epididymis and there is usually coexistent chlamydial urethritis, although this may be asymptomatic (Krieger, 1984). Direct chlamydial infection of the testis occurs rarely, if at all, although this distinction may be difficult to make clinically. If testicular involvement is prominent, alternative infections or testicular torsion should be considered; *N. gonorrhoeae*, coliforms or occasionally *Mycobacterium tuberculosis* are likely pathogens. Chlamydial epididymitis responds promptly to appropriate antibiotic treatment.

The exact role of chlamydial infection in male infertility is uncertain. A recent study of 28 infertile couples in the USA revealed the presence of *C. trachamatis* in the semen of 40% of male partners, detectable only by PCR. There was a statistically significant correlation between this finding and the demonstration of antisperm antibodies in cervical secretions of the corresponding female partner (Witkin *et al.*, 1993).

Prostatitis

The role of *C. trachomatis* in the pathogenesis of prostatitis is controversial; contradictory results have been obtained by different techniques (Schachter, 1985).

It may be that subclinical infection of the prostate does occur, especially in those patients who have evidence of ascending infection, i.e. epididymitis. Such prostatic infection may cause changes detectable on ultrasound, and may become chronic if inadequately treated. There is no place for routine investigations for *C. trachomatis* in patients with prostatitis at present, unless to exclude coexisting urethritis.

Proctitis

Chlamydia trachomatis has been isolated from homosexual men with proctitis, but this is infrequent and usually asymptomatic or associated with minor symptoms (Quinn *et al.*, 1981). Severe chlamydial proctitis is rare, and is caused by *C. trachomatis* of serovars L1–L3.

Adult Paratrachoma

Adult paratrachoma or inclusion conjunctivitis is an STD caused by genital strains of *C. trachomatis*. It is often accompanied by genital chlamydial infection which may be asymptomatic. Affected individuals present with unilateral or bilateral conjunctivitis and pseudoptosis (narrowing of palpebral fissure caused by swollen eyelids). Onset may be acute or subacute, with an incubation period of 2–21 days. There is often a mucopurulent discharge, most noticeable in the morning. Examination of the eyelids reveals papillary hyperplasia and/or follicular hypertrophy. Untreated, the follicular conjunctivitis is chronic, usually lasting about five months. Punctate keratitis and micropannus may occur some weeks after the onset of symptoms, but significant scarring and pannus formation are rare. Vision is not usually impaired and the prognosis is good with prompt treatment. Spread to the middle ear via the Eustachian tube may occur; a history of impaired hearing will usually be elicited in these circumstances. Paratrachoma is readily distinguished from trachoma by the circumstances of its occurrence (sexually active adult in non-trachoma endemic area), and the absence of significant scarring and pannus formation. Paratrachoma may be distinguished from the conjunctivitis of Reiter's syndrome by the presence of follicular hypertrophy, the absence of iritis and the presence of inclusions. The diagnosis is confirmed by the demonstration of *C. trachomatis* of serovars D–K in conjunctival scrapings. Treatment is with appropriate systemic antibiotics; contact tracing is an important part of management.

Neonatal Infections

Up to 50% of women with cervical infections infect their infants at delivery (Schachter *et al.*, 1986). Neonatal infection may be asymptomatic or give rise to ophthalmia neonatorum or pneumonitis (approximately 30% and 10% respectively). Intrauterine chlamydial infection can occur, but infection during passage through the birth canal is the usual mechanism of transmission (Mardh *et al.*, 1984).

Neonatal conjunctivitis

Ophthalmia usually occurs within three weeks of birth and is characterized by mucopurulent conjunctivitis that is characteristically less severe than that caused by *Neisseria gonorrhoeae*, and self-limiting (Ridgway, 1986). There may be associated middle ear involvement with bulging tympanic membranes. Pseudo-membrane formation occurs occasionally; follicle formation and corneal ulceration occur only if treatment is inadequate. Subsequent visual impairment is very uncommon and does not occur if infection is treated promptly and appropriately. Neonatal ophthalmia is quite distinct from trachomatous conjunctivitis in that the causative agent is always serovars D–K even in trachoma endemic areas (Datta *et al.*, 1994).

Neonatal pneumonia

Overall about 10–20% of neonates at risk actually develop pneumonia, and this need not be preceded by conjunctivitis. Up to 50% of those with conjunctivitis will develop pneumonia if untreated. Pneumonitis usually occurs between the ages of four and 12 weeks. Typically there is a paroxysmal cough and tachypnoea without fever, and few signs on auscultation of the chest. Chest X-ray findings are bilateral hyperexpansion and diffuse infiltrates with a variety of radiographic patterns, including interstitial, reticular nodular, atelectasis, coalescence, and bronchopneumonia. An eosinophilia is sometimes present (Beem and Saxon, 1977). Although neonatal chlamydial pneumonitis may be mild and is often self-limiting, it may lead to permanent pulmonary sequelae, especially in premature infants (Attenburrow and Barker, 1985). Treatment of the mother and contact tracing should be part of routine management of neonatal chlamydial infection. *Chlamydia trachomatis* respiratory infection affecting older infants and children has been recorded.

Lymphogranuloma Venereum

The L serovars of *C. trachomatis* cause lymphogranuloma venereum. This uncommon sexually transmitted disease is characterized by inguinal buboes and late complications such as rectal stricture. Transmission is virtually confined to the tropics; when disease occurs in the developed world it has usually been imported (Scieux *et al.*, 1989). The disease progresses through three stages: a primary stage characterized by a small genital ulcer or papule, shortly followed by the secondary stage with granulomatous local inflammation and prominent regional adenopathy, leading ultimately to the third stage with chronic fistulae, sinuses and lymphoedema. The primary lesion is painless and usually unnoticed, occurring on the penis, labia, fourchette or posterior vagina; healing occurs without scarring. The diagnosis of lymphogranuloma venereum is nearly always made in the secondary or tertiary stages of the disease. In the developed world presentation is usually with painful inguinal adenopathy; this may be unilateral or bilateral. The nodes are often matted together with fixation and erythema of the overlying skin; discharging sinuses may be seen. In male homosexuals lymphogranuloma venereum is seen most often presenting as an ulcerative proctitis with regional adenopathy; haemorrhage may be a prominent feature (Bolan *et al.*, 1982). In developing countries genital ulceration is the usual presenting complaint (Bogaerts *et al.*, 1989). Extragenital infections may occur, for example pharyngitis and cervical adenopathy, or papules on the finger or tongue. The secondary stage of disease is accompanied by constitutional disturbance with fever, headache, myalgia and arthralgia. Reactive arthritis, aseptic meningitis, erythema nodosum, hepatitis, pulmonary and cardiac involvement may occur. On investigation there is usually a raised erythrocyte sedimentation rate, leucocytosis and polyclonal increase in γ-globulins. Occasionally patients will present with the late complications of untreated disease. There may be chronic ischiorectal, rectovaginal or rectovesical fistulae; this may be accompanied by lymphoedema of the genitals. Rectal stricture 2–6 cm from the anal margin is a recognized complication of the postinflammatory tissue fibrosis. The diagnosis of lymphogranuloma venereum is usually made clinically and confirmed by serological investigation. If facilities are available then isolation of *C. trachomatis* from bubo aspirate or affected tissue scrapings may be undertaken. The sensitivity of this approach is very low in tertiary disease and less than 50% in secondary disease. Histopathology of lymph nodes shows small stellate abscesses surrounded by histiocytes. The histopathological appearances of proctitis appear similar to Crohn's disease, but may be differentiated by the distal nature of the disease and neuromatous involvement of the submucosal and myenteric plexuses (Quinn *et al.*, 1981).

Sexually Acquired Reactive Arthritis

All chlamydial species have been implicated in the causation of reactive arthritis (Braun *et al.*, 1994). Arthritis occurring together with or soon after nongonococcal urethritis has been termed sexually acquired reactive arthritis (SARA); in about one-third of cases, conjunctivitis and other features characteristic of Reiter's syndrome are seen. SARA usually occurs in males. The exact proportion of SARA preceded by *C. trachomatis* infection is difficult to ascertain, but it seems likely to be a majority. A recent retrospective study in Greenland showed that in untreated or inadequately (penicillin) treated patients with chlamydial urethritis 37% subsequently developed reactive arthritis, compared with 10% of patients treated with tetracycline or erythromycin (Bardin *et al.*, 1992). Despite the good evidence for the presence of chlamydial antigen and DNA, viable organisms have not been isolated from the joints of such patients (Hughes *et al.*, 1991). In a recent study *C.*

trachomatis was isolated from the urethra of nine of 19 men with acute, non-diarrhoeal Reiter's syndrome who had not taken antibiotics (Martin *et al.*, 1984). Earlier studies found *C. trachomatis* was present in up to 70% of patients with urethritis and Reiter's syndrome (Keat *et al.*, 1993). There is also evidence that *C. trachomatis* plays a part in reactive arthritis in women (Martin *et al.*, 1984). Routine bacteriological investigation is largely unhelpful in determining the aetiology of SARA, although swabs should be taken for *C. trachomatis* if the patient has not recently been treated with antibiotics. Serology for *C. trachomatis* is often positive but may be difficult to investigate. Once SARA is established, response to antibiotics is generally disappointing. There is evidence that prolonged (three-month) courses of tetracycline may significantly shorten the duration of arthritis in the subgroup of patients in whom *C. trachomatis* can be isolated from an extra-articular site (Lauhio *et al.*, 1991). Further trials are needed before prolonged antibiotic treatment becomes routine management for all patients with SARA (Svenungsson, 1994). Tissue typing for HLA B27 will identify those patients more likely to have an adverse outcome in terms of severity and chronicity of disease.

Ocular Infections: Trachoma

Trachoma is a chronic keratoconjunctivitis caused by serotypes A, B, Ba and C of *C. trachomatis*. It is believed to affect some 500 million people, of whom 7 million are blind as a consequence, and is the second commonest cause of blindness worldwide, after cataract. Trachoma is now largely confined to developing countries, but this was not always the case. It is a disease of poverty rather than a disease of hot climates.

The active (inflammatory) stage of the disease, a follicular conjunctivitis, affects chiefly the subtarsal conjunctiva. Follicles may be seen elsewhere on the conjunctiva and at the limbus, where they leave characteristic shallow depressions known as Herbert's pits when they resolve. Active trachoma is seen primarily among children in endemic areas. Among older children and adults in trachoma endemic areas, conjunctival fibrosis often develops as the follicles resolve. If this scarring is severe it may distort the upper lid margin, leading to entropion. The lashes rub against the globe (trichiasis), causing continuous discomfort and eventually in some cases blindness due to corneal damage secondary to constant trauma. Trachoma is most usefully classified following World Health Organization guidelines as set out in Table 24.3.

The diagnosis of trachoma is usually made without difficulty based on the geographical location of the patient and clinical assessment. Longitudinal studies have shown that chlamydial antigen is cleared from the affected eye some weeks before resolution of clinical signs. Culture is not a particularly sensitive means of confirming the diagnosis as a consequence. The scarring and subsequent blinding complications of trachoma are thought to result from repeated reinfection and possibly persistent infection. Treatment with appropriate antibiotics is effective in the short term, but long-term benefit for the individual patient is unlikely because of the high incidence of reinfection in trachoma-endemic areas.

Chlamydia pneumoniae

Chlamydia pneumoniae was first detected as a novel ocular serovar in Taiwan in 1976. Since that time it has become apparent that it is a distinct species on genetic, serological, clinical and morphological criteria. It is primarily a respiratory pathogen causing community-acquired pneumonia (Kuo *et al.*, 1986; Grayston *et al.*, 1986). Most infection is subclinical or does not come to medical attention (Hyman *et al.*, 1991), but it can cause severe disease especially in the elderly and those with pre-existing respiratory disease. Patients with *C. pneumoniae* infection often report a sore throat with onset a week or two before their respiratory illness, but there are no other distinguishing features in history, physical examination or radiology that separate *C. pneumoniae* from other causes of community-acquired pneumonia. *Chlamydia pneumoniae* is also a common cause of sinusitis and bronchitis, and occasionally otitis media (Ogawa *et al.*, 1990). Endocarditis and myocarditis are rare manifestations of infection.

Seroepidemiological surveys have shown that the vast majority of the population is exposed to *C. pneumoniae* infection at some stage, with the peak age of seroconversion being 5–15 years. *Chlamydia pneumoniae* tends to cause epidemics of respiratory disease, e.g. in army training camps, and a four- to five-year periodicity has been demonstrated in Seattle and Finland. Seroepidemiological surveys which showed an association between ischaemic heart disease and raised *C. pneumoniae* antibody titres (Saikku *et al.*, 1988) have been confirmed in a prospective study. There have been several independent reports of the identification of *C. pneumoniae* elementary bodies within diseased coronary arteries (Kuo *et al.*, 1993). There is undoubtedly a link between *C. pneumoniae* seropositivity and smoking, but even when this risk factor and others are taken into account there remains a significant association between antibodies to *C. pneumoniae* and ischaemic heart disease. This role of *C. pneumoniae* will be proved if a specific preventative strategy (e.g. vaccination) can be shown to reduce the incidence of atheroma independently.

TABLE 24.3   WHO SIMPLIFIED GRADING OF TRACHOMA

Code	Clinical signs
TF	Trachoma follicles: five or more follicles in the central upper tarsal conjunctiva
TI	Intense trachoma: diffuse infiltration of the upper tarsal conjunctiva that obscures the deep tarsal vessels over 50% or more of the tarsal surface
TS	Trachomatous scarring of the conjunctiva
TT	Trichiasis (inturned eyelashes which touch the eyeball)
CO	Corneal opacity which impairs vision

Chlamydia psittaci

Human infection is acquired primarily from birds, usually psittacines, pigeons, ducks or turkeys; and occasionally from sheep. Individuals exposed to these sources of infection either by occupation or hobby are most at risk of ornithosis. Ornithosis usually affects adults in the 30–60 year age group, causing a non-lobar pneumonia after an incubation period of one to two weeks (Crosse, 1990). Clinical features are usually fever, headache and non-productive cough. Extrapulmonary present- ations are well recognized, including confusion, abdominal pain, hepatitis, endocarditis and Stevens–Johnson syndrome (Crosse, 1990). Physical signs in the respiratory system are usually confined to fine crackles on auscultation without classical evidence of consolidation. Hepato- splenomegaly is a fairly common finding which should suggest the possibility of psittacosis when found in combination with an atypical pneumonia. Hilar lymphadenopathy may be apparent on radio- graphy in up to two-thirds of cases. Although lobar consolidation is not typical of psittacosis, it can occur. Routine haematological and biochemical investigations are generally unhelpful in diagnosis, which is usually established retrospectively on serological criteria. Rarely pregnant women may develop systemic illness with fetal loss if exposed to the ovine abortion agent; this is a hazard in sheep-farming communities during lambing (McKinlay *et al.*, 1985).

Chlamydial Infection in the Immunocompromised

Chlamydial infection is not a common problem in the immunocompromised, although *C. trachomatis* may predispose to the acquisition of HIV as discussed above. *C. pneumoniae* has been reported to cause an illness in AIDS patients resembling *Pneumocystis carinii* pneumonia (Gaydos *et al.*, 1993).

DIAGNOSIS

Laboratory diagnosis of chlamydial infection may be achieved by culture; demonstration of chlamydial antigens, DNA or RNA; or by measur- ing the serological response to infection. No single technique is 100% specific and sensitive; the best diagnostic yield is obtained by using a combi- nation of techniques (see Table 24.4). Generally the direct demonstration of chlamydia is to be preferred to serology if adequate samples of the infected tissue are readily obtainable. Serological techniques are prone to problems caused by cross- reactivity and differentiating current from previous infection, although they have been an invaluable epidemiological tool. In the past chlamydial culture has been regarded as the gold standard of diagnosis, but this is being superseded by the use of batteries of tests including the highly sensitive amplification techniques of polymerase or ligase chain reaction.

Specimen Collection

Specimens collected directly from infected sites (e.g. cervix, urethra, conjunctiva) should be taken with a cotton-tipped plastic swab. Chlamydial infection is intracellular but superficial at these sites, so the aim should be to take a scraping of the endocervical (or equivalent) cells. Cervical swabs should be taken from the endocervix after first wiping away excess secretions on the cervix; urethral swabs should be collected from approxi- mately 2 cm within the male urethra; conjunctival swabs should be taken by gently scraping the everted eyelid. If chlamydial culture is to be attempted the swab should be placed in chlamydial transport medium (sucrose phosphate) unless it is processed immediately. Specimens may be stored for up to 24 hours if refrigerated at 4 °C. If the specimen is to be spread on a slide (e.g. for direct immunofluorescence) the swab should be rolled onto the slide so the maximum quantity of infected material is transferred. Some antigen detection systems come supplied with their own swabs but these may be unsuitable for simul- taneous attempts to isolate chlamydiae in culture. In suspected chlamydial neonatal pneumonia nasopharyngeal aspirates should be collected for antigen detection and culture and cervical swabs taken from the mother. In certain circumstances it

TABLE 24.4 USE OF ROUTINE LABORATORY TESTS FOR DIAGNOSIS OF CHLAMYDIAL INFECTION

Clinical presentation	Specimen	Available laboratory test
Cervicitis (*C. trachomatis* D–K)	Endocervical swab ?Urine–under evaluation	EIA, culture, DIF, PCR, LCR PCR, LCR
Pelvic inflammatory disease/ Fitz-Hugh–Curtis syndrome (*C. trachomatis* D–K)	Endocervial swab Fallopian and peritoneal swabs	EIA, culture, DIF, PCR, LCR EIA, culture, DIF, PCR, LCR
Urethritis (*C. trachomatis* D–K)	Urethral swab Urine (first catch)	EIA, culture, DIF, PCR, LCR EIA, DIF, PCR, LCR
Lymphogranuloma venereum (*C. trachomatis* L1–L3)	Serum Swab of cervix/urethra/rectum/ulcer Lymph node aspirate	MIF, CFT Culture, DIF, EIA Culture
Paratrachoma Ophthalmia neonatorum (*C. trachomatis* D–K) Trachoma (*C. trachomatis* A–C)	Conjunctival swab	EIA, culture, DIF, PCR, LCR
Neonatal pneumonia (*C. trachomatis* D–K)	Serum Nasopharyngeal aspirate	IgM EIA, culture, DIF, PCR, LCR
Ornithosis (*C. psittaci*)	Serum	CFT, MIF, WHIF
Community-acquired pneumonia (*C. pneumoniae*)	Serum Respiratory tract secretions	MIF (not widely available) EIA, DIF

EIA, enzyme immunoassay (for lipopolysaccharide), PCR, polymerase chain reaction; LCR, ligase chain reactions; DIF, direct immunofluorescence; MIF, microimmunofluorescence; CFT, complement fixation test; WHIF, whole cell immunofluorescence.

may be desirable to detect urogenital chlamydial infection using urine samples. Greatest yields of elementary bodies will be obtained in first-catch specimens because these contain the most urethral secretions. Such specimens may be concentrated further by centrifugation, although this is not usually necessary for enzyme immunoassay and DNA amplification techniques. Serological tests are most appropriate for the diagnosis of respiratory illness caused by *C. psittaci* or *C. pneumoniae*. Acute and convalescent sera should be taken, unless the initial titres are very high and consistent with the clinical diagnosis. Seroconversion following *C. pneumoniae* infection may take six to eight weeks, but is not usually long delayed in ornithosis (Wreghitt, 1993). *Chlamydia psittaci* infection of birds thought to be a source of ornithosis is best demonstrated by collection of bird faeces for PCR, thereby avoiding the hazards of *C. psittaci* culture.

Cell Culture

Culture has a sensitivity of 75–90% and high specificity in *C. trachomatis* lower urogenital tract infection, but there are drawbacks in the time-consuming exercise of isolating the organism in cell culture. Culture of *C. trachomatis* is performed by centrifuging EBs from the specimen onto cycloheximide-treated McCoy cells followed by incubation, infection being demonstrated by the presence of inclusions staining with iodine, Giemsa or (for greater sensitivity) appropriate fluorescent monoclonal antibodies 48 hours after inoculation. L serovars of *C. trachomatis* grow better in culture than other serovars, and do not require centrifugation to infect the McCoy cell monolayer. It is important to recognize that occasionally *C. trachomatis* may be present in such large amounts in clinical specimens that it is toxic to cell cultures. The sensitivity of culture may be increased by making an initial blind passage before staining for inclusions on the subsequent passage. *Chlamydia pneumoniae* is relatively difficult to grow in cell culture, growing better in HeLa 229, BHK 21, Hep-2 or HL cells than in McCoy cells. Both *C. pneumoniae* and *C. psittaci* are significant infection hazards to laboratory personnel; *C. psittaci* is a category 3 pathogen. Culture has low sensitivity for *C. pneumoniae* and *C. psittaci* partly because of the difficulty in collecting specimens containing sufficient numbers of infectious elementary bodies.

Enzyme Immunoassay

EIA antigen detection techniques offer advantages in terms of speed and ease of use, and are probably the commonest routine laboratory method for detection of *C. trachomatis* at present. There are several commercial kits available designed to detect the genus-specific lipopolysaccharide (LPS). Sensitivity of these tests now approaches 85–90% of that obtainable by culture for newer commercially available kits, e.g. the Syva MicroTrak EIA and Antigenz EIA (Moncada *et al.*, 1992). The specificity of antigen detection can be improved to over 99% by performing a second confirmatory assay such as blocking tests (monoclonal anti-LPS used to block a repeated EIA) (Moncada *et al.*, 1990) or direct immunofluorescence of a centrifuged deposit of the specimen transport medium. EIA with confirmatory testing is sufficiently sensitive and specific for routine analysis of cervical and urethral swabs, and for antigen detection in urine (Sanders *et al.*, 1994). EIA has been used to detect LPS in respiratory secretions of patients with *C. pneumoniae* infection, but it will not distinguish *C. pneumoniae* from *C. trachomatis*. There are several commercially available bedside or office rapid tests based on EIA; unfortunately these are insufficiently sensitive and specific at the time of writing.

Direct Immunofluorescence

Elementary bodies may be detected directly in clinical specimens using appropriate species-specific fluorescent monoclonal antibodies. This requires access to a fluorescence microscope and staff skilled in interpretation. Smears from cervical, urethral, conjunctival or rectal swabs may be analysed in this way; centrifuged urine, cell culture or transport media may also be used particularly in confirmatory tests. The sensitivity ranges from 70% to 100% and specificity from 80% to 100%, this is in part dependent on the skill of the observer.

DNA Amplification Techniques

The DNA amplification techniques of PCR and ligase chain reaction (LCR) offer theoretical advantages of great sensitivity and specificity. At time of writing commercial kits are available both for PCR (Amplicor, Roche) and LCR (LCX, Abbott) (Dille *et al.*, 1993). The Amplicor PCR technique works by amplifying the DNA sequence of the cryptic chlamydial plasmid, of which there is more than one copy, increasing the sensitivity of the technique. Use of a biotinylated PCR primer permits colorimetric detection of the product, and incorporation of uracil-*N*-glycosylase limits the problem of product carry over into subsequent PCR reactions. The DNA amplification techniques appear to offer a 10% increase in sensitivity when compared with culture for detection of *C. trachomatis* in routine cervical swabs, and much greater sensitivity when used on urine samples (Bassiri *et al.*, 1995; Lee *et al.*, 1995; Dille *et al.*, 1993; Bass *et al.*, 1993). PCR systems have also been described for *C. pneumoniae* and *C. psittaci*, but are not yet available as commercial kits (Tong *et al.*, 1993). The use of PCR for detection of *C. trachomatis* DNA in urine may prove to be particularly significant, because there is preliminary evidence that such a non-invasive test may be sufficient for detection of all lower urogenital tract infections in men and women. These techniques also have particular uses in epidemiological surveys because of the potential to identify minor genetic variants and increased sensitivity in chronic chlamydial infections.

Other Nucleic Acid Detection Techniques

A commercially available chemiluminescent DNA probe for *C. trachomatis* (GenProbe Pace 2,

GenProbe, California) appears as sensitive as EIA (i.e. somewhat less sensitive than culture), but one out of four comparative trials demonstrated lack of specificity (Blanding *et al.*, 1993). The principal advantage of using this technique is the ability to test for *Neisseria gonorrhoeae* at the same time, although routine culture methods are generally considered perfectly adequate. Various other nucleic acid probes have been described but await full evaluation.

Serodiagnosis

The microimmunofluorescence test developed by Wang *et al.* is still the test of choice for determining the species- and serovar-specific antibody response to chlamydial infection (Wang and Grayston, 1970). Humoral immune responses of varying degrees are seen with all chlamydial infections, but difficulties distinguishing current from previous infection and cross-reactivities between various species and serovars means that more direct means of demonstrating infection are preferable. Serodiagnosis is the mainstay for the diagnosis *C. psittaci* and *C. pneumoniae* infections. The serodiagnostic procedure used in the UK has recently been outlined by Wreghitt (Wreghitt, 1993). This is very much biased towards the diagnosis of *C. psittaci* infection on the grounds that *C. psittaci* causes much more severe disease than *C. pneumoniae*, and *C. pneumoniae* will be adequately treated with macrolide antibiotics by

physicians following British Thoracic Society guidelines for the management of community-acquired pneumonia on clinical grounds alone. Under this procedure the genus-specific complement fixation test (CFT) is used and a fourfold or greater rise in CFT titre or a single titre $\geqslant 256$ is taken to be indicative of recent infection. Microimmunofluorescence is impractical because there are at least 11 serovars of *C. psittaci*. Whole cell immunofluorescence (WHIF) is used as a confirmatory test to distinguish *C. pneumoniae* and *C. trachomatis* infection from *C. psittaci*. Unfortunately the eight-fold difference in titre needed to make this species distinction is usually absent during true *C. psittaci* infection, because the genus-specific nature of the immune response obscures any species specificity. High titres against all three species (IgG $\geqslant 512$) in convalescent sera indicate *C. psittaci* infection. This approach to serodiagnosis will undoubtedly miss the majority of *C. pneumoniae* infections, because complement fixation is known to be insensitive. Microimmunofluorescence is the serological test of choice for the detection of *C. pneumoniae* infection but skilled interpretation is necessary because a broad pattern of reactivity is often seen in the sera (Campbell *et al.*, 1990). Better diagnostic methods are needed for *C. pneumoniae* before the clinical significance of this infection is understood. Serodiagnosis has no part to play in the routine diagnosis of *C. trachomatis* infection except for lymphogranuloma venereum.

TABLE 24.5 ANTIBIOTICS IN CLINICAL USE WITH MINIMUM INHIBITORY CONCENTRATION <2 mg/l FOR *CHLAMYDIA TRACHOMATIS* (RIDGWAY *ET AL.*, 1991; HAMMERSCHLAG *ET AL.*, 1992)

Rifampicin
Clarithromycin (most active agent against *C. pneumoniae in vitro* by MIC)
Minocycline
Tetracycline
Doxycycline
Oxytetracycline
Erythromycin
Chlortetracycline
Azithromycin
Clindamycin
Spiramycin
Ofloxacin
Ciprofloxacin

TREATMENT

Antibiotic Choice

Chlamydiae are sensitive to several antibiotics (Table 24.5). In practice only macrolides, tetracyclines, ofloxacin and clindamycin have been shown to be effective in clinical trials. In the past sulphonamides have been used to some benefit, but were abandoned because of the high incidence of side effects. β-Lactam antibiotics are not useful because chlamydiae lack a peptidoglycan cell wall, although they may be sufficiently inhibitory to make chlamydial isolation difficult in patients who are on treatment at the time of specimen collection. Tetracyclines have disadvantages in that they cannot be given to pregnant women or children less than eight years old. The new macrolides (e.g. azithromycin, clarithromycin) are proving to be an important advance on erythromycin because they have improved pharmacokinetic properties and are associated with fewer side effects. In addition the long half-life of azithromycin permits single-dose therapy, improving compliance. We have drawn up recommendations for treatment in Table 24.6 based on published trials and the current recommendations of WHO and CDC. Where doxycycline or lymecycline has been specified, other tetracyclines would almost certainly be equally effective. Important considerations influencing the choice of antimicrobial must be a knowledge of the likely infecting organism(s), cost and compliance.

Treatment regimens

Uncomplicated chlamydial genital tract infection can be treated with single-dose azithromycin 1 g (Martin *et al.*, 1992). In the management of STDs azithromycin and the quinolones have the advantage that they are effective against both *C. trachomatis* and *Neisseria gonorrhoeae*. From the limited data available it appears that in uncomplicated gonorrhoea a single 1 g dose of azithromycin is about 94% effective, versus a near 100% efficacy for most quinolones (Waugh, 1993). Trials comparing single-dose azithromycin and

single-dose ofloxacin alone or in combination for uncomplicated genital tract disease would be particularly useful.

The treatment of PID is a contentious area, particularly the treatment of ambulant patients. PID has a polymicrobial aetiology, including *C. trachomatis*, *Neisseria gonorrhoeae*, vaginal flora, enteric Gram-negative rods and anaerobes. The regimens described in Table 24.6 will treat all the common bacteria found in PID. No specific benefit from anti-inflammatory drugs has been shown. There should be clinical response within three to five days of commencing therapy; in the absence of improvement surgery will often be necessary.

The current WHO recommended treatment for trachoma is tetracycline ointment applied daily for six weeks. Single-dose oral azithromycin has recently been shown to be equally effective (Bailey *et al.*, 1993), but treatment of individual cases is of limited value since early reinfection is the rule in endemic areas.

For symptomatic *C. pneumoniae* infection treatment consists of appropriate supportive measures and a two-week course of macrolide (e.g. erythromycin 500 mg q.d.s.) or tetracycline antibiotics, bearing in mind that relapse may occur. In practice treatment will usually be started before laboratory confirmation of the diagnosis, and should include antibiotics active against the likely causes of community-acquired pneumonia. Treatment of *C. psittaci* is as for *C. pneumoniae*, except that the illness is more likely to require supportive measures should multiple organ involvement occur. Short-course azithromycin therapy may be useful (Schonwald *et al.*, 1990, 1991). Clarithromycin and ofloxacin also have significant antichlamydial activity, but have yet to be validated in large comparative trials.

Antimicrobial resistance

At present chlamydial drug resistance is not a factor influencing therapeutic choice. Chlamydial antibiotic resistance is uncommon; most treatment failures in the sexually transmitted chlamydial infections can be attributed to re-exposure.

TABLE 24.6 RECOMMENDED TREATMENT SCHEDULES FOR CHLAMYDIAL INFECTIONS AND ASSOCIATED DISEASES

Clinical presentation	Antibiotic	Dose schedule	Duration (days)
Chlamydial cervicitis or urethritis Non-gonococcal urethritis	Azithromycin[d,e] or doxycycline or ofloxacin[f]	1 g stat. 100 mg b.d. 300 mg b.d	7 7
Epididymo-orchitis	Cefixime then doxycycline or ofloxacin	400 mg stat. 100 mg b.d. 300 mg b.d.	10 10
Pelvic inflammatory disease Hospitalised	Cefoxitin[a] and doxycycline[g] or gentamicin and clindamycin[g]	2 g i.v. t.d.s. 100 mg i.v. b.d. then oral 2 mg/kg i.v. then 1.5 mg/kg t.d.s. 600 mg i.v. q.d.s. then 450 mg p.o. q.d.s.	≥4 14 (total of i.v. then oral) ≥4 14 (total of i.v. then oral)
Ambulant	Cefoxitin[a] plus probenecid, then doxycycline or ofloxacin plus either metronidazole or clindamycin	2 g i.m. stat. plus 1 g p.o. stat. 100 mg b.d. 400 mg b.d. 400 mg b.d. 450 mg q.d.s	14 14 14 14
Adult paratrachoma[b]	Erythromycin or doxycycline	500 mg q.d.s. 100 mg b.d.	21 21
C. trachomatis-induced reactive arithritis	Lymecycline[h]	300 mg b.d.	3 months
Neonatal infections	Erythromycin syrup	12.5 mg/kg q.d.s.	14
Trachoma	Azithromycin	20 mg/kg stat.	
Lymphogranuloma venereum	Doxycycline or erythromycin	100 mg b.d. 500 mg q.d.s.	≥14 ≥14
C. pneumoniae or *C. psittaci* infections[c]	Doxycycline or erythromycin	100 mg b.d. 500 mg q.d.s.	≥14 ≥14

[a] Third-generation cephalosporins may be used as an alternative, but lack activity against anaerobes.
[b] Single-dose azithromycin as for trachoma probably as effective or better, but no published data.
[c] It would be unusual to establish the diagnosis before starting treatment, so combination therapy will usually be necessary, e.g. as for community-acquired pneumonia.
[d] Martin *et al.* (1992).
[e] Stamm (1991).
[f] Hooton *et al.* (1992).
[g] Walters and Gibbs (1990).
[h] Lauhio *et al.* (1991).

Chlamydial drug resistance has been documented both *in vitro* and *in vivo*, but is only seen when large inocula are screened and is not a stable characteristic when chlamydiae are cultured in the absence of antibiotic (Jones *et al.*, 1990). The molecular and genetic mechanisms underlying chlamydial drug resistance are unknown.

Treatment in pregnancy

Treatment of chlamydial infection in pregnancy should be guided by use of those antibiotics known to be safe. In practice this means erythromycin and clindamycin. Erythromycin is often not tolerated in pregnancy because of gastrointestinal side effects. Clindamycin has the advantage of activity against other pathogens likely to cause puerperal sepsis. Azithromycin is probably safe in pregnancy, but not licensed for this purpose.

We expect that the new macrolides and quinolones will play an important part in future recommendations when further trials have been performed in diseases such as epididymo-orchitis, PID and psittacosis.

PREVENTION

Early treatment and prevention is obviously a desirable objective given the potentially harmful sequelae of chlamydial infection. The expense of screening asymptomatic individuals by laboratory tests means that such measures should be confined to groups with a high prevalence of *C. trachomatis*. Use of barrier contraception, change in sexual behaviour and contact tracing through STD clinics are important control measures for genital strains. Where STD control programmes have been vigorously pursued, most notably in Scandinavia, the incidence of chlamydial genital tract infection has fallen significantly.

Mass treatment programmes have become an option for trachoma control with the advent of an easily administered single-dose treatment in the form of azithromycin. Normally individuals become rapidly reinfected following antibiotic treatment for *C. trachomatis* in endemic areas, but it is hoped that mass treatment programmes will interrupt the transmission cycle by eliminating any infectious reservoir. An important aspect of this intervention is cost, but fortunately the manufacturer has agreed to donate the drug free of charge to countries with organized control programmes. Large-scale trials are underway to determine the efficacy of this approach. The eradication of trachoma is likely to depend ultimately on improved socioeconomic conditions.

No human chlamydial vaccine is available. Preliminary work in the 1960s with crude chlamydial extracts gave disappointing results. This may be because certain chlamydial components (e.g. hsp60) induce hypersensitivity responses, especially in those previously exposed to infection. Recent research has

concentrated on subunit vaccines containing MOMP in the hope of avoiding this problem. Most vaccine candidates are based on the premise that producing a neutralizing IgA response at mucosal surfaces will be protective in humans. There have been some promising results in animal studies, but there is surprisingly little evidence that protective immunity in humans operates in this way, and it may well be that a successful vaccine candidate will have to induce a cell-mediated immune response as well as or instead of humoral or secretory antibodies.

REFERENCES

Attenburrow, A.A. and Barker, C.M. (1985) Chlamydial pneumonia in the low birthweight neonate. *Archives of Disease in Childhood*, **60**, 1169–1172.

Bailey, R.L., Arullendran, P., Whittle, H.C., Mabey, D.C. (1993) Randomised controlled trial of single-dose azithromycin in treatment of trachoma. *Lancet*, **342**, 453–456.

Bardin, T., Enel, C., Cornelis, F. *et al.* (1992) Antibiotic treatment of venereal disease and Reiter's syndrome in a Greenland population. *Arthritis and Rheumatism*, **35**, 190–194.

Barron, A.L. (1988) *Microbiology of Chlamydia*. CRC Press, Boca Raton, FL.

Bass, C.A., Jungkind, D.L., Silverman, N.S. *et al.* (1993) Clinical evaluation of a new polymerase chain reaction assay for detection of *Chlamydia trachomatis* in endocervical specimens. *Journal of Clinical Microbiology*, **31**, 2648–2653.

Bassiri, M., Hu, H.Y., Domeika, M.A. *et al.* (1995) Detection of *Chlamydia trachomatis* in urine specimens from women by ligase chain reaction. *Journal of Clinical Microbiology*, **33**, 898–900.

Beem, M.O. and Saxon, E.M. (1977) Respiratory-tract colonization and a distinctive pneumonia syndrome in infants infected with *Chlamydia trachomatis*. *New England Journal of Medicine*, **296**, 306–310.

Black, C.M., Johnson, J.E., Farshy, C.E. *et al.* (1991) Antigenic variation among strains of *Chlamydia pneumoniae*. *Journal of Clinical Microbiology*, **29**, 1312–1316.

Blanding, J., Hirsch, L., Stranton, N. *et al.* (1993) Comparison of the Clearview Chlamydia, the PACE 2 assay, and culture for detection of *Chlamydia trachomatis* from cervical specimens in a low-prevalence population. *Journal of Clinical Microbiology*, **31**, 1622–1625.

Bleker, O.P., Folkertsma, K. and Dirks Go, S.I. (1989) Diagnostic procedures in vaginitis. *European Journal* of Obstetrics, Gynaecology and Reproductive Biology, **31**, 179–183.

Bleker, O.P., Smalbraak, D.J. and Schutte, M.F. (1990) Bartholin's abscess: the role of *Chlamydia trachomatis*. *Genitourinary Medicine*, **66**, 24–25.

Bogaerts, J., Richart, C.A., Van Dyck, E. *et al.* (1989) The etiology of genital ulceration in Rwanda. *Sexually Transmitted Diseases*, **16**, 123–126.

Bolan, R.K., Sands, M., Schachter, J. *et al.* (1982) Lymphogranuloma venereum and acute ulcerative proctitis. *American Journal of Medicine*, **72**, 703–706.

Braun, J., Laitko, S., Treharne, J. *et al.* (1994) *Chlamydia pneumoniae*: a new causative agent of reactive arthritis and undifferentiated oligoarthritis. *Annals of the Rheumatic Diseases*, **53**, 100–105.

Byrom, N.P., Walls, J. and Mair, H.J. (1979) Fulminant psittacosis. *Lancet*, **i**, 353–356.

Campbell, L.A., Kuo, C.C., Wang, S.P. *et al.* (1990) Serological response to *Chlamydia pneumoniae* infection. *Journal of Clinical Microbiology*, **28**, 1261–1264.

Cates, W., Jr and Wasserheit, J.N. (1992) Genital chlamydial infections: epidemiology and reproductive sequelae. *American Journal of Obstetrics and Gynecology*, **164**, 1771–1781.

Crosse, B.A. (1990) Psittacosis: a clinical review. *Journal of Infection*, **21**, 251–259.

Datta, P., Frost, E., Peeling, R. *et al.* (1994) Ophthalmia neonatorum in a trachoma endemic area. *Sexually Transmitted Diseases*, **21**, 1–4.

De Jong, Z., Pontonnier, F., Plante, P. *et al.* (1988) The frequency of *Chlamydia trachomatis* in acute epididymitis. *British Journal of Urology*, **62**, 76–78.

Dille, B.J., Butzen, C.C. and Birkenmeyer, L.G. (1993) Amplification of *Chlamydia trachomatis* DNA by ligase chain reaction. *Journal of Clinical Microbiology*, **31**, 729–731.

Fukushi, H. and Hirai, K. (1992) Proposal of *Chlamydia pecorum* sp. nov. for *Chlamydia* strains derived from ruminants. *International Journal of Systematic Bacteriology*, **42**, 306–308.

Gatt, D. and Jantet, G. (1987) Perisplenitis and perinephritis in the Curtis–Fitz-Hugh syndrome. *British Journal of Surgery*, **74**, 110–112.

Gaydos, C.A., Quinn, T.C., Bobo, L.D. *et al.* (1992) Similarity of *Chlamydia pneumoniae* strains in the variable domain IV region of the major outer membrane protein gene. *Infection and Immunity*, **60**, 5319–5323.

Gaydos, C.A., Fowler, C.L., Gill, V.J. *et al.* (1993) Detection of *Chlamydia pneumoniae* by polymerase chain reaction–enzyme immunoassay in an immunocompromised population. *Clinical Infectious Diseases*, **17**, 718–723.

Grayston, J.T., Kuo, C.C., Wang, S.P. *et al.* (1986) A new *Chlamydia psittaci* strain, TWAR, isolated in acute respiratory tract infections. *New England Journal of Medicine*, **315**, 161–168.

Halberstaedter, L. and von Prowazek, S. (1907) Uber Zelleinschlusse parasitarer Natur beim Trachom. *Arbeit Gesundheit*, **26**, 44–47.

Hammerschlag, M.R., Qumei, K.K.and Roblin, P.M. (1992) *In vitro* activities of azithromycin, clarithromycin, L-ofloxacin, and other antibiotics against *Chlamydia pneumoniae*. *Antimicrobial Agents and Chemotherapy*, **36**, 1573–1574.

Helm, C.W., Smart, G.E., Cumming, A.D. *et al.* (1989) Sheep-acquired severe *Chlamydia psittaci* infection in pregnancy. *International Journal of Gynaecology and Obstetrics*, **28**, 369–372.

Herring, A.J. (1993) Typing *Chlamydia psittaci*: a review of methods and recent findings. *British Veterinary Journal*, **149**, 455–475.

Hooton, T.M., Batteiger, B.E., Judson, F.N. *et al.* (1992) Ofloxacin versus doxycycline for treatment of cervical infection with *Chlamydia trachomatis*. *Antimicrobial Agents and Chemotherapy*, **36**, 1144–1146.

Hughes, R.A., Hyder, E., Treharne, J.D. *et al.* (1991) Intra-articular chlamydial antigen and inflammatory arthritis. *Quarterly Journal of Medicine*, **80**, 575–588.

Hyman, C.L., Augenbraun, M.H., Roblin, P.M. *et al.* (1991) Asymptomatic respiratory tract infection with *Chlamydia pneumoniae* TWAR. *Journal of Clinical Microbiology*, **29**, 2082–2083.

Ito, J.I., Jr, Lyons, J.M. and Airo Brown, L.P. (1990) Variation in virulence among oculogenital serovars of *Chlamydia trachomatis* in experimental genital tract infection. *Infection and Immunity*, **58**, 2021–2023.

Jones, R.B., Van der Pol, B., Martin, D.H. *et al.* (1990) Partial characterization of *Chlamydia trachomatis* isolates resistant to multiple antibiotics. *Journal of Infectious Diseases*, **162**, 1309–1315.

Keat, A., Thomas, B.J. and Taylor-Robinson, D. (1983) Chlamydial infection in the aetiology of arthritis. *British Medical Bulletin*, **39**, 168–174.

Krieger, J.N. (1984) Epididymitis, orchitis, and related conditions. *Sexually Transmitted Diseases*, **11**, 173–181.

Kuo, C.C., Chen, H.H., Wang, S.P. *et al.* (1986) Identification of a new group of *Chlamydia psittaci* strains called TWAR. *Journal of Clinical Microbiology*, **24**, 1034–1037.

Kuo, C.C., Shor, A., Campbell, L.A. *et al.* (1993) Demonstration of *Chlamydia pneumoniae* in atherosclerotic lesions of coronary arteries. *Journal of Infectious Diseases*, **167**, 841–849.

Laga, M., Manoka, A., Kivuvu, M. *et al.* (1993) Nonulcerative sexually transmitted diseases as risk factors for HIV-1 transmission in women: results from a cohort study. *AIDS*, **7**, 95–102.

Lauhio, A., Leirisalo Repo, M., Lahdevirta, J. *et al.* (1991) Double-blind, placebo-controlled study of three-month treatment with lymecycline in reactive arthritis, with special reference to Chlamydia arthritis. *Arthritis and Rheumatism*, **34**, 6–14.

Lee, H.H., Chernesky, M.A., Schachter, J. *et al.* (1995) Diagnosis of *Chlamydia trachomatis* genitourinary infection in women by ligase chain reation assay of urine. *Lancet*, **345**, 213–216.

Leclerc, A., Frost, E., Collet, M. *et al.* (1988) Urogenital *Chlamydia trachomatis* in Gabon: an unrecognised epidemic. *Genitourinary Medicine*, **64**, 308–311.

Lefevre, J.C., Lepargneur, J.P., Bauriaud, R. *et al.* (1991) Clinical and microbiologic features of urethritis in men in Toulouse, France. *Sexually Transmitted Diseases*, **18**, 76–79.

Lopez Zeno, J.A., Keith, L.G. and Berger, G.S. (1985) The Fitz-Hugh–Curtis syndrome revisited: changing perspectives after half a century. *Journal of Reproductive Medicine*, **30**, 567–582.

Mardh, P.A., Johansson, P.J. and Svenningsen, N. (1984) Intrauterine lung infection with *Chlamydia trachomatis* in a premature infant. *Acta Paediatrica Scandinavica*, **73**, 569–572.

Martin, D.H., Pollock, S., Kuo, C.C. *et al.* (1984) *Chlamydia trachomatis* infections in men with Reiter's syndrome. *Annals of Internal Medicine*, **100**, 207–213.

Martin, D.H., Mroczkowski, T.F., Dalu, Z.A. *et al.* (1992) A controlled trial of a single dose of azithromycin for the treatment of chlamydial urethritis and cervicitis. The Azithromycin for Chlamydial Infections Study Group. *New England Journal of Medicine*, **327**, 921–925.

Masse, R., Laperriere, H., Rousseau, H. *et al.* (1991) *Chlamydia trachomatis* cervical infection: prevalence and determinants among women presenting for routine gynaecologic examination. *Canadian Medical Association Journal*, **145**, 953–961.

McKinlay, A.W., White, N., Buxton, D. *et al.* (1985) Severe *Chlamydia psittaci* sepsis in pregnancy. *Quarterly Journal of Medicine*, **57**, 689–696.

Moncada, J., Schachter, J., Bolan, G. *et al.* (1990) Confirmatory assay increases specificity of the chlamydiazyme test for *Chlamydia trachomatis* infection of the cervix. *Journal of Clinical Microbiology*, **28**, 1770–1773.

Moncada, J., Schachter, J., Bolan, G. *et al.* (1992) Evaluation of Syva's enzyme immunoassay for the detection of *Chlamydia trachomatis* in urogenital specimens. *Diagnosis of Microbiological Infectious Diseases*, **15**, 663–668.

Oakeshott, P., Chiverton, S., Speight, L. *et al.* (1992) Testing for cervical *Chlamydia trachomatis* infection

in an inner city practice. *Family Practitioner*, **9**, 421–424.

Ogawa, H., Fujisawa, T. and Kazuyama, Y. (1990) Isolation of *Chlamydia pneumoniae* from middle ear aspirates of otitis media with effusion: a case report. *Journal of Infectious Diseases*, **162**, 1000–1001.

Oriel, J.D. and Ridgway, G.L. (1983) Genital infection in men. *British Medical Bulletin*, **39**, 133–137.

Oriel, J.D. (1992) Male genital *Chlamydia trachomatis* infections. *Journal of Infection*, **25** (Suppl. 1), 35–37.

Osser, S., Persson, K. and Liedholm, P. (1989) Tubal infertility and silent chlamydial salpingitis. *Human Reproduction*, **4**, 280–284.

Plummer, F.A., Simonsen, J.N., Camerson, D.W. *et al.* (1991) Cofactors in male–female sexual transmission of human immunodeficiency virus type 1. *Journal of Infectious Diseases*, **163**, 233–239.

Quinn, T.C., Goodell, S.E., Mkrtichian, E. *et al.* (1981) *Chlamydia trachomatis* proctitis. *New England Journal of Medicine*, **305**, 195–200.

Ridgway, G.L. (1986) A fresh look at ophthalmia neonatorum. *Transactions of the Ophthalmological Societies of the UK*, **105**, 41–42.

Ridgway, G.L., Mumtaz, G. and Fenelon, L. (1991) The *in vitro* activity of clarithromycin and other macrolides against the type strain of *Chlamydia pneumoniae* (TWAR). *Journal of Antimicrobial Chemotherapy*, **27** (Suppl A), 43–45.

Saikku, P., Leinonen, M., Mattila, K. *et al.* (1988) Serological evidence of an association of a novel *Chlamydia*, TWAR, with chronic coronary heart disease and acute myocardial infarction. *Lancet*, **ii**, 983–986.

Sanders, J.W., Hook, E.W., Welsh, L.E. *et al.* (1994) Evaluation of an enzyme immunoassay for detection of *Chlamydia trachomatis* in urine of asymptomatic men. *Journal of Clinical Microbiology*, **32**, 24–27.

Schachter, J. (1985) Is *Chlamydia trachomatis* a cause of prostatitis? *Journal of Urology*, **134**, 711.

Schachter, J., Grossman, M., Sweet, R.L. *et al.* (1986) Prospective study of perinatal transmission of *Chlamydia trachomatis*. *Journal of the American Medical Association*, **255**, 3374–3377.

Schonwald, S., Gunjaca, M., Kolacny Babic, L. *et al.* (1990) Comparison of azithromycin and erythromycin in the treatment of atypical pneumonias. *Journal of Antimicrobial Chemotherapy*, **25** (Suppl. A), 123–126.

Schonwald, S., Skerk, V., Petricevic, I. *et al.* (1991) Comparison of three-day and five-day courses of azithromycin in the treatment of atypical pneumonia. *European Journal of Clinical Microbiology and Infectious Diseases*, **10**, 877–880.

Scieux, C., Barnes, R., Bianchi, A. *et al.* (1989)

Lymphogranuloma venereum: 27 cases in Paris. *Journal of Infectious Diseases*, **160**, 662–668.

Stacey, C., Munday, P., Thomas, B. *et al.* (1990) *Chlamydia trachomatis* in the fallopian tubes of women without laparoscopic evidence of salpingitis. *Lancet*, **336**, 960–963.

Stamm, W.E. (1991) Azithromycin in the treatment of uncomplicated genital chlamydial infections. *American Journal of Medicine*, **91**, 19S–22S.

Svenungsson, B. (1994) Reactive arthritis. *British Medical Journal*, **308**, 671–672.

Thomas, B.J., Osborn, M.F., Munday, P.E. *et al.* (1990) A 2-year quantitative assessment of *Chlamydia trachomatis* in a sexually transmitted diseases clinic population by the MicroTrak direct smear immunofluorescence test. *International Journal of STD and AIDS*, **1**, 264–267.

Tong, C.Y. and Sillis, M. (1993) Detection of *Chlamydia pneumoniae* and *Chlamydia psittaci* in sputum samples by PCR. *Journal of Clinical Pathology*, **46**, 313–317.

Walters, M.D. and Gibbs, R.S. (1990) A randomized comparison of gentamicin–clindamycin and cefoxitin–doxycycline in the treatment of acute pelvic inflammatory disease. *Obstetrics and Gynecology*, **75**, 867–872.

Wang, S.P. and Grayston, J.T. (1970) Immunologic relationship between genital TRIC, lymphogranuloma venereum, and related organisms in a new microtiter indirect immunofluorescence test. *American Journal of Ophthalmology*, **70**, 367–374.

Wang, S.P. and Grayston, J.T. (1991) Three new serovars of *Chlamydia trachomatis*: Da, Ia, and L2a, *Journal of Infectious Diseases*, **163**, 403–405.

Washington, A.E., Johnson, R.E. and Sanders, L.L.J. (1987) *Chlamydia trachomatis* infections in the United States: what are they costing us? *Journal of the American Medical Association*, **257**, 2070–2072.

Waugh, M.A. (1993) Open study of the safety and efficacy of a single oral dose of azithromycin for the treatment of uncomplicated gonorrhoea in men and women. *Journal of Antimicrobial Chemotherapy*, **31** (Suppl. E), 193–198.

Witkin, S.S., Jeremias, J., Grifo, J.A. *et al.* (1993) Detection of *Chlamydia trachomatis* in semen by the polymerase chain reaction in male members of infertile couples. *American Journal of Obstetrics and Gynecology*, **168**, 1457–1462.

Witkin, S.S., Jeremias, J., Toth, M. *et al.* (1993) Detection of *Chlamydia trachomatis* by the polymerase chain reaction in the cervices of women with acute salpingitis. *American Journal of Obstetrics and Gynecology*, **168**, 1438–1442.

Wreghitt, T. (1993) Chlamydial infection of the respiratory tract. *Communicable Disease Report*, **3**, R119–R124.

Yuan, Y., Zhang, Y.X., Watkins, N.G. *et al.* (1989) Nucleotide and deduced amino acid sequences for the four variable domains of the major outer membrane proteins of the 15 *Chlamydia trachomatis* serovars. *Infection and Immunity*, **57**, 1040–1049.

Zhang, Y.X., Fox, J.G., Ho, Y. *et al.* (1993) Comparison of the major outer-membrane protein (MOMP) gene of mouse pneumonitis (MoPn) and hamster SFPD strains of *Chlamydia trachomatis* with other *Chlamydia* strains. *Molecular Biology and Evolution*, **10**, 1327–1342.

25

RICKETTSIA

James G. Olson and Burt E. Anderson

INTRODUCTION

Members of the order *Rickettsiales* are represented by a diverse group of Gram-negative bacteria that are largely intracellular parasites. Although many species are adapted to existence within arthropods, frequently they are also capable of infecting vertebrates, including humans. At least 13 species in five genera are pathogenic for humans. The diseases caused by these microorganisms have had significant roles in the history of civilization, but recently have been overshadowed by other diseases that have greater epidemic potential and lack effective interventions.

DESCRIPTION OF THE ORGANISMS

Definition

Organisms included in the *Rickettsiales* are Gram-negative and except for *Rochalimaea* are obligate intracellular bacteria The genus *Rickettsia* comprises short, rod-shaped coccobacilli ranging from 0.8 to 2.0 μm in length and from 0.3–0.5 μm in width (Ris and Fox, 1949). *Rickettsia* do not have flagella. They have a five-layered outer envelope and lipopolysaccharide is present in all species (Schramek *et al.*, 1976).

Molecular Characterization

Recent characterizations of species within *Rickettsiales* at the molecular level are causing re-evaluation of phylogenetic relationships. The previous standards for defining rickettsial species include a variety of direct phenotypic features such as morphology and antigenic properties as well as indirect properties such as geographic distribution, host cell type, animal reservoir, and disease characteristics. Restriction fragment length polymorphism (RFLP) analysis of the genome and of amplified genomic fragments has been used to estimate the degree of relatedness among species and in some cases to define new species. However, DNA–DNA hybridizations remain the standard for defining new bacterial species by genetic criteria. Since many members of the order *Rickettsiales* have not yet been cultivated *in vitro*; application of DNA–DNA hybridization techniques to all members of the order is not yet possible. To overcome this obstacle sequencing of polymerase chain reaction (PCR)-amplified 16S rRNA genes has been used to provide genetic data that will accurately reflect the phylogenetic relationships among the rickettsiae. Comparative 16S rRNA gene-sequencing data among all members of a genus has been used to identify new rickettsiae.

Principles and Practice of Clinical Bacteriology. Edited by A.M. Emmerson, P.M. Hawkey and S.H. Gillespie
© 1997 John Wiley & Sons Ltd

coupled with phenotypic data, 16S rRNA gene sequencing can be used to define new species as demonstrated recently with *Bartonella henselae*, and *Ehrlichia chaffeensis*.

Classification

Currently, the order *Rickettsiales* is comprised of three families: Rickettsiaceae containing the genera *Rickettsia, Bartonella, Coxiella, Ehrlichia, Cowdria. Neorickettsia Wolbachia*, and *Rickettsiella*; Bartonellaceae containing the genera *Bartonella* and *Grahamella*; and Anaplasmataceae containing the genera *Anaplasma, Aegyptianella, Haemobartonella*, and *Eperythrozoon* (Weiss and Moulder, 1984). Recently, a proposed change was adopted that included species of the genus *Bartonella* in the genus *Bartonella* and move the family Bartonellaceae to another Order (Brenner *et al.*, 1993). DNA sequence and other molecular analyses might facilitate a number of other changes which could be made to have the order more accurately reflect phylogenetic relationships among the rickettsiae. For example the genus *Ehrlichia* currently contains three serologically and phylogenetically unrelated groups of organisms. By dividing the genus *Ehrlichia* into three genera a more uniform definition of the genus could be achieved.

PATHOGENESIS

Most rickettsiae infect the endothelial cells of the microcirculatory system, especially the capillaries. Damage to the vasculature is the basis for similarities in pathology of rickettsial diseases (Walker and Mattern, 1980). The primary cellular lesion results from dilation and destruction of intracellular membranes, particularly the rough endoplasmic reticulum (Silverman, 1984). As endothelial cells die, necrosis of the blood vessels leads to the formation of hyaline thrombi that manifest themselves clinically as petechiae. Gross and microscopic lesions are found in the brain, heart, kidney and lungs.

Rickettsia rickettsii, unlike the other rickettsiae, are not confined to the capillary endothelium, and invade and destroy smooth muscle cells and vascular endothelium of larger vessels. Spotted fever group (see below) rickettsiae may cause interstitial pneumonia. In fatal cases of RMSF, the distribution of rickettsiae parallels observed pulmonary vasculitis, suggesting that rickettsial invasion of the microcirculation results in the interstitial pneumonitis. The vasculitis, vascular damage and increased vascular permeability results in alveolar septal congestion and oedema, fibrin formation, macrophage accumulation and haemorrhage; and interlobar, septal and pleural effusion (Walker *et al.*, 1980a). Interstitial pneumonitis is more frequent in scrub typhus than in epidemic typhus or spotted fever patients (Allen and Spitz, 1945).

Lesions of the central nervous system play an important role in the clinical manifestations of RMSF and typhus. All portions of the brain and spinal cord may be involved but the midbrain and inferior nucleus are most frequently affected. Focal proliferations of the endothelial and neuroglial cells (once called typhus nodules) are typical. Neurological findings in RMSF are the result of microinfarcts and frequently involve the white matter. Neurological pathology in epidemic and scrub typhus include mononuclear cell meningitis, perivascular cuffing of arteries, focal hemorrhages and degeneration of ganglionic cells (Allen and Spitz, 1945).

Interstitial myocarditis is found in RMSF, epidemic typhus and scrub typhus. RMSF heart lesions are patchy and consist of a mixed mononuclear cell infiltrate. *Rickettsia rickettsii* may be detected in the cardiac vessels by immunofluorescence (Walker *et al.*, 1980b).

The urinary tract is commonly affected in RMSF and typhus. Azotemia is usually prerenal and reflects intravascular volume depletion. Acute renal failure in RMSF is probably due to tubular necrosis that results from systemic hypotension (Allen and Spitz, 1945). Histopathological studies of RMSF, epidemic typhus and scrub typhus have shown testes, epididymis, scrotal skin and adrenals may also be involved. Swollen Kupffer cells of the liver are prominent in typhus and phagocytosis of erythrocytes and inflammatory cells may be noted in the spleen (National Research Council, 1953).

Microscopically the pathology of Q fever is similar to bacterial pneumonia. Severe interalveolar, focally necrotizing haemorrhagic pneumonia that is patchy and involves the alveolar lining cells and is associated with necrotizing bronchitis and bronchiolitis. *Coxiella burnetii* is found in histiocytes of the alveolar exudate. Histiocytic hyperplasia is found in mediastinal lymph nodes, spleen and adrenals. Hepatocellular damage in acute Q fever consists of granulomatous changes in the lobules and occasional involvement of the portal areas (Srigley *et al.*, 1985). Granulomas consist of non-distinctive focal histiocytic and mixed inflammatory cell infiltrates with multinucleated giant cells.

CLINICAL AND EPIDEMIOLOGICAL FEATURES

Most of the illnesses caused by members of order *Rickettsiales* are characterized by acute onset of a fever accompanied by non-specific signs and symptoms. In many diseases a characteristic rash follows the systemic symptoms and may be pathognomonic. Table 25.1 provides a list of agents and a summary of diseases associated with aetiological agents, their geographical distributions and mode of transmission to humans.

Rocky Mountain Spotted Fever

Rocky Mountain spotted fever (RMSF), caused by infection with *Rickettsia rickettsii*, is an acute, tick-borne, potentially fatal disease characterized by fever, headache, rash myalgia and anorexia. Complications include vascular damage, increased permeability, oedema, haemorrhage, disseminated intravascular coagulation, interstitial pneumonitis, central nervous system (CNS) involvement, myocarditis and renal failure (Clements, 1992). The case–fatality ratio (CFR) has been reduced to between 3% and 5% since antibiotic therapy became available but, untreated, the CFR ranged between 23% and 70% (Harrell, 1949). Most of the approximately 600 cases reported annually in the USA are located in the southeast and south central states where the principal vector ticks,

Dermacentor variabilis and *Amblyomma americanum*, are prevalent. The incubation period varies between four and 14 days. The highest incidence occurs in children aged five to nine years and males outnumber females by nearly two to one. Delay in initiating antibiotic therapy and increased age of patients are risk factors that significantly increase complications and death.

Spotted Fevers

A number of other spotted fevers have been described from a wide geographic range. African tick typhus, Kenya tick typhus, Israel tick typhus, Indian tick typhus, Siberian tick typhus, Australian tick typhus and oriental spotted fever are caused by other spotted fever group rickettsiae that are transmitted by ticks. Mediterranean spotted fever (MSF), caused by infection with *R. conorii*, is similar to RMSF but is somewhat milder and is often characterized by a primary necrotic lesion known as an eschar or '*tache noir*' where the site of tick bite occurred. Among hospitalized patients the CFR is 2% (Raoult *et al.*, 1986). The tick vector is *Rhipicephalus sanguineus* in most of Europe.

Louse-borne Typhus

Louse-borne (epidemic) typhus caused by infection with *R. prowazekii* is an acute febrile disease accompanied by headache, myalgia and rash that is transmitted by the human body louse, *Pediculus humanus*. Complications include interstitial pneumonitis, CNS involvement, myocarditis and acute renal failure. During epidemics, the disease may have a CFR between 10% and 66% (Farter, 1981; Megaw, 1942), depending on the health and nutrition of populations afflicted. Outbreaks of louse-borne typhus occur when pediculosis is widespread as a result of the disruption of normal hygiene and lack of adequate water supplies for bathing. Typical settings where louse-borne typhus outbreaks occur include refugee camps, prisons and communities ravaged by war or disaster. An endemic form of the disease occurs in several areas of the world where high altitude and cold

TABLE 25.1   FEATURES OF THE PATHOGENIC RICKETTSIALES SPECIES

Biogroup	Species[a]	Means of transmission Disease in humans	Distribution	To humans
Spotted fever	*R. rickettsii*	Rocky Mountain spotted fever	Western Hemisphere	Tick bite
	R. conorii	Mediterranean spotted fever; also called Boutonneuse fever	Primarily Mediterranean countries, Africa, India, Southwest Asia	Tick bite
	R. siberica	Siberian tick typhus	Siberia, Mongolia, northern China	Tick bite
	R. australis	Australian tick typhus	Australia	Tick bite
	R. akari	Rickettsialpox	USA, USSR	Mite bite
	R. japonica	Oriental spotted fever	Japan	Presumably tick bite
Typhus	*R. prowazekii*	Louse-borne typhus	Primarily highland areas of South America and Africa	Infected louse faeces
		Recrudescent typhus (Brill–Zinsser disease)	Worldwide: follows distribution of persons with primary infections	Reactivation of latent infection
		Sporadic typhus	USA	Contact with flying squirrels *Glaucomys volans*
	R. typhi	Flea-borne typhus	Worldwide	Infected flea faeces
Scrub typhus	*R. tsutsugamushi*	Scrub typhus	Asia, northern Australia, Pacific Islands	Chigger bite
Q fever	*C. burnetii*	Q fever	Worldwide	Infectious aerosols
Ehrlichiosis	*E. sennetsu*	Sennetsu ehrlichiosis	Japan and Malaysia	Unknown
	E. chaffeensis	Human ehrilichiosis	USA, possibly Africa and Europe	Tick bite
	E. phagocytophila	Human granulocytotropic ehrlichiosis?	USA, Europe	Unknown
Bartonellosis	*B. bacilliformis*	Oroyo fever, verruga peruana	South America	Sandfly bite
Bartonella-associated diseases	*B. quintana*	Bacillary angiomatosis	Worldwide	Unknown
	B. henselae	Bacillary angiomatosis	Worldwide	Cat scratch or bite
	B. henselae	Cat-scratch disease	Worldwide	Cat scratch or bite
	B. elizabethae	*Bartonella*-associated endocarditis	USA	Unknown

[a] *B., Bartonella; C., Coxiella; E., Ehrlichia; R., Rickettsia.*

weather combine to promote conditions favouring pediculosis.

Brill–Zinsser Disease

A recrudescent form of the disease (Brill–Zinsser disease) is generally milder than the initial episode but it serves as the mechanism for reintroduction of louse-borne typhus into human populations. Patients who recover from louse-borne typhus may become rickettsemic as a result of diminished immunity due to age, illness or a variety of causes, and transmit rickettsiae to their body lice. If infected lice infest susceptible humans they are capable of beginning an epidemic of louse-borne typhus.

Flea-borne Typhus

Flea-borne (murine) typhus, caused by *R. typhi* infection, is an acute febrile illness typically with associated headache, myalgia anorexia and rash. The disease is mild compared with louse-borne typhus and fatalities are rare (Miller and Beeson, 1946). The worldwide distribution of the disease is attributed to the distribution of the rat flea (*Xenopsilla cheopis*) and the *Rattus rattus* and *R. norvegicus*. The disease is a major cause of febrile illness in the tropics. Populations that are occupationally exposed to rodent contact have increased risk becoming infected, including agricultural workers exposed to rodents and their fleas as a result of harvesting crops.

Scrub Typhus

Scrub typhus (Tsutsugamushi fever), caused by *R. tsutsugamushi*, is a common febrile disease in southeast Asia and south Asia. It is characterized by severe headache, myalgia, arthralgia and maculopapular rash; an eschar is present in about 20% of patients (Berman and Kundin, 1973). Larval mites of the family Trombiculidae serve both as vectors and reservoirs of the rickettsiae. Untreated, the CFR is less than 10% and with antibiotic therapy fatality is rare. Populations at risk of acquiring scrub typhus are those who come

into contact with mite-infested habitats. Military populations and agricultural workers whose occupation require them to spend time in habitats transitional between forest and field have significant risk of infection. Several strains of *R. tsutsugamushi* cause human illness, and infection with one does not confer immunity to subsequent infection with other strains.

Rickettsialpox

Rickettsialpox is caused by infection with *R. akari* and is an uncommon febrile illness characterized by sparse, discrete, maculopapular lesions on the face, trunk and extremities that become vesicular. Eschars occur in most (90%) patients and begin as red papules, developing into shallow, punched-out ulcers. Transmission of *R. akari* occurs to humans via the mite *Liponyssoides sanguineus* when humans come into contact with premises infested with the house mouse, *Mus musculus*. Most cases in the USA are from urban environs of low socioeconomic status. Cases have also been reported from the Ukraine region of the former Soviet Union.

Q Fever

Q fever is a febrile disease caused by infection with *Coxiella burnetii*. Commonly patients have sudden onset of headache, chills, myalgia, arthralgia, photophobia, lymphadenopathy, conjunctivitis, nausea or vomiting, diarrhoea and pharyngitis. Rash is rare and abnormal X-ray findings are present in 50% of cases. The CFR is approximately 1%. Q fever is worldwide in distribution and is usually transmitted from infectious aerosols from animal tissues or products and occasionally from unpasteurized milk. The disease is only rarely reported in the USA. Ticks are infected in nature and may play a role in maintenance and transmission of *C. burnetii* among animal hosts, but probably play little or no role in transmission to humans. Occupational exposure to infected livestock is a major risk factor and abattoir workers, sheep shearers and wool gatherers have highest rates of infection an disease (Bernard *et al.*,

1982). Persons who have contact with sheep, particularly fetuses and birth products, have greatest risk. A rare but frequently fatal chronic form of the disease manifests as endocarditis among patients who have pre-existing heart valve disease (Ellis *et al.*, 1982; Turck *et al.*, 1976).

Ehrlichiosis

Sennetsu ehrlichiosis, caused by *Ehrlichia sennetsu*, is an acute febrile disease characterized by chills, headache, malaise, insomnia, diaphoresis, pharyngitis and anorexia (Misao and Katsuta, 1956). Lymphadenopathy is generalized and characterized by tenderness and is most prominent in the post-auricular and posterior cervical areas. Hepatomegaly and splenomegaly occur in about 33% of cases (Tachibana, 1986). The geographic distribution of confirmed cases include Japan and Malaysia. The disease is self-limiting and no fatalities have been reported. Information on potential vectors and reservoirs is lacking. Risk factors for infection are also unknown.

Human ehrlichiosis in the USA is caused by infection with *E. chaffeensis*. The acute febrile disease is characterized by headache, arthralgia, myalgia, anorexia, nausea or vomiting, chills, pneumonia and, infrequently, rash. Laboratory findings include leukopenia, thrombocytopenia and elevated liver enzymes (Fishbein *et al.*, 1994). The disease is potentially life threatening and complications include disseminated intravascular coagulation and death. The CFR is approximately 3%. More than 300 confirmed cases of human ehrlichiosis have been reported from 25 states in the USA and other countries, including Mali, Portugal and Spain. The south Atlantic and east south central states of the USA account for the vast majority of cases. More than 90% of cases occur between April and September, when vector ticks are actively questing for blood meals. Males account for 75% of the ehrlichiosis cases reported but it is not clear whether the difference in incidence between males and females is due to exposure or other factors. Preliminary evidence suggests that *Amblyoma americanum* may be a vector (Anderson *et al.*, 1993a). The white-tailed

deer is a potential reservoir for maintaining *E. chaffeensis* in nature. Risk factors for infection include occupational and recreational exposure to tick-infested areas.

A new granulocytic form of human ehrlichiosis has been reported from Minnesota and Wisconsin that is caused by infection with an *Ehrlichia* closely related to *E. phagocytophila*. Probably the agent is transmitted by tick bite (Chen *et al.*, 1994). The disease is associated with fever, headache, myalgia, leukopenia, thrombocytopenia and pulmonary interstitial infiltrates. Two of the six laboratory-confirmed patients have died.

Bartonellosis

Bartonellosis is an acute febrile disease caused by infection with *Bartonella bacilliformis*. Most cases exhibit malaise, myalgia and arthralgia. There are two forms of the disease: a cutaneous form, verruga peruana, characterized by red wart-like eruptions on the skin; and a hemolytic anemia, Oroyo fever. Verruga peruana is a mild and self-limiting disease and mortality is rare. On the other hand, Oroyo fever may reach a CFR of 40–70%. The mortality seems to be correlated not with the severity of anemia, but with the frequency of secondary infections with other pathogens, particularly, *Salmonella* spp. (Ricketts, 1949). Humans are the only known reservoir host and sandflies of the genus *Lutzomyia* transmit the bacterium from person to person. Cases are reported from mountainous countries of South America including Peru, Colombia and Ecuador. Risk factors for infection include frequenting areas where the vector sandflies are abundant and outdoor exposure during the evening hours when the peak biting behavior of sandflies occurs.

Bartonella-associated Diseases

Trench fever is caused by infection by *Bartonella* (formerly *Rochalimaea*) *quintana*. Most cases are extremely variable in presentation and may be acute or insidious. The acute disease is characterized by fever, malaise, headache, and pain in bone and body, particularly severe in the shins. Acute disease is mild and no deaths have been reported. An afebrile form of the disease may result in a long debilitating course with numerous relapses. Fever is variable; in some cases a single peak occurs, in others the fever lasts five to seven days, and in others the initial fever is followed by relapses of fever for three or four days at five-day intervals. Relapses may occur months or even years following the initial illness (Vinson, 1973). The vector, *Pediculus humanus*, transmits the agent from bacteraemic humans to uninfected ones via infectious louse faeces rubbed into cuts and abrasions in the skin or through mucous membranes. Risk factors are similar to those of louse-borne typhus, including pediculosis and conditions that increase the frequency of louse burdens and prevalence such as overcrowding, lack of bathing, cold weather and lack of laundering of clothes and bedding. More than one million cases of trench fever were reported among military personnel who served during World War I (Swift, 1920). The disease disappeared following the war, but reappeared among German soldiers serving on the Eastern Front during World War II, causing at least 80 000 cases. Sporadic cases have been reported in Yugoslavia, Poland, Russia, Tunisia, Eritrea, China and Mexico.

Bacillary Angiomatosis

Bacillary angiomatosis, peliosis hepatis and relapsing fever with bacteraemia are caused by infection with *Bartonella henselae* and *B. quintana*. The cutaneous form of disease commonly presents with angiomatous, tender papules or subcutaneous nodules that may resemble Kaposi's sarcoma (LeBoit *et al.*, 1988). Systemic forms of the disease include peliosis hepatis, encephalopathy and septicaemia (Schwartzman, 1992). Patients are almost always immunocompromised and most have acquired immune deficiency syndrome (AIDS) as a consequence of human immunodeficiency virus (HIV) infection. Risk factors for *B. henselae* infections clearly implicate cat scratch, bite, or other cat contact (Tappero *et al.*, 1993; Koehler *et al.*, 1994). No risk factors have been identified for *B. quintana* infections.

Cat-scratch disease (CSD) is characterized by formation of a papule at the site of inoculation, followed by regional lymphadenopathy 7–50 days later. Nodes affected most frequently are head, neck and upper extremities. Nodes are initially tender and suppurate in 15–30% of patients. The episode resolves after two to four months and fatalities have not been reported. Atypical CSD occurs in approximately 10% of cases and includes encephalopathy, lesions of the liver, spleen or bone, and Parinaud's oculoglandular syndrome. CSD has been reported worldwide. An estimated 22 000 CSD cases occur in the USA annually, with an estimated cost for medical services in excess of $12 million per year (Jackson *et al.*, 1993). The incidence in the USA is seasonal, with 80% of cases occurring during the autumn and winter. There is a slight excess of males (53%) over females and most cases are under 20 years of age. The overwhelming risk factor for CSD is contact with cats, specifically being scratched or bitten by kittens (Carithers, 1985). One study suggested that kittens infested with fleas increased the risk of CSD (Zangwill *et al.*, 1993).

Serological evidence that CSD is caused by infection with *Bartonella henselae*, not *Afipia felis*, has repeatedly been demonstrated (Regnery *et al.*, 1992a; Zangwill *et al.*, 1993). Cats are epidemiologically linked to CSD and have been shown to be serologically positive to *B. henselae* (Zangwill *et al.*, 1993; Childs *et al.*, 1994). *Bartonella henselae* has been isolated from the lymph nodes of CSD patients and from the blood of cats (Regnery *et al.*, 1992b; Koehler *et al.*, 1994). *Bartonella henselae* DNA has been detected in lymph node material by PCR (Anderson *et al.*, 1994). Samples of the Hanger–Rose skin test antigen (Margileth, 1968), historically used to confirm suspected CSD cases, contain nucleic acid sequences identical to *B. henselae* but do not have sequences of *A. felis* (Perkins *et al.*, 1992; Anderson *et al.*, 1993).

LABORATORY DIAGNOSIS

Laboratory diagnosis of rickettsial diseases is routinely accomplished by serological assays that detect anti-rickettsial antibodies. Alternative procedures include isolation of rickettsiae from patient tissues and techniques aimed at direct detection of rickettsiae in tissue. However, the latter two methods are generally restricted to research laboratories. Although none of the established techniques reliably provides a diagnosis early enough to affect the outcome of the disease, several new rapid diagnostic techniques have shown promise in research laboratories. Adaptation of some of these new techniques may provide useful tools for early diagnosis of rickettsial diseases in a clinical setting Specifically, PCR assays for the aetiological agents of most rickettsial diseases have been developed. These techniques are undoubtedly the most sensitive means by which rickettsiae can be detected directly in clinical specimens. Additional techniques that have been used successfully to detect rickettsiae early in the course of infection include detection of antigen in peripheral blood cells, and immunoglobulin M (IgM) antibody capture immunoassays. However, serodiagnosis is still the preferred diagnostic approach and testing of serum specimens collected during the acute and convalescent phases of illness is recommended. Preferred techniques for diagnosing rickettsial diseases are shown in Table 25.2.

Serology

Most serological diagnosis of rickettsial diseases is performed by the indirect immunofluorescence assay (IFA) primarily because of the availability of reagents and the ease and economy with which

it can be incorporated into existing antibody screening systems. A variety of other tests have been used for serodiagnosis of rickettsial diseases. A summary of the more common techniques can be found in Table 25.3 and details can be found in the respective references at the end of this chapter. However, relatively few of these techniques are used regularly by most laboratories and laboratories that cannot prepare the needed reagents are limited to techniques that utilize commercially available antigens. Some tests compromise sensitivity (latex agglutination and Weil–Felix) for convenience while other highly sensitive tests (enzyme-linked immunosorbent assay, ELISA) are cumbersome in clinical settings.

Rickettsioses must be distinguished from several viral and bacterial illnesses, including meningococcemia, measles, enteroviral exanthems, leptospirosis, typhoid fever, rubella and dengue fever. The interpretation of serological tests is frequently confounded by the lack of specificity of available rickettsial reagents. Whole rickettsiae are used as antigens for many antibody assays, and since rickettsiae share common antigens (or epitopes) with other bacteria (e.g. *Proteus* spp.), sera from non-rickettsial patients can react at low titers with rickettsial antigens. This has necessitated the designation of minimum positive titers (Table 25.3) to confirm recent rickettsial infections. Since the establishment of minimum positive titers is assigned somewhat arbitrarily, testing of acute- and convalescent-phase serum specimens is recommended.

TABLE 25.2 PREFERRED LABORATORY TECHNIQUES FOR THE DIAGNOSIS OF RICKETTSIAL DISEASES

Infecting organism	IFA (indirect)	ELISA	Isolation	PCR
Rickettsia rickettsii	×	×	×	
Rickettsia conorii	×	×	×	
Rickettsia prowazekii	×	×	×	
Rickettsia typhi	×	×	×	
Rickettsia tsutsugamushi	×		×	
Coxiella burnetii	×		×	
Ehrlichia chaffeensis	×			×
Bartonella bacilliformis	×	×	×	
Bartonella henselae	×		×	×
Bartonella quintana	×		×	×

TABLE 25.3 HIGHLIGHTS OF VARIOUS SEROLOGICAL TECHNIQUES FOR THE DIAGNOSIS OF RICKETTSIAL INFECTIONS

Technique	Minimum positive titre	Time after onset antibody usually detected	Comments
IFA	16–64 depending on investigator	2–3 weeks	Relatively sensitive, requires little antigen; can be used for all rickettsiae and related organisms
CF	8 or 16, depending on investigator	3–4 weeks	Less sensitive than IFA or ELISA but very specific
ELISA	Optical density 0.25 > controls	1 week in some instances	IgM capture assay promising for early diagnosis
Latex agglutination	64	1–2 weeks	Lacks sensitivity for late convalescent sera
IHA	40?	1–2 weeks	Sensitivity ⩾ IFA; more sensitive than CF
Immunoperoxidase	20	7 days	Not evaluated for all rickettsiae; useful in field situations
Microagglutination	⩾8	1–2 weeks	Requires considerable antigen; less sensitive than IFA
Weil–Felix	40–320, depending on investigator	2–3 weeks	Lacks sensitivity and specificity

Recommending a preferred serological technique is not entirely straightforward. Enzyme-linked immunosorbent assay (ELISA) techniques, particularly IgM capture assays, are among the most sensitive procedures available for rickettsial diagnosis, but they require large quantities of purified antigens that are unavailable commercially. ELISAs also are quite amenable for the large-scale screening of serum specimens, but this advantage is usually lost for rickettsial diseases, because with the exception of epidemic typhus rickettsioses usually occur sporadically at a relatively low frequency. A variety of agglutination type assays are in use for serodiagnosis of rickettsial disease. In general these assays require a minimum of specialized equipment but do not compare favorably with the sensitivity of ELISAs or IFA.

Complement fixation

Complement fixation (CF) tests have been used for many years for the diagnosis of most rickettsial diseases. In general these tests, while specific, are less sensitive and more cumbersome than IFA or the agglutination assays and for these reasons are no longer used widely. Group-specific soluble antigens from either typhus or spotted fever group rickettsiae are prepared by methods which employ ether extraction. Antibodies reactive with these group-specific soluble antigens generally appear in the patient's serum 10–14 days after onset of disease and may last a year or longer. Species-specific antigens have been utilized to differentiate infections caused by members within the typhus or spotted fever groups. These specific CF assays rely on differential titres obtained with antigens from individual species of *Rickettsia* (Elisberg and Bozeman, 1969).

The CF assay for diagnosis of Q fever utilizes an ether extract of phase II *C. burnetii*. By the fourth week after the onset of symptoms from Q fever more than 90% of patients have antibodies which fix complement in the presence of phase II antigen (Elisberg and Bozeman, 1969). Antigenic phase variation must be considered for the interpretation of serological results for Q fever. In acute, self-limited Q fever infections, antibodies to the phase II antigen appear first and dominate the humoral immune response. With chronic Q fever infections, however, phase I titers eventually equal or exceed phase II titers. The detection of antibodies that fix complement in the presence of phase I CF antigen has been useful in recognition of subacute Q fever endocarditis. The use of CF assays for the diagnosis of scrub typhus has been met with limited success. The development of CF assays for diagnosis of ehrlichiosis, *Bartonella*-associated infections and bartonellosis have not been reported.

Indirect fluorescent antibody assays

The IFA procedure for the rickettsiae is similar to conventional IFA techniques, with inactivated yolk sac or tissue culture suspensions of rickettsiae being used as antigens (Newhouse *et al.*, 1979). The IFA assay has been almost universally successful for diagnosis of disease caused by rickettsiae and rickettsiae-like organisms. The IFA assays for the diagnosis of infections caused by typhus group, spotted fever group, scrub typhus and Q fever rickettsiae have been utilized for many years with good results. Recently, IFA assays for detecting antibodies to *Ehrlichia chaffeensis* (Dawson *et al.*, 1991) *Bartonella* (Regnery *et al.*, 1992) and *Bartonella bacilliformis* (Knobloch *et al.*, 1985) have been described in the literature and appear to be the method of choice for diagnosis of diseases caused by these organisms. Diagnosis generally depends upon the demonstration of four-fold or greater increase in antibody titer between the acute-phase and convalescent-phase serum samples. IFA tests are reasonably sensitive, although the subjectivity of endpoint determinations is an obvious disadvantage. An additional disadvantage is that serological testing by IFA is generally group reactive, rather than species specific, for the rickettsiae and related organisms.

Enzyme immunoassays

A variety of enzyme immunoassays (or ELISAs) have been developed for the serological diagnosis of rickettsial diseases. These tests offer several major advantages over other assays in that they lend themselves to automation and are not reliant on user interpretation of results. The disadvantages include decreased specificity over some other assays, length of set-up time is not practical for small numbers of sera, and the lack of standardization between laboratories which may give rise to conflicting results.

Generally, the lack of specificity that is associated with rickettsial enzyme immunoassays can usually be avoided by not using whole-cell preparations of rickettsiae as antigens. Enzyme immunoassays that utilize lipopolysaccharide antigens have been successfully developed for spotted fever and typhus group rickettsiae (Jones *et al.*, 1993). The antibody response to this antigen appears to be group specific. Successful use of an immunoassay that utilizes *C. burnetii* lipopoly-saccharide has also been reported (Uhaa *et al.*, 1994). Likewise, an immunoassay for detecting anti-*Bartonella* antibodies has been described (Patnaik *et al.*, 1992).

Agglutination assays

The indirect hemagglutination (IHA) test has received only limited evaluation, but it apparently has a sensitivity equal to that of IFA. An erythrocyte-sensitizing substance (ESS), which can be obtained from typhus and spotted fever group rickettsiae by alkali extraction, is adsorbed onto sheep or human group O erythrocytes, and the coated cells are then used as antigens for simple agglutination tests. The respective ESSs exhibit group-specific antigenic reactivity and appear to be lipopolysaccharide in nature. The convenience of the IHA technique makes it suitable for a clinical setting, although the relatively short shelf life (six months) of sensitized erythrocytes is a disadvantage (Elisberg *et al.*, 1969). Nonetheless, it is potentially valuable as a bedside technique, particularly in the field.

The latex agglutination test has been used with some success in a number of public health laboratories in recent years. Latex spheres are coated with ESS, and the sensitized particles are used as antigens in an agglutination test. The simplicity of the latex agglutination test offers a convenience that is best appreciated at the hospital level, but because it is primarily an IgM assay, it occasionally lacks sensitivity for late-convalescent-phase sera. The convenience of the latex test makes it useful as a bedside diagnostic procedure. It is recommended for that setting over the Weil–Felix test.

The Weil–Felix test became popular in the 1920s after it was observed that certain *Proteus* strains would agglutinate early-convalescent-phase sera from patients with suspected rickettsial disease (Weil and Felix, 1916). The test fell into disfavour because it lacks both sensitivity and specificity (Brown *et al.*, 1983; Hechemy *et al.*, 1979), but it has managed to survive because of its convenience in a clinical setting. Despite its simplicity, it does not reliably provide either early or specific diagnosis of rickettsioses.

Diagnostic criteria

Four-fold rises in titres detected by any technique (Weil–Felix technique excepted) are considered evidence of rickettsial infections. With single serum specimens, CF titres of ⩾16 in a clinically compatible case are also considered positive. With the IFA test, single titres of 64 or higher are considered of borderline significance for typhus and spotted fever group infections, whereas single IFA titres of 256 are considered minimal for confirmation of Q fever. Although these titres are somewhat higher than those recommended by others (see Table 25.2), they usually present no problem in identifying recent infections if appropriately timed sera are available for testing.

The rickettsial species responsible for an infection is difficult to identify by conventional serological tests. Rickettsiae within either the spotted fever or typhus group are antigenically related, resulting in extensive serological cross-reactivity. For example, both flea-borne and louse-borne typhus are endemic in certain areas of the world, and routine IFA tests cannot distinguish between these two infections. Antibody adsorption (Goldwasser and Shepard, 1959) or toxin neutralization (Hamilton, 1945) tests can distinguish patients

who have epidemic or murine typhus infections, but these tests can be performed only by specialized laboratories. In addition, convalescent-phase sera from patients with RMSF or typhus occasionally cross-react with typhus or spotted fever group rickettsiae, respectively (Ormsbee *et al.*, 1978). However, such cross-reactions are infrequent, and the heterologous titres are routinely much lower than in homologous reactions. An ELISA utilizing lipopolysaccharide antigens that eliminates cross-reaction between typhus group and spotted fever group infections has been developed (Jones *et al.*, 1993).

Determining the specific aetiology of spotted fever group infections can be more or less problematic depending on the country of origin. In the Western Hemisphere, RMSF is by far the most prevalent spotted fever group infection. However, in the USA RMSF must occasionally be differentiated from rickettsialpox; differences in the respective clinical and epidemiological features are valuable for determining the likely aetiology. Furthermore, in contrast to RMSF, sera from patients with rickettsialpox are uniformly negative in Weil–Felix tests. Recent data from Europe and Asia suggest that the distributions of *Rickettsia conorii* and *R. siberica* may overlap more than previously known and could confound attempts to identify specific aetiological agents by conventional serological testing. However, because all rickettsiae are susceptible to the tetracyclines, it is not necessary to identify the specific aetiological agent to ensure that individual patients receive proper treatment.

Similar cross-reactivity is seen with patients' sera who have had infections with *Bartonella*. Sera from patients with culture-proven or PCR-positive *B. henselae* infections exhibit strong serological cross-reactivity with *B. quintana* in the IFA assay. Conversely, sera from patients with *B. quintana* infections cross-react with *B. henselae*. This cross-reactivity is also seen within the genus *Ehrlichia*. Sera from humans with PCR-positive *E. chaffeensis* infections, have been shown to have higher IFA titers to *E. canis* (Anderson *et al.*, 1992). This cross-reactivity appears to occur within three groups of serologically and phylogenetically distinct ehrlichiae.

The antigenic diversity of the scrub typhus rickettsiae presents a different problem with respect to serological diagnosis. The most important consideration is an awareness of the antigenic diversity of *R. tsutsugamushi* strains in a given area. Unless an appropriate combination of strains of *R. tsutsugamushi* is included in the battery of test antigens, the titers of some serum specimens could appear falsely low, and some infections could even go undetected (Bougeois *et al.*, 1977).

Laboratory testing is central to the diagnosis of rickettsial diseases although clinical findings can contribute to diagnosis when equivocal serological results are obtained. For the rickettsioses, eschars (at the site of arthropod attachment) are useful indicators of MSF and scrub typhus in endemic areas; the vesicular rash of rickettsialpox is unique among the rickettsioses, and the triad of fever, headache and rash is a useful indicator of RMSF. Because of the hazards of working with living rickettsiae, isolation attempts are usually limited to situations where the outcome is fatal and postmortem tissues are the only specimens available for testing. Even then, direct fluorescent antibody tests of formalin-fixed, paraffin-embedded tissues are faster and safer than rickettsial isolation for diagnosis.

Culture Isolation

Primary isolation

Isolation and identification of members of the genus *Rickettsia* is not recommended for routine diagnosis of rickettsial diseases. These procedures are only recommended for research laboratories that have biosafety containment level 3 facilities and whose personnel have extensive experience in cultivating rickettsiae. Postmortem tissues are usually contaminated with bacteria; therefore, suspensions of these tissues are inoculated into susceptible animals for attempted isolation of rickettsiae. In most cases the guinea-pig is the animal of choice. They are susceptible to infection by *R. typhi*, *R. rickettsii* and *Coxiella burnetii* (Ormsbee *et al.*, 1978) and infection can be monitored by measuring body temperature. Moreover,

male guinea-pigs often present with scrotal swelling when infected with *R. typhi* or *R. rickettsii*. Mice are the species of choice for isolation of *R. akari* and *R. tsutsugamushi*; however, some inbred mice are resistant to infection by scrub typhus rickettsiae (Groves *et al.*, 1980) and outbred mice should be used for isolation of these agents.

Blood specimens are collected from animals that develop overt signs of illness following inoculation; ill animals are then sacrificed, target tissues are harvested aseptically, and blood and tissues are repassaged in animals, embryonated eggs or tissue cultures. Gimenez stain (Gimenez, 1964) or direct immunofluorescence may be used to confirm the isolation of rickettsiae. Further passage into tissue culture or embryonated eggs is necessary to increase the yield of organisms.

Surviving animals are bled 28 days post inoculation and the sera tested for rickettsial antibodies. Animals that were seronegative before inoculation and are positive after 28 days are considered to have been infected with rickettsiae. Seroconversion in the absence of illness likely indicates the presence of a strain of reduced virulence for the animal of choice.

Successful isolation of *Ehrlichia chaffeensis* has only been reported from one patient (Dawson *et al.*, 1991). The technique involves a specialized cell line and has not been used routinely for diagnostic isolation of this agent. The resulting isolate must then be identified. The only methods currently available that permit species-level identification of isolates are PCR-based techniques combined with sequencing (Anderson *et al.*, 1991) or hybridization probes (Anderson *et al.*, 1992). Accordingly, species-level identification of *E. chaffeensis* is best accomplished by specific PCR performed directly on blood specimens (Anderson *et al.*, 1992). Independent confirmation of PCR results by IFA on convalescent serum specimens is desirable. Detection of *E. chaffeensis* in clinical specimens using a species-specific monoclonal antibody has been reported.

Isolates of both *Bartonella henselae* and *B. quintana* have been made from blood and tissue samples of bacteraemic and bacillary angiomatosis patients, respectively (Koehler *et al.*, 1994; Slater *et al.*, 1990; Welch *et al.*, 1992; Regnery *et al.*, 1992). Primary isolates have been recovered using both tissue culture techniques and direct plating on blood or chocolate agar. Although isolates of *B. henselae* have been recovered from the lymph nodes of patients with CSD (Dolan *et al.*, 1993), apparently the diagnostic yield from this sample is disappointing. This may be due in part to the fact that the cellular immune response to the organism may be the primary contributing factor to what is clinically defined as CSD (Gerber *et al.*, 1986). At the point in CSD with which the patient presents with swollen, pus-filled lymph nodes, many of the *Bartonella* may be non-viable. PCR has been used successfully to detect *B. henselae* in the lymph nodes of patients with CSD (Anderson *et al.*, 1994).

Propagation of isolates

Propagation of members of the genus *Rickettsia* is a hazardous procedure that should be attempted only under biosafety level 3 conditions (ACDP containment level 3). Cell cultures provide a convenient method for rickettsial propagation. Numerous cell lines have been used successfully for growing rickettsiae; Vero, primary chicken embryo, WI-38, HeLa, and many others. Infected animal tissues are homogenized thoroughly in sterile diluent and inoculated onto monolayers of susceptible cells. Cultures are incubated at 35 °C and monitored for up to 14 days. No other special growth conditions are necessary, although it is known that *R. rickettsii*, *R. prowazekii*, and *R. typhi* (but not *R. tsutsugamushi*) grow better in an environment with 5% carbon dioxide than they do when exposed to the 0.2–0.3% carbon dioxide that is found in atmospheric air (Kopmans-Gargantiel and Wisseman, 1981). Rickettsial growth can be monitored by scrapping monolayers off the flask with an inoculating loop, and smears are prepared and stained for rickettsiae by the Gimenez technique (Gimenez, 1964) and by the direct fluorescent-antibody procedure, if appropriate. Rickettsiae also grow quite well in the yolk sac of embryonated hen eggs although this technique is quite labour intensive.

Final confirmation of *Rickettsia* isolation requires that the isolate be morphologically similar to rickettsiae, grow intracellularly, fail to grow on bacteriological media, and react with appropriate immune serum but not with non-immune sera. Species-level identification of *Rickettsia* can be performed by restriction endonuclease digestion of PCR-amplified products from isolates. Additional details concerning the procedures for rickettsial isolation can be found in the review by Weiss (Weiss, 1981). Several genetic as well as biochemical tests can be performed on *Bartonella* isolates that allow species-level identification.

Direct Detection of Organisms

Immunofluorescence

Rickettsia have been detected by immunofluorescence in tissue biopsies obtained from the site of tick attachment and from cutaneous lesions (Woodward *et al.*, 1976). Technical improvements in the biopsy assay have resulted in a highly specific assay for confirming MSF. Evaluations of this technique indicate that it will detect *R. rickettsii* or *R. conorii* in about 50% of patients with RMSF or MSF. All of the factors that contribute to the lack of sensitivity are not known, although most false negative results were from patients who had received specific antibiotic therapy before the biopsy was performed.

Rickettsia are also present in circulating endothelial cells. Because of their relatively low number, detection by direct fluorescence microscopy was not feasible until Drancourt and his colleagues (1992) utilized monoclonal antibody-coated beads to concentrate circulating endothelial cells from patients with MSF and then detected rickettsiae in the cells by direct immunofluorescence. The procedure had a sensitivity of 66% in initial evaluation. It takes less than 3 hours to perform, and shows promise as a rapid diagnostic assay for MSF and other rickettsial infections.

Directing fluorescent antibody testing of tissues collected post mortem is a useful approach for the retrospective diagnosis of rickettsial diseases. This technique was first applied to the rickettsiae by Walker and Cain (1978), who successfully detected them in kidney tissue of seven of 10 patients who had died of suspected RMSF.

Polymerase chain reaction

Studies by Tzianabos *et al.* (1989) showed that rickettsial DNA can be detected in blood during rickettsial infections. Using PCR to amplify a 264 bp portion of the 17 kDa antigen, they successfully diagnosed *R. rickettsii* infection in seven of nine patients with confirmed cases of RMSF. Additional testing with clinical specimens indicated that the technique is highly specific but lacks sensitivity; PCR detected rickettsiae best in patients who were seriously ill with RMSF and is of potential importance in the early diagnosis of RMSF and other rickettsial infections.

PCR for the specific detection of *Ehrlichia chaffeensis* in the blood of patients with ehrlichiosis has been described (Anderson *et al.*, 1992). Blood collected in ethylenediaminetetraacetic acid (EDTA) is used to prepare a DNA template for amplification using an *E. chaffeensis* primer pair specific for a 389 bp fragment of 16S rRNA gene. The identity of the PCR-amplified products is confirmed with an oligonucleotide probe. Broad-range PCR, a technique were PCR primers from a conserved region of the 16S rRNA gene are used to amplify a product that is subsequently sequenced, has been valuable in detecting a variety of *Ehrlichia*. This technique was used to identify the agent of human ehrlichiosis and for its detection in patients blood samples. Broad-range PCR coupled with sequencing has also been recently used to identify *E. phagocytophila* or a closely related organism in blood samples from patients with a granulocytic form of ehrlichiosis (Chen *et al.*, 1994).

PCR methods have been particularly valuable for the detection and identification of *Bartonella*. Broad-range PCR coupled with sequencing provided the first association between *Bartonella* and bacillary angiomatosis (Relman *et al.*, 1990) as well as identifying only *B. henselae* DNA in skin test antigens used for the diagnosis of CSD (And-

erson *et al.*, 1993b). A more specific PCR assay for the detection of both *B. henselae* and *B. quintana* has been developed and the resulting PCR product is used as the target for species-specific oligonucleotide hybridization probes. This specific assay has been used to detect *B. henselae* in lymph node tissue from patients with CSD.

In general PCR has been invaluable for the detection, characterization and diagnosis of rickettsiae and related organisms. The difficulty in isolating *Rickettsia*, *Ehrlichia* and *Bartonella* make PCR-based methods more practical than with more easily cultivated non-fastidious bacteria. Although PCR should be regarded as an experimental technique, its role in diagnosis of rickettsial diseases will undoubtedly increase in the future.

TREATMENT

Antibiotic therapy is, in general, of great benefit to patients infected with rickettsiae. RMSF cases when treated with doxycycline, tetracyclines, or chloramphenicol have a CFR much reduced from untreated patients (Harrell, 1949) and show rapid evidence of clinical improvement, including defervescence and cessation of constitutional signs and symptoms. Other spotted fevers, most notably MSF, have been successfully treated with erythromycin and ciprofloxacin (Beltran and Herrero, 1992). Tetracyclines, doxycycline and chloramphenicol are the antibiotics of choice for treatment of most rickettsial illnesses and are also effective in the treatment of acute Q fever. In contrast, chronic Q fever requires combination therapy of both doxycycline and ciprofloxacin for long periods up to years to prevent episodic illness (Levy *et al.*, 1991).

Bartonella infections among immunocompromised patients are treatable with antibiotics, including erythromycin, doxycycline and rifampicin, and must be continued for four to six weeks to prevent relapse (Tappero *et al.*, 1993; Slater *et al.*, 1992; Leong *et al.*, 1992). Intravenous administration of gentamicin and ceftriaxone followed by ciprofloxacin has also been effective in eradicating fever and resolution of lesions (Slater *et al.*, 1992; Lucey *et al.*, 1992).

Antibiotic treatment of CSD is not usually recommended as clinical experience suggests that the resolution of symptoms occurs with or without therapy (Schwartzman, 1992; Carithers, 1985). However, anecdotal studies (Bogue *et al.*, 1989; Lewis and Wallace, 1991) suggest that gentamicin sulfate may have some beneficial affect on CSD patients. A recent retrospective study (Margileth, 1992) suggests the efficacy of rifampicin, ciprofloxacin, gentamicin and trimethoprim-sulfamethoxazole in the treatment of CSD.

PREVENTION

Prevention of the arthropod-borne diseases caused by rickettsiae and rickettsia-like agents includes a variety of measures that reduce the likelihood of contact between vector and susceptible humans. In general, avoiding exposure to habitats known to be endemic for the diseases and/or infested with vectors of the diseases is prudent advice but not usually practicable. Persons who are exposed to vector-infested endemic areas must rely on personal protective measures to minimize contact with potentially infected vectors. Recommendations for prevention of tick-borne *Rickettsiae* and *Ehrlichiae* infections include avoidance of tick-infested habitats and, when that is not feasible, taking personal precautions that prevent tick bite. Wearing long trousers and shirts that fit tightly around ankles and wrists may reduce tick infestation. Clothing impregnated with permethrin or other repellents may also prevent tick infestation. Early removal of ticks either before they imbed their mouthparts into the skin or within hours of imbedding may prevent infection. Similar precautions for preventing louse-borne infections include prevention of louse infestations by regular bathing and washing clothes with soap and hot water. Disinfestation of human populations infested with body lice is an effective measure to contain epidemics. The use of a formalin-killed vaccine may also have been a factor in limiting the spread of louse-borne typhus during World War II. Prevention of scrub typhus depends on avoiding the habitat infested by vector chiggers. Elimination of vegetation that supports mites and their small

mammal hosts may be an effective means of reducing human infections. Prophylactic administration of antibiotics has been shown to be effective among populations occupationally exposed to risk (Olson *et al.*, 1980). Prevention of flea-borne typhus depends on measures similar to those of plague control and include use of insecticides to reduce populations of fleas on rodents, followed by rodent control programs. Avoidance of areas where sandfly vectors of *Bartonella bacilliformis* occur and limiting exposure to hours of the day when biting activity of sandflies is minimal may reduce the frequency of human infections. The effectiveness of repellent-impregnated clothing remains to be evaluated for the prevention of most diseases.

Q fever can be prevented by avoidance of contact with potentially infectious animal tissues and products. Occupationally exposed persons may reduce their risk of infection with *Coxiella burnetii* by wearing respirators that prevent aerosol infections. A vaccine used in Australia is highly effective in preventing illness among abattoir workers (Marmion *et al.*, 1984). CSD and *Bartonella henselae* infection prevention depends on avoidance of bites or scratches from cats (particularly kittens). The mode of transmission of *B. quintana* in cases of bacillary angiomatosis and of *B. elizabetheae* is unknown.

PREVENTION

Immune Mechanisms

Immunity to both spotted fever group and typhus group *Rickettsia* infections (like other intracellular bacteria) involves both the cellular and humoral arms of the immune response. Several vaccines for rickettsial disease have been produced although none has been completely effective. A vaccine to prevent Q fever has shown some promise (Marmion *et al.*, 1984) in preventing this disease. Vaccines for human ehrlichiosis, *Bartonella*-associated diseases and bartonellosis have not yet been developed.

In the case of spotted fever group *Rickettsia*, vaccines have been developed but have not been effective in preventing RMSF. Individual antigens have been identified that play a role in eliciting immunity in both the mouse toxin neutralization assay and the guinea-pig model. Two high molecular weight surface proteins, rOMPA (also termed the 190 or 155 kDa antigens based on differing molecular mass estimates) and rOMPB (also termed 135 or 120 kDa antigen) have been shown to contain protective epitopes. Both rOMPA and rOMPB proteins from *Rickettsia rickettsii* contain amino acid sequence homology with the species protective antigen (SPA) of *R. typhi*. These surface proteins show promise as candidates for subunit vaccines (McDonald *et al.*, 1987). The identification of such protective epitopes in *Ehrlichia chaffeensis* and *Bartonella* has not yet been accomplished.

The mechanisms of immunity to infection with *Bartonella* have not yet been well described. Patients with CSD elicit a strong cellular immune response, as witnessed by the strong granulomatous histopathology observed with this disease. Additionally, the Hanger–Rose skin test used for the diagnosis of CSD is based upon a delayed hypersensitivity-type reaction to a heat-inactivated extract from a lymph node aspirate of a histologically confirmed case of CSD. In general skin testing for diagnosis of CSD has fallen into disfavour because of safety concerns. Gerber *et al.* (1986) have suggested that the strong cellular response observed with CSD result in an exaggerated, prolonged inflammation that contributes to the pathogenesis of this disease. No vaccine has yet been developed for preventing *Bartonella* infections.

REFERENCES

Allen, A.C. and Spitz, S. (1945) A comparative study of the pathology of scrub typhus (tsutsugamushi disease) and other rickettsial diseases. *American Journal of Pathology*, **21**, 603–680.

Anderson, B.E., Dawson, J.E., Jones, D.C. *et al.* (1991) *Ehrlichia chaffeensis*, a new species associated with human ehrlichiosis. *Journal of Clinical Microbiology*, **29**, 2838–2842.

Anderson, B.E., Sumner, J.W., Dawson, J.E. *et al.* (1992) Detection of the etiologic agent of human ehrlichiosis by polymerase chain reaction. *Journal of Clinical Microbiology*, **30**, 775–780.

Anderson, B.A., Kelly, C., Threlkel, R. *et al.* (1993) Detection of *Rochaliniaea henselae* in cat-scratch disease skin test antigen. *Journal of Infectious Diseases*, **168**, 1034–1036.

Anderson, B.E., Sims, K.G., Olson, J.G. *et al.* (1993a) *Amblyomma americanum*: a potential vector for human ehrlichiosis. *American Journal of Tropical Medicine and Hygiene*, **49**, 239–244.

Anderson, B., Kelly, C., Threlkel, R. *et al.* (1993b) Detection of *Rochaliniaea henselae* in cat-scratch disease skin test antigens. *Journal of Infectious Diseases*, **168**, 1034–1036.

Anderson, B., Sims, K., Regnery, R. *et al.* (1994) Detection of *Rochaliniaea henselae* DNA in specimens from cat scratch disease patients by PCR. *Journal of Clinical Microbiology*, **32**, 942–948.

Beltran, R.R. and Herrero, J.I.H. (1992) Evaluation of ciprofloxacin and doxycycline in the treatment of Mediterranean spotted fever. *European Journal of Clinical Microbiology and Infectious Diseases*, **11**, 427–431.

Berman, S.J. and Kundin, W.D. (1973) Scrub typhus in South Vietnam. *Annals of Internal Medicine*, **79**, 26–30.

Bernard, K.W., Parham, G.L. Winkler, W.G. *et al.* (1982) Q fever control measures: recommendations for research facilities using sheep. *Infection Control*, **3**, 461–465.

Bogue, C.W., Wise, J.D., Gray, G.F. *et al.* (1989) Antibiotic therapy for cat-scratch disease? *JAMA*, **262**, 813–816.

Bourgeois, A.L., Olson, J.G., Fang, R.C.Y. *et al.* (1977) Epidemiological and serological study of scrub typhus among Chinese military in the Pescadores Islands of Taiwan. *Transactions of the Royal Society of Tropical Medicine and Hygiene*, **71**, 338–342.

Brenner, D.J., O'Connor, S.P., Winkler, H.H. *et al.* (1993) Proposals to unify the genera *Bartonella* and *Rochaliniaea*, with descriptions of *Bartonella quintana* comb. nov., *Bartonella vinsonii* comb. nov., *Bartonella henselae* comb. nov., and *Bartonella elizabethae* comb. nov., and to remove the family *Bartonellaceae* from the order Rickettsiales. *International Journal of Systematic Bacteriology*, **43**, 77–786.

Brown, G.W., Shirai, A., Rogers, C. *et al.* (1983) Diagnostic criteria for scrub typhus: probability values for immunofluorescent antibody and *Proteus* OXK agglutinin titers. *American Journal of Tropical Medicine and Hygiene*, **32**, 1101–1107.

Carithers, H.A. (1985) Cat-scratch disease: an overview based on a study of 1,200 patients. *American Journal of Diseases of Children*, **139**, 1124–1133.

Chen, S.-M., Dumler, J.S., Bakken, J.S. *et al.* (1994) Identification of a granulocytotropic *Ehrlichia* species as the etiologic agent of human disease. *Journal of Clinical Microbiology*, **32**, 589–595.

Childs, J.E., Rooney, J.A., Cooper, J.L. *et al.* (1994) Epidemiologic observations on infection with *Rochaliniaea* among cats living in Baltimore, MD. *Journal of the American Veterinary Medical Association*, **204**, 1775–1778.

Clements, M.L. (1992) Rocky Mountain spotted fever. In *Infectious Diseases* (ed. S.L. Gorbach, J.G. Bartlett and N.R. Blacklow), pp. 1304–1312. Saunders, Philadelphia.

Dawson, J.E., Anderson, B.E., Fishbein, D.B. *et al.* (1991) Isolation and characterization of an *Ehrlichia* sp. from a patient with human ehrlichiosis. *Journal of Clinical Microbiology*, **29**, 2741–2745.

Dolan, M.J., Wong, M.T., Regnery, R.L. *et al.* (1993) Syndrome of *Rochaliniaea henselae* suggesting cat scratch disease. *Annals of Internal Medicine*, **118**, 331–336.

Drancourt, M., George, F., Brouqui, P. *et al.* (1992) Diagnosis of Mediterranean spotted fever by indirect immunofluorescence of *Rickettsia conorii* in circulating endothelial cells isolated with monoclonal antibody-coated immunomagnetic beads. *Journal of Infectious Diseases*, **166**, 660–663.

Elisberg, B.L. and Bozeman, F.M. (1969) Rickettsiae. In *Diagnostic Procedures for Viral and Rickettsial Infections* (ed. E.H. Lennette and N.J. Schmidt), pp. 826–868. American Public Health Association, New York.

Ellis, M.E., Smith, C.C. and Moffat, M.A.J. (1982) Chronic or fatal Q fever infection: a review of 16 patients seen in north-east Scotland (1967–80). *Quarterly Journal of Medicine* (new series), **205**, 54–66.

Fishbein, D.B., Dawson, J.E. and Robinson, L.E. (1994) Human ehrlichiosis in the United States, 1985–1990. *Annals of Internal Medicine*, **120**, 736–743.

Foster, G.M. (1981) Typhus disaster in the wake of war: the American–Polish relief expedition 1919–1920. *Bulletin of the History of Medicine*, **55**, 221–232.

Gerber, M.A., Rapacz, P., Kalter, S.S. *et al.* (1986) Cell-mediated immunity in cat-scratch disease. *Journal of Allergy and Clinical Immunology*, **78**, 887–890.

Gimenez, D.F. (1964) Staining rickettsiae in yolk-sac cultures. *Stain Technology*, **39**, 135–140.

Goldwasser, R.A. and Shepard, C.C. (1959) Fluorescent antibody methods in the differentiation of murine and epidemic typhus fever: specificity changes resulting from previous immunization. *Journal of Immunology*, **82**, 373–380.

Groves, M.G., Rosenstreich, D.L., Taylor, B.A. *et al.* (1980) Host defences in experimental scrub typhus: mapping the gene that controls nature resistance in mice. *Journal of Immunology*, **125**, 1395–1399.

Hamilton, H.L. (1945) Specificity of toxic factors associated with epidemic and murine strains of typhus rickettsiae. *American Journal of Tropical Medicine and Hygiene*, **25**, 391–395.

Harrell, G.T. (1949) Rocky Mountain spotted fever. *Medicine*, **28**, 333–370.

Hechemy, K.E., Stevens, R.W., Sasowski, S. *et al.* (1979) Discrepancies in Weil–Felix and micro-immunofluorescence test results for Rocky Mountain spotted fever. *Journal of Clinical Microbiology*, **9**, 292–293.

Jackson, L.A., Perkins, B.A. and Wenger, J.D. (1993) Cat scratch disease in the United States: an analysis of three national databases. *American Journal of Public Health*, **83**, 1707–1117.

Jones, D., Anderson, B., Olson, J. *et al.* (1993) Enzyme-linked immunosorbent assay for detection of human immunoglobulin G to lipopolysaccharide of spotted fever group rickettsiae. *Journal of Clinical Microbiology*, **31**, 138–141.

Knobloch, J.L., Solano, M.O., Alverez, G. *et al.* (1985) Antibodies to *Bartonella bacilliformis* as determined by fluorescence antibody test, indirect haemagglutination and ELISA. *Tropical Medicine and Parasitology*, **36**, 183–185.

Koehler, J.E., Glaser, C.A. and Tappero, J.W. (1994) *Rochaliniaea henselae* infection: a new zoonosis with the domestic cat as reservoir. *Journal of the American Medical Association*, **271**, 531–553.

Kopmans-Gargantiel, A.I. and Wisseman, C.L., Jr (1981) Differential requirements for enriched atmospheric carbon dioxide content for intracellular growth in cell culture among selected members of the genus *Rickettsia*. *Infection and Immunity*, **31**, 1277–1280.

LeBoit, P.E., Berger, T.G., Egbert, B.M. *et al.* (1988) Epithelioid haemangioma-like vascular proliferation in AIDS: manifestation of cat scratch disease bacillus infection? *Lancet*, **i**, 960–963.

Leong, S.S., Cazen, R.A., Yu, G.S.M. *et al.* (1992) Abdominal visceral peliosis associated with bacillary angiomatosis. *Archives of Pathology and Laboratory Medicine*, **116**, 866–871.

Levy, P.Y., Drancourt, M., Etienne, J. *et al.* (1991) Comparison of different antibiotic regimes for therapy of 32 cases of Q fever endocarditis. *Antimicrobial Agents and Chemotherapy*, **135**, 533–537.

Lewis, D.E. and Wallace, M.R. (1991) Treatment of adult systemic cat scratch disease with gentamicin sulfate. *Western Journal of Medicine*, **154**, 330–331.

Lucey, D., Dolan, M.J., Moss, C.W. *et al.* (1992) Relapsing illness due to *Rochaliniaea henselae* in immunocompetent hosts: implication for therapy and new epidemiological associations. *Clinical Infectious Diseases*, **14**, 638–683.

Margileth, A.M. (1968) Cat scratch disease: non-bacterial regional lymphadenitis. *Pediatrics*, **42**, 803–818.

Margileth, A.M. (1992) Antibiotic therapy for cat-scratch disease: clinical study of therapeutic outcome in 268 patients and a review of the literature. *Pediatric Infectious Diseases*, **11**, 474–478.

Marmion, B.P., Ormsbee, R.A., Kyrkou, M. *et al.* (1984) Vaccine prophylaxis of abattoir-associated Q fever. *Lancet*, **ii**, 1411–1414.

McDonald, G.A., Anacker, R.L. and Garjian, K. (1987) Cloned gene of *Rickettsia rickettsii* surface antigen: candidate vaccine for Rocky Mountain spotted fever. *Science*, **235**, 83–85.

Megaw, J.W.D. (1942) Louse-borne typhus fever. *British Medical Journal*, **ii**, 401–403, 433–435.

Miller, E.S. and Beeson, P.B. (1946) Murine typhus fever. *Medicine*, **25**, 1–15.

Misao, T. and Katsuta, K. (1956) Epidemiology of infectious mononucleosis. *Japanese Journal of Clinical and Experimental Medicine*, **33**, 73–82.

National Research Council, Division of Medical Sciences, Committee on Pathology (1953) Pathology of epidemic typhus. Report of fatal cases studied by the United States of America Typhus Commission in Cairo, Egypt during 1943–1945. *Archives of Pathology*, **56**, 397–435.

Newhouse, V.F., Shepard, C.C., Redus, M.D. *et al.* (1979) A comparison of the complement fixation, indirect fluorescent antibody and microagglutination test for the serological diagnosis of rickettsial diseases. *American Journal of Tropical Medicine and Hygiene*, **28**, 387–395.

Olson, J.G., Bourgeois, A.L., Fang, R.C.Y. *et al.* (1980) Prevention of scrub typhus: prophylactic administration of doxycycline in a randomized double-blind trial. *American Journal of Tropical Medicine and Hygiene*, **29**, 989–997.

Ormsbee, R., Peacock, M., Philip, R. *et al.* (1978) Antigenic relationships between the typhus and spotted fever groups of rickettsiae. *American Journal of Epidemiology*, **108**, 53–59.

Ormsbee, R., Peacock, M., Gerloff, R. *et al.* (1978) Limits of rickettsial infectivity. *Infection and Immunity*, **19**, 239–245.

Patnaik, M., Schwartzman, W.A., Barka, N.E. *et al.* (1992) Possible role of *Rochaliniaea henselae* in pathogenesis of AIDS encephclopathy. *Lancet*, **340**, 971.

Perkins, B.A., Swaminathan, B., Jackson, L.A. *et al.* (1992) Pathogenesis of cat scratch disease (letter). *New England Journal of Medicine*, **327**, 1599–1600.

Raoult, D., Weiller, P.J., Chagnon, A. *et al.* (1986) Mediterranean spotted fever: clinical, laboratory and epidemiological features of 199 cases. *American Journal of Tropical Medicine and Hygiene*, **35**, 845–850.

Regnery, R.L., Olson, J.G., Perkins, B.A. *et al.* (1992a) Serologic response to *Rochalimaea henselae* antigen in suspected cat scratch disease. *Lancet*, **339**, 1443–1445.

Regnery, R.L., Martin, M. and Olson, J.G. (1992b) Naturally occurring '*Rochalimaea henselae*' infection in domestic cat. *Lancet*, **340**, 557–558.

Regnery, R.L., Anderson, B.E., Clarridge, J.E. *et al.* (1992) Characterization of a novel *Bartonella* species, *R. henselae* sp. nov., isolated from blood of a febrile human immunodeficiency virus-positive patient. *Journal of Clinical Microbiology*, **30**, 265–274.

Relman, D.A., Loutit, J.S., Schmidt, T.M. *et al.* (1990) The agent of bacillary angiomatosis. *New England Journal of Medicine*, **323**, 1573–1580.

Ricketts, W.E. (1949) Clinical manifestations of Carrion's disease. *Archives of Internal Medicine*, **84**, 751–781.

Ris, H. and Fox, J.P. (1949) The cytology of rickettsiae. *Journal of Experimental Medicine*, **89**, 681–686.

Schramek, S.R., Brezina, R. and Tarasevich, I.V. (1976) Isolation of a lipopolysaccharide antigen from Rickettsia species. *Acta Virologica*, **20**, 270.

Schwartzman, W.A. (1992) Infections due to *Bartonella*: the expanding clinical spectrum. *Clinical Infectious Diseases*, **15**, 893–902.

Silverman, D.J. (1984) *Rickettsia rickettsii*-induced cellular injury of human vascular endothelium in-vitro. *Infection and Immunity*, **44**, 545–553.

Slater, L.N., Welch, D.F., Hensel, D. *et al.* (1990) A newly recognized fastidious Gram-negative pathogen as a cause of fever and bacteremia. *New England Journal of Medicine*, **323**, 1587–1593.

Slater, L.N., Welch, D.F. and Min, K.W. (1992) *Rochaliniaea henselae* causes bacillary angiomatosis and peliosis hepatitis. *Archives of Internal Medicine*, **152**, 602–606.

Srigley, J.R., Geddie, W.R., Vellend, H. *et al.* (1985) Q-fever: the liver and bone marrow pathology. *American Journal of Surgical Pathology*, **9**, 752–758.

Swift, H.F. (1920) Trench fever. *Archives of Internal Medicine*, **26**, 76–98.

Tachibana, N. (1986) Sennetsu fever: the disease, diagnosis, and treatment. In *Microbiology* (ed. H. Winkler and M. Ristic), pp. 205–208. American Society for Microbiology, Washington, DC.

Tappero, J.W., Mohle-Boetani, J., Koehler, J.E. *et al.* (1993) The epidemiology of bacillary angiomatosis and bacillary peliosis. *Journal of the American Medical Association*, **269**, 770–775.

Turck, W.P.G., Howitt, G., Turnberg, L.A. *et al.* (1976) Chronic Q fever. *Quarterly Journal of Medicine* (new series), **45**, 193–217.

Tzianabos, T., Anderson, B.E. and McDade, J.E. (1989) Detection of *Rickettsia rickettsii* DNA in clinical specimens by using polymerase chain reaction technology. *Journal of Clinical Microbiology*, **27**, 2866–2868.

Uhaa, I.J., Fishbein, D.B., Olson, J.G. *et al.* (1994) Evaluation of the specificity of the indirect enzyme-linked immunosorbent assay for diagnosis of human Q fever. *Journal of Clinical Microbiology*, **32**, 1560–1565.

Vinson, J.W. (1973) Louse-borne diseases worldwide: trench fever. *Proceedings of the International Symposium on Lice and Louse-borne Diseases*, pp. 76–79. Pan American Health Organization Scientific Publication No. 263, Washington, DC.

Walker, D.H. and Cain, B.G. (1978) A method for specific diagnosis of Rocky Mountain spotted fever on fixed, paraffin-embedded tissue by immunofluorescence. *Journal of Infectious Diseases*, **137**, 206–209.

Walker, D.H. and Mattern, W.D. (1980) Rickettsial vasculitis. *American Heart Journal*, **100**, 896–906.

Walker, D.H., Crawford, G.C. and Cain, B.G. (1980a) Rickettsial infection of the pulmonary microcirculation: the basis for interstitial pneumonitis in Rocky Mountain spotted fever. *Human Pathology*, **11**, 263–272.

Walker, D.H., Palletta, C.E. and Cain, B.G. (1980b) Pathogenesis of myocarditis in Rocky Mountain spotted fever. *Archives of Pathology and Laboratory Medicine*, **104**, 171–174.

Weil, E. and Felix, A. (1916) Zur serologischen Diagnose des Fleckfiebers. *Wiener Klinische Wochenschrift*, **29**, 33–35.

Weiss, E. (1981) The family Rickettsiaceae: human pathogens. In *The Prokaryotes* (ed. M.P. Starr *et al.*), pp. 2137–2160. Springer-Verlag, Berlin.

Weiss, E. and Moulder, J.W. (1984) *Rickettsiales*. In *Bergey's Manual of Systematic Bacteriology*, Vol. 1 (ed. N.R. Krieg), pp. 687–704. Williams & Wilkins, Baltimore.

Welch, D.F., Pickett, D.A., Slater, L.N. *et al.* (1992) *Rochaliniaea henselae* sp. nov., a cause of septicemia, bacillary angiomatosis, and parenchymal bacillary peliosis. *Journal of Clinical Microbiology*, **30**, 275–280.

Woodward, T.E., Pedersen, C.D., Jr, Oster, C.N. *et al.* (1976) Prompt confirmation of Rocky Mountain spotted fever: identification of rickettsiae in skin tissues. *Journal of Infectious Diseases*, **134**, 297–301.

Zangwill, K.M., Hamilton, D.H., Perkins, B.A. *et al.* (1993) Cat scratch disease in Connecticut: epidemiology, risk factors and evaluation of a new diagnostic test. *New England Journal of Medicine*, **329**, 8–13.

Zangwill, K.M., Hamilton, D.H., Perkins, B.A. *et al.* (1993) Cat scratch disease in Connecticut. *New England Journal of Medicine*, **329**, 8–13.

26

GARDNERELLA

A. M. Emmerson

HISTORY

In 1953, Leopold isolated an organism from the cervical swabs of women with 'signs of cervicitis' and from the urine of the husbands of women with positive cervical cultures. Leopold described this organism as a previously unrecognized *Haemophilus*-like organism associated with prostatitis and cervicitis. Two years after these results were published, Gardner and Dukes (1955) assigned the name *Haemophilus vaginalis* to a bacillus cultured from 92% (127 of 138) of women with 'bacterial vaginitis' and also from the urethra of 96% (45 of 47) of males. There seems little doubt that the two reports independently described the same organism. However, the organism did not require haemin (factor X) or nicotinamide adenine dinucleotide (factor V) and because it sometimes appeared to be Gram positive and formed 'Chinese letters' it was removed from the genus *Haemophilus* and renamed *Corynebacterium vaginale* (Zinneman and Turner, 1963). Others believed that *H. vaginalis* was a dissociated form of certain lactobacillus strains, such was the thinking of the time. Regardless of the name, there was ample support, during the 1950s, that this organism was the principal aetiological agent in cases of 'non-specific' bacterial vaginitis, albeit a 'mixed bacterial' infection of the vagina.

Seventeen years after Zinneman and Turner (1963) proposed that *H. vaginalis* should be renamed *C. vaginale*, Greenwood and Pickett (1980) proposed that *H. vaginalis* should be transferred to a new eponymous genus, *Gardnerella*. *Gardnerella vaginalis* remains the sole species in this genus.

DESCRIPTION OF THE ORGANISM

Dunkelberg in 1965 was the first to evaluate the Gram stain for the diagnosis of bacterial vaginosis (BV) by using it to detect *G. vaginalis*. A standardized method for use of the direct Gram stain for the diagnosis of BV has been described by Spiegel (1983), encompassing the Kopeloff modification of the Gram stain and using basic fuchsin as the counterstain. Nevertheless, *G. vaginalis* commonly stains Gram negative or Gram variable, which probably accounts for the early taxonomic controversies. It is more likely to stain Gram positive when stained with the Kopeloff modification of the Gram stain. However, because of its taxonomic uncertainty, *G. vaginalis* is currently grouped with the Gram-negative bacteria in the 9th edition of *Bergey's Manual* (Greenwood and Pickett, 1986).

Gardnerella vaginalis is a facultatively anaerobic, non-spore-forming, Gram-variable bacillus (Greenwood and Pickett, 1980). It ferments

---

Principles and Practice of Clinical Bacteriology. Edited by A.M. Emmerson, P.M. Hawkey and S.H. Gillespie

various carbohydrates, e.g., glucose, maltose and sucrose, with the production mainly of acetic acid, and it is catalase, oxidase, indole and urease negative. The cell wall contains alanine, glutamic acid, glycine and lysine; the G + C composition of the DNA is 42–44 mol% (different from *Coryne-bacterium*, at 55–60 mol%). The organism is a small (1.5–2.5 μm × 0.5 μm) pleomorphic bacillus showing metachromatic granules when stained using Albert's method.

Gardnerella vaginalis grows between 25 and 40 °C, with an optimum of 35–37 °C. It produces β-haemolysis on rabbit and human blood agar but not on sheep blood agar. It will grow in air but the yield is improved by the addition of 5% carbon dioxide or under anaerobic conditions. It can be grown routinely on human blood bilayer – Tween 80 agar after 48 hours of incubation in 5% carbon dioxide. Colonies are pinpoint size at 24 hours and approximately 1 mm at 48 hours. Although most strains are facultatively anaerobic, obligate anaerobic strains have been described.

PATHOGENICITY

Most women without an abnormal vaginal discharge have few or no *G. vaginalis* or anaerobic bacteria in their vaginal flora and the vaginal pH is 4.5 or less. The normal vaginal flora consists predominantly of lactobacilli. Large numbers of *G. vaginalis* and anaerobic bacteria are cultured from many patients with an offensive vaginal discharge of pH 5.0 or more.

Convenient animal models for investigating pathogenicity of *G. vaginalis* do not exist. The weak local polymorph inflammatory response suggests only low pathogenicity compared with that of *Candida albicans*. Gardner and Dukes (1955) monitored an unspecified number of their 11 patients for four months. These patients had acquired experimental BV by vaginal fluid transfer: none showed spontaneous cure or improvement. Several other studies have shown, however, that spontaneous remission of the signs of BV occurs in 25–43% of adults. Lactobacilli appear to play an important role in controlling the composition of the vaginal flora. The mean vaginal pH

before therapy of BV is 5.1 which falls to a mean of 4.2 after therapy.

Endotoxin activity has been detected in cell extracts by using the *Limulus* amoebocyte assay but lipid A has not been found. The concentration of endotoxin is higher in the vaginal fluid of women with BV than in that of women in whom the vagina appears normal on examination; however, it is unlikely that the detection of vaginal endotoxin will prove to be a useful diagnostic test!

Because attachment is the first step in infection and because 'clue cells' (see below) are such a prominent feature of BV the adherence of *G. vaginalis* and *Mobiluncus* spp. have been studied. *Gardnerella vaginalis* organisms which have pili adhere better to vaginal epithelial cells at pH 5–6 than at 4.0.

Amines associated with BV and malic acid produced by *Mobiluncus* spp. can cause irritation of mucous membranes, and volatile fatty acids, *G. vaginalis* and succinate from vaginal fluid anaerobes inhibit granulocyte chemotaxis. The source of amines is yet to be determined.

EPIDEMIOLOGY

Normal Habitat

Gardnerella vaginalis can be isolated from the human genital/urinary tract and appears to have a worldwide distribution. It is a common member of the endogenous vaginal flora. Totten *et al.* (1982), using a semi-quantitative technique, showed that the organism could be isolated from 91% of women with BV compared with 26% of BV negative women. While detection or quantification of *G. vaginalis* in vaginal fluid cannot be used as a routine diagnostic test for BV, the increased prevalence and concentration of the organism in patients with this syndrome suggests that *G. vaginalis* plays a role in BV even though it is not the *sole* aetiological agent.

In patients with BV, lactobacilli are replaced by *G. vaginalis* and a mixed, predominantly anaerobic flora including *Bacteroides* spp., *Prevotella* spp. *Peptostreptococcus* spp., *Mobiluncus* spp., *Eubacterium* spp., *Fusobacterium* spp. and *Veillonella parvula*. *Mobiluncus* spp. are the most recently recognized member of the vaginosis-associated flora. There is a significant decrease in the number of hydrogen peroxide-producing strains of lactobacilli.

Gardnerella vaginalis can be isolated from the male urethra and from semen but rarely causes disease in men.

In the course of quantifying the microbiological flora of the vaginal secretions from 82 selected women Taylor *et al.* (1982) stressed that the major problems in investigating non-specific vaginal discharge are those of patient selection and evaluation of discharge. Other factors, including varying methods of contraception, the stage of the oestrous cycle, pregnancy, age, promiscuity and personal hygiene, have all been considered as possible explanations for conflicting results. The results of this very careful study (Taylor *et al.*, 1982) with exacting microbiological methods conclude that *G. vaginalis* and anaerobic bacteria are infrequently present in large numbers in the normal vagina, but they are cultured from many women with non-specific vaginal discharge. However, *G. vaginalis* can be isolated in smaller numbers from the vagina in 30–40% of 'normal' women and must be considered part of the normal flora (Ison *et al.*, 1983).

Gardnerella vaginalis infection is probably transmitted sexually although infectivity appears to be low. Whilst *Gardnerella* infection of the male urethra is unlikely, colonization of this site may be an important factor in the epidemiology of non-specific vaginitis. There is an association between the use of intrauterine contraceptive devices (IUCDs) and BV.

CLINICAL FEATURES

Characteristic clinical features of *G. vaginalis*-associated BV is a mild but common condition of the vagina characterized by a foul-smelling discharge, which is thin, homogeneous and usually grey or white; it is usually not profuse. The smell is caused by anaerobes but large numbers of *G. vaginalis* organisms are also found. The term vaginosis was introduced to indicate that in BV,

unlike the specific vaginitides, there is an increased discharge without significant inflammation, as indicated by a relative absence of polymorphonuclear leucocytes. The pH of the discharge is higher (4.5–6.0) than in normal controls (4.0–4.7) but usually not as high as in patients with trichomoniasis (5.0–6.0). More than half of the patients with demonstrable evidence of BV are unaware of the malodorous discharge.

Gardnerella vaginalis can also cause urinary tract infections, amnionitis and intra- and postpartum pyrexia with bacteraemia in women; it is associated with pelvic inflammatory disease (PID). It is a rare cause of neonatal infection.

LABORATORY DIAGNOSIS

Investigation of vaginal discharge is commonly unrewarding. It is relatively easy to exclude the diagnosis of *Candida albicans* and *Trichomonas vaginalis* infection but many lower genital tract infections remain unexplained and are loosely referred to as non-specific vaginitis. Samples of vaginal secretions and swabs from the cervix should be sent to the laboratory without delay. Strong clinical suspicion of BV can be substantiated by performing direct Gram stain (with modification) on the secretions and the demonstration of 'clue' cells on a saline wet mount. If 'clue' cells are seen, then there is a strong possibility (>70%) that *G. vaginalis* and non-sporing anaerobes will be cultured. 'Clue' cells are vaginal epithelial cells so heavily coated with coccobacillary organisms that the cell borders are obscured. On the Gram stain there is a striking lack of polymorphs, few lactobacilli and many small Gram-negative/Gram-variable bacilli (i.e., *Gardnerella* or *Bacteroides*) (Nugent *et al.*, 1991). The addition of 0.1% methylene blue to wet smears stains bacteria deep blue and distinguishes lactobacilli readily.

Vaginal pH is easy to measure by simply inserting, via a speculum, a Whatman BDH pH paper. Although the pH is frequently higher in BV than under normal conditions a raised pH is not proof of BV.

Some women with BV are aware of a fishy malodour associated with a vaginal discharge which is made worse following intercourse, possibly because semen, having a relatively high pH, releases amines. The 'amine' test is readily performed by exposing 10% potassium hydroxide to vaginal fluid, thus releasing volatile polyamines giving off a fish-like odour. Because of its subjectivity the 'amine' test has a variable sensitivity of 40–80%.

Ansel *et al.* (1983) proposed that clinical diagnosis should require the presence of three of the following signs: (1) vaginal fluid with a pH of >4.5, (2) homogeneous adherent discharge, (3) fishy odour with the amine test and (4) 'clue' cells seen on a saline wet mount.

Because *G. vaginalis* produces small nondescript colonies on routine media, it is helpful to use one of the differential media that have been developed for primary isolation.

Taylor *et al.* (1982) used pre-reduced thioglycollate broth as a transport media and cultured samples in anaerobic cabinets using freshly made, prereduced enriched selective blood agar media (containing 10 mg/l nalidixic acid). 'Vaginalis' (V) agar contains Columbia agar base (BBL), 1% Proteose Peptone Number 3 (Difco) and 5% human blood. Ison *et al.* (1982) used Proteose Peptone Number 3 with human blood plus nalidixic acid, amphotericin B and gentamicin, which inhibited endogenous flora apart from lactobacilli. Totten *et al.* (1982) used human blood bilayer–Tween 80 agar with supplements, thus enhancing the β-haemolysis of *G. vaginalis*.

Gardnerella vaginalis can also be detected in vaginal secretions or identified in pure culture with immunofluorescence and enzyme immunoassay. Biotyping and serotyping systems are available but not widely used. Several non-culture laboratory techniques are available, including the use of gas–liquid chromatography (GLC) to detect acetic acid. There is also an increased quantity of succinic acid and a decreased quantity of lactic acid.

ANTIMICROBIAL SUSCEPTIBILITY

Gardnerella vaginalis is sensitive to penicillin, ampicillin, vancomycin and clindamycin. Surprisingly for a facultative anaerobe *G. vaginalis* is sensitive to metronidazole. Clinical trials have shown the efficacy of a single 2 g dose of metronidazole compared with seven days therapy of 500 mg b.d. Inhibition of *G. vaginalis* by metronidazole may be due in part to its increased susceptibility to the hydroxy metabolite. Tetracycline, although active against *G. vaginalis*, is not an effective therapy for BV. Topical clindamycin cream benefits some patients.

Management of Infection

Clinical evidence shows that metronidazole is effective against BV but its activity is very much greater against the anaerobes, e.g. *Bacteroides*, than it is against *G. vaginalis*. Since there is a reservoir of *G. vaginalis* among men, the treatment of BV should be directed towards eradication of the infecting organism(s) from both partners, as with other sexually transmitted pathogens.

Other treatment strategies include intravaginal metronidazole, lactate gel and hydrogen peroxide-producing lactobacilli. Relapses or reinfections occur after 'successful' treatment which may be due to the mixed nature of the infection or to the increase in minimal inhibitory concentration of metronidazole above 32 mg/ml. Single-dose therapy is to be preferred because it can be given under supervision, which promotes patient compliance, and there are fewer side effects due to the disulfiram effect of metronidazole.

Infection Control

There are no cross-infection problems.

REFERENCES

Amsel, R., Totten, P.A., Spiegel, C.A. *et al.* (1983) Non-specific vaginitis: diagnostic criteria and microbial and epidemiologic associations. *American Journal of Medicine*, **74**, 14–22.

Dunkelberg, W.E. (1965) Diagnosis of *Haemophilus vaginalis* vaginitis by Gram-stained smears. *American Journal of Obstetrics and Gynecology*, **91**, 998–1000.

Gardner, H.L. and Dukes, C.D. (1955) *Haemophilus vaginalis* vaginitis: a newly defined specific infection previously classified 'non-specific' vaginitis. *American Journal of Obstetrics and Gynecology*, **69**, 962–976.

Greenwood, J.R. and Pickett, M.J. (1980) Transfer of *Haemophilus vaginalis* Gardner and Dukes to a new genus, *Gardnerella*: *G. vaginalis* (Gardner and Dukes) comb. nov. *International Journal of Systematic Bacteriology*, **30**, 170–178.

Greenwood, J.R. and Pickett, M.J. (1986) Genus *Gardnerella* Greenwood and Pickett 1980. In *Bergey's Manual of Determinative Bacteriology*, 9th edn, Vol. 2 (ed. P.H.A. Sneath), pp. 1283–1286. Williams & Wilkins, Baltimore.

Ison, C.A., Dawson, S.G., Hilton, J. *et al.* (1982) Comparison of culture and microscopy in the diagnosis of *Gardnerella vaginalis* infections. *Journal of Clinical Pathology*, **35**, 550–554.

Ison, C.A., Easmon, C.S.F., Dawson, S.G. *et al.* (1983) Non-volatile fatty acids in the diagnosis of non-specific vaginitis. *Journal of Clinical Pathology*, **36**, 1367–1370.

Leopold, S. (1953) Heretofore undescribed organism isolated from genitourinary system. *US Armed Forces Medical Journal*, **4**, 263–266.

Nugent, R.P., Krolin, M.A. and Hillier, S.L. (1991) Reliability of diagnosing bacterial vaginosis is improved by a standardised method of Gram stain interpretation. *Journal of Clinical Microbiology*, **29**, 297–301.

Spiegel, C.A. (1983) Diagnosis of bacterial vaginosis by direct Gram stain of vaginal fluid. *Journal of Clinical Microbiology*, **18**, 170–177.

Taylor, E., Barlow, D., Blackwell, A.L. and Phillips, I. (1982) *Gardnerella vaginalis*, anaerobes and vaginal discharge. *Lancet*, **i**, 1376–1379.

Totten, P.A., Amsel, R., Hale, J. *et al.* (1982) Selective differential human blood bilayer media for isolation of *Gardnerella vaginalis*. *Journal of Clinical Pathology*, **15**, 141–147.

Zinneman, K. and Turner, G.C. (1963) The taxonomic position of *Haemophilus vaginalis* (*Corynebacterium vaginale*). *Journal of Pathology and Bacteriology*, **85**, 213–219.

FURTHER READING

Spiegel, C.A. (1991) Bacterial vaginosis. *Clinical Microbiological Reviews*, **4**, 485–502.

27

AEROBIC ACTINOMYCETES

Stephen H. Gillespie and A. Michael Emmerson

INTRODUCTION

The aerobic actinomycetes form a heterogeneous group of more than genera of which only a few are important in human infection. They are classified together on morphological criteria: they are Gram-positive organisms which can grow as branching filamentous cells (see Figure 27.1). Although once thought to be Fungi Imperfecti they are prokaryotes and there is little evidence to suggest that they are 'higher bacteria' – a link between bacteria and fungi. They are closely related to the corynebacteria and the mycobacteria (see Chapters 4 and 6) (Ruimy *et al.*, 1996). Mycobacteria are acid fast by virtue of long-chain mycolic acid present in their cell wall. Some strains of corynebacteria contain mycolic acids with a much shorter chain length and may be acid fast when grown under appropriate conditions. Organisms of the genera *Nocardia*, *Rhodococcus*, *Gordona* and *Tsukamurella* possess mycolic acids of intermediate chain length and consequently express a degree of acid fastness.

NOCARDIA SPP.

HISTORY

Edmond Nocard, a veterinarian working on the island of Guadeloupe, described a filamentous organism as the cause of bovine farcy (Nocard, 1888). In the following year the organism was characterized and named *Nocardia farcinica*, although later it was recognized that a *Mycobacterium* is the cause of bovine farcy and that the organism that Nocard had isolated was probably *M. farcinoges*. The first human case of nocardiosis was reported one year later in a patient with pneumonia and a brain abscess: this organism was classified as *Nocardia asteroides* (Blanchard, 1896). *Nocardia transvalensis* was first described in 1927, having been isolated from an African patient with Madura foot (Pijper and Pullinger, 1921). More than 12 different species have now been described. Nocardiae are regularly, but uncommonly, implicated in human infections of immunocompetent subjects but they are being

Principles and Practice of Clinical Bacteriology. Edited by A.M. Emmerson, P.M. Hawkey and S. Gillespie
© 1996 John Wiley & Sons Ltd

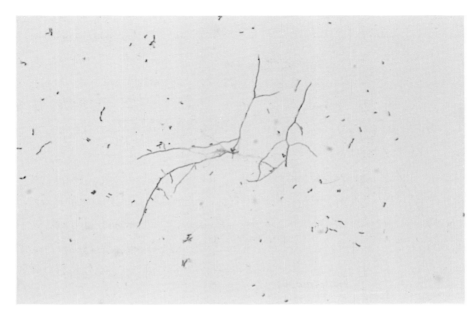

Figure 27.1. Gram stain of pus from a nocardial brain abscess showing long branched filaments and coccal forms.

increasingly recognized in patients on immunosuppressive regimens and in those infected with the human immunodeficiency virus (Beaman and Beaman, 1994; McNiel and Brown, 1994; Miralles, 1994; Schiff *et al.*, 1993).

DESCRIPTION OF THE ORGANISM

Morphological and Physiological Characteristics

Nocardia are Gram-positive, aerobic, catalase-positive, non-motile filamentous bacteria which exhibit branching. The filaments break up into rods and coccal forms and aerial filaments (hyphae) are always produced. The cell wall contains *meso*-diaminopimelic acid, arabinose and galactose and is naturally resistant to degradation by lysozyme: the G + C mol% ranges from 64 to 72 (McNiel and Brown, 1994). Like other members of the *Corynebacterium*, *Mycobacterium*, *Nocardia* (CMN) group *Nocardia* spp. contain mycolic acid in the cell wall. The carbon chain length ranges between C_{44} and C_{60} and is responsible for the

weak acid fastness these organisms exhibit when grown on appropriate lipid-containing media (Beaman and Beaman, 1994; Butler *et al.*, 1987). Peptidoglycan makes up as little as 25% of the cell wall mass, rising to 45% during the stationary phase of growth (Beaman and Moring, 1988). As in mycobacterial cell walls the peptidoglycan is attached to the arabinogalactan polymer by way of a phosphodiester link (see Chapter 6a).

Taxonomy

The nocardiae are phylogenetically related to *Mycobacterium*, *Corynebacterium*, *Gordona* and *Tsukamurella* using 16S rRNA genes (Chun and Goodfellow, 1995) (see Figure 27.2). At the time of writing there are 11 recognized species in the genus *Nocardia*: *N. asteroides*, *N. carnea*, *N. brasiliensis*, *N. farcinica*, *N. brevicatena*, *N. otidiscaviarum*, *N. nova*, *N. seriolae*, *N. transvalensis*, *N. vacinii*. This includes a new species, *N. pseudobrasiliensis*, which has recently been recognized among isolates previously identified as *N. brasiliensis* (Wallace *et al.*, 1995; Ruimy *et al.*,

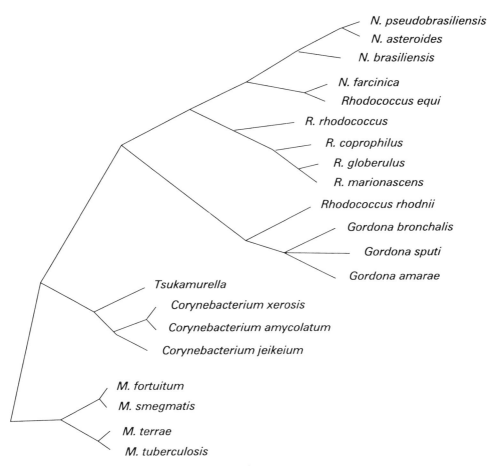

Figure 27.2. Schematic representation of the taxonomy of the *Corynebacterium, Mycobacterium* and *Nocardia* group. (Redrawn from data presented in Ruimy *et al.*, 1996.)

1996). The species previously named as *N. amarae* has been transferred to the genus *Gordona* on the basis of chemical microbiological and sequencing methods (Goodfellow *et al.*, 1994) and the species *N. pinensis* has been excluded (Blackail *et al.*, 1995).

PATHOGENESIS

Experiments with T cell-deficient mice and the experience of immunocompromised patients indicates an important role for T cells in immunity from *Nocardia*.

Nocardial Antigens

During the phases of growth the composition of the nocardial cell wall changes significantly and the virulence of *Nocardia* appears to vary with the growth phase of the organism with logrithmically growing filamentous cells being more virulent than stationary phase cells of the same organism (Beaman and Sugar, 1983; Beaman and Moring, 1988). The cell wall also contains a number of antigens which have been associated with pathogenicity in mycobacteria: tuberculostearic acid and trehalose-6–6'-dimycolate (cord factor). The latter substance is thought to play a role in preventing phososmal–lysosomal fusion (see below) (Spargo et al., 1991).

Nocardia possess a superoxide dismutase which is expressed on the surface of the organism and protects the organism from the toxic effects of superoxide radicals (Beaman et al., 1983). This effect is added to by the action of the organism's catalase (Beaman et al., 1985). Several studies have reported the presence of toxins including a haemolysin in strains of N. asteroides, N. brasiliensis and N. otidiscaviarum.

Interaction with Phagocytes

Nocardia spp. are readily phagocytosed by macrophages and although the majority of organisms are killed some are able to survive as L-forms multiplying inside macrophages. This may explain reports of relapsing infection after apparently successful therapy. L-forms have also been shown to induce fatal infection in mice (Beaman, 1980).

Virulent N. asteroides is able to inhibit phagosomal lysosomal fusion and this effect appears to be mediated by cord factor (Spargo et al., 1991). There is also evidence that virulent strains of the organism (e.g, GUH-2) are capable of blocking the acidification of phagosome whereas avirulent strains are unable to do this. The mechanism whereby this occurs is not known (Black et al., 1986). Nocardia asteroides is also able to utilize acid phosphatase as a carbon source, inhibiting the effect of this toxic macrophage enzyme. Nocardia spp. also possess mycolic acids which have been implicated in Mycobacterium pathogenesis (see Chapter 6a).

EPIDEMIOLOGY

Habitat

The nocardiae are environmental organisms found in soil and vegetation and they are thought to have a role in the decay of organic plant material. Nocardiae have been isolated from marine environments and freshwater sources, including tap water (Beaman and Beaman, 1994). Nocardia

asteroides is more frequently isolated in temperate countries and N. brasiliensis in tropical and subtropical regions (Beaman and Beaman, 1994). Isolation of Nocardia from human specimens may occur as a result of colonization and one study from Australia suggested that only 20% of isolations were clinically significant (Georghiou and Blacklock, 1992).

Animal Infection

Nocardia spp. are reported to cause infection in a wide variety of animals, including cattle (Dohoo, 1989), horses (Biberstein et al., 1985), dogs and pigs (McNiel and Brown, 1994). These infections take the form of bovine mastitis which results in decreased milk production. Equine infection is rarely reported and most commonly takes the form of bronchopneumonia which may develop into disseminated disease. This syndrome is associated with foals with combined immunodeficiency and adult horses with hyperadrenalism secondary to pituitary tumours. Localized abscesses are also rarely reported.

Human Infection

It is normally assumed that nocardial infections are rare but a number of studies have indicated that the number of cases is underestimated (Beaman et al., 1976; Boiron et al., 1992; Georghiou and Blacklock, 1992). With the rise in patients who are severely immunocompromised the number of cases of Nocardia infection is likely to rise. Organisms of the Nocardia genus may act as primary pathogen in adults without evidence of immunocompromise or can act as invaders in patients who are severely immunocompromised. The strongest associations with immunocompromising conditions are found in patients with organ transplantation, malignant neoplasms, lymphomas, sarcoidosis, collagen vascular disease or infection with HIV (McNiel and Brown, 1994).

In immunocompetent patients cutaneous infection is usually caused by N. asteroides, N. brasiliensis and N. otidiscaviarum. There are a wide variety of cutaneous clinical syndromes including lymphocutaneous infection, skin abscesses and skin infection with general dissemination (Georghiou and Blacklock, 1992; Goodfellow *et al.*, 1994; Sachs, 1992). Mycetoma is a chronic granulomatous subcutaneous infection of the foot which occurs in tropical countries and is thought to be secondary to minor local trauma. Infection is usually in the foot and is associated with walking barefoot but mycetoma of the hand has been reported (Beaman and Beaman, 1994). The infection can be caused by aerobic actinomycetes including *N. brasiliensis*, *Actinomadura madurae*, *Streptomyces somaliensis*, or other *Nocardia* spp. Ocular infection is usually secondary to minor corneal trauma or through inadequately sterilized contact lenses or ocular surgery. This may lead to keratitis and later ophthalmitis (Douglas *et al.*, 1991). Ocular infection may be seeded haematogenously in immunocompromised patients with another infective focus.

Colonization of the respiratory tract of immunocompetent patients is not uncommon and may even result in a mild self-limiting infection (Georghiou and Blacklock, 1992). *Nocardia asteroides* is implicated in invasive disease which takes the form of a subacute or chronic cavitatory pneumonia. Common predisposing conditions include local compromise of pulmonary defences such as chronic obstructive airways disease, pulmonary fibrosis, healed tuberculosis, hydatid disease or bronchiectasis or general immunosuppression such as steroid therapy, AIDS, diabetes or severe combined immunodeficiency (Georghiou and Blacklock, 1992). Rarely pulmonary nocardiosis may take an acute fulminating course (Neu *et al.*, 1967).

Disseminated infection can occur in any patient but more usually presents in patients with immunocompromise and is associated with a poor prognosis. It can arise late in the natural history of the infective process and may be caused by any of the species of *Nocardia* (Esteban *et al.*, 1994; Poonwan *et al.*, 1995; McNeil *et al.*, 1992; Georghiou and Blacklock, 1992; Miralles, 1994). Dissemination of infection may result in secondary lesions in the brain and the eyes. Central nervous system infection most often takes the form of an isolated brain abscess and nocardial meningitis is very rarely reported (Bross and Gordon, 1991).

HIV Infection

Nocardiosis is a relatively rare complication of infection with HIV in comparison with other pathogens such as *Pneumocystis carinii or Toxoplasma gondii*. This may be because non-T cell mechanisms are more important for defence against this organism. *Nocardia asteroides* is the commonest species isolated (McNiel and Brown, 1994), but there are a number of case reports with infection by *N. farcinica* and *N. nova* (McNiel and Brown, 1994; Schiff *et al.*, 1993).

CLINICAL FEATURES

Although species of *Nocardia* may occasionally be found in healthy persons, they are not considered part of the normal flora.

Pulmonary Disease

The majority of cases of pulmonary nocardiosis are caused by *N. asteroides*. The first case of primary pulmonary nocardiosis occurring in a patient in the USA was described by Flexner in 1898. The pathological feature of pulmonary nocardiosis is usually a suppurative lesion, e.g. lung abscess, but a granulomatous response or a mixture of these two may occur. The clinical and radiological features are very variable and non-specific, thus making diagnosis difficult without the use of invasive techniques. In the 'usual' course of events, one or more lung abscesses may develop and enlarge to form cavities similar to those seen in chronic tuberculosis; therein lies the diagnostic difficulty. Pulmonary nocardiosis may also mimic carcinoma, actinomycosis or fungal infection. *Nocardia brasiliensis* possesses considerably higher virulence than *N. asteroides* and may cause primary pulmonary infection in otherwise healthy individuals.

The manifestations within the lungs may vary from a mild, diffuse infiltration to a lobar or multilobar consolidation. There may be solitary masses, reticulonodular infiltrates, large irregular nodules, interstitial infiltrates and pleural effusions. In many cases the correct diagnosis is not made until autopsy when *Nocardia* can be seen under microscopy and grown in heavy culture. From the lung the organisms may spread by way of the bloodstream, where they seem to have a predilection for the brain and kidneys, but can establish infections in any part of the body. Unlike actinomycosis or tuberculosis, bone destruction is rare.

Cutaneous Nocardiosis

Primary cutaneous nocardiosis usually occurs following traumatic introduction of *Nocardia* spp., usually *N. brasiliensis*, into the skin. Following inoculation, the organism grows, leading to accumulation of pus which may result in either cellulitis or pyodema. Although the infection remains local and self-limiting (e.g., *N. asteroides*), it may progress and on occasion can spread via the lymphatics, resulting in lymphocutaneous lesions, as with *N. brasiliensis*. Since local lesions may resemble those due to *Staphylococcus aureus*, the true diagnosis

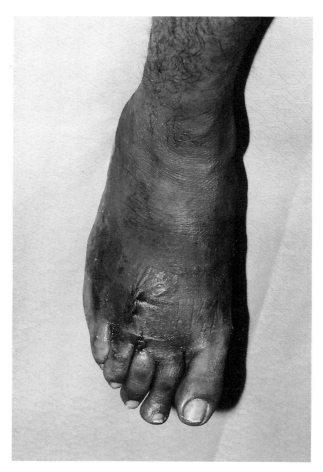

Figure 27.3. Swollen foot of a patient with madura foot also showing that a biopsy has been taken to make the diagnosis.

may not be made unless the lesions are cultured. Most of the skin lesions are found in patients in the USA or in Australia, and rarely in Europe.

Infections may result in fungating tumour-like masses termed *mycetomas*. These are chronic, subcutaneous infections in which the abscesses extend by destruction of soft tissue, sometimes the bone, with eventual eruption through the skin. In equatorial Africa the mycetomas are caused by *Actinomadura pellitieri* and *Streptomyces somaliensis* (see below), but in Mexico the majority of infections are due to *N. brasiliensis*. This infection occurs most commonly in developing countries and is rarely seen in the USA and Europe. It is important to differentiate between actinomycotic and eumycotic mycetoma forms because the latter requires complete excision (i.e. amputation of the foot) to effect a cure, but the actinomycotic form may respond to aggressive medical treatment and conservative surgical excision.

Madura foot is a chronic granulomatous infection of the bones and soft tissue of the foot resulting in mycetoma formation and gross deformity. It occurs in the Sudan, north Africa and the west coast of India, principally among those who walk barefoot and are prone to contamination of foot injuries by soil-derived organisms. One of the causative organisms is *N. madurae*, but it is also caused by other nocardiae and by fungi as mentioned previously (see Figure 27.3).

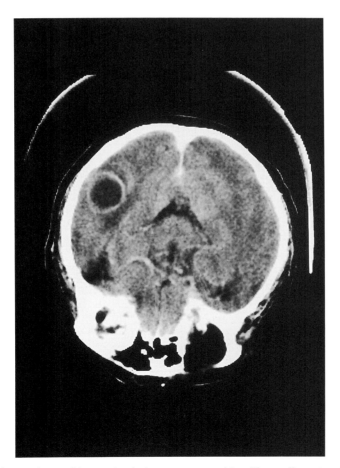

Figure 27.4. CT scan of a patient with cerebral abscess caused by *Nocardia asteroides*.

Systemic Infection

Nocardial lesions in the lungs or elsewhere in the body frequently erode into blood vessels. In systemic nocardiosis, the nocardiae behave as pyogenic bacteria and infection becomes relentlessly progressive. Infection of the central nervous system occurs frequently, but this is often insidious in onset and difficult to diagnose and treat successfully. It often takes the form of a cerebral abscess which may be confused with a pyogenic or fungal abscess or with cerebral toxoplasmosis (see Figure 27.4).

Nocardia farcinica is microbiologically related but distinct from *N. asteroides* and is noted for its propensity to cause serious systemic infection in both normal *and* immunocompromised hosts and for its marked degree of resistance to multiple antimicrobial agents. *Nocardia farcinica* may cause a variety of clinical presentations including cerebral abscess, pulmonary and cutaneous infections. Because of the close similarity that *N. farcinica* has with *N. asteroides* great care has to be exercised in differentiating the two (Wallace *et al.*, 1990). Schiff *et al.* (1992) reported a case of cutaneous *N. farcinica* in a non-immunocompromised patient who developed a facial abscess with underlying osteomyelitis.

Severely immunocompromised patients are predisposed to *N. transvalensis* infections and are at risk from pneumonia or disseminated disease, the lung being the main portal of entry. *Nocardia transvalensis*, a rare *Nocardia* sp., has previously been recognized as a cause of actinomycotic mycetoma. McNeil *et al.* (1992) have reviewed 16 cases of *N. transvalensis* infection.

LABORATORY DIAGNOSIS

Nocardiae are difficult to recognize and identify in the routine diagnostic laboratory, and this is made more difficult by the slow growth on primary isolation from clinical samples.

Collection of Specimens

In pulmonary cases, a single specimen of sputum or bronchial washings should be sent to the laboratory in a sterile screw-cap container. Biopsy and autopsy specimens, exudate, pus and scrapings from skin lesions should be collected in tightly stoppered bottles and sent to the laboratory without delay. Specimens held in storage or delayed in transit should be kept at 4 °C. Preserving fluids are not necessary, but if the laboratory is some distance the specimen should be inoculated onto blood agar locally prior to despatch.

Direct Examination

A presumptive diagnosis of pulmonary nocardiosis may be made by microscopical examination of sputum or bronchoalveolar lavage, for example. Pus and other exudates should be diluted in sterile water if necessary and examined for the presence of microcolonies. These are best seen in an unstained wet mount between slide and cover slip under greatly reduced light or phase-contrast light. In many cases the sputum contains numerous lymphocytes and macrophages, some of which contain pleomorphic Gram-positive and weakly acid-fast bacilli and occasionally extracellular branching filaments. Differentiation of the microcolonies is difficult and requires specialist attention. Branched hyphal filaments may belong to any of a number of genera, e.g., *Nocardia*, *Actinomadura* and *Streptomyces*.

Nocardia are Gram positive, with a variety of shapes and sizes, but they stain irregularly and their filaments are generally beaded (Figure 27.1). Acid fastness is variable in *N. asteroides*, *N. brasiliensis* and *N. caviae*, both in clinical specimens and in culture. The usual Ziehl–Nielsen staining procedure may be employed, but the period of decolonization with acid alcohol must not exceed 5–10 seconds.

Tissue sections

The microcolonies (granules) show up well in sections stained with haematoxylin and eosin, but this stain often fails to demonstrate other morphological forms of nocardiae. The Grocott–Gomori silver methanamine method stains the granules very well. The Gram–Weigert technique is effective for both granules and filaments.

Culture and Isolation

Nocardiae grow on most standard bacteriological media in 2–30 days. Suitable media include brain–heart infusion agar and trypticase soy agar enriched with blood. *Nocardia asteroides* grows well on Sabouraud's dextrose agar in a humid atmosphere at 37 °C aerobically, producing the classic wrinkled pigmented colonies. Colonies are cream, orange or pink coloured and their surfaces may develop a dry chalky appearance which adhere firmly to the medium. Colonies with abundant aerial growth have a 'cotton wool ball' appearance that may resemble many *Streptomyces* spp. The colours are due to various carotenoid-like pigments and their intensity depends on the specific culture conditions used to grow the nocardiae.

The recovery of *Nocardia* spp. from mixed cultures can be facilitated by the use of a selective medium. Garrett *et al.* (1992) described a buffered charcoal–yeast extract medium (similar to *Legionella* media) containing polymyxin, anisomycin and vancomycin. Sabouraud's dextrose agar with chloramphenicol has been used to isolate *Nocardia* spp. from sputum, but many isolates are susceptible to chloramphenicol. Media containing paraffin as the sole source of carbon have also been shown to be effective for the selection of *Nocardia* from sputum. Since *N. asteroides* grows well at 45 °C initial incubation at temperatures above 37 °C may help to separate this species from other bacteria. Cultures are examined at intervals from two days to two weeks. *Nocardia* spp. grow well on Lowenstein–Jensen media and produce moist and glabrous colonies and must be differentiated from mycobacteria.

Identification

The only constant morphological feature of nocardiae is a tendency of the aerial or vegetative mycelium to fragment. The consistency and composition of the growth medium can affect the growth and stability of both aerial and substrate hyphae (Williams *et al.*, 1976). *Nocardia* spp. are Gram positive, weakly acid fast, non-mobile, aerobic and catalase positive and oxidize a number of sugars. They are ONPG positive, reduce nitrate and utilize urea. With few exceptions all *Nocardia* spp. grow in nutrient broth supplemented with lysozyme, whereas most *Rhodococcus*, *Actinomadura* and *Streptomyces* spp. do not. In general the *N. farcinica* type strain (ATCC 3318) is differentiated from *N. asteroides* type strain (ATCC 19247) by the ability of the former to grow and produce acid from rhamnose, to grow on 2,3-butylene glycol (1% vol./vol.) and at 45 °C and to utilize acetamide as a carbon and nitrogen source. The standard Gordon series of tests (involving 40 different physiological properties) are unable to differentiate between *N. asteroides* and *N. farcinica* (Le Chevalier, 1989). Wallace *et al.* (1990) have reported that resistance to cefotaxime, tobramycin and erythromycin is a useful adjunct to biochemical tests in the identification of *N. farcinica*. More recently Carson and Hellyer (1994) have confirmed the finding that all of their 18 strains of *N. farcinica* opacified Middlebrook 7H10 agar (Difco Laboratories, Detroit, Michigan) whilst none of their 23 strains of *N. asteroides* did. Coupled with the ability of *N. farcinica* to grow at 45 °C and its resistance to cefotaxime etc., this test should prove of great value. Differentiation tests are summarized in Table 27.1.

Serodiagnostic Tests

Currently there is no single serodiagnostic test that is routinely used to identify patients with nocardial infections. Patients infected with nocardiae develop only a minimal antibody response that is non-specific. Serological detection of nocardial infection has been attempted, with inconclusive results, in part because of the low sensitivity of the immunodiffusion techniques used and the lack of specificity of the antigen mixtures, producing extensive cross-reactivity with sera from *Mycobacterium*-infected patients (Humphreys *et al.*, 1975). More recently, Salinas-Carmona and col-

TABLE 27.1   DIFFERENTIATION OF *NOCARDIA* SPECIES

Characteristic	*N. asteroides*	*N. brasiliensis*	*N. transvalensis*	*N. farcinica*
Decomposition of:				
Adenine	–	–	–	–
Casein	–	+	–	–
Hypoxanthine	–	+	+	–
Tyrosine	–	+	–	–
Xanthine	–	–	+	–
Growth in lysozyme	+	+	+	+
Acetamide utilization	17%			80%
Acid from rhamnose	10%	–	–	80%
Growth at 45 °C for 3 days[a]	43%	–	–	100%
Resistance to:				
Cefamandole	5%			93%
Tobramycin	17%			100%

[a] See Wallace *et al.* (1990).
% = percentage of 40 strains reacting positive.

leagues (1993) have developed an enzyme-linked immunosorbent assay (ELISA) using two immunodominant antigens, the 26 and 24 kDa proteins. The absorbance values for the ELISA in mycetoma patients (30) were higher than patients with tuberculosis (29), leprosy (24) and healthy individuals (31). The specificity is not 100% because of the cross-reactivity between *N. asteroides* and *N. brasiliensis*, but the former rarely causes skin lesions. However, the best single marker to date for active infection by *Nocardia* spp. is the presence of antibodies to a 55/54 kDa protein which is secreted into the culture medium during nocardial growth (Boiron and Steynem, 1992). However, Kjelstrom and Beamon (1993) have improved on this by developing a panel of tests for recognition of nocardial infections based on reactivity to a variety of antigens by using ELISA and cytoplasmic, culture filtrate and cord factor antigens, immunofluorescence assay against whole cells of *N. asteroides*, and Western blot analysis of secreted protein antigens of *N. asteroides* GUH-2. When this diagnostic panel was applied to human sera, there was excellent sensitivity and specificity for culture-proven cases of clinical disease caused by nocardiae.

ANTIMICROBIAL SUSCEPTIBILITY

Nocardia farcinica has a high degree of resistance to various antibiotics, especially the third-generation cephalosporins, e.g. cefotaxime. Fortunately, strains are usually susceptible to ciprofloxacin (88%) and imipenem (82%), and all are sensitive to amikacin and sulphamethoxazole (Wallace *et al.*, 1990). Most strains are resistant to ampicillin, cefamandole, ceftriaxone (80%), erythromycin, gentamicin and tobramycin. The drug of choice for the treatment of most *Nocardia* strains is sulphamethoxazole. Whilst the sulphonamides work *in vivo* they often appear resistant with *in vitro* testing because of difficulties of testing. Disc testing of sulphonamide sensitivity is notoriously variable and more reliable results are obtained using both microdilution (MICs) provided the inoculum is standardized.

Nocardia transvalensis, like *N. farcinica*, has a high degree of *in vitro* resistance to many antibiotics. McNeil *et al.* (1992) found that more than one-half of 11 isolates were resistant to amoxycillin–clavulanate, ampicillin and doxycycline. Two of the strains were resistant to amikacin and half were resistant to cefotaxime and ceftriaxone. Antimicrobial susceptibility tests performed by a reference laboratory should help to guide therapeutic choice.

The choice of empirical therapy prior to susceptibility testing is sulphamethoxazole with or without trimethoprim for an extended period, often three months or more. The prognosis is poor particularly if the organisms have metastasized to other organs of the body. The *in vitro* activities of new quinolones, new aminoglycosides, a new cephamycin and a new spectinomycin analogue have been reported by Khardori *et al.* (1993). The new quinolones and the cephamycin cefmetazole look promising.

MANAGEMENT OF INFECTION

There are no specific clinical signs diagnostic for pulmonary nocardiosis and the clinical presentation of disease may run the full spectrum of either acute or chronic pulmonary infection. Thus pulmonary infections caused by *Nocardia* spp. are often misdiagnosed as pyogenic infections, tuberculosis, actinomycosis, mycoses of various aetiologies, benign tumours and various forms of cancer. Difficulties in diagnosis are compounded when coexistent disease such as nocardiosis *and* tuberculosis occur to such a large extent (6–30% of cases of *Nocardia* infections) (Kim *et al.*, 1991). In many of these instances the correct diagnosis can only be established by both visualization of nocardiae within the tissue and isolation of the organisms in pure culture from the affected area.

Nocardia spp. show species-specific drug resistance and good identification plus carefully controlled MICs and MBCs should point the way for directed and prolonged therapy. Whilst the sulphonamides or co-trimoxazole are the drugs of choice, because many patients. particularly those with AIDS, are unable to tolerate them (approximately 20%), alternative drugs such as minocycline, erythromycin, amikacin or imipenem may have to be used. Symptomatic treatment of mild to moderate allergic reactions should be attempted before the drug is discontinued.

PREVENTION AND CONTROL

Because of the widespread occurrence of *Nocardia* spp. in soil, control is impossible. These organisms are ubiquitous in the environment and although inhalation of microorganisms may lead to pulmonary disease, in many cases of *N. transvalis* infection, no environmental source has been identified. Superficial infections with other *Nocardia* spp. are often the result of local trauma and soil contamination of the wound. One can only suggest that all wounds are thoroughly cleaned, and debrided if necessary. The use of prophylactic antibiotics is controversial since several of the nocardial strains are resistant to the usual oral drugs. Humans undoubtedly possess considerable resistance to infection because most cases of nocardiosis occur in debilitated or immunocompromised patients.

INFECTION CONTROL

Whilst patient-to-patient transmission would seem to occur very rarely, two nosocomal outbreaks of *N. asteroides* infection in renal transplant recipients have been reported (Houang *et al.*, 1980). If surveillance techniques were more sophisticated, nocardial transmission between immunocompromised patients attending outpatient clinics would be documented more frequently.

ACTINOMADURA SPP.

Vincent first isolated an organism responsible for Madura foot which he named *Streptothrix madurae*. It is now known that many organisms can give rise to this syndrome, including other aerobic actinomycetes such as *Nocardia* spp. (see above) and fungi. The organism which Vincent described was renamed *Nocardia* then transferred to *Actinomadura* together with *A. pellettieri* (McNiel and Brown, 1994). It has been clearly separated from the other aerobic actinomycetes by 16S rRNA cataloguing (Stackebrandt and Schleifer, 1984). The genus is defined on the basis of its cell wall chemotype, the morphology of its aerial hyphae and the presence of a specific sugar, madurose, which has been identified as 3-*O*-methyl-D-galactose. It does not possess mycolic acid in its cell wall and fails to grow in the presence of lysozyme (McNiel and Brown, 1994). There have been as many as 26 species defined but only two of these are important in human infections: *A. madurae* and *A. pellettieri*.

Actinomadura is one of the most frequent bacterial causes of madura foot (see above). It has also been associated with infection of long-standing indwelling catheters and wounds but these are rare. Microscopy of specimens reveals the organism in the form of branched filaments with short chains of spores. Colonies have a molar tooth appearance after 48 hours in culture and aerial hyphae are sparse and may only be seen after two weeks in culture Speciation within the genus is on the basis of biochemical tests: amino acid and aesculin hydrolysis and oxidation of sugars (McNiel and Brown, 1994).

Most isolates of *A. madurae* are susceptible to amikacin, imepenem, and many are resistant to ampicillin. Cephalosporins, trimethoprim–sulphamethoxazole and penicillins have limited activity (McNiel *et al.*, 1990).

DERMATOPHILUS CONGOLENSIS

Dermatophilosis was first recognized as a cattle disease in the Belgian Congo in 1915 by van Saceghem. It is a chronic dermatitis damaging skins and wool and more rarely causing foot rot. The causative organism, *Dermatophilus congolensis*, is the only member of the genus. Humans acquire infection by close contact with infected animals or their products. The diagnosis of dermatophilosis depends on visualizing the organism in wet mounts or specimens stained with methylene blue or Giemsa. Gram stain is not an effective method as some of the detail of the organism is obscured. *Dermatophilus congolensis* may be isolated with difficulty in brain–heart infusion agar containing horse blood, but may require animal passage (McNiel and Brown, 1994). Colonies are small, grey-white, they pit the agar and β-haemolysis may be seen. The organism is motile, catalase positive and urease positive, and

hydrolyses casein slowly. Glucose is fermented producing acid but no gas, but lactose, sucrose, xylose, dulcitol, sorbitol and salicin are not fermented and maltose and galactose results are variable (McNiel and Brown, 1994). The organism is susceptible to penicillin, streptomycin, chloramphenicol, tetracycline, erythromycin and trimethoprim–sulphamethoxazole.

GORDONA SPP.

Gordona spp. are rarely isolated from human subjects but have been associated with primary cutaneous infection, catheter-related sepsis and a pulmonary infection resembling tuberculosis. The genus was defined in 1988 on the basis of 16S rRNA and includes species previously ascribed to the genus *Rhodococcus*. The following species are found in the genus: *G. bronchialis*, *G. ruboperticus*, *G. sputi* and *G. terrae*. *Gordona* spp. have mycolic acids with a shorter chain length than *Mycobacterium* spp., but longer than those of *Rhodococcus*. *Gordona* produces mycobactins under conditions of iron limitation. Wrinkled, dry, beige colonies grow after three to seven days' incubation on blood agar. Microscopically the organisms are small, Gram-positive, weakly acid-fast beaded bacilli. Species within the genus cannot be fully differentiated on the basis of hydrolysis of amino acids and casein, acid production from sugars or high-performance liquid chromatography for mycolic acid (Chun and Goodfellow, 1995; Buchman *et al.*, 1992). Species identification requires the use of ribotyping (Buchman *et al.*, 1992; Lasker *et al.*, 1992).

OTHER AEROBIC ACTINOMYCETES

Organisms from a number of other genera of aerobic actinomycetes which are rarely associated with human infection include *Oerksovia* spp., *Rothia dentocariosa*, *Streptomyces* spp. and *Tsukamurella* spp. The main characteristics, pathology and microbiology of these organisms have been reviewed in detail (McNiel and Brown, 1994).

REFERENCES

Beaman, B.L., Burnside, J., Edwards, B. and Causey, W. (1976) Nocardial infections in the United States 1972–1974. *Journal of Infectious Diseases*, **134**, 286–289.

Beaman, B.L. (1980) Induction of L-phase variants of *Nocardia caviae* within intact murine lungs. *Infection and Immunity*, **29**, 244–251.

Beaman, B.L., Scates, S.M, Moriing, S.E., Deem, R. and Misra, H.P. (1983) Purification and properties of a unique superoxide dismutase from *Nocardia asteroides*. *Journal of Biological Chemistry*, **258**, 91–96.

Beaman, B.L., Black C.N., Doughty, F. and Beaman, L. (1985) Role of superoxide mutase and catalase as determinants of pathogenicity of *Nocardia asteroides*: importance in resistance to microbicidal activities of human polymorphonuclear neutrophils. *Infection and Immunity*, **47**, 135–141.

Beaman, B.L. and Beaman, L. (1994) Nocardia species: host–parasite relationships. *Clinical Microbiology Reviews*, **7**, 213–264.

Beaman, B.L. and Moring, S.E. (1988) Relationship among cell wall composition, stage of growth, and virulence of *Nocardia asteroides* GUH-2. *Infection and Immunity*, **56**, 557–563.

Beaman, B.L. and Sugar, A.M. (1983) *Nocardia* in naturally acquired and experimental infections in animals. *Journal of Hygiene*, **91**, 393–419.

Biberstein, E.L., Jang, S.S. and Hirsh, D.C. (1985) *Nocardia asteroides* infection in horses: a review. *Journal of the American Veterinary Association*, **186**, 273–277.

Black, C.M., Palieschesckey, M., Beaman, B.L., Beaman, R.L., Donovan, R.M. and Goldstein, E. (1986) Acidification of phagosomes in murine macrophages: blockage by *Nocardia asteroides*. *Journal of Infectious Diseases*, **54**, 917–919.

Blackail, L.L., Barker, S.C. and Hugenholtz, P. (1995) Phylogenetic analysis and taxonomic history of *Nocardia pinensis* and *Nocardia amarae*. *Systematic Applied Microbiology*, **17**, 519–526.

Blanchard, R. (1896) Parasites végétaux a l'exclusion de bacteries. In *Traite de Pathologie Generale* (ed. C. Bouchard), pp. 811–913. Masson, Paris.

Boiron, P. and Stynen, D. (1992) Immunodiagnosis of nocardiosis. *Gene*, **115**, 219–222.

Boiron, P., Provost, F., Chevrier, G. and Dupont, B. (1992) Review of nocardial infections in France 1987–1990. *European Journal of Clinical Microbiology and Infectious Diseases*, **11**, 709–714.

Bross, J.E. and Gordon, G. (1991) Nocardial meningitis: case reports and review. *Reviews of Infectious Diseases*, **13**, 160–165.

Buchman, A.L., McNiel, M.M., Brown, J.M., Lasker, B.A. and Ament, M.E. (1992) Central venous catheter sepsis caused by unusual *Gordona* (*Rhodococcus*) species: identification with a digoxigenin-labelled rDNA probe. *Clinical Infectious Diseases*, **15**, 694–697.

Butler, W.R., Kilburn, J.O. and Kubica, G.P. (1987) High performance liquid chromatography analysis of mycolic acids as an aid in laboratory identification of *Rhodococcus* and *Nocardia* species. *Journal of Clinical Microbiology*, **25**, 2126–2131.

Carson, M. and Hellyer, A. (1994) Opacification of Middlebrook agar as an aid in distinguishing *Nocardia farcinica* within the *Nocardia asteroides* complex. *Journal of Clinical Microbiology*, **32**, 2270–2271.

Chun, J. and Goodfellow, M. (1995) A phylogenetic analysis of the genus *Nocardia* with 16S rRNA gene sequences. *International Journal of Systematic Bacteriology*, **45**, 240–245.

Dohoo, I. (1989) *Nocardia*, spp., mastitis in Canada. *Canadian Veterinary Journal*, **30**, 969.

Douglas, R.M., Grove, D.I., Elliot, J., Looke, D.F. and Jordan, A.S. (1991) Corneal ulceration due to *Nocardia asteroides*. *Australian and New Zealand Journal of Ophthalmology*, **19**, 317–320.

Esteban, J., Ramos, J.M., Fernandez-Guerrero, M.L. and Soriano, F. (1994) Isolation of *Nocardia* sp. from blood cultures in a teaching hospital. *Scandinavian Journal of Infectious Diseases*, **26**, 693–696.

Flexner S. (1898) Pseudo-tuberculosis hominis streptotthricha. *Journal of Experimental Medicine*, **3**, 435–450.

Garrett, M.M., Homes, H.T. and Nolte, F.S. (1992) Selected buffered charcoal–yeast extract medium for isolation of Nocardiae from mixed cultures. *Journal of Clinical Microbiology*, **30**, 1891–1892.

Georghiou, P.R. and Blacklock, Z.M. (1992) Infection with *Nocardia* species in Queensland: a review of 102 clinical isolates. *Medical Journal of Australia*, **156**, 692–697.

Goodfellow, M., Chun, J., Stubbs, S. and Tobili, A.S. (1994) Transfer of *Nocardia amarae* Lechevalier and Lechevalier 1974 to the genus *Gordona* as *Gordona amarae* comb. nov. *Letters in Applied Microbiology*, **19**, 401–405.

Houang, E.T., Lovett, I.S., Thompson, F.D. *et al.* (1980) *Nocardia asteroides* infection: a transmissible disease. *Journal of Hospital Infection*, **1**, 31–40.

Humphreys, D.W., Crowder, J.G. and White, A. (1975) Serological reactions to *Nocardia* antigens. *American Journal of Medical Science*, **269**, 323–336.

Kim, J., Minamoto, G.Y. and Grieco, M.H. (1991) *Nocardial* infection as a complication of AIDS:

report of six cases and review. *Reviews of Infectious Diseases*, **13**, 624–629.

Kjelstrom, J.A. and Beaman, B.L. (1993) Development of a serologic panel for the recognition of nocardial infections in a murine model. *Diagnostic Microbiology of Infectious Diseases*, **16**, 291–301.

Lasker, B.A., Brown, J.M. and McNiel, M.M. (1992) Identification and epidemiological typing of clinical and environmental isolates of the genus *Rhodococcus* with use of digoxigenin rDNA gene probe. *Clinical Infectious Diseases*, **15**, 223–233.

Le Chevalier, H.A. (1989) Nocardioform actinomycetes. In *Bergey's Manual of Systematic Bacteriology*, Vol. 4, 9th edn. (ed. S.T. Williams, M.E. Sharp and J.G. Holt), pp. 2348–2404.

McNeil, M.M., Brown, J.M., Georghiou, P.R., Allworth, A.M. and Blacklock, Z.M. (1992) Infections due to *Nocardia transvalensis*: clinical spectrum and antimicrobial therapy. *Clinical Infectious Diseases*, **15**, 453–463.

McNiel, M.M., Brown, J.M., Jarvis, W.R. and Ajello, L. (1990) Comparison of species distribution and antimicrobial susceptibilities of aerobic actinomycetes from clinical specimens. *Reviews of Infectious Diseases*, **12**, 778–783.

McNiel, M.M. and Brown, J.M. (1994) The medically important aerobic Actinomycetes: epidemiology and microbiology. *Clinical Microbiology Reviews*, **7**, 357–417.

Miralles, G.D. (1994) Disseminated *Nocardia farcinica* infection in an AIDS patient. *European Journal of Clinical Microbiology and Infectious Diseases*, **13**, 497–500.

Neu, H.C., Silva, M., Hazen, E. and Rosenhein, S.H. (1967) Necrotizing nocardial pneumonitis. *Annals of Internal Medicine*, **66**, 274–284.

Nocard, M.E. (1888) Note sur la maladie des boeufs de la Guadeloup connue sous le nom de farçin. *Annales de l'Institut Pasteur*, **2**, 293–303.

Pijper, A. and Pullinger, B.D. (1927) South African nocardiasis. *Journal of Tropical Medicine and Hygiene*, **30**, 153–156.

Poonwan, N., Kusum, M., Mikami, Y., Yazawa, K., Tanaka, Y., Gonoi, T., Hasegawa, S. and Konyama, K. (1995) Pathogenic *Nocardia* isolated from clinical specimens including those of AIDS patients in Thailand. *European Journal of Epidemiology*, **11**, 507–512.

Ruimy, R., Riegel, P., Carlotti, A., Boiron, P., Bernardin, G., Monteil, H., Wallace, R.J., Jr and Christen, R. (1996) *Nocardia pseudobrasiliensis* sp.

nov., a new species of *Nocardia* which groups bacterial strains previously identified as *Nocardia brasiliensis* and associated with invasive diseases. *International Journal of Systematic Bacteriology*, **46**, 259–264.

Sachs, M.K. (1992) Lymphocutaneous *Nocardia brasiliensis* infection acquired from a cat scratch: case report and review. *Clinical Infectious Diseases*, **15**, 710–711.

Salinas-Carmona, M.C., Welsh, O. and Casillas, S.M. (1993) Enzyme-linked immunosorbent assay for serological diagnosis of *Nocardia brasilensis* and clinical correlation with mycetoma infections. *Journal of Clinical Microbiology*, **31**, 2901–2906.

Schiff, T.A., McNeil, M.M. and Brown, J. (1992) Cutaneous *Nocardia farcinica* infection in a non immunocompromised patient: case report and review. *Clinical Infectious Diseases*, **16**, 756–760.

Schiff, T.A., Sanchez, M., Moy, J., Klirsfeld, D., McNeil, M.M. and Brown, J.M. (1993) Cutaneous nocardiosis caused by *Nocardia nova* occurring in an HIV-infected individual: a case report and review of the literature. *Journal of Acquired Immune Deficiency Syndromes*, **6**, 849–851.

Spargo, B.J., Crowe, L.M., Ioneda, T., Beaman, B.L. and Crowe, J.H. (1991) Cord factor (α α-trehalose 6,6'-dimycolate) inhibits fusion between phospholipid vesicles. *Proceedings of the National Academy of Science USA*, **88**, 737–740.

Stackebrandt, E. and Schleifer, K.H. (1984) Molecular systematics of actinomyces and related organisms. In *Biological, Biochemical and Biomedical Aspects of Actinomycetes* (ed. L. Ortriz-Ortiz, L.F. Bojalil and V. Yakoleff), pp. 485–504. Orlando, FL, Academic Press.

Wallace, R.J., Tsukamara, M., Brown, B.A. *et al.* (1990) Cefotaxime-resistant *Nocardia asteroides* strains are isolates of the controversial species *Nocardia farcinica*. *Journal of Clinical Microbiology*, **28**, 2721–2732.

Wallace, R.J., Jr., Brown, B.A., Blacklock Z., Ulrich, R., Jost, K., Brown, J.M., McNeil, M.M., Onyi, G., Steingrube, V.A. and Gibson, J. (1995) New *Nocardia* taxon among isolates of *Nocardia brasiliensis* associated with invasive disease. *Journal of Clinical Microbiology*, **33**, 1528–1533.

Williams, S.T., Sharples, G.P., Serrano, J.A. *et al.* (1976) The micromorphology and fine structure of nocardioform organisms. In *The Biology of the Nocardiae* (ed. Goodfellow, Brownell and Serrano), pp. 103–140. Academic Press, London.

INDEX

Index compiled by Geoffrey C. Jones